CHOOSING HEALTH'S STUDENT ADVISORY BOARD

96 Student Story Contributors   **1750** Student Class Testers!   **175** Student Advisory Board Members

We would like to thank the following students at: University of California at Berkeley, Stanford University, East Carolina University, Central Piedmont Community College, East Mecklenburg High School, The University of Texas at Austin, New York University, University of Pennsylvania, University of Texas at San Antonio, Clemson University, University of Massachusetts at Amherst, University of Windsor, The University of Alabama at Birmingham, University of Florida, University of Central Florida, Franklin W. Olin College of Engineering, University of Ottawa, University of Michigan, Palm Beach State College, Vanderbilt University, San Francisco State University, University of California at Davis, California Polytechnic State University San Luis Obispo, and Georgia Southern University for their help in developing the text and media for *Choosing Health*.

- Warren Adderley
- Stephany Aguilar
- Anuella Alexander
- Raquel Alleyne
- Samantha Alridge-Taylor
- Miroslava Alvarado
- Erika Amaya
- Yeani Anthony
- Elizabeth Ann Arline
- Janine Armstrong
- Syed Azfar
- Paige Baratta
- Abbey Barber
- Stephen Barbieri
- Shelby Barry
- Tabitha B. Bednarczyk
- Ombria Bell
- Antonio Bellocchio
- Addison Benson
- Karen Anne Bernatavitz
- Kenneth Bethea Jr.
- Tarmeshia Bivins
- Paulette Blanc
- Steven Briones
- Allen Brooks
- Mark Brooks
- Ryan Burnside
- Melissa Ann Byrum
- Cara Elizabeth Carr
- Jessica Lynne Carr
- Jaketa Cash
- Brendan Chan
- Amelia Carolyn Chappell
- Jephthe Louis Charles
- Jessica Cocke
- Joshua Cole
- Michael Cooper
- Joan Craig
- Lorriane Crook
- Molly Crowther
- Logan Cuddington
- Viege Delva
- Sarah Dobbs
- Carrie Grey Downing
- Emily Ehlers
- Aaron Evans
- Taeilor Evans
- Corey Fletcher
- Joshua Fletcher
- Betty S. Foh
- Akoye O. Gamory
- David Garcia
- Javier Garcia
- Marvin Gary
- Natashia George
- Nick Geraine
- Andrew Gines
- Danielle Goldman
- Danielle Gonzalez
- Nancy Greene
- Morgan P. Grissom
- Katherine Guzman
- Rachel Halverson
- Derek V. Hampton Jr.
- Jasmine Harris
- Monique Heath
- Lauren Heather Helms
- Danon Elora Hirsch
- Ted Hoffman
- Martin Hogarty
- Amanda Jane Holland
- Caleb Hopkins
- Allison Huberlie
- Curt Hughes
- Amanda Humphrey
- Holly Christine Ipock
- Seresa'u Ivey
- Molly Jack
- Douglas Jackson
- Stefani M. Janvier
- Sara Jaramillo
- Caitlin Jensen
- Ahmed Kabore
- Bryson Keen
- D'Jillisser Kelly
- Reza Kermani
- Angela Maria Korleski
- Danuel Laan
- Steven Le
- Chloe Anne Lebatard
- Stephanie Jane Leibfried
- Terri Lewis
- Munir Limant
- Michael Lopez
- Claudia-Regina Lopez-Ferrer
- Hilary Louis
- Courtney Lugo
- Lauraine Lynch
- Stephen Malone
- Samantha Mandel
- Margot Markman
- Ashley Marie Mason
- Brittany Rae Massey
- Whitney Allison McCall
- Jonathan McClure
- Michelle McGovern
- Katherine McGrath
- Courtney A. Meier
- Madonna Messana
- Chris Morris
- Cody Morris
- Christy Nance
- Seeta Nath
- Elizabeth Negrete
- Linda Nguyen
- Nidya Ortiz
- Brittney Nicole Partridge
- Joseph Patterson
- Daleine Paulinis
- Eboni Peoples
- Bruce Pittman
- Brianna Pomatico
- Raven A. Pritchett
- Jasmine Raeford
- Christopher Rahim
- Camille Reynolds
- Yessica Rivas
- Ally Rodgers
- Krystal Rodriguez
- Rebecca L. Rooks
- Rachel Rozier
- Diana Salazar
- Julius Scott
- Emmanuel Seide
- Alexandra Rose Seidman
- Freeman Senecharles
- Jessica Seracino
- John Michael Sheahan
- Evan Skinner
- Annie Snodgrass
- Christopher Sorianao
- Bryon Spencer
- Demauria Arielle Squires
- Jessica Stark
- Brandon J. Staton
- Corinne Steiner
- Tara Sterling
- Lamin Subaneh
- Lee Tavasso
- David Theologou
- Catina T. Thrasher
- Bradford Threlkeld
- Greg Toner
- Michael Torres
- Ashley Traywick
- Christian Tripp
- Sandra A. Trybus
- Daniel Udo
- Melissa Updyke
- Luis Urrea
- Ana von Son
- Briana Verdugo
- Christine Vo
- Jerri Ashley Waller
- Annie Wang
- Brian Watson
- Lydia Wearden
- Freddie Weinberg
- Laura White
- Kaitlin Emily Wiggins
- Shana Wilkins
- Kristina Nicole Williamson
- Charles H. Wilson
- Katherine D. Wilson
- Ceili R. Wonilowicz

BEHAVIOR CHANGE CONTRACT

My behavior change: _____

1. Three important short-term benefits I've discovered from my research about my behavior change are:
   1. _____
   2. _____
   3. _____

2. My SMART goal for this behavior change is:
   _____
   _____
   _____

3. Keeping my current stage of behavior change in mind, these short-term goals and rewards will make my SMART goal more attainable:

   _____ _____ _____
   Short-term goal   Target date   Reward

   _____ _____ _____
   Short-term goal   Target date   Reward

   _____ _____ _____
   Short-term goal   Target date   Reward

4. Barriers I anticipate to making this behavior change are:
   1. _____
   2. _____
   3. _____

   The strategies I will use to overcome these barriers are:
   1. _____
   2. _____
   3. _____

5. Resources I will use to help me change this behavior include:
   a friend, partner, or relative: _____
   a school-based resource: _____
   a health-care resource: _____
   a community-based resource: _____
   a book or reputable website: _____

6. When I achieve the long-term behavior change described above, my reward will be:
   _____   _____
   Reward   Target date

7. I intend to make the behavior change described above. I will use the strategies and rewards above to achieve the goals that will contribute to a healthy behavior change.

   Signed: _____

When it comes to health, what will your students choose?

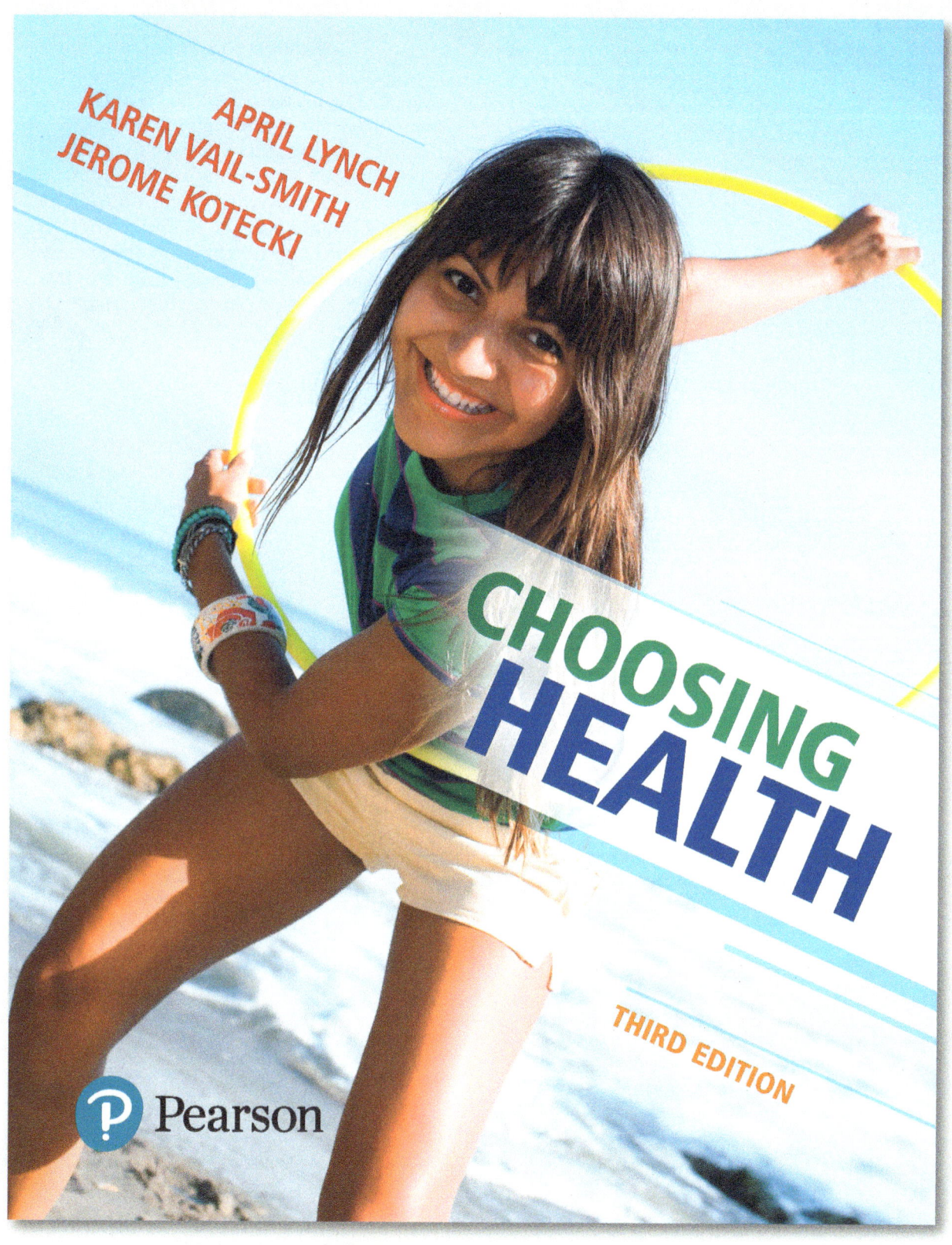

Helping Students Understand That Their Actions

CHAPTER 2 STUDY PLAN

CHAPTER SUMMARY

LO 2.1
- Psychological health encompasses both mental and emotional health. Its six facets are self-acceptance, positive relations with others, autonomy, environmental mastery, a sense of purpose in life, and ongoing personal growth.
- Maslow's hierarchy of needs models the theory that people experience ever-higher levels of psychological health as they meet ever-higher levels of needs. Those with high emotional intelligence can process information of an emotional nature and use it to guide their thoughts, actions, and reactions.
- Optimism is the psychological tendency to have a positive interpretation of life's events.

LO 2.2
- Psychological health is influenced by complex genetic factors interacting with aspects of environment.
- Childhood abuse or neglect can prompt the development of maladaptive coping patterns that are carried through adulthood. Current level of social support can also strongly influence response to psychological challenges.
- Religion and spirituality can contribute to psychological health. Spiritual well-being is said to rest on three pillars: a strong personal value system, connectedness and community in relationships, and a meaningful purpose in life.

LO 2.3
- Common psychological challenges include shyness, loneliness, and anger.

LO 2.4
- Mental disorders are common and can cause long-term disruptions in thoughts and feelings that reduce an individual's ability to function in daily life.
- The United States has the highest rate of mental disorders in the world. About 25% of U.S. college students report being treated for or diagnosed with some type of mental disorder; the actual prevalence may be much higher.
- The chemical imbalance theory of mental illness arose in the 1950s; however, the American Psychiatric Association acknowledges that the causes of mental disorders are complex or unknown.

LO 2.5
- Depressive disorders and bipolar disorder are mood disorders. Depression is considered one of the most treatable mental disorders.
- A variety of forms of psychotherapy are successful in treating depression. Regular exercise can help. Antidepressant medications are often effective; however, they can prompt serious side effects.
- Bipolar disorder is characterized by periods of mania followed by periods of depression.

MasteringHealth™
Build your knowledge—and health!—in the Study Area of MasteringHealth™ with a variety of study tools.

LO 2.6
- The most common mental disorders among college students are anxiety disorders, such as generalized anxiety disorder, panic disorder, and social anxiety disorder.
- Psychotherapy and antidepressant medications are common treatments.

LO 2.7
- Other mental disorders common in young adults are obsessive compulsive disorder (OCD), post-traumatic stress disorder (PTSD), attention disorders, such as ADHD, and schizophrenia.

LO 2.8
- Non-suicidal self-injury is the act of cutting, burning, bruising, or otherwise injuring yourself in an effort to cope with negative, intrusive thoughts or feelings of dissociation.
- Suicide is the second most common cause of death in young adults. If a friend makes a statement indicating suicidal thoughts, offer to call a crisis hotline together, accompany your friend to your campus health services or a counseling center, or head to the nearest emergency room.

LO 2.9
- Common options in psychotherapy include cognitive-behavioral therapy (CBT), behavior therapy, psychodynamic therapy, positive psychotherapy, and acceptance and commitment therapy. Some therapists use a combined approach.

LO 2.10
- Self-care can be a good place to start if you are experiencing psychological distress. Self-care includes eating well, getting the right amount of sleep, exercising, setting realistic goals, and taking steps to build your self-esteem.
- A desire to isolate yourself is a common symptom of psychological distress; reaching out is an important coping strategy.
- Meditation can help increase relaxation and positive feelings.
- To help a friend with psychological distress or a diagnosed mental disorder, listen objectively and compassionately. Don't try to fix things for your friend but do offer your presence and support.
- There are many ways to promote psychological well-being on campus, from joining an organization such as Active Minds to volunteering to become a peer counselor.

NEW! Study Plan Tied to Learning Outcomes Numbered learning outcomes now introduce every chapter and are associated with every section heading, giving students a roadmap for their reading. Each chapter concludes with a Study Plan, which summarizes key points of the chapter and provides review questions to check understanding, all tied to the chapter's learning outcomes. A Study Plan item covering all learning outcomes in the chapter is assignable in **MasteringHealth**.

UPDATED! Chapter on Sleep, Your Body, and Your Mind Previously available as an electronic chapter, the topic of sleep has been thoroughly updated and expanded and now follows the Stress Management chapter. The extensively revised chapter covers everything from how sleep affects health to how to get your best night's sleep and includes the most up-to-date research on sleep.

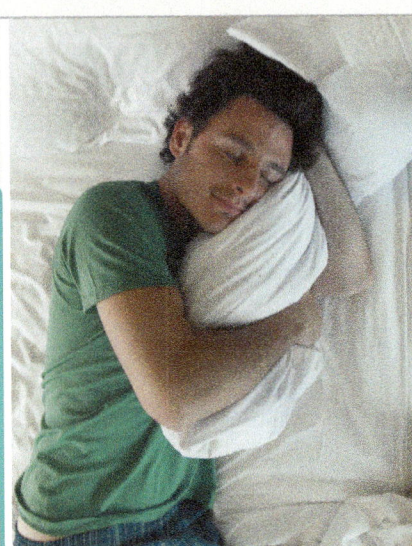

4

> More than half of American adults say they experience a sleep problem almost every night.[1]

> About 15% of American adults say they sleep fewer than 6 hours on weeknights.[1]

> Americans aged 19–29 have the latest bedtime of any age group: on average, two minutes before midnight.[1]

SLEEP, YOUR BODY, AND YOUR MIND

and Behavior Matter

UPDATED! Choose This, Not That boxes highlight good vs. bad choices students make about common health issues. Each box promotes the healthy choice and explains why the poor choice is problematic. New Choose This, Not That boxes include "Sleep: Ample Sleep vs. Sleep Deprived" and "Your Body: Fit and Active vs. Unfit and Sedentary."

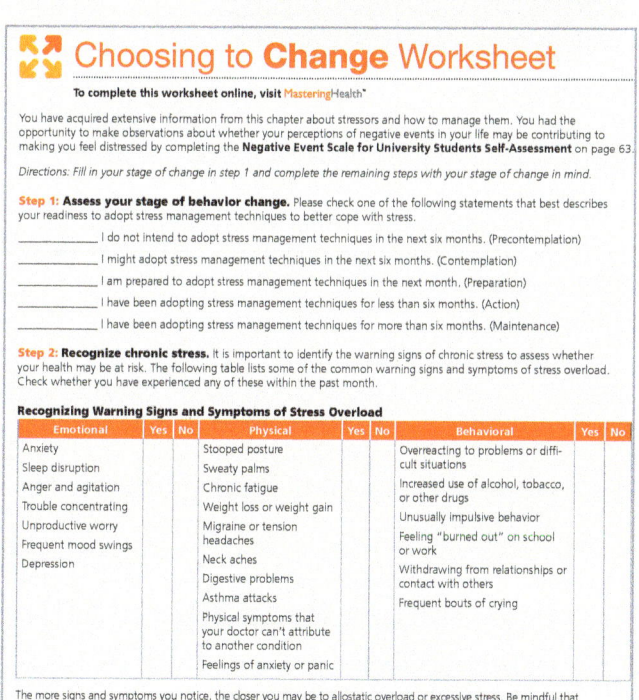

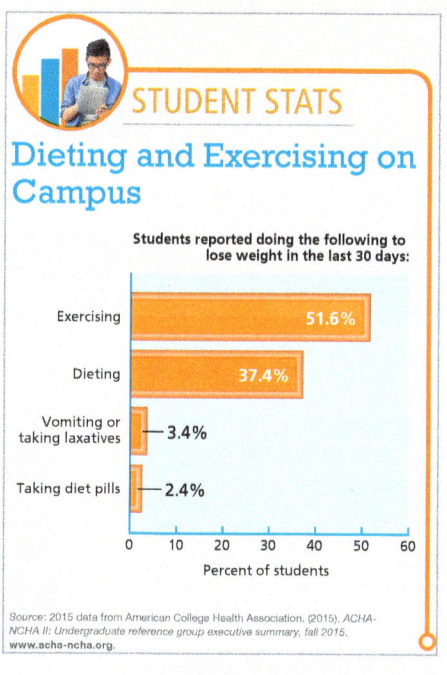

UPDATED! Student Stats What do students across the nation think about pertinent health topics? Do they think differently than your students do? Student Stats throughout the book present up-to-date national statistics and research on key health topics that apply to today's college population.

HALLMARK! Choosing to Change Worksheets help students target a behavior they want to change, determine the stage of behavior change based on the transtheoretical model of behavior change, think through the steps necessary to make positive change, and put themselves on a path to success.

Continuous Learning
Before, During, and After Class

BEFORE CLASS
Mobile Media and Reading Assignments Ensure Students Come to Class Prepared

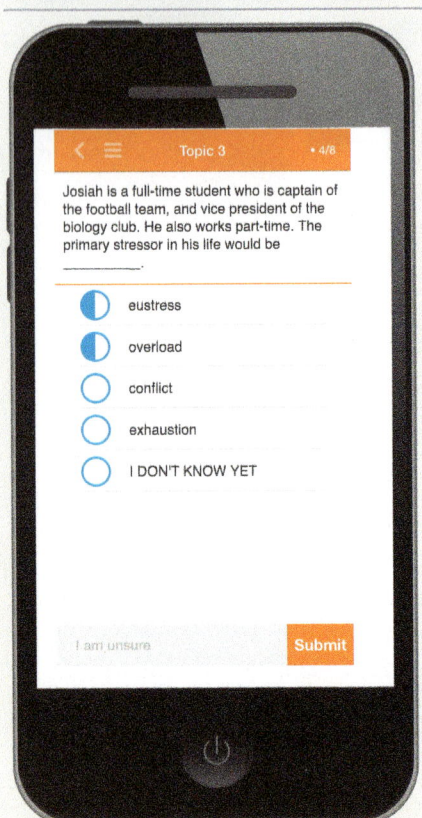

NEW! Dynamic Study Modules help students study effectively by continuously assessing student performance and providing practice in areas where students struggle the most. Each Dynamic Study Module, accessed by computer, smartphone, or tablet, promotes fast learning and long-term retention.

NEW! Interactive eText 2.0 gives students access to the text whenever they can access the internet. eText features include:
- Now available on smartphones and tablets.
- Seamlessly integrated videos and other rich media.
- Accessible (screen-reader ready).
- Configurable reading settings, including resizable type and night-reading mode.
- Instructor and student note-taking, highlighting, bookmarking, and search.
- Now available for offline use via the Pearson eText 2.0 app.

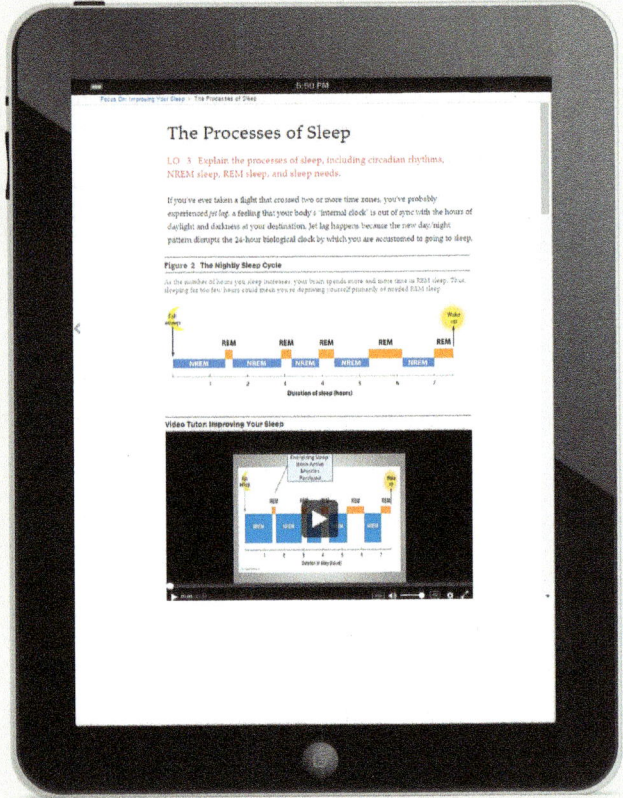

Pre-Lecture Reading Questions are easy to customize and assign

Reading Questions ensure that students complete the assigned reading before class and stay on track with reading assignments. Reading Questions are 100% mobile ready and can be completed by students on mobile devices.

with MasteringHealth™

DURING CLASS

Engage Students with Learning Catalytics

Learning Catalytics, a "bring your own device" student engagement, assessment, and classroom intelligence system, allows students to use their smartphone, tablet, or laptop to respond to questions in class.

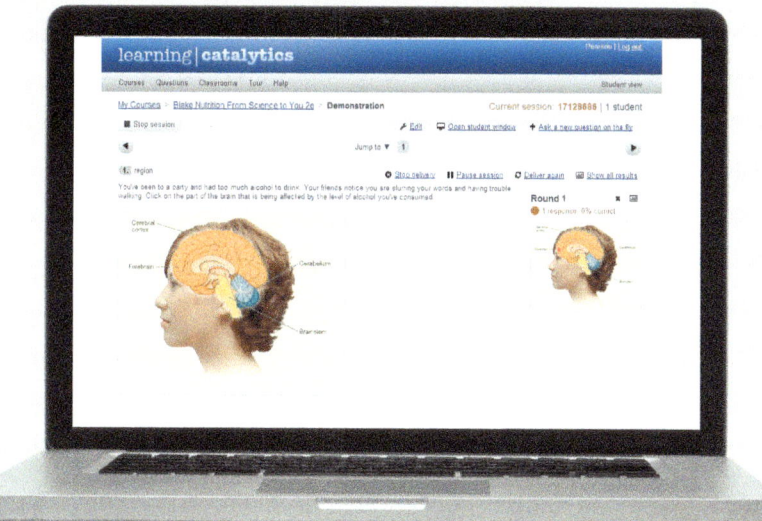
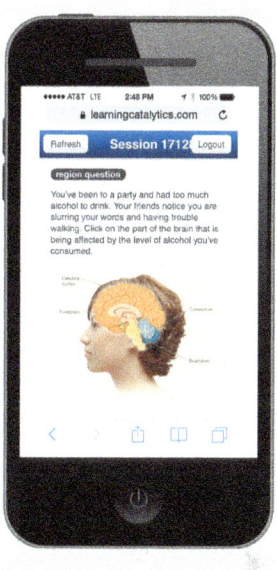

AFTER CLASS

MasteringHealth Delivers Automatically Graded Health and Fitness Activities

NEW! Interactive Behavior Change Activities—Which Path Would You Take? Students explore various health choices through an engaging, interactive, low-stakes, and anonymous experience. These activities show students the possible consequences of various choices they make today on their future health. These activities are assignable in **MasteringHealth** with follow-up questions.

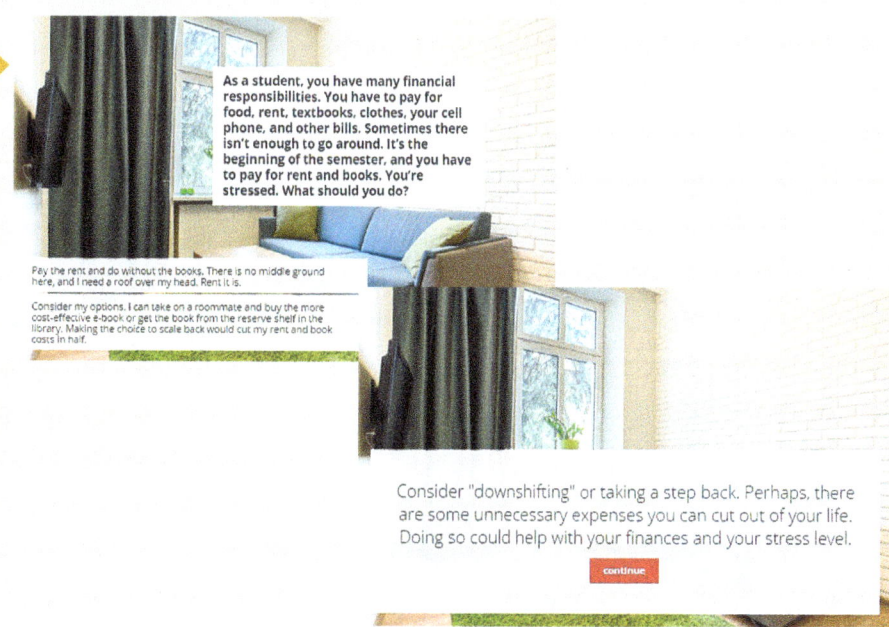

Continuous Learning
Before, During, and After Class

AFTER CLASS
Easy to Assign, Customize, Media-Rich, and Automatically Graded Assignments

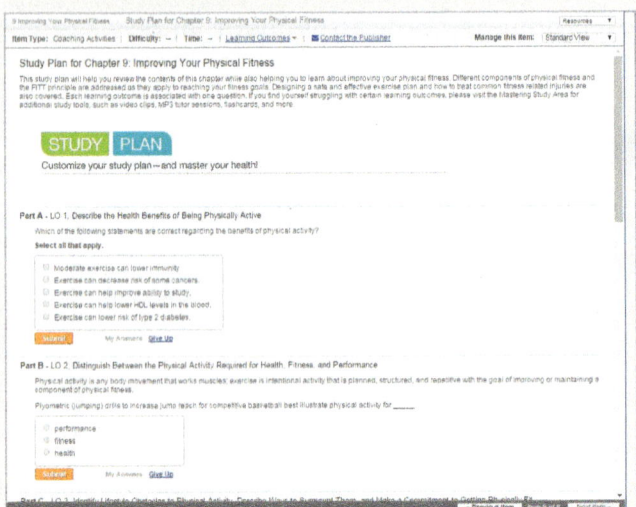

NEW! Study Plans tie all end-of-chapter material to specific numbered Learning Outcomes and **MasteringHealth** assets. Assignable study plan items contain at least one multiple choice question per Learning Outcome and wrong-answer feedback.

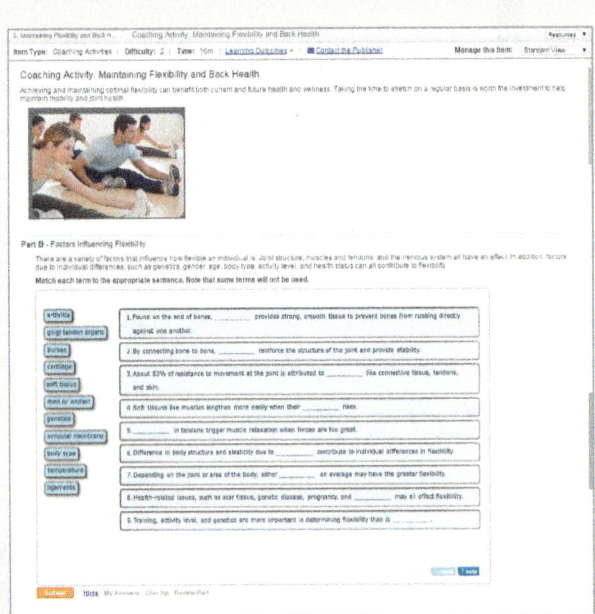

NEW! Coaching Activities guide students through key health and fitness concepts with interactive mini-lessons that provide hints and feedback.

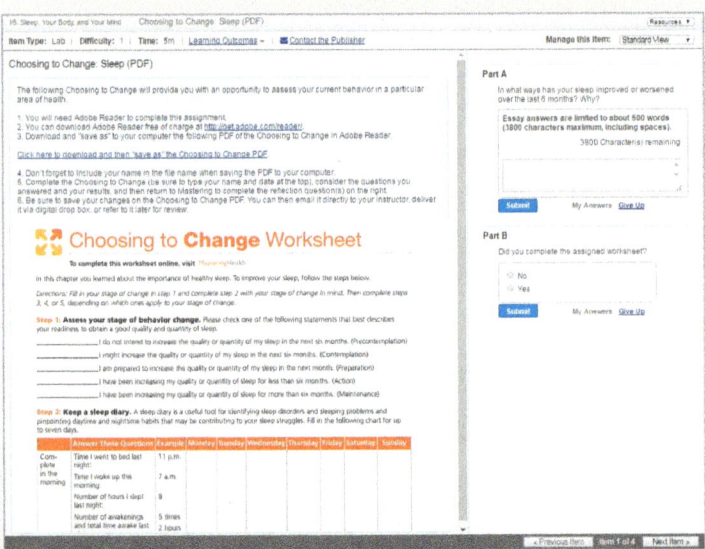

UPDATED! Choosing to Change Worksheets are available as assignable labs within **MasteringHealth**.

with MasteringHealth™

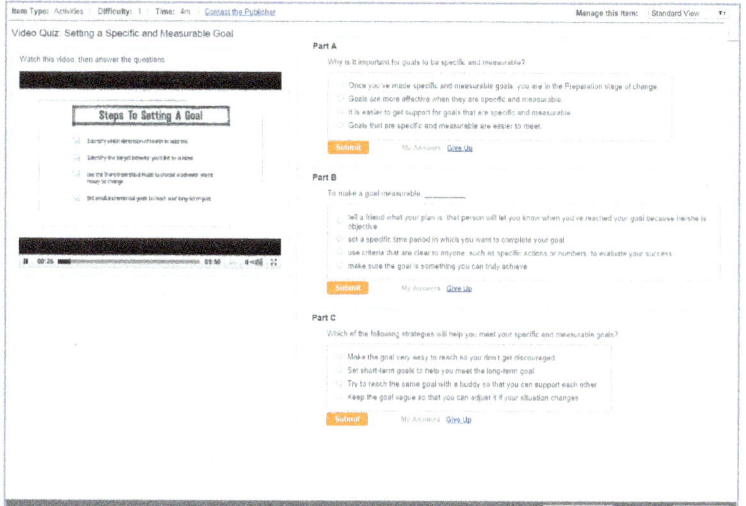

Behavior Change Videos are concise whiteboard-style videos that help students with the steps of behavior change, covering topics such as setting SMART goals, identifying and overcoming barriers to change, planning realistic timelines, and more. Additional videos review key fitness concepts such as determining target heart rate range for exercise. All videos include assessment activities and are assignable in MasteringHealth™

NEW! ABC News Videos bring health to life and spark discussion with up-to-date hot topics from 2012–2015. Activities tied to the videos include multiple choice questions that provide wrong-answer feedback to redirect students to the correct answer.

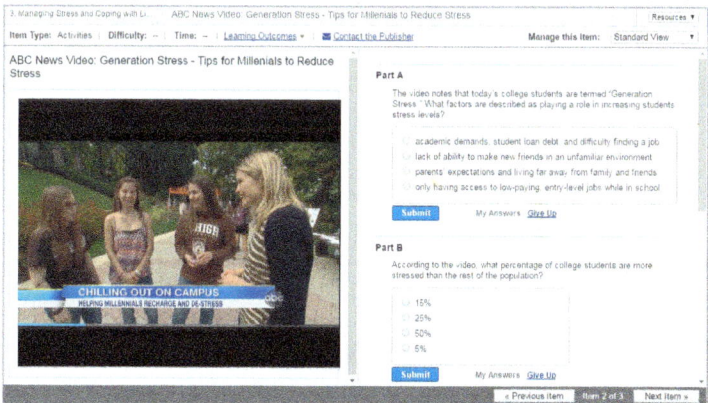

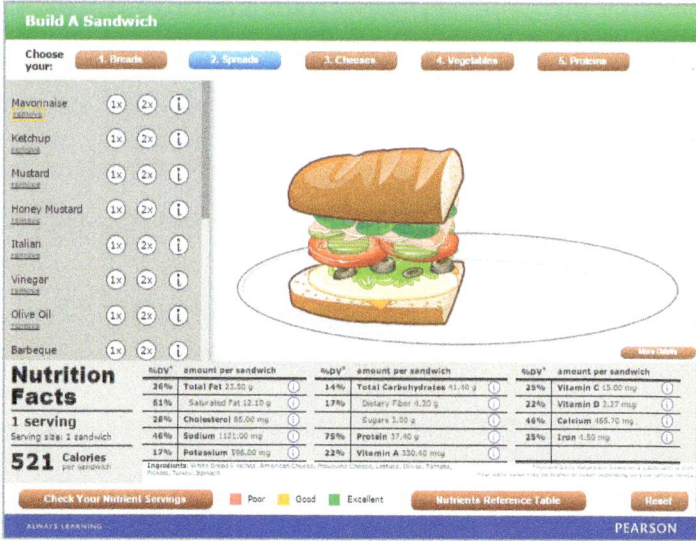

UPDATED! NutriTools Coaching Activities in the nutrition chapter allow students to combine and experiment with different food options and learn firsthand how to build healthier meals.

Resources for YOU, the Instructor

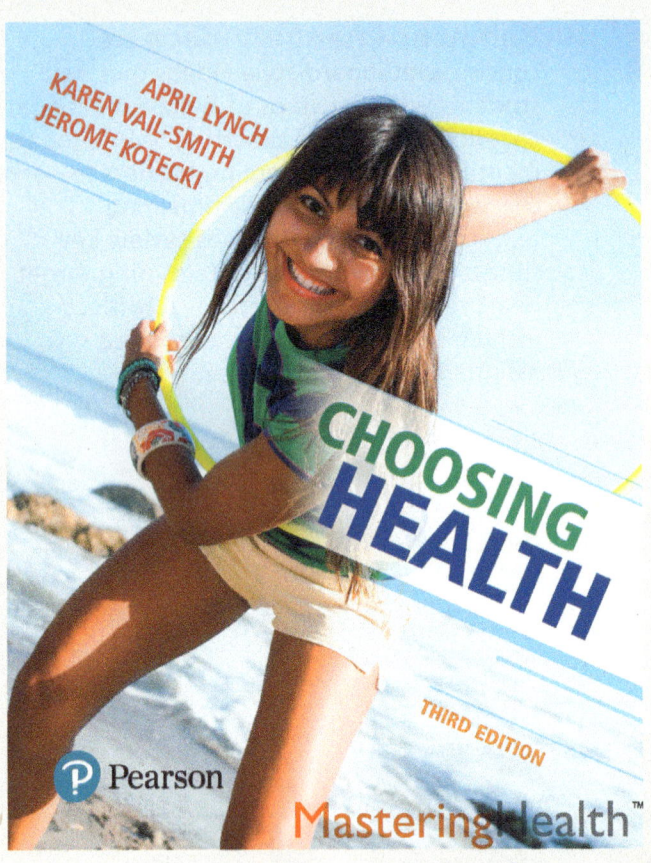

MasteringHealth provides you with everything you need to prep for your course and deliver a dynamic lecture, in one convenient place. Resources include:

MEDIA ASSETS FOR EACH CHAPTER

- *ABC News* Lecture Launcher videos
- Behavior Change videos
- PowerPoint Lecture Outlines
- PowerPoint clicker questions and Jeopardy-style quiz show questions
- Files for all illustrations and tables and selected photos from the text

TEST BANK

- Test Bank in Microsoft Word, PDF, and RTF formats
- Computerized Test Bank, which includes all the questions in a format that allows you to easily and intuitively build exams and quizzes.

TEACHING RESOURCES

- Instructor Resource and Support Manual in Microsoft Word and PDF formats
- Teaching with Student Learning Outcomes
- Teaching with Web 2.0
- Learning Catalytics: Getting Started
- Getting Started with MasteringHealth

STUDENT SUPPLEMENTS

- Take Charge of Your Health Worksheets
- Behavior Change Log and Wellness Journal
- Eat Right! Healthy Eating in College and Beyond
- Live Right! Beating Stress in College and Beyond
- Food Composition Table

Measuring Student Learning Outcomes? All of the MasteringHealth assignable content is tagged to book content and to Bloom's Taxonomy. You also have the ability to add your own learning outcomes, helping you track student performance against your learning outcomes. You can view class performance against the specified learning outcomes and share those results quickly and easily by exporting to a spreadsheet.

CHOOSING HEALTH

THIRD EDITION

April Lynch, M.A.

Karen Vail-Smith, M.S., M.P.A.
EAST CAROLINA UNIVERSITY

Jerome Kotecki, H.S.D.
BALL STATE UNIVERSITY

With contributions by
Laura Bonazzoli

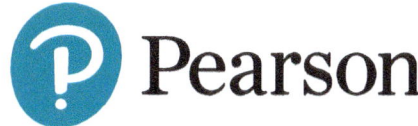

Vice President, Editor-in-Chief, HIED: Adam Jaworski
Vice President, Production & Digital Studio, STEM: Lauren Fogel
Portfolio Manager: Michelle Yglecias
Content Producers: Lauren Bakker and Martha Steele
Portfolio Management Assistant: Nicole Constantine
Courseware Director, Content Development: Barbara Yien
Development Editors: Cathy Murphy, Tanya Martin
Managing Producer, Science: Nancy Tabor
Executive Content Producer: Laura Tommasi
Mastering Content Producer, Science: Lorna Perkins
Senior Mastering Media Producer: Katie Foley
Associate Mastering Media Producer: Lucinda Bingham
Production Management and Composition: Cenveo Publisher Services
Illustrators: Lachina
Design Managers: Marilyn Perry and Mark Ong
Interior Designer: Elise Lansdon
Cover Designer: Elise Lansdon
Photo Researcher: Danny Meldung
Senior Procurement Specialist: Stacey Weinberger
Executive Product Marketing Manager: Neena Bali
Senior Marketing Manager: Mary Salzman
Cover Illustration Credit: Stellapictures/Blend Images/Alamy Stock Photo

Credits and acknowledgments borrowed from other sources and reproduced, with permission, in this textbook appear on the appropriate page within the text or on page CR-1.
Copyright © 2018, 2015, 2012 by Pearson Education, Inc. Published by Pearson Education, Inc. All rights reserved. Manufactured in the United States of America. This publication is protected by Copyright and permission should be obtained from the publisher prior to any prohibited reproduction, storage in a retrieval system, or transmission in any form or by any means, electronic, mechanical, photocopying, recording, or likewise. To obtain permission(s) to use material from this work, please submit a written request to Pearson Education, Inc., Permissions Department, 1900 E. Lake Ave., Glenview, IL 60025. For information regarding permissions, call (847) 486-2635.

Many of the designations used by manufacturers and sellers to distinguish their products are claimed as trademarks. Where those designations appear in this book, and the publisher was aware of a trademark claim, the designations have been printed in initial caps or all caps. PEARSON, ALWAYS LEARNING, MasteringHealth®, are exclusive trademarks, in the United States and/or other countries, of Pearson Education, Inc. or its affiliates.

Library of Congress Cataloging-in-Publication Data on file.

ISBN 10: 0-134-49367-2; ISBN 13: 978-0-134-49367-1 (Student edition)
ISBN 10: 0-134-63624-4; ISBN 13: 978-0-134-63624-5 (Instructor's Review Copy)
ISBN 10: 0-134-55421-3; ISBN 13: 978-0-134-55421-1 (Books A La Carte edition)

2 2022

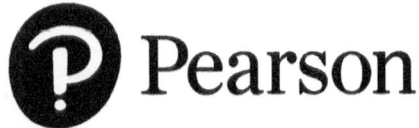

" *This book is dedicated to my husband, Colin, daughter, Ava, and son, Van. In the ever-changing love and laughter project that is our family, I'm inspired to reach for better choices, every single day.*"

—April Lynch

" *I dedicate this book to my loving family, William, Alex, Mary-Brett, and Zan. I thank my colleagues, who always provide support and good counsel, and my students, who teach me every day.*"

—Karen Vail-Smith

" *This book is dedicated to my friends and family for their continued support and love. They allowed me the time and energy to focus my passion and write this book.*"

—Jerome Kotecki

ABOUT THE AUTHORS

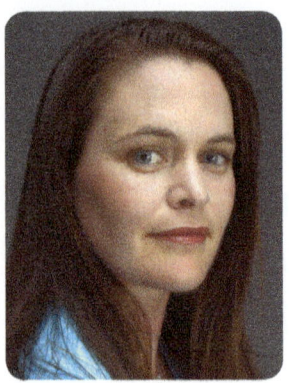

April Lynch, M.A.

April Lynch is an award-winning author and journalist who specializes in health, the medical and biological sciences, and human genetics. During her tenure with the *San Jose Mercury News*, the leading newspaper of Silicon Valley, she served as the science and health editor, focusing the paper's coverage on personal health and scientific developments in the field of disease prevention. She has also worked as a writer and editor for the *San Francisco Chronicle*. April has written numerous articles on personal health, medical and scientific advances, consumer issues such as health insurance, and the ways that scientific breakthroughs are redefining our understanding of health. She has been a frequent contributor to leading university textbooks covering applied biology, nutrition, and environmental health and science. Along with *Choosing Health*, April has co-authored *Health: Making Choices for Life,* an innovative personal health textbook for instructors who desire a more detailed, in-depth book for students majoring in health-related subjects. Together with a leading genetic counselor, April is also the co-author of *The Genome Book*, a hands-on guide to using genetic information in personal health decisions. Her work has won numerous awards from organizations such as the Society of Professional Journalists, the California Newspaper Publishers Association, and the Associated Press. Her current interests include a focus on how people receive and interact with health information online as well as how complex scientific and medical information is best shared compellingly and effectively in digital media. She lives in the San Francisco Bay Area with her husband and children.

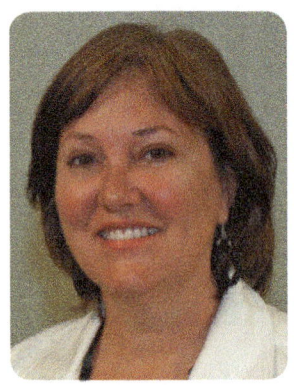

Karen Vail-Smith, M.S., M.P.A.
East Carolina University

Karen Vail-Smith received a B.S. from The University of North Carolina at Chapel Hill and an M.S. and an M.P.A. from East Carolina University. She has been a faculty member in East Carolina University's Department of Health Education and Promotion for 27 years and has taught more than 10,000 college students how to lead healthier lives. She specializes in personal health, alcohol and other drugs, and human sexuality. She has received numerous teaching awards, including the prestigious UNC Board of Governor's Distinguished Professor for Teaching award. During her career she has published more than 30 articles in health professional journals, produced 50 nationally distributed health promotion videos, and contributed to several personal health textbooks.

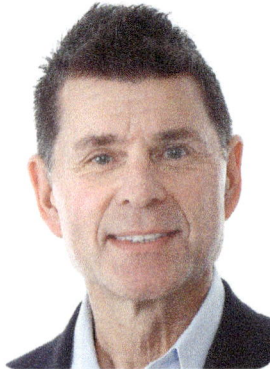

Jerome Kotecki, H.S.D.
Ball State University

Jerome E. Kotecki is a professor of health science in the Department of Nutrition and Health Science, located within the College of Health, at Ball State University. Jerome earned his doctorate in health education and his master's degree in exercise science from Indiana University. He has published more than 40 scientific research papers on the prevention, arrest, and reversal of the most common chronic diseases facing Americans today. Jerome has authored and co-authored multiple textbooks on the importance of healthy lifestyle habits to enhance the multidimensional components of human health and prevent cardiovascular disease, diabetes, cancer, and other chronic conditions. Jerome has extensive experience in health promotion, with particular focus on physical activity and health. An experienced teacher and researcher, he is devoted to helping students adopt and maintain healthy lifestyles. Jerome has been recognized for his contributions to the scholarship of teaching and learning by his department, college, and university. He is an avid fitness participant and enjoys cycling, resistance training, running, mountain biking, hiking, swimming, and yoga.

ABOUT THE CONTRIBUTOR

Laura Bonazzoli

Laura Bonazzoli has been writing and editing in the health sciences for over 20 years. Her early work in human anatomy and physiology, chemistry, and other core sciences laid the foundation for writing projects in nursing, pathology, nutrition, complementary and alternative medicine, and personal health. Her commitment as a writer is to help her readers appreciate the power of small choices to improve their health and the health of their communities. In her free time, Laura and her daughter enjoy exploring the gardens, byways, and beaches of mid-coast Maine.

BRIEF CONTENTS

1	HEALTH IN THE 21ST CENTURY	1
2	PSYCHOLOGICAL HEALTH	25
3	STRESS MANAGEMENT	51
4	SLEEP, YOUR BODY, AND YOUR MIND	74
5	NUTRITION	96
6	PHYSICAL ACTIVITY FOR FITNESS AND HEALTH	126
7	BODY IMAGE, BODY WEIGHT	154
8	ADDICTIONS AND DRUG USE	181
9	ALCOHOL AND TOBACCO USE AND ABUSE	205
10	SOCIAL RELATIONSHIPS AND COMMUNICATION	234
11	SEXUALITY, CONTRACEPTION, AND REPRODUCTIVE CHOICES	255
12	PREVENTING INFECTIOUS DISEASES AND SEXUALLY TRANSMITTED INFECTIONS	291
13	DIABETES, CARDIOVASCULAR DISEASE, AND CANCER	318
14	CONSUMER HEALTH	352
15	PERSONAL SAFETY AND INJURY PREVENTION	376

Additional Electronic Chapters
Access these chapters online through MasteringHealth™

16	YOUR ENVIRONMENT, YOUR HEALTH	400
17	AGING WELL	430

CONTENTS

Preface xxiii | Acknowledgments xxix

CHAPTER 1
HEALTH IN THE 21ST CENTURY 1

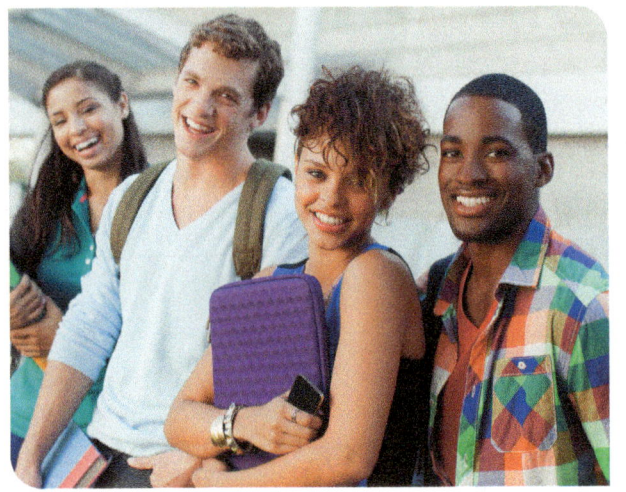

What Is Health? 2
Health Versus Disease 2
Health Versus Wellness 3

Dimensions of Health 3

Current Health Challenges 4
Health Across America 4
Health on America's Campuses 7
Health Around the World 7

Determinants of Health 8
Biology and Genetics 9
Individual Behaviors 9
Social Determinants 10
Physical Determinants 10
Health Services 11
Policy-Making 11

What Factors Influence Behavior Change? 13
Predisposing Factors 13
Enabling Factors 13
Reinforcing Factors 13

How Does Behavior Change Occur? 14
The Transtheoretical Model 14
The Health Belief Model 14
Ecological Models 14

Change Yourself, Change Your World 15
Personal Choices 15
Campus and Community Advocacy 18

Choosing to Change Worksheet 21
Chapter Summary 22
Get Connected 23
Test Your Knowledge 23
What Do You Think? 24

CHAPTER 2
PSYCHOLOGICAL HEALTH 25

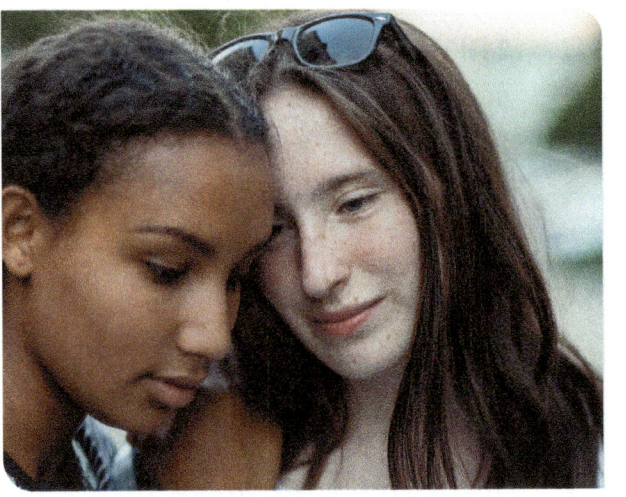

What Is Psychological Health? 26
Components of Psychological Health 26
Facets of Psychological Health 26
Maslow's Hierarchy of Needs 28
The Role of Emotional Intelligence 28
The Value of Optimism 29

Factors Affecting Psychological Health 29
Family History 29
Social Support 29
The Role of Spiritual Health 29

Common Psychological Challenges 31
Shyness 31
Loneliness 32
Anger 32

Mental Disorders in the United States: An Overview 33

Prevalence of Mental Disorders 33
Diagnosis and Treatment of Mental Disorders 33

Mood Disorders 34
Depressive Disorders 34
Bipolar Disorder 36

Anxiety Disorders 37
Generalized Anxiety Disorder (GAD) 37
Panic Attacks and Panic Disorder 37
Social Anxiety Disorder 37
Phobias 37
Treating Anxiety Disorders 38

Other Disorders 38
Obsessive-Compulsive Disorder (OCD) 38
Post-Traumatic Stress Disorder (PTSD) 38
Attention Disorders 39
Schizophrenia 40

Self-Injury and Suicide 40
Non-suicidal Self-Injury 40
Suicide 41

Getting Help for a Psychological Problem 42
Options on Campus 42
Clinical Options 42

Change Yourself, Change Your World 45
Taking Care of Yourself 45
Helping Others 45

Choosing to Change Worksheet 46
Chapter Summary 48
Get Connected 49
Test Your Knowledge 49
What Do You Think? 50

CHAPTER 3
STRESS MANAGEMENT 51

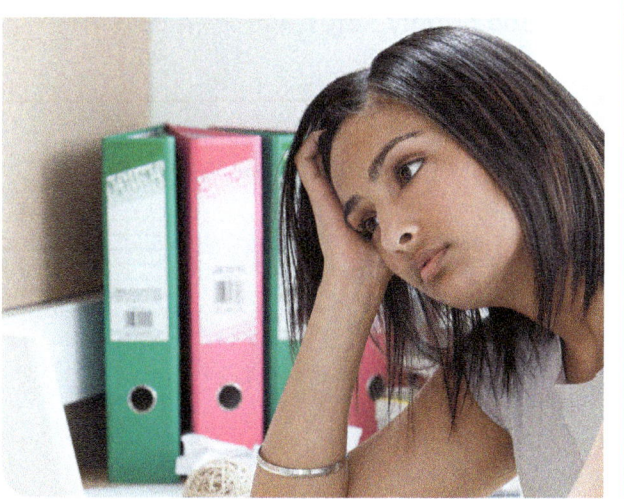

What Is Stress? 52

The Body's Stress Response 52
Alarm Stage: The Fight-or-Flight Response 53
Resistance Stage 54
Exhaustion Stage and Allostatic Overload 54

Health Effects of Chronic Stress 54
Effects on the Cardiovascular System 55
Effects on Digestion, Glucose Regulation, and Body Weight 55
Effects on the Immune System 56
Stress and Headaches 56
Effects on Sleep 56
Effects on Relationships and Sexual Functioning 57
Effects on Mind and Mental Health 57

What Influences the Stress Response? 57
The Role of Personality Types 57
The Role of Personality Traits 58
The Role of Biology 58

What Are College Students' Common Stressors? 59
Academic Pressure 59
Financial Stressors 59
Job-Related Stressors 59
Social Stressors 59
Minor Hassles and Major Life Changes 61
Environmental Stressors 62
Internal Stressors 62

Resources for Managing Stress 62
Social Support 62
Help on Campus 62
Medical Options 64

Change Yourself, Change Your World 64
Manage Your Time Effectively 64
Improve Your Test-Taking Skills 65
Live a Healthier Lifestyle 65
Relieve Your Tensions 66
Change Your Thinking 67
Create a Personalized Stress Management Plan 68

Choosing to Change Worksheet 69
Chapter Summary 71
Get Connected 72
Test Your Knowledge 72
What Do You Think? 73

CHAPTER 4
SLEEP, YOUR BODY, AND YOUR MIND 74

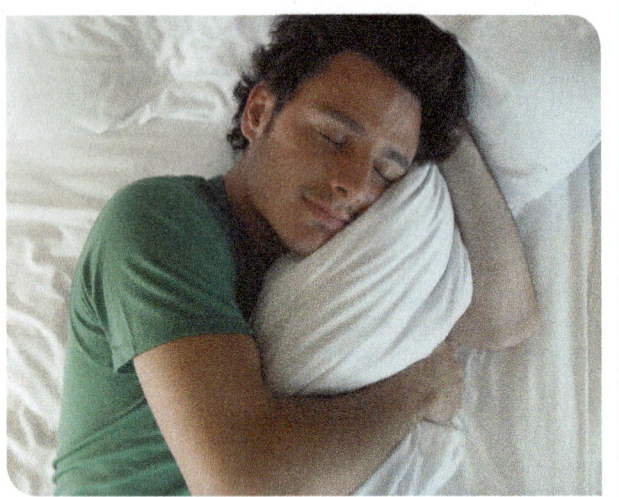

What Is Sleep? 75
Regions and Rhythms of Sleep 75
Stages of Sleep 76
Cycles of Sleep 77

Sleep: How Much and Why It Matters 77
Research on Short and Long Sleep 78
Short Sleep: The American Way? 79
Why Is Ample Sleep Important? 79

What Factors Influence Sleep? 81
Biology and Genetics 81
Individual Behaviors 81
Factors in the Environment 83

Sleep Disorders 83
Insomnia 83
Snoring 83
Sleep Apnea 84
Narcolepsy 85
Parasomnias 85

Getting Help for a Sleep Disorder 86
Campus and Community Support 86
Clinical Diagnosis and Treatment 86
Complementary and Alternative Therapies 88

Change Yourself, Change Your World 88
Personal Choices 88

Choosing to Change Worksheet 91
Chapter Summary 93
Get Connected 94
Test Your Knowledge 94
What Do You Think? 95

CHAPTER 5
NUTRITION 96

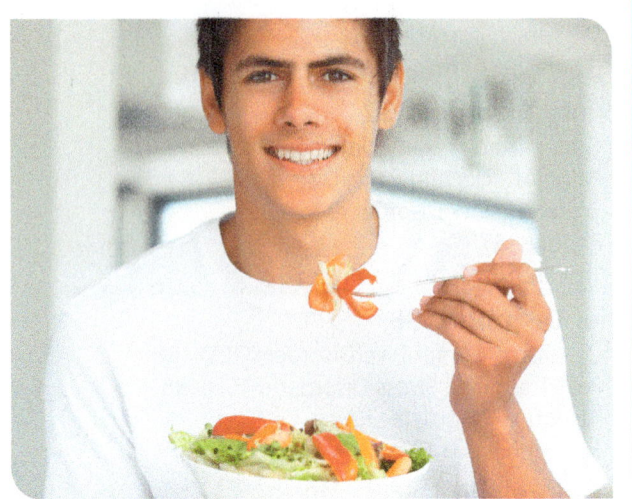

What Are Nutrients? 97
Energy and Calories 97
Carbohydrates 98
Fats 100
Proteins 102
Vitamins 103
Minerals 104
Water 104

What About Functional Foods and Dietary Supplements? 106
Phytochemicals 107
Probiotics and Prebiotics 108
Dietary Supplements 108

What Tools Can Help You Eat Right? 110
Dietary Reference Intakes (DRIs) 110
Food Labels 111
Dietary Guidelines for Americans 113
MyPlate 113

Is Our Food Supply Safe? 116
Foodborne Illness 116
Food Allergies and Intolerances 117
Food Residues 118

Change Yourself, Change Your World 118
Think Smart When Making Choices 120
Eat Smart When Eating Out 120
Shop Smart When Money's Tight 120
Campus Advocacy 121

Choosing to Change Worksheet 122
Chapter Summary 123
Get Connected 124
Test Your Knowledge 124
What Do You Think? 125

CHAPTER 6
PHYSICAL ACTIVITY FOR FITNESS AND HEALTH 126

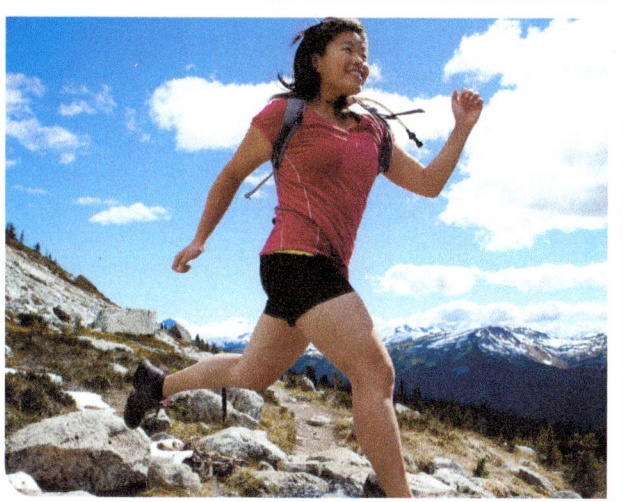

What Is Physical Fitness? 127
- Cardiorespiratory Fitness 127
- Muscular Strength 127
- Muscular Endurance 128
- Flexibility 128
- Body Composition 128

What Are the Benefits of Physical Activity? 129
- Stronger Heart and Lungs 129
- Management and Prevention of Type 2 Diabetes 130
- Reduced Risk of Some Cancers 130
- Increased Immune Function 130
- Stronger Bones 130
- Reduced Risk of Injury 130
- Healthful Weight Management 130
- Benefits to Psychological Health, Stress Management, and Sleep 130

Principles of Fitness Training 131
- Overload 131
- Specificity 131
- Reversibility 131
- Individuality 132
- Diminishing Returns 132

What Types of Physical Activity Should You Consider? 132
- Aerobic Exercise 132
- Exercise for Muscular Strength and Endurance 135
- Exercises for Improving Flexibility 136

How Much Physical Activity Do You Need? 142
- Guidelines for Health Maintenance 142
- Avoid Sustained Sitting 144
- Increase Your Level of Activity 144

Exercise Safe, Exercise Smart 145
- Get Medical Clearance and Be Prepared 145
- Warm Up and Cool Down 145
- Get Training 145
- Eat Right 145
- Stay Hydrated 145
- Prepare for Hot or Cold Weather 146
- Start Slowly and Watch Out for Red Flags 146
- Care for Injuries 147
- Be Wary of Performance-Enhancing Drugs 148

Change Yourself, Change Your World 148
- Personal Choices 148

Choosing to Change Worksheet 151
Chapter Summary 152
Get Connected 152
Test Your Knowledge 152
What Do You Think? 153

CHAPTER 7
BODY IMAGE, BODY WEIGHT 154

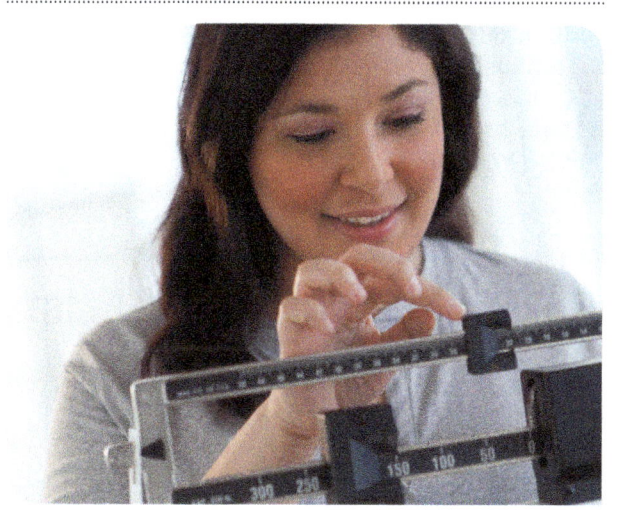

Body Image and Body Weight 155
- Many Factors Influence Body Image 155
- Defining a Healthful Body Weight 156

Alarming Trends in Body Weight 158
- Weight Trends in the United States 158
- Weight Trends Around the World 158
- Weight Trends on Campus 159

Risks and Costs of Obesity 159
- Health Risks 159
- Financial Burden of Obesity 160

Factors that Contribute to Weight Gain 161
- Biology and Genetics 161
- Individual Behaviors 163
- Social Factors 163

Physical Factors 164
Public Policy 164

Reducing Excess Body Weight 164
Can Dieting Work 164
Comparing Diets 166
Diet "Aids"? 167
Clinical Options for Obesity 168
The Importance of Physical Activity 169
What If You Want To Gain Weight? 169
How Do You Maintain a Healthful Weight? 170

Change Yourself, Change Your World 170
Campus Resources for Maintaining a Healthy Weight 171

Body Image and Eating Disorders 171
Body Image Disorders 171
Eating Disorders 172
Other Unhealthful Eating Behaviors 174
Getting Help for a Body Image or Eating Disorder 175
Personal Choices: Develop a More Positive Body Image 176

Choosing to Change Worksheet 176
Chapter Summary 178
Get Connected 179
Test Your Knowledge 179
What Do You Think? 180

CHAPTER **8**

ADDICTIONS AND DRUG USE 181

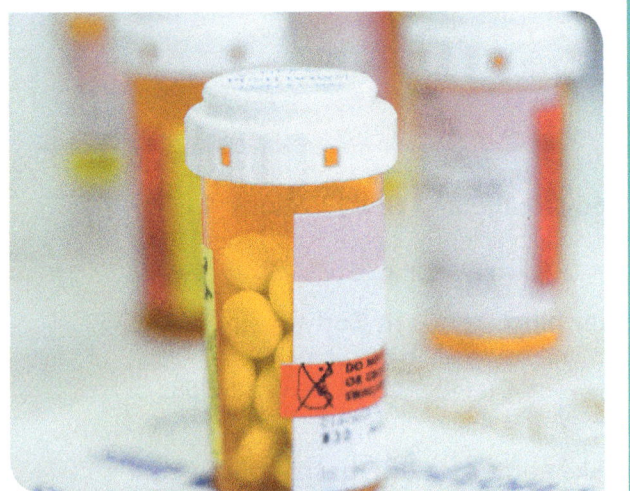

An Overview of Addiction 182
What Is Addiction? 182

What Are Behavioral Addictions? 183
Pathological Gambling 183
Hypersexual Disorder 183

Compulsive Spending 183
Technology Addiction 183

Patterns of Drug Use 184

How the Body Responds to Drugs 185
Drug Misuse and Abuse 185
Initial Effects on the Brain 185
Effects of Chronic Use 185
How Drugs Leave the Body 187

Commonly Abused Drugs 187
Prescription and Over-the-Counter Medications 187
Heroin 188
Marijuana 190
Stimulants 191
Hallucinogens 193
Club Drugs 193
Inhalants 194
Depressants 194

Preventing Drug Abuse 195

Getting Help for a Drug Problem 195
Campus and Community-Based Options 197
Clinical Options 197

Change Yourself, Change Your World 198
Personal Choices 198
Helping a Friend 199

Choosing to Change Worksheet 200
Chapter Summary 202
Get Connected 203
Test Your Knowledge 203
What Do You Think? 204

CHAPTER **9**

ALCOHOL AND TOBACCO USE AND ABUSE 205

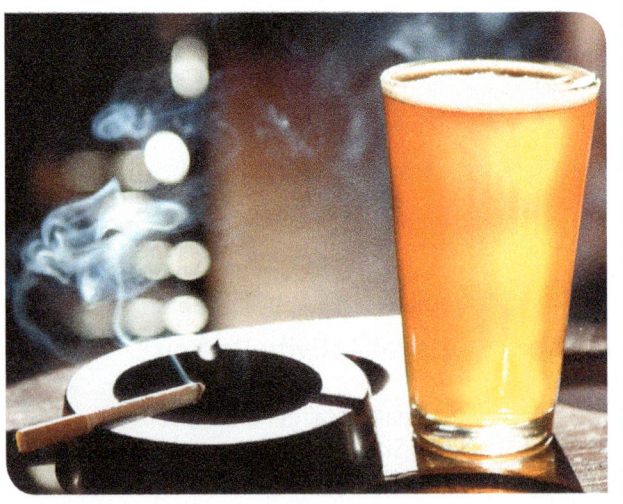

xii CONTENTS

Alcohol Use in the United the States 206
    Alcohol Use and Binge Drinking on Campus 206
    The Makeup of Alcohol 208

How the Body Absorbs and Metabolizes Alcohol 209
    Blood Alcohol Concentration 209

The Effects of Alcohol on the Body 211
    Intoxication 211
    Immediate Effects of Alcohol on the Body 211
    Long-Term Effects of Alcohol on the Body 212
    Alcohol and Pregnancy 213
    Health Benefits of Alcohol? 214

The Effects of Alcohol on Behavior 214
    Drinking and Driving 214
    Alcohol and Sexual Activity 215
    Alcohol and Other Problems 216

Alcohol Abuse 216
    Alcoholism 216

Alcohol Abuse: Treatment and Prevention 217
    Treatment Options 218
    Dealing with Relapse 218
    Prevention Strategies 218

Smoking in the United States 220
    Smoking on Campus 220
    What's in a Cigarette? 221

Effects of Smoking on Health 221
    Short-Term Health Effects 221
    Long-Term Health Effects 223
    Smoking and Pregnancy 223
    Secondhand Smoke 224

Other Forms of Tobacco 225
    Cigars 225
    Clove Cigarettes 225
    Bidis 225
    Hookahs 226
    Smokeless ("Spit") Tobacco 226
    Electronic Cigarettes 226

Getting Help to Quit Smoking 227
    Treatment Options 227
    Dealing with Relapse 228

Change Yourself, Change Your World 228
    Personal Choices 228
    Campus Advocacy 229

Choosing to Change Worksheet 230
Chapter Summary 231
Get Connected 232
Test Your Knowledge 232
What Do You Think? 233

CHAPTER **10**

SOCIAL RELATIONSHIPS AND COMMUNICATION 234

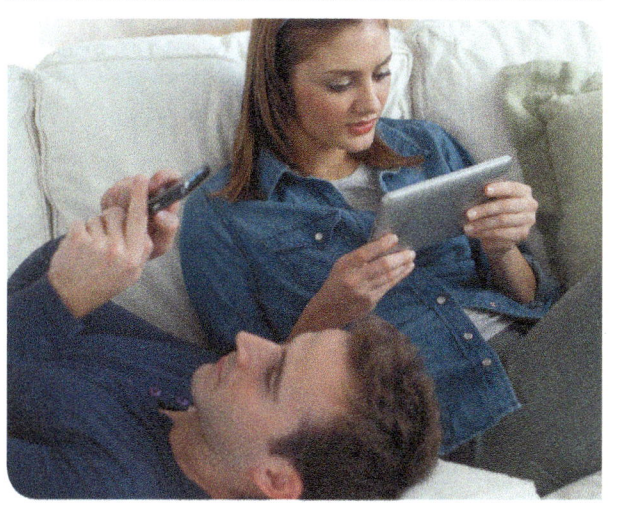

Communication in Relationships 235
    Communicating Feelings 235
    Being a Good Listener 236
    Resolving Conflicts 236
    Gender Roles and Communication 237

Developing Relationships 238
    Self-Perception 238
    Early Relationships 238
    Gender Roles 238

Friendships 239
    Maintaining Old Friendships 239

Intimate Relationships 240
    Sternberg's Triangular Theory of Love 240
    What Causes Attraction? 242
    Dating 242
    Same-Sex Relationships 243
    Healthy Relationships 243
    Dysfunctional Relationships 244
    When Relationships End 245

Committed Relationships 245
    Cohabitation 246
    Marriage 246
    Domestic Partnerships 248
    Staying Single 248

Starting a Family 248
    Choosing to Have Children 249
    Stepfamilies 249
    Single Parenthood 249
    Characteristics of Happy Families 250

Change Yourself, Change Your World 250
    Personal Choices 250
    Campus Advocacy 250

Choosing to Change Worksheet 251
Chapter Summary 253
Get Connected 253
Test Your Knowledge 254
What Do You Think? 254

CHAPTER 11

SEXUALITY, CONTRACEPTION, AND REPRODUCTIVE CHOICES 255

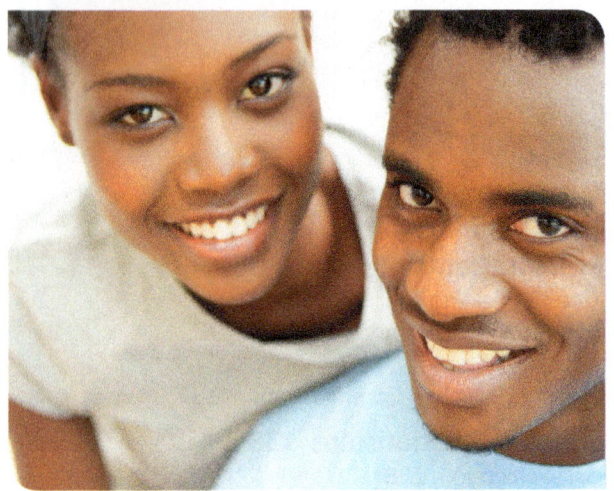

Sexual Anatomy and Health 256
Female Sexual Anatomy and Sexual Health 256
Male Sexual Anatomy and Sexual Health 258

The Menstrual Cycle 259
Phases of the Menstrual Cycle 260
Disorders Associated with the Menstrual Cycle 261

The Sexual Response Cycle 262
Sexual Dysfunctions 262

Sexual Behavior 264
Abstinence and Celibacy 264
Sexual Intercourse 264
Oral Sex 264
Communicating About Sex 265
Non-Intercourse Sexual Activity 265

Sexual Orientation and Gender Identity 267
Heterosexuality 267
Homosexuality 267
Bisexuality 268
Gender Identity 268

Conception and Contraception 268
Conception 269
Contraceptive Options 269
Which Method Is the Best? 276

Abortion 277

Methods of Abortion 278
Physical and Psychological Complications of Abortion 279
Legal Status of Abortion 279

Pregnancy and Childbirth 280
Pregnancy 280
Childbirth 284

Infertility 285
Causes of Infertility 285
Options for Infertile Couples 286

Change Yourself, Change Your World 286
Personal Choices 286
Campus Advocacy 287

Choosing to Change Worksheet 287
Chapter Summary 288
Get Connected 289
Test Your Knowledge 290
What Do You Think? 290

CHAPTER 12

PREVENTING INFECTIOUS DISEASES AND SEXUALLY TRANSMITTED INFECTIONS 291

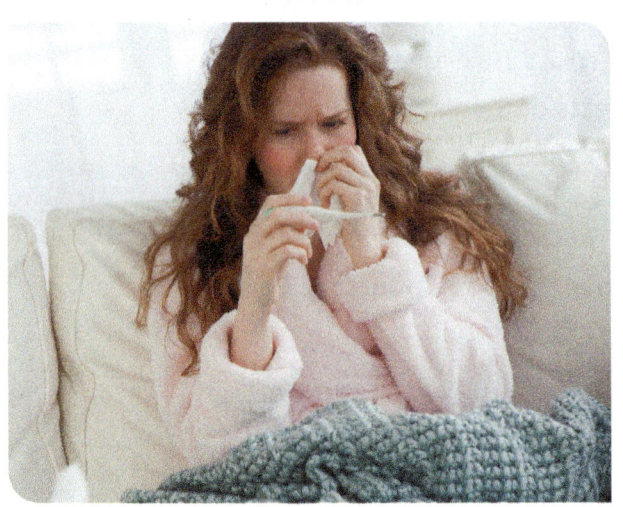

How Are Infections Spread? 292

Protecting Against Infections 293
The Body's First Line of Defense 293
The Body's Immune Response 293
Immunization 294
Immune Disorders 296

Infectious Diseases 297
Viral Infections 297
Bacterial Infections 299
Fungal Infections 303
Protozoan Infections 303
Parasitic Worm Infections 304

xiv   CONTENTS

Sexually Transmitted Infections 304
　Risk Factors for STIs 304
　HIV and AIDS 305
　Hepatitis B 307
　Genital Herpes 308
　Human Papillomavirus 308
　Chlamydia 309
　Gonorrhea 309
　Pelvic Inflammatory Disease 309
　Syphilis 311
　Pubic Lice and Scabies 311
　Trichomoniasis 311

Change Yourself, Change Your World 312
　Personal Choices 312

Choosing to Change Worksheet 313
Chapter Summary 315
Get Connected 316
Test Your Knowledge 316
What Do You Think? 317

CHAPTER 13
DIABETES, CARDIOVASCULAR DISEASE, AND CANCER 318

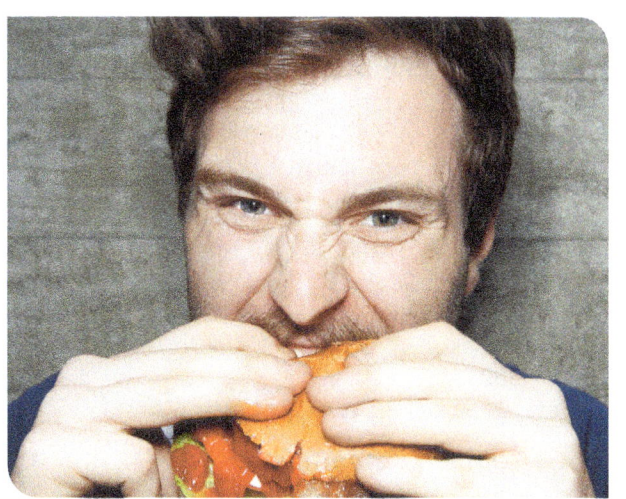

Overview of Chronic Diseases 319
　Scope of the Problem 319
　Influence of Four Key Behaviors 319

Diabetes 320
　Types of Diabetes 320
　Detecting Diabetes 323
　Complications of Diabetes 323
　Risk Factors for Type 2 Diabetes 324
　Clinical Management of Diabetes 325

Cardiovascular Disease 326
　The Healthy Cardiovascular System 326
　Atherosclerosis 327
　Hypertension (High Blood Pressure) 328
　Coronary Heart Disease 329
　Heart Failure 331
　Stroke 332
　Other Forms of Cardiovascular Disease 334
　Risk Factors for Cardiovascular Disease 334

Cardiometabolic Risk 336

Cancer 337
　What Is Cancer? 338
　Risk Factors for Cancer 338
　Detecting Cancer 340
　Types of Cancer 341
　Common Cancers in Men and Women 341
　Common Cancers in Men 344
　Common Cancers in Women 344
　Treating Cancer 346

Change Yourself, Change Your World 346

Choosing to Change Worksheet 348
Chapter Summary 349
Get Connected 350
Test Your Knowledge 351
What Do You Think? 351

CHAPTER 14
CONSUMER HEALTH 352

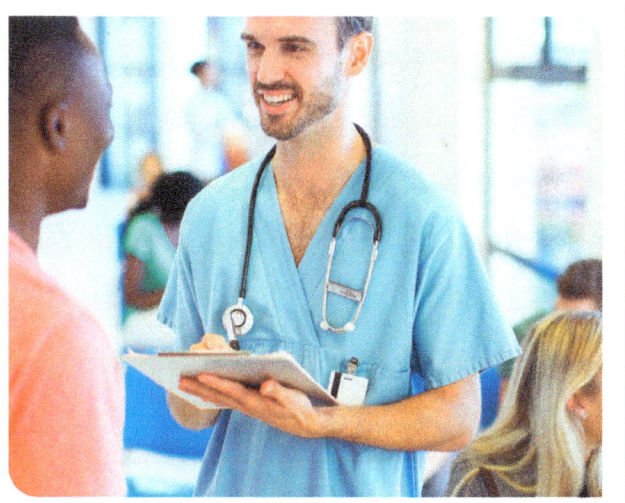

Choosing Self-Care 353
　Practicing Prevention 353
　Finding Accurate Health Information 354
　Options for Self-Care 355

When to See a Doctor 356
　Checkups and Preventive Care 357
　Health Problems Beyond Self-Care 357

Conventional Medicine 358
　Where to Find Conventional Health Care 359

Choosing a Provider 360
Being a Smart Patient 360
Handling Prescription Medications Properly 361

Complementary and Alternative Medicine (CAM) 362
Evaluating Complementary and Alternative Therapies 364

Paying for Health Care 364
Discount Programs 365
Health Insurance 365
Health Savings Accounts and Flexible Spending Accounts 368
Students and Health Insurance 368
What Happens When I Graduate? 368

"Personalized Medicine" and the Future of Consumer Health 369
A Short Course in Genetics and Genomics 369
Uses of Genomic Information 370
Ethical, Social, and Legal Implications of Genomic Advances 371

Change Yourself, Change Your World 371

Choosing to Change Worksheet 372
Chapter Summary 373
Get Connected 374
Test Your Knowledge 374
What Do You Think? 375

CHAPTER **15**

PERSONAL SAFETY AND INJURY PREVENTION 376

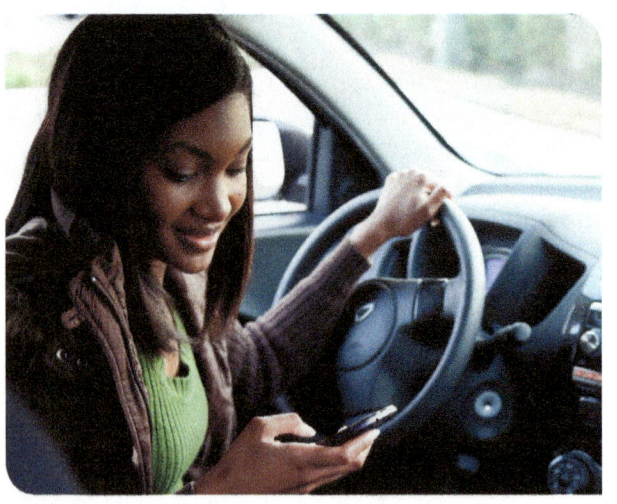

Overview of Unintentional Injuries 377

Motor Vehicle Accidents 378
What Factors Increase the Risk for Motor Vehicle Accidents? 378
Motorcycle Accidents 380

Pedestrian and Cyclist Safety 381
Accidents Involving Pedestrians and Cyclists 381

Residential, Recreational, and Occupational Injuries 382
Unintentional Poisoning 382
Choking and Suffocation 382
Drowning and Other Water Injuries 383
Fire Injuries 384
Work-Related Injuries 384

Intentional Injuries and Violence 385

Violence Within Communities 388
Assault 388
Homicide 388
School and Campus Violence 388
Hate Crimes 389
Terrorism 389

Violence Within Relationships 389
Intimate Partner Violence 389
Stalking and Cyberstalking 390
Addressing Violence Within Relationships 391

Sexual Violence 391
Risk Factors for Sexual Violence 391
Sexual Harassment 391
Rape 392
Effects of Sexual Violence 394

Change Yourself, Change Your World 395
Personal Choices 395
Helping a Friend 395
Campus Advocacy 396

Choosing to Change Worksheet 396
Chapter Summary 397
Get Connected 398
Test Your Knowledge 398
What Do You Think? 399

Additional Electronic Chapters

Access these chapters online through MasteringHealth™

CHAPTER 16
YOUR ENVIRONMENT, YOUR HEALTH 400

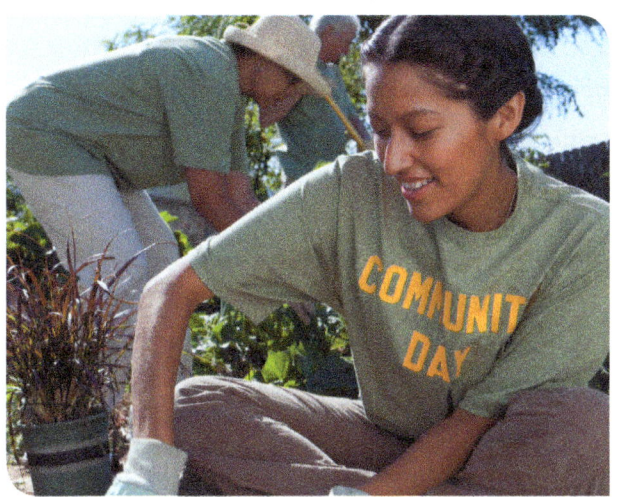

Overview of Environmental Health 401
  Defining Your Environment 401
  Environmental Health Is a
  Global Concern 402
  The Evolution of Environmental Health 402
  Toward Sustainability 403

Overpopulation 403
  Factors Contributing to Population Growth 404
  Effects of Overpopulation 404
  Reversing Population Growth 405

Air Pollution and Climate Change 405
  Air Pollutants, Global Warming, and Climate Change 406
  Air Pollutants, Ozone, and Smog 407
  Air Pollutants and Production of Acid Rain 408
  What Can Be Done to Reduce
  Air Pollution? 409

Water Pollution 411
  Pollutants Found in Water 412
  Is Bottled Water Worth It? 413

Land Pollution 414
  Municipal Waste and Its Management 414
  Hazardous Waste and Its Management 415

Pollution at Home 416
  Pollutants in Foods and Beverages 416
  Pollutants in Packaging 418
  Pollutants in Indoor Air 419

Noise Pollution 420

Radiation 422
  Types and Health Effects of Radiation 422
  What Can You Do to Reduce Your Exposure to Radiation? 422

Change Yourself, Change Your World 424
  Campus Advocacy 424

Choosing to Change Worksheet 425
Chapter Summary 426
Get Connected 427
Test Your Knowledge 428
What Do You Think? 429

CHAPTER 17
AGING WELL 430

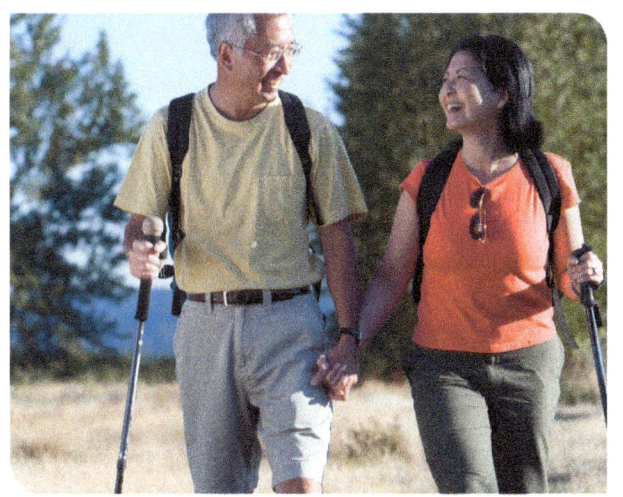

Aging in the United States 431
  Trends in Health and Health Care 431
  Life Expectancy 432
  Gender and Longevity 432

What Happens as You Age? 433
  Physical Changes 433
  Psychosocial Changes 437

What Are the Keys to Successful Aging? 438
  Physical Activity 439
  Good Nutrition 439
  Weight Management 439
  Avoiding Tobacco 441
  Mental Exercise 441
  Meaning, Purpose, and Connection 441

Understanding Death and Dying 441
  What Is Death? 441
  How Do We Develop Our Concepts of Death and Dying? 443

Planning for the End of Life 444
- Complete Advance Directives 444
- Consider Organ Donation 444
- Write a Will 444
- Research Your Options for End-of-Life Care 444
- Clarify Your Beliefs and Values 445

After a Death 446
- Autopsy 446
- Care of the Body 446
- Planning a Service 446
- Experiencing Grief 447

Change Yourself, Change Your World 448
- Supporting a Loved One Who Is Dying 448
- Supporting a Loved One Who Is Grieving 448
- Campus Advocacy 448

Choosing to Change Worksheet 450
Chapter Summary 452
Get Connected 453
Test Your Knowledge 453
What Do You Think? 454

QUICK CHECK ANSWERS AN-1

TEST YOUR KNOWLEDGE ANSWERS AN-2

CREDITS CR-1

GLOSSARY GL-1

REFERENCES RF-1

INDEX I-1

FEATURE BOXES

STUDENT STORIES

Corey: Proud of My Scars 11
Javier: Dealing with Depression 36
Kristina: A Friend's Suicide 41
David: The Stress of Responsibility 55
Jessica: The Pressure to Succeed 64
Remy: Sleep Apnea 85
Jasmine: Sleep Deprived 87
Peter: What Should I Do? 108
Nidya: Why I'm Vegetarian 112
Sean: Cardiorespiratory Fitness 132
Molly: Adapting Exercise to My Needs 150
Josh: Active Loser 163
Viege: Eating Disorders: Regrets About a Friend 176
Ana: Coping with Addiction 197
Courtney: Drinking's Darker Side 214
Addison: Quitting Cold Turkey 228

Brittany: A New BFF 239
Jonathan and Yeani: Talk It Out 242
Betty: Choosing the Pill 269
Abbey: Open Talk About STIs 278
Jessica: Germaphobe 295
Gabe: Unprotected Sex 313
Michael: Diabetes in the Family 326
Amanda: Surviving Cancer 345
Holly: The Cost of Being Uninsured 366
Caleb: Seat Belt Saved Me 381
Jenny: From Control to Abuse 390
Toby: Car vs. Campus Shuttle 412
Camille: Recycling Cell Phones 415
Stephen: Handling Aging 437
Michelle: Grieving 447

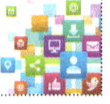

MEDIA AND …

Media and Health: Evaluating Health Information in the Media 12
Media and Fitness: Do Fitness Apps Work? 147
Media and Alcohol and Tobacco Use: How Entertainment and Ads Drive Drinking and Smoking 222

Media and Sexuality: Is Porn a Problem? 266
Media and Aging: Do High-Tech Games Boost the Brain? 442

CHOOSE THIS.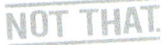

Stress: Exercise vs. Alcohol 68
Sleep: Ample Sleep vs. Sleep Deprived 80
Hunger: A Healthful Lunch vs. An Empty-Calorie Lunch 116
Your Body: Fit and Active vs. Unfit and Sedentary 129

Weight Loss: A Pound or Two Each Week vs. Crash Diet 172
Conflict: A Fair Fight vs. Full-On "Fight Club" 237
Motor Vehicle Accidents: Attentive and Defensive Driving vs. Distracted, Impaired, or Aggressive Driving 380

 SPECIAL FEATURE

Procrastination: Sabotaging Your Future Self   60
Starting Right for a Restful Night   90
Feeding Your Bones   106
Dietary Guidelines: A Blueprint for Better Nutrition   114
Core Concerns: Why You Should Strengthen Your Core   135
Are "Study Drugs" Smart—or Safe?   189
Peer Pressure: Resisting the Pitch   219
Social Media, Communication, and Cyber-Bullies   241
Emerging Mosquito-Borne Diseases: Zika Virus   302
Helping Someone in a CVD Emergency   333
Reducing Your Risk for Chronic Disease   347
What the Affordable Care Act Means for You   367
Title IX: Know Your Rights   393

 SELF-ASSESSMENT

How Healthy Is Your Current Lifestyle?   19
Anxiety Assessment   39
Negative Event Scale for University Students   63
Are You Getting Enough Sleep?   89
Do You Follow a Healthful Eating Pattern?   120
Determining Your Maximum Heart Rate and Target Heart Rate Range   133
Assessing Your Weight-Related Health Risks   158
Could I Have an Eating Disorder?   175
Should You Seek Drug Treatment?   198
Alcohol Use Disorders Identification Test (AUDIT)   217
Is My Relationship Healthy?   245
Are You and Your Partner Ready for Sex?   265
Are You at Risk for an STI?   305
Are You at Risk for Type 2 Diabetes?   324
What's Your Risk for a Heart Attack?   336
What's Your Risk for Cancer?   339
How Proactive Are You About Preventive Health Care?   371
Are You an Aggressive Driver?   379
Is Loud Music Damaging Your Hearing?   422
Are You Comfortable with Death?   449

 Choosing to **Change** Worksheet

Behavior Change Contract   21
Improving Psychological Health   46
Adopting Stress Management Techniques   69
Increasing the Quantity or Quality of Sleep   91
Improving Diet   122
Improving Overall Fitness   151
Changing Body Weight and Improving Body Image   176
Reducing or Eliminating Drug Use   200
Quitting or Cutting Back on Drinking or Tobacco Use   230
Building Healthy Relationships   251
Practicing Safer Sex   287
Reducing STI Risk   313
Reducing the Risk of Chronic Disease   348
Taking Part in Preventive Care   372
Reducing Aggressive Driving Behavior   396
Improving Environmental Health   425
Aging Well   450

PRACTICAL Strategies

Building Self-Efficacy   17
Building Self-Esteem   27
Questions to Ask Before Starting a Medication for Mental Health Issues   36
Spotting Destructive Thoughts   44
Recognizing the Signs of Stress Overload   58
Coping with Financial Stress   60
Exercising for Stress Management   67
Naps: When and How?   78
Choosing Fiber-Rich Carbohydrates   100
Choosing Healthful Fats   102
Go Lean with Protein   103
Finding Nutrient-Dense Fast Foods   121
Safe Weight Lifting   136
Cutting Calories, Not Nutrition   169
Warning Signs of Addiction   183

How to Protect Yourself from Risky Alcohol-Related Behavior 215
Quitting Smoking 229
Tips for Maintaining a Strong Relationship 244
Communicating Effectively About Sex and Birth Control 277
Protecting Yourself Against Infectious Diseases 303
Reducing Your Risk of STIs 307
Tips for Affordable Health Care 369

Reducing Your Risk of Injury While... 382
Preventing Tech Injuries 386
10 Tips for Campus Safety 395
Choosing to Combat Climate Change 409
Promoting Clean Water 414
Limiting Household Hazardous Waste 416
Reducing Pollution at Home 420
Coping with Grief 449

STUDENT STATS

Common Health Problems Reported by College Students 7
Psychological Health on Campus 32
Top 10 Impediments to Academic Performance 57
Sleepless on Campus 79
Top Supplements Used by Students 109
Physical Activity on College Campuses 144
Overweight, Obesity, and Dieting on Campus 160
Dieting and Exercising on Campus 164
Drug Use Among Young Adults 185
Alcohol Use on Campus 208
Smoking on Campus 220
Students and Relationships 248

Sex and the College Student 264
Contraception and College Students 273
STIs in People Aged 15–24 312
College Students' Reported Participation in Key Health Behaviors 320
CAM Use Among College Students 362
An Improving Insurance Picture for Young American Adults 368
Top Five Causes of Death in the United States Among People Aged 15–24 378
Top Seven Causes of Death from Unintentional Injury in the United States Among People Aged 15–24 383
How Many College Students Think Green? 403

MYTH OR FACT?

Can Stress Give You an Ulcer? 56
Is It Safe to Mix Alcohol and Caffeine? 213
Should Boys Be Circumcised for Health Reasons? 259
Do Vaccines Cause Autism? 296

Do Electric Vehicles Merit Their Hype? 411
Does Using a Cell Phone Fry Your Brain? 423

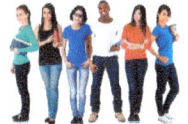

DIVERSITY & HEALTH

Health Disparities Among Different Racial and Ethnic Groups 6
Stress in Minority Populations 61
Sleep Habits Vary 82
Vegetarian Diets 111
Safe Exercise for Special Populations 149
Drug Use and Overdose 186
Alcohol and Tobacco Use: Breaking It Down 207

Same-Sex Marriage: The State of Our Current Debate 247
STIs Among Different Sexes, Races, and Sexual Orientations 310
Disparities in Chronic Disease 322
Injuries and Violence: Special Concerns for Young Men 387
Working for Environmental Justice 417
Aging in the Blue Zones 440

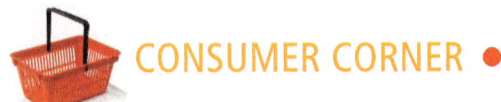

CONSUMER CORNER

Choosing a Therapist Who's Right for You   43
Should You Try OTC Sleep Aids?   88
Drinking Calories: What's in Your Bottle?   107
Organic, Non-GMO, Local, Fair Trade: What to Choose?   119

Choosing Athletic Shoes   146
Are "Light" Cigarettes Safer to Use?   225
Using an Over-the-Counter Medication Safely   356
What's in That Bottle?   413

PREFACE

When it comes to your health, what will you choose? You might think that question pertains to something in your future, such as who your next doctor should be or how you can avoid illness down the road.

But the truth is you have already answered that question several times today, in ways both large and small. Did you get enough sleep last night? What will you have for lunch? Will you really hit the gym this afternoon or just think about it? Are you waiting until the last minute to begin that paper due next week, or are you planning ahead so that you don't get overwhelmed?

In an era filled with medical innovations and high-tech health care, it's easy to overlook the fact that much of your health still rests in your hands. We all have to live with some factors we can't immediately control, such as our genetics and the physical environment that surrounds us. But beyond these fixed elements, your decisions and lifestyle habits count for a lot. This book is called *Choosing Health* to underscore that your actions and behavior *matter*. You can consciously make decisions now that greatly reduce your chances of developing health problems later. The health you choose is an essential part of creating the life you want, both on campus now and in the years ahead.

Key Features of This Text

We wrote this book to help you make the best possible health choices, using the most recent and scientifically accurate information available. Other textbooks provide plenty of health information but offer little guidance for actively improving your health. *Choosing Health,* third edition, makes health information more relevant to you, with unique features such as these:

- **New! MasteringHealth with eText 2.0** This product features all of the resources of MasteringHealth in addition to the new Pearson eText 2.0. Now available on smart phones and tablets and ADA accessible, Pearson eText 2.0 comprises the full text, including videos and other rich media. Students can configure reading settings, including resizable type and night-reading mode; take notes; and highlight, bookmark, and search the text.
  - A Robust MasteringHealth course: Find new ABC news videos and updated Nutritools activities and associated coaching activities, Tough Topics Coaching activities, Which Path Would You Take? decision-making activities, and auto-graded self-assessments, reading quizzes, and more!
  - Increased mobile offerings with Interactive eText 2.0:
    - Embedded interactive self-assessment worksheets that students can anonymously fill out and receive feedback on
    - Embedded media such as ABC News videos, Student Story videos, nutrition animations, behavior change videos, and Which Path Would You Take? decision-making activities
- **New! Chapter 4: Sleep, Your Body, and Your Mind** covers the most up-to-date research on sleep, its effects on health, and how to get your best night's rest. Previously available as an electronic chapter, the topic of sleep has been thoroughly updated and expanded and now follows the Stress Management chapter.
  - Also available as electronic chapters are Chapter 16: Your Environment, Your Health and Chapter 17: Aging Well.
- **New, clear learning path and study plan:** The third edition includes achievable learning outcomes that are linked to chapter sections and end-of-chapter material to create a clear learning path and study plan. Learning outcomes are called out after each main section and listed (by number) next to the relevant chapter summary and Test Your Knowledge and new critical thinking questions in the end-of-chapter study plan. Study plan items in MasteringHealth allow instructors to assign one assessment item that covers all key learning outcomes in a chapter.
- **New end-of-section review questions:** Each main section in a chapter ends with review questions that help students confirm that they have achieved an understanding of the learning outcome for that section.
- **Updated Choose This, Not That** boxes highlight good and poor choices students make about common health issues. Each box promotes the healthy choice and explains why the poor choice is problematic. New Choose This, Not That boxes include "Sleep: Ample Sleep vs. Sleep Deprived" and "Your Body: Fit and Active vs. Unfit and Sedentary."
- **Updated Media and ...** boxes discuss how today's media—everything from TV commercials to phone apps—affect our actions and feelings concerning a variety of health topics.
- **Updated Choosing to Change Worksheets** (also available online through MasteringHealth™) in every chapter help you target a behavior you want to change, determine your stage of behavior change based on the transtheoretical model of behavior change, think through the steps necessary to make a positive change, and put yourself on a path to success.

- **Updated Change Yourself, Change Your World** sections at the end of each chapter show you how to implement the health information you've just learned. Each section offers advice on personal choices, and in some cases, suggestions on helping friends, family, or your community.
- **Updated "What Do You Think?" questions** prompt you to think deeply and appear throughout each chapter.
- **Student Stories** appear throughout the text. QR codes next to select Student Stories in the text link directly to that student's video. These stories reveal how students have dealt with health challenges and may inspire you to make changes in your own life.
- **Updated and additional Student Stats** throughout the book show you how health issues affect the college student population. Colorful graphs display statistics compiled by national surveys of college students.
- **Health Online** links throughout the book guide you to relevant health-related quizzes, tools, websites, videos, and podcasts. These links can also be found on MasteringHealth™, where they will be updated as needed.
- **Self-Assessments,** also available online through MasteringHealth™ and in interactive form in eText 2.0, enable you to evaluate your current health behaviors and identify areas you may wish to work on.
- **A thoroughly updated book design** makes the book fun to read and easier to navigate.
- **The lively, engaging writing** is informative, scientifically reliable, and authoritative.
- **Practical Strategies** boxes provide concrete tips you can use to develop and maintain healthful behaviors.
- **Consumer Corner** boxes examine consumer-related issues such as using over-the-counter medications safely, choosing athletic shoes, and deciding whether to purchase organic produce.
- **Diversity & Health** boxes highlight how health issues can affect certain populations disproportionately, depending on sex, racial/ethnic background, socioeconomic class, and other factors.
- **Myth or Fact?** boxes provide scientific evidence supporting or refuting common health-related claims.
- **Updated and additional Special Feature** boxes highlight hot topics in health, including subjects like how procrastination sabotages your future, the importance of getting enough calcium in your diet, the benefits of strengthening your core, the Zika virus, reducing your risk for chronic disease, and your rights under Title IX.

New in the Third Edition

The entire text has been reviewed and updated for the most current research, data, and statistics. In addition, the organization of many chapters has been updated to promote readability and clarity. The presence of Choose This, Not That features, Change Yourself, Change Your World sections, and Choosing to Change Worksheets enhance an already robust behavior change emphasis throughout the text. The expanded What Do You Think? questions encourage students to use their higher thinking skills. Above and beyond these improvements, each chapter has undergone specific changes.

Chapter 1:
- Introduced several pairs of key terms related to health, such as incidence and prevalence, morbidity and mortality, and causes and risk factors.
- Updated Figure 1.2, on dimensions of health, to make it more readable.
- Expanded information on emerging infectious diseases, such as the Zika virus.
- Added overview of genetics and discussion of determinants of health, including Figure 1.4 on genes, DNA, and chromosomes.
- Expanded information on the influence of economic inequality on life expectancy.

Chapter 2:
- Added information about the effects of bullying on psychological health.
- Updated stats on the number of college students experiencing mental health issues.
- Included recent discoveries about the causes of depression.
- Revised and updated information about the treatment of ADHD.
- Expanded section of non-suicidal self-injury.
- Reorganized sections to comply with designations in DSM-5.

Chapter 3:
- Reorganized and clarified the discussion of the physiology of the stress response, including the neural and hormonal phases.
- Increased the discussion of the health benefits of moderate stress and added a brief discussion of the concept of underload.
- Expanded the discussion of stress and body weight.
- Added a discussion of stress and headaches.
- Discussed the ambiguity surrounding the associations between stress and academic performance.
- Expanded the discussion of stress and age.
- Changed the discussion "Common Causes of Stress" to "What Are College Students' Common Stressors?" focusing the discussion on college students.
- Included new section called "Resources for Managing Stress," which identifies social support, campus support, and medical options, and integrates some of the material formerly under "Campus Advocacy."
- Added a Special Feature, called Procrastination: Sabotaging Your Future Self, on procrastination as a source of stress.

Chapter 4:

- Moved the sleep chapter from online into the printed book to follow the stress chapter and heavily revised and expanded coverage of sleep topics.
- Updated the scientific information that covers the stages and cycles of sleep, in both the related text and graphics.
- Created a new Choose This, Not That feature on the benefits of ample sleep.
- Updated the scientific and medical information on the topic of sleep apnea.
- Created a new Practical Strategies feature on effective approaches to napping that don't disrupt night-time sleep.
- Expanded information and statistics on the sleep-disrupting properties of electronic devices.

Chapter 5:

- Changed terminology for the type of carbohydrates recommended to consume from complex to fiber-rich carbohydrates.
- Changed lean proteins discussion to a Practical Strategies box, Go Lean with Protein.
- Significantly altered the discussion of the role of calcium supplements in bone health.
- Updated the discussion of the concerns about sugary drinks to include the information that calories as fluid don't trigger the sensation of satiety in the brain.
- Reorganized for clarity the discussion of functional foods, including foods rich in phytochemicals, some of which act as antioxidants, and probiotics and prebiotics.
- Discussed recent state and federal actions against the makers of fraudulent and dangerous dietary supplements.
- Updated the discussion of the new FDA Nutrition Facts panel.
- Updated the discussion of the Dietary Guidelines for Americans to the 2015–2020 Guidelines.
- Removed separate discussion called "How Do Nutrition Guidelines Vary for Different Groups?"
- In addition to celiac disease, mentioned non-celiac gluten sensitivity.
- Integrated discussion of genetically modified foods in the Consumer Corner called Organic, Non-GMO, Local, Fair Trade: What to Choose?
- Mentioned how to support developing an on-campus food bank.

Chapter 6:

- Added a new table and information on the Metabolic Equivalent of Task (METs) scale.
- Added a new chart and information on the Rated Perceived Exertion (RPE) scale.
- Updated the "Self-Assessment" feature to include the Karvonen equation.
- Added information on the idea of "diminishing returns" in fitness.
- Added information on additional types of stretching exercises.
- Expanded information on safe weight-lifting techniques.
- Expanded and updated information on performance-enhancing drugs.

Chapter 7:

- Included updated statistics and information on the global obesity crises and alarming trends in weight gain among American children.
- Added discussion of the effects of social media on body image.
- Removed the Diversity & Health box about the thrifty gene theory of weight loss.
- Added updated statistics on the financial burden of obesity.
- Revised the section on the role genes play in promoting obesity.
- Expanded the section on prescription weight loss medications to include two new drugs.
- Added sections on two additional disordered eating problems: anorexia athletic and orthorexia nervosa.

Chapter 8:

- Updated scientific and medical information about addiction in general, both in the main text and in a new Choose This, Not That feature on the effects of drugs on the brain.
- Expanded a section on behavioral addictions.
- Significantly expanded and updated the topic of opioid abuse, addictions, overdose, including both prescription opioids and heroin.
- Significantly expanded and updated the topic of marijuana, including legalization and medical use.
- New information on the topic of drugged driving.

Chapter 9:

- Updated statistics on alcohol and tobacco use on campus.
- Included a new section evaluating health benefit claims of alcohol use.
- Included discussion explaining why scientists believe that alcohol use leads to an increase risk of certain cancers.
- Updated alcohol use and drunk driving statistics.
- Included most recent findings and statistics on the health effects of tobacco use.
- Updated information and statistics about smoking on campus and why some students smoke.
- Revised section on electronic cigarettes to included latest information on risks and regulation.
- Added a section on hookahs.

Chapter 10:
- Updated demographic data and statistics throughout the chapter.
- Extensive updates to the information on the state of same-sex marriage legalization.
- Updated the Special Feature about social media, communication, and cyberbullies to include newer forms of social media, such as Instagram.
- Updated the "Student Stats" feature to provide a detailed demographic look at the numbers of students who are married or who are parents.
- Updated the single parenthood section.

Chapter 11:
- Added updated ACOG guidelines for pelvic and pap exams.
- Added updated PMDD diagnostic criteria from DSM-5.
- Updated sexual behavior statistics.
- Revised section on sexting to include practical information about avoiding negative consequences.
- Added extensive revision of gender identity section.
- Revised IUD and emergency contraception sections to include information on currently available products.

Chapter 12:
- Updated and focused the Special Feature box entirely on Zika virus to provide in-depth information on this growing public health concern, including a new U.S. vector map.
- Merged and streamlined information on reducing risk of contracting infections by moving information on hand sanitizer use to the Practical Strategies box.
- Updated and merged information on MRSA as a topic within the overall discussion of bacterial infections.
- Extensive updates to the information on HIV/AIDs and the ongoing global campaign against the virus.

Chapter 13:
- Improved Figure 13.1 on the mechanisms of diabetes.
- Added a Student Stats figure on college students' participation in key health behaviors linked to chronic disease.
- Eliminated the Diversity & Health box on gender differences in heart disease, while still discussing the key points in the narrative.
- Included a more comprehensive discussion of the role of proto-oncogenes and tumor-suppressor genes in cancer.
- Altered the Self-Assessment on cancer risk to reflect new understanding of the more limited role of specific nutrients and foods in cancer risk.
- Removed the feature boxes on testicular self-exam and breast self-exam as these self-exams are no longer recommended by the American Cancer Society or the U.S. Preventive Services Task Force.
- Covered the steps students can take to reduce their risks for type 2 diabetes, cardiovascular disease, and cancer in a Special Feature called Reducing Your Risk for Chronic Disease. This replaces narrative paragraphs and the former Practical Strategies called Healthy Food Choices.

Chapter 14:
- Extensive updates to information on the Affordable Care Act, including health insurance options after graduation.
- Updated information on handling prescription medications properly, especially in the context of prescription opioid abuse and overdose.
- Expanded key information on interacting with the medical system, including an expanded section on when to seek professional medical care and a new section on patient rights.
- Moved information about vaccinations into the infectious disease chapter.
- Updated all health screenings information and reorganized the table on screenings to make the information easier to use.
- Updated all information about CAM use among college students, as well as information about evaluating CAM practitioners and treatments.

Chapter 15:
- Revised Practical Strategies box to include preventing tech injuries from using mobile devices.
- Added a Special Feature on students' rights and protections under Title IX and also added updated information in the text.
- Included extensive updates to all injury and crime statistics.
- Updated figure on types of distracted driving
- Included new information on opioids as the leading cause of drug overdose deaths.
- Removed the feature on purchasing bicycle helmets.
- Removed section on injuries from backpack use.

Chapter 16:
- Included a discussion of the effects of China's one-child policy.
- Completely reorganized and rewrote the third main section of the chapter, Air Pollution and Climate Change, to update research into evidence, long-lived greenhouse gases, etc., and to eliminate former redundancies.
- Revised graph showing the association between increased global surface temperature and increased atmospheric CO_2 levels between 1880 and 2015.
- Included a discussion of the landmark Paris Agreement on climate change.
- Entirely rewrote the Myth or Fact feature box on electric vehicles.

- Deleted the table on air pollutants because it repeated information already in the narrative.
- Completely reorganized and rewrote the discussion of types of water pollutants, including the discussion of arsenic in rice, lead in Flint, Michigan, and other communities, dioxins, and agricultural chemicals.
- Entirely rewrote the Diversity & Health feature box on working for environmental justice.
- Included a brief discussion of the hazards associated with phthalates in plastic products and personal care items, and of perfluorinated compounds (PFCs) used in food packaging and other materials.
- Deleted the table on pollutants at home because a significant portion of it repeated information already in the narrative.
- Entirely rewrote the Myth or Fact feature box on the potential link between use of cell phones and brain cancer.

Chapter 17:

- Added statistical information on centenarians.
- Replaced discussion of "eight Americas," which was becoming outdated, with new information on troubling disparities in life expectancy.
- Modestly expanded information on:
  - Andropause and the risks and benefits of testosterone therapy
  - Benefits of exercise in moderating age-related changes, including cognitive decline
  - Risks of smoking in brain changes affecting cognition
  - Benefits of mental exercises such as engaging in hobbies or learning a new language
  - Opposition to and advocacy of physician aid in dying
  - The grief experience
- Completely rewrote the Media and Aging box on brain fitness games.
- Added a new discussion on the contributions of meaning, purpose, and connection to longevity.
- Replaced Tufts University MyPlate for Older Adults with a plate based on the ChooseMyPlate.gov recommendations.

Student Supplements

The student supplements for this textbook include:

- **MasteringHealth™ (www.masteringhealthandnutrition.com)** is the most effective and widely used online homework, tutorial, and assessment system for the sciences. It delivers self-paced tutorials that focus on course objectives, provides individualized coaching, and responds to your progress. Through MasteringHealth™, access:
  - Health Coaching Activities that guide you through key health and fitness concepts with interactive mini-lessons that provide hints and feedback.
  - NutriTools Build-a-Meal Activities, which allow you to combine and experiment with different food options and learn firsthand how to build healthier meals.
  - Dynamic Study Modules that enable you to study effectively on your own in an adaptive format. You receive an initial set of questions with a unique answer format asking you to indicate your confidence level. Once completed, reviews include explanations using materials taken directly from the text. These modules can be accessed on smart phones, tablets, and computers.
  - eText 2.0 is a mobile friendly and ADA accessible version of the textbook included at no additional cost in MasteringHealth. eText 2.0, accessible via computers, smart phones, and tablets, comes complete with embedded ABC News videos, Student Story videos, and interactive self-assessment worksheets and includes instructor and student note taking, highlighting, bookmarking, and search functions.

MasteringHealth™ also contains a complete set of student videos; health-related *ABC News* videos; online behavior change tools; Choosing to Change Worksheets and Self-Assessments; practice tests and additional self-assessments; links to updated websites, videos, and podcasts; and a rich suite of additional study tools, including MP3 audio files, mobile tips you can access on your smart phone, audio case studies, an online glossary, and flashcards.

- **Mobile Tips!** Now you can access health tips covering everything from stress management to fitness wherever you go, via your smart phone. A set of four different tip "cards" per chapter are available. Access them by navigating to **http://chmobile.pearsoncmg.com** on any mobile device. Or go straight to each chapter's cards by scanning the QR code provided at the end of the chapter.
- **A YouTube channel (www.youtube.com/ch00sing health)** features selected student videos as well as videos from around the web.
- ***The Behavior Change Log Book and Wellness Journal*** is a booklet you can use to track your daily exercise and nutritional intake and create a long-term nutrition and fitness prescription plan.
- **A Digital 5-Step Pedometer** measures steps, distance (miles), activity time, and calories.
- **MyDietAnalysis (www.pearsonhighered.com/mydietanalysis)** is an online tool powered by ESHA Research, Inc., that features a database of nearly 20,000 foods and multiple reports. It allows you to track your diet and physical activity, receive analyses of what nutrients you may be lacking, and generate and submit reports electronically.
- ***Eat Right! Healthy Eating in College and Beyond*** is a guidebook that provides practical tips, shopper's guides, and recipes so that you can start putting healthy principles into action. Topics include healthy eating in the cafeteria, dorm room, and fast food restaurants; eating on a budget; weight-management tips; vegetarian alternatives; and guidelines on alcohol and health.

- ***Live Right! Beating Stress in College and Beyond*** is a guidebook that provides useful strategies for coping with a variety of life's challenges, during college and beyond. Topics include sleep, managing finances, time management, coping with academic pressure, relationships, and being a smart consumer.
- ***Take Charge of Your Health! Worksheets*** is a collection of 50 self-assessment exercises that you can fill out to assess your health and wellness. Worksheets are available as a gummed pad and can be packaged at no additional charge with the main text.

Instructor Supplements

This textbook comes with a comprehensive set of supplemental resources to assist instructors with classroom preparation and presentation.

- **MasteringHealth™ (www.masteringhealthandnutrition.com)** helps instructors maximize class time with easy-to-assign, customizable, and automatically graded assessments that motivate students to learn outside of the class and arrive prepared for lecture. Through MasteringHealth™, access:
  - Publisher-provided problems with easy-to-edit questions and answers. It is also easy to import your own questions or quickly add images or links to further enhance the student experience.
  - Learning Outcomes that are tied to Bloom's Taxonomy and are designed to let Mastering do the work in tracking student performance against your learning outcomes. Mastering offers a data-supported measure to quantify students' learning gains and to share those results quickly and easily.
  - Learning Catalytics that let you use a wide variety of question types to engage students and understand what they do or don't know.

MasteringHealth™ also has a new Calendar View displaying upcoming assignments and due dates and allows instructors to easily schedule assignments.

- **The Teaching Toolkit Online Resources** replaces the former printed Teaching Toolbox and DVD set and provides everything you need to prep for your course and deliver a dynamic lecture. These resources are downloadable from the Instructor Resources section in MasteringHealth as well as from Pearson's Instructor Resource Center. The Teaching Toolkit Resources include more than 50 *ABC News* Lecture Launcher videos, PowerPoint Lecture Outlines, PowerPoint clicker questions and *Jeopardy*-style quiz show questions, files for all illustrations and tables and selected photos from the text, the Test Bank in Word and PDF formats, the Computerized Test Bank, the Instructor's Resource Support Manual, Introduction to MasteringHealth™, Introductory video for Learning Catalytics, *Great Ideas! Active Ways to Teach Health and Wellness, Teaching with Student Learning Outcomes, Teaching with Web 2.0, Take Charge of Your Health! Worksheets, Behavior Change Log Book and Wellness Journal, Eat Right! Healthy Eating in College and Beyond,* and *Live Right! Beating Stress in College and Beyond.*

We are a team of health educators and communicators whose work reflects our deeply held belief that discussions of health are always a dialogue in progress. We hope this book will help you make changes toward better health. We also hope you'll let us know how those changes are going, and how we can make *Choosing Health* even more useful. Go to MasteringHealth™ and share your stories with us!

April Lynch
Karen Vail-Smith
Jerome Kotecki
Laura Bonazzoli

ACKNOWLEDGMENTS

Authoring a textbook can feel like a solitary job during countless hours alone, researching topics or drafting chapters. But in reality, we as authors were supported not only by each other but by an amazing team of editors, publishing professionals, content contributors, supplement authors, and reviewers.

Collectively, the authors would like to thank everyone at Pearson for their support and belief in our vision and our book, and call out a few of the key players for special thanks. First off, this book would not be possible without the support of Pearson Science's vice president and editor-in-chief, Adam Jaworski, and former vice president and editorial director, Frank Ruggirello (now retired), who was always there to provide backing and funds for the project and to be our advocate to the highest reaches of the organization. Another lifeline for the book is Michelle Yglecias, senior acquisitions editor, who joined our team enthusiastically, provided creative guidance for the book as a whole, and really fosters our student-centric approach to teaching health. This book would not be what it is today without the razor-sharp, insightful, and deeply knowledgeable edits, feedback, and management of two amazing development editors: Cathy Murphy and Tanya Martin, as well as Barbara Yien, courseware director of content development. Additional editorial vision, direction, coordination, and management was provided by Content Producers Lauren Bakker and Martha Steele. Lauren and Martha kept us in good cheer in the fact of tight schedules and kept us all happy and on track. We'd also like to thank editorial assistant Nicole Constantine; Mastering content producer Lorna Perkins; and Mastering editorial content producers Lucinda Bingham, Libby Reiser, and Tim Hainley, who worked tirelessly to develop a robust MasteringHealth course and interactive eText 2.0 for the third edition. We must also thank everyone at Cenveo Publisher Services, especially project manager Heidi Allgair, for their wonderful work on the production and composition of the book; no matter how tight the schedule, they were always able to turn out the next round of page proofs. Senior procurement specialist Stacey Weinberger researched all types of paper and printing methods for us, to help us produce the most beautiful printing of the book possible. And speaking of beautiful, a million thanks to Elise Lansdon, who designed the modern, engaging, and lively cover and interior for the book. Kathleen Zander of Cenveo Publisher Services and Danny Meldung of Photo Affairs, Inc., provided invaluable expertise in the researching and coordinating of hundreds of photos for the book. A huge thanks goes out to Neena Bali, executive product marketing manager, and Mary Salzman, senior marketing manager, who have worked tirelessly to get the message of *Choosing Health* out to instructors across the country.

We would also like to thank Laura Bonazzoli, whom we can't thank enough for her time and expertise. Without Laura Bonazzoli, this book would not have been made. Her creativity, attention to detail, and passion for explaining complex health issues show throughout the entire text.

The creation of the instructor and student supplements for *Choosing Health*, third edition, could not have been completed without the excellent work of our supplement authors. The Test Bank was created by Lisa Tunks. The PowerPoint Lecture Outlines and *Jeopardy*-style quiz shows were written by Sloane Burke-Winkelman and Autumn Hamilton, respectively. Nicole George-O'Brien authored the Instructor Resource and Support Manual. Many thanks to all of them.

We'd also like to acknowledge the contributions of Barry Elmore.

And, finally, we'd like to thank all the reviewers who spent their time reading and commenting on our chapters—we listened to each and every one of your comments and are extremely grateful for your feedback. A full list of reviewers begins on the next page.

From April Lynch

I have countless people to thank, beginning with all those who have helped with the heavy lifting required to turn ideas into a new way to teach the subject of health, and helped put words to page for each edition of this book. This project has thrived thanks to the consistent, long-term support of the Pearson editorial team, and has grown and thrived in this edition thanks to the invaluable contributions of co-authors Jerome Kotecki, Laura Bonazzoli, and Karen Vail-Smith, who have brought new levels of expertise and polish to our team and been helpful sounding boards every step of the way. It has taken a talented team, past and present, to bring this book to life and help it grow, and I'd like to thank everyone who has been a part of the effort.

From Karen Vail-Smith

I'd like to thank my East Carolina University colleagues who always provide the best advice, expertise, and unconditional support. I am especially thankful for the Health 1000 team: Debra Tavasso, Brian Cavanaugh, and Charla Blumell. They are hands-down the most dedicated health advocates and talented teachers imaginable. A million thanks to an unsung hero, my department chair, Dr. Don Chaney. He works tirelessly to make all of our jobs easier. I could not have worked on this book without his support. Thank you to all my new and old friends at Pearson and of course, to April, Jerome, and Laura. You are truly the best at what you do! I'm convinced that it takes a village of a talented individuals to bring a book to press—and to all involved with this one, I extend my heartfelt thanks.

From Jerome Kotecki

First, I am privileged to have had the opportunity to work with the extremely gifted team of April Lynch, Karen Vail-Smith, Laura Bonazzoli, and Pearson Education. Second, I am deeply grateful to those who continue to teach me on a daily basis: my students. The way in which they embrace learning—by being intellectually curious and inquisitive—provides a feedback loop that helps keep me focused on my own research and on investigating the latest findings in health research to expand my perspicacity as a professor. Third, I am fortunate to work with administrators and faculty who maintain that a well-written and researched textbook, based on expert knowledge, reflects an important faculty contribution when it comes to the scholarship of translational health research that links the latest health science discoveries to effective behavioral interventions that enhance health and well-being. Knowledge and best practice in health are constantly changing and new research and experience broaden our understanding. I appreciate the support of Dr. Mitchell Whaley, dean of the College of Health, my colleagues in the Department of Nutrition and Health Science, and Dr. Terry King, interim president of Ball State University. Finally, I wish to extend my gratitude to my mentors. Thank you to Dr. James Stewart, my undergraduate advisor, for having faith in my abilities and encouraging me to stretch myself academically; and to Dr. Budd Stalnaker, Dr. John Seffrin, Dr. Mohammad Torabi, and Dr. Morgan Pigg, my graduate advisors, for your expertise and high standards and for guiding me on a path of enlightenment during my years at Indiana University and beyond.

THIRD EDITION REVIEWERS

Michelle Alexander
Thomas Nelson Community College

Krisztina Beni
Clarion University of Pennsylvania

Rebecca Brey
Ball State University

Ryan Donovan
Colorado State University

Kathy Finley
Indiana University—Bloomington

LaNita Harris
University of Central Oklahoma

Karla Jones
Central Piedmont Community College

Dena Pistor
Rollins College

Chris Repka
Northern Arizona University

Natascha Romeo
Wake Forest University

Giovanna Sabatini-Key
Western Michigan University

Dana Sherman
Ozarks Technical Community College

Melissa Thomas
University of Mobile

Debra Trigoboff
Palm Beach State College

eTEXT 2.0 REVIEWERS

Trevor Burns
Daytona State College

Daniel Czech
Georgia Southern University

Jennifer Dearden
Morehead State University

Amanda Divin
Western Illinois University

Karen Edwards
University of Delaware

Dina Hayduk
Kutztown University

SECOND EDITION REVIEWERS

Ni Bueno
Cerritos College

Lisa Shanti N. Chaudhari
Northern Arizona University

Max Faquir
Palm Beach State College

Autumn Hamilton
Minnesota State University

Kim Heffernan
University of Maryland

Annette Carrington Johnson
North Carolina Central University

Cheryl A. Kerns-Campbell
Grossmont College

Ayanna Lyles
California University of Pennsylvania

Debbie Lynch
Rose State College

Donna McGill-Cameron
Woodland Community College

Grace Pokorny
Long Beach City College

Andrea S. Salis
Queensborough Community College—CUNY

Terese A. Sheridan
University of Nebraska—Kearney

Kelly Fisher Shobe
Georgia Perimeter College

Amanda Tapler
Elon University

Iva Toler
Prince George's Community College

Ladona Tornabene
University of Minnesota, Duluth

Cody Trefethen
Palomar College

Gayle Truitt-Bean
Clarion University of Pennsylvania

MasteringHealth REVIEWERS

Steve Hartman
Citrus College

Kris Jankovitz
California Polytechnic State University, San Luis Obispo

Ayanna Lyles
California University of Pennsylvania

Karla Rues
Ozarks Technical and Community College

Debra Smith
Ohio University

FIRST EDITION REVIEWERS

Katherine Lewis Allen
Northern Arizona University

Elizabeth Barrington
San Diego Mesa College

Linda Beatty
McLennen Community College

R. Cruz Begay
Northern Arizona University

Robin Benton
Salem State College

James Brenner
West Chester University

Liz Brown
Rose State College

Jocelyn Buck
Wake Technical Community College

Ni Bueno
Cerritos College

Sloane Burke
East Carolina University

Angela Burroughs
North Carolina Central University

Annette Carrington
North Carolina Central University

Dusty Childress
Ozarks Technical Community College

Fay Cook
Lock Haven University of Pennsylvania

Jane Curth
Georgia Perimeter College

Dan Czech
Georgia Southern University

Asad Dalia
University of Cincinnati

Brent Damron
Bakersfield College

Kathleen Dayton
Montgomery College, Rockville

Jennifer Dearden
Morehead State

Jacqueline Dove
Baylor University

Maureen Edwards
Montgomery College

Paul Finnicum
Arkansas State University

Ari Fisher
Louisiana State University

Kelly Fisher Shobe
Georgia Perimeter College

Autumn Hamilton
Minnesota State University

Chris Harman
California University of Pennsylvania

Valarie L. Hilson
Arkansas State University

Yvonne Hilton
Lincoln University

Kathy Hixon
Northeastern State University

Angela D. Holley
Georgia Perimeter College

Jane House
Wake Technical Community College

Guoyuan Huang
University of Southern Indiana

Hollie Huckabee
Arkansas State University

Emogene Johnson-Vaughn
Norfolk State University

Aaron Junta
Shasta College

Patricia Kearney
Bridgewater College

Bill Kernan
William Patterson University

Brian Kipp
Grand Valley State University

John Kowalczyk
University of Minnesota, Duluth

Gary Ladd
Southwestern Illinois College

Ellen Larson
Northern Arizona University

Ayanna Lyles
California University of Pennsylvania

Debbie Lynch
Rose State College

Bridget Melton
Georgia Southern University

Roseann Poole
Tallahassee Community College

Mary Jo Preti
MiraCosta College

Elizabeth Ridings
Montgomery College

Albert Simon
Jackson State University

Becky Slonaker
McLennen Community College

Carol Smith
Elon University

Deborah Stone
Louisiana State University

Nancy Storey
Georgia Perimeter College

Cody Trefethen
Palomar College

Sandra Walz
West Chester University

Lesley Wasilko
Montgomery College

Linda White
Metropolitan State College

Sharon Woodard
Wake Forest University

PERSONAL HEALTH FORUM AND FOCUS GROUP PARTICIPANTS

Kim Archer
Stephen F. Austin State

Brian Barthel
Utah Valley University

Laura Blitzer
Long Island University

Dan Czech
Georgia Southern University

Jennifer Dearden
Morehead State University

Joel Dering
Cameron University

Joyce Fetro
Southern Illinois University

Paul Finnicum
Arkansas State University

Teresa Hardman
Moorehead University

Emogene Johnson-Vaughn
Norfolk State University

Andrew Kanu
Virginia State University

Patricia Marcum
University of Southern Indiana

Bridget Melton
Georgia Southern University

Maria Okeke
Florida A&M University

Dana Sherman
Ozarks Technical Community College

CLASS TESTERS

Fran Babich
Butte College

Elizabeth Bailey
Elon University

Stephanie Bennett
University of Southern Indiana

Tina Cummings
Bakersfield College

Dan Czech
Georgia Southern University

Kathy Deresinski
Triton College

Melody Durrenberger
Georgia Perimeter College

Max Faquir
Palm Beach State College

Renee Fenwick-Frimming
University of Southern Indiana

Kendra Guilford
University of Alabama, Tuscaloosa

Essam Hamido
Tennessee State University

Chris Harman
California University of Pennsylvania

Guoyuan Huang
University of Southern Indiana

Hollie Huckabee
Arkansas State University

Emogene Johnson-Vaughn
Norfolk State University

Tim Jones
Tennessee State University

Walt Justice
Southwestern College

September Kirby
South Dakota State University

Ayanna Lyles
California University of Pennsylvania

Bridget Melton
Georgia Southern University

Susan Milstein
Montgomery College

Kim Queri
Rose State College

Lesley Rennis
Borough of Manhattan Community College

Bernard Smolen
Prince George's Community College

Resa Walch
Elon University

Sharon Woodard
Wake Forest University

INTERVIEWEES

Duro Agbede
Southwestern College

Mike Basile
Borough of Manhattan Community College

Philip Belcastro
Borough of Manhattan Community College

Rebecca Brey
Ball State University

Elaine Bryan
Georgia Perimeter College

Ni Bueno
Cerritos College

Laura Burger-Simm
Grossmont College

Lynda Butler-Storsved
Elon University

Michael Calhoun
Elon University

Cheryl Campbell
Grossmont College

Doug Casey
Georgia Perimeter College

Steve Chandler
Florida A&M University

Kim Clark
California State University, San Bernardino

Mary Conway
Sierra College

Marianne Crocker
Ozarks Technical Community College

Paula Dahl
Bakersfield College

Brent Damron
Bakersfield College

James Deboy
Lincoln University

Eva Doyle
Baylor University

Melanie Durkin
Southwestern College

Maureen Edwards
Montgomery College

Kelly Falcone
Palomar College

Paul Finnicum
Arkansas State University

Barb Francis
Metropolitan State College

Valerie Goodwin
Southwestern College

Michelle Harcrow
University of Alabama, Tuscaloosa

Chris Harrison
Montgomery College

Bryan Hedrick
Elon University

Casie Higginbotham
Middle Tennessee State University

Valerie Hilson
Arkansas State University

Yvonne Hilton
Lincoln University

Kris Jankovitz
California Polytechnic State University, San Luis Obispo

Carol Jensen
Metropolitan State College

David Jolly
North Carolina Central University

Shannon Josey
Middle Tennessee State University

Beth Kelley
Grossmont College

Aaron Krac
Queensborough Community College

Randy Maday
Butte College

Rick Madson
Palm Beach State College

Vance Manakas
Moorpark College

Patricia Marcum
University of Southern Indiana

Mitch Mathias
Arkansas State University

Connie Mettille
Winona State University

Gavin O'Connor
Ozarks Technical Community College

Maria Okeke
Florida A&M University

Kevin Petti
San Diego Miramar College

Rod Porter
San Diego Miramar College

Regina Prodoehl
James Madison University

Elizabeth Ridings
Montgomery College

Karla Rues
Ozarks Technical Community College

Todd Sabato
James Madison University

Dana Sherman
Ozarks Technical Community College

Agneta Sibrava
Arkansas State University

Jeff Slepski
Mt. San Jacinto College

Nancy Storey
Georgia Perimeter College

Debra Sutton
James Madison University

Amanda Tapler
Elon University

Karen Thomas
Montgomery College

Silvea Thomas
Kingsborough Community College

Iva Toler
Prince George's Community College

Tim Wallstrom
Riverside Community College

Lesley Wasilko
Montgomery College

Patti Waterman
Palomar College

Linda White
Metropolitan State College

Susanne Wood
Tallahassee Community College

LaShawn Wordlaw-Stinson
North Carolina Central University

Bonnie Young
Georgia Perimeter College

Thank You to Our Student Advisory Board

The *Choosing Health* Student Advisory Board consists of students who submit stories, videos, questions, or feedback to us about *Choosing Health*.

1

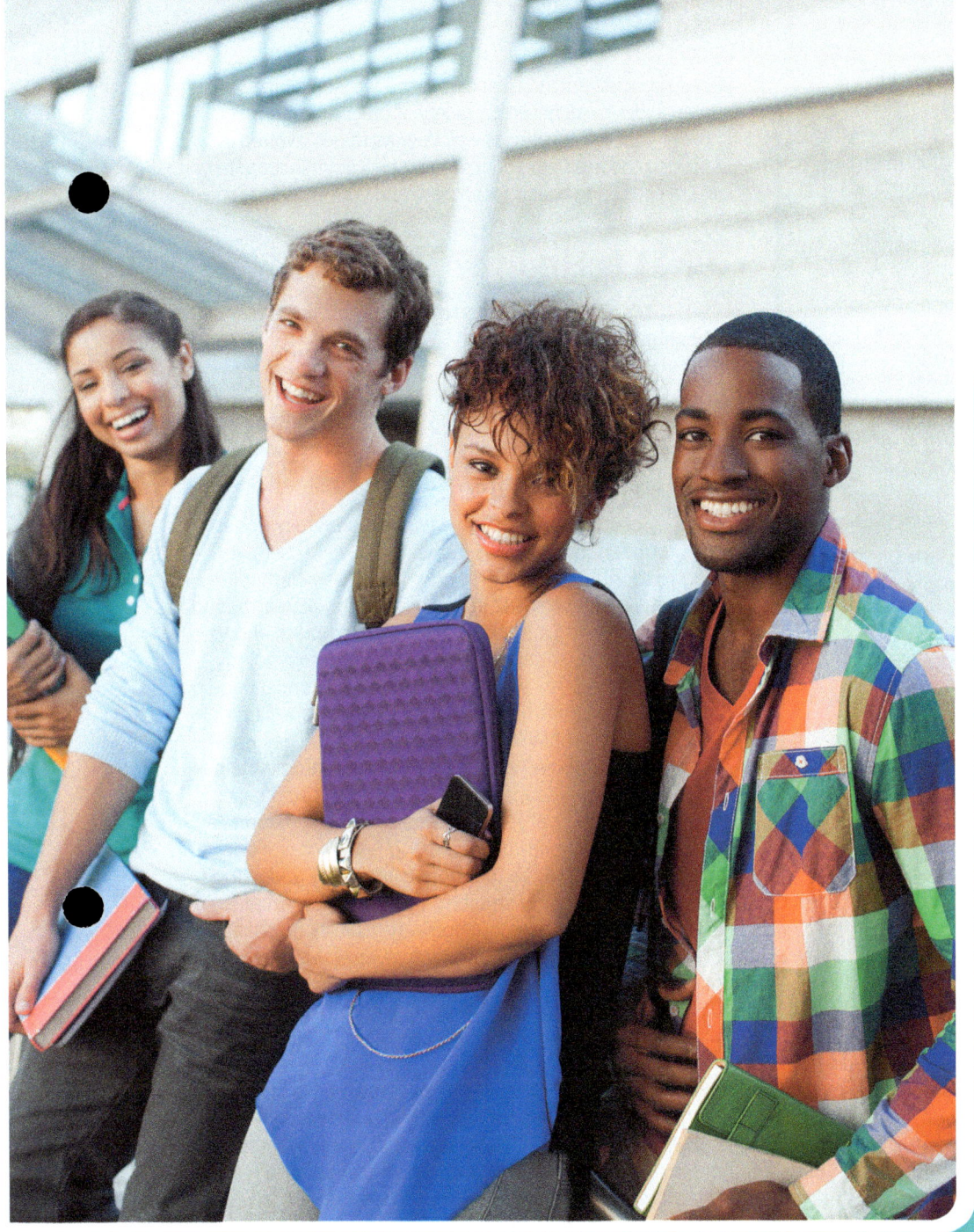

> The current life expectancy at birth in the United States is 78.8 years.[i]

> Heart disease and cancer are responsible for nearly half of all deaths in the United States.[i]

> Poor nutrition, inadequate physical activity, obesity, tobacco use, and alcohol abuse are the factors most strongly linked to premature death.[ii]

HEALTH IN THE 21ST CENTURY

LEARNING OUTCOMES

LO 1.1 Discuss the evolution of our current understanding of health.

LO 1.2 Identify and describe seven dimensions of health.

LO 1.3 Discuss health challenges across America and around the world.

LO 1.4 Classify determinants of health into six broad groups, identifying the group that is most strongly within an individual's control.

LO 1.5 Explain how predisposing, enabling, and reinforcing factors can promote or hinder behavior change.

LO 1.6 Compare three models of behavior change.

LO 1.7 List seven steps for achieving successful behavior change and two strategies for preventing relapse.

Health matters.

disease An alteration in body structure or biochemistry that is significant enough to cause the body's regulatory mechanisms to fail. Symptoms may or may not be present.

illness A subjective state in which a person feels unwell. Disease may or may not be present.

signs Objective, often visible or measurable, indications that disease or injury is present.

symptoms Subjective experiences such as pain or fatigue that indicate disease or injury is present.

health More than merely the absence of disease, a state of well-being that encompasses physical, social, psychological, and other dimensions and is a resource for everyday life.

Have you ever noticed that, when you're ill, stressed, or sleep deprived, you're more likely to doubt yourself, argue with your roommate, and feel overwhelmed by even simple tasks? But when you're bursting with strength and stamina, even daunting challenges—like hiking a grueling trail or solving a calculus proof—can seem like fun.

Intuitively, you know health matters. But do your choices each day—what to eat, how much to sleep, whether to exercise, smoke, or abuse alcohol—really make health a priority? A theme of this text is that these *lifestyle choices* can have a profound influence on your health. Over many years, the cumulative effects of lifestyle choices can greatly increase or decrease your risk for disease and early death. If health matters, then your choices matter, too.

This text provides the facts you need to begin evaluating your current lifestyle choices. But information is just a first step. Each chapter concludes by identifying a variety of practical strategies to improve your own health, as well as ways to get involved in improving the health of your community. With this support, you can start choosing health for yourself and your world.

What Is Health?

LO 1.1 Discuss the evolution of our current understanding of health.

If health matters, then it's worth taking a moment to explore what the term means.

Health Versus Disease

For many centuries, the term *health* was generally understood to mean the absence of disease. Disease itself was recognized, fundamentally, as an imbalance, whether in temperature (hot versus cold), elements (fire, air, earth, and water), or *humors* (body fluids referred to as black and yellow bile, phlegm, and blood). As science and technology advanced in the 19th and 20th centuries, our understanding of the nature of this imbalance shifted. Physicians came to recognize that, in a state of health, the body has a variety of regulatory mechanisms that enable it to maintain stable internal conditions. The healthy body continually maintains this internal stability, even as external factors—environmental temperature, food and water intake, and so forth—change. **Disease** therefore came to be understood as an alteration in body structure or biochemistry that is significant enough to cause the body's regulatory mechanisms to fail. This failure is often temporary—as when we experience congestion for several days before throwing off a cold. But in many cases, the body is unlikely to be able to return to a balanced state without medical care.

With this understanding, you can probably appreciate that the traditional definition of health as "the absence of disease" is problematic. People can and do experience **illness**, a subjective state in which a person feels unwell, whether or not true disease is present. Should we describe such a person as healthy? Conversely, people can experience themselves as entirely well despite having a serious disease. For example, certain types of cancer can go unrecognized until they are in a very advanced stage because they produce no obvious **signs**—objective clues such as dramatic weight loss—or **symptoms**—subjective feelings such as pain or fatigue. Moreover, some people who have a diagnosed disease live highly productive lives and do not perceive themselves as unwell. Are they healthy?

In 1948, the newly formed World Health Organization (WHO)—the global health unit of the United Nations—published a radical new definition of **health** as "a state of complete physical, mental, and social well-being, and not merely the absence of disease or infirmity."[1] This holistic view was praised for acknowledging that, in a healthy person, many different dimensions of life work together harmoniously. However, the WHO definition's insistence upon "complete" physical well-being led to charges that it excluded people who are positive, fulfilled, and even vibrant despite having a disability or disease. This concern led to the introduction of a broader concept of health we now know as wellness.

Health Versus Wellness

Although the term *wellness* can be traced back to the 17th century, its first modern use was by Halbert L. Dunn, M.D., in a 1959 article in the *American Journal of Public Health*. Influenced by the WHO definition of health, Dunn argued that health-care providers should stop focusing so narrowly on disease and begin studying the factors that support good health. He proposed thinking about disease and health as a "graduated scale" with death at one extremity and "peak wellness" at the other. He defined "peak wellness" as "performance at full potential in accordance with an individual's age and makeup."[2]

Dunn's work directly influenced that of John W. Travis, M.D., who founded the first "wellness center" in the United States in 1975. Travis developed a model of wellness he called the *illness–wellness continuum*, which has two extremes: premature death at one end and high-level wellness on the other **(Figure 1.1)**. At any given moment, most of us fall somewhere in between these extremes, shifting between states of feeling sick, "neutral," and vibrantly healthy. Your general direction on the continuum (either toward high-level wellness or toward premature death) matters more than your place on it at any given time. You may have an **acute** condition—an illness or injury that comes on suddenly and is usually brief, such as a cold or a sprained ankle—but if you are taking care of yourself and have a positive attitude, your general direction will be toward greater wellness. Moreover, people who have a **chronic** disease—a disease that tends to persist despite medical treatment—can experience high-level wellness, if they feel they are learning, growing, and contributing creatively to their world.

Today, the National Wellness Institute defines **wellness** as "an active process through which people become aware of, and make choices toward, a more successful existence."[3] People who have a high level of wellness make decisions that promote health in multiple areas of their lives.

acute Characteristic of an illness or injury that comes on suddenly, progresses and resolves rapidly, and may or may not require medical treatment.

chronic Characteristic of a disease that typically comes on slowly, progresses gradually, and tends to persist despite medical treatment.

wellness An active process through which people become aware of, and make choices toward, a more successful existence.

LO 1.1 QUICK CHECK

Over the past century, both in the United States and elsewhere around the world, our understanding of health has

a. narrowed from a focus on imbalances to a focus on the presence or absence of disease.
b. broadened from a focus on alterations in body structure or biochemistry to a focus on the subjective experience of illness.
c. broadened to incorporate not only the absence of disease or infirmity but also the ability to make life-enhancing choices.
d. not changed significantly.

Dimensions of Health

LO 1.2 Identify and describe seven dimensions of health.

Recall that the WHO definition of health identifies three dimensions—physical, mental, and social—all of which are working harmoniously. Though some public health experts accept these three dimensions as adequate, others have identified more or different dimensions appropriate for the populations they serve. In this text, we acknowledge the following seven dimensions of health: physical, intellectual, psychological, spiritual, social, environmental, and occupational **(Figure 1.2**, next page**)**.

Physical health focuses on the body: how well it functions and how well you care for it. Optimal physical health includes being physically active; eating nutritiously; getting enough sleep; making responsible decisions about sex, drinking, and drugs; and taking steps to avoid injuries and infectious diseases.

Intellectual health is marked by a willingness to take on new intellectual challenges, an openness to new ideas and skills, a capacity to think critically, and a sense of humor and curiosity. People who have a high level of intellectual health not only recognize problems quickly but also seek and create solutions.

Psychological health is a broad category encompassing autonomy, self-acceptance, and the ability to respond appropriately to the environment. It also includes the ability to maintain nurturing relationships and to pursue meaningful goals. Finally, people who are psychologically healthy sense that they are continually growing as individuals.

Spiritual health is influenced by your beliefs and values and the ways in which you express them—for instance, in humanitarian activities, religious practices, or efforts on behalf of nature and the environment. Spiritual health contributes to a sense of place and purpose in life and can be a source of support when you face challenges.

Social health describes the quality of your interactions and relationships with others. Good social health is characterized

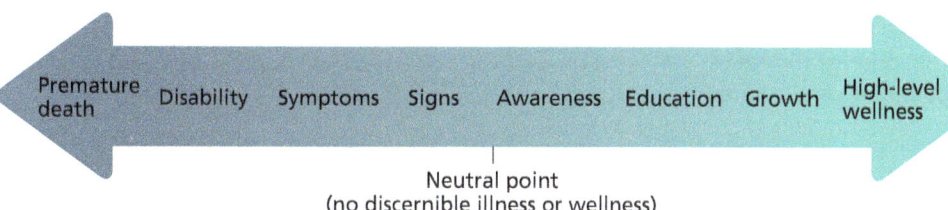

FIGURE 1.1 **The Illness–Wellness Continuum.** Your general direction on the continuum matters more than your specific point on it at any given time. *Source:* Adapted from "Illness–Wellness Continuum" from *Wellness Workbook: How to Achieve Enduring Health and Vitality*, 3rd edition, by John W. Travis, MD, and Regina Sara Ryan. Copyright © 1981, 1988, 2004 by John W. Travis. Adapted and reprinted with permission.

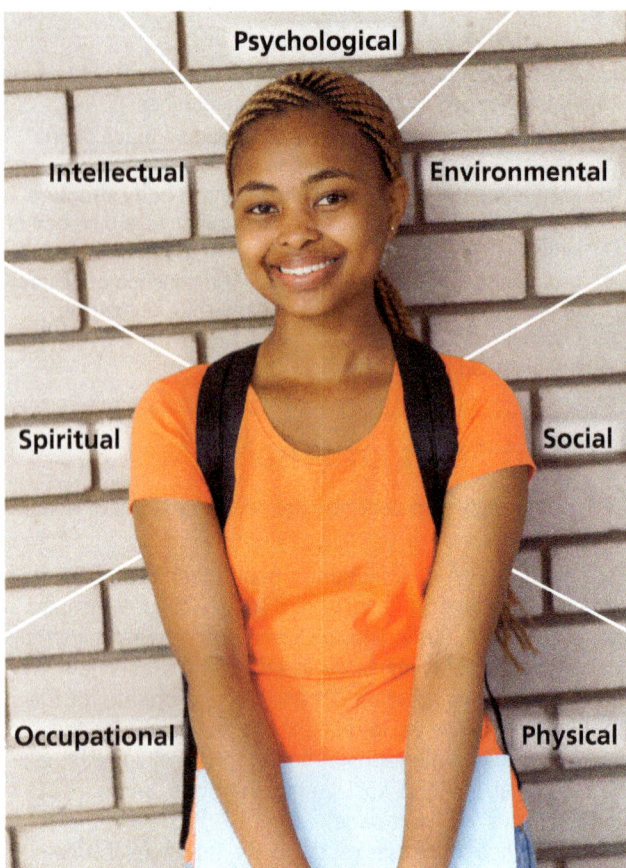

FIGURE 1.2 **Dimensions of Health.** More than just the absence of disease, health encompasses multiple dimensions of life.

by satisfying relationships, an ability to fulfill social roles—whether as a family member, friend, or community member—and an ability to provide support to others and receive it in return.

Environmental health describes the quality of your home, work, school, and social environments—as well as the health of our planet. Air quality, availability of clean water and nutritious food, crime rates, weather, pollution, and exposure to chemicals are just a few of the variables that factor into environmental health.

Occupational health describes the quality of your relationship to your work. Rather than a paying job, your "work" may consist of your studies, an athletic endeavor, or an artistic pursuit—whatever you consider your primary occupation. Challenges to occupational health include stress, lack of fulfillment in the work, poor relationships with colleagues, inadequate compensation, and sudden unemployment.

LO 1.2 QUICK CHECK

The seven dimensions of health include
a. financial health.
b. intellectual health.
c. artistic health.
d. heredity.

Current Health Challenges

LO 1.3 Discuss health challenges across America and around the world.

In the past century, dramatic technological advances have enabled people worldwide to enjoy longer, healthier lives. Advances in public health, such as municipal water purification, sanitation, and food service inspection, have decreased the **prevalence** (the percentage of the population affected) of infectious disease. At the same time, new diagnostic techniques such as MRI scans and genetic testing, as well as vaccines, medications, and new types of surgery have helped us to find and treat disease earlier and more successfully. Despite such progress, many health challenges remain.

> **prevalence** The proportion of a total population found to have a disease or other condition.
>
> **life expectancy** The average number of years a person may expect to live.
>
> **mortality** Clinical term for death, typically the number of deaths in a certain population due to a certain cause.

Health Across America

By one very basic measure of health—how long the average person born in the United States can expect to live—we are in far better shape than our predecessors. The current **life expectancy** at birth in the United States is a record 78.8 years—more than 15 years longer than it was in 1940.[4] The causes of **mortality** (the term used in public health for deaths within a population) have also changed dramatically over the years. In 1900, the leading causes of mortality were infectious diseases such as pneumonia, influenza, and tuberculosis.[5] Today, the leading causes are chronic diseases (see **Table 1.1**).

>> Want to know your life expectancy? Try an online longevity calculator like the one at **www.northwesternmutual.com**.

TABLE 1.1 Top Five Causes of Death in the United States

	Cause of Death
All ages	1. Heart disease 2. Cancer 3. Chronic lower respiratory disease 4. Accidents/unintentional injuries 5. Stroke
15–24 years old	1. Accidents/unintentional injuries 2. Suicide 3. Assault/homicide 4. Cancer 5. Heart disease

Source: Data from *Deaths: Final Data for 2013*, by J. Xu, S. L. Murphy, K. D. Kochanek, & B.A. Bastian, 2016, *National Vital Statistics Reports, 64*(2), pp. 38–42.

America's Health Challenges

In 2013, just two chronic diseases—heart disease and cancer—were responsible for almost half of all deaths

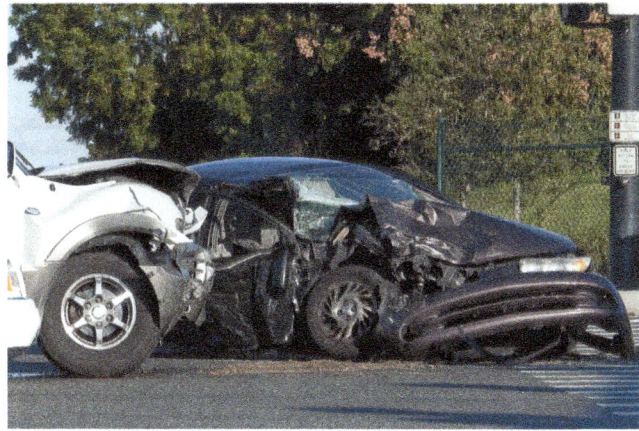

Unintentional injuries, including motor vehicle accidents, are the leading cause of death among people aged 15–24 in the United States.

(46.5%) in the United States.[4] Moreover, our chronic disease **morbidity**—the rate of chronic disease within our population—is about 50%.[6] These statistics are all the more shocking when you realize that chronic diseases are among the most preventable of all health problems in the United States.[6] That's why one of the world's oldest and largest public health agencies—the U.S. Centers for Disease Control and Prevention (CDC)—is sponsoring a national initiative to reduce our rate of chronic disease. As part of this initiative, the CDC has identified four common behaviors that are responsible for most of the suffering and early death related to chronic diseases **(Figure 1.3):**[6]

- Lack of physical activity
- Poor nutrition
- Tobacco use
- Drinking too much alcohol

Some of these behaviors can act as direct **causes** of disease. For example, tobacco use is known to cause lung cancer. Others act as **risk factors;** that is, factors that increase the chance that the person will develop a disease. Lack of physical activity, for example, increases an individual's risk for cardiovascular disease.

Are Americans changing their behaviors to reduce their risk for disease? Consider these trends among U.S. adults:

- Fewer than half (49%) meet the 2008 *Physical Activity Guidelines.*[7]
- More than one-third of all adults (34.9%) are obese.[8]
- 20.5% of males and 15.3% of females smoke.[9]
- One in six admits to binge drinking four or more times a month.[10]

As these statistics suggest, it's time for Americans to make healthful lifestyle choices a priority.

Organizations That Promote America's Health

The U.S. Department of Health and Human Services (HHS) is the U.S. government's principal agency for enhancing and protecting the health of all Americans.[11] Its primary division is the U.S. Public Health Service (PHS), which is directed by the Office of the Surgeon General. The PHS includes a dozen operating divisions that work together to promote and protect the health of Americans. Among these are the CDC and the following:[11]

- The *Food and Drug Administration (FDA)* is responsible for assuring the safety, efficacy, and security of medications, medical devices, the food supply, cosmetics, and products that emit radiation.
- The *National Institutes of Health (NIH)* is the primary center for medical research in the United States.
- The *Substance Abuse and Mental Health Services Administration* is an agency whose mission is to reduce the impact of substance abuse and mental illness on America's communities.

The Healthy People Initiative

In 1979, HHS launched the **Healthy People initiative** with a report of the surgeon general on health promotion and disease prevention efforts in the United States. **Health promotion** includes information, programs, and services such as employee fitness centers that help populations improve their health. **Disease prevention** includes activities such as vaccinations

> **morbidity** Clinical term for disease, specifically the level of disease within a population.
>
> **cause** In health, a factor such as a genetic defect or virus that is directly responsible for a certain resulting condition.
>
> **risk factor** A factor such as advanced age or alcohol abuse that increases the likelihood that an individual will experience a certain disease or injury.
>
> **Healthy People initiative** A federal initiative to facilitate broad, positive health changes in large segments of the U.S. population every 10 years.
>
> **health promotion** Information, programs, and services provided to help populations improve their health.
>
> **disease prevention** Activities such as vaccinations and cancer screenings to help prevent disease.

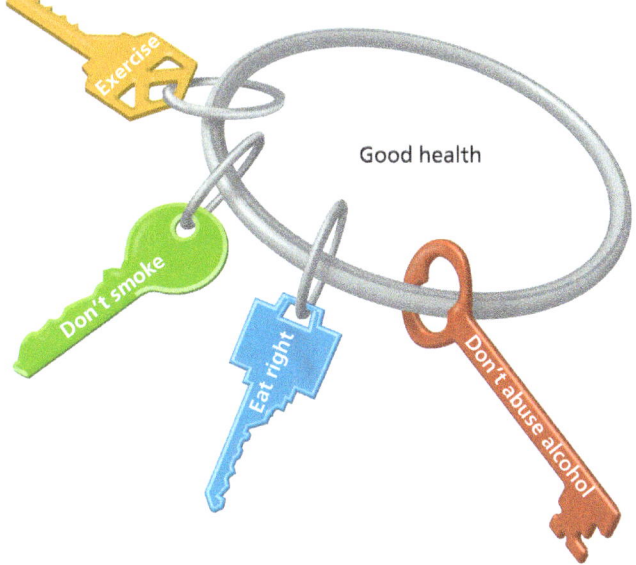

FIGURE 1.3 **Four Keys to Good Health.**
These four behaviors can significantly reduce your risk of chronic disease and early death.

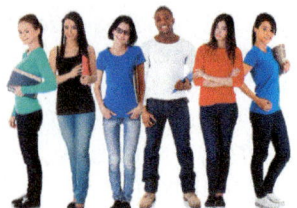

DIVERSITY & HEALTH

Health Disparities Among Different Racial and Ethnic Groups

Whether the causes are socioeconomic, biological, cultural, or still not well understood, health disparities exist among different racial and ethnic populations in the United States. For example, Asian Americans, overall, have lower rates of most chronic diseases, such as heart disease. Their risk for fatal injuries (from homicides, suicides, and motor vehicle accidents) also tends to be lower. Native Americans also experience lower-than-average rates of some common chronic diseases, but they share with Caucasian Americans more than double the rates of motor vehicle fatalities and suicides seen in other racial/ethnic groups. They also have the highest rate of diabetes. Hispanic Americans have average rates of chronic disease and lower risks for injury deaths.[1]

The racial/ethnic group with consistently high rates of chronic disease is African Americans. For example:[1]

- **Obesity.** Just over half (51%) of African American women are obese, a rate 20% higher than for Caucasian women. Obesity in African American girls is 9% higher than in Caucasian girls.
- **Hypertension (high blood pressure).** African Americans have the highest prevalence of hypertension, 41% compared to 27%–29% for Hispanic and Caucasian Americans.
- **Heart attacks and strokes.** African Americans are at much higher risk of death from a heart attack or stroke. Their death rate from these causes is 20% higher than for Caucasian Americans, nearly 75% higher than for Hispanic Americans, and more than 200% higher than for Asian Americans.
- **Diabetes.** Although Native American adults have the highest rates of diabetes (approximately 14%), more than 11% of African and Hispanic American adults also have been diagnosed with diabetes, as compared to 6.8% of Caucasian and 7.9% of Asian Americans.

In addition, although African Americans have lower rates of motor vehicle fatalities and suicides, the homicide rate among African Americans is more than double that of Native Americans, triple that of Hispanic Americans, and seven times that of Caucasian or Asian Americans.[1]

What Do You Think?

1. Nearly 11% of the poorest Americans have been diagnosed with diabetes, as compared to about 6% of affluent Americans. Similarly, hypertension affects 33% of poor Americans and 28% of affluent Americans. Do you think there could be a link between income disparities, racial and ethnic disparities, and health disparities? Why or why not?
2. Despite the fact that African American women are less likely to develop breast cancer than Caucasian women, they are more likely to die from it.[2] Why might this be?
3. Health disparities are complex problems with multiple contributing factors. What could you do as an individual—independently or on campus or in your community—to contribute to reducing health disparities?

References: 1. "CDC Health Disparities and Inequalities Report—United States, 2013," by the Centers for Disease Control and Prevention, November 22, 2013, *Morbidity and Mortality Weekly Report*, vol. 62 (Supplement) No. 3. Available at www.cdc.gov/mmwr. 2. "Cancer Facts & Figures, 2016," by the American Cancer Society, Atlanta, 2016, retrieved from www.cancer.org.

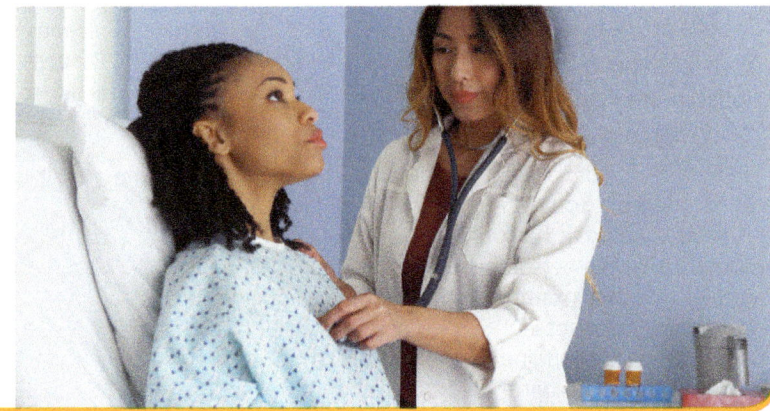

---

and cancer screenings to help prevent disease. In 1980, HHS published Healthy People 1990, a set of 10-year objectives for building a society in which all people live long, healthy lives. Every decade since, HHS has updated Healthy People to include both new objectives and a report of the progress made over the previous decade. The most recent effort, Healthy People 2020, was released in December 2010.[12]

One of the primary goals of the Healthy People initiative is to achieve *health equity*—the attainment of the highest level of health for all people—and to eliminate **health disparities**—differences in the rate and burden of disease and the access to and quality of health care among various population groups. These include groups based on race or ethnicity, disability, **gender** (social, cultural, or psychological traits associated with male or female identity), sexual orientation, socioeconomic status, and other characteristics historically linked to discrimination or exclusion.[12] The **Diversity & Health** box identifies key health disparities specific to race and ethnicity, and we'll examine the role of poverty and other disparities as we continue in this chapter.

health disparities Gaps in the rate and burden of disease and the access to and quality of health care among various population groups.

gender Social, cultural, or psychological traits associated with identification as either male or female.

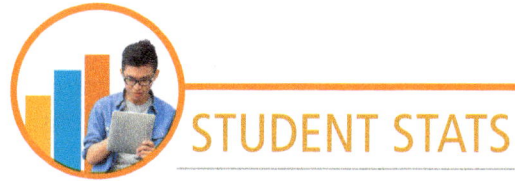

STUDENT STATS

Common Health Problems Reported by College Students

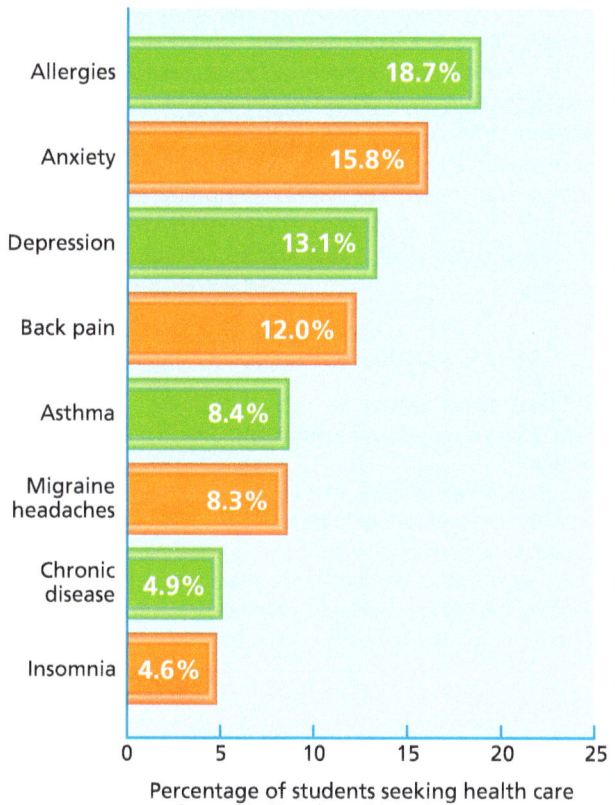

Percentage of students seeking health care for each disorder within the past year

Data from *American College Health Association National College Health Assessment (ACHA-NCHA II) Reference Group Executive Summary, Spring* 2015, by the American College Health Association, 2015, retrieved from **www.acha-ncha.org**.

>> For more information on Healthy People 2020, visit **www.healthypeople.gov**.

Health on America's Campuses

Centers of higher learning, as microcosms of our larger society, have come to recognize that promoting students' health helps the institution meet its goal of providing the best education possible. Stress, sleep deprivation, poor nutrition, depression, anxiety, alcohol and tobacco use, and sexually transmitted infections are just a few of the health issues that can affect academic performance and achievement.

Campus Health Challenges

Each year, the American College Health Association (ACHA) conducts national surveys of college students' health concerns. In the spring 2015 survey, 86.5% of college students described their health as good, very good, or excellent. Still,

> *"The behaviors that increase the risk of developing chronic diseases—including unhealthy eating habits and a lack of physical activity—are common among college students."*

students routinely visit their health care provider for treatment of acute conditions such as injuries and infections, and a surprising number for treatment of persistent health problems, as shown in the **Student Stats** box.[13]

Among Americans aged 15–24, the leading causes of death are accidents, suicide, and homicide (see Table 1.1). These sudden, traumatic deaths lead mortality in this age group because young people don't experience the high rates of chronic diseases (such as heart disease and cancer) that increase mortality among the adult population as a whole. However, the behaviors that increase the risk of developing chronic diseases—including unhealthy eating habits and a lack of physical activity—are common among college students. Although 60% of students report being at a healthy weight, nearly 5% are underweight, 22.5% are overweight, and 12.5% are obese.[13] Furthermore, although 46% of college students meet national recommendations for physical activity (moderate exercise for at least 30 minutes at least 5 days per week or vigorous exercise for at least 20 minutes at least 3 days per week), over half do not.[13]

Interestingly, research has shown that students tend to vastly overestimate how many of their peers are regularly using alcohol, tobacco, or other drugs.[13] For example, students believed that over 75% of their peers had smoked cigarettes and over 80% had used marijuana within the past 30 days. In reality, only 11% had smoked and 17% had used marijuana. The lesson here: When it comes to substance use, it's simply not true that "everyone is doing it."

The Healthy Campus Initiative

In conjunction with the Healthy People initiative, the ACHA has developed an initiative called **Healthy Campus** for use in student settings. Colleges and universities participating in this program can choose to focus on achieving health goals most relevant to them, such as:

- Reducing rates of anxiety and depression
- Decreasing substance abuse
- Increasing on-campus opportunities for physical activity
- Improving sexual health among students

Healthy Campus An offshoot of the Healthy People initiative specifically geared toward college students.

>> More information on Healthy Campus 2020 is available at **www.acha.org**.

Health Around the World

In spring 2014, the WHO reported a limited outbreak of the potentially fatal Ebola virus disease in the West African nation of Guinea. The disease soon spread to bordering nations, and before the end of the year, patients had been diagnosed worldwide, including in both Europe and North America. Similarly, in early 2016, the WHO reported a surge in severe birth defects attributed to the Zika virus, declaring it a public health emergency of international concern. Zika was discovered decades ago in Uganda and slowly spread—primarily via the bite of an infected mosquito or the semen of an infected man—throughout Africa, Asia, and more recently, to South America and, via travelers, to the United States. These outbreaks are a grim reminder that, in our increasingly mobile and connected world, limiting the spread of infectious disease is an urgent concern.

Other significant global infectious disease threats are cholera, which is transmitted via contaminated water; malaria, which is transmitted by mosquitoes; and influenza, which is transmitted person to person. Although the rate of new infections from the human immunodeficiency virus (HIV), which causes AIDS, dropped by 38% between 2001 and 2014, the United Nations Programme on HIV/AIDS reports that 35 million people are living with HIV, and fewer than 40% of these are receiving the recommended antiretroviral therapy. Over 70% of infected people (25 million) live in sub-Saharan Africa.[14]

Some infections are now resisting conventional treatment with antimicrobial drugs. For example, the bacteria that cause tuberculosis have become increasingly resistant to conventional antibiotics. As a result, infections with extensively drug-resistant TB (XDR-TB) are on the rise worldwide.[15] Although these infections can be cured, the cure rate is lower than with other forms of TB.[15]

>> For more information on infectious diseases around the world, visit the World Health Organization website at www.who.int.

Undernourishment is still a concern in developing nations: In 2015, 795 million people in the world remained chronically undernourished. Nearly 98% of these hungry people live in the developing world.[16] Deficiency of certain vitamins and minerals causes a variety of diseases, such as night blindness, which develops when vitamin A is deficient, and a form of intellectual disability called cretinism, which is due to iodine deficiency. Malnutrition also increases an individual's susceptibility to infection, as well as the risk that infection will result in death.

To address global health concerns, a number of privately funded health organizations have joined with international agencies such as the WHO to support immunizations, mosquito nets, water filters, vitamin drops, and the addition of iodine to salt. These efforts are improving global health.

A third global health concern is the rising rates of chronic diseases—including heart disease, diabetes, and certain types of cancer—related to obesity. Two trends contribute to the rising prevalence of "globesity": A greater percentage of the world's population now has access to low-cost, processed foods high in added sugars and calories and, at the same time, more people have access to motorized transportation, labor-saving devices, and sedentary forms of entertainment. These trends have contributed to an alarming statistic: The WHO estimates that worldwide obesity has more than doubled since 1980, and 600 million people are now obese.[17]

LO 1.3 QUICK CHECK

Heart disease and diabetes
a. are diseases of affluence, prevalent only in developed nations.
b. prompt more than 20% of college students to visit their health care provider at least once each year.
c. have decreased in prevalence worldwide because of advances in sanitation, food inspection, and vaccination.
d. are increasing in prevalence worldwide along with increased rates of obesity.

Determinants of Health

LO 1.4 Classify determinants of health into six broad groups, identifying the group that is most strongly within an individual's control.

The WHO, the HHS, and other public health organizations recognize that individuals are not solely responsible for the state of their health. They acknowledge that health is influenced by a range of personal, social, economic, and environmental factors collectively referred to as **determinants of health.** Any steps taken to improve health—both for individuals and for populations—are likely to be more successful when they target multiple determinants of health.[18]

> **determinants of health** The range of personal, social, economic, and environmental factors that influence health status.

>> To watch a video explaining and providing examples of how determinants influence an individual's health, go to www.healthypeople.gov and type in the search bar "determinants of health."

Determinants of health fall into six broad categories, all of which overlap to a greater or lesser extent. Let's take a closer look.

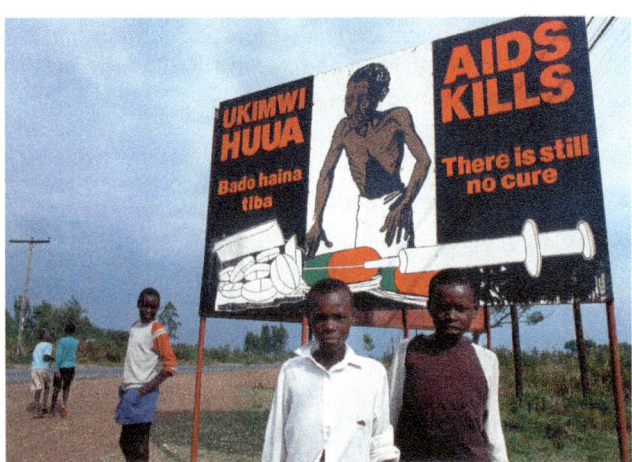

HIV/AIDS continues to be a serious concern worldwide, especially in sub-Saharan Africa.

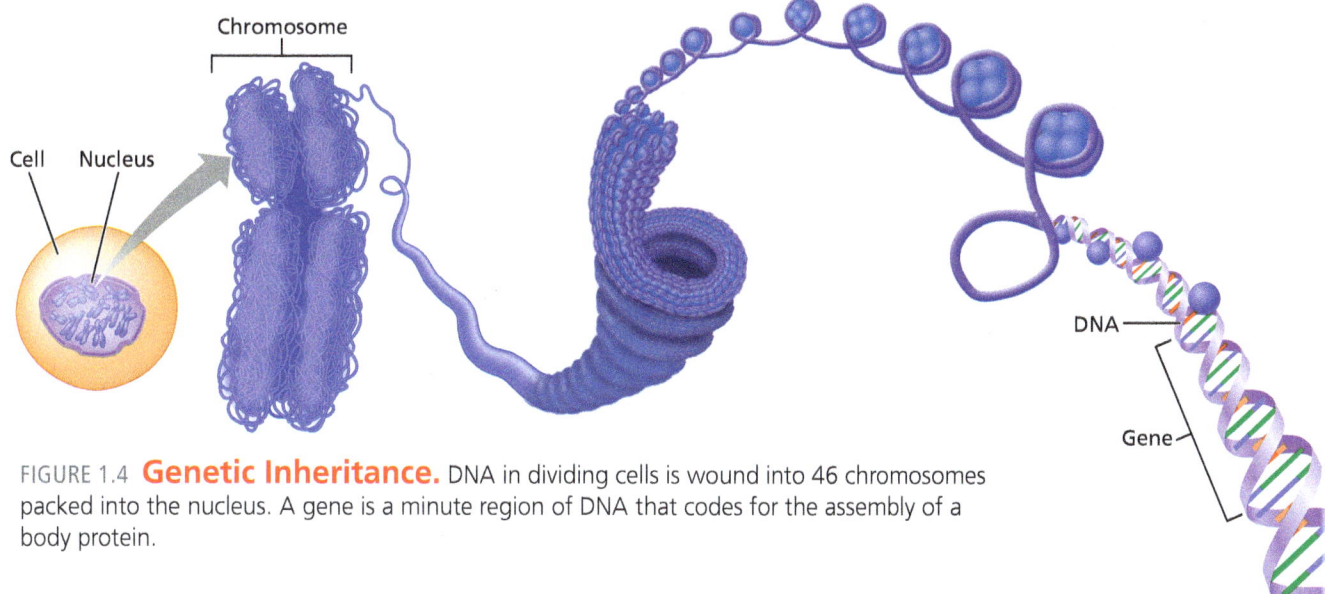

FIGURE 1.4 **Genetic Inheritance.** DNA in dividing cells is wound into 46 chromosomes packed into the nucleus. A gene is a minute region of DNA that codes for the assembly of a body protein.

Biology and Genetics

Biological and genetic determinants influence your health but are beyond your control. Because one of the most significant of these determinants is the DNA—the genetic material—you inherited from your parents, it's worth taking a moment to review some key concepts in genetics:

- Most of your body cells have a nucleus stuffed with a compound called **DNA (deoxyribonucleic acid)** that resembles a twisted ladder known as a double helix **(Figure 1.4).**
- Some segments of DNA carry the instructions—or code—your cells use to assemble the proteins that build body tissues and participate in body functions. A protein-coding segment of DNA is called a **gene.**
- When cells are dividing, their DNA forms tight bundles called **chromosomes.** Your **genome** is your entire collection of genes on your 46 chromosomes (23 pairs). You inherited one set of 23 chromosomes from each of your parents. Although all human beings share mostly the same DNA, everyone's genome contains a few unique differences, or *genetic variants*. Your variants make you distinct in many ways, including in some aspects of your health.

The 23rd chromosome you inherited from your father at conception determined your **sex**—that is, the anatomical and physiological features that differentiate males from females. These biological differences between men and women strongly influence health. Women tend to live about four years longer than men, for example, but have higher rates of arthritis and osteoporosis (low bone density). Men have a higher prevalence of heart disease and diabetes.[19]

Other biological and genetic determinants include the following:

- **Age.** Incomplete growth and development make children more susceptible to certain health problems, such as infectious diseases. At the other end of the age spectrum, the physical and cognitive effects of aging increase an older adult's vulnerability to poor health.[18]

- **Race/ethnicity.** Certain population groups have a higher risk for certain diseases than the general population. (See the **Diversity & Health box** on page 6.) Knowing about these differences can prompt you to make better lifestyle choices and can prompt your physician to provide more targeted care. For example, because African Americans have higher rates of hypertension (high blood pressure), informed doctors may encourage more frequent blood pressure screenings for their African American patients at an earlier age.

- **Health history.** Some conditions that you experienced in the past may still be influencing your health today. For instance, some sexually transmitted infections can reduce your fertility many years later. Past injuries can also continue to affect health.

- **Family history.** You—and your children—are at increased risk for developing some of the same diseases that members of your family have experienced. This is true not only for recognized genetic diseases but also for many chronic diseases such as hypertension and diabetes, and even for some psychological disorders such as depression. It's important to know your family health history so that you and your health-care provider can take steps to reduce any risks.

> **DNA (deoxyribonucleic acid)** A compound in the nucleus of living cells that transfers genetic information.
>
> **gene** A segment of DNA that codes for the assembly of a protein.
>
> **chromosome** In humans, one of 46 bundles of DNA carrying genes that determine heredity.
>
> **genome** The genetic material of a living organism.
>
> **sex** Biological characteristics of males and females based on their genetic inheritance.

▶▶ Create and print out your own family health history tree by using the interactive tool My Family Health Portrait from the U.S. Surgeon General, at **https://familyhistory.hhs.gov**.

Individual Behaviors

Although you can't select different genes or turn back the clock on aging, you can control your lifestyle choices. The

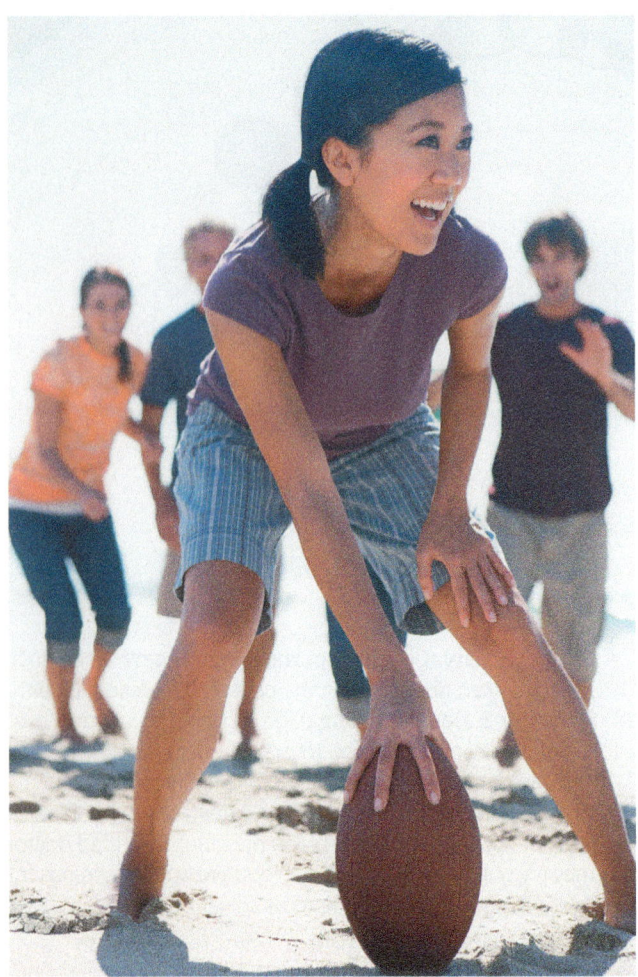

Engaging in regular physical activity is one of the keys to good health.

NIH has identified five modifiable behaviors that are responsible for the majority of premature deaths in the United States. In order of significance, these are tobacco use, poor diet, physical inactivity, alcohol abuse, and drug abuse.[20] The first four of these behaviors contribute to premature deaths because, as we noted earlier, they strongly increase your risk for chronic disease (see Figure 1.3).

Other behavioral determinants of health include the steps you take to manage your stress, the quantity and quality of your sleep, the choices you make to develop supportive relationships, your sexual decision making, and the ways you promote your personal safety, such as by wearing a seat belt. These behaviors are discussed later in this text.

Social Determinants

Social determinants are the economic and societal conditions in which people live. They include, for example, interpersonal and community relationships, discrimination, poverty, educational and job opportunities, transportation, and public safety.[18] You can work to improve these conditions, but no individual can fully control them.

Research over the past two decades has increasingly acknowledged the significant influence of social determinants on health. For example, a family may understand the value of regular physical activity but may live in a high-crime area where they're afraid to go out walking and lack the resources to pay for membership in a fitness club. If you're getting the sense that poverty is a fundamental social determinant of health, you're right: Socioeconomic disparities lead to higher levels of "biological dysregulation" that in turn promote disease.[21] Called the **status syndrome,** this disparity has traditionally been attributed to a poor person's reduced access to quality health care; nutritious foods; safe, adequate shelter; and opportunities for physical activity. However, some researchers now believe that it occurs in part because people who are poor are less likely to feel in control of their circumstances and more likely to perceive themselves as unequal in the workplace and in their communities. These perceptions dramatically increase stress, causing physiological changes that can lead to disease.[19] A 2016 analysis found that, for Americans born in 1950, males in the lowest income bracket have an average life expectancy of 73.6 years, whereas males in the highest income bracket have an average life expectancy of 87.2 years, a gap of 14 years. For females, the corresponding gap in life expectancy is 13 years.[22]

> **status syndrome** The disparity in health status and rates of premature mortality between the impoverished and the affluent within any given society.

Physical Determinants

Physical determinants are physical conditions in the environment. Examples include:[18]

- Aspects of the natural environment, such as plants and climate
- Aspects of the *built environment*, which includes all buildings, spaces, and products that are made or modified by people
- Presence or absence of toxic substances and other physical hazards

For example, climate extremes, air pollution, and other hazards are aspects of the physical environment that threaten health, whereas nearby parks, community swimming pools, and farmers' markets support health.

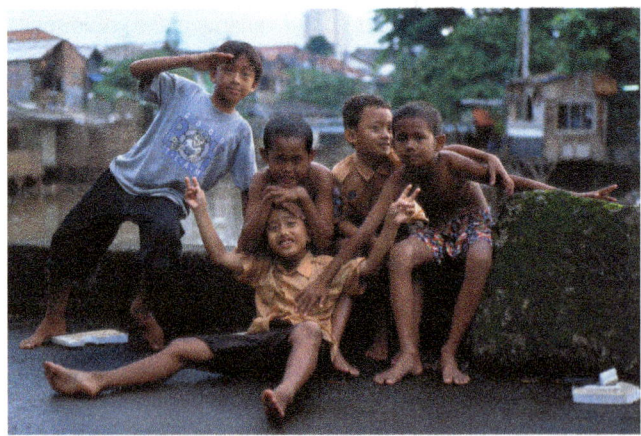

These boys live in a poor area of Jakarta, Indonesia, that lacks parks, playgrounds, and other safe and stimulating places to play. These are aspects of the physical environment that strongly influence a child's health.

STUDENT STORY

Proud of My Scars

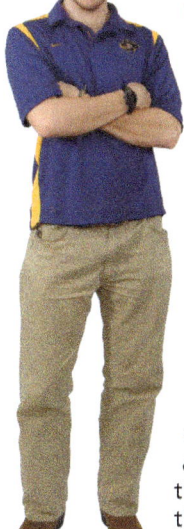

"HI, I'M COREY. I'm 19, and I'm a sophomore park and rec management major. I was born with a skeletal condition where the left side of my body is bigger than the right side. The doctors had to even out my legs so that I could walk flat-footed and wouldn't have back problems later in life. I've had a total of three surgeries, which left me with some scars. I also have a scar from my belly button all the way to the side of my rib cage. Growing up, I was always self-conscious, especially during the summer, when everybody was out at the beach in swimsuits, and all these guys had six-pack abs. I knew I'd never be able to have abs like that because I have this scar running straight through my abdominal muscle.

Now, though, I've realized that my scars are a great conversation starter. People will see me and ask, 'Oh, cool scar, how'd you get it?' I've learned over the years that everybody has a fail point and mine just happens to be physical. I've just learned to live with it. Those scars are what make me 'me.' I also have friends who don't really care what I look like or whether I'm the strongest or best-looking guy in the world. My friends are there whether I'm having surgeries or I'm on top of the world."

What Do You Think?

1. Where do you think Corey falls on the illness–wellness continuum?
2. Assess how Corey is doing in at least three different dimensions of health.
3. Discuss the role of biological determinants of health and access to health services in shaping Corey's health.

Health Services

Health services include availability of quality health care as well as access to that care. Health literacy is also included in health services.

Access to Health Services

In countries with a national health service, access to care is not typically a determinant of health. But in the United States, lack of health insurance reduces access to health services, which in turn threatens health. The uninsured (or underinsured) are less likely to have a regular doctor or to receive preventive care. They are also more likely to delay medical treatment, waiting until a condition has advanced to a crisis stage before visiting a local hospital emergency room—a habit that greatly increases the level of care required as well as the cost of that care.

In 2010, the U.S. Congress passed into law a set of comprehensive health-care reforms. Called the Affordable Care Act, the legislation has reduced the number of uninsured Americans by about one-third—almost 16 million people—since it took effect.[23] Among other measures, it provides subsidies that help families pay for private insurance and that enable states to enroll eligible families in Medicaid. Still, 20 states have failed to accept federal subsidies to expand Medicaid, and nearly 29 million Americans remain uninsured.[23]

>> For updates on the Affordable Care Act, visit **www.healthcare.gov**.

health literacy The ability to evaluate and understand health information and to make informed choices for your health care.

Health Literacy

In the 21st century, quality health care increasingly depends upon **health literacy,** the ability to obtain and understand basic health information and services in order to make appropriate decisions for your own care. It includes the ability to read, understand, and follow medical instructions such as prescription drug labels; listen to health-care providers, ask good questions, and analyze the information you receive; and navigate an often-complex health-care system.[24] Increasingly, health literacy also requires a degree of computer literacy and media awareness.

A goal of this text is to increase your health literacy by providing you with strategies to evaluate all the health information that you are exposed to—whether from print media, television, or the Internet. Online searches are increasingly popular for people seeking health information, but search results don't distinguish between sites that provide scientifically sound information and sites that contain inaccurate or misleading content. The accompanying **Media and Health** box will help you evaluate health information in the media.

Policy-Making

Policies at the local, state, and federal levels affect health. Local and state taxes on cigarettes improve health by reducing the number of people who smoke. State regulations to increase motor vehicle safety—for example, establishing speed limits, mandating seat belt use, and outlawing texting while driving—reduce traumatic injuries and deaths. At the federal level, HHS funds health insurance for older Americans (Medicare) and Americans in need (Medicaid); the FDA works to improve food safety; and the U.S. Environmental Protection Agency (EPA) regulates air, water, and soil quality.

Policy-making also includes corporate initiatives. For example, many large companies provide employee fitness centers and a variety of incentives to use them.

LO 1.4 QUICK CHECK

The determinants of health most strongly within your control are
a. biology and genetics.
b. individual behaviors.
c. social determinants.
d. physical determinants.

MEDIA AND Health
Evaluating Health Information in the Media

Is the health information you just researched on the Internet accurate? Can you trust a celebrity endorsement for a weight-loss product? How can you make sense of the endless stream of media headlines trumpeting health studies with contradictory findings?

The term *media* can mean a variety of things. We use it here to include print (books, newspapers, magazines), television and radio, Internet websites, and even mobile apps. Whether you're in Midtown Manhattan or a campsite in Montana, media can be your ally, as long as you understand how to use it.

When you come across an article about the results of the latest health-related study, answer the following questions:

- Was the study conducted by an unbiased source, or was it carried out by an individual or organization with a vested interest in the outcome?
- Have the results been replicated by other researchers?
- Was the sample size of the study large or small, and were the study participants similar to or different from you in age, sex, health habits, and other factors?
- Was the study conducted over a short or long period of time?
- Perhaps most importantly, is the study only showing a *correlation* between two things, or is it truly showing that one variable is the direct result of another variable? For example, a study may find that populations consuming a vegetarian diet have a higher average life expectancy. However, many behaviors common to people who eat a vegetarian diet (such as engaging in physical activity, avoiding tobacco use, and so forth) also play a role in life expectancy. Thus, you should not assume that the study results suggest that eating a vegetarian diet increases longevity.

When you're evaluating health information online, how can you tell whether the information is credible? Answer the following questions:

- Who is the sponsor of the site? Agencies of the U.S. government have sites with URLs ending in .gov, and educational institutions use .edu. These sites are more likely to provide credible information than those that end in .com, which designates a commercial site. The domain .org is used by many credible, nonprofit, noncommercial sites, but it is sometimes used by commercial entities as well.
- What is the purpose of the site? Is it to inform and educate, or is it to sell you something? If it is to sell you something, be aware that the information presented is more likely to be biased.
- Does the site tell you where the information it presents is coming from? If so, is the content based on scientific evidence, or was it written by someone hired by the site to produce marketing information? Sites that are able to provide citations and links to scientific studies and journals are more likely to be credible than sites lacking these references.
- Does the site specify when its content was last updated? Health information can sometimes change quickly, so you want to seek out information that is as current as possible.

Throughout this text, the **Get Connected** feature at the end of each chapter lists health-related websites where you can obtain reliable health information. Still, keep in mind that information on the Internet is never a substitute for consulting a health-care professional. After you've conducted your own online research, make an appointment with your doctor and ask questions to make sure you receive the most accurate information about any health issue you may be facing.

What Do You Think?

1. Log onto your favorite online news source. Click on an article describing a health-related research study. As you read the article, try to determine whether the study found a correlation or a cause–effect relationship. In your view, has the journalist presented the study results accurately? Is the article potentially misleading? If so, in what ways?

2. How often have you seen advertisements promoting prescription drugs—for everything from weight loss to social anxiety? Do these ads affect the way you think about the role of prescription drugs in maintaining your health? Do you think seeing advertisements makes you more or less likely to take prescription drugs, or do ads have no effect?

3. Identify a health-related topic (such as the benefits of a low-carb diet or the ideal amount and type of physical activity) for which the advice of experts seems to have frequently changed. Why do you think health recommendations often do change? How might an awareness of the apparent contradictions in some health-related research influence the way you explore a health topic of interest to you?

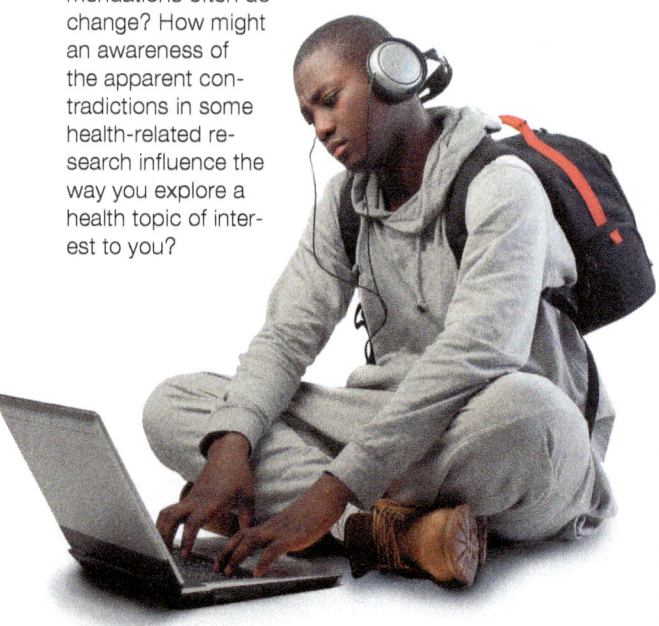

What Factors Influence Behavior Change?

LO 1.5 Explain how predisposing, enabling, and reinforcing factors can promote or hinder behavior change.

We often have a good idea of what choices we *ought* to be making—for instance, eating more fruits and vegetables or setting aside time each day to exercise—but actually doing these things and achieving lasting **behavior change** is the hard part. Let's take a look at some factors that can help you make positive change or hinder your efforts to change.

Predisposing Factors

Predisposing factors are the physical, mental, emotional, social, and environmental factors that affect the likelihood that you will decide to change a current behavior. These factors exert their influence beforehand, by increasing or decreasing your motivation to change. They include your knowledge of health issues, your beliefs about how susceptible you are to injury or disease, and your attitude toward how a behavior change might benefit your health. Let's say, for instance, that although you know the health dangers of smoking, you haven't tried to quit. Anything that might increase or decrease the likelihood of your taking action to quit—whether it's the increasing cost of cigarettes, or your memory of a relative who "smoked two packs a day and lived to be 100"—would qualify as a predisposing factor.

The values you hold are predisposing factors that can and do influence motivation—but what if you hold conflicting values? For instance, most people value a long life free of disease and disability. But what if you so highly value a slender appearance that you smoke cigarettes in order to suppress your appetite?

Your peer and family relationships can also be predisposing factors. For instance, having a partner who finds smoking disgusting might increase your motivation to quit.

Enabling Factors

Enabling factors are the skills, social supports, and resources that make it possible (or easier) for your change efforts to succeed. The knowledge and skills you'll acquire in your personal health course, for instance, will support you. Other examples of enabling factors include access to health-care resources, such as a low-cost weight-loss clinic; environmental factors, such as living in a neighborhood that shares a community garden; and financial resources, which can enable an affluent individual, for example, to pay for sessions with a personal trainer. Even physical and psychological health are resources that can enable you to maintain a program of change, such as regular exercise.

Your peers are key enablers: If you're trying to stop smoking, hanging out with nonsmokers is likely to help you succeed. Of course, peer pressure often works the other way, prompting you to give up on a desired change. In such

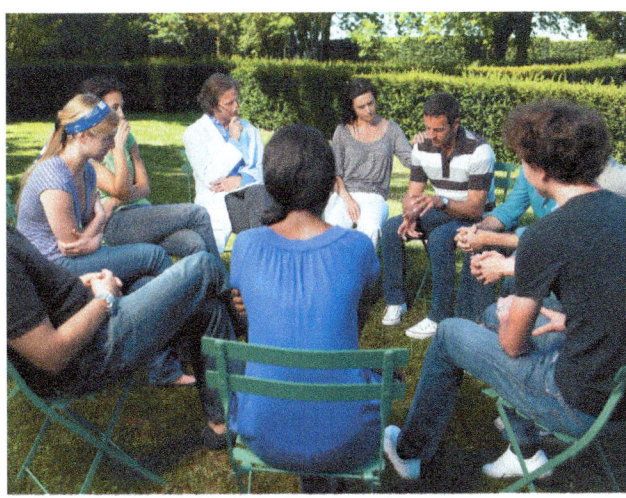

Support groups for quitting smoking or drinking can play a key role in lasting behavior change.

cases, policy-making can sometimes help; for instance, attending a college with a smoke-free campus would strongly enable your smoking-cessation efforts.

Reinforcing Factors

Positive **reinforcing factors** are encouragements and rewards that promote successful behavior change. In other words, these factors motivate you to "keep up the good work." An end-of-year bonus for employees who have logged a certain number of hours in the company's fitness center is an example. Negative reinforcing factors are barriers that can oppose, impede, or entirely derail your efforts to change. Perhaps you've begun a strength-training program to increase your level of fitness. All goes well for the first three weeks—but then you prematurely increase the weights and throw out your lower back. You'll need persistence and determination to overcome this negative reinforcer.

> **behavior change** A sustained change in a habit or pattern of behavior that affects health.
>
> **predisposing factor** A physical, mental, emotional, or surrounding influence that affects the likelihood that a person will decide to change a current behavior.
>
> **enabling factor** A skill, social support, or resource that makes it possible (or easier) to succeed in changing a targeted behavior.
>
> **reinforcing factor** An influence that either rewards or opposes a change effort in progress. Positive reinforcers encourage individuals to continue their efforts to change; negative reinforcers discourage or block change.

LO 1.5 QUICK CHECK

Kendra, who is obese, just learned that a blood test shows she is at high risk for developing diabetes. Her physician told her she could probably reduce this risk by losing 15–20 pounds. Kendra has finally decided it's time to get serious about losing weight. Her diagnosis is

a. a predisposing factor.
b. an enabling factor.
c. a positive reinforcer.
d. a negative reinforcer.

How Does Behavior Change Occur?

LO 1.6 Compare three models of behavior change.

transtheoretical model of behavior change A model of behavior change that focuses on decision-making steps and abilities. Also called the *stages of change* model.

health belief model A model of behavior change that emphasizes the influence of personal beliefs on the process of creating effective change.

ecological models Behavior-change models that acknowledge the creation of a supportive environment as being equally important to achieving change as an individual's acquisition of health information and development of new skills.

A *model* is a description that helps you understand something you can't directly observe. If you've ever attended a five-year sobriety celebration or discovered that a formerly obese friend from high school has lost a lot of weight, you might have wondered how—exactly—these people did it. And would the methods they used work for you?

Over many decades, public health researchers have proposed various models of processes by which they believe lasting behavior change happens. Two of the oldest and most established of these are the transtheoretical model and the health belief model. More recently, researchers have developed a variety of ecological models of behavior change. Let's take a look.

The Transtheoretical Model

The **transtheoretical model of behavior change**, also called the *stages of change* model, was developed by psychologist James O. Prochaska and his colleagues. Its basic premise is that behavior change is a process and not an event, and individuals are at varying levels of readiness to change. The model identifies six stages of change that a person progresses through before achieving sustained behavior change **(Figure 1.5)**:[25]

- **Precontemplation.** During this stage, a person may or may not recognize a health challenge, and in either case has no intention of making changes to address it in the near future (that is, within the next six months).
- **Contemplation.** During this stage, a person acknowledges the health challenge and thinks about making a change within the next six months. At this stage, the person is still not ready to take action but is thinking about it.
- **Preparation.** During this stage, a person intends to change the behavior within the next month and has a plan of action in mind (such as enrolling in a class or joining a support group).
- **Action.** During this stage, a person modifies the behavior in an observable way—for example, quits smoking, begins jogging each week, etc. In this stage, the change is initiated but is not yet consistent over time.
- **Maintenance.** During this stage, a person has maintained the new behavior for six months or more and continues to actively work to prevent relapse (reverting to old habits). Maintenance can last months or even years, and relapse is not unusual.
- **Termination.** During this stage, a person has successfully achieved behavior change to the point where he or she is completely confident that relapse will not occur.

The transtheoretical model is widely used as a framework for research studies in public health and can be useful to consider when you think about embarking on a behavior-change plan in your own life.

The Health Belief Model

In the 1950s, researchers at the U.S. Public Health Service introduced the **health belief model** of behavior change. This model identifies four factors as instrumental in predicting behavior change:

- **Perceived threat.** You perceive a threat (such as injury or disease) and that this threat is real.
- **Perceived severity.** You understand that this threat could have serious consequences in terms of pain, lost work time, financial loss, etc.
- **Perceived benefit.** You believe that the benefits of making the behavior change will outweigh the costs, inconveniences, and other challenges and that the change is possible for you to make and maintain.
- **Cues to action.** You have an experience that causes you to commit to making the change. For example, a young person at risk for diabetes might witness a parent attempting to cope following a foot amputation that resulted from the disease.

You might find it helpful to consider the health belief model when you assess your own readiness for changing a health behavior: Do you perceive a serious threat to your health? If so, can you identify real benefits to making changes—benefits that outweigh the time and other costs involved?

Ecological Models

A criticism of most models of behavior change is that they highlight the role of individual thoughts and actions and downplay the contributions of social and physical determinants, access to health services, and policy-making. This has led to the development of a variety of **ecological models** of behavior change, in which the creation of a supportive

Precontemplation → Contemplation → Preparation → Action → Maintenance → Termination

FIGURE 1.5 The Transtheoretical Model of Behavior Change. Developed by James Prochaska, this model outlines six stages of behavior change.

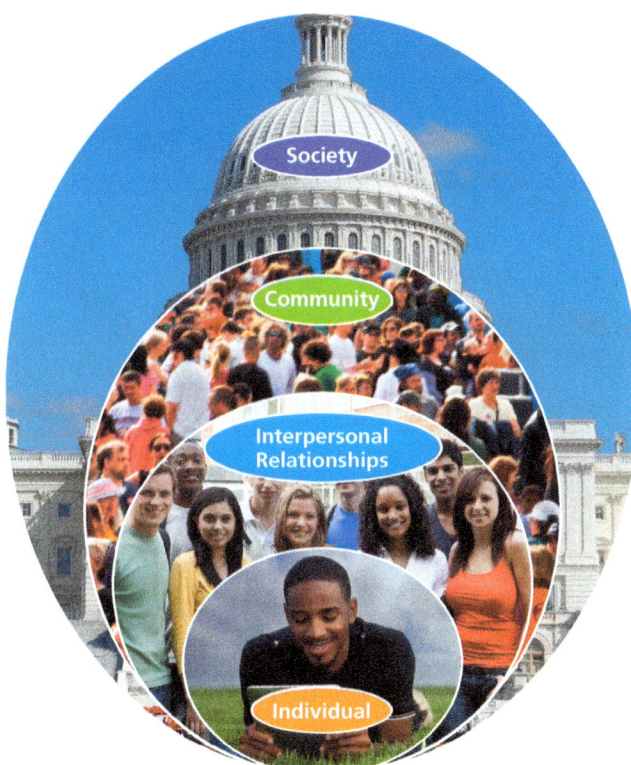

FIGURE 1.6 An Ecological Model of Behavior Change. The coordination of multiple factors at different levels, from individual to societal, promotes successful behavior change.

environment is acknowledged to be as important to achieving change as is an individual's acquisition of health information and development of new skills.

Ecological models emphasize these principles:

- Multiple levels of factors—from individual behavior to family values, community support, and public policy—influence health behaviors **(Figure 1.6)**.
- Influences at different levels interact to promote or impede change.
- For successful behavior change, interventions at multiple levels are most effective.

For example, an individual's motivation to lose weight might interact positively with a physician's advice to exercise, an employer's financial incentive for logging time at the company gym, and a city's construction of a new bike path. On the other hand, personal motivation is less effective when environments and policies make it difficult to choose healthful behaviors.

This means that, if you want to make lasting change, you shouldn't try to go it alone. You're more likely to succeed if you reach out for support from your health-care provider, your campus health services, and other resources in your community. In the next section, we talk more about recruiting support for your change. If the resources you need don't currently exist, advocate for them! Every chapter of this text concludes with ideas on campus advocacy for health-related change.

LO 1.6 QUICK CHECK

An individual's readiness to change a behavior is a key aspect of the

a. ecological models of behavior change.
b. ecological and health belief models of behavior change.
c. health belief and transtheoretical models of behavior change.
d. precontemplation stage of the transtheoretical model of behavior change.

Change Yourself, Change Your World

LO 1.7 List seven steps for achieving successful behavior change and two strategies for preventing relapse.

By enrolling in a personal health course and reading this text, you've already taken the initial step toward achieving better health and wellness. Throughout this text you'll find **Self-Assessments** that will help you assess your current health status, as well as **Choosing to Change Worksheets** that guide you on how to set appropriate goals and implement plans for behavior change. Each Choosing to Change Worksheet will prompt you to list your level of readiness for change—also known as your stage of behavior change—based on the transtheoretical model you read about earlier in this chapter. The worksheets will then walk you through behavior-change techniques appropriate for your stage of change, promoting a greater chance of success. To find electronic versions of the Self-Assessments and Choosing to Change Worksheets, online practice quizzes and activities, videos of real health students talking about their health issues, *ABC News* videos about current health news, and more, visit **MasteringHealth™**.

This chapter's **Self-Assessment** on pages 19–20 is a general self-survey evaluating your current health behaviors. Complete the survey and then read the instructions for interpreting your score. Now, is there a particular area of health you'd like to turn around? Once you've identified the health behavior you most want to change, how do you begin? Let's look at the personal choices that help people succeed in making behavior change.

Personal Choices

Changing your targeted behavior will require more than a quick decision to "just do it." Effective change is a seven-step process that starts with information.

Step 1: Get Informed

You've identified a goal—"Get fit!"—but how much do you really know about the behavior you want to change? For instance, what are the components of fitness, what are the benefits, how is it achieved, and how is it measured? If you're going to set a fitness goal and create a plan for reaching it, you need to be able to answer these questions. So your first step is to do some homework. The information in this text, together with the **Get Connected** links at the end of each chapter, are good resources for researching your health concerns. You can also find information at your campus health services center, from your health-care provider, and from reputable professional journals. Answering specific questions will, among other things, help you identify a more effective behavior-change goal—that is, a SMART goal.

Step 2: Set a SMART Goal

If you don't know precisely where you're going, how will you know when you've arrived? Experts in business, health care, and personal development agree that goals are more likely to be achieved when you put them in writing, following the acronym SMART. SMART stands for the five qualities of an effective goal:[26]

- **Specific.** When writing your goal, include specific details. For example, "I want to get more sleep" is not a SMART goal. How many hours of sleep do you want to get each night?
- **Measurable.** Include objective criteria for evaluating your success. What data would make it clear to anyone that you have succeeded? For instance, "By the end of this semester, I'll have paid off my credit card debt."
- **Attainable.** Does the research you did earlier convince you that you can achieve your goal? If not, you probably won't. So make sure your goal is attainable. For instance, for most people who are overweight, it's sensible to aim to lose about ½–1 pound of body weight per week; however, 3 pounds a week is not attainable without putting your health at risk.
- **Relevant.** Don't borrow somebody else's health goal! Make sure that the goal you've written feels right for you. For instance, let's say you can't even climb a flight of stairs without feeling winded. You've been looking for some inspiration to get fit when a friend invites you to join him in training for a local marathon. Your friend has been running cross-country since middle school. The goal is relevant for him, but it's not SMART for you.
- **Time based.** A SMART goal has a time frame. For instance: "For the next six months, each time I weigh myself—on the 15th and the 30th of each month—I'll have lost at least one pound. In five months' time, by December 30th, I'll have lost 10 pounds."

> **shaping** A behavior-change technique based on breaking broad goals into more manageable steps.
>
> **self-efficacy** The conviction that you can successfully execute the behavior required to make the change you desire.

The National Institutes of Health also advises that your goal be *forgiving*.[27] That is, it should allow for the occasional intervention of unforeseen events. A goal of walking for 30 minutes a day, 5 days a week, is forgiving. A goal of walking for 30 minutes a day, every day, is not.

Step 3: Make a Plan

A SMART goal is like a guiding vision, but to make it happen, you need an action plan, and that means you need to break down your goal into day-to-day actions that will enable you to achieve it. In doing this, it helps to use a technique called **shaping**, which involves breaking a big goal into a series of smaller, measurable steps. If you'd like

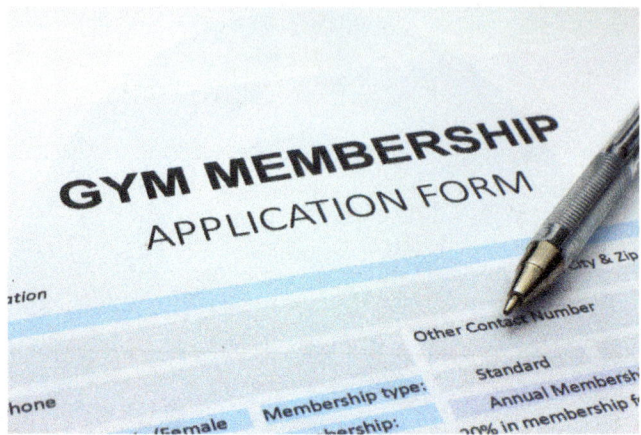

Set a goal that is relevant and attainable, and you're more likely to reach it.

to eventually run a 10K, for instance, set yourself a goal of a shorter distance at first and then gradually increase your distance a little each week.

When shaping, it can be helpful to ask yourself questions like who? what? when? where? why? how? and how long? Here is an example:

- On Sunday morning, I'll weigh myself and write down my weight.
- Monday to Friday, whenever I'm thirsty, I'll have diet soda or water instead of a regular soft drink or juice.
- Also, after my last class on M/W/F, I'll walk to the fitness center. I'll do at least 15 minutes on the stationary bike and 15 minutes on the treadmill. On Saturday morning, I'll take the drop-in power yoga class.
- On Sunday morning, I'll weigh myself again. If I've lost 1 pound or more, I'll continue with my plan for another week. And I'll call my best friend to celebrate! If I haven't, I'll increase my exercise next week to 20 minutes per machine.

Step 4: Identify Barriers and How You'll Overcome Them

Barriers are factors that stand in the way of successful change. One of the most important psychological barriers to change is a characteristic known as low self-efficacy. Psychologist Albert Bandura of Stanford University was the first to recognize the importance of self-efficacy in behavior change. In a 1977 paper, he described **self-efficacy** as the conviction that you can successfully execute the behavior required to make the change you desire.[28] Bandura explained that your expectations of personal efficacy determine whether you'll initiate a behavior change process, how much effort you'll expend, and how long you'll sustain it in the face of obstacles. If you believe in your ability to get in better shape, for example, you'll keep exercising, even if a few workouts leave you tired or sore. This persistence will further reinforce your sense of efficacy. In contrast, if you have low self-efficacy, you may give up quickly and, as a result, you're likely to retain your self-defeating expectations.

PRACTICAL Strategies

Building Self-Efficacy

Try these strategies to build self-efficacy:[1]

- **Start small and repeat.** If a behavior change seems beyond your ability, set a modest goal you're confident you can achieve. For instance, maybe you'd love to lose 20 pounds but are confident only that you can lose 2. Follow your weight-loss program for as long as it takes to lose those 2 pounds and then celebrate your success. Then set a new goal—another 2 pounds? 3? Repeated accomplishment of small goals helps build self-efficacy.
- **Model others who have made the same change.** Bandura points out that our expectations are often derived from vicarious experiences. That is, seeing others perform challenging activities successfully helps us realize that we can improve if we behave in the same way. If you'd like to eat less junk food, for example, observe and copy the habits of a health-conscious friend.
- **Seek constructive feedback.** When someone in authority—a health instructor, physician, personal trainer, etc.—informs you that you have everything it takes to make a change, that affirmation alone can build your self-efficacy. But it's even more helpful to solicit the expert's feedback on your change process: What details of your actions might be undermining your efforts? Are there any gaps? What improvements would they suggest?
- **Engage in self-monitoring.** As you begin to achieve your small goals, find a way to record your progress. If you're trying to increase your sleep time, for instance, keep a log of exactly how many hours of sleep you get each night. Written evidence of improvement helps build your self-efficacy. Your record can also show you when it's time to shift your change plan into higher gear.

References: Bandura, A. (1977). Self-efficacy: Toward a unifying theory of behavior change. *Psychological Review 84*(2), 191–215.

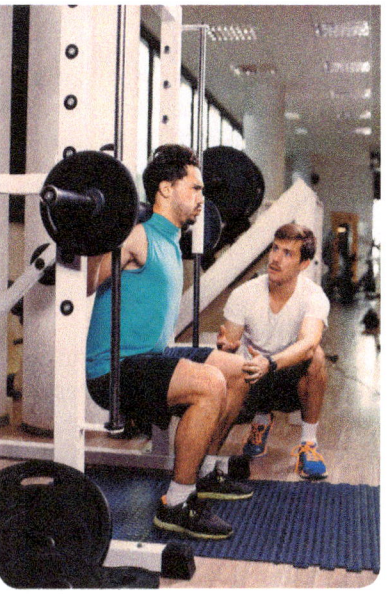

Your sense of self-efficacy is closely tied to your **locus of control,** a concept first developed by psychologist Julian B. Rotter in 1954.[29] If you have an *internal* locus of control, you are more likely to believe that you are the master of your own destiny. When a barrier presents itself, you'll look for ways to overcome it. If you have an *external* locus of control, you are more likely to believe that events are out of your hands—that there's little you can do to overcome barriers.

Barriers can also emerge from your social environment. Let's say you want to lose weight, but your roommate is constantly baking the most delectable treats—and asking you to try them. You might overcome this barrier by telling your roommate about your weight-loss plan and inviting him or her to create some low-calorie snacks. Self-advocacy is an essential—though sometimes uncomfortable—skill to practice in demonstrating self-efficacy.

Aspects of your physical environment can act as barriers, too. But with some ingenuity, you can often find ways to overcome them. For example, if you struggle with binge eating, make sure you go through your apartment or dorm room and get rid of any junk foods.

The significant disparity in access to quality health services in the United States is a barrier to change for millions of Americans. Fortunately, as a college student, you may have access to low-cost health services and programs.

People with a high level of self-efficacy may be able to overcome most barriers to behavior change. You can increase your own sense of self-efficacy by using the techniques identified in the accompanying **Practical Strategies** box.

Step 5: Recruit Some Support

According to the ecological models of behavior change, your plan for change will be more likely to succeed if you have different levels of support. Start with your family members and friends. With whom do you feel comfortable sharing your plans for change? Give your support group members specific instructions about how they can help, and when your motivation wanes, call

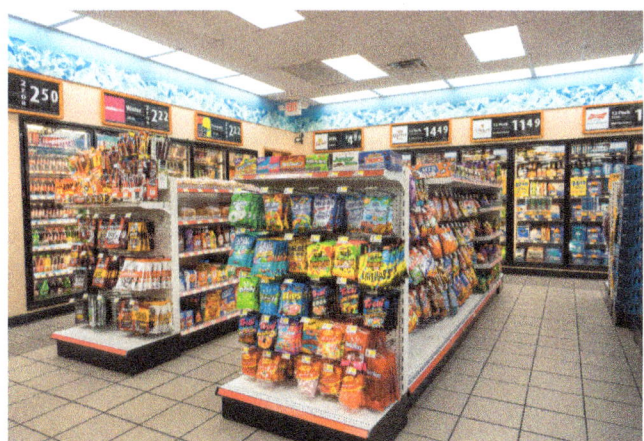

Factors in your environment can be barriers to behavior change.

> **locus of control** A person's belief about where the center of power lies in his or her life; it can be external or internal.

on them to cheer you on. If family members and friends can't provide the consistent support you need, consider joining a campus or community self-help group.

Step 6: Promise Yourself Rewards

Rewards keep you motivated to sustain change. For example, you might promise yourself new clothing after you've reached a target weight goal. However, rewards don't have to be material objects. For instance, the natural "high" people often feel after physical exercise can be its own positive reinforcement.

End-goal rewards are important, but it's also important to reward yourself for small steps along the way. For instance, if you enroll in an aerobics class that meets Tuesdays and Thursdays, you might promise yourself that, in the weeks that you attend both sessions, you'll reward yourself with an act of "self-kindness," such as a call to a loved one.[27]

Step 7: Commit in Writing

Many people find it helps to write out and sign their name at the bottom of a behavior-change contract—indicating that they've made a pact with themselves that they intend to keep. So if you're ready to take the plunge, turn to the **Choosing to Change Worksheet** on page 21 for a form you can use. Notice that the steps in this contract follow those just discussed. Make copies of your behavior-change contract and place them anywhere you want support.

relapse A return to the previous state or pattern of behavior.

cue control A behavior-change technique in which the individual learns to change the stimuli that provoked the lapse.

counter-conditioning A behavior-change technique in which the individual learns to substitute a healthful or neutral behavior for an unwanted behavior triggered by a cue beyond his or her control.

advocacy Working independently or with others to directly improve aspects of the social or physical environment or to change policies or legislation.

Preventing Relapse

When people attempt to change a long-term behavior, a lapse—a temporary "slip" back to the previous behavior—is highly likely. For instance, a person trying to quit smoking who takes a drag on a friend's cigarette is experiencing a lapse. Unfortunately, a **relapse**, a complete return to the previous pattern of behavior, is also common. For example, according to the American Cancer Society, a majority of the people who successfully quit smoking have tried to quit—and relapsed—several times before.[30]

Preventing a relapse is easy if you can prevent a lapse in the first place! Cue control and counter-conditioning are two strategies for preventing lapses.

With **cue control,** you learn to change the stimuli that provoke your unwanted behavior. For example, you may recognize that you're more likely to overeat while you're watching television, or whenever your mom leaves her latest batch of homemade cookies on the kitchen counter, or when you're around a certain friend. With cue control, you could change the behavior by:[27]

- Separating the behavior from the cue (don't eat while watching television)
- Taking action to avoid or eliminate the cue (ask your mom to put her cookies in a closed container out of sight)
- Changing the environment or other circumstances surrounding the cue (plan to meet your friend in a nonfood setting)

Counter-conditioning is a technique in which you learn to substitute a healthful or neutral behavior for an unwanted behavior when it's triggered by a cue beyond your control. One of the simplest examples is the urge to have something in their mouths that strikes most smokers repeatedly in the first few weeks after they quit. With counter-conditioning, the person replaces cigarette smoking with chewing on something, whether gum, licorice, or even a toothpick. Counter-conditioning can help you cope with peer pressure as well. Write out and memorize a short, assertive statement such as, "No thanks, I've had enough." Then, in situations in which you'd usually say, "Okay," substitute your assertion.

Campus and Community Advocacy

When a barrier to change exists in your social or physical environment or results from poor health services or policy-making, your best chance for change might just be in **advocacy**—that is, working independently or with others to directly improve aspects of your world. You may think of advocacy as lobbying to legislators, and while that's one form, there are many others available to you in your role as a college student, including the following:

- Get better informed about the issue, especially what's happening on campus and within your community.
- Meet with campus faculty or staff members or community leaders to learn more about the issue and share your concerns.
- Use social networking to heighten awareness of the issue among your contacts.
- Write about the issue for campus and community news services.
- Speak about the issue at campus and community gatherings.
- Organize a letter-writing campaign to your dean of students or other decision makers.
- Join a campus organization that is already working on the issue. If none exists, found an organization of your own.

Concluding many chapters of this text, you'll find suggestions for advocacy specific to the topics addressed in that chapter, from nutrition to discrimination to climate change. These suggestions may or may not be appropriate for your campus. Still, we hope they'll provide you with examples of strategies that have worked for others and some inspiration for advocacy of your own.

LO 1.7 QUICK CHECK

After writing down your SMART goal, the next step in successful behavior change is to

a. develop a plan of day-to-day actions that will enable you to achieve your goal.
b. develop an external locus of control that will enable you to advocate on campus and in your community.
c. reward yourself.
d. get out there and make it happen!

▶▶ Watch videos of real students discussing their health at **Mastering**Health™

SELF-ASSESSMENT
How Healthy Is Your Current Lifestyle?

Directions: Answer the following questions regarding each dimension of health. Indicate how often you think the statements describe you using the scale below.

1 = Rarely, if ever
2 = Sometimes
3 = Most of the time
4 = Always

Physical health:

1. I accumulate at least 150 minutes (2 hours and 30 minutes) of moderate-intensity aerobic activity or 75 minutes (1 hour and 15 minutes) of vigorous-intensity aerobic activity every week or an equivalent mix of moderate- and vigorous-intensity aerobic activity.   1 2 3 4
2. I include muscle-strengthening activities on 2 or more days a week that work all major muscle groups (legs, hips, back, abdomen, chest, shoulders, and arms).   1 2 3 4
3. I maintain a healthy body weight, which includes evaluating my waist circumference periodically to ensure that fat is not accumulating around my waist.   1 2 3 4
4. I consume five or more servings of fruits and vegetables each day. In particular, I select from all five vegetable subgroups—dark green, orange, legumes, starchy vegetables, and other vegetables—several times a week.   1 2 3 4
5. To limit my intake of less healthful fats and increase my intake of beneficial fats, I eat fish at least twice a week and at least half of my remaining meals are vegetarian.   1 2 3 4
6. I avoid smoking cigarettes.   1 2 3 4
7. If I choose to drink alcohol, I do so in moderation.   1 2 3 4
8. I have regular check-ups and age-appropriate health screenings completed by health care providers to identify potential health problems early.   1 2 3 4
9. I regularly take steps to avoid injuries (e.g., wearing a safety belt while riding in a car, wearing a helmet while riding a bike).   1 2 3 4
10. I get 7–9 hours of sleep most nights.   1 2 3 4

1 = Rarely, if ever
2 = Sometimes
3 = Most of the time
4 = Always

Social health:

11. When I meet people, I feel good about the impression I make on them.   1 2 3 4
12. I am open, honest, and get along well with other people.   1 2 3 4
13. I participate in a wide variety of social activities and enjoy being with people who are different from me.   1 2 3 4
14. I try to be a "better person" and work on behaviors that have caused problems in my interactions with others.   1 2 3 4
15. I get along well with the members of my family.   1 2 3 4
16. I am a good listener.   1 2 3 4
17. I am open and accessible to a loving and responsible relationship.   1 2 3 4
18. I have someone I can talk to about my private feelings.   1 2 3 4
19. I consider the feelings of others and do not act in hurtful or selfish ways.   1 2 3 4
20. I consider how what I say might be perceived by others before I speak.   1 2 3 4

Emotional health:

21. I find it easy to laugh about things that happen in my life.   1 2 3 4
22. I avoid using alcohol as a means of helping me forget my problems.   1 2 3 4
23. I can express my feelings without feeling silly.   1 2 3 4
24. When I am angry, I try to let others know in nonconfrontational and nonhurtful ways.   1 2 3 4
25. I am not a chronic worrier and do not tend to be suspicious of others.   1 2 3 4
26. I recognize when I am stressed and take steps to relax through exercise, quiet time, or other activities.   1 2 3 4
27. I feel good about myself and believe others like me for who I am.   1 2 3 4
28. When I am upset, I talk to others and actively try to work through my problems.   1 2 3 4
29. I am flexible and adapt or adjust to change in a positive way.   1 2 3 4
30. My friends regard me as a stable, emotionally well-adjusted person.   1 2 3 4

Environmental health:

31. I am concerned about environmental pollution and actively try to preserve and protect natural resources.   1 2 3 4
32. I report people who intentionally hurt the environment.   1 2 3 4
33. I recycle my garbage.   1 2 3 4
34. I reuse plastic and paper bags and tin foil.   1 2 3 4
35. I vote for pro-environment candidates in elections.   1 2 3 4
36. I write my elected leaders about environmental concerns.   1 2 3 4
37. I consider the amount of packing covering a product when I buy groceries.   1 2 3 4
38. I try to buy products that are recyclable.   1 2 3 4
39. I use both sides of the paper when taking class notes or doing assignments.   1 2 3 4
40. I try not to leave the faucet running too long when I brush my teeth, shave, or bathe.   1 2 3 4

Spiritual health:

41. I believe life is a precious gift that should be nurtured.   1 2 3 4
42. I take time to enjoy nature and the beauty around me.   1 2 3 4

		1	2	3	4
43.	I take time alone to think about what's important in life—who I am, what I value, where I fit in, and where I'm going.	1	2	3	4
44.	I have faith in a greater power, be it a God-like force, nature, or the connectedness of all living things.	1	2	3	4
45.	I engage in acts of caring and good will without expecting something in return.	1	2	3	4
46.	I feel sorrow for those who are suffering and try to help them through difficult times.	1	2	3	4
47.	I feel confident that I have touched the lives of others in a positive way.	1	2	3	4
48.	I work for peace in my interpersonal relationships, in my community, and in the world at large.	1	2	3	4
49.	I am content with who I am.	1	2	3	4
50.	I go for the gusto and experience life to the fullest.	1	2	3	4

1 = Rarely, if ever
2 = Sometimes
3 = Most of the time
4 = Always

Intellectual health:

51.	I think about consequences before I act.	1	2	3	4
52.	I learn from my mistakes and try to act differently the next time.	1	2	3	4
53.	I follow directions or recommended guidelines and act in ways likely to keep myself and others safe.	1	2	3	4
54.	I consider the alternatives before making decisions.	1	2	3	4
55.	I am alert and ready to respond to life's challenges in ways that reflect thought and sound judgment.	1	2	3	4
56.	I do not let my emotions get the better of me when making decisions.	1	2	3	4
57.	I actively learn all I can about products and services before making decisions.	1	2	3	4
58.	I manage my time well rather than let time manage me.	1	2	3	4
59.	My friends and family trust my judgment.	1	2	3	4
60.	I think about my self-talk (the things I tell myself) and then examine the evidence to see if my perception and feelings are sound.	1	2	3	4

Occupational health:

61.	I am happy with my career choice.	1	2	3	4
62.	I look forward to working in my career area.	1	2	3	4
63.	The job responsibilities/duties of my career choice are consistent with my values.	1	2	3	4
64.	The payoffs/advantages in my career choice are consistent with my values.	1	2	3	4
65.	I am happy with the balance between my work time and leisure time.	1	2	3	4
66.	I am happy with the amount of control I have in my work.	1	2	3	4
67.	My work gives me personal satisfaction and stimulation.	1	2	3	4
68.	I am happy with the professional/personal growth provided by my job.	1	2	3	4
69.	I feel my job allows me to make a difference in the world.	1	2	3	4
70.	My job contributes positively to my overall well-being.	1	2	3	4

Personal checklist:

Now total your scores in each of the health dimensions and compare them to the ideal scores. Which areas do you need to work on?

	Ideal Score	Your Score
Physical health	40	_____
Social health	40	_____
Emotional health	40	_____
Environmental health	40	_____
Spiritual health	40	_____
Intellectual health	40	_____
Occupational health	40	_____

WHAT YOUR SCORES MEAN

Scores of 35–40 points: Excellent. Your answers show that you are aware of the importance of this area to your health. More important, you are putting your knowledge to work for you by practicing good health habits. As long as you continue to do so, this area should not pose a serious health risk. It's likely that you are setting an example for your family and friends to follow. Although you reported a very high score on this part of the assessment, you may want to consider areas where your scores could be improved.

Scores of 30–34 points: Your health practices in this area are good, but there is room for improvement. Look again at the items you answered that scored one or two points. What changes could you make to improve your score? Even a small change in behavior can often help you achieve better health.

Scores of 20–29 points: Your health practices need improvement. Find information on how you could change these behaviors. Perhaps you need help deciding how to make the changes you desire. Assistance is available in this book, from your professor, and from resources on your campus.

Scores of 19 and lower: Your health practices need serious improvement and you may be taking unnecessary risks with your health. Perhaps you are not aware of the risks and what to do about them. In the textbook you will find the information you need to help improve your scores and your health.

To complete this Self-Assessment online, visit **Mastering**Health™

Source: Adapted and modified from *Healthstyle: A Self-Test*, by USDHHS Publication Number (PHS) 8150155.

Choosing to **Change** Worksheet

To complete this worksheet online, visit MasteringHealth™

The **Choosing to Change Worksheets** guide you on how to implement your behavior-change plans based on the stages of change identified by the transtheoretical model.

Stages of Behavior Change:

Precontemplation: I do not intend to make a change in the next six months.

Contemplation: I might make a change in the next six months.

Preparation: I am prepared to make a change in the next month.

Action: I have been making a change for less than six months.

Maintenance: I have been maintaining a change for more than six months.

After you have completed the **Self-Assessment** in this chapter, consider what stage of change you are in for each of the categories listed. Remember, it is common to be at various stages of change for different behaviors. Then, select one behavior in which you are at either the contemplation or preparation stage that you would like to target for change over the next few months. Next, fill out the **Behavior-Change Contract** below. Make sure you sign it and either display it where you'll see it often or discuss it with your health instructor as part of your work toward your long-term goal.

Behavior-Change Contract

My behavior change: _____

1. Three important short-term benefits I've discovered from my research about my behavior change are:

    1. _____
    2. _____
    3. _____

2. My SMART goal for this behavior change is:

    _____
    _____

3. Keeping my current stage of behavior change in mind, these short-term goals and rewards will make my SMART goal more attainable:

Short-term goal	Target date	Reward
Short-term goal	Target date	Reward
Short-term goal	Target date	Reward

    Barriers I anticipate to making this behavior change are:

    _____
    _____

4. The strategies I will use to overcome these barriers are:

    _____
    _____

5. Resources I will use to help me change this behavior include:
   - a friend, partner, or relative: _____
   - a school-based resource: _____
   - a health-care resource: _____
   - a community-based resource: _____
   - a book or reputable website: _____

6. When I achieve the long-term behavior change described above, my reward will be:

   _____   _____
   Reward   Target date

   I intend to make the behavior change described above. I will use the strategies and rewards above to achieve the goals that will contribute to a healthy behavior change.

   Signed: _____

CHAPTER 1 STUDY PLAN

CHAPTER SUMMARY

LO 1.1
- For centuries, the term *health* was generally understood to mean the absence of disease, which is an alteration in the body's structure or biochemistry that causes its natural regulatory mechanisms to fail.
- In 1948, the World Health Organization recognized health as a state of physical, mental, and social well-being, not just the absence of disease.
- Our understanding of health now includes the concept of *wellness*, defined by the National Wellness Institute as an active process through which people become aware of, and make choices toward, a more successful existence.

LO 1.2
- Public health experts have identified a variety of dimensions of health appropriate for the populations they serve.
- In this textbook, we acknowledge seven dimensions of health: physical, intellectual, psychological, spiritual, social, environmental, and occupational.

LO 1.3
- Life expectancy in the United States is 78.8 years. Heart disease and cancer cause almost 47% of all deaths.
- The four behaviors responsible for most suffering and early death related to chronic disease in the United States are lack of physical activity, poor nutrition, tobacco use, and drinking too much alcohol.
- The U.S. Department of Health and Human Services (HHS) Healthy People initiative is a set of 10-year objectives for building a society in which all people live long, healthy lives. One of the HHS's key goals is to eliminate health disparities and increase access to and quality of health care among various populations.
- Among Americans aged 15–24, the leading causes of death are accidents, suicide, and homicide. Anxiety, depression, allergies and asthma, alcohol and tobacco use, and sexual health are all common health concerns faced by college students.
- Three significant global health problems are infection, especially the growth of drug-resistant strains of infectious microbes; undernourishment; and obesity and obesity-related chronic diseases.

LO 1.4
- Determinants of health are a broad range of biological, economic, and other factors that influence health.
- The six broad categories of determinants of health are biology and genetics, individual behaviors, social determinants, physical determinants, health services—including access to quality health care and health literacy—and policy-making.

LO 1.5
- Predisposing factors are influences that increase or decrease the likelihood that a person will decide to change a health-related behavior.

MasteringHealth™

Build your knowledge—and health!—in the Study Area of **MasteringHealth**™ with a variety of study tools.

- Enabling factors are skills, social contacts, or other resources that make it easier or more difficult to change.
- Positive reinforcing factors are encouragements or rewards that keep you going; negative reinforcers are barriers that arise as a result of trying to change.

LO 1.6
- The *transtheoretical model of behavior change* proposes six stages, from precontemplation, contemplation, and preparation, to action, maintenance, and termination, that a person progresses through before achieving sustained behavior change.
- The *health belief model* identifies four factors as instrumental in predicting health-related behavior change: perceive the existence of a threat, recognize the threat is severe, determine that the benefits of addressing the threat outweigh the costs of changing, and witness or experience one or more cues to action.
- Ecological models of behavior change acknowledge that creating a supportive environment is as important to achieving change as is an individual acquiring health information and developing new skills.

LO 1.7
- Seven steps for implementing a health-related behavior change include becoming informed, setting a SMART goal, breaking down your goal into a sequential action plan, identifying barriers to change and how you'll overcome them, recruiting support, promising yourself rewards, and committing in writing.
- To reduce risk of relapse, take inventory of the full ecological spectrum of factors that might trigger a relapse. Then identify strategies for coping, including cue control and counter-conditioning.
- Campus or community advocacy can be effective when a barrier to change exists in your social or physical environment or results from poor health services or policy-making.

GET CONNECTED

>> Visit the following websites for further information about the topics in this chapter:

- Centers for Disease Control and Prevention
  www.cdc.gov
- Go Ask Alice (answers to health questions, sponsored by Columbia University)
  http://goaskalice.columbia.edu
- U.S. Department of Health and Human Services' healthfinder.gov
  http://healthfinder.gov
- U.S. Department of Health and Human Services' Healthy People 2020
  www.healthypeople.gov

MOBILE TIPS!
Scan this QR code with your mobile device to access additional health tips. Or, via your mobile device, go to **http://chmobile.pearsoncmg.com** and choose by topic: health tips.

- Medline Plus
  www.nlm.nih.gov/medlineplus
- Mayo Clinic
  www.mayoclinic.org
- World Health Organization
  www.who.int/en
- Media Literacy Project
  www.medialiteracyproject.org

Website links are subject to change. To access updated web links, please visit MasteringHealth™

TEST YOUR KNOWLEDGE

LO 1.1
1. An appreciation of the capacity of people with a disability or chronic disease to make choices toward a more successful existence contributed to
   a. the concept of disease as a state of imbalance.
   b. the 1948 WHO definition of health.
   c. the development of the concept of wellness.
   d. the recognition of the importance of self-efficacy in behavior change.

LO 1.2
2. Which dimension of health is characterized by the quality of your interactions and relationships with other people?
   a. intellectual health
   b. psychological health
   c. spiritual health
   d. social health

LO 1.3
3. Which of the following statements about current health challenges is true?
   a. Heart disease and diabetes are responsible for almost half of all deaths in the United States.
   b. Among Americans aged 15–24, cancer is the leading cause of death.
   c. The rate of new infections from the human immunodeficiency virus (HIV) increased by 38% between 2001 and 2014.
   d. Worldwide, more people are undernourished than are obese.

4. The CDC recognizes several behaviors as being responsible for much of the suffering and early death related to chronic disease:
   a. lack of physical activity, overeating, and substance abuse.

b. lack of physical activity, poor nutrition, tobacco use, and excessive alcohol consumption.
c. failing to meet current physical activity guidelines, a high-fat diet, smoking, and alcohol consumption.
d. a high-fat, high-sugar diet, tobacco use, alcohol consumption, and driving without a seatbelt.

LO 1.4

5. Health literacy is an example of which type of health determinant?
   a. individual behaviors
   b. social determinants
   c. health services
   d. policy-making

LO 1.5

6. You're determined to get fit and have begun to walk from your apartment to campus daily. The fact that you live in a warm, sunny climate is an example of
   a. a predisposing factor for behavior change.
   b. an enabling factor for behavior change.
   c. a positive reinforcing factor for behavior change.
   d. a negative reinforcing factor for behavior change.

LO 1.6

7. In the transtheoretical model of behavior change, which stage indicates the period during which a person has modified the behavior in an observable way?
   a. precontemplation
   b. contemplation
   c. preparation
   d. action

8. Which of the following is a principle of ecological models of behavior change?
   a. The individual's belief that making a change will reduce a threat to his or her health is the primary factor in behavior change.
   b. Interventions at multiple levels—from individual to society—are most effective in making health-related behavior change.
   c. The individual must be able to admit the potential environmental consequences of changing a behavior.
   d. Individuals cannot succeed in making and maintaining behavior change unless all aspects of their environment are supportive of the change.

LO 1.7

9. Damian's strength-training program hits a snag when he pulls a muscle in his thigh. After a course of physical therapy, he resumes his program, modifying it as prescribed. Damian's behavior *best* exemplifies
   a. self-efficacy.
   b. a strong external locus of control.
   c. a forgiving SMART goal.
   d. counter-conditioning.

10. Relapse is
    a. less likely when the person learns to change the stimuli that typically provoke a lapse.
    b. almost always due to circumstances beyond the person's individual control.
    c. a temporary "slip" back to the previous behavior.
    d. uncommon.

WHAT DO YOU THINK?

LO 1.1

1. Willa has inherited a genetic defect that significantly increases her risk for the most serious form of skin cancer. It does not, however, cause any pain, rash, or other symptoms. Willa strictly limits her sun exposure; eats a nourishing diet; exercises regularly; does not use tobacco, alcohol, or illegal drugs; and sees her dermatologist every six months for skin checks. Does Willa have a disease? Where would you place Willa on the illness–wellness continuum (Figure 1.1), and why?

LO 1.2

2. Go online to map.feedingamerica.org to find a map of the United States indicating levels of food insecurity (lack of dependable access to food). Compare your state's rate of food insecurity to rates in other parts of the United States. Click on your state, find a breakdown of food security rates for your county, and compare your county's rate to that of counties nearby. How might food insecurity influence an individual's physical, intellectual, or other dimensions of health?

LO 1.5

3. Fernando has been walking nightly in his neighborhood to lose weight. Provide one example illustrating how each of the following types of factors might have influenced his initiating or maintaining his behavior change program: a positive predisposing factor, a negative predisposing factor, an enabling factor, a positive reinforcer, and a negative reinforcer.

LO 1.6

4. Because of a family history of obesity and diabetes, Grady is concerned about his own obesity, and he has scheduled an appointment with his physician to discuss strategies for weight loss. According to the transtheoretical model of behavior change, what stage of change is Grady in? Which of the four factors of the health belief model might be influencing Grady at this time?

LO 1.7

5. Trish currently eats no more than one serving of fruits and vegetables a day. She would like to increase her fruit and vegetable consumption so that, within one month, she has met the national guidelines of at least five servings a day. Write a SMART goal appropriate for Trish. Why is shaping important? How might she use shaping in her action plan?

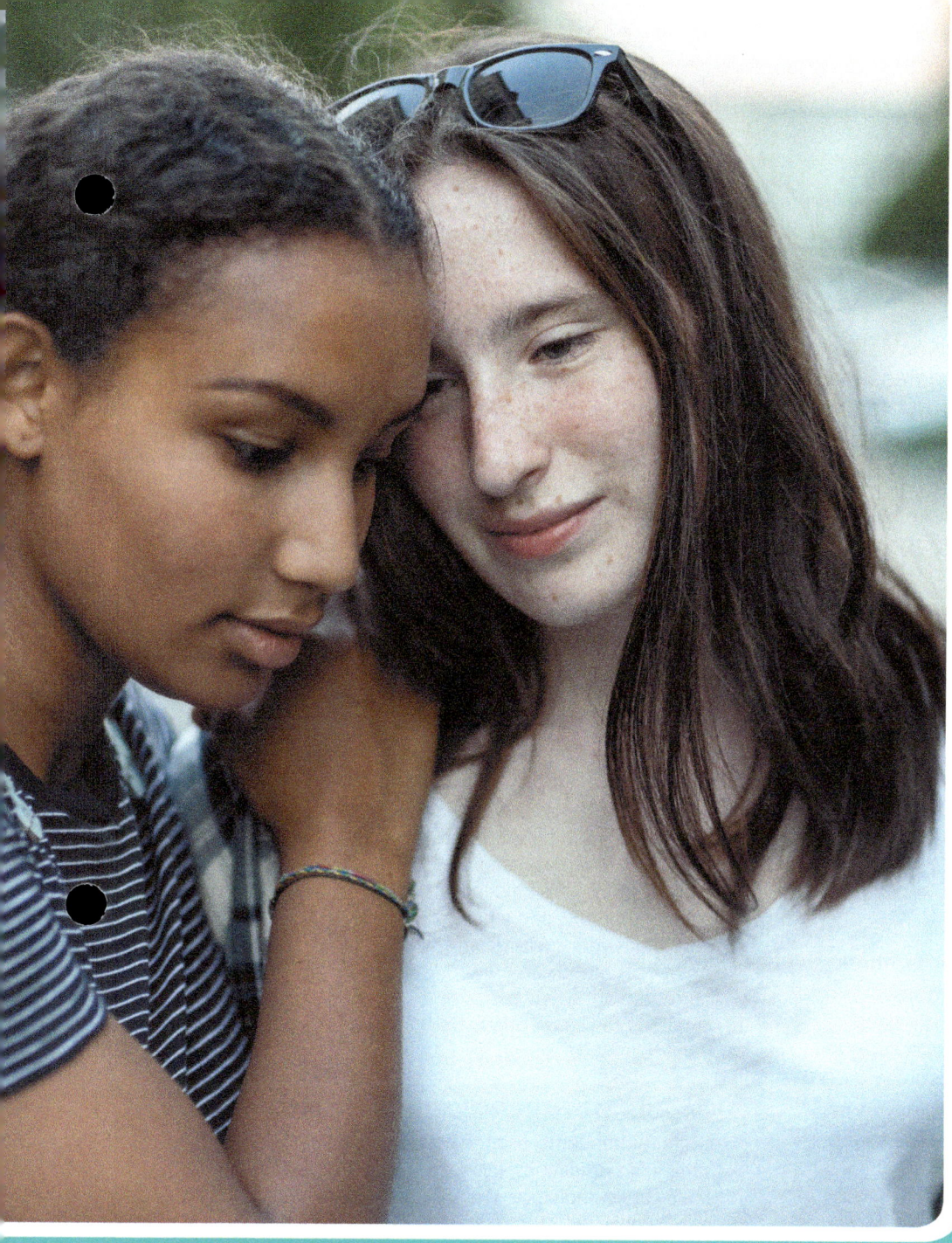

2

PSYCHOLOGICAL HEALTH

> About 58% of college students report having felt overwhelming anxiety at some time within the past year.[i]

> During the college years (late adolescence/young adulthood) the first symptoms of panic disorder, bipolar disorder, and obsessive-compulsive disorder may begin to appear.[ii]

> More than 1 in 10 college students report having been recently diagnosed or treated for depression.[i]

> The second leading cause of death among 15- to 24-year-olds is suicide.[iii]

LEARNING OUTCOMES

LO 2.1 Identify two components and six facets of psychological health.

LO 2.2 Discuss a variety of factors that influence psychological health.

LO 2.3 Describe common psychological challenges and ways to address them.

LO 2.4 List reasons for the high prevalence of mental disorders in the United States.

LO 2.5 Discuss the characteristics, possible causes, and treatments of mood disorders.

LO 2.6 Discuss the characteristics, possible causes, and treatments of anxiety disorders.

LO 2.7 Discuss the characteristics, possible causes, and treatments of other disorders.

LO 2.8 Define non-suicidal self-injury and discuss suicide warning signs and prevention strategies.

LO 2.9 Describe different options for the treatment of mental disorders.

LO 2.10 Identify strategies for improving your psychological health and for helping a friend.

Look at a brochure

advertising any college in the country, and you'll find photos of happy students enjoying their studies and having fun. But as you know, real life for college students is more complicated than such images suggest. When worry, anger, or loneliness arises, good psychological health can help you maintain your balance and resolve the challenge effectively.

So what does it mean to have "good" psychological health? How do you develop it? We discuss these questions in this chapter.

What Is Psychological Health?

LO 2.1 Identify two components and six facets of psychological health.

The field of psychology emerged in the late 19th century, when German and American scientists began conducting experiments to try to discover a physical basis for mental disorders. At the same time, the Austrian neurologist Sigmund Freud began exploring the role of past traumas in prompting unconscious conflicts that lead to mental disorders. But decades passed before researchers began to study the question of what constitutes psychological health. Here, we explore a few of the key concepts such work has revealed.

Components of Psychological Health

At its most basic, **psychological health** can be defined as the dimension of health and wellness that encompasses both mental and emotional components. **Mental health** can be described as the "thinking" component of psychological health—your ability to perceive reality accurately and respond to its challenges rationally and effectively. **Emotional health** refers to the "feeling" component of psychological health—how you react emotionally to the ups and downs of life. People with good emotional health are able to "roll with the punches" and keep less happy times in perspective.

Mental and emotional health affect other dimensions of health. Your physical health—for example, your breathing, heart rate, and immune response—is influenced by your thoughts and emotions. So is your social health: An upbeat mood can draw others to you, whereas stormy emotions can cause others to disengage.

> **psychological health** A broad dimension of health and wellness that encompasses both metal and emotional health.
>
> **mental health** The "thinking" component of psychological health that allows you to perceive reality accurately and respond rationally and effectively.
>
> **emotional health** The "feeling" component of psychological health that influences your interpretation of and response to events.
>
> **self-acceptance** A sense of positive and realistic self-regard, which results in elevated levels of self-confidence and self-respect.
>
> **intimacy** A close relationship with another person.

Facets of Psychological Health

One tool frequently used to assess psychological health in a variety of populations, including college students, is the Ryff Scales of Psychological Well-Being. Developed by psychologist Carol D. Ryff, the tool identifies six key facets of psychological health **(Figure 2.1)**[1].

Self-Acceptance

Ryff states that the characteristic most common among psychologically healthy people is **self-acceptance** (also called *self-esteem*): having a positive regard for oneself. Self-accepting people tend to respond effectively to challenges, have optimistic outlooks, and even enjoy better physical health.[2] They are realistic, acknowledging their positive and negative qualities. They focus on what they can control and accept what they cannot. Self-esteem can be improved. For tips on doing so, see the **Practical Strategies** box on page 27.

Positive Relations with Others

Psychologically healthy people have empathy and affection for all human beings and are consequently concerned about their welfare. Moreover, they are capable of **intimacy**—that

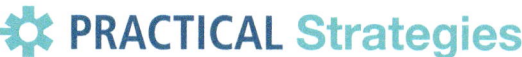

Building Self-Esteem

- **Listen to yourself.** What do you really want, need, and value? If you want others to listen to you, you need to understand and respect your own thoughts and feelings first.
- **Stretch your abilities.** Decide to learn something new, whether it's a school subject that seems intimidating or a sport you've never tried. Give yourself time to learn your new skill piece by piece and then watch your talents grow.
- **Tackle your "to do" list.** Think about tasks you've been putting off, like calling a relative with whom you haven't spoken for a while or cleaning out your closet. Get a couple of them done each week. You'll be reminded of how much you can accomplish and feel less distracted by loose ends.
- **Pat yourself on the back.** Notice when something you've done turns out well and take a moment to congratulate yourself.
- **Schedule some fun.** In your drive to finish your "to do" list, make sure to leave time in your schedule for fun. Don't wait for others to invite you to a party or a film—invite them first. If money is tight, suggest hitting the bike paths or hiking trails and get the added feel-good benefit of exercise.
- **Serve others.** There is no simpler, or more generous, way to build self-esteem than by doing something nice for someone else. You'll both benefit.

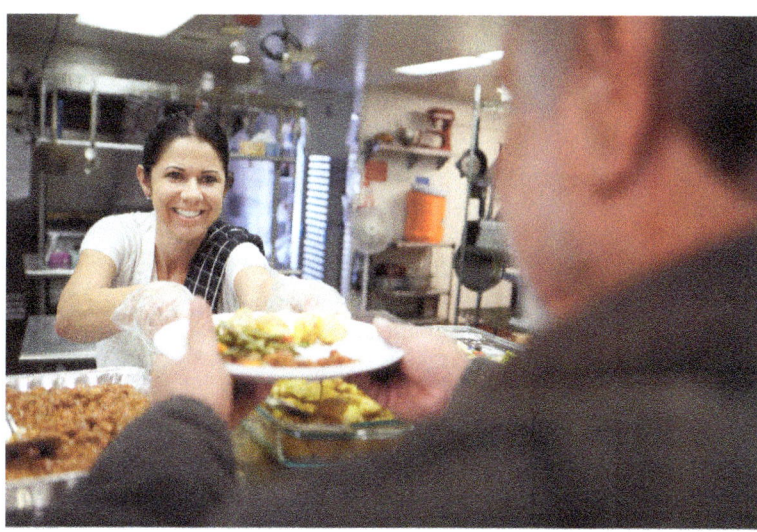

Participating in volunteer activities is a great way to boost **self-esteem.**

is, maintaining close relationships with family members, romantic partners, and/or friends.

Autonomy

Autonomy is your capacity to make informed, uncoerced decisions and to regulate your behavior internally. Autonomous people tend to base their decisions on their own judgments and values. They are also likely to take responsibility for the results of their actions. Autonomy does not devalue the opinions of others. It simply keeps them in perspective.

Autonomy is usually expressed in **assertiveness,** or making your decisions clear to others. Unlike anger or aggression, assertiveness means you express yourself calmly and clearly in ways that respect yourself and others.

autonomy The capacity to make informed, uncoerced decisions.

assertiveness The ability to clearly express your needs and wants to others in an appropriate way.

environmental mastery The ability to choose or create environments that suit you.

Environmental Mastery

Your chemistry instructor is a bore. What do you do? **Environmental mastery** is the ability to choose or create environments that suit you. Sometimes, environmental

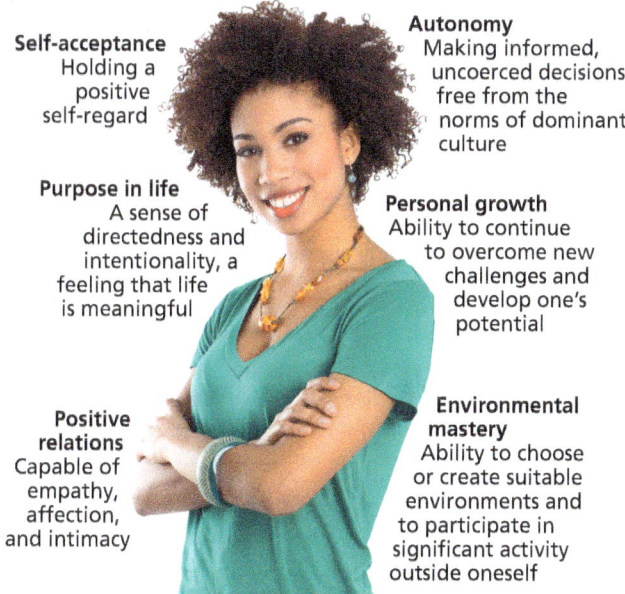

FIGURE 2.1 **Ryff's Facets of Psychological Health.** Each of these characteristics is a hallmark of psychological health.

mastery requires you to change your thoughts about a situation; for instance, you might recognize that you're not all that happy with your instructor, but you accept that switching out of the course wouldn't be worth the stress and instead, you use other resources to succeed.

Purpose in Life

Because you're in college, you probably don't feel that you're wandering aimlessly through life. But are your choices—in classes, relationships, and other aspects of your life—aligned with a larger purpose, one you could readily articulate? People who clearly comprehend their life's purpose and take actions to achieve that purpose feel productive—they feel as though they are actively creating their lives.

Personal Growth

Peak psychological health requires that you continue to grow and expand as a person, opening yourself to new experiences that challenge how you think about yourself and the world. Rather than settle for a fixed state in which all your problems are solved, you accept a certain level of anxiety as you move outside your comfort zone to accept challenges and develop your full potential.

Maslow's Hierarchy of Needs

Humanistic psychologist Abraham Maslow began publishing his ideas about positive psychological health in the 1940s. Maslow proposed that a key factor in achieving psychological health is our drive to meet our needs.[3] That is, people experience increased levels of psychological health as they meet and master ever-higher levels of innate needs via successful interactions with their environment. Maslow modeled this *hierarchy of needs* as a pyramid **(Figure 2.2)**.

The base of Maslow's pyramid represents our physiological needs (for air, food, water, shelter, etc.). If you've ever been truly hungry or shivered uncontrollably from prolonged exposure to the cold, then you know that your survival needs for food or warmth can become all-consuming, driving you to meet those needs to the exclusion of almost anything else. Your success or failure will then determine whether you progress to perceive—and work on meeting—the next level of needs. This means, of course, that the struggle to put food on the table and pay the rent could block individuals from experiencing peak psychological health.

On the other hand, once your physiological needs are reliably and consistently met, you will experience an inner drive to meet progressively less urgent needs. For instance, whereas a partner in an abusive relationship may be driven to meet the need for safety, those already in loving relationships can work toward self-esteem.

When you finally master the four lower levels, you recognize and work toward fulfilling your need for **self-actualization**—that is, your need to become everything you're capable of becoming, to realize your "full humanness." In later work, Maslow added one higher goal—selfless actualization, or self-transcendence, a "going beyond oneself" to work toward a values-driven goal in service to others or to an ideal.[4]

The Role of Emotional Intelligence

In 1985, Wayne Leon Payne published the first study of **emotional intelligence (EI),** which he defined as the ability to accurately sense, assess, and manage emotions.[5] In the decades since then, psychologists have come to characterize EI as encompassing four key abilities:[6]

- Perceive and express emotion
- Incorporate emotion in thought
- Understand and reason with emotion
- Regulate emotion in oneself and others

People with higher levels of EI tend to be both self-aware and socially adept. They conduct themselves in a balanced way, neither denying their emotions nor being overwhelmed by them. They also tend to be more productive, less prone to stress, and happier overall than those with lower EI.[7]

Whereas some propose that EI is an inborn trait, others claim that it is a skill anyone can develop by consciously recognizing and naming emotions when you feel them, thinking about other people's feelings and motivations in specific situations, and accepting your emotions without allowing them to control you.

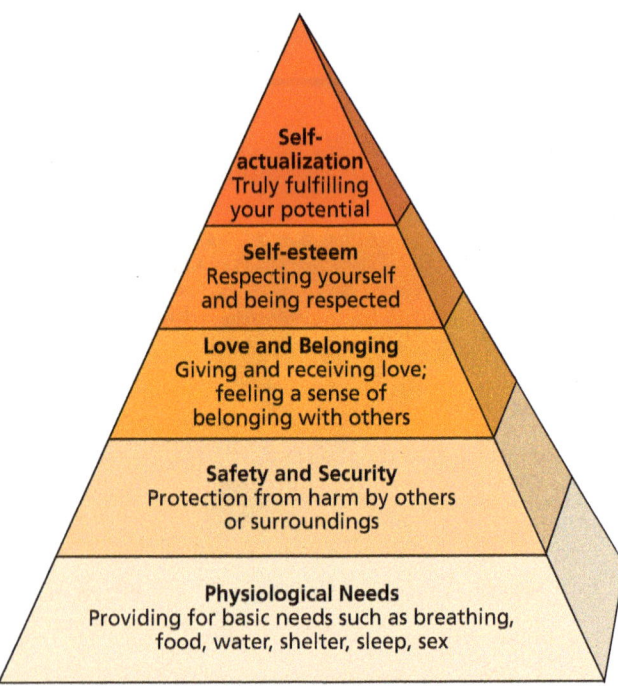

FIGURE 2.2 Maslow's Hierarchy of Needs Pyramid. Basic, physiological needs appear at the base of the pyramid. As you move upward, you address needs that are less urgent to satisfy, developing greater psychological health, until you realize self-actualization.

Source: Maslow, Abraham H.; Frager, Robert D.; Fadiman, James, *Motivation and Personality*, 3rd ed., ©1987. Adapted and electronically reproduced by permission of Pearson Education, Inc., Upper Saddle River, New Jersey.

self-actualization The pinnacle of Maslow's hierarchy of needs, which indicates truly fulfilling your potential.

emotional intelligence (EI) The capacity to perceive, express, and reason accurately with emotion and emotional information.

The Value of Optimism

Optimism is the psychological tendency to interpret life's events positively. Psychologist Martin Seligman explains that optimistic people embrace the belief that positive outcomes are more probable than negative ones. People with optimistic outlooks are more likely to view problems as challenges within their power to solve; thus, they are motivated to take action. On the other hand, they are unlikely to see bad events as long-lasting or as capable of damaging other aspects of their lives.[8] In contrast, pessimists tend to believe that bad events will have long-lasting negative effects, undermining everything else they do, and are their own fault. They also give up easily and have higher rates of depression than optimists.

Optimism helps us in a broad range of situations. Optimists tend to exceed the predictions of aptitude tests and are more likely than pessimists to succeed academically.[8] Among college students, optimism has been found to be the best predictor of both psychological well-being and reduced levels of psychological distress.[9] Especially following traumatic stress, optimism is also a strong predictor of **resiliency**—the innate capacity to adapt to a changing environment.[10] It may even reduce pain. In one study, among subjects given a *placebo* (a substance with no active ingredients) for pain, optimists reported greater pain relief.[11] And optimism helps patients fighting serious disease maintain a positive outlook during treatment and avoid anxiety and depression.[12] Fortunately, you can learn to be more optimistic at any age.

> **optimism** The psychological tendency to have a positive interpretation of life's events.
>
> **resiliency** The innate capacity to experience success and satisfaction following trauma or other stressors.
>
> **social support** A sufficient quantity of relationships that provide emotional concern, help with appraisal, information, and even goods and services.

▶▶ How optimistic are you? Take Seligman's free "Happiness Quiz" at **www.pursuit-of-happiness.org/science-of-happiness/happiness-quiz/**.

LO 2.1 QUICK CHECK ✔

Katherine has difficulty expressing her feelings and "rolling with the punches" in her everyday life. These issues are examples of which component of psychological health?

a. spiritual
b. emotional
c. social
d. mental

Factors Affecting Psychological Health

LO 2.2 Discuss a variety of factors that influence psychological health.

What makes someone psychologically healthy? Recent genetic studies link variants of certain genes directly to specific "psychological resources," including optimism and self-esteem. But researchers acknowledge that these genes are just one factor affecting psychological resources, and that "there is plenty of room for environmental factors as well."[13]

Family History

Rejection. Abuse. Abandonment. Shaming. More than a century ago, Sigmund Freud recognized that experiences such as these during childhood could prompt unconscious conflicts that could result in adult mental disorders. Today, psychologists theorize that such experiences exert their effect by causing us to develop "early maladaptive" patterns that we then carry into adulthood.[14] As a result, we might become less successful in meeting our needs, mastering our environment, and learning the appropriate lessons for each stage of life.

In one study, the presence of such patterns among college students was shown to significantly impair their adjustment to college life. It reduced the students' academic success, their social and emotional adjustment, and their attachment to the institution in which they were enrolled.[14]

Social Support

Do you have friends you can count on if things ever got really tough? If so, then you have **social support.** A person with social support has a variety of relationships that can and do provide emotional concern, assistance with realistic appraisal of situations, information, and even goods and services if necessary. Social support can help by eliminating, changing, or helping you adjust to conditions that cause you distress. Just as social support is essential to good mental health, lack of early social support in extreme forms, like bullying, can be devastating. A recent study concluded that bullying by peers negatively affects the mental health of children later in life even more significantly than having been mistreated by adults.[15]

In a recent study of college students, social support was identified as a significant factor in improving the psychological adjustment of students to college life. Compared to students with higher levels of social support, students with lower levels of support were more likely to experience psychological health problems, including a six-fold risk of depression.[16]

The Role of Spiritual Health

Spiritual health contributes to psychological health by providing a sense of connection to a larger purpose coupled with a system of core values that provide direction and meaning in life. For many, that connection takes the form of religion.

> **❝** *In a recent study of college students, social support was identified as a significant factor in improving the psychological adjustment of students to college life.* **❞**

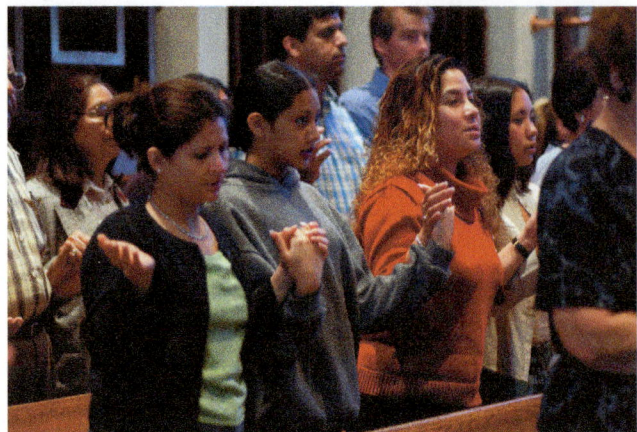

Religion can benefit psychological well-being.

Defining Religion

A **religion** is a system of beliefs and practices related to the existence of a transcendent (*otherworldly*) power or presence. Religious beliefs are typically expressed in acts of service and devotion, either through an organized group or independently.

In a 2014 survey, 76.5% of American adults said that they are affiliated with a particular religion. Here's the breakdown:[17]

- About 71% of respondents identify themselves as Christians.
- About 6% of respondents practice another religion.
- The remaining 23% of respondents identify themselves as atheist, *agnostic* (that is, they claim neither belief nor disbelief in a divine being), nothing in particular, or uncertain.

The statistics for religious affiliation for young adults are somewhat lower: 36% of Americans aged 18–24 say they have no religious affiliation. This is up over 10% in seven years.[17]

Benefits of Religion

A recent Gallup poll found that people who identify themselves as "very religious" have higher levels of well-being than people who describe themselves as only moderately religious or not religious at all.[18] Similarly, in a study of university students, participants who scored high on "religiousness"—adherence to religious values and practices in daily living—demonstrated higher-than-average levels of psychological well-being and lower levels of psychological distress.[9]

Defining Spirituality

Affiliation with an organized religion is just one expression of a broader approach to life commonly referred to as **spirituality.** The term is difficult to define, in part because spirituality is inclusive of just about everything. According to Brian Luke Seaward, a pioneer in the field of health psychology, spirituality is ageless and timeless; it knows no bounds and has no allegiances.[19] The World Health Organization defines spirituality as "that which is in total harmony with the perceptual and non-perceptual environment."[20] For many, spirituality is a lifelong quest for the answers to life's biggest questions.

Seaward suggests that spiritual well-being rests upon three main "pillars" **(Figure 2.3)**:[19]

- A strong personal value system
- Relationships, connectedness, and community
- A meaningful purpose in life

Let's take a closer look at each.

Personal Values. Your term paper is due tomorrow and you haven't even started it. Should you buy one from an online site, stay up all night writing, or go to your instructor's office empty-handed, apologize, and ask for an extension? A decision such as this forces you to reflect on our **values,** the internal guidelines you use to make decisions and evaluate the world around you. Building your spirituality starts with knowing your values and putting them into practice. Your answers to questions like these will help reveal your values:

> **religion** A system of beliefs and practices related to the existence of a transcendent power.
>
> **spirituality** A lifelong quest for the answers to life's biggest questions.
>
> **values** Internal guidelines used to make decisions and evaluate the world around you.

- What is important to me?
- What principles do I want to live by?
- What do I stand for?

Values evolve over the course of a lifetime. Many college students arrive on campus with values very similar to those of their parents. However, with new relationships and experiences, values often change. Throughout adult life, a wide array of influences and circumstances requires you to refine your values repeatedly.

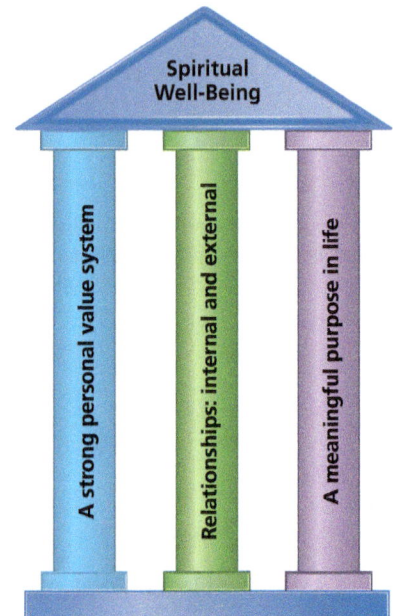

FIGURE 2.3 Seaward's Pillars of Spiritual Well-being. A strong sense of values, meaningful relationships, and a sense of purpose together support spiritual well-being.

Source: Adapted from *Health of the Human Spirit: Spiritual Dimensions for Personal Health,* 2nd ed., by B. L. Seaward, 2013, Burlington, MA: Jones & Bartlett Learning.

"Living your values" means reflecting them in the choices you make. For example, if you value the dignity of all human beings, you may be compelled to take action to reduce homelessness in your community. This might lead you to join a homeless outreach program.

Relationships. Your first relationship is with yourself. How comfortable are you with your own company? Through reflection, prayer, or meditation, you can begin to develop a relationship with your "higher self," whatever you conceive this to be.[19] This in turn can help you understand how you relate to everyone and everything in your environment: people, nature, institutions, and even concepts such as principles and laws.

> **altruism** The practice of helping and giving to others out of genuine concern for their well-being.
>
> **shyness** The feeling of apprehension or intimidation in social situations, especially in reaction to unfamiliar people or new environments.

Spiritual well-being also rests upon your connectedness with others. For a college student, peer relationships are very important. However, you may also find spiritual support in your relationships with parents and siblings, old friends, romantic partners, or a spouse and children. These loved ones can help you explore your spiritual questions.

As you work to clarify your internal and external relationships, avoid focusing on flaws. Instead, try starting from a place of gratitude. Adopting an "attitude of gratitude" can brighten your outlook on life. This, in turn, can lead to **altruism,** the practice of giving to others out of selfless concern for their well-being. Acts of altruism can also provide benefits to you. For example, helping others might help you develop perspective, build self-esteem, manage stress, sleep better, and even live longer.[21]

Purpose. Why do we exist? Throughout history, the world's great thinkers have provided various answers to this question, most of which focus on service to humanity. But of utmost importance to you is how you would personally answer this question. Is it important to you to conduct yourself in such a way that you know your life has made some difference? If so, given your unique values and gifts, how will you express your purpose?

Benefits of Spirituality

Studies of the benefits of spirituality on psychological health yield conflicting results. These differences may be due primarily to the differing ways studies define the terms associated with religion and spirituality.

Studies that differentiate between religion and spirituality have found that respondents who score high on "religiousness" experience significantly lower rates of psychological distress than average, whereas respondents who score high on "spirituality" tend to have higher rates of psychological distress. This finding might reflect the potential for people to turn to spirituality as a form of self-treatment for psychological challenges. It's also possible that some people scoring high on spirituality have turned away from organized religion and are thus experiencing psychological distress caused by a "crisis of faith."

Studies that consider "religion and spirituality" as a single variable consistently find it strongly associated with greater psychological health.[22] Moreover, this benefit is not correlated with the frequency of participation in religious activities. Specific effects include decreased anger, anxiety, depression, and substance abuse, as well as increased hope, optimism, sense of satisfaction with life, and inner peace.[22,23] Moreover, many studies have associated spirituality with increased physical health and self-healing.[24,25]

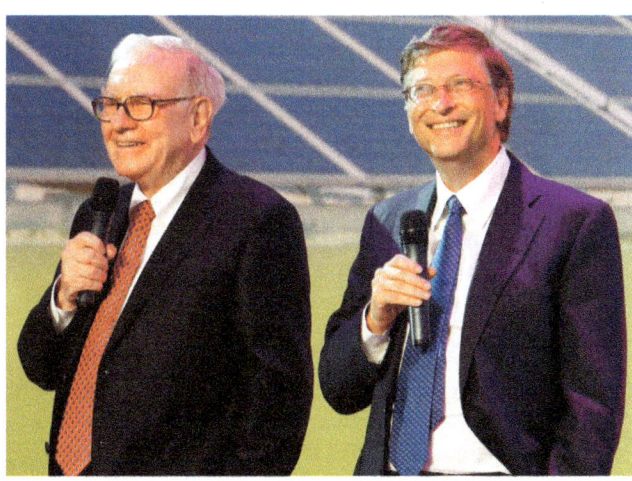

In 2010, investor Warren Buffet and Microsoft founder Bill Gates challenged fellow billionaires with "The Giving Pledge." As a result of these acts of **altruism**, 137 of the world's richest people have pledged at least half of their fortunes to charity.

LO 2.2 QUICK CHECK

Values, relationships, and purpose are three pillars of
a. religiosity.
b. spirituality.
c. safety and security.
d. social support.

Common Psychological Challenges

LO 2.3 Describe common psychological challenges and ways to address them.

There may come times when you face challenges to your psychological well-being, just as you do to your physical health. This vulnerability does not mean there is something "wrong" with you. These challenges are common, and some simple strategies can help you overcome them.

Shyness

Shyness is characterized by a feeling of apprehension or intimidation in social situations, especially in reaction to unfamiliar people or new environments. In a survey of more than 25,000 college students, 5% said that the statement "I am shy around others" was extremely like them.[26]

Unlike introverts, who prefer to keep to themselves, shy people actually want to participate in social interactions but have difficulty doing so because of self-consciousness, fear of embarrassment, or a negative self-image. Shyness can vary in severity from a slight feeling of discomfort to a pattern of avoidance that can be disabling. It can also lead to *social isolation,* a general withdrawal from or avoidance of social contact or communication.

A common belief is that people are "born" shy, and one variation of a gene that helps regulate brain chemistry has been linked to some cases of shyness.[27] But this "shy gene" doesn't work alone. Life experiences and other environmental factors contribute.

Mild forms of shyness can usually be overcome with practice. Try making small talk with someone you'll probably never see again, like a person in line at the airport. If that feels reasonably comfortable, then try it again with a person you barely know, like the clerk at the bagel shop. In short, ease out of your comfort zone slowly. In addition, cognitive-behavioral therapy, discussed later in this chapter, can help.

Loneliness

Recently, more than 60% of college students reported that they felt very lonely during the past year.[26] This could be due in part to recent trends in socializing among college students. In 1987, about 38% of college freshman spent at least 16 hours per week socializing, but in 2014, only 18% of freshmen spent that much time socializing.[28]

Loneliness is not a synonym for being alone. Many people are content to spend much of their time alone. In contrast, **loneliness** is a feeling of isolation from others, a sense that you don't have—and don't know how to make—meaningful connections. In fact, loneliness can be particularly acute when you're with others.

If you feel as though you need more meaningful connections in your life, you have many options:

- **Take advantage of the social and volunteer opportunities offered on campus or in your community.** Seek out groups that share your interests, such as in sports, politics, or theatre, where you are more likely to meet others who share your passions and values—and to form meaningful relationships.
- **Express yourself openly and honestly.** Sharing your true feelings with someone can foster a feeling of connection that mere socializing cannot.

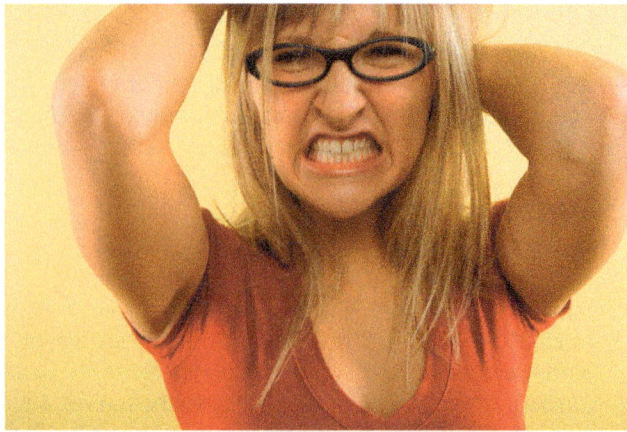

Although it may not feel like it, you can modify **anger**.

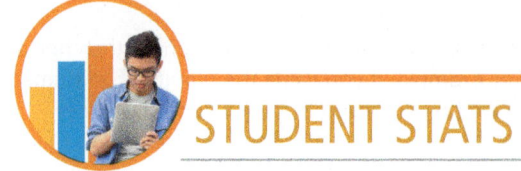

Psychological Health on Campus

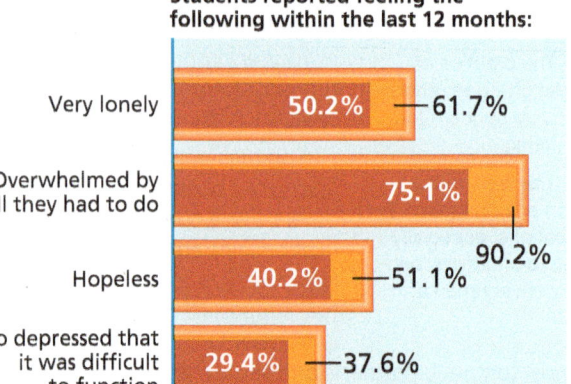

Students reported feeling the following within the last 12 months:

- Very lonely: Men 50.2%, Women 61.7%
- Overwhelmed by all they had to do: Men 75.1%, Women 90.2%
- Hopeless: Men 40.2%, Women 51.1%
- So depressed that it was difficult to function: Men 29.4%, Women 37.6%
- Overwhelming anxiety: Men 45.3%, Women 63.6%
- Overwhelming anger: Men 34.4%, Women 41.0%

Percent of students who reported feeling

Data from *ACHA-NCHA II: Undergraduate reference group executive summary, fall 2015,* by the American College Health Association, 2015.

- **Look into college counseling center resources.** Campus counseling centers usually offer a variety of resources that can help you build your social skills and develop more meaningful relationships.

Anger

Anger is a completely normal and even healthy human emotion. Recognizing factors that make you angry can help you understand your values and assert yourself. Expressing anger is an important facet of the communication process.

However, anger that is out of control can be destructive. It can damage your relationships and may make it difficult for you to hold a job or participate in group activities. It can even damage your heart. The exploding rage you feel when you get really angry raises your blood pressure and appears to be associated with abnormal heart rhythms that can lead to sudden cardiac arrest.[29] An analysis of 44 separate studies concluded that anger increases the risk for developing heart disease even in otherwise healthy people.[30]

Anger that remains bottled up can also be harmful. The key is to express your anger in a constructive way. When you find yourself getting angry, take a step back and assess the

> **loneliness** A feeling of isolation from others, often prompted by a real or perceived loss.

situation objectively. Try to relax—a few deep breaths can often do the trick. Then explain, as calmly as you can, what's upsetting you. Speak honestly but avoid criticism, blame, and threats. If necessary, walk away from the person or situation and give yourself time to think. Once you're calmer, you may see solutions to the problem that you didn't notice before.

LO 2.3 QUICK CHECK

Charlotte is very shy. She sometimes avoids people, especially in new situations. Such a pattern of avoidance could lead to

a. a negative self-image.
b. self-actualization.
c. social isolation.
d. self-consciousness.

Mental Disorders in the United States: An Overview

LO 2.4 List reasons for the high prevalence of mental disorders in the United States.

Everyone occasionally feels sad, worried, or "spaced out." The feelings may last a few hours or a few weeks, but eventually we get over it and move on with our lives. In contrast, **mental disorders** cause long-term disruptions in thoughts and feelings that reduce an individual's ability to function in daily life. A disorder that substantially interferes with or limits one or more major life activities is considered to be a *serious mental illness* (SMI).

Since 1952, mental health professionals across the United States have used the *Diagnostic and Statistical Manual of Mental Disorders* (DSM) to diagnose specific mental illnesses. The DSM contains a listing of the diagnostic criteria for every psychiatric disorder recognized by the American Psychiatric Association (APA) and the U.S. health-care system.

> **mental disorders** Significant behavioral and psychological disorders that disrupt thoughts and feelings, impair ability to function, and increase risk of pain, disability, or even death.
>
> **psychoactive drugs** Drugs that affect the user's mood, perceptions, or other aspects of the mental state.
>
> **neurotransmitters** Chemicals that enable the transmission of messages from one neuron to another across synapses.

Prevalence of Mental Disorders

Mental disorders are common. The National Institute of Mental Health (NIMH) estimates that more than 1 in 4 Americans over the age of 18 have experienced a DSM-diagnosable mental disorder at some time in the past year—a figure that translates to more than 57 million people.[31,32] Fortunately, most of these cases are mild. Annually, about 4% of Americans suffer from a serious mental illness.[31,32]

College students face distinct academic and social pressures that can challenge their psychological health. Today's college freshmen have the lowest ever self-rating of emotional health compared to freshmen from the past 50 years, and significantly more students are coming to campus with a history of mental illness.[33]

> *"A World Health Organization survey of 17 countries found that the United States has the highest lifetime prevalence of DSM-diagnosable mental disorders."*

In 2015, approximately 1 in 4 U.S. college students reported being treated for or diagnosed with some type of mental disorder in the past year.[34] However, because many students fail to seek treatment, the actual statistics are thought to be much higher. In one large national survey, almost half of all college students met the diagnostic criteria for at least one mental disorder in the previous 12 months.[35]

>> Search for "depression on rise in college students" at this site to find a National Public Radio program that discusses rising rates of mental health issues on campus: **www.npr.org**.

A comparison of the rate of mental disorders in the United States with that of other countries is troubling. A World Health Organization survey of 17 countries found that the United States has the highest lifetime prevalence of DSM-diagnosable mental disorders: Over 47% of Americans have one or more at some point in their lives. This rate was dramatically higher than the average (27%) of the 16 other countries surveyed.[36] However, despite the fact that antidepressant use has risen substantially in the past three decades, with 13% of Americans taking them currently, the United States does not lead the world in antidepressant use.[37] Antidepressant use in other developed countries has nearly doubled since 2000, with Iceland having the highest rate of antidepressant consumption.[38]

Diagnosis and Treatment of Mental Disorders

Clinicians are required to use a DSM diagnostic code for reimbursement of mental health services, including prescription of **psychoactive drugs** (drugs that affect the patient's mental state). Because it provides a standardized and detailed description of every recognized disorder, the DSM is also an effective tool for collecting and communicating accurate national mental health statistics. Released in 2013, the current edition, DSM-5, includes some new disorders, including hoarding, gambling disorder, premenstrual dysphoric disorder, binge eating disorder, and caffeine withdrawal.[39]

In the 1950s, use of psychoactive drugs became the primary form of treatment for mental disorders as physicians began to accept the *chemical imbalance theory* of mental disorders.[40] The theory arose as drugs initially used to treat certain physical disorders were found to have psychological side effects.[41] Initially, researchers could not explain these effects, but over time, it became clear that the drugs were flooding the brain with chemicals called **neurotransmitters.** These chemicals—including serotonin, dopamine, and others—are called neurotransmitters because they enable the transmission of messages from one nerve cell (called a *neuron*) to another across microscopic gaps called *synapses*.

Researchers theorized that mental disorders might occur because a patient's brain was producing an excess or a deficit of neurotransmitters. Thus, psychoactive drugs were prescribed to "correct the imbalance." However, despite decades of research, scientists have failed to find the evidence to support this theory. Neurotransmitter levels and functioning appear to be normal in people with mental disorders before drug treatment.[40,41] Thus, the current thinking among experts is that the causes of most mental disorders are unknown and complex, and researchers have begun to investigate gene–environment interactions as the source.[41]

We discuss the most common mental disorders, including individual characteristics and treatment options, in the next sections.

LO 2.4 QUICK CHECK

Which of the following statements best summarizes what the DSM concludes about the cause of most mental illness?
a. The cause of mental illness is genetic.
b. The imbalance of neurotransmitters is the mostly likely cause of mental illness.
c. Early childhood trauma causes most mental illness.
d. The causes of mental disorders are unknown and complex.

Mood Disorders

LO 2.5 Discuss the characteristics, possible causes, and treatments of mood disorders.

Mood disorders are chronic, pervasive emotional states that significantly alter the person's thoughts, behavior, and normal functioning.

Depressive Disorders

Though most of us have felt sadness from time to time, the feeling is usually temporary and in reaction to a disappointment or loss. However, in a person diagnosed with a **depressive disorder,** the sadness is more profound and long term, and it interferes with daily life. Approximately 18 million adult Americans suffer from a depressive disorder every year.[42] In 2015, 14.5% of college students reported that they had been diagnosed with or treated for depression.[34]

Although the most basic symptom of depressive disorders is persistent sadness, other symptoms include the following:[39]

- A feeling of being slowed down or lacking energy
- Feelings of helplessness, hopelessness, meaninglessness, or "emptiness"
- Feelings of worthlessness or guilt
- Loss of interest in school, work, or activities once enjoyed
- Social withdrawal
- Difficulty thinking clearly or making decisions
- Sleep disturbances
- Changes in eating habits, eating more or less than formerly
- Restlessness, irritability
- In the most severe cases, recurring thoughts of death or suicide

Depressive disorders also often occur in conjunction with anxiety disorders and substance abuse.

Types of Depressive Disorders

Two of the most common forms of depressive disorder are major depressive disorder and dysthymic disorder.

Major Depressive Disorder. Also called **unipolar depression, major depressive disorder** affects approximately 6.7% of American adults in a given year.[31,32] It is diagnosed when someone consistently experiences five or more depressive symptoms for at least two weeks straight.[39] These symptoms impair a person's ability to study, work, eat, sleep, maintain relationships, and feel pleasure. An episode of major depression may occur only once in a person's life, or it may occur several times.

Dysthymic Disorder. Also called **dysthymia, dysthymic disorder** is characterized by the depressive symptoms listed earlier; however, the symptoms tend to be milder and are chronic, occurring on a majority of days for at least two years in adults (one year in children). The person may experience several days or weeks without symptoms but not longer than two months. Those with dysthymia are more likely to suffer a major depressive episode in their lifetime. This type of depression is less common, affecting about 1.5% of American adults in a given year.[31,32]

Causes of Depressive Disorders

Research continues to explore the complex question of what causes depression. Two recent studies have each identified the same region of DNA as involved in major depression.[43,44] And a 2015 discovery of an excess amount of a protein in the brains of those with depression provides more evidence that at its core, depression is a physical illness.[45] However, biochemistry and genetics alone are not to blame. The pattern is likely influenced by the interactions of genetic and biochemical factors with environmental factors, such as certain learned behaviors passed by family members from one generation to the next.

Physical factors such as chronic pain can also contribute to depressive disorders. Irregular hormone levels can also be a factor, which is why doctors often test a patient's thyroid, a gland that secretes

> **mood disorder** Any chronic, pervasive emotional state that significantly alters the person's thoughts, behaviors, and normal functioning.
>
> **depressive disorder** A mental disorder usually characterized by profound, persistent sadness or loss of interest that interferes with daily life and normal functioning.
>
> **major depressive disorder (unipolar depression)** A type of depressive disorder characterized by experiencing five or more symptoms of depression, including either depressed mood or loss of interest or pleasure, for at least two weeks straight.
>
> **dysthymic disorder (dysthymia)** A milder, chronic type of depressive disorder that lasts two years or more.

regulatory hormones, before diagnosing a depressive disorder. Certain medications for physical illnesses can prompt major depressive episodes, and substance abuse is also a common trigger.[46]

External events such as the loss of a relationship, financial problems, and academic and career pressures can lead to depression. If a person's network of emotional support is limited, or if it changes following the loss of a loved one, the person may be especially vulnerable.[46]

Depressive Disorders in Men and Women

About twice as many women suffer from depressive disorders as men in any given year.[46]

The causes and symptoms may vary between sexes.

Women and Depression. Until adolescence, girls and boys experience depressive disorders at about the same rate. But after puberty, there is an increased rate in women.[46] One factor may be the hormonal changes women experience in connection with the menstrual cycle, pregnancy, childbirth, the postpartum period, the years just before menopause, and menopause. These hormonal shifts appear to increase the risk of depressive disorders, but no precise cause for this increased risk is known.[46]

A number of social and interpersonal factors increase women's stress, which contributes to depression. Women still tend to play a larger role than men in child care, while also pursuing professional careers. Women also experience higher rates of poverty and sexual abuse than men do.

For about 12% to 20% of new mothers, the combination of wildly shifting hormonal and physical changes, a radical change in lifestyle, the responsibility for a new baby, and a lack of sleep may contribute to *postpartum depression*. This disorder can make it difficult for a mother to bond with her new baby or, in the most serious cases, can promote thoughts of harming herself or her newborn.[47]

Men and Depression. Depressive disorders in men are often underdiagnosed and undertreated. Therefore, the disparity in rates of depressive disorders between men and women may not be as large as reported. Some of the lack of recognition may arise from the different ways men express their illness. Rather than appearing sad, they may be irritable, angry, or even abusive. Men with a depressive disorder are also prone to physical effects like fatigue and difficulty sleeping.[46]

Depressed men are more likely than women to self-medicate through destructive behaviors such as drug and alcohol abuse or to engage in reckless, risky behavior.[46] Also, depression is a risk factor for suicide, and although women are more likely to attempt suicide, men are much more likely to succeed. In 2012, 78% of all suicides in the United States were committed by males.[48]

Treatment of Depressive Disorders

For several decades, psychiatrists have acknowledged that many people recover spontaneously from depressive episodes—if given adequate time.[49,50] Still, many people benefit greatly from treatment, and for some, it can be life-saving. One of the first steps in getting treatment should be an evaluation by a health-care provider to check for any physical causes. If physical sources have been ruled out, several types of treatment can help depressed people get their lives back on track.

Psychotherapy. Talking with a trained counselor or psychologist can make a difference for many people with depressive disorders. Talk therapies (described shortly) encourage depressed people to open up about their thoughts, feelings, relationships, and experiences in order to recognize problems that underlie their depression and work to improve them. Talk therapy may be the best treatment option for mild to moderate depressive disorders.[46]

Antidepressants. For those who are severely depressed or suicidal, a health-care provider may suggest medication as an adjunct to talk therapies. Like most psychoactive drugs, antidepressants prompt a change in the levels of neurotransmitters—typically serotonin—in the brain. Antidepressants do not relieve symptoms immediately, and patients must take regular doses for at least two to four weeks before experiencing an effect.

These medications are not addictive, but abruptly stopping them can cause withdrawal symptoms or lead to a relapse of depression. It's very important that if you decide to stop taking antidepressants, you taper them off gradually and under a physician's supervision.

Common side effects of antidepressants include headache, insomnia, tremors, anxiety, and sexual dysfunction. Severe side effects are less common but include panic attacks, hostility, delusions, and suicidal thoughts.

In the 1990s, studies began warning of the increased risk of suicide in young people taking certain antidepressants. Since 2004, the U.S. Food and Drug Administration (FDA) has required that all antidepressant labels carry a warning that alerts consumers about the suicide risk among teens and young adults up to the age of 24. Since then, the number of antidepressant prescriptions for adolescents has decreased;[51] however, there has also been a corresponding increase in suicide in this age group.[52] Since untreated

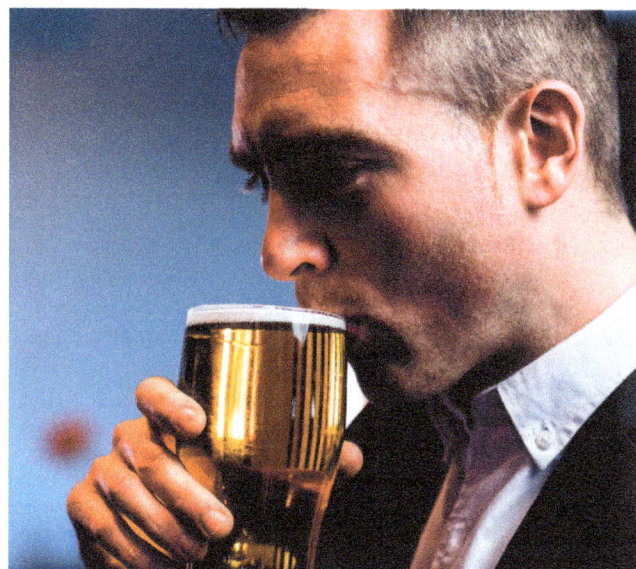

Depressed men are more likely than women to self-medicate through alcohol or drug use.

depression is the biggest risk factor for suicide, mental health experts warn that a decrease in the use of one form of treatment, such as antidepressants, must be countered with an increase in the use of other treatments.[53]

Although many experts have concluded that, for people suffering from severe depression, a course of supervised drug therapy can be helpful, researchers have questioned the effectiveness of antidepressants in cases of mild to moderate depression.[54-56] They suggest that the best path forward is for psychiatrists and patients to weigh carefully the risk–benefit equation for any treatment. If your doctor suggests that an antidepressant or another medication may help you, check out the **Practical Strategies** box for some important questions to discuss together. If you decide against taking medication, talk to your doctor about other treatment options. These are discussed in detail later in this chapter.

Bipolar Disorder

Bipolar disorder, also known as **manic-depressive disorder,** is characterized by occurrences of abnormally elevated mood (or *mania*) alternating with depressive episodes, with periods of normal mood in between. Mania can cause

PRACTICAL Strategies

Questions to Ask Before Starting a Medication for Mental Health Issues

If your doctor or mental health professional thinks you might benefit from taking medication to address a mental health issue, discuss the following questions to help decide whether it's the right option for you:

- Why do you believe that medication is the right choice for me?
- Why do you suggest this particular medication for me?
- How would I know if the medication is really working and I'm not feeling better for other reasons?
- When would I feel its effects? What should I do while I wait for it to work?
- What are the side effects? Am I at risk for them? What should I do if I decide to take this drug and start experiencing side effects?
- What is your practice for following up with your patients on the effects of the medication you prescribe?
- When do you anticipate that I could stop taking it? What would the withdrawal process entail?

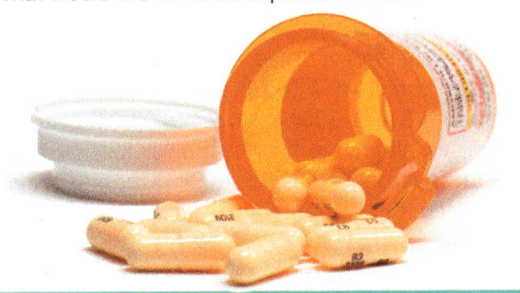

increased energy and decreased need for sleep, an expansive or irritable mood, impulsive behavior, and unrealistic beliefs or expectations. Manic people's thoughts race, their speech is rapid, their attention span is low, and their judgment is poor. Extreme manic episodes can include aggression or delusions and hallucinations. The alternating depressive episodes can lead to thoughts of suicide.

Bipolar disorder affects approximately 5.7 million American adults, about 2.6% of the U.S. population.[31,32] It occurs equally among both sexes and in all races and ethnic groups.[57] It usually develops in the late teens or early adult years and, until the 1980s, was not recognized in children. Over the past two decades, diagnoses of bipolar disorder in children have increased by 4,000%.[58] Approximately 1.7% of a national sample of American college students indicated that they had been diagnosed with or treated for bipolar disorder in the past year.[34]

Bipolar disorder has a tendency to run in families, and scientists are looking for genes that may increase a person's likelihood of developing the illness.

bipolar disorder (manic-depressive disorder) A mental disorder characterized by occurrences of abnormally elevated mood (or mania), often alternating with depressive episodes, with periods of normal mood in between.

STUDENT STORY

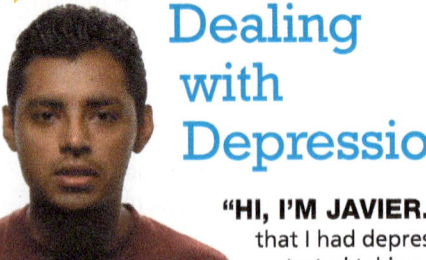

Dealing with Depression

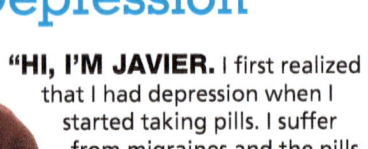

"HI, I'M JAVIER. I first realized that I had depression when I started taking pills. I suffer from migraines and the pills make me go to sleep so I was kind of addicted to them. I took them all the time and I was practically asleep 24-7. I stopped going to school and I failed a lot of classes because of that. And so I went to a doctor and he told me that I suffer from mild depression and that I needed to do something about it. I needed to stop the medication I was on and take the medication that he prescribed. It was pretty hard for me to accept it. I mean, most guys don't think that there's something wrong with them until, you know, life hits them."

What Do You Think?

1. Javier self-medicated with his migraine pills when he was depressed. What are some other signs that can indicate depression in men?
2. What options does Javier have to deal with his depression?
3. If you had a friend who was experiencing symptoms like Javier's, would you say something to him? What would you say?

However, most agree that many different genes are likely to act along with environmental factors to produce the illness.

The most common treatment for bipolar disorder is a mood-stabilizing drug such as lithium. Anticonvulsant medications, antidepressants, and antipsychotics may be prescribed as well.

>> Hear people with bipolar disorder discuss their condition: **www.webmd.com**. (Search for "bipolar tv.")

LO 2.5 QUICK CHECK ✔

What is the primary difference between major depressive disorder and dysthymic disorder?

a. Major depressive disorder lasts longer than dysthymic disorder.
b. Dysthymic disorder is more likely to be diagnosed in men than women.
c. Major depressive disorder and dysthymic disorder have different symptoms.
d. Dysthymic disorder has milder but more chronic symptoms than major depressive disorder.

Anxiety Disorders

LO 2.6 Discuss the characteristics, possible causes, and treatments of anxiety disorders.

anxiety disorders A category of mental disorders characterized by persistent feelings of fear, dread, and worry.

generalized anxiety disorder (GAD) An anxiety disorder characterized by chronic worry and pessimism about everyday events that lasts at least six months and may be accompanied by physical symptoms.

panic attacks Episodes of sudden terror that strike without warning.

panic disorder A mental disorder characterized both by recurring panic attacks and the fear of a panic attack occurring.

social anxiety disorder (social phobia) An anxiety disorder characterized by an intense fear of being judged by others and of being humiliated by your own actions, which may be accompanied by physical symptoms.

phobia An extreme, disabling, irrational fear of something that poses little or no actual danger.

Anxiety disorders cover a wide range of conditions characterized by persistent feelings of fear, dread, and worry. They are the most common mental health problems among American adults, affecting more than 40 million adults each year.[31,32] They are also the most common mental disorder among college students; nearly 17.3% reported being diagnosed or treated for anxiety in 2015.[34] Anxiety disorders frequently occur in conjunction with depressive disorders or substance abuse problems.

Generalized Anxiety Disorder (GAD)

People who suffer from **generalized anxiety disorder (GAD)** feel chronic anxiety, exaggerated worry, and pessimism, even when there is little or nothing to provoke it. Physical symptoms that often accompany the anxiety include fatigue, headaches, muscle tension, muscle aches, difficulty swallowing, trembling, and nausea. The condition is diagnosed when symptoms last at least six months. GAD affects about 6.8 million adult Americans and about twice as many women as men.[31,32] It usually develops gradually and is often accompanied by depression, other anxiety disorders, or substance abuse.

> **"** *Although people experiencing panic attacks often truly fear that they might die, panic attacks will not kill you.*"

Panic Attacks and Panic Disorder

Panic attacks are sudden feelings of terror that strike without warning. Symptoms include chest pain, shortness of breath, dizziness, weakness, and nausea. Panic attacks usually induce a sense of unreality and fears of impending doom or losing control, even though there is no rational reason for the person to believe something bad might happen. While people experiencing panic attacks often truly fear that they might die, panic attacks will not kill you. They usually go away on their own in less than 10 minutes.

Many people have just one panic attack and never have another, but those experiencing repeated panic attacks may have **panic disorder**. Panic disorder affects about 6 million adults in the United States and is twice as common in women as men.[59] It often begins in late adolescence or early adulthood, and the susceptibility appears to be inherited.

About one-third of people who suffer from panic disorder go on to develop *agoraphobia*, the fear of being in places where they cannot quickly leave or get help should they have a panic attack.[59] This often occurs because people who have experienced panic attacks have excess fear of them happening again when they are away from their homes. Agoraphobia can eventually leave victims virtually housebound.

Social Anxiety Disorder

Social anxiety disorder, also called **social phobia**, typically involves an intense fear of being judged by others and of being humiliated by your own actions. It can be accompanied by physical symptoms such as sweating, blushing, increased heart rate, trembling, and stuttering. It may strike only in certain situations—for instance, when called on in class—but in its most severe form, a person might experience the symptoms any time he or she is around other people.[60] Social anxiety disorder affects about 15 million adults in the United States, and women and men are equally likely to develop it.[31,32]

Phobias

Many people have an irrational fear of something—such as mice or spiders—that poses little or no actual danger. A **phobia** is similarly irrational but so extreme as to be disabling. Nearly 9% of American adults experience some type of phobia, with the age of onset around 10 years old.[59] The American Psychiatric Association classifies simple phobias into five categories: animal phobias; natural environment phobias (e.g., heights, water); situational phobias (e.g.,

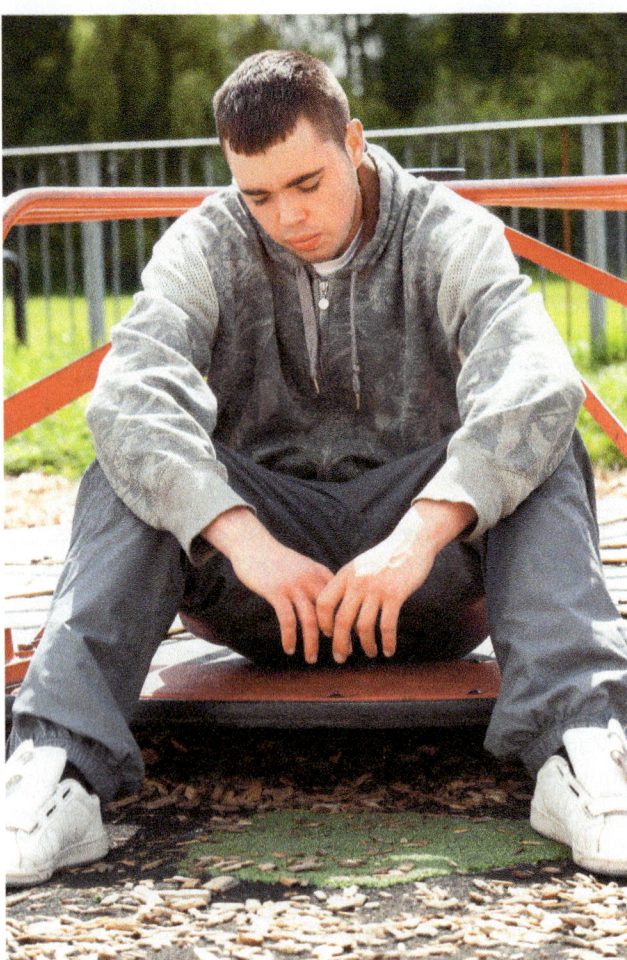

Social anxiety disorder can cause people to isolate themselves from others.

confined spaces, darkness); blood, injection, or injury phobias; and other phobias.[39]

Treating Anxiety Disorders

Cognitive-behavioral therapy (discussed later) is effective at teaching people with anxiety to recognize and redirect anxiety-producing thought patterns. One effective treatment, called *exposure therapy* or *systematic desensitization*, encourages patients to face their fears head-on. For instance, part of the therapy for a student with social phobia about public speaking might be for him to make a presentation to just one person and then progressively add more people to his audience. The therapist will help him work through his anxiety as his audience grows, and eventually his reaction will become less severe.

Biofeedback is increasingly being integrated with cognitive-behavioral therapy for patients with anxiety. Biofeedback is discussed in more detail later in the chapter.

While a class of medications known as benzodiazepines (Valium, Xanax, etc.) exert an immediate calming effect, they also have a high rate of dependence and are therefore not recommended as a long-term treatment for anxiety disorders.[61] Instead, antidepressants are the first-choice medication for the treatment of most anxiety disorders.[62]

LO 2.6 QUICK CHECK

Anxiety disorders
a. are the most common mental health problem among American adult
b. are typically treated with a class of medications called antidepressants
c. include depression and bipolar disorder
d. have symptoms such as hallucinations, delusions and thought disorders

Other Disorders

LO 2.7 Discuss the characteristics, possible causes, and treatments of other disorders.

In this section, we discuss 4 more of the 157 mental disorders recognized by the APA in the most recent edition of the DSM.[39]

Obsessive-Compulsive Disorder (OCD)

People with **obsessive-compulsive disorder (OCD)** have repeated and unwanted thoughts (obsessions) that cause them to develop rituals (compulsions) in an attempt to control the anxiety produced by these thoughts. The obsessions tend to be overblown, such as extreme concern about contamination by germs, fear of home intruders, or death of a loved one. The rituals provide brief relief from anxiety, even though the sufferer often knows they are meaningless.

The rituals can ultimately control the person's life. For example, a student obsessed with germs may develop hand-washing rituals that are so extensive that she is unable to leave her apartment to get to class on time. Other common rituals include repeatedly checking things, touching things in a certain order or a certain number of times, or hoarding unnecessary items. Occurring equally in men and women, OCD affects 2.2 million adults in the United States.[31,32] First symptoms frequently appear in childhood or adolescence. OCD is often diagnosed concurrently with eating disorders, anxiety disorders, or depression.

> **obsessive-compulsive disorder (OCD)** An anxiety disorder characterized by repeated and unwanted thoughts (obsessions) that lead to rituals (compulsions) in an attempt to control the anxiety.
>
> **post-traumatic stress disorder (PTSD)** An anxiety disorder characterized by recurrent fear, anger, and depression occurring after a traumatic event.

▶▶ Sufferers of OCD tell their stories: www.nytimes.com. (Search for "patient voices: O.C.D.")

Post-Traumatic Stress Disorder (PTSD)

After a traumatic event, people sometimes feel recurrent fear, anger, and depression, a condition known as **post-traumatic stress disorder (PTSD).** Experiences that commonly cause PTSD include child abuse, natural disasters, automobile accidents, being the victim of a violent crime, or military service, primarily in combat zones.

People with PTSD often startle easily, feel numb emotionally, and can become irritable or even violent. They

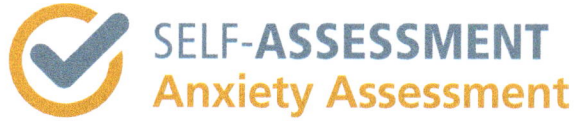

SELF-ASSESSMENT
Anxiety Assessment

Instructions: How has each of these symptoms disturbed or worried you during the past seven days? Circle the most appropriate score relating to your state.

0 = Never 1 = A little 2 = Moderately 3 = A lot 4 = Extremely

1.	Nervousness or shaking inside	0	1	2	3	4
2.	Nausea, stomach pain, or discomfort	0	1	2	3	4
3.	Feeling scared suddenly and without any reason	0	1	2	3	4
4.	Palpitations or feeling that your heart is beating faster	0	1	2	3	4
5.	Significant difficulty falling asleep	0	1	2	3	4
6.	Difficulty relaxing	0	1	2	3	4
7.	Tendency to startle easily	0	1	2	3	4
8.	Tendency to be easily irritable or bothered	0	1	2	3	4
9.	Inability to free yourself of obsessive thoughts	0	1	2	3	4
10.	Tendency to awaken early in the morning and not go back to sleep	0	1	2	3	4
11.	Feeling nervous when alone	0	1	2	3	4

HOW TO INTERPRET YOUR SCORE If you indicated scores of 3 or 4 to five or six questions, your anxiety level is significant, and you should consider different strategies such as better health practices or adding relaxation techniques or physical exercise to your daily routine. If you indicated scores of 3 or 4 in all your answers, your level of anxiety is critical, and you should consult your doctor.

To complete this Self-Assessment online, visit MasteringHealth™

Source: "Anxiety Self-assessment Questionnaire" used by permission of the Mental Illness Foundation, Montreal.

---

attention disorders A category of mental disorders characterized by problems with mental focus.

attention deficit/hyperactivity disorder (ADHD) A type of attention disorder characterized by inattention, hyperactive behavior, fidgeting, and a tendency toward impulsive behavior.

tend to relive the trauma in flashbacks or dreams, and they avoid places or experiences that might remind them of the traumatic event. PTSD can be accompanied by depression, anxiety disorders, and substance abuse.

About 7.7 million adults in the United States experience PTSD each year, but it can strike children as well.[63] The condition is more common in women than men. The likelihood of developing PTSD increases with intense, long-lasting trauma involving personal injury or death of a loved one, especially if the victim had little control over the event and received little support afterward.[63] Because of the increasing number of American military service personnel returning to school, many colleges are offering veterans specialized counseling services for PTSD.

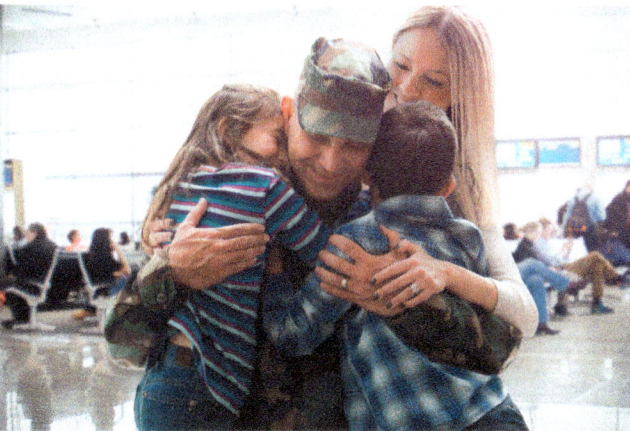

Soldiers returning home from war can often suffer from **PTSD**.

>> Listen to soldiers talk about PTSD in their own words at **www.pbs.com**. (Search for "frontline: the soldier's heart.")

Attention Disorders

Attention disorders create difficulty with jobs that require sustained concentration, such as completing a single task over a long period of time or sitting still for extended periods. The most common form of attention disorder is **attention deficit/hyperactivity disorder (ADHD),** which is characterized by inattention, hyperactive behavior, fidgeting, and poor impulse control. The majority of diagnoses in children are based on teacher complaints, with more than twice as many boys being diagnosed as girls.[64]

Although attention disorders usually become evident by age 7, many cases continue into adulthood. ADHD is diagnosed in about 4.4% of adults.[65] In a 2015 study of college students in the United States, 5.8% reported having ADHD.[34] Although research hasn't conclusively identified social or psychological effects of ADHD among college students, there is consistent evidence that ADHD reduces academic performance.[65] Adults with ADHD can have difficulty following directions, remembering information, and meeting deadlines; they may be chronically late, anxious, unorganized, or irritable. People with attention disorders are also at increased risk for tobacco use and substance abuse. Furthermore, ADHD can have a negative impact on employment and earning potential throughout adulthood, especially for minorities and economically disadvantaged people.[66]

> *There is consistent evidence that ADHD reduces academic performance."*

Options for treating attention disorders include cognitive-behavioral therapy and prescription stimulants such as methylphenidate (Ritalin or Concerta) or amphetamine/dextroamphetamine (Adderall). These drugs affect how the brain controls impulses and regulates attention.[67] Side effects include agitation, irritability, and anxiety, as well as insomnia, headache, nausea, and loss of appetite.

The number of children taking these medications has soared from 600,000 in 1990 to more than 3.5 million today. A Centers for Disease Control and Prevention–funded study found that up to 11% of all 5- to 13-year-olds were taking ADHD medications; however, fewer than half of them met the diagnostic criteria for ADHD.[68] Some experts contend that these drugs are overprescribed as a result of a successful two-decade marketing campaign by the pharmaceutical companies that produce them.[69]

In 2015, a national survey found that 5.7% of college students reported using Adderall, Ritalin, and other stimulants without a prescription.[34] Typically, students use these drugs to help them study longer; however, research evidence suggests that nonmedical use among college students doesn't confer any substantial academic benefit. In fact, users have lower GPAs on average than nonusers and are more likely to abuse other drugs as well.[70] The illicit use of stimulants, part of a larger problem of prescription drug abuse, is discussed in Chapter 8.

Schizophrenia

Schizophrenia is a severe, chronic, and potentially disabling mental disorder that is characterized by *psychosis*, abnormal thinking and loss of contact with reality. It affects about 1% of adults in the United States, usually appearing in the late teens through early 30s.[31,32] Research has shown that schizophrenia affects both sexes equally and occurs in similar rates in all ethnic groups. Because it occurs in 10% of people who have a first-degree relative (parent or sibling) with the disorder, and in 40% to 65% of people whose identical twin has it, researchers are studying the role of genes in the disorder.[71] Although no specific gene or genes have yet been identified, it is known that people with schizophrenia have higher rates of genetic mutations overall. These mutations may disrupt brain functioning.[71] Nevertheless, researchers conclude that it is doubtful that genetics alone cause the disease to develop.

> **schizophrenia** A severe mental disorder characterized by delusions, hallucinations, and other aspects of psychosis.

The following are the primary symptoms of schizophrenia:[71]

- **Delusions.** False beliefs, such as thinking you possess unusual powers or believing that others are plotting against you.
- **Hallucinations.** False perceptions of reality, such as hearing or seeing things—most often voices—that are not there.
- **Thought disorders.** Often called *disorganized thinking*—problems with thinking or speaking clearly or maintaining focus.
- **Movement disorders.** Agitated or repetitive body movements, or in some extreme cases becoming catatonic (immobile).
- **Reduction in professional and social functioning.** Social withdrawal, unpredictable behavior, poor hygiene, or paranoia that impair social and professional function.
- **Inappropriate emotions.** Aloofness, a so-called flat affect, or inappropriate or bizarre reactions to events.

Any of a variety of antipsychotic medications may be prescribed to manage these symptoms. Their long-term use can be problematic for patients, however, because of a wide range of adverse effects, from weight gain to inability to control muscle movements. Promising new research suggests that talk therapy may also be effective in treating schizophrenia.[72]

Although schizophrenia has a reputation for being incurable, both historic records and contemporary research studies have shown that many people do recover and go on to lead independent, satisfying lives.[71]

>> People with schizophrenia tell their stories: **www.nytimes.com**. (Search for "patient voices: schizophrenia.")

LO 2.7 QUICK CHECK

Since surviving a sexual assault, Sharon sometimes feels recurrent fear, anger, and depression. She startles easily, feels numb emotionally, and has flashbacks. Her symptoms are characteristic of

a. post-traumatic stress disorder.
b. social anxiety disorder.
c. panic disorder.
d. generalized anxiety disorder.

Self-Injury and Suicide

LO 2.8 Define non-suicidal self-injury and discuss suicide warning signs and prevention strategies.

When people experience deep and persistent anguish, they may consider self-harm. Two common types are non-suicidal self-injury and suicide.

Non-suicidal Self-injury

Included for the first time in the latest version of the DSM, non-suicidal self-injury (NSSI) occurs in the form of intentional, self-inflicted cuts, burns, bites, bruises, or other injuries, without the desire to die.[73] Studies suggest that NSSI is used as a means of coping with overwhelming tension; negative, intrusive thoughts; or feelings of dissociation—of being detached from one's body and emotions.[74] Although the behavior provides the injurer with a moment of calm, it is usually followed by feelings of guilt and shame.

NSSI often begins in adolescence. Overall, 17% to 18% of adolescents and 13% of young adults injure themselves intentionally; females are significantly more likely to self-injure than males.[75,76] In a nationwide 2015 study, approximately 6.5% of college students in the United States reported engaging in NSSI in the past year, but this may be an underestimate because many who injure themselves conceal it.[34]

STUDENT STORY

A Friend's Suicide

"HI, I'M KRISTINA. In my senior year of high school one of my good girlfriends decided to take her own life. It was pretty devastating—emotionally, mentally, physically even. I don't think anyone expects, as a high-schooler, that one of their peers will commit suicide. At first I felt angry, and then it gradually hit me and I was very upset and cried all the time. I guess, after that all happened, the positive thing that came out of it was I had a closer relationship with my girlfriends and my family; we really watch out for each other and we say 'I love you' more.

I just want people to know that nothing is bad enough to take your own life. Even if you feel like nothing's going right in your life, it doesn't mean that you can't turn those negative things into positive things. There are many problems that people have in their teenage years that they can't help, but they end up stronger people because of it."

What Do You Think?

1. Is Kristina right that young people don't expect one of their peers to commit suicide? Why or why not?
2. What does Kristina mean about turning negative things into positive things? Have you ever turned a negative into a positive?
3. Do you agree that what might be seen as an overwhelming problem today might one day be considered a turning point for possible change?

Therapy and medications can help self-injurers learn to deal with their difficult feelings more appropriately and stop their self-abuse. On the other hand, the use of certain medications, such as antidepressants, is associated with an increased risk for self-injury.[54]

Suicide

More than 41,000 people in the United States took their own lives in 2013. For every death there are at least another 11 attempted suicides, and U.S. hospitals treat almost 500,000 people for self-inflicted injuries per year.[77] College students are more likely than the general population to try to take their own lives, and suicide is the second leading cause of death on college campuses. Approximately 9.6% of students said they had seriously considered attempting suicide in the past year.[34] Although women attempt suicide more often than men, men are four times more likely to actually die by suicide, possibly because they choose more lethal means.[32,77]

Multiple studies have suggested that lesbian, gay, bisexual, and transgender (LGBT) students have a higher-than-average risk for suicide.[78] Factors contributing to this risk include experiences of prejudice and discrimination, verbal or physical harassment, violence, and rejection by family members or peers.[78]

Native Americans and Caucasians have a rate of suicide more than double that of other ethnic groups, and Caucasian males over age 85 have the highest suicide rate of any group in the United States.[79] Recent reports reveal, however, that the suicide rate of white middle-aged Americans is at an all-time high.[80]

>> Watch a video explaining this surge in the death rate among white middle-aged men at **www.sciencedaily.com**. (Search for "middle aged white men dying.")

Causes and Warning Signs of Suicide

Several factors clearly play a role in driving up suicide risk. More than 90% of people who commit suicide in the United States have a diagnosable mental health or substance use disorder.[79] In addition, financial problems, serious illness, and the loss of a loved one are frequent catalysts. A family history of suicide, previous suicide attempts, and having access to guns in the home also increase suicide risk.

The following are among the signs that a person may be considering suicide:

- Statements that indirectly imply suicidal thoughts, such as "I don't have much to live for" or "You won't have to worry about me much longer"
- An inability to let go of grief
- Changes in behavior and personality that focus on hopeless, negative thoughts and feelings
- A noticeable downturn in mood within the first few weeks of starting a new antidepressant medication
- Loss of interest in classes, work, hobbies, or spending time with friends and loved ones
- Expressions of self-hatred, excessive risk taking, or apathy toward one's own well-being
- Disregard for personal appearance
- Changes in sleep patterns or eating habits
- A preoccupation with thoughts or themes of death

Preventing Suicide

Don't assume that a person who talks of suicide is just having a bad day or seeking attention. Instead, let the person know you care and that you are there to help. Never be afraid to raise the subject. Offer to be there with the person as he or she calls a crisis hotline, goes to a counseling center, or heads to the nearest emergency room (**Figure 2.4**, next page).

>> Find links to all of National Public Radio's mental health podcasts at **www.npr.org/sections/mental-health**.

LO 2.8 QUICK CHECK

If a friend talks to you about committing suicide, what should you do?
a. Try to cheer him up.
b. Take him seriously and offer to help.
c. Change the subject to get his mind off it.
d. Let him know that you aren't trained to deal with this and ask him to talk with someone else.

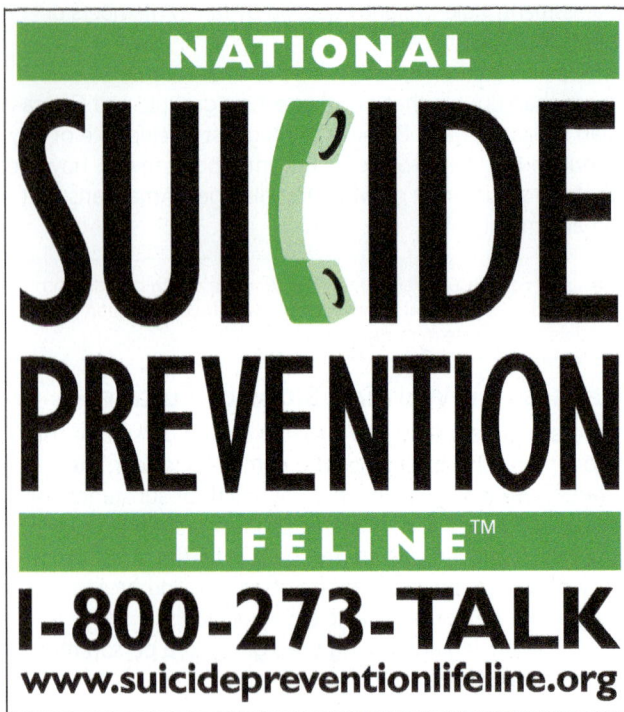

FIGURE 2.4 **National Suicide Prevention Lifeline.**
Source: U.S. Department of Health and Human Services, Substance Abuse and Mental Health Services Administration.

Getting Help for a Psychological Problem

LO 2.9 Describe different options for the treatment of mental disorders.

A recent survey found that the number-one reason college students fail to get help for a psychological problem is personal *stigma*, an internalized feeling of shame about the condition.[81,82] However, if you're in distress, remember that anxiety, depression, and other problems are common among college students, are treatable conditions, and are not signs of weakness or deficiency! In fact, seeking help is a sign of psychological health; it shows that you esteem yourself enough to reach out and that you trust your community to respond effectively.

Options on Campus

Approximately 1 in 5 students utilizes psychological services in the first year of college, with male students being more likely to seek counseling than their female peers.[82,83] However, more than 60% of all students who stop attending college do so because of a mental health–related reason. Of these, half drop out without even trying to access mental health services.[81] Don't be among them. Most campuses offer a range of options to help address the mental and emotional pressures students face. These services are usually provided free or at low cost or are covered by your insurance plan. Your campus health clinic or counseling center is a good place to start looking for help.

Clinical Options

In addition to campus and community services, it's important to be aware of the full range of your clinical options.

Types of Mental Health Professionals

The following are the types of licensed professionals who most commonly work with people experiencing psychological distress:

- **Counselors.** Counselors have a master's degree in counseling, social work, or marriage and family therapy. They primarily focus on talk therapy. Counselors may lead group, family, or individual therapy sessions, as well as recommend services available within your community.
- **Psychologists.** Psychologists have a doctoral degree and provide talk therapy. Many have particular specialties, and they may lead group, family, or individual therapy sessions.
- **Psychiatrists.** Psychiatrists have a medical degree and usually focus on the medical aspects of psychological issues. Unlike counselors or psychologists, psychiatrists can prescribe medication and may have admitting privileges at local hospitals. Psychiatrists and psychologists often work together to provide a full range of care.

See the **Consumer Corner** box on page 43 for information about what to discuss before choosing a therapist.

Once you have found a mental health professional, the real work begins. Your treatment can succeed only if you are open and honest about your thoughts, emotions, and what is going on in your life. Therapy can sometimes bring up uncomfortable feelings, but that isn't necessarily a bad thing; it can be a sign that you are working through issues. However, if at any point something happens in therapy that you don't like, say so. Therapists should be eager to work with you to resolve any problems that come up.

Types of Therapy

The type of therapy you choose should depend on your specific condition and your preferences. Some people benefit from a combination of several types of therapy.

Cognitive-Behavioral Therapy. A form of psychotherapy that emphasizes the role of thinking (cognition) in how we feel and what we do, **cognitive-behavioral therapy (CBT)** is usually short term and focused. There are many approaches to CBT, but all are based on the idea that our *thoughts* cause our feelings and behaviors, not external things, such as people, situations, and events. The benefit of this acknowledgement is that when we can change the way we think, we end up feeling and acting better even if our situation does not change.[84]

> **cognitive-behavioral therapy (CBT)** A form of psychotherapy that emphasizes the role of thinking (cognition) in how we feel and what we do.

CONSUMER CORNER
Choosing a Therapist Who's Right for You

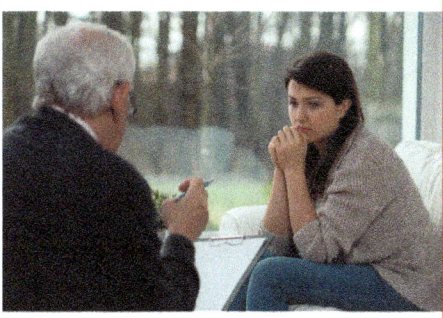

Therapy can help people with a variety of issues, but it's important to find a therapist with whom you feel comfortable and who is qualified to address your needs.
Discuss these key points in your first meeting with a potential therapist:

- Cost. Make sure you understand what the costs are and how they will be covered. If you are paying for care yourself, therapists will sometimes offer a sliding scale for fees, so be sure to ask.
- The therapist's credentials, education, and approach to therapy.
- Areas of specialization that the therapist has or that you would prefer—for example, specializations in bipolar disorder, childhood trauma, cognitive therapy, and so on.
- An overview of the problems you are experiencing and your goals for therapy.
- The experience the therapist has in helping people with similar problems.
- Whether you are taking or are interested in taking antidepressants or other medication. Keep in mind that psychologists and counselors cannot prescribe medication.
- Frequency and length of therapy sessions.

The information you get from this preliminary conversation, as well as your overall impression of the therapist, will help you determine whether you would like to undertake therapy with that person. Don't be afraid to have initial consultations with a few different therapists or to switch to someone else if, after a few sessions, you don't feel comfortable.

One premise of CBT is that consistent dysfunctional thinking, sometimes called *cognitive distortion*, results in unwanted feelings and behaviors. See the **Practical Strategies** box on page 44 for tips on how to notice cognitive distortions that you may have.

In CBT, the therapist and patient work collaboratively to identify distorted, negative thinking and replace it with more positive, reinforcing thinking. This occurs within the treatment setting, but the patient is also typically given homework. Gradually, the patient learns to think and behave in more healthful ways. Cognitive therapy is most effective in treating mood and anxiety disorders. Researchers have recently discovered that supplementing CBT with antidepressants is a very effective treatment combination for those suffering from the hardest-to-treat forms of OCD.[85]

Behavior Therapy. Either under the umbrella of CBT or alone, **behavior therapy** focuses on changing learned behaviors as efficiently and effectively as possible. The core idea behind behavior therapy is that once our behavior changes, our thoughts, feelings, attitudes, and moods will follow. Techniques include exposure therapy, which is gradual exposure to an anxiety-provoking situation paired with relaxation techniques; positive reinforcement, which encourages desired behaviors; and aversion therapy, negative reinforcement that discourages unwanted behaviors. Behavioral therapy is often used for anxiety and attention disorders.

Psychodynamic Therapy. Also called *psychoanalysis*, **psychodynamic therapy** is founded on the idea that there are unconscious sources for a person's behavior and psychological state. Although originating in the work of Sigmund Freud about a century ago, contemporary psychodynamic therapy focuses broadly on the exploration and discussion of the patient's emotions, past experiences, and coping patterns. Together, patient and therapist unearth unresolved conflicts buried in the unconscious and then talk through these conflicts in order to understand them and to change the ways in which they affect the patient today.

Positive Psychotherapy. **Positive psychotherapy** focuses on identifying psychological strengths and using them in new ways rather than dwelling on "fixing" psychological problems. This type of therapy aims to nurture in patients traits such as kindness, originality, humor, generosity, and gratitude and to help patients learn optimism. In positive psychotherapy, you perform a variety of activities—such as noting three good things that happen to you each day—with the goal of increasing your happiness.[84]

>> Hear prominent positive psychologist Martin Seligman explain his approach at **www.ted.com**. (Search for "Martin Seligman new era.")

Acceptance and Commitment Therapy. In contrast to positive psychotherapy, **acceptance and commitment therapy (ACT)** views happiness not as a goal but as a by-product of living according to one's values. An outgrowth

---

behavior therapy A type of therapy that focuses on changing a patient's behavior and thereby achieving psychological health.

psychodynamic therapy A type of therapy that focuses on the unconscious sources of a patient's behavior and psychological state.

positive psychotherapy A recent field of psychology that focuses on increasing psychological strengths and improving happiness rather than on psychological problems.

acceptance and commitment therapy (ACT) An outgrowth of cognitive-behavioral therapy that increases patients' ability to engage in values-based, positive behaviors while experiencing difficult thoughts, emotions, or sensations.

CHAPTER 2 ■ Psychological Health

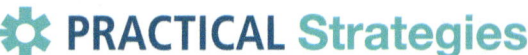
PRACTICAL Strategies

Spotting Destructive Thoughts

Do you ever find yourself thinking thoughts like "I *never* get things right!" or "I'm such a failure!"? If so, these cognitive distortions may be the sources of a bad mood or even serious depression. Here are some thought patterns to watch out for:

- **All-or-nothing thinking.** In all-or-nothing thinking, there is no middle ground. You think of situations or yourself as either perfect or a complete failure.
- **Overgeneralization.** You make a general conclusion based on a single event or experience from the past. You see one negative event as a never-ending pattern of defeat.
- **Mental filter.** You dwell excessively on a single negative detail, although everything else is positive.
- **Disqualifying the positive.** You reject positive experiences because they "don't count" for one reason or another.
- **Jumping to conclusions.** Without any definite facts to support it, you assume that other people are thinking or feeling negatively toward you. Or you predict that a situation will turn out badly and feel convinced that it is an already-established fact.
- **Magnification (catastrophizing) or minimization.** You exaggerate the importance of something minor (such as a poor grade on a quiz). Or you minimize a significant positive event (such as acing the final exam), predicting that "it won't make any difference."
- **Emotional reasoning.** You assume that your negative emotions reflect the way things really are: "I feel it, so it must be true."
- **Should statements.** You tell yourself what you "should" do, and if you don't perform, you feel guilty. This can also be applied to other people; if they don't live up to the "should" statement, you can feel angry, frustrated, or resentful.
- **Labeling and mislabeling.** Instead of thinking of something in a balanced way, you attach labels to yourself or others, such as "I'm a loser" or "He's no good." Mislabeling involves describing an event with highly colored or emotionally loaded language.
- **Personalization.** You think that everything people do or say is in reaction to you; you think you are the cause of a negative external event that, in reality, you had nothing to do with.

Source: Based on *The Feeling Good Handbook*, by D. D. Burns, 1999, New York: Plume.

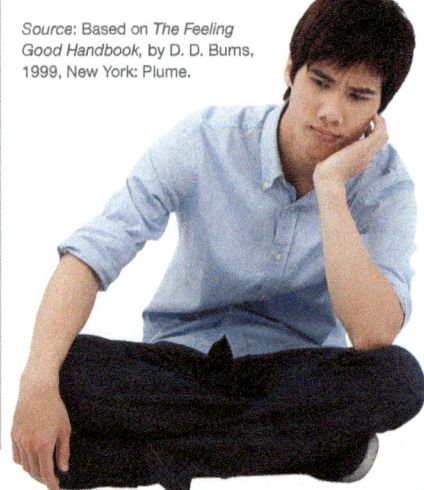

of cognitive-behavioral therapy, ACT uses mindfulness and behavioral techniques to help patients clarify their values, set goals guided by these values, and take committed action to achieve these goals while experiencing difficult thoughts, emotions, or sensations.[86] Although a reduction in symptoms may indeed occur as a result of taking committed action, ACT makes no attempt at symptom control. Rather, it points out that patients' efforts to control their symptoms through alcohol abuse, overeating, and other destructive choices impede achievement of their goals. Thus, patients learn to take action to create a meaningful life while accepting the pain that inevitably accompanies such a pursuit.

Other Clinical Options

One of the most commonly prescribed clinical options is of course, pharmacologic therapy, which we have discussed with specific disorders.

Another option is *biofeedback* therapy. Biofeedback patients are trained to monitor and change physiological activity in their own bodies. They are connected to instruments that provide feedback about their muscle tension, breathing rate, skin temperature, and other aspects of their body's functioning. They then make subtle changes, such as relaxing their muscles or breathing more slowly, that help them manage their symptoms. Biofeedback is increasingly being integrated with cognitive-behavioral therapy for patients with anxiety and PTSD. In a recent study of college students receiving treatment for anxiety, those who had biofeedback as an adjunct to cognitive-behavioral therapy experienced a greater reduction in anxiety symptoms than those who had therapy alone.[87] In addition, although you might associate it with horror films, electroconvulsive therapy (ECT) is still sometimes used for severely ill patients who are not responsive to counseling or drug treatment. Formerly called *electroshock therapy*, ECT is administered using devices that transmit a jolt of electricity that induces seizures in the anesthetized patient. No one knows precisely how ECT produces therapeutic effects.

The FDA classifies ECT machines as high-risk devices because of the potential for significant adverse effects, including memory loss and cognitive impairment that may last several months.[88] Despite controversy over ECT, some psychiatrists support its use in patients with resistant suicidal depression and other severe mental disorders.

LO 2.9 QUICK CHECK

Michael has had a difficult first semester and is at risk of becoming one of the 60% of students who leave college for mental health reasons. What is the most likely reason he will fail to get help for his psychological problem?

a. lack of mental health resources on campus

b. his inability to pay for mental health services on campus
c. personal stigma associated with seeking help for a psychological problem
d. no effective treatments available for the types of problems experienced by college students

Change Yourself, Change Your World

LO 2.10 Identify strategies for improving your psychological health and for helping a friend.

There are many steps you can take independently, among friends, and on campus to promote psychological well-being. Let's start with you.

Taking Care of Yourself

When you're experiencing mental or emotional distress, the basic tasks of daily life can feel overwhelming, yet it's at just such times that self-care becomes more important than ever. If you are feeling mentally or emotionally on edge, be sure to do the following:

- **Eat well.** Don't skip meals or binge on junk food. Scientific evidence points to an undisputable relationship between nutrition and mental health.[89]
- **Get the right amount of sleep.** Sleeping seven to nine hours every night is important to both physical and mental well-being. In your busy schedule as a college student, make sure you make sleep a priority. (For more on sleep, see Chapter 4.) If you're depressed and find yourself sleeping more than usual, know that the very act of getting out of bed can be an instant boost. Once you're up, open the curtains and windows; letting in light and air will help improve your mood.
- **Get some exercise.** Exercise releases body chemicals that boost mood. Even a half-hour walk is likely to improve your mood, clear your head, and make you feel better. Daytime exercise will also help make it easier to sleep at night.
- **Set realistic goals.** Don't expect yourself to function at your regular level. Set smaller goals and break big jobs up into small ones.
- **Take steps to build your self-esteem.** CBT recognizes that there are things you can do to change the way you think and the way you act that will, as a result, change the way you feel. For suggestions, see the **Practical Strategies** box on page 44.
- **Reach out.** Feelings of anxiety and despair can often cause you to prefer to be alone. If this is the case for you, it's important to recognize a desire for isolation as a symptom of your distress. Defy it—and reach out. Talk to someone you trust, or if you'd prefer to confide in a professional, visit your campus counseling center. Support groups are also good options. Often free or low cost, they are usually led by a trained professional who can steer the group's conversations and interactions in positive ways.

>> Find online support at one of these websites: www.patientslikeme.com, www.dailystrength.org.

- **Chill out.** Psychological health thrives when you withdraw your thoughts from the chaos of everyday life, and meditation can help you do that. For some, the practice is as simple as sitting quietly and focusing attention on a single idea, word, or symbol, or on the breath. Others find meditative contemplation in nature. This might mean a solitary walk through the park or getting up early to watch the sun rise.

>> Don't know how to meditate? Try one of these tools: www.mayoclinic.com (search for "video need to relax") or http://health.howstuffworks.com. (Search for "relieve stress daily life")

Helping Others

How do you support a friend who's feeling sad, anxious, or angry? How would you respond if a friend told you he or she was diagnosed with a mental illness? The following are some suggestions:

- **Get informed.** Find out about what's going on. Did your friend's arms get scratched when she tried to pet a neighbor's cat, as she claims, or is she cutting herself? Is your friend holing up in his dorm room because he's trying to finish a project, or is he depressed? You might decide to check your own observations against those of mutual friends. If you agree that your friend's behavior is a cause for concern, then you need to have the courage to ask him or her about it.
- **Listen.** Listen without judging. Acknowledge that your friend's pain—even if it's difficult for you to understand—is real for him or her. Don't dismiss it with assertions such as, "But your parents seem so understanding!" Such comments might only cause your friend to lose trust in you. On the other hand, if your friend refuses to say what's up, accept that and simply affirm that you'll be there if needed.
- **Offer your help.** Don't put pressure on yourself to fix things. An open-ended question—Is there anything I can do to help?—is fine, or you can offer specific assistance, like driving your friend to a scheduled appointment. You can also help your friend by modeling healthy behavior (see Chapter 1). Trust that maintaining your own balance will help your friend realize his or her own capacity to navigate life's challenges successfully.

>> Want to be an advocate on your campus for mental health? Find out how at Active Minds, a national student-founded and student-led advocacy organization at www.activeminds.org or learn more about "NAMI on Campus," campus-based advocacy clubs sponsored by the National Alliance on Mental Health, at www.nami.org.

>> Watch videos of real students discussing psychological health at MasteringHealth™

LO 2.10 QUICK CHECK

When you're experiencing mental or emotional distress, what becomes more important than ever?
a. addressing problems in your relationships
b. keeping up with your school work
c. practicing self-care
d. fulfilling all your commitments

Choosing to **Change** Worksheet

To complete this worksheet online, visit MasteringHealth™

PART I. Building the Qualities of Psychological Health

Directions: Fill in your stage of behavior change in step 1 and complete the rest of Part I with your stage of change in mind.

Step 1: Assess your stage of behavior change. Please check one of the following statements that best describes your readiness to improve your psychological health.

_____I do not intend to improve my psychological health in the next six months. (Precontemplation)

_____I might improve my psychological health in the next six months. (Contemplation)

_____I am prepared to improve my psychological health in the next month. (Preparation)

_____I have been improving my psychological health for less than six months but need to do more. (Action)

_____I have been improving my psychological health for more than six months. (Maintenance)

Step 2: Identify a facet of psychological health to improve. The Ryff Scale of Psychological Well-Being identifies six key facets of psychological health (see Figure 2.1 on page 27). With this in mind, think about one facet of your psychological health that is important to you and needs improvement. Write it down.

_____

Step 3: Make a plan to improve psychological health. Keeping your current stage of behavior change in mind, describe what you might do or think about as a "next step" to improve that quality of psychological health. You can use the strategies presented in this chapter for ideas. Also write down your timeline for making your next step.

_____

_____

_____

_____

Step 4: Overcome challenges to psychological health. In our daily lives, we sometimes experience challenging situations that can put our psychological health to the test. What techniques can you use to counter roadblocks to developing your psychological health to the fullest? Again, you can refer to the information provided in this chapter.

_____

_____

_____

_____

Step 5: Set a SMART goal. Keeping your current stage of change in mind, set a SMART goal, including a timeline, for improving your psychological health.

Goal: _____

_____

_____

Timeline: _____

PART II. Reducing Cognitive Distortions and Increasing Positive Thinking

Directions: Far too often we engage in negative self-talk and destructive thinking patterns. If you have thoughts that consistently weigh you down, work through the steps below to unravel that harmful pattern of thinking.

Step 1: Identify cognitive distortions. Take a look at the types of cognitive distortions discussed in the **Practical Strategies** box on page 44. Do any of these thinking patterns sound familiar to you? Write down any negative thoughts you have and list which category each fits into.

Thoughts	Categories
_____	_____
_____	_____
_____	_____
_____	_____
_____	_____

Step 2: Dispute your negative thoughts. Pick one of these thoughts to focus on. Do the facts of your current situation back up your negative perception? Write down all the facts that go against your current negative interpretation.

Example:

Thought: I am going to fail my English class.

Facts that go against the negative interpretation: Although I did poorly on my last test, I received good grades on the tests before that one.

Thought: _____

Facts that go against the negative interpretation: _____

_____

_____

Step 3: Change your perspective. Imagine that a friend or a family member was thinking the thought that you wrote down in step 2. What would you say to cheer up that person? Would things seem so bad if they weren't happening to you?

_____

_____

_____

Step 4: Create a more optimistic viewpoint. Taking into account the evidence above that goes against your negative self-talk, can you think about the situation in a more optimistic way?

Example: Instead of thinking "I received a bad grade on this test; I'm going to flunk out of school!" you could think "I did poorly on this test, but I've done well on tests before. Now I know to create a study plan and attend review sessions before the next test."

_____

_____

_____

_____

_____

CHAPTER 2 STUDY PLAN

CHAPTER SUMMARY

LO 2.1
- Psychological health encompasses both mental and emotional health. Its six facets are self-acceptance, positive relations with others, autonomy, environmental mastery, a sense of purpose in life, and ongoing personal growth.
- Maslow's hierarchy of needs models the theory that people experience ever-higher levels of psychological health as they meet ever-higher levels of needs. Those with high emotional intelligence can process information of an emotional nature and use it to guide their thoughts, actions, and reactions.
- Optimism is the psychological tendency to have a positive interpretation of life's events.

LO 2.2
- Psychological health is influenced by complex genetic factors interacting with aspects of environment.
- Childhood abuse or neglect can prompt the development of maladaptive coping patterns that are carried through adulthood. Current level of social support can also strongly influence response to psychological challenges.
- Religion and spirituality can contribute to psychological health. Spiritual well-being is said to rest on three pillars: a strong personal value system, connectedness and community in relationships, and a meaningful purpose in life.

LO 2.3
- Common psychological challenges include shyness, loneliness, and anger.

LO 2.4
- Mental disorders are common and can cause long-term disruptions in thoughts and feelings that reduce an individual's ability to function in daily life.
- The United States has the highest rate of mental disorders in the world. About 25% of U.S. college students report being treated for or diagnosed with some type of mental disorder; the actual prevalence may be much higher.
- The chemical imbalance theory of mental illness arose in the 1950s; however, the American Psychiatric Association acknowledges that the causes of mental disorders are complex or unknown.

LO 2.5
- Depressive disorders and bipolar disorder are mood disorders. Depression is considered one of the most treatable mental disorders.
- A variety of forms of psychotherapy are successful in treating depression. Regular exercise can help. Antidepressant medications are often effective; however, they can prompt serious side effects.
- Bipolar disorder is characterized by periods of mania followed by periods of depression.

MasteringHealth™
Build your knowledge—and health!—in the Study Area of **MasteringHealth**™ with a variety of study tools.

LO 2.6
- The most common mental disorders among college students are anxiety disorders, such as generalized anxiety disorder, panic disorder, and social anxiety disorder.
- Psychotherapy and antidepressant medications are common treatments.

LO 2.7
- Other mental disorders common in young adults are obsessive compulsive disorder (OCD), post-traumatic stress disorder (PTSD), attention disorders, such as ADHD, and schizophrenia.

LO 2.8
- Non-suicidal self-injury is the act of cutting, burning, bruising, or otherwise injuring yourself in an effort to cope with negative, intrusive thoughts or feelings of dissociation.
- Suicide is the second most common cause of death in young adults. If a friend makes a statement indicating suicidal thoughts, offer to call a crisis hotline together, accompany your friend to your campus health services or a counseling center, or head to the nearest emergency room.

LO 2.9
- Common options in psychotherapy include cognitive-behavioral therapy (CBT), behavior therapy, psychodynamic therapy, positive psychotherapy, and acceptance and commitment therapy. Some therapists use a combined approach.

LO 2.10
- Self-care can be a good place to start if you are experiencing psychological distress. Self-care includes eating well, getting the right amount of sleep, exercising, setting realistic goals, and taking steps to build your self-esteem.
- A desire to isolate yourself is a common symptom of psychological distress; reaching out is an important coping strategy.
- Meditation can help increase relaxation and positive feelings.
- To help a friend with psychological distress or a diagnosed mental disorder, listen objectively and compassionately. Don't try to fix things for your friend but do offer your presence and support.
- There are many ways to promote psychological well-being on campus, from joining an organization such as Active Minds to volunteering to become a peer counselor.

GET CONNECTED

>> Visit the following websites for further information about the topics in this chapter:

- American Psychological Association Help Center
  www.apa.org/helpcenter
- National Institute of Mental Health
  www.nimh.nih.gov
- Beliefnet
  www.beliefnet.com
- ScienceDaily: Mind & Brain
  www.sciencedaily.com/news/mind_brain
- Anxiety and Depression Association of America
  www.adaa.org

MOBILE TIPS!

Scan this QR code with your mobile device to access additional tips about psychological health. Or, via your mobile device, go to **http://chmobile.pearsoncmg.com** and choose by topic: psychological health.

- National Suicide Prevention Lifeline
  www.suicidepreventionlifeline.org
- American Psychological Association Psychologist Locator
  http://locator.apa.org
- Mental Health America
  www.mentalhealthamerica.net
- The Jed Foundation
  www.jedfoundation.org

Website links are subject to change. To access updated web links, please visit MasteringHealth

TEST YOUR KNOWLEDGE

LO 2.1
1. One of Ryff's six facets of psychological health is
   a. having a romantic relationship.
   b. achieving a fixed state of wellness.
   c. happiness.
   d. environmental mastery.

LO 2.2
2. Values, relationships, and purpose are three pillars of
   a. religiosity.
   b. spirituality.
   c. generativity.
   d. ego integrity.

LO 2.3
3. Loneliness is
   a. the experience of being alone.
   b. sometimes prompted by a real loss.
   c. rarely experienced when you're with others.
   d. all of the above.

LO 2.4
4. Mental disorders are
   a. more common in developing nations than in the United States.
   b. caused by an underlying chemical imbalance in the brain.
   c. classified in the *Diagnostic and Statistical Manual of Mental Disorders* (DSM).
   d. diagnosed in about 6% of Americans.

LO 2.5
5. Depressive disorders
   a. are more common in men than in women.
   b. are typically treated by a class of medications called benzodiazepines.
   c. include dysthymic disorder and bipolar disorder.
   d. are none of the above.

LO 2.6
6. Anxiety disorders
   a. are often treated with antidepressants.
   b. are the second most common mental health problem among American adults.
   c. are characterized by mania, delusions, and hallucinations.
   d. are classified as mood disorders.

LO 2.7
7. Schizophrenia is
   a. a disabling and irrational fear of something that poses little or no actual danger.
   b. associated with compulsive behaviors such as hand washing.
   c. characterized by psychosis.
   d. incurable.

LO 2.8
8. A suicidal person
   a. is not making idle threats.
   b. needs help immediately.
   c. wants relief from a situation that feels unbearable.
   d. All of the above

LO 2.9
9. Psychiatrists
   a. specialize in group therapy.
   b. only see patients with severe mental illness.
   c. can prescribe medication.
   d. All of the above

LO 2.10

10. Which of the following is a sensible strategy for psychological self-care?
    a. Eat nourishing foods and don't skip meals.
    b. On days when you have no early-morning commitments, get as many hours of sleep as possible.
    c. Allow yourself lots of alone time each day so that you can figure things out.
    d. Do all of the above.

WHAT DO YOU THINK?

LO 2.2

1. In what specific ways do you think your upbringing influenced your mental health, both positively and negatively?

LO 2.3

2. In what ways can social media sites be effective in helping people deal with shyness and loneliness? What are some examples of how participating in social medial sites might be harmful to a person's mental health?

LO 2.4

3. Why do you think today's college students have the lowest ever self-rating of emotional health?

LO 2.7

4. There are more than five times as many adolescents and young adults taking stimulants for attention disorders today than 30 years ago. Why?

LO 2.8

5. If you were worried about the possibility of a friend committing suicide, what signs would you look for? If your suspicions were confirmed, how would you help your friend?

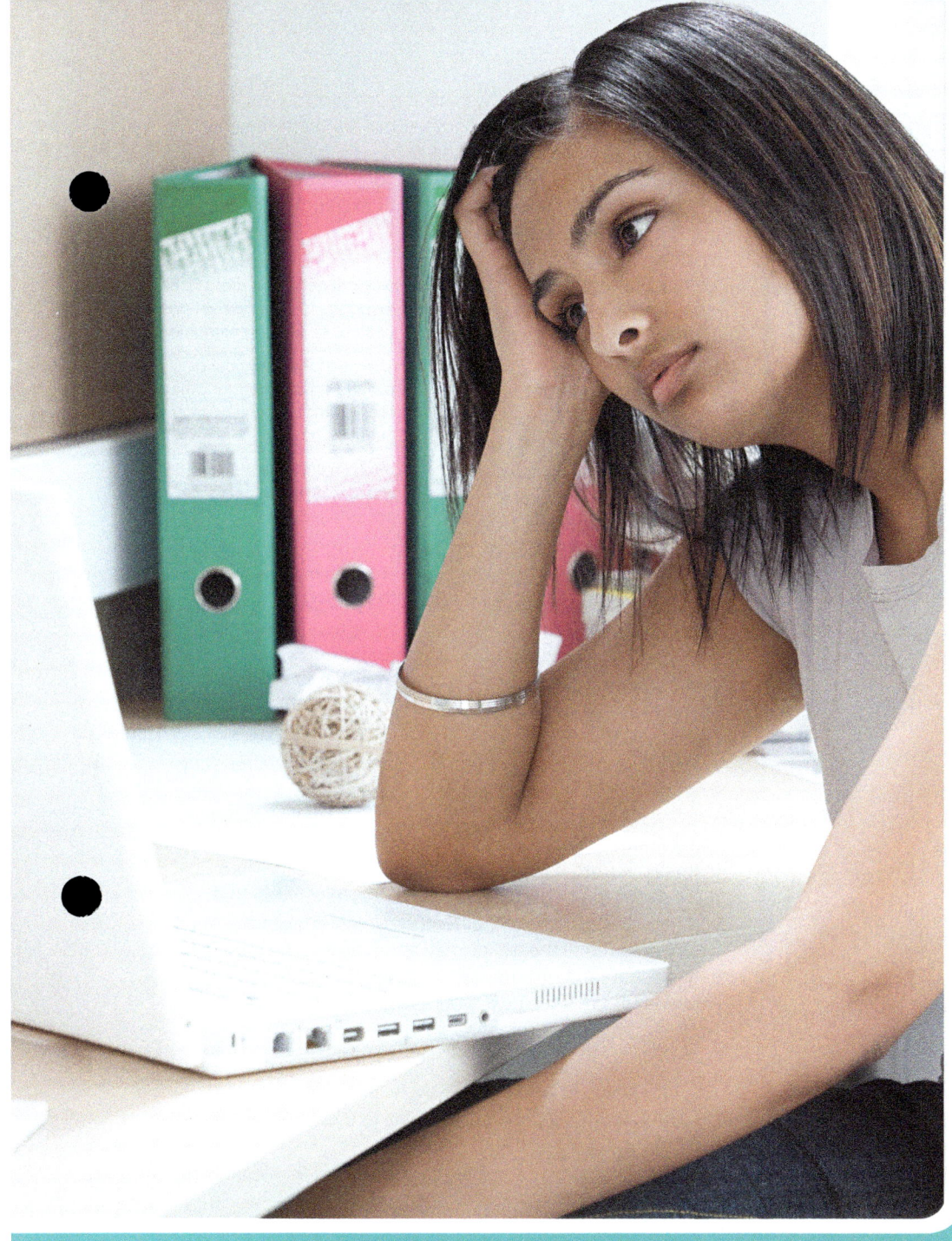

3

STRESS MANAGEMENT

> Year after year, college students report stress as the number-one obstacle to their academic achievement.[i]

> Money is the greatest source of stress among American adults in general, and the second greatest source of stress (after academics) among college students.[i,ii]

> Millennials (those aged 18–35) report the highest levels of stress of any age group in the United States.[ii]

LEARNING OUTCOMES

LO 3.1 Distinguish between stress, stressor, eustress, and distress.

LO 3.2 Describe the body's stress response.

LO 3.3 Explain why severe, longstanding stress is harmful.

LO 3.4 Discuss the influence of personality and biology on the stress response.

LO 3.5 Distinguish common sources of stress among college students.

LO 3.6 Identify social, campus, and medical resources for managing stress.

LO 3.7 Summarize strategies for effectively managing stress.

As a student, you live with stress every day.

Assignments, exams, financial challenges, relationships, concerns about the future . . . sometimes the pressure can feel overwhelming. Although you may not always be able to control these challenges, you *can* control how you deal with the stress they bring.

In this chapter, we describe the body's physical response to stress, explain why uncontrolled, long-term stress is harmful, and introduce strategies for reducing and managing stress. By the end of the chapter, you'll have the tools to analyze the sources of stress in your own life and to create a personalized action plan for better stress management.

What Is Stress?

LO 3.1 Distinguish between stress, stressor, eustress, and distress.

Each year, the American Psychological Association conducts a survey called Stress in America. The most recent survey reveals that, overall, Americans are stressed out! Nearly 30% of American adults say their stress increased over the previous year, 25% say their stress is affecting their health, and 75% report having experienced at least one symptom of stress in the previous month.[1] But what, precisely, do Americans mean when they say they're stressed?

People use the term *stress* to identify different things. They might be referring to a past, present, or anticipated event—such as an argument with a partner or an upcoming exam—that causes anxiety, or to the symptoms—such as distracting thoughts or sleep loss—that tell them they're anxious. For the purposes of this textbook, we define **stress** as the collective psychobiological condition that occurs in response to a disruptive, unexpected, or exciting stimulus. We use the term **stressor** to refer to any physical or psychological event or other change that stimulates stress.

When you think of a stressor, a major event such as a friend's death might initially come to mind. But stressors can be day-to-day demands—for instance, having to commute to school in heavy traffic or living in a crowded, noisy neighborhood. Drugs such as nicotine, alcohol, and caffeine can also be stressors, as can a junk-food diet.

Hans Selye, a pioneering stress scientist, recognized that both positive and negative stimuli can be stressors. He coined the term **eustress** (*eu-* = "good") for stress resulting from changes that are perceived as advantageous. He called stress resulting from changes that feel threatening **distress**.[2] Think about how you felt the last time your favorite sports team came from behind at the last minute to win. Then think about the last time you got a lower test grade than you had hoped. The likely differences in your feelings—excitement in the first case, dismay and worry in the second—help illustrate the distinctions between *eustress* and *distress*. However, as we'll see next, your body's response to both types of stress is the same.

> **stress** The collective psychobiological condition that occurs in response to a disruptive, unexpected, or exciting stimulus.
>
> **stressor** Any physical or psychological event or other change that causes positive or negative stress.
>
> **eustress** Stress resulting from changes that are perceived as advantageous.
>
> **distress** Stress resulting from changes that are perceived as threatening.
>
> **homeostasis** The physiological processes by which the body maintains its internal conditions within a narrow, healthful range.

LO 3.1 QUICK CHECK

Downing an energy drink on your way to morning class is an example of
a. a psychobiological condition that occurs in response to a stimulus.
b. eustress.
c. distress.
b. a stressor.

The Body's Stress Response

LO 3.2 Describe the body's stress response.

The human body has a remarkable ability to respond to change in a way that enables it to maintain its internal conditions within a narrow, healthful range. In 1932, American physiologist Walter B. Cannon named this ability **homeostasis,** from the Greek words *homios,* meaning "similar," and *stasis,* indicating a "stance." For example, let's say you eat a sundae or similar large, sweet dessert. As you digest it, a load of sugar surges into your bloodstream. In response, homeostatic control mechanisms spring into action. These include release of a chemical called *insulin* that speeds the transport of sugar into your body cells, bringing your blood sugar level back into a healthful range.

Like eating a super-sweet dessert, experiencing a stressor—whether a quarrel with a friend or a lost credit card—triggers a characteristic homeostatic response. One of the best-known explanations of this response is the **general adaptation syndrome (GAS),** developed by Hans Selye **(Figure 3.1).** Commonly called the *stress response*, the GAS includes three stages: alarm, resistance (also called adaptation), and exhaustion.[3] All three stages are not inevitable: it's only when the alarm stage continues without successful resistance that exhaustion typically occurs. In the decades since Selye introduced the GAS, further research has led to refinements in our understanding of the physiology of the stress response, as noted in the following discussion.

Alarm Stage: The Fight-or-Flight Response

Imagine that you're rock climbing. You're reaching for your next handhold when the narrow shelf of rock beneath your boots crumbles. As you scramble to find a new foothold, you're likely to experience a set of physical reactions characteristic of the alarm stage and shown in **Figure 3.2.**

What's causing all these changes? Your body, perceiving a threat, has generated two types of responses: a rapid response generated by nerves and a slower response generated by hormones.

Nervous System Response

First, your nervous system has prompted the release of two *neurotransmitters* (chemicals that transmit messages along nerves) called norepinephrine and epinephrine. Norepinephrine is released by the nerves themselves, and epinephrine is released by your adrenal glands (sitting on top of your kidneys), but they work together to quickly and dramatically alter your body's activities:

- Your lung passages widen and your breathing rate increases, boosting oxygen delivery to your body tissues.
- Your liver releases into your bloodstream its stores of a simple sugar called *glucose*, which your cells use for fuel.
- Your heart rate and blood pressure rise to increase the flow of blood—and its oxygen and glucose—to your brain, muscles, and other tissues, enhancing their response to the stressor. Your pulse quickens, too.
- Blood vessels in your body core constrict, slowing your digestion, while blood vessels serving your muscles dilate, further boosting the delivery of oxygen and glucose.
- Nerve stimulation to your muscles also increases, enabling bursts of power but making your smaller muscles—like those in your hands—tremble.
- Your pupils dilate to let in more light.
- Your circulatory system, anticipating injury, starts producing blood-clotting proteins.

Hormonal Response

Whereas the effects of the body's nervous system response are nearly instantaneous, the hormonal response requires some "travel time." **Hormones** are chemicals released by glands into the bloodstream, which transports them to their target organs elsewhere in the body. When hormones reach their target, they act in a way that regulates its activity. The second wave of the alarm stage begins when a region of your brain called the hypothalamus signals the nearby pituitary gland to release into the bloodstream a hormone called ACTH. This acronym stands for *adrenocorticotropin hormone,* reflecting the fact that

> **general adaptation syndrome (GAS)** A homeostatic response to a stressor consisting of three stages: alarm, resistance, and exhaustion.
>
> **hormone** A chemical secreted by a gland and transported through the bloodstream to a distant target organ, the activity of which it then regulates.

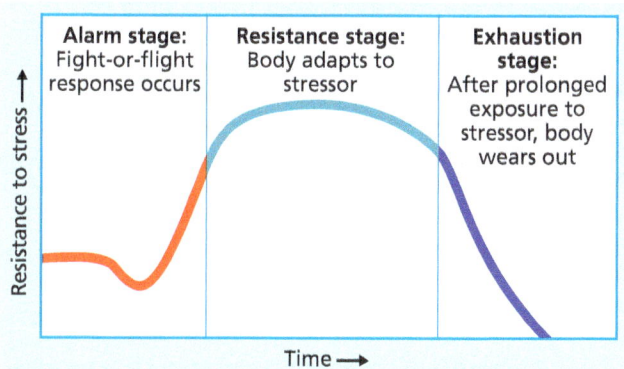

FIGURE 3.1 **The General Adaptation Syndrome.** The general adaptation syndrome, developed by Hans Selye, is a theory that attempts to explain the biology of stress.

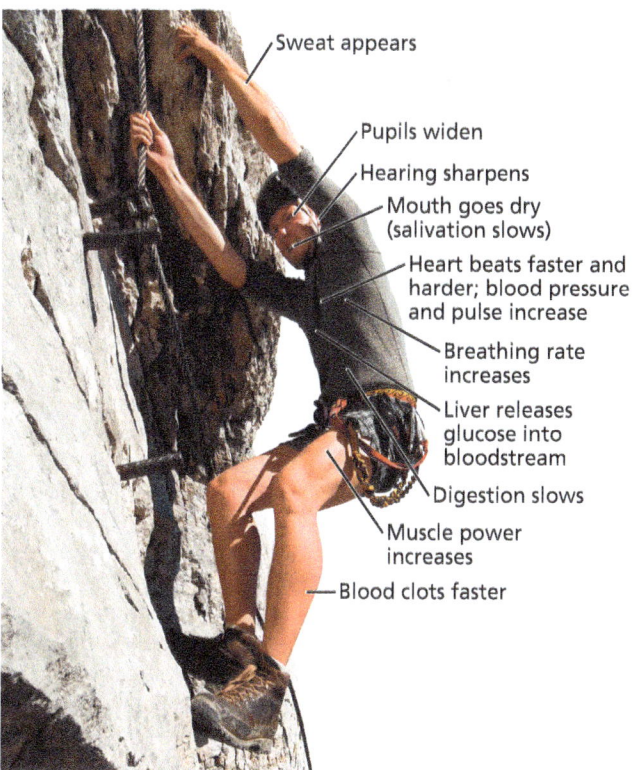

FIGURE 3.2 **The Fight-or-Flight Response.** The fight-or-flight response is a set of physical reactions that prepares you to deal with a perceived threat.

CHAPTER 3 ■ Stress Management

ACTH targets the adrenal glands, causing them to release an important stress hormone called **cortisol.** The flood of cortisol acts to both support glucose production and inhibit tissue building, leaving more of your body's raw materials to be used for generating fuel. Cortisol thereby sustains your ability to respond to the threat.

An Evolutionary Response in a Modern World

Like homeostasis, the complex set of reactions characteristic of the alarm stage was first described by Walter B. Cannon, who named it the **fight-or-flight response.** Cannon theorized that it evolved as a survival mechanism to help early humans fight an enemy or escape from a predator; probably our ancestors could not have survived in their dangerous "eat-or-be-eaten" world without it.

Even today, your fight-or-flight response can enable you to fight off a would-be assailant or flee a smoke-filled building. But it can also be unhelpful or even harmful. Most of our day-to-day stressors are not the extreme physical threats that our ancestors faced. Yet a fight-or-flight response kicks in *any* time you face a stressor—even when that stressor is mostly emotional or psychological, such as ongoing concerns about your grades, finances, or relationships. If you experience fight-or-flight reactions too often, or find yourself unable to resist them successfully, then in a sense you remain perpetually in the alarm stage. Such "high-alert" living can take a powerful toll on your body and your health.

>> Stress researcher Robert Sapolsky explains the evolution of the stress response and how it affects us today. Search for "Stress Response: Savior to Killer," at www.youtube.com.

Resistance Stage

As a stressor continues, the body mobilizes homeostatic mechanisms that help it adapt to the stressor. For example, the first time you hike a strenuous trail, you're likely to experience significant physical distress. But if you were to hike that trail twice weekly, you'd soon adapt to its demands, and it would no longer set off the alarm stage.

Even with stressors that aren't primarily physical, you can develop strategies that increase your level of resistance and help you adapt. For instance, if you're a college freshman, you might feel stress hormones pouring into your bloodstream as you sit down to take your first midterm exam. But over time, repetition helps you perceive the situation as more familiar (and thus less like a "change"). Moreover, you learn that, when you study thoroughly, you do well. Building this "track record" of success also helps calm your nerves. Finally, over time, you may learn a set of stretches, breathing techniques, or motivational phrases to keep you relaxed during exams. As a result of your growing familiarity with the situation, your confidence in your preparation, and your use of coping mechanisms, the jolt of stress you feel as you walk toward the exam room is likely to actually improve your performance by keeping you alert and focused. That's right: A little stress actually helps you do better.

This phenomenon was first identified in 1908 by psychologists Robert Yerkes and John Dodson. According to the Yerkes–Dodson law, performance improves with moderate physiological or mental arousal—which today we call stress. Similarly, in 1982, cardiologist Peter Nixon described a human function curve according to which a manageable degree of stress improves a performance . . . but too much stress leads to illness.[4]

Exhaustion Stage and Allostatic Overload

When the degree of stress is not manageable—when stressors are severe and persistent—the homeostatic mechanisms that formerly helped you adapt become depleted. Both Selye and Nixon recognized that, at this point, your body enters the exhaustion stage and, as a result, you experience stress-related disease and **burnout.**

Recently, some researchers have introduced the term **allostatic overload** to describe the exhaustion stage. The prefix *allo-* means "variability," so an allostatic overload is a harmful state resulting from the cumulative burden of adapting, again and again, to stress.[5] But whether researchers call it exhaustion or allostatic overload, most agree that the result of chronic, excessive stress is a failure of homeostasis, which manifests as disease.

An even more recent topic of stress research is underload! Increasingly, researchers are finding that boredom—for example, working a tedious job all day—can lead to headaches, stomachaches, and other problems usually associated with overload. In one recent study, participants watching a boring movie experienced greater surges in cortisol and other signs of stress than participants watching an emotionally engaging movie.[6] Thus, as we noted earlier, moderate stress can be beneficial.

cortisol An adrenal gland hormone that is secreted at higher levels during the stress response.

fight-or-flight response A series of physiological reactions to a stressor designed to enable the body to stand and fight or to flee.

burnout A phenomenon in which increased feelings of stress and decreased feelings of accomplishment lead to frustration, exhaustion, lack of motivation, and disengagement.

allostatic overload A harmful state resulting from the cumulative burden of adapting, again and again, to stress.

LO 3.2 QUICK CHECK

You're on vacation in the Bahamas when you wake up in the middle of the night to your hotel's fire alarm. As you leap out of bed, you are in

a. the nervous-system phase of the alarm stage.
b. the hormonal phase of the alarm stage.
c. the resistance stage of the GAS.
d. allostatic overload.

Health Effects of Chronic Stress

LO 3.3 Explain why severe, longstanding stress is harmful.

Physical symptoms associated with acute stress include fatigue, lying awake at night, headache, upset stomach,

STUDENT STORY

The Stress of Responsibility

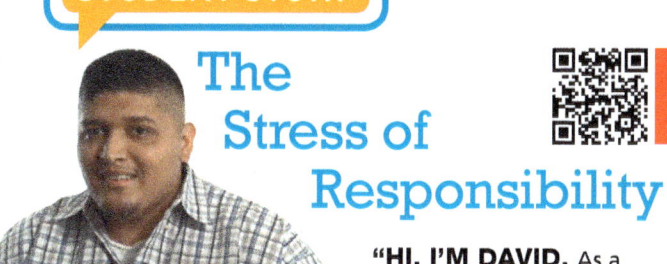

"HI, I'M DAVID. As a nontraditional student, some of the things that stress me out are maybe a little bit different than what other students go through. I own a house. I have to pay a mortgage, bills, and taxes. I have to put food on my kids' table, clothing on their backs, and spend time with my wife. These things really stress me out! And on top of all of that, I'm a full-time college student.

One of the ways that I balance being a family man and college student is to try to keep both worlds separate. I know that when I go to school, that's what I need to concentrate on. I try to do all my homework and everything else at school. And when I go home, I try to leave the school behind. Sometimes the two blend together, but that's a good thing, I think."

What Do You Think?

1. Identify at least three stressors that David is dealing with. Do these stressors cause *eustress* or *distress*?
2. How well do you think David is managing his stress load?
3. If David's stress were to increase so much that he felt unable to cope, what negative health effects could he experience?

---

muscle tension, change in sex drive, teeth grinding, dizziness, feeling a tightness in the chest, and, for women, a change in the menstrual cycle. The feelings most commonly attributed to acute stress include anger, irritability, nervousness, lack of motivation, a sense of being overwhelmed, and depression or sadness.[1]

You're unlikely to become seriously ill simply because of a few days of acute stress. In contrast, most researchers acknowledge that severe, longstanding stress—that is, stress that continues for months to years—increases your risk for a variety of health problems **(Figure 3.3)**.

Effects on the Cardiovascular System

Stress causes the heart to pump harder and faster, raising blood pressure. Studies have shown that chronically elevated cortisol levels significantly increase an individual's risk for cardiovascular disease, including experiencing a heart attack or stroke.[7] This is in part because chronically elevated cortisol intensifies the nervous system phase of the alarm stage whenever you encounter a new stressor. This intensified response includes, for example, a dramatic increase in blood pressure.[8]

> *"Both children and adults who are overweight or obese report greater stress levels compared with people of normal weight."*

Chronic stress is also an important risk factor for atherosclerosis—that's the buildup of deposits in blood vessels that can lead to a heart attack or stroke. Stress appears to increase the risk of inflammation in blood vessel walls, which is the first step in the development of atherosclerotic deposits.[9] In a recent laboratory study, a group of mice given cortisol for 13 weeks developed significant atherosclerosis.[10]

Effects on Digestion, Glucose Regulation, and Body Weight

Your digestive tract has its own network of nerves called *enteric nerves*. In response to norepinephrine, the activity of these nerves is inhibited. In addition, when the fight-or-flight response causes blood vessels in the body core to constrict, the stomach and intestines don't get the fuel they need to perform their functions. Both of these factors can contribute to stomachache, constipation, or diarrhea. You might be wondering whether stress can trigger the formation of ulcers. Check out the nearby **Myth or Fact?** box to find the answer.

As noted earlier, the neurotransmitters and hormones released during the alarm stage prompt increased blood glucose, which is helpful in responding to a threat. However, when cells are continually confronted with high blood

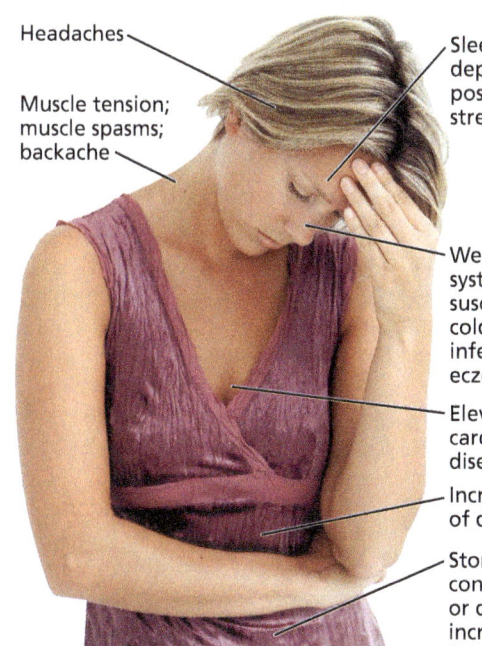

FIGURE 3.3 **Health Effects of Severe, Long-Term Stress.**

MYTH OR FACT?

Can Stress Give You an Ulcer?

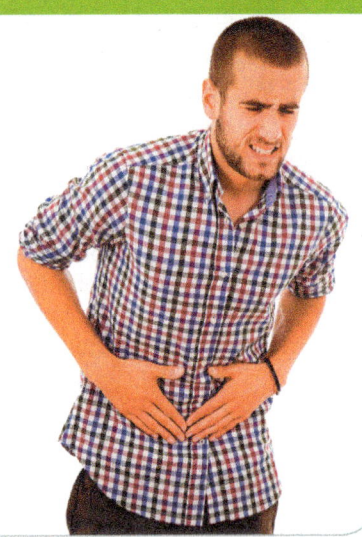

You've got a huge set of lab problems to solve for class, and you're way behind on getting it done. After a quick dinner of cold, old pizza, you head for the library. Your stomach is killing you—again. Yes, the pizza was nasty. But you still wonder if all the pressure this term is giving you an ulcer.

Ulcers are lesions in the lining of the stomach or small intestine that can cause pain, bloating, and nausea. But though your stress could be affecting your digestion, it probably isn't directly causing an ulcer. Researchers have found that most ulcers are caused by a species of bacteria called *Helicobacter pylori* that thrives in the acidic environment of the stomach. Ulcers not due to *H. pylori* infection most likely result from overuse of anti-inflammatory pain medications such as aspirin or ibuprofen. Smokers also have an increased risk of ulcers, and their ulcers are especially resistant to healing.

Although researchers no longer believe that stress directly causes ulcers, studies have shown that chronic stress can increase stomach acid production, impair your immune system, and make the symptoms of an ulcer worse. If you suffer from ongoing stomach pain, visit your campus health center or personal doctor.

References: **1.** Mayo Clinic. (2013, July 26). *Peptic ulcer: Causes.* www.mayoclinic.org. **2.** DiMarino, M. C. (2014, May). Peptic ulcer disease. *Merck Manual Professional Version.* www.merckmanuals.com.

---

glucose, they begin to resist the effects of insulin, the hormone mentioned earlier that helps them take up the glucose from the bloodstream. This insulin resistance is a key factor in the development of diabetes. Thus it's not surprising that some studies associate longstanding elevated cortisol levels with an increased diabetes risk.[11,12]

Several recent studies support a link between longstanding stress and increased storage of so-called visceral fat, a layer of fat covering your abdominal organs.[13,14] Visceral fat is known to increase your risk for both cardiovascular disease and diabetes. Of course, stress can also contribute to overall weight gain by inducing a longing for sweets, chips, or other "comfort foods" high in calories.[15] In addition, both children and adults who are overweight or obese report greater stress levels compared with people of normal weight.[16]

Effects on the Immune System

Do you always seem to get sick during finals week? At the end of the term, a quarter or semester's worth of stress may weaken your body's ability to fight off viruses and other infections. **Psychoneuroimmunology** is the study of interactions among psychological processes, the nervous system, hormones, and the immune system. When acute stress activates the fight-or-flight response, your body's release of neurotransmitters and hormones may actually strengthen your immune system. Even stress from relatively minor events such as academic exams can cause temporary increases in white blood cell counts, a sign that the immune system has been activated to ward off a threat.[17] However, longstanding stress can decrease your immune cells' number and function, reducing their ability to protect you from infection. It can also increase the negative effects of the immune response, such as low-grade inflammation.[18]

psychoneuroimmunology The study of interactions among psychological processes, the nervous system, hormones, and the immune system.

Stress and Headaches

Any chemical activity affecting either your brain tissue or the nerves, blood vessels, or muscles serving your head and neck can trigger headaches. As you've learned, the stress response releases a surge of such chemicals.

The most common headaches are tension headaches. They're mild to moderate in severity, typically last less than a day, and often feel as if a tight band were around your head. Migraines, in contrast, are severe and tend to last hours to a few days. They are often described as throbbing and can be accompanied by nausea and extreme sensitivity to light and sound.

In two recent studies, one involving adults and one with teens, a high stress or anxiety score was significantly associated with an increased incidence of both recurrent tension headaches and chronic migraines.[19,20]

Effects on Sleep

Adequate sleep is essential to conserve body energy; grow, repair, and restore your body's cells and tissues; maintain your immune system; and organize and synthesize new learning and memories. Unfortunately, many college students are not experiencing the benefits of enough sleep: A national survey found that 4.6% of college students had been diagnosed with insomnia in the past year, and 20% said that sleep problems affected their academic performance.[21] Although many factors can interfere with sleep, stress is a common culprit.[22] In turn, not getting enough sleep increases the physical stress placed on your body. (You'll learn more about sleep and its many health benefits in Chapter 4.)

Effects on Relationships and Sexual Functioning

Next time you're stressed out, check your human connections! As you probably know instinctively, supportive relationships can help you cope with stress. But chronic stress can damage relationships, causing you to feel irritable, impatient, or too fatigued to accommodate a partner's needs. Stress "spilling over" from a partner's job or academic pressures, for example, is widely acknowledged as a threat to happiness within a marriage.[23]

Chronic stress can also have a negative effect on sexual functioning, frequency, and satisfaction—for both men and women.[24] It can also reduce fertility. In one study, women whose saliva samples showed a high level of an enzyme strongly linked to chronic stress had more than double the risk of infertility.[25]

Effects on Mind and Mental Health

In a national survey, college students rated stress as their top impediment to academic performance.[21] But the association between stress and grades is ambiguous. Some studies associate moderate stress with higher class attendance and better performance.[26] Others find that it's our interpretation of our anxiety that matters; that is, when faced with an upcoming exam or presentation, students who view their anxiety as motivating typically perform better than students who experience their anxiety as threatening. The lesson may be that you shouldn't worry about your worry![27]

Chronic stress is an important risk factor for many mental disorders. For example, major life stressors, especially those prompting interpersonal stress, are recognized as the primary risk factors for depression.[28] And some researchers theorize that an inappropriate activation of the alarm stage may partly underlie panic attacks (sudden episodes of intense fear), which feature the same neurotransmitter and hormonal responses.[29] Unfortunately, stress and mental health problems often form a vicious cycle; when an individual experiencing severe long-term stress develops depression, for example, that condition can strain their relationships, threaten their employment and finances, and increase other stressors in their lives.

As a college student, you're bound to feel some degree of stress. So how do you know whether a few signs and symptoms you might be experiencing are normal—or increase your risk for illness? Check out the **Practical Strategies** box on page 58 for help recognizing the signs of stress overload.

LO 3.3 QUICK CHECK

The risk of developing both cardiovascular disease and diabetes is increased in people who have a chronically high level of what hormone circulating in their bloodstream?
a. cholesterol
b. cortisol
c. glucose
d. caffeine

What Influences the Stress Response?

LO 3.4 Discuss the influence of personality and biology on the stress response.

We said earlier that our perception of a change as advantageous, neutral, or threatening influences whether we experience distress. But two people can perceive the same change in different ways. Why is this the case? Stress researchers believe that personality, sex, and age can all play a part.

The Role of Personality Types

A **personality type** is a set of behavioral tendencies. For instance, if you tend to analyze situations, someone might refer to you as a left-brain type, as opposed to a right-brain type who makes creative leaps. In 1959, cardiologists Meyer Friedman and Ray Rosenman proposed a relationship between personality type and risk for cardiovascular disease.[30] They described a *type A* personality characterized by impatience,

> **personality type** A set of behavioral tendencies.

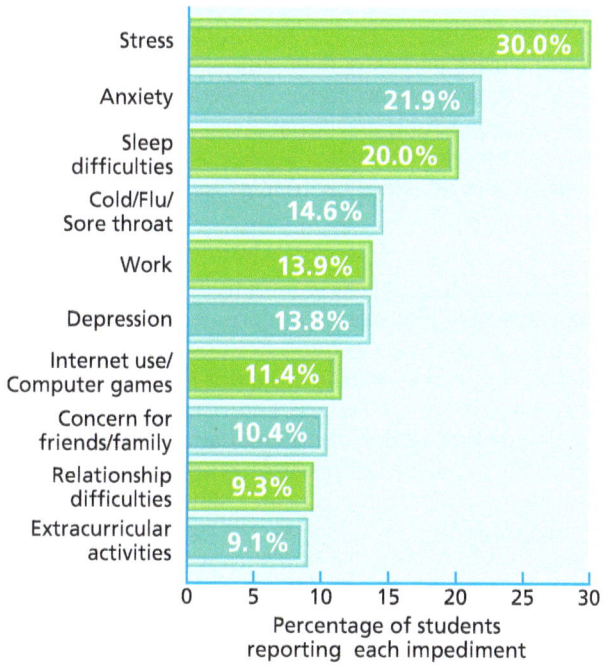

STUDENT STATS

Top 10 Impediments to Academic Performance

- Stress — 30.0%
- Anxiety — 21.9%
- Sleep difficulties — 20.0%
- Cold/Flu/Sore throat — 14.6%
- Work — 13.9%
- Depression — 13.8%
- Internet use/Computer games — 11.4%
- Concern for friends/family — 10.4%
- Relationship difficulties — 9.3%
- Extracurricular activities — 9.1%

Percentage of students reporting each impediment

Data from *ACHA-NCHA II undergraduate reference group executive summary, spring 2015*, by the American College Health Association, 2015, www.acha-ncha.org.

PRACTICAL Strategies

Recognizing the Signs of Stress Overload

It's important to be able to recognize the warning signs of too much stress before they add up to a serious health problem. While many people find the following symptoms common, keep in mind that stress affects different individuals in different ways. You may have less-typical signs of stress, but they still merit the same attention.

Emotional warning signs
- Anxiety
- Sleep disruption
- Anger and agitation
- Trouble concentrating
- Unproductive worry
- Frequent mood swings
- Depression

Physical warning signs
- Stooped posture
- Sweaty palms
- Chronic fatigue
- Weight loss or weight gain
- Migraine or tension headaches
- Neck aches
- Digestive problems
- Asthma attacks

- Physical symptoms that your doctor can't attribute to another condition

Behavioral warning signs
- Overreacting to problems or difficult situations
- Increased use of alcohol, tobacco, or drugs
- Unusually impulsive behavior
- Withdrawing from relationships or contact with others
- Feeling "burned out" on school or work
- Frequent bouts of crying

If you're experiencing the warning signs of stress overload, use the stress management techniques outlined in this chapter. Also, consult your college health center, which may offer classes, workshops, or individual or group counseling to further help you cope with stress.

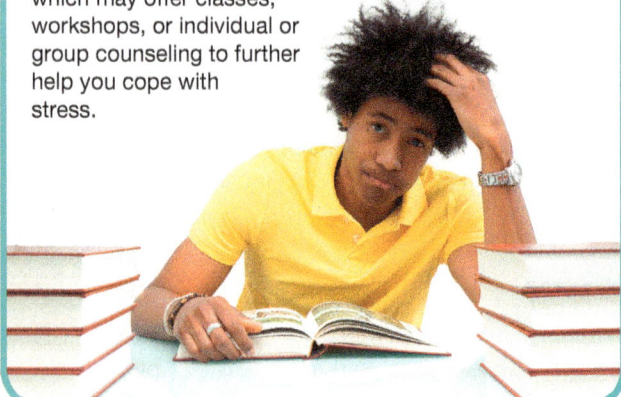

irritability, hostility, low self-esteem, and a competitive drive. Their research found that type A people had twice the risk for cardiovascular disease as people with a *type B* personality, who are patient, tolerant, and friendly, with a realistic sense of self-esteem.[30]

Two additional personality types have been proposed: *Type C* people are said to be stoic and to internalize stress, whereas *type D* people are described as responding to stressful situations either with resignation or withdrawal. These types may also be linked to certain health risks.

In thinking about these various personality types, it's important to recognize that there is a great deal of debate among researchers as to whether the types have any real validity. Although they may be useful in theory, they cannot explain the complexity of human personality or behavior, and they cannot fully capture how each of us responds to stress over the course of our lives.

The Role of Personality Traits

Some stress researchers have linked certain personality traits to an improved ability to adapt to stress. Primary among these are optimism, hardiness, and resilience:[31]

- **Optimism.** People who are optimistic are likely to see stressors as transient and specific and, therefore, within their power to change and control. At the same time, they are less likely to view stressors as a consequence of internal faults. (For more on optimism, see Chapter 2.)

- **Hardiness.** Social psychologist Suzanne Kobasa identified a quality she called *hardiness* as important in enabling a person to successfully navigate the resistance stage of the stress response.[32] Hardiness is an ability to respond to the challenges of life and turn them into opportunities for growth. It includes a strong commitment to yourself, a sense of meaningfulness, an attitude of vigorousness toward your environment, and an internal locus of control (see Chapter 1).[32] A recent study of nursing students found that hardiness training improved stress management and increased GPA.[33]

- **Resilience.** The American Psychological Association defines *resilience* as the process of adapting well to adversity.[34] Resilient people are typically able to make realistic plans and carry them out, and they are confident in their power to do so. They communicate well, can manage strong feelings and impulses, and are skilled at solving problems. Studies of college students suggest that resilience contributes to mental health and a higher GPA.[35]

Other personality traits have been associated specifically with an increased ability to manage day-to-day stressors. For example, conscientiousness—a principled carefulness in one's actions—is strongly linked to reduced reactivity to minor stressors overall, and agreeableness—kindness and consideration of others—appears to protect people against the effects of stressful social situations.[36] Although personality traits might seem fixed, you can change your patterns of thinking and responding, as we discuss later in this chapter.

The Role of Biology

Year after year, the Stress in America survey mentioned earlier finds that sex and age strongly influence our experience of stress.[1] For example, women report higher levels of stress than men, and they are more likely than men to report experiencing a wide variety of symptoms of stress, including worry, depression, and fatigue. More than 50% of women versus 32% of men report that they have lain awake at night in the past month because of stress. The factors contributing to these variations may include differences in the sex chromosomes, in socialization of girls versus boys, or in the types of and susceptibility to stressors in women's and men's lives.

Growing older appears to mean growing wiser when it comes to stress. Millennials (those aged 18–35) report the highest levels of stress (5.5 on a scale of 1 to 10) of any age group in the United States, and Americans aged 36 to 50 are close behind (5.4). In contrast, Americans aged 51 to 70 report lower stress levels (4.5), and those over 70 report levels even lower (3.5). Moreover, 51% of Millennials say they have lain awake at night during the past month because of stress, versus only 27% of Americans over 70.[1] A recent study combining data from nearly 200,000 individuals from 83 countries points to increasing levels of trust as a key factor in reducing stress as we age.[37] The study also identified as factors the greater ability of older adults to shake off minor frustrations and insults and to give back to others.

LO 3.4 QUICK CHECK

Mara's belongings were destroyed when her apartment building caught fire. For a few weeks, she lived with friends who let her borrow what she needed, and when her insurance money came through, she rented a new apartment. Mara is exhibiting

a. type A personality.
b. type C personality.
c. resilience.
d. an external locus of control.

What Are College Students' Common Stressors?

LO 3.5 Distinguish common sources of stress among college students.

Among college students, academic pressure, money, work, and relationships are common stressors.

Academic Pressure

A recent national survey of college students found that, within the prior 30 days, two-thirds (67.3%) of students had felt overwhelmed by all they had to do.[21] Much of this overload is academic; 45% of students reported that their academic responsibilities had been traumatic or very difficult to handle, making academic pressure the most significant stressor in students' lives.[21] A key contributor to many college students' academic struggles is procrastination. You might think dragging your feet on assignments and studying is simply a "bad habit," but new research suggests that there's more to it. See the nearby **Special Feature** to learn more.

Financial Stressors

More than one-third of U.S. college students report that, within the past year, their finances have been traumatic or very difficult to handle.[21] Moreover, a recent national survey found that 72% of college students feel stressed about money.[38] Students commonly worry about their ability to pay for tuition, books, and fees, but some struggle even to pay for food. Like low-income Americans overall, struggling college students are often disproportionately burdened by stress and stress-related illness. For example, studies have associated lower socioeconomic status with higher levels of circulating cortisol, which in turn promotes the stress-related health problems discussed earlier.[39] Moreover, financial stress may be self-perpetuating: Anxiety about money is thought to lead to short-sighted and risk-averse decision making that limits a person's ability to achieve long-term goals, including better health and greater financial security.[40]

Many people, especially students, find it difficult to manage money. The **Practical Strategies** box on page 60 provides some tips.

Job-Related Stressors

In addition to academics and finances, you may also be stressed about work responsibilities. About 72% of American undergraduates hold a job, and more than half of these students work at least 20 hours a week.[41] About 20% of undergraduates actually work full-time, year-round! Although employment can of course ease your financial stress, it brings stress of its own when it cuts into your time for classwork. Not surprisingly, more than one-fourth of college students report being stressed out by work-related issues.[21]

Social Stressors

Supportive relationships with family members, friends, and romantic partners can act as buffers against stress.[42] On the other hand, a growing body of behavioral and neurological research suggests that the absence of strong social ties—essentially, loneliness—can promote a level of stress that can be harmful to your health.[43] As compared to socially connected people, lonely people have higher levels of circulating stress hormones as well as greater evidence of cellular stress and a weaker immune response. Loneliness is unfortunately common among college students: In a 2015 national survey, more than 37% of students reported having felt "very lonely" within the past 30 days.[21]

Although social networks can do a great deal to help carry you through tough times, research into the effects of social networking using sites like Facebook is mixed. For example, a recent study that examined 1.5 million college students' Facebook messaging found that the formation of social relationships helps students cope with high-stress situations and build resilience.[44] But the number and type of postings matter; another recent study links frequent social networking on sites like Facebook with increased levels of distress due to both communication overload and reduced self-esteem.[45]

SPECIAL FEATURE

Procrastination
Sabotaging Your Future Self

You got the syllabus in September, so why is it Thanksgiving weekend, and you still haven't started working on a term paper that's due in December? The simple answer is procrastination—but it's a more complex problem than merely poor time management.

Procrastination is commonly defined as delaying a task you view as unpleasant even though you know that doing so will cause you suffering. Research suggests that it's fundamentally a failure to recognize and regulate your emotions in the moment. From an evolutionary perspective, the anxiety you experience when facing a threat is motivational. Your fight-or-flight response is telling you to tackle it or flee it. When threatened by a wild animal, your primitive ancestors might have chosen either response, but as a college student, the only way to deal with that research paper is to get it done. Delaying and denying might soothe your anxiety in the short term, but over time, procrastination sabotages the security and happiness of your "future self."[1]

So what can you do about it? Here's where acceptance and commitment therapy (introduced in Chapter 2) can help.[2] When task anxiety arises, acknowledge that you're freaking out! Accept your emotions without judgment. Then redirect your attention onto your values and goals, the reasons you're willing to face your fears. Maybe you want to teach low-income kids or help reduce climate change. Remind yourself, aloud or in writing, of these goals and what you have to do to achieve them: Writing the paper is necessary to pass the course, which you must do to get your degree, which will qualify you for the career you seek. Finally, get practical. Make a schedule that breaks up the task into discrete, smaller steps, and stick to it. You'll get more help with managing tasks and time later in this chapter.

Sources: **1.** Sirois, F. M., & Pychyl, T. A. (2013). Procrastination and the priority of short-term mood regulation: Consequences for future self. *Social and Personality Psychology Compass, 7*(2), 115–127. doi: 10.1111/spc3.12011.

2. A-Tjak, J. G., Davis, M. L., Morina, N., Powers, M. B., Smits, J. A., & Emmelkamp, P. M. (2015). A meta-analysis of the efficacy of acceptance and commitment therapy for clinically relevant mental and physical health problems. *Psychotherapy and Psychosomatics, 84*(1), 30–36. doi: 10.1159/000365764.

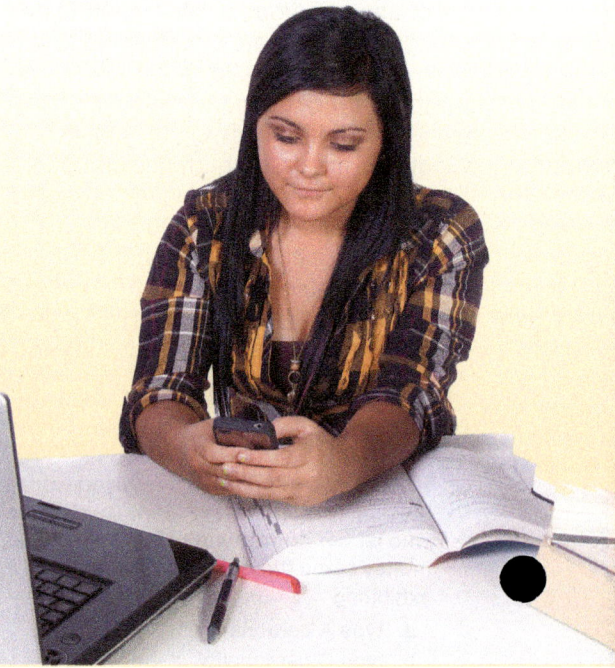

✱ PRACTICAL Strategies

Coping with Financial Stress

Surveys over many years reveal money as among the top stressors reported by college students.

The following are some strategies for coping with financial stress:

- To get a realistic handle on your finances, make a budget. How much money do you have coming in from your family, your job, and/or financial aid? How much money does it take to pay your rent, groceries, books and tuition, clothing, transportation, utilities, and day-to-day expenses? Try a (free) online budget tracker, such as the ones listed in the **Get Connected** section on page 72, which makes it easy for you to input information and identify where you can cut back.
- If you're carrying any credit card debt, develop a plan for paying it off. Reserve a set amount of money each month for paying off debt and *stick to it*. You will feel less stress just by having a plan in place than if you do nothing and watch your debt mount.
- Increase your income by taking on or increasing your hours in a part-time job—no matter how small. If there are no jobs to be found, get entrepreneurial! Consider your skills and advertise your services—for example, tutoring, babysitting, lawn mowing, housecleaning . . . you get the picture.
- Take an honest look at your current lifestyle. Do you pay for cable/premium TV or a cell phone plus a land line? How much money do you spend each month on eating out, or on small but daily expenses like bottled water or expensive coffee drinks? Distinguish luxuries from true necessities and *pare back*. You might be surprised at how all the "little things" can add up to a sizable chunk of change.
- Talk to a financial aid advisor to make sure you've explored all the aid options available to you. This is especially important if your family's financial circumstances—due to job loss, illness, or divorce, for instance—have recently changed. Ask for information about private scholarships available to students in their second and subsequent years of college. Consider additional student loans only if you feel certain you will be able to pay them back.

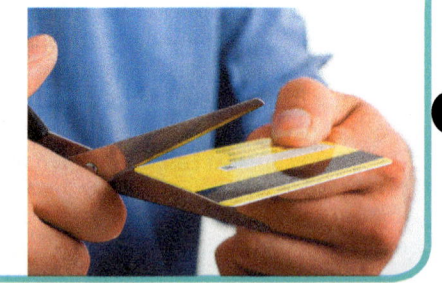

DIVERSITY & HEALTH

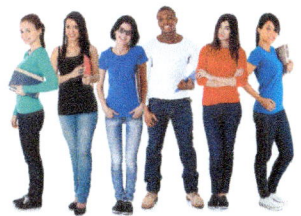

Stress in Minority Populations

Prejudice and discrimination are daily realities for many people whose gender identity, sexual orientation, religious beliefs or non-beliefs, race or ethnicity, or other factors distinguish them from the populations among which they live or work. The *minority stress model* proposes that day-to-day exposure to prejudice and discrimination causes higher stress levels within minority populations as compared to non-minorities, and it negatively affects their well-being.[1,2]

For example, the model recognizes that the increased risk of mental disorders and suicide in LGBT individuals is in part a consequence of living in a threatening environment.[3] Similarly, an extensive review study found that a primary source of stress for atheists and agnostics was the negative perceptions others hold about them.[4] And in a study of Mexican American teens, higher levels of circulating cortisol were strongly associated with self-reports of higher levels of perceived discrimination.[5]

Another disturbing consequence of minority stress is its influence on health-related choices: Among African Americans, everyday discrimination has been associated with increased rates of smoking, eating a low-quality diet, and sleeping fewer hours—behaviors strongly associated with cardiovascular disease.[6] In fact, the risk of premature death from a heart attack or stroke is nearly double among African Americans compared to among Caucasians. And overall, racial and ethnic minorities are more likely than Caucasian Americans to report fair or poor physical and mental health.[7]

What Do You Think?

1. In Chapter 1, we discussed determinants of health. What type of determinant is discrimination? In addition to its association with harmful lifestyle choices such as smoking, how might discrimination contribute to health disparities?

2. Do you experience minority stress? Explain your answer.

3. Have you observed instances of discrimination toward others on your campus or in your community? How are individuals or organizations responding to this discrimination? In your opinion, are these responses effective? If not, what changes would you suggest?

References **1.** Sawyer, P. J., Major, B., Casad, B. J., Townsend, S. S., & Mendes, W. B. (2012). Discrimination and the stress response: Psychological and physiological consequences of anticipating prejudice in interethnic interactions. *American Journal of Public Health, 102*(5), 1020–1026. **2.** Bijleveld, E., Scheepers, D., & Ellemers, N. (2012). The cortisol response to anticipated intergroup interactions predicts self-reported prejudice. *PLOS One, 7*(3), e33681. **3.** Pandya, A. (2014). Mental health as an advocacy priority in the lesbian, gay, bisexual, and transgender communities. *Journal of Psychiatric Practice, 20*(3), 225–227. doi: 10.1097/01.pra.0000450322.06612.a1. **4.** Weber, S. R., Pargament, K. I., Kunik, M. E., Lomax, J. W. II, & Stanley, M. A. (2012). Psychological distress among religious nonbelievers: A systematic review. *Journal of Religion and Health, 51*(1), 72–86. doi: 10.1007/s10943-011-9541-1. **5.** Zeiders, K. H., Doane, L. D., & Roosa, M. W. (2012). Perceived discrimination and diurnal cortisol: Examining relations among Mexican American adolescents. *Hormones and Behavior, 61*(4), 541–548. **6.** Sims, M., Diez-Roux, A. V., Gebreab, S. Y., Brenner, A., Dubbert, P., et al. (2015). Perceived discrimination is associated with health behaviours among African-Americans in the Jackson Heart Study. *Journal of Epidemiology & Community Health*. doi: 10.1136/jech-2015-206390. **7.** U.S. Centers for Disease Control and Prevention. (2013, November). *CDC Health Disparities & Inequalities Report—U.S. 2013*. www.cdc.gov.

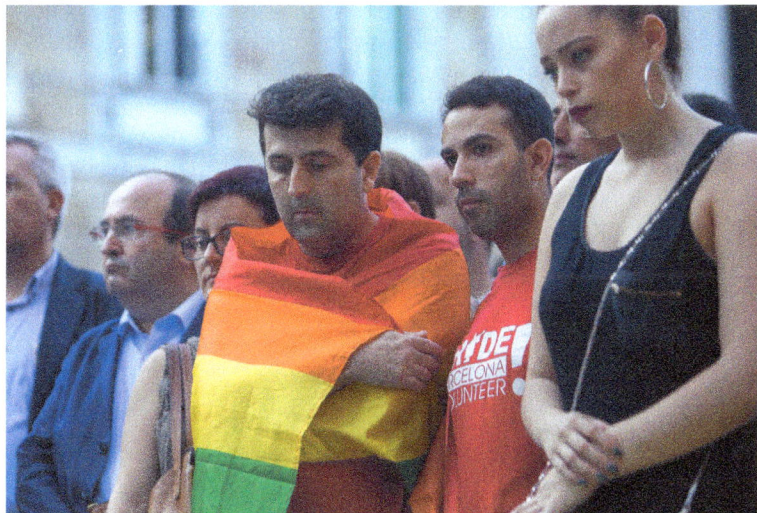

LGBT students, like those belonging to other minority groups, face unique stressors.

Different population groups can perceive or experience stress in varying ways. Discrimination, for example, may be a source of stress for members of minority groups. Minority stress is examined in more detail in the **Diversity & Health** box above.

Minor Hassles and Major Life Changes

Yesterday the bursar's office said they couldn't find evidence you'd paid your tuition this term, even though your bank says the check has been cashed. Today the subway you take to campus broke down, and you missed your morning class. These stressors may sound small, but daily hassles can lead to "stressor pile-up," which in turn can have multiple negative effects on your health.[46]

Traumas such as a bad breakup or a death in the family are obvious stressors. But positive, exhilarating events such as starting college or getting married can also bring heavy doses of stress. In 1967, psychiatrists Thomas Holmes and Richard Rahe published what has come to be known as Holmes and Rahe's Social Readjustment Rating

> *"Digital technologies (such as cell phones) that beep to alert you to text messages or voicemails can also be a subtle source of environmental stress."*

Scale (SRRS), an inventory of 43 stressful life events that can increase the risk of illness.[47] The scale assigns "life change units" from 1 to 100 for each stressful event, such as the death of a spouse (100 units), personal injury or illness (53 units), and marriage (50 units). The scale also includes more minor stressors, such as a change in living conditions (25 units). According to this scale, the higher the number of "life change units" a person accumulates over a given year, the greater that person's risk of illness. More recently, researchers have developed a similar "Negative Event Scale" for college students. Complete the **Self-Assessment** on page 63 to gauge the stress load in your own life.

Environmental Stressors

Environmental stressors are factors at home, on campus, or on the job that you find disruptive. Examples include pollution, noise, and severe weather—as well as having an annoying roommate and living in an unsafe neighborhood or in housing where you're concerned that the security is lax. Digital technologies (such as cell phones) that beep to alert you to text messages or voicemails can also be a subtle source of environmental stress.

Internal Stressors

In an era when few of our stressors are physical, some of our most constant stressors are worries, critical thoughts, and the demands we place on ourselves. Researchers have long recognized, for example, a correlation between perfectionism and high stress levels, and studies have shown that methods for reducing perfectionistic attitudes among college students decrease stress.[48]

Do you find yourself overreacting to small problems? Do you view every task as critical when many of them really aren't? When you make a mistake, do you feel ashamed? Are you often imagining horrific consequences for your actions that will probably never come to pass? Later in this chapter we explore ways you can change your thinking and thereby reduce your stress.

LO 3.5 QUICK CHECK ✔

College students report that their most significant stressor is their
a. academic workload.
b. finances.
c. job.
d. relationships.

Resources for Managing Stress

LO 3.6 Identify social, campus, and medical resources for managing stress.

Sometimes we face stress that feels truly overwhelming. If you find yourself having trouble managing stress on your own, seek help from your social network, campus community, or health-care providers.

Social Support

We noted earlier that social support offers protection against distress throughout the life span, but this is especially true during times of intense change, such as when you're transitioning from dependence on your family to independent adulthood.[42] The Stress in America survey mentioned earlier found that self-reported stress levels are much higher (on a scale from 1 to 10, 6.2 versus 4.8) among people who say they have no one to rely on for emotional support.[1] In contrast, a recent study of college students found that while unhealthful coping mechanisms like drinking or drug use harm well-being, positive social support brings a major boost.[49] So calling your family and making time for your friends, especially old friends who know you well, can help you keep the stress in your life in perspective. At the same time, building a new network of friends in your residence hall, classes, or social clubs will let you find support in a group that knows the pressures you face firsthand.

When you're under stress yourself, it may seem impossible to fit in time for others. But taking a few minutes each day to support a friend can benefit both of you. When friends are stressed, even a brief text or a supportive email can make a big difference. Invite someone to take a break for coffee or play a fast game of basketball. And if a friend seems dangerously stressed, help him or her find professional support through your campus health center.

Help on Campus

Confused about course materials or assignments? Ask your instructors for help. Visit them in person during office hours to get a new perspective on material you don't understand, to voice your concerns, or to get advice on how to prepare for exams.

Your campus might also offer peer tutoring, peer counseling, or support groups and programs for various stressors, from illness to discrimination. For example, making the transition from home to campus—a huge stressor for first-year students—can be easier if students have access to stress management information and services. A new program aims to give students exactly that. Called *The Transition Year*, it's jointly sponsored by the American Psychiatric Association and the Jed Foundation, a nonprofit established by Donna and Phil Saltow, who lost their son Jed to suicide. The campaign includes a website that offers tools and links to help students manage their stress.

▶▶ Check out the Jed Foundation's website at **www.transitionyear.org**.

SELF-ASSESSMENT
Negative Event Scale for University Students

Below is a list of items that can be negative events. **Please remember that it is important that you** circle one number for each item even if there was no hassle **and consider each item with** only the last month in mind.

How much of a *hassle* was this negative event?
- 0 = Did not occur
- 1 = Event occurred but there was no hassle
- 2 = Event occurred and was a little bit of a hassle
- 3 = Event occurred and was somewhat of a hassle
- 4 = Event occurred and was a lot of a hassle
- 5 = Event occurred and was an extreme hassle

In the past month:

Problems with Friends
1. Negative feedback from your friend/s   0 1 2 3 4 5
2. Negative communication with friend/s   0 1 2 3 4 5
3. Conflict with friend/s   0 1 2 3 4 5
4. Disagreement with friend/s   0 1 2 3 4 5

Problems with Your Spouse/Partner (Boyfriend/Girlfriend)
5. Negative communication with your spouse/partner (boyfriend/girlfriend)   0 1 2 3 4 5
6. Conflict with spouse/partner (boyfriend/girlfriend)   0 1 2 3 4 5
7. Disagreement with spouse/partner (boyfriend/girlfriend)   0 1 2 3 4 5
8. Rejection by your spouse/partner (boyfriend/girlfriend)   0 1 2 3 4 5
9. Your spouse/partner (boyfriend/girlfriend) let you down   0 1 2 3 4 5

Work Problems
10. The nature of your job/work (if employed)   0 1 2 3 4 5
11. Your work load   0 1 2 3 4 5
12. Meeting deadlines or goals on the job   0 1 2 3 4 5
13. Use of your skills at work   0 1 2 3 4 5

Money Problems
14. Not enough money for necessities (e.g., food, clothing, housing, health care, taxes, insurance, etc.)   0 1 2 3 4 5
15. Not enough money for education   0 1 2 3 4 5
16. Not enough money for emergencies   0 1 2 3 4 5
17. Not enough money for extras (e.g., entertainment, recreation, vacations, etc.)   0 1 2 3 4 5

Problems with Children
18. Negative communication with your child(ren)   0 1 2 3 4 5
19. Conflict with your child(ren)   0 1 2 3 4 5
20. Disagreement with your child(ren)   0 1 2 3 4 5

School Problems
21. Your study load   0 1 2 3 4 5
22. Study/course deadlines   0 1 2 3 4 5
23. Time pressures   0 1 2 3 4 5
24. Problems getting assignments/essays finished   0 1 2 3 4 5

Problems with Teachers/Lecturers
25. Negative communication with teacher/s, lecturer/s   0 1 2 3 4 5
26. Negative feedback from teacher/s, lecturer/s   0 1 2 3 4 5
27. Conflict with teacher/s, lecturer/s   0 1 2 3 4 5
28. Disagreement with your teacher/s, lecturer/s   0 1 2 3 4 5

Problems with Other Students
29. Negative communication with other student/s   0 1 2 3 4 5
30. Conflict with other student/s   0 1 2 3 4 5
31. Disagreement with other student/s   0 1 2 3 4 5
32. Doing things with other student/s   0 1 2 3 4 5

Problems with Relatives
33. Negative communication with relative/s   0 1 2 3 4 5
34. Conflict with relative/s   0 1 2 3 4 5
35. Disagreement with relative/s   0 1 2 3 4 5
36. Doing things with relative/s   0 1 2 3 4 5

Health Problems
37. Your health   0 1 2 3 4 5
38. Your physical abilities   0 1 2 3 4 5
39. Your medical care   0 1 2 3 4 5
40. Getting sick (e.g., flu, colds)   0 1 2 3 4 5

Problems with Your Work Supervisor/Employer
41. Negative feedback from your supervisor/employer   0 1 2 3 4 5
42. Negative communication with your supervisor/employer   0 1 2 3 4 5
43. Conflict with your supervisor/employer   0 1 2 3 4 5
44. Disagreement with your supervisor/employer   0 1 2 3 4 5

Hassles Getting a Job
45. Finding a job (e.g., interviews, placements)   0 1 2 3 4 5
46. Finding work   0 1 2 3 4 5
47. Problems with finding a job   0 1 2 3 4 5
48. Employment problems (e.g., finding, losing a job)   0 1 2 3 4 5

Academic Limitations
49. Not getting the marks (results) you expected   0 1 2 3 4 5
50. Your academic ability not as good as you thought   0 1 2 3 4 5
51. Not understanding some subjects   0 1 2 3 4 5

School Interest
52. Courses not relevant to your future career   0 1 2 3 4 5
53. Your courses are boring   0 1 2 3 4 5

HOW TO INTERPRET YOUR SCORE Any negative events for which you score a 4 or 5 would be considered significant stressors. You can use the *Choosing to Change Worksheet* at the end of the chapter to help you modify your perceptions of these stressors and reduce the amount of hassle you feel.

To complete this Self-Assessment online, visit MasteringHealth™

Source: "Negative Event Scale" by Dr. Darryl Maybery, Monash University, Melbourne, Australia. Reprinted with permission.

If your stress starts to feel overwhelming, visit your campus health center. You may be eligible for free or low-cost individual or group therapy, which can help you manage the stressors in your life and reframe how you perceive them.

Medical Options

If you're experiencing a serious stress-related condition such as depression, persistent anxiety, or panic attacks, make an appointment with your physician, who may refer you to a psychotherapist or psychiatrist. You may be advised to begin prescription medication to help you get your symptoms under control. Antidepressants and anti-anxiety medications are discussed in Chapter 2. Don't try to "tough it out" on your own: A recent report shows that people who do not receive stress or behavioral management help from a health-care provider are more likely to say their stress increased in the past year than those who do get help.[50]

>> View videos of stress management techniques at http://health.howstuffworks.com/wellness/stress-management.

LO 3.6 QUICK CHECK

If you're experiencing a serious stress-related condition such as depression, persistent anxiety, or panic attacks, your best resource is
a. a family member.
b. a peer counselor.
c. your health instructor.
d. your physician.

Change Yourself, Change Your World

LO 3.7 Summarize strategies for effectively managing stress.

You can't expect to eliminate stress overnight. But by managing your time effectively, improving your test-taking skills, choosing a healthier lifestyle, and thinking in more productive ways, you can tackle your stressors and get more fun out of your college years.

Manage Your Time Effectively

For many students, a 24-hour day seems about 10 hours too short. If this describes you, the **Choosing to Change Worksheet** at the end of this chapter offers a way to evaluate where your time goes. The following are additional strategies you can employ for better time management:

- **Plan, even just a little.** Use a daily planner to remind yourself of big events and track your to-do list. Even a simple paper-based scheduler can keep important tasks from sneaking up on you.

STUDENT STORY

The Pressure to Succeed

"HI, I'M JESSICA. The biggest source of stress in my life would probably be school and just the pressure to succeed in the future. My family doesn't really put pressure on me but I think I put a lot of pressure on myself, just based on the economy and based on the amount of money I feel I need to make to give myself a good future.

To minimize stress, exercise really is important to me. I don't do it as often as I would like but the days I do it, it does make me feel a lot better. I, unfortunately, relieve stress in other ways like drinking, like a lot of college students do. Not in any dangerous sense or any excess, maybe once a week at most. And, you know, I stress in typical other ways like crying, too."

What Do You Think?

1. Jessica uses several methods to manage stress. Which are healthy and which are less so? What advice would you give Jessica about how to handle her stress?
2. What does Jessica identify as the biggest source of stress in her life? What would you choose as your own top stressor?
3. Jessica mentions the economy as a source of stress. Does the economy affect your stress levels? If so, what can you do to address that now and in the future? Do you track your spending? How much of what you spend money on are true essentials (versus luxuries)?

- **Stay prepared.** When you find out the dates of big assignments at the start of the term, make note of them in your planner and begin to tackle them ahead of time. Also, read assignments before class and review your class notes shortly after class ends. These steps will help you get more out of class and make study sessions a lot easier.
- **Break down big jobs.** In Chapter 1, you learned about shaping a behavior-change program, and it works for assignments, too. Write down all the steps required to get a project done and then tackle them one at a time.
- **Focus on one task at a time.** You might think you're multitasking, but after only about *half a second* of parallel processing, your brain reverts to sequential

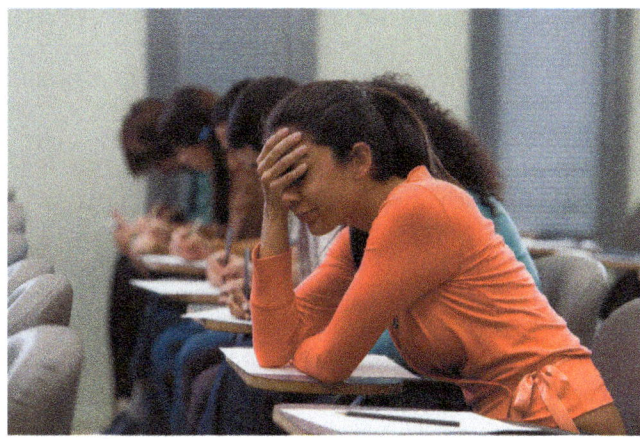

Stress less when preparing for and taking exams.

processing—handling only one task at a time. Multitasking actually forces your brain to switch rapidly from one task to another, expending great mental effort and time.[51]

- **Hate it? Do it first.** If you can get the task you dread out of the way, everything that follows will feel easier.
- **Leave time for surprises.** If every hour of your schedule is always booked, you won't have room to deal with the unexpected turns life takes, like your car breaking down or the electricity going out.
- **Reward yourself.** Been wrestling with a challenging assignment for an hour? Take a break. Finish a paper early for a change? Let your laundry slide and watch a movie. If you're working hard in college, you've more than earned a reward.

Improve Your Test-Taking Skills

The following steps can help get you ready for success *before* your next test:

- Many colleges offer classes on test-taking skills. Sign up for one!
- Learn about the test ahead of time. Find out not only what topics the test will cover but also what format it will be in. If your instructor provides practice tests, use them.
- Schedule your study time over a series of days or weeks. Avoid cramming at the last minute or pulling an "all-nighter."
- Talk with your instructor in advance if you experience test anxiety. He or she may be able to offer suggestions or help.
- Prepare yourself mentally. Think positively. In the days leading up to the test, visualize yourself calmly taking the test and knowing the answers.
- Prepare yourself physically. Get enough sleep the night before.

When test day arrives, get up early so that you avoid having to rush. Before the test, eat a light meal so you're not hungry. Once you're in the testing room, choose a seat in a place that seems comfortable—for instance, near a window so you can get some fresh air, or away from a classmate whose mannerisms you find distracting. During the test, follow these strategies:

- Read the directions carefully.
- Answer the easy questions first. This will give you confidence and allow you to budget your remaining time on the more difficult questions.
- If you get stuck on a question, move on. You can turn back to the question later.
- Stay calm. If you find yourself getting anxious: (1) Relax and remind yourself that you are in control and are well prepared for this test. (2) Take slow, deep breaths. (3) Concentrate on the questions, not on your fear. (4) Remind yourself that some anxiety is natural.
- Even if you don't know the final answer, show your work. Graders may give you partial credit.
- Don't be alarmed if others turn in their tests before you. They might have left several questions unanswered. Use all the time you need.
- When you have finished, check your work. However, don't second-guess yourself or change an answer unless you've remembered new information.

What if you've finished the test and then start to stress out about your grade? Try these three post-test strategies:

- **Focus on the positive.** Think about all the things you did right either before or during the test.
- **Evaluate your test preparation.** Which strategies were helpful and which were not? Did you neglect anything? For instance, perhaps you were distracted because your mouth was dry during the test and wished you had brought a bottle of water or some mints.
- **Develop a plan for your next test.** Base your new plan on what worked and what didn't work for this test.

Live a Healthier Lifestyle

Practicing the following basic wellness habits can help you reduce your stress level:

- **Get adequate sleep.** Sleep is a naturally restorative process that is essential for healthy physical and psychological functioning—and reducing your body's stress. For information on how to get a better night's sleep, see Chapter 4.
- **Eat well.** Food and stress have a reciprocal relationship. The higher your cortisol levels, the greater your attraction to rich, pleasing foods.[52] Yet a nutritious diet helps keep you focused and energized and thereby better able to manage your stressors.
- **Exercise.** Exercise, especially activities such as walking, cycling, weight training, or running that work your large muscles and build sustained strength, is an effective stress reducer.[53] Scientists theorize that physical activity

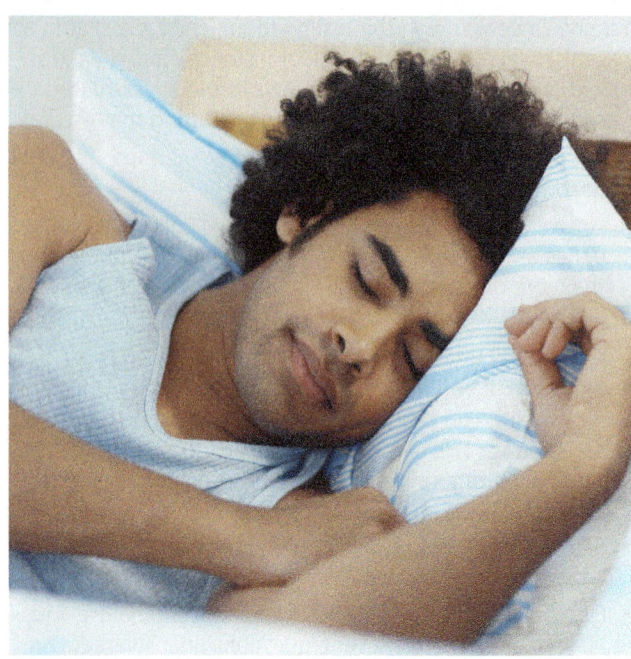

Sleep can refresh and revive you and help you feel less stressed.

allows the body to complete the fight-or-flight response by actually doing what it has been prepared to do. After all, whether you are running around a track or running from a bear, you are still "fleeing" and thereby helping your body return to balance. As little as 20 to 30 minutes of aerobic activity has been shown to help you feel calmer, and the effect can last for several hours.[54] For tips on exercising for stress management, see the **Practical Strategies** box on page 67.

- **Avoid alcohol, nicotine, and other drugs.** They can seem to offer a brief vacation from stress, but their long-term health risks far outweigh the few moments of relief they offer. If you find yourself drawn to potentially addictive substances to relieve stress, seek help from a healthcare professional.
- **Take time for hobbies and leisure.** It probably feels like you have no time for dance class, mountain biking, or helping design T-shirts for friends' bands. But time spent away from school and work will reduce your stress and renew your energy. Breaks can also improve learning, giving you time to consider the material you've been studying in new ways.
- **Keep a journal.** Make time to record what's going on in your life and how you feel about it. If you don't feel like toting around a traditional diary, you can keep a journal by writing an online blog or a personal web page (with privacy controls).

Relieve Your Tension

For centuries, people have practiced a variety of physical and mental techniques to relieve their tension, including the following:

- **Progressive muscle relaxation (PMR).** In PMR, you contract and relax each major muscle group in your body, one by one, until your whole body feels relaxed. Studies have established that PMR is effective in reducing not only people's self-reported stress but also their cortisol levels.[55] Start by choosing one part of your body, such as your left foot. Inhale and contract all the muscles of that foot. Then exhale as you relax it. Repeat this once or twice. Then move on to your left leg and repeat the process. Slowly move through all the major muscle groups of your body, contracting and releasing, until your whole body is relaxed.
- **Yoga.** Fundamental to the ancient Indian healing system called *ayurveda*, yoga is a mind–body practice that includes three main components: physical postures and stretches, breathing techniques, and quiet contemplation. Growing evidence suggests that yoga not only relaxes your muscles but may also relieve stress, depression, and anxiety.[56]
- **Massage.** A professional massage therapist uses pressure, stretching, friction, heat, cold, and other forms of manipulation to stimulate skin and muscles and relieve tension. Some studies have associated massage with short-term relief of stress, anxiety, and pain.[57] Check with your campus wellness center to see if it offers reduced-price massages on campus.
- **Deep breathing.** Research suggests that deep breathing can reduce stress.[58] Try the following technique: With your mouth closed, inhale slowly through your nose. Exhale through your mouth. Inhaling and exhaling should each take about six seconds. Notice that, while you are inhaling, your chest wall and upper abdomen move outward—away from your core. They relax back in again as you empty your lungs. Throughout, your shoulders should remain stationary. Rising and falling shoulders indicate breathing that is high and shallow. If this is happening, just focus on expanding your rib cage outward with each inhalation and letting it relax back inward with each exhalation. Continue the exercise for several minutes.
- **Meditation.** Studies over many years have supported the effectiveness of meditation for reducing stress and anxiety.[59] Meditation commonly includes the following steps: Choose a quiet location free of distractions. Assume a posture that will be comfortable for you to maintain for several minutes, whether sitting, standing, lying down, or slowly walking. Focus your attention on a word, phrase, object, or your breathing. Observe without judgment each thought or feeling that arises, then set it aside, gently bringing your attention back to your point of focus.
- **Music.** Taking a break can be as close as your MP3 player. A large review study suggests that listening to slow-tempo music can reduce heart rate, blood pressure, anxiety, and pain as well as improve the quality of sleep.[60] It does this in part by helping to induce the body's relaxation response.

⚙ PRACTICAL Strategies
Exercising for Stress Management

Having trouble getting moving? Consider the following tips:

- Think of exercise as "recess"—not as a chore but as a chance to break up an otherwise routine day with a fun, active, recreational activity.
- Vary your exercise activity. You might go swimming one day and bicycling another day. This way, you will have more options to choose from, depending on your mood on any given day.
- Pick activities you genuinely enjoy. If you hate jogging but love to dance, by all means, dance!
- Remember that any activity that gets your body moving can ease stress. If you're not into sports, consider a brisk walk around campus, walking your dog, or even walking up and down the flights of stairs in your residence hall. Any physical activity is better than none!
- Consider exercise classes such as yoga or tai chi that focus on breathing and relaxation.
- Enlist a friend as an exercise partner. You can keep each other encouraged and have more fun while you exercise.
- Make exercise a regular part of your schedule. Prioritize it the same way you would prioritize your schoolwork or a job.
- Exercise releases endorphins in the body, which makes you feel good. So the next time you find yourself resisting it, remind yourself of how great you'll feel afterward!

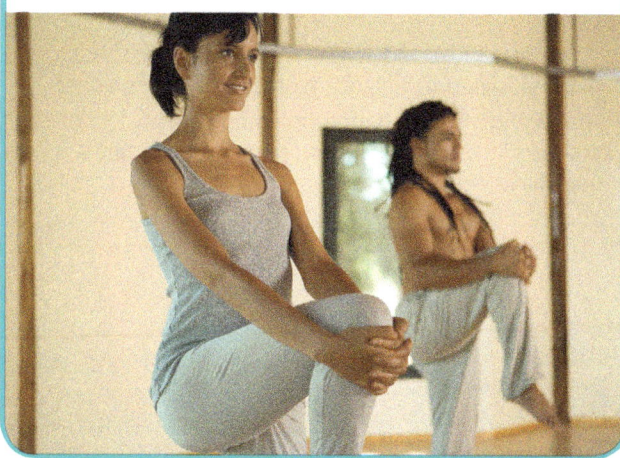

So make yourself a relaxation playlist of music you find soothing and listen to it regularly.

▶▶ This university website offers information about various mind and body relaxation techniques: **www.uhs.uga.edu/stress/relax.html**.

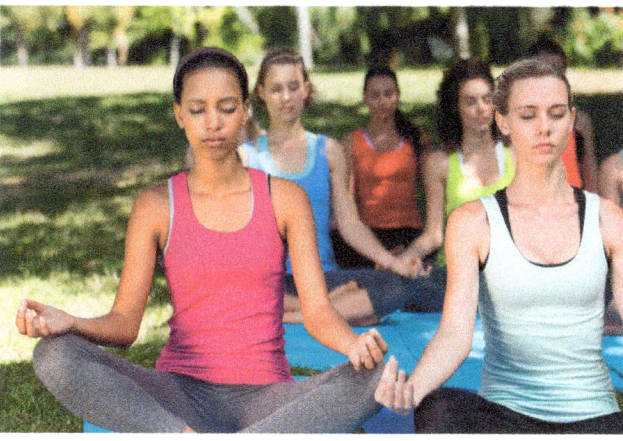

Meditating for even a few minutes can help you feel refreshed and less stressed.

Change Your Thinking

Changing the way you think about the stressors in your life can help hold stress at bay. To keep your everyday stressors from turning into mountains of tension, consider the following:

- **Rewrite internal messages.** If you tend to tell yourself negative messages, first identify them and then restate them as positive, solution-oriented, constructive messages. For example, when you have a test coming up, remind yourself that with consistent study, you can do well.
- **Set realistic expectations.** Regardless of how ambitious you are, give yourself permission to set realistic goals that, with your best effort, you can achieve.
- **Build your self-esteem.** Review the self-esteem-boosting tips we discussed in Chapter 2. These can help you build the inner strength and confidence to handle stressful situations when they come along.
- **Have a sense of humor.** A little laughter can go a long way toward reducing stress. Laughter increases your intake of oxygen, improves your circulation, relaxes your muscles, and reduces tension. So watch some funny YouTube videos or talk to your most hilarious friend. Humor can help you get a better perspective on which stressors are really important and which ones are overblown.
- **Take the long view.** Are most of the stressors in your life right now going to matter to you in a few years? Cultivating patience and a sense of what matters in the long term can help you keep problems in perspective.
- **Accept that, although you can't control everything, you *can* control how you respond to less-than-ideal situations.** Just reminding yourself of this simple fact can help you deal with stressors. For instance, if you play team sports, consciously acknowledge that the final score or season ranking isn't up to you alone.

When you're stressed, the way you choose to cope with it can help—
or set you up for more problems. To de-stress in a healthy way:

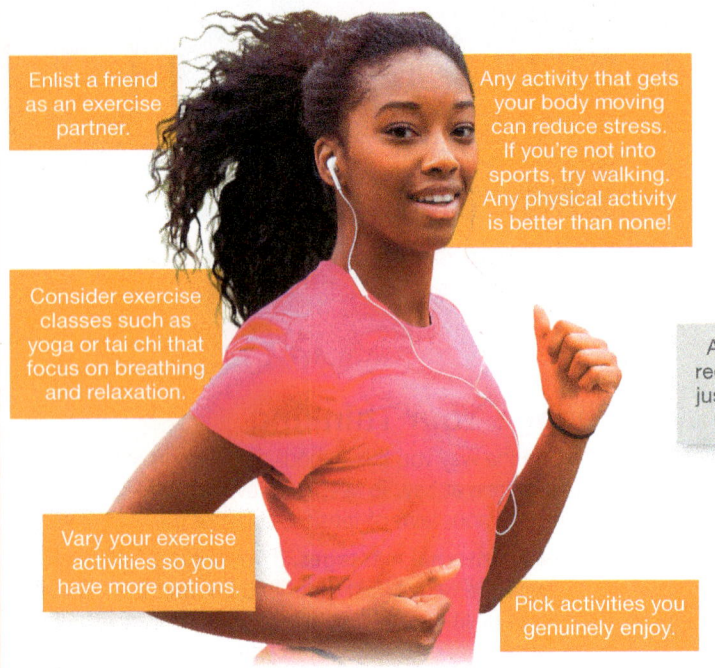

CHOOSE THIS.

- Enlist a friend as an exercise partner.
- Any activity that gets your body moving can reduce stress. If you're not into sports, try walking. Any physical activity is better than none!
- Consider exercise classes such as yoga or tai chi that focus on breathing and relaxation.
- Vary your exercise activities so you have more options.
- Pick activities you genuinely enjoy.

Exercise:
Exercise releases endorphins in the body, which make you feel good and help reduce stress. As little as 20 minutes per day can have an effect on your stress level.

NOT THAT.

- Using alcohol to deal with stress can lead to alcohol dependence.
- Alcohol is a depressant, and excessive alcohol use over time can make it harder for you to deal with stress.
- Alcohol won't reduce stress; it just covers it up temporarily.
- A hangover the next day will increase your feelings of stress and limit your ability to effectively manage it.
- Drinking can lead to behaviors such as fights, unprotected sex, or injuries.

Alcohol:
You may think that having a drink, or several, is a good stress reliever. But alcohol's negative effects can actually make stress worse.

Create a Personalized Stress Management Plan

You can create a personalized stress management plan by first identifying the stressors in your life. To realistically assess your current stressors, complete the **Self-Assessment** on page 63. Next, turn to the **Choosing to Change Worksheet** found at the end of this chapter to evaluate your readiness for behavior change and to take steps to reduce the controllable stressors.

Once you have done everything you can to minimize the controllable stressors in your life, it's time to think about how you can better respond to (and manage) the stress that remains. Review this chapter's strategies for managing stress and select a few that seem the most comfortable and natural for you. Keep the following guidelines in mind:

- **Not all stress is harmful.** You may find one of your classes tough, for example, but intellectually stimulating and even fun. Use the stress to motivate you to participate fully in the class and work hard on assignments and studying.
- **If the stress management technique that you pick requires adjusting your schedule, do it.** For example, if you've decided to shake some of your stress through exercise, schedule time for workouts in your planner.
- **Managing stress is a lifelong commitment.** Tackle your stressors little by little, and over time, you'll create a college experience that's not only more rewarding but more fun.

▶▶ This video from Dartmouth College provides tips on how to incorporate stress management into your life:
www.dartmouth.edu/~acskills/videos/video_sm.html

▶▶ Watch videos of real students discussing stress management at Mastering Health™

LO 3.7 QUICK CHECK

To manage your stress, it may be helpful to
a. remind yourself that everything in your life really is in your control.
b. set realistic, achievable goals.
c. recognize that all stress is harmful, so you need to get serious about avoiding it.
d. work out at least once a week to the point of exhaustion.

Choosing to **Change** Worksheet

To complete this worksheet online, visit MasteringHealth™

You have acquired extensive information from this chapter about stressors and how to manage them. You had the opportunity to make observations about whether your perceptions of negative events in your life may be contributing to making you feel distressed by completing the **Negative Event Scale for University Students Self-Assessment** on page 63.

Directions: Fill in your stage of change in step 1 and complete the remaining steps with your stage of change in mind.

Step 1: Assess your stage of behavior change. Please check one of the following statements that best describes your readiness to adopt stress management techniques to better cope with stress.

_____ I do not intend to adopt stress management techniques in the next six months. (Precontemplation)

_____ I might adopt stress management techniques in the next six months. (Contemplation)

_____ I am prepared to adopt stress management techniques in the next month. (Preparation)

_____ I have been adopting stress management techniques for less than six months. (Action)

_____ I have been adopting stress management techniques for more than six months. (Maintenance)

Step 2: Recognize chronic stress. It is important to identify the warning signs of chronic stress to assess whether your health may be at risk. The following table lists some of the common warning signs and symptoms of stress overload. Check whether you have experienced any of these within the past month.

Recognizing Warning Signs and Symptoms of Stress Overload

Emotional	Yes	No	Physical	Yes	No	Behavioral	Yes	No
Anxiety			Stooped posture			Overreacting to problems or difficult situations		
Sleep disruption			Sweaty palms			Increased use of alcohol, tobacco, or other drugs		
Anger and agitation			Chronic fatigue			Unusually impulsive behavior		
Trouble concentrating			Weight loss or weight gain			Feeling "burned out" on school or work		
Unproductive worry			Migraine or tension headaches			Withdrawing from relationships or contact with others		
Frequent mood swings			Neck aches			Frequent bouts of crying		
Depression			Digestive problems					
			Asthma attacks					
			Physical symptoms that your doctor can't attribute to another condition					
			Feelings of anxiety or panic					

The more signs and symptoms you notice, the closer you may be to allostatic overload or excessive stress. Be mindful that the signs and symptoms of stress can also be caused by other psychological and physiological medical problems. If you're experiencing any of the warning signs of stress overload, it's important to see a health-care professional for a full evaluation.

Step 3: Identify stressors. What were your top five stressors, based on your completion of the **Negative Event Scale for University Students Self-Assessment** on page 63? Choose those for which you scored as a 4 (a lot of a hassle) or 5 (an extreme hassle).

My Top 5 Stressors	How Much of a Hassle Was This Stressor? (4 or 5)
1.	
2.	
3.	
4.	
5.	

Now that you have completed steps 2 and 3, you can begin to take action about changing the way you think about the primary stressors in your life and reduce or eliminate stress by completing steps 4 and 5.

Step 4: Choose stress management techniques. For each of the stressors listed in step 3, write down a stress management technique from the **Change Yourself, Change Your World** section of the chapter that can reduce this stressor. On a scale of 1 (lowest) to 5 (highest), what is your confidence in your ability to implement the stress management technique the next time you experience the stressor?

Stressor	Stress Management Technique	How Confident Are You in Your Ability to Employ This Technique?				
		Low Confidence (1)			High Confidence (5)	
1.		1	2	3	4	5
2.		1	2	3	4	5
3.		1	2	3	4	5
4.		1	2	3	4	5
5.		1	2	3	4	5

Step 5: Use effective time management to reduce daily hassles. You can reduce some of your daily stress and handle the hassles in your life more effectively by rethinking how you use your time. Start by taking a closer look at your schedule. Using the following chart, fill in your activities every day for a week.

Time	Monday	Tuesday	Wednesday	Thursday	Friday	Saturday	Sunday
5:00 a.m.							
6:00 a.m.							
7:00 a.m.							
8:00 a.m.							
9:00 a.m.							
10:00 a.m.							
11:00 a.m.							
12:00 p.m.							
1:00 p.m.							
2:00 p.m.							
3:00 p.m.							
4:00 p.m.							
5:00 p.m.							
6:00 p.m.							
7:00 p.m.							
8:00 p.m.							
9:00 p.m.							
10:00 p.m.							
11:00 p.m.							
12:00 a.m.							
12 a.m.–5 a.m.							

Now examine the chart and consider the following: Which tasks are most important to your goals in school and in your personal life? Which tasks are needed to keep you healthy, such as eating, sleeping, and making time to relax? Which tasks are unnecessary time-busters—that is, activities that eat away at your time or waste it (be honest)? Decide how you can kick a time-buster or two out of your schedule. Mark these areas with red pencil and see how much more time you have for important tasks.

Step 6: Set a SMART goal for how you can manage stress, including a timeline.

_____

_____

_____

CHAPTER 3 STUDY PLAN

CHAPTER SUMMARY

LO 3.1
- Stress is the collective psychobiological condition that occurs in response to a disruptive, unexpected, or exciting stimulus.
- A stressor is any physical or psychological event or other change that stimulates stress, which can be either of two types: Eustress results from changes that are perceived as advantageous; distress results from changes that are perceived as threatening.

LO 3.2
- The stress response is set of specific psychobiological changes that occurs as the body attempts to cope with a stressor and return to homeostasis, a balanced state.
- The most common explanation of the stress response is the general adaptation syndrome (GAS). It consists of three stages: alarm, resistance, and exhaustion.
- The alarm stage, also called the fight-or-flight response, begins with the release of the neurotransmitters norepinephrine and epinephrine, which prepare the body to deal with a stressor. A hormonal response follows, in which the secretion of cortisol maintains the production of glucose.
- During the resistance stage, the body mobilizes homeostatic mechanisms that help it adapt to the stressor.
- Exhaustion, also referred to as allostatic overload, is a harmful state resulting from the cumulative burden of adapting, again and again, to stress.

LO 3.3
- Severe, longstanding stress can increase your risk of a heart attack or stroke, inhibit digestive functions, and promote insulin resistance, weight gain, and storage of visceral fat.
- Short-term stress can boost the immune response, but chronic stress impairs immunity, contributes to headaches, disrupts sleep, and negatively affects sexual functioning, frequency, and satisfaction.
- Severe, uncontrolled stress can also reduce academic performance and increase the risk for depression, panic attacks, and other mental disorders.

LO 3.4
- How you think about your stressors can have a critical impact on how stress affects your health.
- People with a type B personality may be more tolerant of stressors than those with a type A personality.

MasteringHealth™
Build your knowledge—and health!—in the Study Area of **MasteringHealth**™ with a variety of study tools.

- Optimism, hardiness, and resilience are personality traits that help individuals manage and recover from stress. Conscientiousness and agreeableness also appear to help people manage day-to-day stressors.
- Biology also influences stress: Women report more stress and more symptoms of stress than men, and young adults have higher stress levels than older adults.

LO 3.5
- Academic pressure is the most significant stressor in college students' lives. Finances are not far behind: over 70% of students feel stressed about money.
- Work responsibilities and relationships are also common sources of stress for college students. Social relationships can produce stress when they are too numerous or negative, and discrimination may be a source of stress for members of minority groups.
- Minor daily hassles can contribute to "stressor pile-up," and major life changes such as the death of a loved one or transferring to a new college can be key stressors.
- Aspects of your environment, such as noise or pollution, can be sources of stress, as can worry, perfectionism, and self-critical thoughts.

LO 3.6
- Social support offers protection against distress throughout the life span. On campus, instructors, peer tutors and counselors, and the services of your campus health center can help you manage stress.
- If you're experiencing a serious stress-related condition such as depression, persistent anxiety, or panic attacks, make an appointment with your physician.

LO 3.7
- General strategies for reducing stress include managing your time effectively, improving your test-taking skills, getting enough sleep, eating well, exercising, avoiding substance abuse, taking time for hobbies and leisure, keeping a journal, relieving your tension by practicing a variety of relaxation techniques, and changing your thinking.

GET CONNECTED

>> Visit the following websites for further information about the topics in this chapter:

- American Psychological Association
  www.apa.org
- Time Management for Students
  www.dartmouth.edu
- Stress Management Techniques
  www.mindtools.com

MOBILE TIPS!
Scan this QR code with your mobile device to access additional stress-management tips. Or, via your mobile device, go to http://chmobile.pearsoncmg.com and choose by topic: stress-management.

- Budget Worksheet for College Students
  http://financialplan.about.com
- Kiplinger.com Build-Your-Budget Worksheet
  www.kiplinger.com

  Website links are subject to change. To access updated web links, please visit MasteringHealth™

TEST YOUR KNOWLEDGE

LO 3.1
1. The psychobiological response that Petra and Danek experienced during the month before their wedding is called
   a. eustress.
   b. distress.
   c. a stressor.
   d. allostatic overload.

LO 3.2
2. The fight-or-flight response
   a. is characteristic of the resistance stage.
   b. involves both nervous system and hormonal mechanisms.
   c. is a sign of allostatic overload.
   d. is a failure of homeostasis.

3. A harmful state resulting from the cumulative burden of adapting, again and again, to stress is called
   a. homeostasis.
   b. burnout.
   c. allostatic overload.
   d. distress.

LO 3.3
4. The effects of severe, longstanding stress can include
   a. increased risk of a heart attack or stroke.
   b. increased responsiveness of body cells to insulin.
   c. sweaty palms.
   d. reduced storage of visceral fat.

LO 3.4
5. When his roommate accused him of stealing his cell phone, Ayo smiled and gently reminded him that he'd been charging it in the outlet by his desk. What personality trait is Ayo exhibiting?
   a. type A personality
   b. optimism
   c. hardiness
   d. agreeableness

LO 3.5
6. Financial stress
   a. is the most common type of stress experienced by college students.
   b. is experienced by nearly one-third of college students.
   c. is most commonly due to an inability to make timely payments on student loans.
   d. may be self-perpetuating.

7. Worries, critical thoughts, and perfectionism are examples of
   a. environmental stressors.
   b. internal stressors.
   c. social stressors.
   d. post-traumatic stress disorder.

LO 3.6
8. Which of the following resources is the most appropriate for managing mild stress?
   a. solitude
   b. prescription antidepressants
   c. old and new friendships
   d. the Internet

LO 3.7
9. Janie just found out she failed her midterm. To relieve her stress, she should
   a. treat herself to a caramel latte and a slice of chocolate cake.
   b. go for a 20- to 30-minute walk.
   c. plan a shopping trip for the coming weekend.
   d. listen to some loud, heavy-metal music.

10. Progressive muscle relaxation involves
    a. systematically contracting and relaxing muscle groups.
    b. taking naps of longer and longer lengths.
    c. stretching your muscles a little more each day.
    d. quietly focusing on relaxing only your body's tiniest muscles.

WHAT DO YOU THINK?

LO 3.2

1. You're driving home one night when your wheels hit ice and your car spins out of control. You manage to steer out of the skid, but you're still shaking when you arrive home. Describe in chronological order the physiological events that have occurred in your body over these few minutes.

LO 3.3

2. Identify at least two mechanisms by which severe, chronic stress can increase your risk for a heart attack or stroke.

LO 3.5

3. Why do you think that loneliness is itself a stressor? Propose at least two reasons.

LO 3.7

4. List at least five strategies for improving your test-taking skills.
5. Explain the mechanism by which exercise is believed to help the body cope with stress.

4

> More than half of American adults say they experience a sleep problem almost every night.[i]

> About 15% of American adults say they sleep fewer than 6 hours on weeknights.[i]

> Americans aged 19–29 have the latest bedtime of any age group: on average, two minutes before midnight.[i]

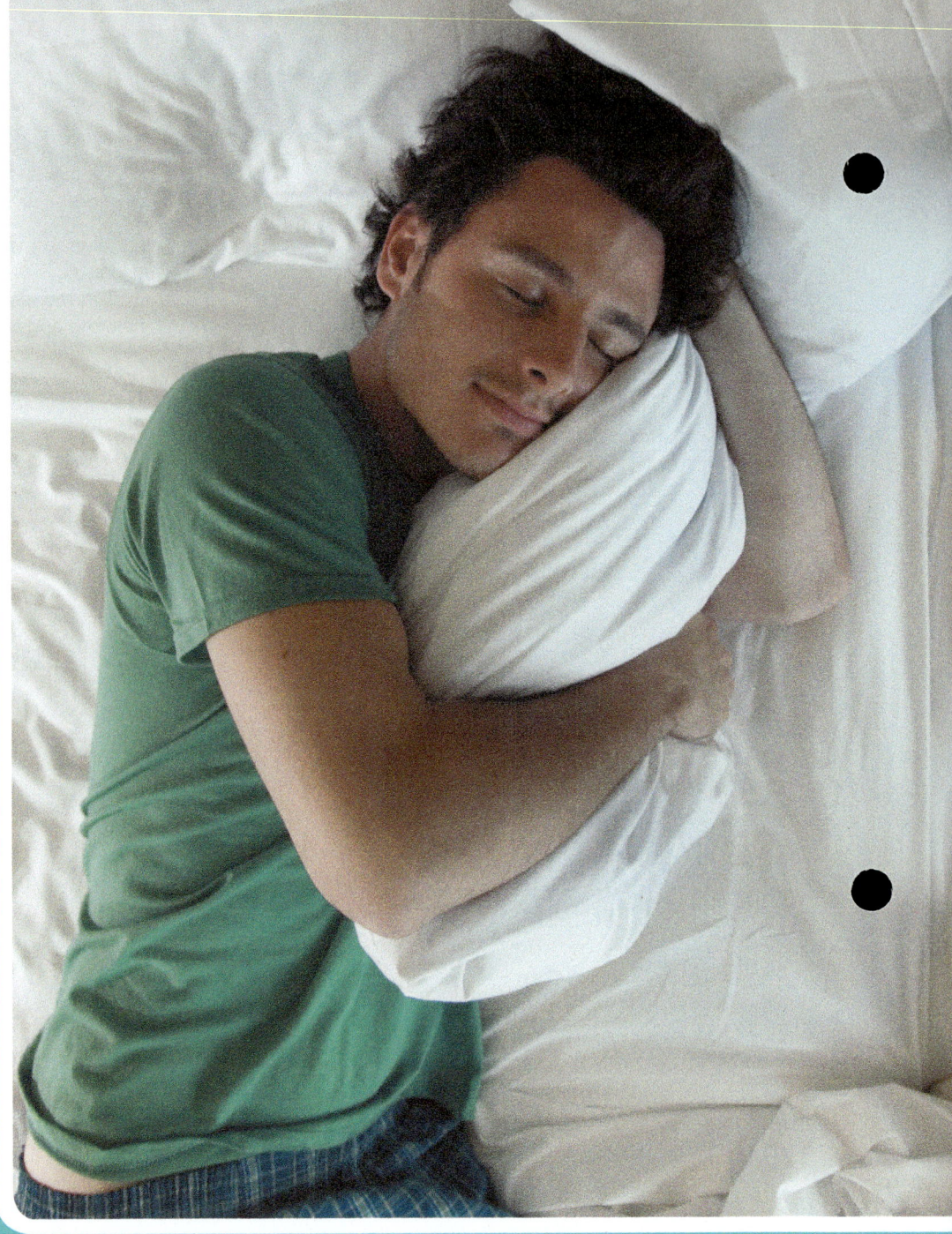

SLEEP, YOUR BODY, AND YOUR MIND

LEARNING OUTCOMES

LO 4.1 Describe the stages of a full night's sleep.

LO 4.2 Identify the benefits of ample sleep and the risks of sleep deprivation.

LO 4.3 Discuss a variety of factors that influence sleep.

LO 4.4 Define and describe sleep disorders such as insomnia, sleep apnea, and parasomnias.

LO 4.5 Discuss the clinical diagnosis and treatment of sleep disorders.

LO 4.6 Identify strategies for improving the quantity and quality of your sleep.

Troubled sleep.

Few experiences in life can match its power to hijack your health and drive you to despair. In a recent survey of more than 1,000 college students, about 60% said they feel tired and sleep deprived three or more days each week.[1] What makes college students vulnerable to troubled sleep? And if you're among the sleep deprived, what can you do about it? Before we address these questions, let's define the strange phenomenon we call sleep.

What Is Sleep?

LO 4.1 Describe the stages of a full night's sleep.

Until the middle of the 20th century, sleep was thought to be a state of "global shutdown," prompted by darkness, silence, and other reductions in stimulation from the environment. Then, experiments using a medical device called an **electroencephalograph (EEG)** revealed that sleep is induced by distinctive patterns of nerve cell communication involving several brain regions. Researchers also learned that during sleep, all major organs continue to function, and some activities of the brain and endocrine glands actually increase. As a result, we now recognize **sleep** as a physiologically prompted, dynamic, and readily reversible state of reduced consciousness essential to human survival.

Regions and Rhythms of Sleep

Sleep is generated and maintained by structures in the three primary regions of your brain (**Figure 4.1** on page 76).

The Brain Stem

The *brain stem* is the lowest part of your brain. It connects to your spinal cord and sends signals from your spinal cord to higher regions of your brain. Running through the core of the brain stem is a group of nerve cells called the *reticular activating system* (*RAS*), which helps regulate sleep. Active signaling of the RAS keeps you awake, whereas inactivity induces sleep.[2] Another region of the brain stem, called the *pons*, sends signals upward to initiate REM sleep—a stage of dreaming sleep discussed shortly—and sends signals downward to the spinal cord to paralyze your muscles so that you won't act out your dreams.

The Diencephalon

The *diencephalon*, the region above the brain stem, contains two structures especially important in sleep. These are the *hypothalamus* and the *pineal gland*, both of which help regulate your body's **circadian rhythm**—its distinctive 24-hour pattern of wakefulness and sleep.

The hypothalamus contains a distinct region of tissue that functions as your "body clock," synchronizing with changing patterns of darkness and light in your environment to prompt you to feel sleepy and to wake up. The same region also regulates other body functions according to these changes in darkness and light—for instance, your body temperature and the release of certain hormones.

Meanwhile, the pineal gland responds to changing levels of darkness and light by altering its production of a hormone called *melatonin*. As dusk begins to fall, melatonin secretion begins to rise. Eventually, levels increase enough to make you sleepy.

Jet lag is thought to occur in part because, when you travel across time zones, you're subjected to a sudden change in the habitual pattern of darkness and light. Most people need two or three days to "reset" their circadian rhythm according to the dark–light cycle in the new location.

The Cerebrum

The *cerebrum* consists of the tissue located immediately beneath your skull. The cerebrum's outermost "bark," called the *cerebral cortex*, is the thinking area of your brain. When it's time to solve an equation or write a short story, your cerebral cortex goes into action. This part of your brain is also essential to a wakeful state, receiving chemical signals from the hypothalamus that promote waking you up from sleep and keeping you awake. And when your circadian rhythm says it's time to sleep, the cerebral cortex continues to stay active: Patterns of electrical activity generated by the cerebral cortex distinguish each of the different stages of sleep, identified next.

---

electroencephalograph (EEG) A device that monitors the electrical activity of different regions of the cerebral cortex of the brain, using electrodes placed on or in the scalp; a tracing of brain activity is called an *electroencephalogram*.

sleep A physiologically prompted, dynamic, and readily reversible state of reduced consciousness essential to human survival.

circadian rhythm A pattern of physical and behavioral changes that follows a 24-hour cycle, in accordance with the hours of darkness and light.

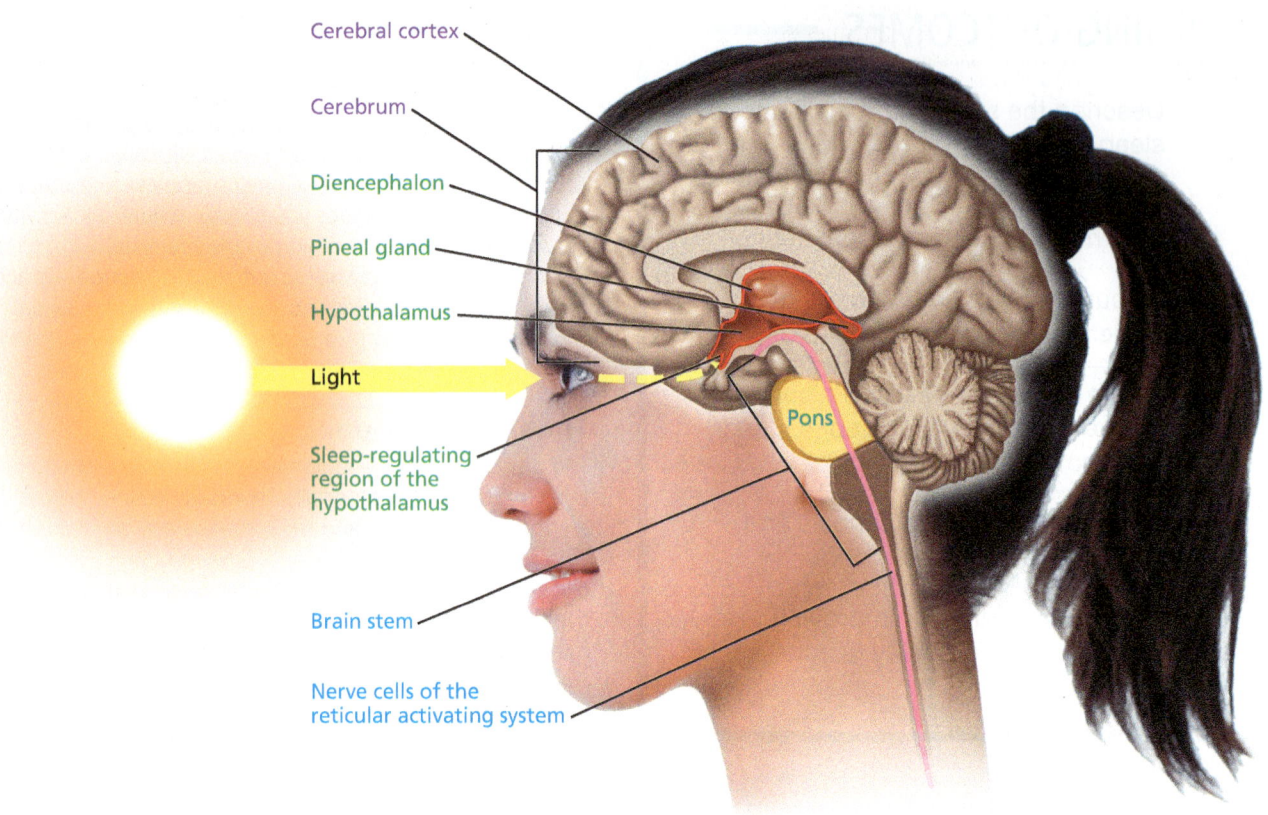

FIGURE 4.1 **Brain Regions and Structures Involved in Sleep.**

Stages of Sleep

Have you ever felt drowsy in an afternoon class, tried to stay alert, and had your whole body jerk and startle as if you were about to fall off a cliff? This jarring sensation, a very common phenomenon that sleep scientists call *hypnic myoclonia*, signals that you've entered the first stage of sleep.[3]

Decades ago, sleep researchers using EEGs to study brain activity during rest began to distinguish five stages of true sleep **(Figure 4.2)**. They grouped these into two primary types characterized by the absence or presence of a key physiological sign: *rapid eye movement* (*REM*), a hallmark of dreaming sleep. During several hours of sleep, you progress through several cycles of sleep, each of which includes some or all of the following stages.

During Non-REM Sleep, You Rest

Rapid eye movement does not occur during **non-REM (NREM) sleep.** Instead of dreaming, you rest. NREM sleep is also called *slow-wave sleep* because it's characterized by EEG waves that gradually get slower and broader as you move from light sleep to deep sleep. The four stages of NREM sleep are as follows (see Figure 4.2):

non-REM (NREM) sleep A type of restful sleep during which the rapid eye movement characteristic of dreaming does not typically occur.

- **Stage 1.** You're drifting off. Brain activity, as measured on an EEG, begins to slow. Your muscles may twitch, and you are easily awakened. This light stage of sleep typically lasts just a few minutes.
- **Stage 2.** You're truly—but lightly—asleep. Your body temperature cools. Your breathing rate and pulse slow. You are less easily aroused. This stage of sleep may initially last about 15 minutes, but over the course of a night, you spend more time in this stage than in any other. EEG waves become slower and broader.
- **Stages 3 and 4.** These stages of NREM sleep—which some researchers consider a single stage—are characterized by tall, slow brainwaves. In stage 3, these waves are just beginning to appear, and you are falling into deep sleep. By stage 4, more than half of the brain waves are the tall, slow waves characteristic of deep sleep. Your breathing rate and pulse slow even more, and your blood pressure drops. You are sleeping deeply and are very difficult to rouse. Talking and sleepwalking, though uncommon, typically occur in this stage. Also during stage 4 sleep, the pituitary gland (located in the brain near the hypothalamus) releases *growth hormone,* which among other functions is important in the repair of wear and tear on body tissues. You may spend half an hour or more in stage 4 early in the night, but as the night goes on, you spend less and less time in this stage of deep sleep.

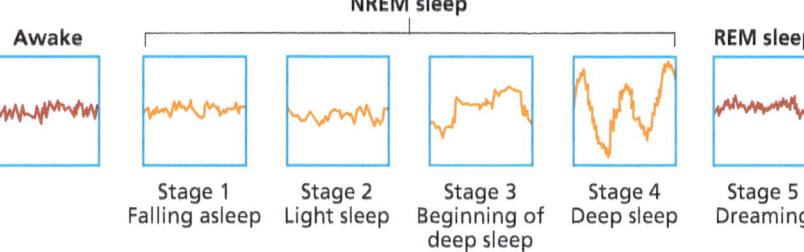

FIGURE 4.2 **Stages of Sleep.** Drowsiness is followed by four stages of NREM sleep and a fifth stage of REM sleep. Brain activity gradually slows and lengthens in NREM sleep, only to speed up again in REM sleep.

During REM Sleep, You Dream

The fifth stage of sleep, **REM sleep,** is prompted by signals from the pons in the brain stem. The pons also inhibits the release of neurotransmitters necessary for muscle movement; as noted earlier, this protective mechanism means you're not able to act out your dreams. When this mechanism fails, the sleeper experiences a rare and potentially dangerous sleep disorder called *REM behavior disorder*.

Although the pons inhibits movements of most of your body's muscles, three groups remain active: Your respiratory muscles allow you to continue to breathe; the tiny muscles of your inner ear still function; and your eye muscles generate the rapid eye movements that give this sleep stage its name.[4] Sleep researchers have noticed that these darting eye movements appear to follow the activities sleepers later say they were engaging in during their dreams.

Brain wave activity during REM sleep is somewhat similar to types of activity measured when someone is awake. Moreover, the brain's oxygen consumption is higher than it is even when you're performing complex tasks. In general during REM sleep, the brain appears to be doing everything but resting.[4] So why do we experience REM sleep? We'll discuss its importance shortly.

REM sleep A type of sleep characterized by brain waves similar to those that occur while awake, during which rapid eye movement and dreaming occur.

sleep debt An accumulated amount of sleep loss that develops when the amount of sleep you routinely obtain is less than the amount you need.

Cycles of Sleep

A graph of brain activity during a full night's sleep looks like a plot of an 8-hour earthquake (**Figure 4.3**). After you first fall asleep, you progress through each of the four stages of NREM sleep. After 20 to 40 minutes in deep sleep, you cycle back to stages 3 and 2 before entering a short phase of REM sleep. However, as the night continues, the duration of NREM sleep decreases, and the duration of REM sleep increases. After about 4 hours of sleep, stage 4 sleep all but disappears, and the sleeper cycles back quickly into longer and longer periods of REM. Most researchers believe that 7 to 8 hours of sleep allow for adequate REM sleep. This is especially important during your college years because REM is thought to increase the capacity to learn new material, consolidate memories, and improve creativity—as we discuss in detail shortly.

>> Sleep Cycle is an iPhone app that tracks your sleep cycles and wakes you up during the lightest cycle of sleep closest to your wake-up alarm time. Find it where you download apps or at **www.sleepcycle.com**.

LO 4.1 QUICK CHECK

What is melatonin?
a. A hormone related to skin tone and eye color
b. Something that your body stops making when you have jet lag
c. A hormone related to sleep and drowsiness
d. None of the above

Sleep: How Much and Why It Matters

LO 4.2 Identify the benefits of ample sleep and the risks of sleep deprivation.

Sleep experts report that most adults need 7 to 9 hours of sleep each night to feel alert and well rested.[5] Any amount less than 7 hours is referred to as *short sleep*, whereas any amount more than 9 hours is considered *long sleep*.

Many college students develop a **sleep debt,** an accumulated amount of sleep loss prompted by short sleep.

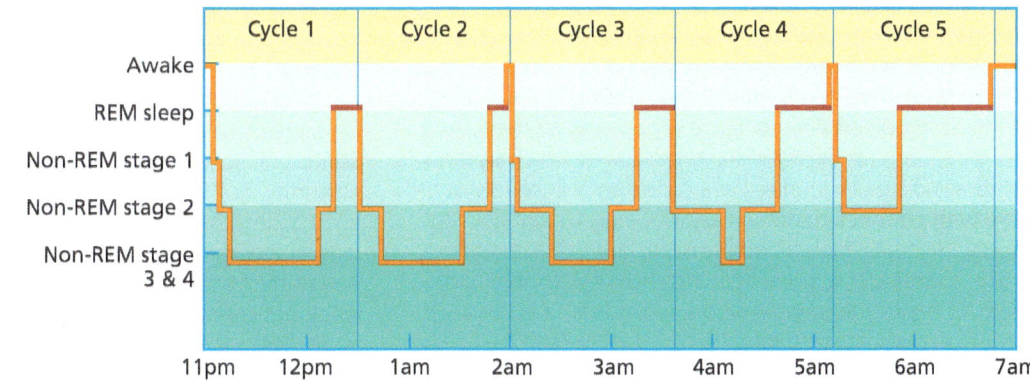

FIGURE 4.3 **Cycles of Sleep.** Sleep comes in cycles in which the stages of sleep shift in order and length throughout the night. A person who has been asleep for several hours may go straight from REM sleep to NREM stage 2, for example, or spend more time in REM sleep later.

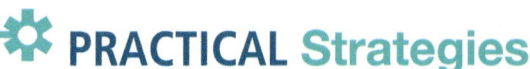

PRACTICAL Strategies

Naps: When and How?

Napping can certainly help you feel less tired, especially if you are sleep deprived. One study found that daytime napping after a night of sleep loss not only reduced feelings of tiredness and improved mental performance but led to reduced levels of stress-related hormones such as cortisol in the blood.[1] But napping remains most effective when it's a support for healthy sleep habits, not a substitute for them. To get the most from a short daytime rest, be sure to:[2,3]

- **Keep it short.** About 20 to 30 minutes is ideal, and even naps of 10 minutes can help improve alertness. Longer naps may leave you feeling groggy throughout the day.
- **Make a plan.** If you know you are likely to need a nap on a particular day, set aside time in advance rather than waiting until you are too cross-eyed to function.
- **Set a pattern.** There is a biological reason for the regular nap habits of babies and toddlers. If you find yourself seeking a nap a few times a week, try to nap at a consistent time (early afternoon is best) and for a regular duration of 20 to 30 minutes.
- **Avoid using naps as a crutch.** If you consistently deprive yourself of night-time sleep and then try to get by on day-time naps, you may set off a cycle of exhaustion. Frequent, long, random daytime naps can harm the quality of nighttime sleep, which in turn has negative health consequences. If you feel like you need a long nap every day, try adjusting your nighttime sleep before you shift your daytime schedule to accommodate more napping.

References: **1.** "Daytime napping after a night of sleep loss decreases sleepiness, improves performance, and causes beneficial changes in cortisol and interleukin-6 secretion," by A. N. Vgontzas, S. Pejovic, E. Zoumakis, H. M. Lin, E. O. Bixler, et al., January 2007, *American Journal of Physiology: Endocrinology and Metabolism*, doi: 10.1152/ajpendo.00651.2005. **2.** "Naps, cognition and performance," by G. Ficca, J. Axelsson, D. J. Mollicone, V. Muto, & M. V. Vitiello, 2010, *Sleep Medicine Reviews*, 14, pp. 249–258. **3.** "Napping may not be such a no-no," by Harvard Health Publications, November 2009, www.health.harvard.edu.

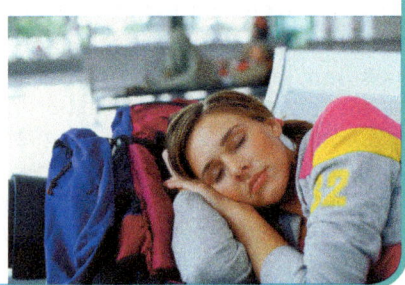

Although it may sound logical to reduce sleep debt by sleeping late on weekends, doing so may disrupt your sleep schedule and bring on insomnia. What about napping? Certainly a short nap—20 to 30 minutes in the early afternoon—can be refreshing. But longer or later naps can leave you feeling groggy during the day and can sometimes disturb your nighttime sleep.[6] (For a closer look at napping, see the **Practical Strategies** box above.) Sleep experts agree that the best way to make up sleep debt is gradually, by getting just a little extra sleep each night.

Research on Short and Long Sleep

Sleep researchers do not simply ask people how much they sleep and assume that the average must be the amount most people need. Researchers conduct two types of studies to determine sleep needs. In one type, they compare the number of hours of sleep patients report—when they visit their physician, for example—and the age at which patients eventually die. Such studies have consistently linked short sleep with poor health outcomes, including weight gain and obesity, diabetes, high blood pressure, heart disease and stroke, depression, and even an increased risk for premature death.[5] On average, people who sleep at least 7 hours a night experience greater longevity.

The second method for determining sleep needs is to conduct sleep-lab experiments. In one type of study, participants who normally sleep 7 to 8 hours are tested for their performance on specific tasks—often computerized activities requiring quick decision making. They're then allowed to sleep for only 6 hours a night—or less—for a period of several days or weeks, during which time they again perform the same tasks. Researchers compare their performances. Over many years, such studies have shown significant reductions in performance among subjects getting less than 7 hours of sleep.[7]

Some studies even show significant reductions in performance with exactly 7 hours of sleep.[8] One researcher explained that the impairment doesn't show up after a single night but appears consistently within five to seven nights of 7 hours of sleep a night. Thus, if you're short-changing your sleep, what you gain in time you lose in performance. Moreover, study subjects don't appear to be aware of their impairment: They report that sleepiness is not affecting them even as their performance scores plummet.[8]

What about long sleep? Does it reduce or improve performance? We don't really know for sure because people don't tend to sustain long sleep even when given the opportunity. For instance, in one study, researchers encouraged college students to "sleep as much as possible" over several weeks. The participants increased their average sleep time from 7.5 hours to nearly 10 hours for the first week but then "settled in" at an average of 8.5 hours a night. This increased sleep was associated with improved alertness and reaction time.[9] Several other studies have also shown that a moderate increase in sleep duration (to more than 8 hours) improves not only alertness and performance but also mood.[7]

Short Sleep: The American Way?

A national poll conducted in 2013 found that American adults typically experience short sleep every night of the work and school week, sleeping slightly less than 7 hours per night Monday through Friday. As shown in **Figure 4.4**, 1 in 5 American adults experiences *very* short sleep—less than 6 hours—on weeknights. The *average* number of hours American adults sleep on weeknights is 6.8—which also qualifies as short sleep. Even on weekends, the average creeps up only to 7.5 hours, barely edging into the range considered ample sleep.[10]

It might surprise you to learn that Americans of college age (19 to 29) tend to get more sleep than average. Only 23% experience short sleep, and most sleep about 7 hours, typically from midnight until about 7:00 a.m.[11] That said, no comparable data exist for young adults actually attending college, and a large national survey of college students found that more than 40% feel that daytime sleepiness presents a moderate to significant problem.[1] See **Student Stats** for more detail on sleepiness in college students.

Why Is Ample Sleep Important?

The link between ample sleep and increased longevity and functioning has been recognized for decades. Recently, researchers have been uncovering additional benefits of ample sleep—and some serious risks of short sleep.

Health Effects

Sleep influences your physical and psychological health in a variety of ways:

- Ample sleep can help you ward off colds and other infectious diseases. At the same time, short sleep reduces the number of functioning immune cells that help you respond to invaders.[12] One study in young men found that going without sleep for more than 24 hours triggered an immune response similar to that of physical stress, leading to abnormal white blood cell counts.[13]

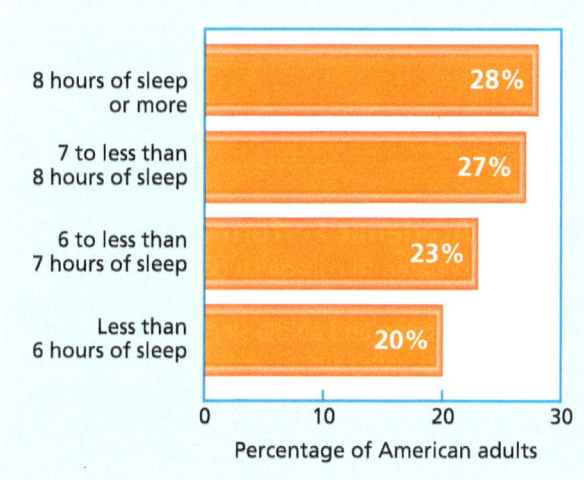

FIGURE 4.4 **Sleep in America.** Only 28% of American adults get 8 or more hours of sleep a night.
Source: Data from the *2009 Sleep in America Poll: Health and Safety*, from the National Sleep Foundation website, 2009.

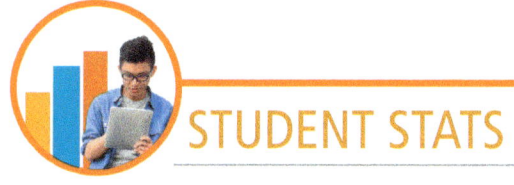

STUDENT STATS
Sleepless on Campus

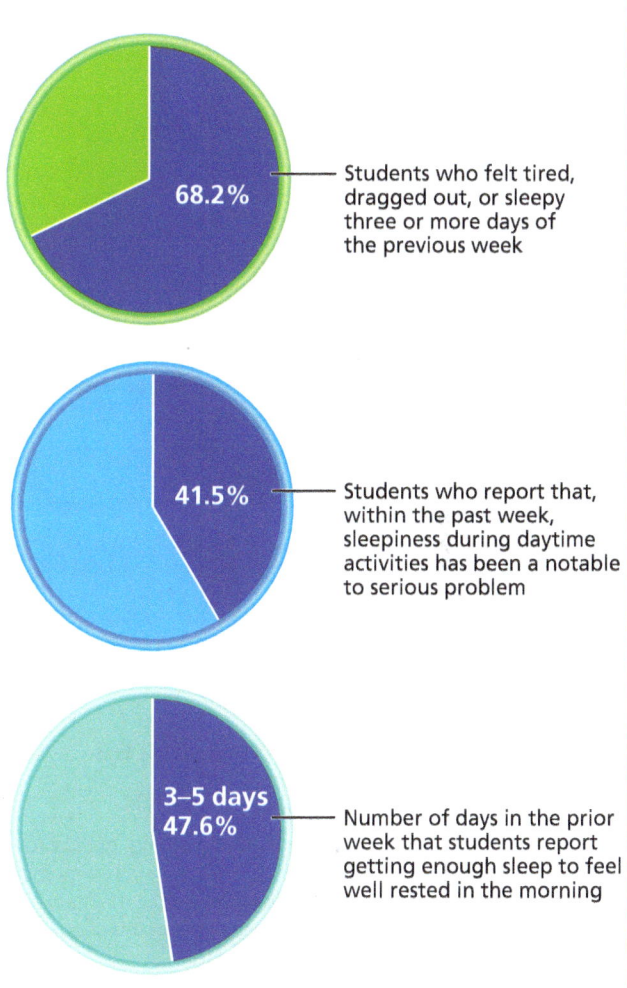

Source: American College Health Association. (2015). *ACHA-NCHA II: Undergraduate reference group executive summary, spring 2015*. www.acha-ncha.org.

- The U.S. Centers for Disease Control and Prevention (CDC) links short sleep to an increased risk for a variety of chronic diseases, including type 2 diabetes, heart disease, and obesity.[14] Several major studies have found that between increasing risk of both chronic disease and injuries such as fatigue-related driving accidents, less sleep can mean a shorter life span.[15]

- The CDC also associates short sleep with depression.[14] Among college students specifically, more than one study has found that those experiencing either a sleep debt or significant daytime sleepiness are at increased risk for depression.[16,17] Excessive sleeping, technically called *hypersomnia*, is also associated with depression. Another study has found that college students experiencing poor-quality sleep have increased levels of physical aggression and thoughts of suicide.[18]

Live better—get some rest! To get rid of those dark circles under your eyes:

CHOOSE THIS.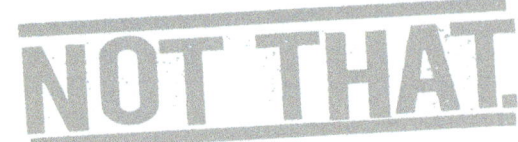

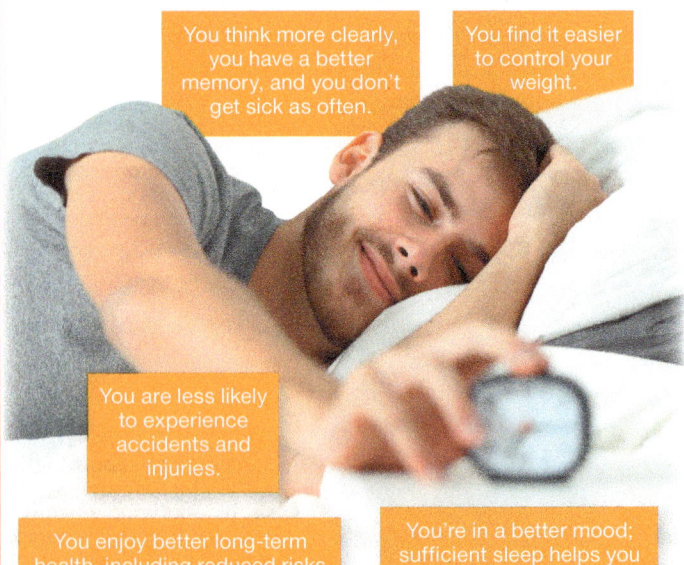

- You think more clearly, you have a better memory, and you don't get sick as often.
- You find it easier to control your weight.
- You are less likely to experience accidents and injuries.
- You enjoy better long-term health, including reduced risks of serious diseases such as diabetes or heart disease.
- You're in a better mood; sufficient sleep helps you weather challenges and have more energy for fun and laughter.

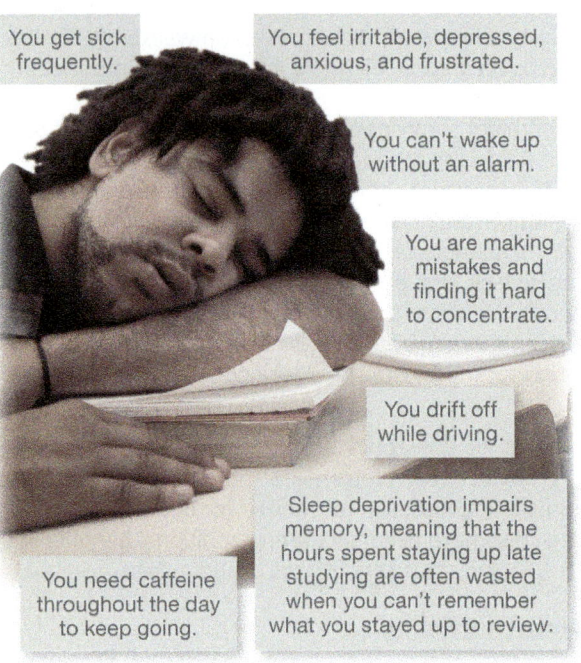

- You get sick frequently.
- You feel irritable, depressed, anxious, and frustrated.
- You can't wake up without an alarm.
- You are making mistakes and finding it hard to concentrate.
- You drift off while driving.
- You need caffeine throughout the day to keep going.
- Sleep deprivation impairs memory, meaning that the hours spent staying up late studying are often wasted when you can't remember what you stayed up to review.

What Life Look Likes With Ample Sleep:

Ample sleep not only makes for a great morning, but improved long-term health. When you are well rested, you remember more, enjoy better moods, find it easier to maintain a healthy weight, and reduce your risk of infectious and chronic disease.

Source: WebMD. (2011, December 27). *9 surprising reasons to get more sleep.* www.webmd.com.

You, Sleep Deprived:

Sleep deprivation may seem like the only path to better grades, but it's actually counterproductive. A chronic lack of sleep makes it harder to study effectively, impairs memory, dampens your mood, and leaves you more vulnerable to getting sick.

Source: American Academy of Sleep Medicine. (2013, January 1). *Seven signs you need sleep.* www.sleepeducation.org.

- Recently, researchers conducting a review of 36 studies of obesity found—across continents, ethnicities, and ages—that short sleep was strongly and consistently associated with current and future obesity.[19] One study of teenagers, for example, found that increasing nightly sleep from about 7 to 10 hours per night reduced the proportion of teens classified as overweight or obese by almost 5%.[20] One factor underlying reduced sleep and increased weight might be the effect that fatigue has on the brain, food cravings, and food choices. One recent study found a connection between shorter sleep, junk food consumption, and weight gain.[21]

Effects on Academic Performance

Sleep is closely related to college students' capacity for learning. Studies have consistently associated short sleep with impaired learning and ample sleep with improved academic and test-taking success.[22,23] In one study of college students, sleep quality was the strongest predictor of academic performance.[24] This link may be driven by an area at the very front of the cerebral cortex (called the *prefrontal cortex*) that is associated with complex thinking and decision making and that especially benefits from adequate sleep.

In light of this, it's not surprising that college students experiencing insomnia and other sleep concerns are significantly

> **"Drowsy driving is involved in 1 in 6 fatal motor vehicle accidents in the United States."**

overrepresented among students in academic jeopardy (GPA less than 2.0).[25] More specifically, college students who report pulling all-nighters to help them get their work done have, on average, lower GPAs than those who don't.[26]

On the other hand, students who report good sleep are more likely to succeed academically.[27] Why? One factor is that ample sleep after studying dramatically improves recall.[28] Recent research indicates that when it comes to memory, sleep is a highly active state in which memories undergo a process of consolidation, which is critical to long-term memory formation.[29]

During REM sleep, the brain transfers short-term memories from a temporary holding region to a long-term storage site at the sides of the cerebral cortex (called the *temporal lobes*). This process is known as *memory consolidation*. Because you build up most of your REM sleep only after you've been asleep for 6 hours, short sleep means you won't be able to consolidate memories as effectively.[30] REM sleep also allows the brain to replenish its stores of certain neurotransmitters that participate in memory, learning, performance, and problem solving.[30]

Risk for Traumatic Injury

Drowsy driving is involved in 1 in 6 fatal motor vehicle accidents in the United States, resulting in more than 1,500 American deaths each year.[31] In a national poll, more than one-third of adults admitted to having fallen asleep behind the wheel at least once in the past year.[10] Short sleep is associated with other kinds of traumatic injury, including work-related injuries, athletic injuries, and recreational injuries, with one study finding that about 13% of workplace injuries could be attributed to sleep problems.[32] Remember, if you're drowsy, you're within seconds of falling asleep. And if you're driving drowsy, you may be within seconds of a potentially fatal crash.

LO 4.2 QUICK CHECK

How much sleep do experts recommend for the average person each night?
a. At least 8 hours
b. At least 9 hours
c. Whatever feels practical for you, given everything else you have to do
d. At least 7 hours

What Factors Influence Sleep?

LO 4.3 Discuss a variety of factors that influence sleep.

The last time you lay awake at 3:00 a.m., did you think about the reasons? Maybe you blamed the energy drink you had while you were studying, or the hot weather, or anxiety about an upcoming exam. Or maybe, if you often have trouble sleeping, you wondered if it's just the way you are. Although no one can say for sure what keeps you awake on any particular night, researchers have identified the factors that most commonly influence sleep.

Biology and Genetics

Over many years, numerous twin studies have shown a genetic influence on sleep patterns, including sleep-time brain activity, tendencies toward timing and length of sleep, and tendencies toward sleep disorders.[33] Nonetheless, environmental and behavioral factors are considered more important than genetics. Similarly, although gender and ethnic differences in sleep patterns exist, they are thought to be due to factors such as socioeconomic differences and discrimination, stressors with the potential to affect sleep, rather than gender and ethnicity themselves.[34] For more on sleep differences across genders and ethnicities, see the **Diversity & Health** box.

Poor health commonly disrupts sleep, especially when it's accompanied by pain, stress, impaired breathing, fever, or other distressing symptoms. A medical condition called sleep apnea, discussed shortly, causes frequent waking and restless sleep. In women, both pregnancy and the hormonal shifts of the normal menstrual cycle can contribute. In one recent national survey, people experiencing chronic pain experienced both poorer sleep quality and a greater sleep debt than those not living with pain.[35] Psychological conditions, including depression and anxiety, can also disturb sleep. Some medications, including antidepressants and drugs for asthma and high blood pressure, can interfere with sleep as well.

Individual Behaviors

If you're having trouble sleeping, any of the following factors may be contributing:

- **Presleep use of technology.** A recent national survey of families found that almost 90% of adults and 75% of children have at least one electronic device in the bedroom, and the vast majority of households have such devices, with many of them often left on at night.[36] If you're part of this majority, you might be interested to know that researchers have identified two problems with your behavior: First, use of such devices can be "alerting," provoke anxiety, or disrupt sleep, making it difficult to disengage, fall asleep, and stay asleep. Second, the screens of these devices emit a particular type of blue light that researchers believe is especially disruptive to sleep. Focusing on "blue light" devices just before trying to sleep may limit your body's melatonin production and shift your circadian rhythm. So in the hour before bedtime, choose an activity that will help you unwind, like reading a calming book—and not on your iPad or Kindle.

- **Hunger.** Food stays in your stomach about 2 to 4 hours before it is released, a little at a time, into the small intestine.[37] You should stay upright during this time. If you lie down, the acid your stomach naturally produces to help break down the food can seep backward into the lower portion of your esophagus, irritating its lining and giving you the sensation commonly known as heartburn. Gastroesophageal reflux disease (GERD), the technical name for persistent heartburn, commonly provokes sleepless

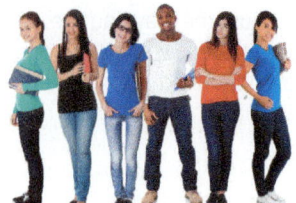

DIVERSITY & HEALTH

Sleep Habits Vary

The National Sleep Foundation has been conducting a *Sleep in America* poll annually for the past decade, with surveys that have focused on women and sleep and ethnicity and sleep. Here are key findings:

Sex

- Overall, American men sleep better than American women.
- Men are about 11% more likely than women to say they get more sleep than they need, whereas women are about 11% more likely to say they get less sleep than they need.
- Men are about 13% more likely than women to have their sleep needs met both on weekdays and weekends.

Ethnicity

- Overall, Asian Americans have fewer sleep problems than any other ethnic group.
- Asian Americans are the ethnic group most likely to say that they had a good night's sleep at least a few nights or more a week (84%).
- Asian Americans are also the least likely to report using sleep medication (5%). In contrast, 13% of Caucasians, 9% of African Americans, and 8% of Hispanics report using sleep medication.
- At least one-third of Hispanics (38%) and African Americans (33%) report that financial, employment, relationship, and/or health-related concerns disturb their sleep at least a few nights a week. These concerns disturbed the sleep of 28% of Caucasians and 25% of Asian Americans.
- African Americans report getting the lowest amount of sleep each night—at least half an hour less than the amount of sleep reported by other ethnic groups.
- Caucasians are much more likely (14%) than any other ethnic group (2% each) to say they usually sleep with a pet.

What Do You Think?

1. What are some of the reasons that men might report getting more of the sleep they need than women?
2. Given what you've learned about the health effects of sleep, what might be some of the long-term health consequences for women related to getting relatively less sleep?
3. What are some of the factors (cultural, economic, social) that might lead certain groups to use sleep medication more than others?

Source: Data from *Sleep in America* by the National Sleep Foundation, 2010 and 2007, retrieved from **www.sleepfoundation.org**.

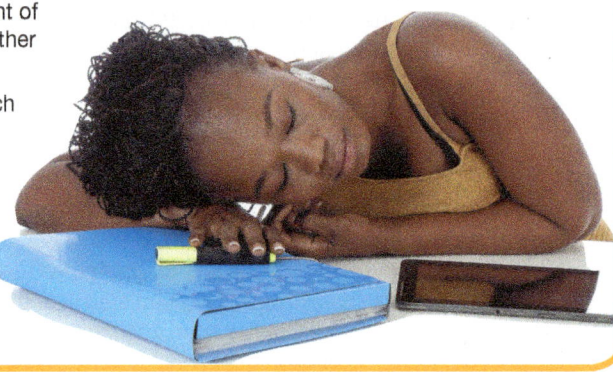

nights, and recent research has found that poor sleep can in turn trigger further GERD-related symptoms.[38] But although you should definitely avoid eating a full meal before going to bed, you should also avoid trying to sleep if you are physically hungry. So go for a light snack. Some experts recommend a banana and a small glass of milk—a snack that not only takes away your hunger pangs but also provides amino acids, carbohydrates, and minerals in combinations that are thought to be relaxing.

- **Spicy foods.** Is it a myth that spicy foods keep you awake? Several studies over the years suggest that it's true. A classic study involving young, healthy males found that on nights when the participants had Tabasco sauce and mustard with their evening meals, it took longer for them to fall asleep, and their sleep was more fitful throughout the first sleep cycle. Indigestion was not thought to be the culprit. Instead, the researchers believe that the spices elevated the participants' body temperature enough to disturb the nervous and hormonal mechanisms that normally initiate sleep.[39]
- **Smoking.** While some people believe that a smoke before sleep is relaxing, exactly the opposite is true: Nicotine, the psychoactive drug in tobacco, is a stimulant. Moreover, the adverse physical effects of smoking, including the so-called smoker's cough, can disrupt sleep throughout the night. Finally, smoking in bed can be dangerous! Falling asleep with a lit cigarette can start a fire, and every year, almost 1,000 Americans die in residential fires caused by smoking.[40] Bottom line: If you smoke, stop.
- **Caffeine.** The stimulant most commonly associated with sleep troubles is caffeine. Teenagers who consume a relatively high amount of caffeine, for example, have reported both having trouble sleeping at night and feeling tired in the morning.[41] But both the amount and the timing of intake matter. Studies suggest that the amount of caffeine in as many as 4 cups of coffee or 8 cups of tea per day confers little health risk.[42] However, your body gets rid of caffeine only slowly, taking about 5 to 7 hours, on average, to eliminate *half* of it. Even after 8 to 10 hours, 25% of the caffeine is still present.[43] This means that, if you plan to get to bed at 11:00 p.m., you might be okay enjoying coffee or a cola at lunch but not afterward.
- **Stimulant medications.** In 2014, about 1 million Americans abused prescription stimulants, usually Ritalin,

Adderall, and other drugs developed for people with attention disorders.⁴⁴ Abuse of these drugs on college campuses is an increasing concern among public health experts because of the drugs' potential for addiction, adverse effects on students' creativity, and relationship to sleep problems—which in turn reduce learning. In one study involving nearly 500 college students, those who reported stimulant abuse also reported lower sleep quality and greater sleep disturbance. Moreover, although the primary reason these students gave for abusing stimulants was to improve their concentration and academic performance, the students reporting high GPAs were actually the least likely to abuse stimulants.⁴⁵

- **Alcohol.** Because alcohol is a sedative—a drug that promotes calm and drowsiness—drinking before bedtime can help you fall asleep. The problem is what happens a few hours later: In the second, deeper sleep cycle, the drowsiness wears off.⁴⁶ As a result, you are likely to awaken from periods of REM sleep and find it difficult to return to sleep.

Incidentally, if you're wondering whether or not vigorous exercise close to bedtime can disturb your sleep, the jury is still out. Although some health-care experts still advise against nighttime exercise, recent studies have not found that it disturbs sleep.⁴⁷

Factors in the Environment

Nearly any sensory disturbance in your environment—noise in the dorm hallway, prickly bedding, a sagging mattress, or a bedroom that's too hot or too bright—can disturb your sleep. So can a disturbance in your schedule—a shift in your work hours, travel, or transitioning from summer back into the academic year.

Other external stressors that commonly disrupt sleep are financial problems, academic concerns, relationship conflicts, and feelings of being overwhelmed—that there just aren't enough hours in a day for all you have to do. In one national sleep survey, those with severe or very severe stress were more than twice as likely to report poorer sleep quality than people with little or no stress (83% versus 35%).³⁵ Also, 67% of those with severe or very severe stress reported difficulty sleeping in the past seven days, compared with only 25% of those with no or mild stress.³⁵

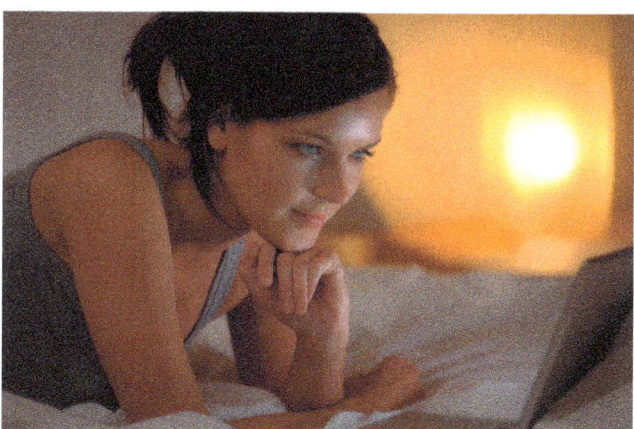

Using a laptop in bed can make getting to sleep difficult.

Unfortunately, the connection between stress and sleep is reciprocal: Stress affects the quality and duration of your sleep, and poor sleep reduces your ability to manage stress. Moreover, stressing out about your inability to sleep can actually reinforce your sleep problem!

LO 4.3 QUICK CHECK

Why does technology use an hour or two before bed hinder sleep?

a. The information viewed or used may be stressful or upsetting.
b. The bright light emitted by many devices may limit melatonin production.
c. Even when set aside, devices often emit noise if not shut off.
d. All of the above

Sleep Disorders

LO 4.4 Define and describe sleep disorders such as insomnia, sleep apnea, and parasomnias.

In a recent, large-scale study, 27% of students at a public university were found to be at risk for at least one sleep disorder.²⁵ The American Academy of Sleep Medicine identifies dozens of such disorders, divided into six major categories related to everything from sleeping too little or too much to breathing difficulties and abnormal sleep times.⁴⁸ Here, we discuss only the most common.

Insomnia

Insomnia—a term that literally means "no sleep"—is a condition characterized by difficulty falling or staying asleep, a pattern of waking too early, or poor-quality sleep. Although 30% to 35% of American adults occasionally suffer from insomnia in any given year, about 10% experience chronic insomnia—that is, insomnia that lasts more than a month.⁴⁹

> **insomnia** A condition characterized by difficulty falling or staying asleep, a pattern of waking too early, or poor-quality sleep.
>
> **snoring** A ragged, hoarse sound that occurs during sleep when breathing is obstructed.

There are two types of insomnia. *Secondary insomnia* is by far the most common and is due to a behavior such as substance abuse or another medical disorder such as heart disease. *Primary insomnia* occurs in only about 20% of people with insomnia and almost always develops as a result of stress. Before diagnosing primary insomnia, a physician will conduct an interview and a series of tests to rule out behaviors (such as alcohol or caffeine intake) and medical disorders that could be causing secondary insomnia. Treatment of insomnia and other sleep problems is discussed shortly.

Snoring

If you've ever been kept awake by someone's **snoring**, you know how irritating the sound can be. It occurs when breathing is obstructed during sleep. As many as half of all Americans snore at least occasionally.⁵⁰ Alcohol consumption,

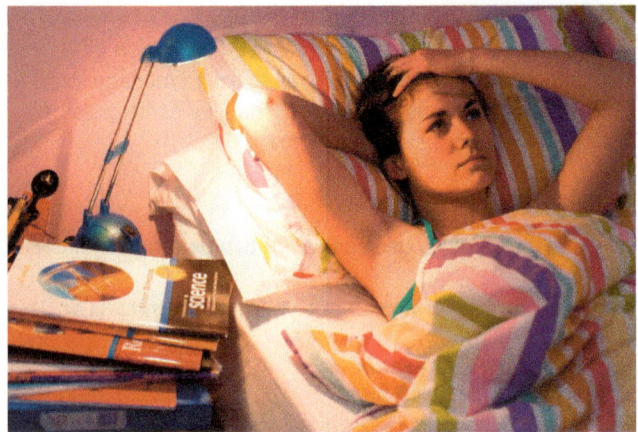

Insomnia can sometimes be caused by stress.

overweight, and colds and allergies all contribute to narrowing of your airways and can result in snoring. Occasional light snoring is nothing to be concerned about; however, if your snoring is chronic, if it is loud enough to waken your roommate, or if you wake up in the middle of the night feeling as if you are choking, you may have sleep apnea.

>> For tips on reducing snoring, search for "7 easy fixes for snoring" at **webmd.com**.

Sleep Apnea

sleep apnea A disorder in which one or more pauses in breathing occur during sleep.

Sleep apnea (AP-nee-ah) is a disorder in which one or more pauses in breathing occur during sleep. These breathing pauses can last from a few seconds to minutes. They often occur 5 to 30 times an hour.[51] Typically, normal breathing then starts again, sometimes with a loud snort or choking sound.

Although it can develop at any age, sleep apnea becomes more common as you get older. At least 1 in 10 people over age 65 has sleep apnea. It is most common in men, in people who are overweight, and in people who smoke.[52]

As you can imagine, sleep apnea significantly disrupts sleep, jerking the person out of deep sleep and into light sleep, or even waking the person up. This results in overall poor-quality sleep. The pauses in breathing also increase the person's risk for heart attack or stroke, and the poor sleep can lead to daytime drowsiness that sets the stage for traumatic injury. Any of these can be deadly: A comprehensive, long-term study found that Americans with sleep apnea have a threefold greater risk of premature death than those without the disorder.[52]

There are two types of sleep apnea. In *obstructive sleep apnea*, the airway collapses or becomes blocked during sleep (**Figure 4.5**). When the sleeper tries to breathe, any air that squeezes past the blockage can cause loud snoring. Breathing pauses may occur, and choking or gasping may follow the pauses. In *central sleep apnea*, which is less common, the area of the brain that controls breathing doesn't send the correct signals to the respiratory muscles. As a result, breathing stops for brief periods. Snoring doesn't typically happen with central sleep apnea.[52]

Diagnosis and Treatment of Sleep Apnea

To check for sleep apnea, a physician looks for structural abnormalities—such as excessive tissue—in the back of the mouth and throat. The physician might also order a *polysomnogram*, a test conducted in a sleep lab that records brain wave activity, breathing, and other signs while the patient sleeps. Alternatively, the physician may suggest testing at home using a sleep monitor.

For mild cases of sleep apnea, taking care of contributing factors may solve the problem. For example, the patient may need to lose weight, quit smoking, avoid all alcohol, or use nasal decongestants. Patients are also advised to sleep on their side.

For moderate cases, an orthodontist can fit the patient with a plastic mouthpiece that adjusts the lower jaw and tongue to keep the airways open during sleep. Or the patient can sleep with a CPAP machine. *CPAP* stands for *continuous positive airway pressure:* Through a mask that fits over the sleeper's nose and mouth, the device sends air into the sleeper's throat at a pressure just high enough to keep the airways open (see **Figure 4.5c**).

In cases of severe sleep apnea, surgery to widen the breathing passages may be necessary. It usually involves shrinking, stiffening, or removing excess tissue in the mouth and throat or resetting the lower jaw.

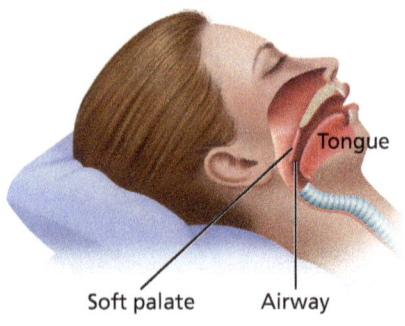
(a) Normal sleep

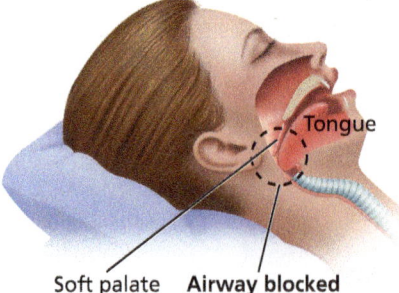
(b) Obstructive sleep apnea

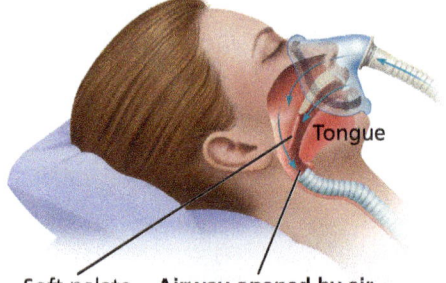
(c) Treatment of sleep apnea with CPAP machine

FIGURE 4.5 **Obstructive Sleep Apnea.** (a) During normal sleep, the airways at the back of the mouth and throat remain open. (b) In obstructive sleep apnea, tissues at the back of the mouth and throat are collapsed, blocking the airways. (c) CPAP generates a wave of air that continuously presses against the sleeper's tissues, keeping the airways open.

STUDENT STORY

Sleep Apnea

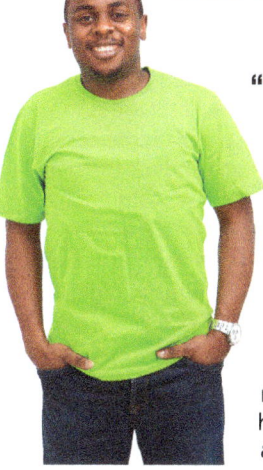

"HI, I'M REMY. I was diagnosed with sleep apnea about six months ago. I had been feeling really tired every day, even though I thought I was getting enough sleep, and there were a few times when I almost fell asleep when I was driving. I went to the doctor and at first he wasn't sure what was wrong but when I told him that my roommate says I snore really badly, he arranged for me to get a sleep apnea testing kit to take home with me. Now I sleep every night with a CPAP machine. It's a little weird to get used to, but it's worth it to not feel so tired."

What Do You Think?

1. Untreated sleep apnea increases Remy's risk for which physical problems? How might it affect his schoolwork?
2. Does Remy have obstructive sleep apnea or central sleep apnea? How can you tell? What's the difference between the two?
3. What factor in Remy's life increases his risk for sleep apnea? Which factor makes his case less common?

Narcolepsy

Narcolepsy is a disorder in which the brain fails to regulate sleep–wake cycles normally. Patients sleep a normal amount but cannot control the timing of their sleep. During the day, they may experience sudden attacks of sleepiness combined with a loss of muscle tone and sometimes hallucinations and brief paralysis. The disorder is also associated with insomnia. Although the precise cause of narcolepsy is still unknown, genetic, biological, and environmental factors all may play a part. About 1 in 200 people have some form of narcolepsy.[53]

Treatment for narcolepsy includes the use of certain medications, such as stimulants and antidepressants, to control sleep–wake cycles. Behavioral therapies are also important and include scheduling regular naps, avoiding heavy meals, and avoiding alcohol.

Parasomnias

The prefix *para-* can mean both "along with" and "abnormal," so a **parasomnia** is a condition in which unusual events accompany sleep. The most common example is nightmares, frightening dreams that wake you from REM sleep. About 50% of children and 50% to 85% of adults occasionally experience nightmares. Nightmares are not considered a sleep disorder unless they become chronic, in which case they may cause short sleep because the person fears falling asleep. Psychotherapy and stress management are among the most common treatments.[54]

Sleep Terrors

Sleep terrors (also called *night terrors*) are similar to nightmares in that they involve either dreams or feelings of intense fear. However, nightmares tend to occur during one of the later cycles of REM sleep, toward morning, whereas sleep terrors typically occur during one of the first NREM periods of the night. To observers, the sleeper appears to awaken from a dream screaming and often thrashing; however, the sleeper is not awake, and the episode may persist for 10 minutes or more, despite attempts at arousal, such as calling or shaking. Often the terror subsides on its own, and the person drifts back into restful sleep. If the person does wake up, he or she is usually very confused. Sleep terrors are much less common than nightmares, occurring in more than 6% of children and about 2% of adults.[55]

Sleepwalking

Sleepwalking occurs during stages 3 and 4 of NREM sleep, usually early in the night. Although it can occur at any age, it is most common in childhood. Up to 17% of children sometimes sleepwalk, and about 4% of adults do so as well.[56] Episodes can last from several seconds to 30 minutes. The person rises out of bed, eyes open, but with a blank look, and typically begins walking or performing another activity, such as dressing or going to the bathroom. If the person talks, the words make no sense. Because injury during sleepwalking is common, the sleeper should be gently guided back to bed or awakened. Sleepwalking is generally not serious and needs no treatment.[56]

> **narcolepsy** A disorder in which the brain fails to regulate sleep–wake cycles normally.
>
> **parasomnia** A condition in which unusual events accompany sleep.
>
> **sleep terror** Parasomnia characterized by the appearance of awakening in terror during a stage of NREM sleep.
>
> **sleepwalking** Parasomnia in which a person walks or performs another complex activity while still asleep.
>
> **sleep bruxism** Clenching or grinding the teeth during sleep.

Sleep Bruxism

If you ever awaken with a sore jaw, it's possible that you may have been clenching or grinding your teeth during sleep—a behavior called **sleep bruxism.** It can also cause earache, headache, and damage to your tooth enamel and the soft tissues of your mouth. Although the cause of sleep bruxism is not known, possible factors include stress, substance abuse (especially abuse of stimulants, including nicotine), and misalignment. If you suspect that you're grinding your teeth at night, a first step is to see your dentist, who may prescribe a mouth guard or refer you to another specialist.[57]

Nocturnal Eating

Sleep and hunger are both fundamental physiological drives regulated by the hypothalamus and other regions

nocturnal eating disorder A condition characterized by significant food consumption at night and typically accompanied by depression, insomnia, and a daytime eating disorder.

REM behavior disorder (RBD) Parasomnia characterized by failure of inhibition of muscle movement during REM sleep.

restless legs syndrome (RLS) A nervous system disorder characterized by a strong urge to move the legs, accompanied by creeping, burning, or other unpleasant sensations.

involved in circadian rhythms.[58] When the coordination of these two drives is impaired, a **nocturnal eating disorder** can occur. Although two such disorders are recognized, they have more similarities than differences. In *night-eating syndrome,* a person awakens from sleep and eats a significant amount of food before returning to sleep. In *sleep-related eating disorder,* the person typically reports that he or she is half asleep or even fully asleep while eating. In both conditions, more than one eating episode may occur each night, and sufferers are at increased risk for obesity. Both conditions are more common in women than men, and depression, insomnia, and daytime eating disorders are typically seen in people with either diagnosis.[59] Treatment usually involves psychotherapy and medication.

REM Behavior Disorder

Recall that, normally, a region of the brain stem called the pons inhibits almost all muscle movement during REM sleep. In **REM behavior disorder (RBD),** this inhibition fails to occur, and the sleeper acts his dreams, sometimes with punching, kicking, or jumping. RBD is a rare parasomnia, occurring in less than 1% of the population, almost always in males, and has been linked to several health behaviors or medical conditions, including tobacco use and having a prior head injury. It's typically treated with medications, and the patient must also avoid alcohol.[60]

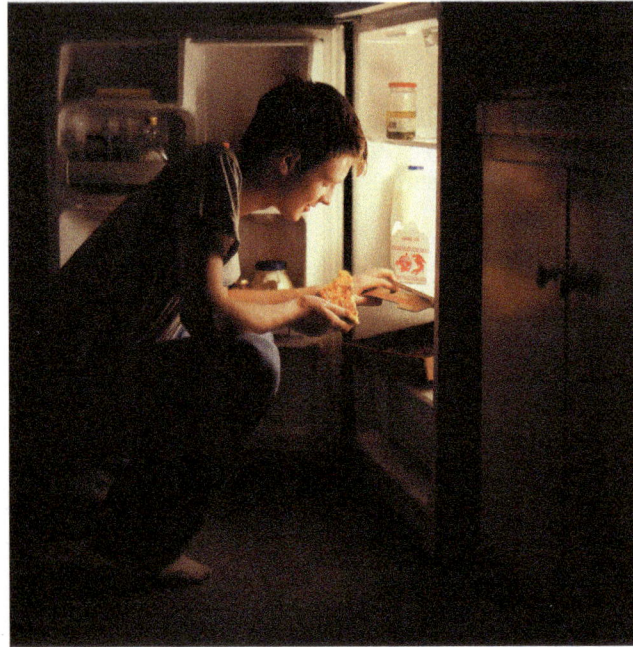

Those who suffer from a **nocturnal eating disorder** can be at risk for obesity.

Restless Legs Syndrome

Although it might not sound like a sleep disorder, **restless legs syndrome (RLS)** only comes on when a person is inactive, so it commonly disrupts sleep. RLS causes a strong urge to move the legs, accompanied by creeping, burning, itching, or otherwise unpleasant feelings in the legs—and sometimes in the arms. Getting up and walking or stretching or massaging the legs can help. Although no one knows the precise causes of RLS, both alcohol and tobacco can trigger episodes, so both should be avoided. Some cases appear to be associated with iron deficiency, and for them an iron supplement may be prescribed, while other cases appear to have a genetic component. About 1 in every 10 people experience RLS. People with RLS may find that vigorous physical activity during the day reduces their symptoms at night.[61]

LO 4.4 QUICK CHECK

Which of the following is not a cause of insomnia?
a. stress
b. exercise
c. substance abuse
d. large amounts of caffeine

Getting Help for a Sleep Disorder

LO 4.5 Discuss the clinical diagnosis and treatment of sleep disorders.

Fortunately, both campus health services and the medical community have become increasingly aware of the importance of addressing sleep problems early and aggressively, and effective help is available.

Campus and Community Support

Administrators and health-care providers on campuses across the United States are beginning to wake up to the need for programs and services to address sleep deprivation among their students.[62] Some campuses have delayed the start of the academic day, rescheduling all 8:00 a.m. classes to 9:00 a.m. or later. Some are instituting quiet hours and noise ordinances in dorms. Some are offering seminars, workshops, and extended programs to teach students the importance of sleep and strategies to improve their sleep. In a study of one such program, the Sleep Treatment and Education Program for Students (STEPS), participants reported significantly improved sleep quality.[63] College students may be especially likely to benefit from in-person sleep behavior classes and other assistance because adult sleep patterns are just being formed and are likely to respond well to guidance and behavior change efforts.[64] So if you're having trouble sleeping, stop off at your campus health center. Chances are the staff there will be able to help.

Clinical Diagnosis and Treatment

If sleep problems persist beyond one month, it's time to see your doctor. Usually, a primary care provider is able to diagnose and treat sleep disorders following an interview and certain lab tests, but in some cases, referral to a sleep clinic may be necessary.

Sleep Studies

Sleep studies are tests conducted while you sleep—usually in a sleep lab within a hospital or at a specialized sleep clinic. Prior to the test, electrodes (small metal discs) are attached to your scalp and body. While you sleep, these send feedback to a device that records data such as your brain waves, eye movements, heart rate, and snoring. A soft belt around your torso records your breathing rate, and a clip on one fingertip records the level of oxygen in your blood. Although these devices may feel unusual, they do not cause pain.

The results of a sleep study may reveal, for example, blocked airflow or limb muscle movement. Typically, a sleep specialist reviews the findings and recommends appropriate treatment.

>> Search youtube.com for "Shaq attacks sleep apnea" to view a video by Harvard Medical School on how NBA star Shaquille O'Neal underwent a sleep study and received treatment for sleep apnea.

Medications

Twenty-five percent of Americans take some type of medication every year to help them sleep.[65] However, the American Academy of Sleep Medicine recommends that you avoid sleeping pills, if possible, and suggests taking them only under a doctor's care for either occasional or short-term use.[66] One analysis of sleep therapy among college students also discouraged the use of medications because behavior-based approaches can deliver both effective short- and long-term improvements without the side effects of sleeping pills.[67]

These warnings reflect the fact that some types of sleep medications—benzodiazepines such as Valium—are highly addictive, and even the newer drugs—the so-called z-drugs, such as Ambien—are habit forming, with some studies showing an addictive potential similar to that of the older drugs.[68,69]

In addition, the z-drugs are associated with side effects that can be distressing or even dangerous. For example, the uncommon but severe side effects of Ambien include confusion, memory loss, hallucinations, new or worsening depression, thoughts of suicide, agitation, aggressive behavior, and anxiety. Rarely, after taking Ambien, people have gotten out of bed and sleepwalked, prepared and eaten food, made phone calls, and even driven a car while not fully awake.

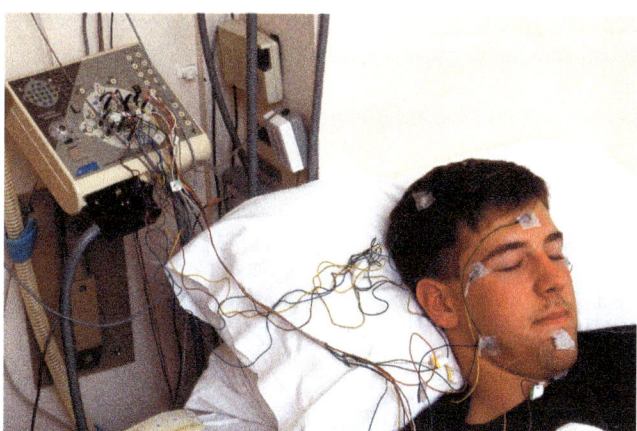

Sleep studies can determine the sources of sleep problems.

STUDENT STORY

Sleep Deprived

"HI, I'M JASMINE. I'm a freshman and I'm a child development major. Each night, I'm very lucky if I get 4 hours of sleep. I'm just a night owl. I like staying up at night. My father's the exact same way. It's like 3 o'clock in the morning and we'll still be up watching the food channel. Around exam time, I find myself awake at 7:30 in the morning, still up—knowing that I have a test at 9:30. Why, I don't know.

I don't think I'm doing my best right now because when I drag myself to class, I'm half asleep. I do need to change and get better rest so that I can do better in school. I don't think I've gotten 8 hours of sleep since I was 13. I'm 19, so that's six years of not getting a full night's sleep. That takes a toll on your body and your mind."

What Do You Think?

1. How ready do you think Jasmine is to make a change? Think back to the stages of health behavior change from Chapter 1. What stage of would you guess that Jasmine is in?
2. What factors in Jasmine's environment are reinforcing her late-night behavior? What factors are going against it?
3. What are three constructive steps that Jasmine can take to get more sleep? (Don't just critique her current routine; rather, suggest concrete alternatives.)

Often the person does not recall these events in the morning. One recent study even linked a popular z-drug with a nearly five-fold increased risk of early death.[68]

Due to such risks, in 2013 the U.S. Food and Drug Administration required the makers of Ambien and similar z-drugs to reduce the recommended dose. The FDA also issued a warning against driving the morning after taking these medications.[70]

What about over-the-counter sleep aids? Are they effective—and safe? See the **Consumer Corner** on page 88 for answers.

Cognitive-Behavioral Therapy

Several studies of college students have supported the effectiveness of cognitive-behavioral interventions in changing the thought patterns and behaviors that may be contributing to troubled sleep.[71] Techniques may include muscle relaxation, deep breathing, changes to your sleep routine, and psychotherapy to help you identify and cope with the anxieties or other thoughts that disturb your sleep. In one study, students learned a "worry control" procedure consisting of identifying worries keeping them awake and writing down possible solutions to the worries. The study found that the

CONSUMER CORNER
Should You Try OTC Sleep Aids?

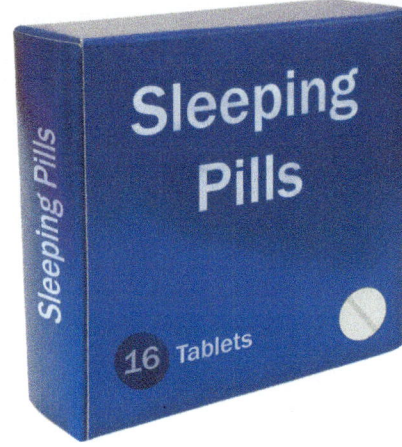

A variety of over-the-counter (OTC) sleep remedies have been available for decades, but do they work, and are they safe?

The most popular OTC sleep drugs are antihistamines. That's right: Their active ingredient is the same thing you might take for hay fever or an allergic skin rash. That's because the same drug that blocks the release of histamine in allergic reactions also causes drowsiness—which is why you're not supposed to drive or operate any type of machinery when you're taking allergy medications. OTC antihistamines for sleep include Excedrin PM, Tylenol PM, Sominex, and others, including generic brands.

Sleep experts say that the safety and effectiveness of such sleep aids aren't well understood.[1] You build up tolerance quickly, so the more often you take the drugs, the less effective they become. Moreover, they're notorious for leaving you feeling groggy and tired when you wake up—not exactly the best start for your hectic day. And, because they're identical to antihistamines sold for hay fever, they dry out your nose and mouth.[1,2] In general, the long-term safety and effectiveness of OTC antihistamine sleep remedies has not been well studied, and many authorities recommend against their use, even in the short term.[2–3]

So if you're having trouble sleeping, what should you do? First, make sure you've tried all of the sleep-hygiene suggestions in this chapter. Then, if you're still tossing and turning, make an appointment to see your doctor.

References: 1. "Sleep aids: Understand over-the-counter options," by the Mayo Foundation, November 20, 2014, www.mayoclinic.org. 2. "Safety of over-the-counter sleeping pills," by Harvard Health, August 2005, *The Harvard Medical School Family Health Guide*, www.health.harvard.edu. 3. "Sleep complaints: Whenever possible, avoid the use of sleeping pills," October 2008, *Prescrire International*, *17*(97), 206–212.

---

procedure significantly reduced the time it took for students to fall asleep.[72]

Complementary and Alternative Therapies

Although over a million Americans use complementary and alternative therapies for sleep problems each year, the research into their effectiveness is limited. Both chamomile and valerian—two herbs commonly used for insomnia—are safe to use in moderation, but neither has been proven in clinical trials to be effective for sleep problems.[73] The evidence is somewhat stronger for melatonin supplements, which are typically used by travelers to ward off jet lag: Studies suggest that melatonin may be able to help elderly people with insomnia fall asleep a few minutes faster and may also relieve jet lag. However, side effects have been reported, and more research is needed.[73]

In contrast, various forms of physical activity do appear to help reduce sleep problems. In one review study of 12 clinical trials involving patients with insomnia, cognitive-behavioral therapy was found most effective. However, both yoga and *t'ai chi* (a slow, meditative movement therapy from China) also significantly improved sleep. Another study of college students found improvement in sleep with both *t'ai chi* and a form of body exercise called Pilates.[74]

LO 4.5 QUICK CHECK
Which of the following cognitive-behavior techniques may be helpful with insomnia?
a. Muscle relaxation
b. Deep breathing
c. A "worry control" writing exercise
d. All of the above

Change Yourself, Change Your World

LO 4.6 Identify strategies for improving the quantity and quality of your sleep.

Have you ever woken up from a good night's sleep feeling as if you're ready for anything? When you're well rested, you manage stress more easily, solve problems more effectively, and make more realistic assessments of yourself and your world. In one study, a single night of sleep deprivation seriously impaired subjects' abilities to make accurate assessments of risks versus benefits and effective decisions about their well-being.[75]

Personal Choices

In college, sleep may feel like the last thing you can fit into your schedule. But investing in sufficient, regular sleep will pay off with improvements in your academic performance and your health. If you're ready to give your sleep the time and attention it merits, a first step is to identify where you're starting from. Once you know that, you'll be able to recognize the sleep-boosting strategies that are right for you.

Self-Monitor Your Sleep

Earlier in this chapter, we listed seven signs that you're sleep deprived. If one or more of those signs applies to you, you might want to ask yourself some questions about the quality and quantity of your sleep. Take the **Self-Assessment** to find some answers.

Improve Your Ability to Fall Asleep and Stay Asleep

Sleep experts recognize two tasks required for a good night's sleep. First, you have to be able to fall asleep! You

SELF-ASSESSMENT
Are You Getting Enough Sleep?

How likely are you to doze off or fall asleep in the following situations, in contrast to feeling just tired? As you complete this Self-Assessment, think about your usual way of life in recent times. Even if you have not done some of these things recently, try to gauge how they would have affected you. Use the following scale to choose the most appropriate number for each situation:

0 = no chance of dozing
1 = slight chance of dozing
2 = moderate chance of dozing
3 = high chance of dozing

Situation	Chance of Dozing
1. Sitting and reading	0 1 2 3
2. Watching TV	0 1 2 3
3. Sitting inactive in a public place (e.g., a theater or a meeting)	0 1 2 3
4. Being a passenger in a car for an hour without a break	0 1 2 3
5. Lying down to rest in the afternoon when circumstances permit	0 1 2 3
6. Sitting and talking with someone	0 1 2 3
7. Sitting quietly after a lunch without alcohol	0 1 2 3
8. Driving a car, while stopped for a few minutes in traffic	0 1 2 3

Total Score: _____

How To Interpret Your Score
1–6: Congratulations, you are getting enough sleep!
7–8: Your score is average.
9 and up: Seek the advice of a sleep specialist without delay.

To complete this Self-Assessment online, visit **MasteringHealth™**

Source: "A new method for measuring daytime sleepiness: The Epworth sleepiness scale," by M. W. Johns, 1991, *Sleep, 14*(6), 540–545. © 1991 American Academy of Sleep Medicine. Republished with permission conveyed through Copyright Clearance Center, Inc.

---

can increase your success in this task, technically called *sleep initiation*, by paying attention to certain aspects of your **sleep hygiene**—the behaviors and environmental factors that together influence the quantity and quality of your sleep. The material in the **Special Feature** on page 90 identifies several steps to help get you off to sleep.

sleep hygiene The behaviors and environmental factors that together influence the quantity and quality of sleep.

Some people drift off to sleep quite easily, only to waken again in a few minutes—or in the middle of the night—unable to get back to sleep. Other people sleep 5 or 6 hours but still wake too early to be fully rested. Sleep experts consider such problems of *sleep maintenance* a form of insomnia. If they characterize your nights, here are some aspects of your sleep hygiene that just might be contributing to the problem.

Are you haphazard about the time you get to bed and the time you wake up—shifting your sleep schedule according to the tasks of the day? If so, this one bad habit could be the sole cause of your sleep problem. To solve it, set a regular sleep–wake schedule and stick to it. It might sound challenging, but going to bed and getting up at roughly the same time every day is the most important step you can take to help your body get into a regular sleep pattern.[76] If you're sure you're carrying a sleep debt and long to sleep in next weekend, set your alarm for no more than 1 hour later than your usual wake-up time. Paying back sleep debt gradually will help your body get back to a healthful sleep–wake cycle and maintain it all week long.

Try not to depend on random naps. If you are consistently sleep deprived, you may often feel like grabbing a nap when you can during the day, but you run the risk of leaving yourself feeling groggy later on, especially if you take long naps. Napping can also make you feel less sleepy at night and throw off your regular bedtime. Napping should be a refresher, not a crutch that helps you limp along without consistent, adequate sleep. If you do need to nap, 20 to 30 minutes before 3 p.m. is ideal.

As noted earlier in this chapter, avoid alcohol for at least 6 hours before bedtime. Steer clear of caffeine starting in the afternoon. And watch your intake of other fluids, too. If you drink too much of any fluid right before bedtime, you'll almost certainly wake up in the middle of the night, needing to use the bathroom.

Finally, make an all-out effort to avoid all-nighters, which leave you exhausted the next day and throw off your normal sleep cycle. Plan study time in advance to make all-nighters unnecessary, especially since sleep improves one mental capability essential to studying: memory. Encourage your friends and classmates to do the same by organizing group study sessions when collaborative study time suits the work at hand. You'll not only get more rest but help your fellow students do the same.

LO 4.6 QUICK CHECK ✓

Which of the following is a benefit of going to bed at the same time every night?
a. It helps your body get into a regular sleep pattern.
b. It stops your melatonin production.
c. It makes it easier to know when to take a sleeping pill.
d. It speeds up your brain waves.

>> Watch videos of real students discussing their sleep at **MasteringHealth™**

SPECIAL FEATURE

Starting Right for a Restful Night

The faster you get to sleep, the more hours of total sleep you can accrue. Here are some general tips for getting off to sleep more quickly:[1,2]

- **Think of your bedroom as your "sleep cave."** Make it as dark as possible, using room-darkening shades, if necessary, to block out streetlights. Avoid working or studying in bed. Try to reserve your bed only for sleep.
- **Aim for a warm bed in a cool room.** Many people find it difficult to fall asleep in a hot, stuffy room. In winter, turn down the thermostat a few degrees—to 65°F or below—and put an extra blanket on the bed. In summer, use air conditioning or fans to cool the room as much as possible. And make sure the room has adequate ventilation. If appropriate, crack open a window.
- **Keep it quiet.** Many campuses are instituting quiet hours in dorms. But if you can't control noise in your building or out on the street, at least try to block it out with white noise, either by using the white-noise setting on your clock radio or downloading a free audio "soundscape" app to play on your MP3 player or phone. And, of course, there are always ear plugs.
- **Cut caffeine.** Avoid caffeinated drinks after lunchtime because caffeine can stay in your system for hours. Bear in mind that some energy drinks contain as much caffeine as a similar amount of brewed coffee. Moreover, bottled teas, iced-tea mixes, premium brands of coffee ice cream, hot cocoa, and chocolate all contain caffeine.
- **Watch your food intake.** Although a small snack before bed can help make you sleepy, avoid large meals, which can prompt heartburn. Also avoid spicy foods, which can raise your body temperature enough to cause you to lie awake.
- **Hit the gym or try lighter exercise later in the day.** Getting exercise during the day—even just 10 to 20 minutes of walking—improves your likelihood of a good night's sleep. In a national poll about sleep quality, those who engaged in light to vigorous exercise daily were much more likely to say they enjoyed a good night's sleep on a regular basis.[3] Although vigorous exercise within a few hours of bedtime hasn't been proven to disturb sleep, you may still want to opt for more gentle exercise, such as yoga or tai chi, in the evening hours to prepare for sleep.
- **Get adequate exposure to natural light throughout the day.** This helps provide your brain with stimuli that help keep your body clock in sync with the environment. As a result, you'll find it easier to nod off.
- **Set aside stressors until morning.** Try to deal with stressors—anything from paying your bills to asking your roommates to clean up their act—as early in the day as possible. If you can't resolve your worries entirely before bedtime, at least try to set them aside—for instance, by writing them down along with two strategies for addressing them the next day. Sleep is your chance to rest and recover.
- **Try to limit nighttime technology use.** An emerging body of research indicates that bright light from devices such as laptops, tablets, and phones may make you less drowsy and perhaps limit sleep-inducing melatonin production. One small study, for example, found that wearing orange-tinted, light-blocking glasses during pre-bed screen time resulted in more natural evening sleepiness.[4]
- **Don't stare at the ceiling.** If you've gone to bed and can't fall asleep within 20 minutes, get up and do something relaxing until you feel sleepy again and can head back to bed.

Sources: 1. *Sleep hygiene tips*, by Centers for Disease Control and Prevention, 2012, www.cdc.gov; 2. *Healthy sleep habits*, by the American Academy of Sleep Medicine, 2014, www.sleepeducation.org; 3. *National Sleep Foundation Poll Finds Exercise Key to Good Sleep*, by the National Sleep Foundation, March 2013, www.sleepfoundation.org; 4. "Blue blocker glasses as a countermeasure for alerting effects of evening light-emitting diode screen exposure in male teenagers," by van der Lely, S., Frey, S., Garbazza, C., Wirz-Justice, A., Jenni, O., et al., January 2015, *Journal of Adolescent Health, 56*(1), 113–119.

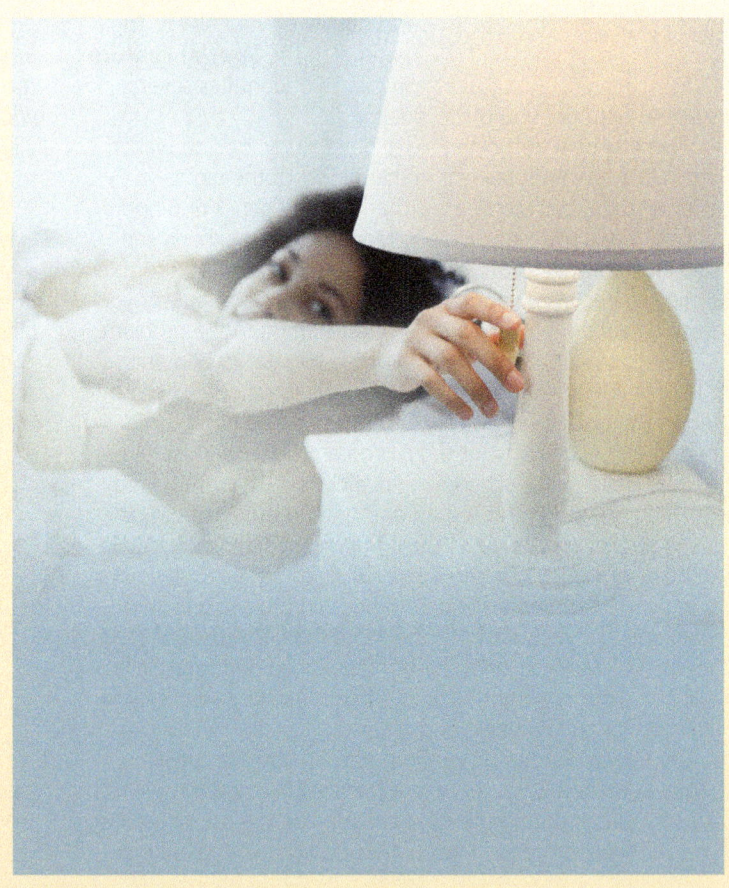

Choosing to **Change** Worksheet

To complete this worksheet online, visit MasteringHealth™

In this chapter you learned about the importance of healthy sleep. To improve your sleep, follow the steps below.

Directions: Fill in your stage of change in step 1 and complete step 2 with your stage of change in mind. Then complete steps 3, 4, or 5, depending on which ones apply to your stage of change.

Step 1: Assess your stage of behavior change. Please check one of the following statements that best describes your readiness to obtain a good quality and quantity of sleep.

_____I do not intend to increase the quality or quantity of my sleep in the next six months. (Precontemplation)

_____I might increase the quality or quantity of my sleep in the next six months. (Contemplation)

_____I am prepared to increase the quality or quantity of my sleep in the next month. (Preparation)

_____I have been increasing my quality or quantity of sleep for less than six months. (Action)

_____I have been increasing my quality or quantity of sleep for more than six months. (Maintenance)

Step 2: Keep a sleep diary. A sleep diary is a useful tool for identifying sleep disorders and sleeping problems and pinpointing daytime and nighttime habits that may be contributing to your sleep struggles. Fill in the following chart for up to seven days.

	Answer These Questions	Example	Monday	Tuesday	Wednesday	Thursday	Friday	Saturday	Sunday
Complete in the morning	Time I went to bed last night:	11 p.m.							
	Time I woke up this morning:	7 a.m.							
	Number of hours I slept last night:	8							
	Number of awakenings and total time awake last night:	5 times 2 hours							
	How long I took to fall asleep last night:	30 mins.							
	Medications taken last night:	None							
	How awake I felt when I got up this morning: 1 – Wide awake 2 – Awake but a little tired 3 – Sleepy	2							
Complete in the evening	Number of caffeinated drinks and time I had them today:	1 drink at 8 a.m.							
	Number of alcoholic drinks and time I had them today:	1 drink at 9 p.m.							
	Naptimes and lengths of naps today:	3:30 p.m. 45 mins.							

(continued)

Answer These Questions	Example	Monday	Tuesday	Wednesday	Thursday	Friday	Saturday	Sunday
Exercise times and lengths today:	None							
How sleepy I felt during the day today:	1							
1 – So sleepy I had to struggle to stay awake during much of the day								
2 – Somewhat tired								
3 – Fairly alert								
4 – Wide awake								

Source: *Your Guide to Healthy Sleep*, by the National Heart, Lung, and Blood Institute, 2011. NIH Publication No. 11-5271.

After filling in the sleep diary, do you notice any habits, such as drinking alcohol or caffeine, taking medications, lack of exercise, or napping, that could be negatively affecting your sleep?

_____
_____
_____

Step 3: Work within the precontemplation or contemplation stage of change. Answer the questions below to move toward improving your sleep patterns.

What are some reasons to improve your sleeping habits?

_____
_____
_____

What is holding you back from improving your sleeping habits?

_____
_____
_____

How can you overcome these obstacles to improving your sleep?

_____
_____
_____

Step 4: Work within the preparation or action stage of change. The tips for getting to sleep more quickly provided on page 90 are listed below. On a scale of 1–5 (1 being the lowest and 5 the highest), rate your confidence in your ability to implement each strategy.

Strategy	How Confident Are You in Your Ability to Employ This Technique?				
	Low Confidence				High Confidence
Think of your bedroom as your "sleep cave."	1	2	3	4	5
Maintain a warm bed in a cool room.	1	2	3	4	5
Keep it quiet.	1	2	3	4	5
Cut caffeine.	1	2	3	4	5

(continued)

Strategy	How Confident Are You in Your Ability to Employ This Technique?				
	Low Confidence			High Confidence	
Avoid large meals close to bedtime.	1	2	3	4	5
Participate in a regular exercise program.	1	2	3	4	5
Get adequate exposure to natural light throughout the day.	1	2	3	4	5
Set stressors aside until morning.	1	2	3	4	5
Don't work or study in bed.	1	2	3	4	5
Give yourself time to wind down.	1	2	3	4	5
Don't stare at the ceiling. Get up if you're still awake after 20 minutes.	1	2	3	4	5
Other	1	2	3	4	5

Your confidence may be low for all strategies but pick the one you feel may be the most helpful. How might you begin to implement that strategy?

_____

_____

Select one strategy that you feel highly confident in implementing and set a start date. Start date:

_____

Tell someone what you plan to do. Being accountable to others motivates you and also offers you the support and encouragement of others. Who did you tell?

_____

Step 5: Work within the action and maintenance stages. For three days, keep track of your sleep quality and quantity. Evaluate your sleep and explain whether you plan to modify your plan to improve your sleep.

CHAPTER 4 STUDY PLAN

CHAPTER SUMMARY

LO 4.1
- Sleep is a physiologically prompted, dynamic, and readily reversible state of reduced consciousness essential to human survival.
- All three regions of the brain are involved in sleep. In the diencephalon, the hypothalamus and the pineal gland together help regulate your body's circadian rhythm.
- A full night of sleep includes several cycles of non-REM and REM sleep. REM (rapid eye movement) sleep helps the brain store memories and process information.

LO 4.2
- Most adults need 7 to 9 hours of sleep each night to feel alert and well rested. Less than 7 hours is referred to as short sleep, whereas more than 9 hours is considered long sleep.
- College students are prone to sleep debt, routinely getting short sleep. Ample sleep is associated with increased longevity and increased cognitive functioning. Short sleep reduces the immune response; increases the risk for chronic disease, depression, and death; and impairs complex thinking and decision making.
- Drowsiness, including drowsy driving, is a major cause of traumatic injuries and deaths.

LO 4.3
- Although genetics appears to play a part in sleep patterns, environmental and behavioral factors are thought to be more important. Stress is a primary cause of troubled sleep.
- Frequent, extended use of media and technology devices shortly before bedtime can also make it harder to fall asleep.

MasteringHealth™
Build your knowledge—and health!—in the Study Area of **MasteringHealth™** with a variety of study tools.

LO 4.4

- Insomnia is characterized by difficulty falling or staying asleep, a pattern of waking too early, or poor-quality sleep. Primary insomnia occurs in only about 20% of people with insomnia and almost always develops as a result of stress. Secondary insomnia is caused by behaviors or an underlying medical condition.
- Sleep apnea is a potentially life-threatening disorder in which one or more pauses in breathing occur during sleep. In narcolepsy, the person is not able to regulate the timing of sleep appropriately and may fall asleep frequently during activities of daily living.
- Parasomnias, conditions in which sleep is accompanied by an unusual event, include sleep terrors, sleepwalking, sleep bruxism, nocturnal eating, REM behavior disorder, and restless legs syndrome.

LO 4.5

- Sleep disorders may be diagnosed with the help of a sleep study conducted overnight in a sleep lab.
- Over-the-counter and prescription sleep remedies are not necessarily more effective than behavior-based sleep therapies, should be avoided if possible, and should never be used for longer than three weeks.
- Cognitive-behavioral therapy can be effective in the treatment of troubled sleep.

LO 4.6

- You can improve the quality and quantity of your sleep by following good sleep hygiene, helping your ability to initiate and maintain sleep.

GET CONNECTED

▸▸ Visit the following websites for further information about the topics in this chapter:

- National Sleep Foundation
  www.sleepfoundation.org
- American Academy of Sleep Medicine's Consumer Information Site
  www.sleepeducation.org
- MedlinePlus at the National Library of Medicine (search for Sleep Disorders)
  www.nlm.nih.gov

MOBILE TIPS!
Scan this QR code with your mobile device to access additional sleep tips. Or, via your mobile device, go to **http://chmobile.pearsoncmg.com** and choose by topic: sleep.

- Stanford University's Center for Sleep and Dreams's Sleep Guide
  www.end-your-sleep-deprivation.com

Website links are subject to change. To access updated web links, please visit MasteringHealth™

TEST YOUR KNOWLEDGE

LO 4.1

1. The pineal gland responds to changing levels of darkness and light by changing its level of production of a hormone called
   a. growth hormone.
   b. insulin.
   c. melatonin.
   d. adrenaline.

LO 4.1

2. Which of the following statements about REM sleep is true?
   a. REM sleep is the deepest stage of sleep.
   b. As the night continues, the duration of REM sleep increases.
   c. As the night continues, REM sleep entirely ceases.
   d. It is extremely difficult to waken someone from REM sleep.

LO 4.2

3. Which of the following statements about short sleep is true?
   a. Short sleep is any amount of total nightly sleep below 7 hours.
   b. Half of all American adults experience short sleep every night.
   c. Short sleep is another name for stage 1 of non-REM sleep.
   d. Short sleep is associated with increased longevity.

LO 4.2, 4.4

4. Daytime drowsiness and difficulty concentrating are classic signs of
   a. long sleep.
   b. sleep deprivation.
   c. hypersomnia.
   d. sleep bruxism.

LO 4.3

5. The stimulant most commonly associated with sleep problems is
   a. nicotine.
   b. alcohol.
   c. cocaine.
   d. caffeine.

LO 4.4

6. Secondary insomnia is
   a. far less common than primary insomnia.
   b. almost always a result of stress.
   c. prompted by an underlying medical disorder.
   d. treated with a CPAP machine.

7. Obstructive sleep apnea
   a. is the medical name for snoring.
   b. is typically diagnosed in underweight women.
   c. is less common than central sleep apnea.
   d. increases the risk for a heart attack, stroke, or traumatic injury.

8. REM behavior disorder is
   a. characterized by movements suggesting that the sleeper is acting out a dream.
   b. one of the most common types of parasomnia.
   c. likely to occur in the first sleep cycle of the night.
   d. accompanied by an unpleasant feeling in the legs.

LO 4.5

9. As a first step in addressing sleep problems, health experts recommend
   a. herbal sleep remedies containing either chamomile or valerian.
   b. prescription sleep medications.
   c. vigorous exercise 1 to 2 hours before bedtime.
   d. assessing and altering aspects of your sleep hygiene.

LO 4.2, 4.6

10. The most important strategy for improving your sleep maintenance is
   a. taking a late-afternoon nap of no more than 10–20 minutes daily.
   b. setting and keeping a regular sleep–wake schedule.
   c. drinking a small glass of water just before bed.
   d. maintaining a bedroom temperature of at least 68°F.

WHAT DO YOU THINK?

LO 4.3

1. Despite busy, often tiring lives, young adults have the latest bedtime of any age group in the United States. What are some reasons for this?

LO 4.5

2. Should the manufacturers of prescription sleeping pills be held responsible for driving violations, injuries, and fatalities involving patients taking these drugs?

LO 4.1, 4.2

3. What are three important health or academic benefits that college students gain from getting ample sleep on a regular basis?

LO 4.1, 4.6

4. Why is frequent daytime napping a poor substitute for regular nighttime sleep?

LO 4.5, 4.6

5. If you were experiencing persistent insomnia and had tried changing aspects of your sleep hygiene without success, would you consider trying a prescription or over-the-counter sleep aid? If so, what precautions would you take to avoid any adverse effects?

5

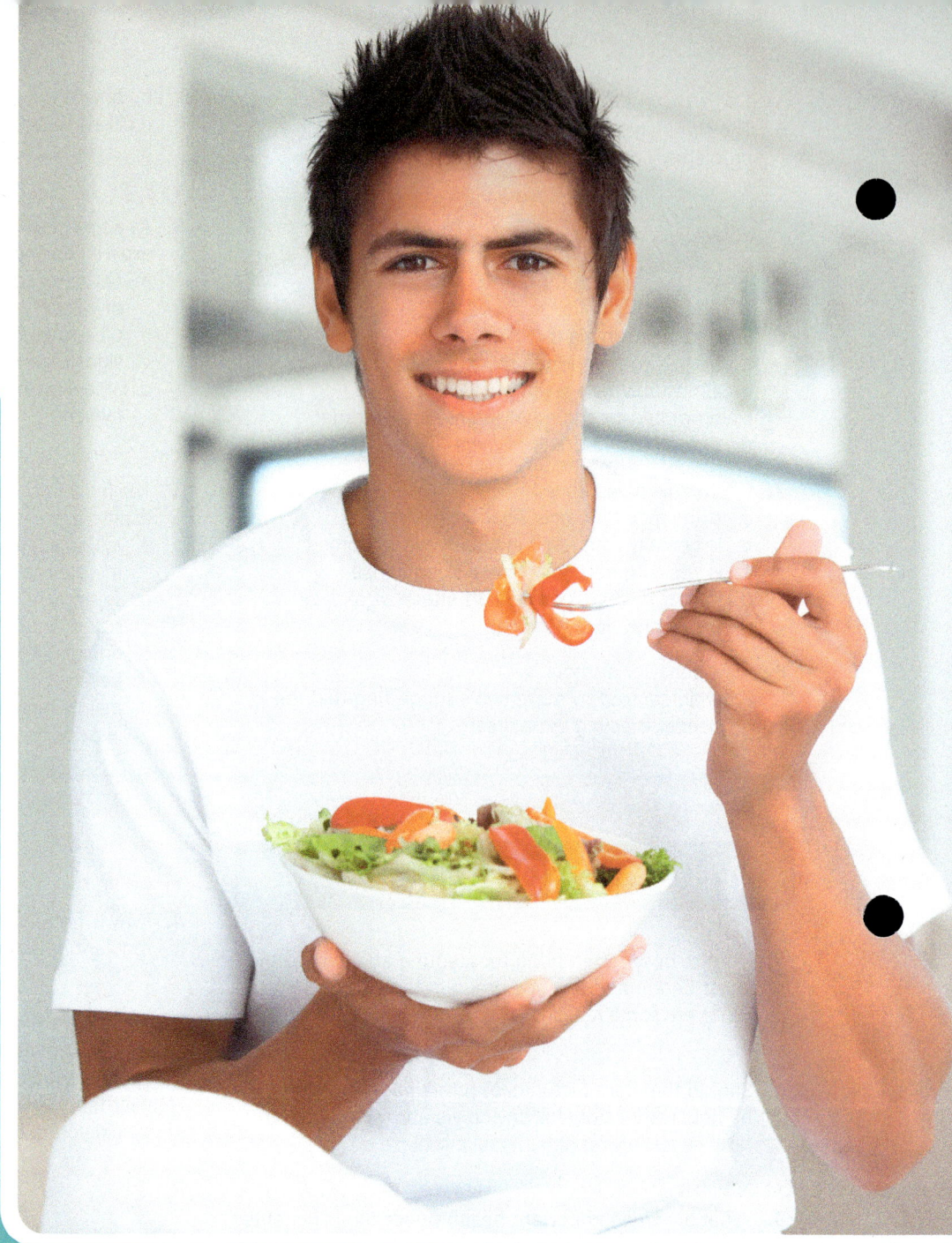

> The average person in the United States consumes 23 teaspoons of added sugars every day.[i]

> A meal consisting of a McDonald's Big Mac, large fries, and small iced mocha contains 1,340 calories, 13% of which are from saturated fat.[ii]

> Eight foods cause more than 90% of all food allergies: milk, eggs, peanuts, tree nuts, soy, wheat, fish, and shellfish.[iii]

NUTRITION

LEARNING OUTCOMES

LO 5.1 Describe the six classes of nutrients and explain their functions in the body.

LO 5.2 Discuss the potential benefits and concerns related to consumption of functional foods and dietary supplements.

LO 5.3 Demonstrate how to use the DRIs, MyPlate, and other resources to design a healthful diet.

LO 5.4 Describe ways to reduce your risk for foodborne illness, manage food allergies and intolerances, and avoid environmental contaminants.

LO 5.5 Identify strategies for making nutritious, inexpensive choices when shopping, cooking, and eating out.

Why is an orange more nutritious than orange soda?

Why does a baked potato beat French fries? Why is fat from a fish better than fat from a cow? In short, what foods should you limit, and what foods should you favor? Most importantly, why does it matter?

The science of **nutrition** investigates the effects of diet on body and health. A nutritious **diet** provides you with energy, helps you stay healthy, and allows you to function at your best. Whether you're in line at the deli or your dining hall, knowing the basic principles of good nutrition can help you make choices that will benefit your health for a lifetime.

What Are Nutrients?

LO 5.1 Describe the six classes of nutrients and explain their functions in the body.

Your body relies on food to provide chemicals called **nutrients**. In the process of digestion, the food you eat is broken down into nutrients that are small enough to be absorbed into your bloodstream (**Figure 5.1**, next page). Once in your body, nutrients work together to provide energy; support growth, repair, and maintenance of body tissues; and regulate body functions.

Six major classes of nutrients are found in food:

- Carbohydrates
- Fats (more appropriately called *lipids*)
- Proteins
- Vitamins
- Minerals
- Water

Nutrients your body needs in relatively large quantities are called *macronutrients* (*macro-* means "large"). These are carbohydrates, fats, proteins, and water. Nutrients you need in relatively small quantities are called *micronutrients* (*micro-* means "small"). These are vitamins and minerals.

Energy and Calories

Three of the four macronutrients—carbohydrates, fats, and proteins—are also known as *energy-yielding nutrients* because the body breaks them down to provide you with the energy you need to move, to think, and simply to survive. Although vitamins, minerals, and water assist this process, they don't supply you with energy.

If you've ever thought that you felt warmer after eating a meal, you weren't imagining it! Scientists determine the amount of energy that a food provides by measuring how much heat it generates. They calculate that heat in units called *kilocalories*. You're probably more familiar with the simpler term **calorie,** which we will use throughout this text.

The energy-yielding nutrients differ in their calorie content. Carbohydrates and proteins each provide 4 calories per gram. (A gram is a very small amount; for instance, a teaspoon of sugar contains 4 grams.) Fats provide 9 calories per gram—more than twice the amount in carbohydrates or proteins. Alcohol is not a nutrient because it doesn't provide any substance you need to grow or survive. However, alcohol does provide energy, 7 calories per gram, which explains why consuming alcohol regularly can pack on the pounds. Regardless of their source, calories consumed in excess of energy needs are converted to and stored in the body as fat.

Vitamins, minerals, and water provide no energy, but they are essential to **metabolism,** the term for all of the chemical reactions that take place in your body, including those by which your body converts foods into energy.

People vary in how many calories they need to eat each day to meet their energy needs yet avoid gaining weight. For instance, women, on average, need fewer calories than men. And because vigorous activity burns more calories than sitting still, athletes need many more calories than people who don't exercise.

> **nutrition** The scientific study of food and its physiological functions.
>
> **diet** The food you regularly consume.
>
> **nutrients** Chemicals the body derives from food and requires for energy, growth, and survival.
>
> **calorie** Common term for *kilocalorie*. The amount of energy required to raise the temperature of 1 kilogram of water by 1° Celsius.
>
> **metabolism** The sum of all chemical reactions occurring in body cells, including those that break large molecules down into smaller molecules.

▸▸ How many calories do *you* need each day? Find out in seconds at **www.cancer.org**. From the home page, type "calorie counter" in the Search bar.

Carbohydrates

Carbohydrates are compounds that contain three common elements: carbon, hydrogen, and oxygen. Plants manufacture carbohydrates using energy from the sun, and we derive the carbohydrates in our diets predominantly from plant foods. Milk and other dairy products are exceptions, but even the carbohydrates in these foods come from the plants that the cow, goat, or sheep consumed.

Carbohydrates are sometimes called the body's universal energy source because most body cells, especially during high-intensity activities, prefer carbohydrates for energy. Some body cells, including those in your brain, can use only carbohydrates for fuel.

There are two categories of carbohydrates: *simple carbohydrates* and *complex carbohydrates*. Both are composed of the same basic building blocks: sugar molecules, whose names usually end in "ose."

Simple Carbohydrates

Simple carbohydrates are constructed from just one or two sugar molecules. That means they are easily digested.

> *"Some body cells, including those in your brain, can use only carbohydrates for fuel."*

We commonly refer to simple carbohydrates as *sugars*, and six are important in nutrition: glucose, fructose (fruit sugar), galactose, maltose (malt sugar), sucrose (table sugar), and lactose (milk sugar). Of these, the most important is glucose. It is the most abundant sugar in foods and in our bodies, and it is our most important energy source.

carbohydrates A macronutrient class composed of carbon, hydrogen, and oxygen that is the body's universal energy source.

simple carbohydrates The most basic unit of carbohydrates, consisting of one or two sugar molecules.

added sugars Sugars not naturally present in foods or beverages but added during processing or preparation.

Sugars provide much of the sweetness found naturally in fruits, some vegetables, honey, and milk. **Added sugars** are those used in the production of soft drinks and other sweetened beverages, desserts, and many other processed foods. They also include sugar sprinkled on cereal or stirred into coffee or tea. In fact, Americans consume an average of 23 teaspoons of added sugars every day.[1]

Although the fructose present in an orange is the same, chemically, as the fructose in the high-fructose corn syrup (HFCS) used to sweeten orange soda, this doesn't mean that eating an orange is the same as drinking orange soda! Foods with naturally occurring sugars provide many other nutrients and healthful compounds. Foods high in added sugars generally provide little more than calories. Moreover, population studies have demonstrated that the higher a group's intake of added sugars, the greater their risk for cardiovascular disease.[2] In addition, an experimental study found that reducing intake of added sugars by obese children—without altering their intake of total calories—dramatically improved several risk factors for both cardiovascular disease and diabetes.[3]

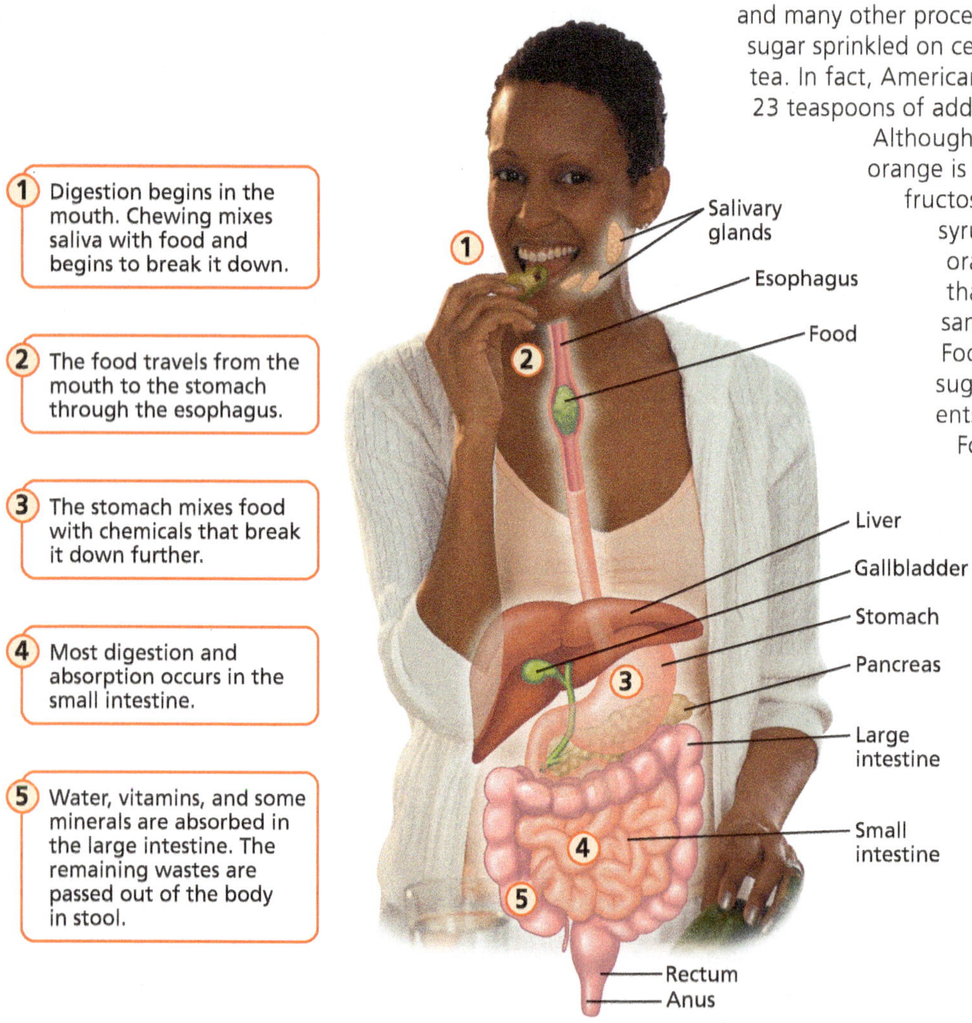

1 Digestion begins in the mouth. Chewing mixes saliva with food and begins to break it down.
2 The food travels from the mouth to the stomach through the esophagus.
3 The stomach mixes food with chemicals that break it down further.
4 Most digestion and absorption occurs in the small intestine.
5 Water, vitamins, and some minerals are absorbed in the large intestine. The remaining wastes are passed out of the body in stool.
Salivary glands
Esophagus
Food
Liver
Gallbladder
Stomach
Pancreas
Large intestine
Small intestine
Rectum
Anus

FIGURE 5.1 **The Digestive Process.** Digestion is the process of breaking food down into nutrients that can be used by the body for energy.

Complex Carbohydrates

Complex carbohydrates are made up of long chains of glucose molecules; therefore, they take longer to digest than do simple carbohydrates. There are three forms of complex carbohydrate: *Starches* are found in a variety of plants, especially grains (oats, rice, wheat, etc.) and legumes (dried beans, lentils, and peas) and other vegetables. A few fruits, including bananas and dates, also provide starch. *Glycogen* is a storage form of glucose in animal tissues, including the liver and muscles. We consume very little glycogen from meat, however, because it typically breaks down when an animal is slaughtered. **Fiber** is a tough (fibrous) complex carbohydrate that gives structure to plants. Although it's not a nutrient, it's a very important component of a healthful diet. Let's see why.

Facts About Fiber

Whereas starch is readily digested and its components absorbed, fiber passes through the intestines without being digested or absorbed. Nevertheless, it has many health benefits:

- **Weight control.** Fiber can make you feel full before you've consumed lots of calories. In this way, a high-fiber diet can help you avoid weight gain.

- **Bowel health.** As it moves through your large intestine, fiber provides bulk for feces. Because it absorbs water along the way, it also softens feces, making stools easier to pass. A diet rich in fiber can help you to avoid hemorrhoids, constipation, and other bowel problems.

- **Cardiovascular health.** No doubt you've heard of cholesterol, a waxy substance that can clog blood vessels, including those that serve your heart and brain, increasing your risk for a heart attack or stroke. A diet rich in fiber can help lower the level of cholesterol in your blood. It's thought that this happens because fiber binds to bile, a cholesterol-containing substance that your liver makes. When fiber is excreted from your body in feces, bile—and its cholesterol load—is excreted along with it. This leaves less cholesterol in your bloodstream.

- **Blood glucose control.** By slowing the transit of food through your intestines, fiber promotes a more gradual absorption of nutrients, including glucose, into your bloodstream. This can help prevent wide fluctuations in blood glucose levels, which is important in managing diabetes.

These are all good reasons to maintain a high-fiber diet. For adults to age 50, men need 38 grams of fiber per day, and women need 25 grams per day.[4] Because fiber absorbs water, a high-fiber diet should be accompanied by plenty of fluids to keep the digestive mass moving through your intestines.

Fiber is plentiful in legumes and other vegetables, many fruits, nuts, and seeds, as well as whole grains. But what exactly qualifies as a whole grain food?

Choose Whole Grains

Unrefined grains, or **whole grains,** include three parts—bran, germ, and endosperm—and generally can be sprouted **(Figure 5.2)**. Common examples are whole wheat, whole oats, popcorn, and brown rice. Whole grains are especially nutritious because the bran and germ provide valuable vitamins, minerals, and fiber. Like any other fiber-rich food, whole grains

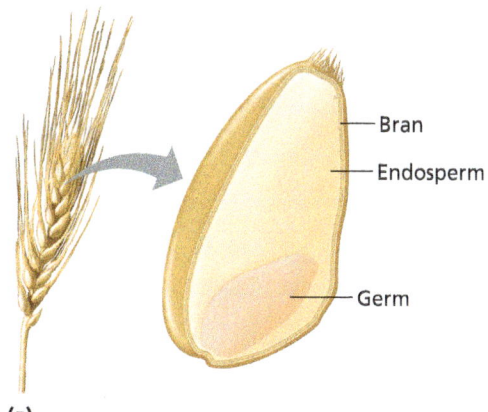

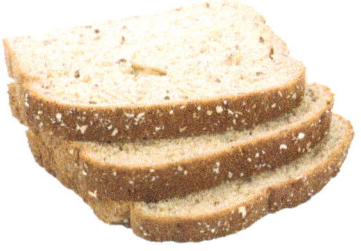

FIGURE 5.2 **Whole Grains.** (a) A whole grain includes the bran, endosperm, and germ. (b) Whole wheat bread is an excellent source of whole grain.

are bulky, and the body digests them slowly, using the energy they provide more efficiently, and helping people to feel full sooner and for a longer time.

In contrast, refined grains are stripped of their bran and germ during processing, reducing both their fiber and nutrients. Only the starchy endosperm is retained. Examples are white bread, white rice, and pastries. Despite having fewer nutrients, these products usually retain all the calories of their unrefined counterparts.

Many refined carbohydrates, including white bread, are "enriched" after processing, meaning that some of the lost vitamins and minerals are replaced. However, many other important nutrients are not replaced, nor is the fiber.

More than 92% of adults in the United States fail to eat the recommended three servings of whole grains a day.[5] If you're among them, you may be missing out on nutrients and fiber. Next time you're debating between white or whole grain toast, go for the whole grain.

> **complex carbohydrates** Carbohydrates that contain chains of multiple sugar molecules; commonly called *starches* but also come in two non-starch forms: *glycogen* and *fiber*.
>
> **fiber** A nondigestible complex carbohydrate that aids in digestion.
>
> **whole grains** Unrefined grains that contain bran, germ, and endosperm.
>
> **glycemic index** A measure of the potential of foods to raise the level of blood glucose.

Does Glycemic Index Matter?

The **glycemic index** is a measure of the potential of foods to raise the level of glucose in your bloodstream. Foods and

CHAPTER 5 ■ Nutrition **99**

beverages with a high glycemic index, such as breads made with refined flour or sugary drinks, are quickly broken down into glucose, which then flows rapidly from your small intestine into your bloodstream. Your pancreas detects this excessive blood glucose and, in response, releases a flood of insulin, a hormone that acts to get the glucose out of your blood and into your cells. This surge in insulin prompts a dramatic clearing of glucose out of your bloodstream, leaving you feeling hungry again very quickly. This may lead to overeating and weight gain. In fact, high-glycemic-index foods prompt a sugar rush similar to the "high" associated with drugs of abuse, and some researchers believe they are implicated in so-called food addictions.[6] In addition, a 2013 review study suggests that a high-glycemic-index diet may aggravate acne.[7]

In contrast, when you eat low-glycemic-index foods, glucose seeps more slowly into your bloodstream, and your pancreas releases a smaller amount of insulin to move it into your cells. As a result, your blood glucose level falls gradually, and you feel satisfied much longer. A low-glycemic index diet has also been linked to a reduced risk for cardiovascular disease.[8] Fiber-rich carbohydrates typically have a low glycemic index.

>> For an online list of the glycemic index of more than 100 foods, go to **www.health.harvard.edu** and type "glycemic index 100 foods" in the Search bar.

Recommended Carbohydrate Intake

Adults 19 years of age or older should consume an absolute minimum of 130 grams of carbohydrates each day.[4] This amount—which you'd get from eating about three slices of whole wheat bread—is estimated to supply adequate fuel to your brain. But you also need carbohydrates to fuel physical activity, and they're an excellent source of other nutrients, as well as fiber. For these reasons, nutrition experts recommend that you consume about half (45–65%) of your total daily calories as carbohydrates. Focus on fiber-rich carbohydrates from whole grains, fruits, and legumes and other vegetables. The **Practical Strategies** box shows you how.

Fats

Fats are one type of a huge group of compounds called *lipids* that are found throughout nature. Like carbohydrates, lipids are made up of carbon, hydrogen, and oxygen. But these elements are arranged in a way that gives lipids their key characteristic: They are not soluble in water, which is why olive oil will float to the top of your salad dressing. This insolubility enables your cells to function. Lipids also cushion and insulate your organs, enable your body to absorb fat-soluble vitamins, and supply your body with energy both while you're active and while you sleep. For all of these reasons, lipids are critical to your health.

Fats Are One of Three Types of Food Lipids

Three types of lipids are present in foods.

Phospholipids. The least common dietary lipids are *phospholipids*. They are found only in peanuts, egg yolk, and a few processed foods such as salad dressing. Phospholipids are made up of lipid molecules attached to a compound called phosphate. They're a key component of the cell membrane—the flexible "wall" that keeps the contents of your cells in place. But your body can make them from other substances, so you don't need to consume them.

Sterols. *Sterols* are ring-shaped lipids found in both plant- and animal-based foods. Plant sterols are not very well absorbed by the body but are thought to have an important health benefit: They appear to block the absorption of **cholesterol,** the animal sterol most common in the American diet. Cholesterol

cholesterol An animal sterol found in the fatty part of animal-based foods such as meat and whole milk.

PRACTICAL Strategies

Choosing Fiber-Rich Carbohydrates

A diet high in fiber-rich carbohydrates keeps your digestive tract running smoothly and reduces your risk of obesity, heart disease, and type 2 diabetes. So how can you focus on fiber? Here are some tips:

- Start your day with whole grain cereal and a piece of fresh fruit.
- Switch to whole grain bread for morning toast and lunchtime sandwiches.
- Choose vegetarian chili or a bean burrito for lunch.
- Instead of a side of French fries or potato chips, choose a small salad, carrot sticks, or slices of sweet red pepper.
- For an afternoon snack, mix dried fruits with nuts, sunflower seeds, and whole grain pretzels.
- If dinner includes rice, pasta, pizza crust, or tortillas, choose whole grain versions.
- Include a side of beans, peas, or lentils with dinner, along with a leafy green vegetable, sweet potato, or vegetable soup.
- For an evening snack, choose popcorn, popcorn cakes, peanut butter on whole grain toast, or a bowl of whole grain cereal with milk.

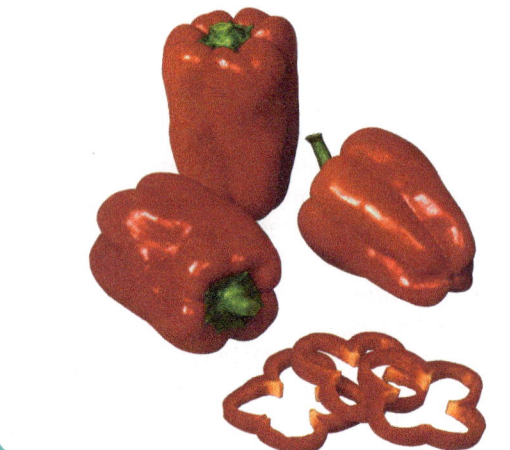

is found in animal-based foods such as meats, eggs, shellfish, butter, lard, and whole milk. As we mentioned earlier, a high level of cholesterol circulating in your bloodstream can increase your risk for a heart attack or stroke. Still, some cholesterol is essential for your survival because it's a component of cell membranes, certain hormones, and many other compounds. But you don't have to consume it because your liver can make all the cholesterol you need.

Fats. The most abundant lipids in your diet, **fats** are present in a wide variety of plant and animal foods. Food scientists refer to dietary fats as **triglycerides** because they are made up of three fatty acid chains (*tri-* means "three") attached to a compound called glycerol (a type of alcohol). Depending on the structure of the fatty acid chains, one of three different types of fats is formed: saturated, monounsaturated, or polyunsaturated. Each type has different characteristics and different effects on your health.

Saturated Fats

Saturated fats are so named because their fatty acid chains are "saturated" with hydrogen. This makes them solid at room temperature.

Although not all experts agree, researchers from the American Heart Association state that saturated fats can contribute to cardiovascular disease and should be limited in an overall healthful diet.[9] So what foods should you avoid? Saturated fats generally are found in animal-based foods such as meat, cream, whole milk, cheese, lard, and butter. Red meats tend to have more saturated fat than poultry or fish. Fried meats are higher in saturated fat than meats that are broiled, grilled, or baked. Processed foods, including prepared meals, are often loaded with saturated fat. Palm, palm kernel, and coconut oils, although derived from plants, also are highly saturated.

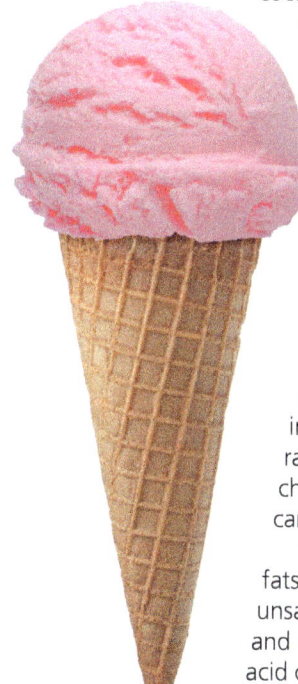

Ice cream, unfortunately, is loaded with saturated fat.

Unsaturated Fats

In **unsaturated fats,** the fatty acid chains have one or more areas that are not "saturated" with hydrogen. This structure makes them more flexible, and they are typically liquid at room temperature. Unsaturated fats are abundant in most plant oils and fatty fish. Replacing saturated fats with unsaturated fats can lower your blood cholesterol level and your risk for cardiovascular disease.[10]

The two types of unsaturated fats are monounsaturated and polyunsaturated. *Mono-* means "one," and monounsaturated fats have fatty acid chains with one unsaturated region. Sources of monounsaturated fats include canola oil, olive oil, peanut oil, nuts, avocado, and sesame seeds. *Poly-* means "many," and polyunsaturated fats have fatty acid chains with two or more unsaturated regions. Sources of polyunsaturated fats include corn oil, safflower oil, fatty fish, many salad dressings, mayonnaise, nuts, and seeds.

Two polyunsaturated fats—*omega-6 fatty acids* and *omega-3 fatty acids*—are essential to your body's functioning and are thought to provide some protection against cardiovascular disease. As they cannot be assembled by your body and must be obtained from your diet or from supplements, they are also known as the **essential fatty acids (EFAs).**

Most people in the United States get plenty of omega-6 fatty acids from plant oils, seeds, and nuts. However, most people need to increase significantly their consumption of omega-3 fatty acids, which are found in fatty fish (like salmon and mackerel), walnuts, flaxseed, canola oil, and dark green, leafy vegetables. Two omega-3 fatty acids found in fish, EPA and DHA, are thought to be particularly effective in reducing your risk for cardiovascular disease. Eating fish twice a week (a total of 8 ounces) is recommended for most adults.[11]

> **fats (triglycerides)** Lipids made up of three fatty acid chains attached to a molecule of glycerol; the most common types of food lipid.
>
> **saturated fats** Fats that are typically solid at room temperature and that are generally found in animal-based foods.
>
> **unsaturated fats** Fats that are typically liquid at room temperature and that generally come from plant sources.
>
> **essential fatty acids (EFAs)** Polyunsaturated fatty acids that cannot be synthesized by the body but are essential to body functioning.
>
> ***trans* fat** A type of fat produced through the process of hydrogenation, which converts an oil into a solid.

Avoid *Trans* Fats

So far, we've been discussing fats that occur naturally in foods. Now let's turn our attention to a particularly harmful form of fat that occurs almost exclusively in processed foods containing partially hydrogenated oils (PHOs). During hydrogenation, an unsaturated fat such as corn oil is saturated with hydrogen. This process changes the oil into a solid fat—such as corn oil margarine—that is less likely to spoil. However, the process creates a unique type of fatty acid chain called a ***trans* fat** that is worse for your health than saturated fats! For this reason, the U.S. Food and Drug Administration (FDA) in 2015 declared that PHOs are no longer recognized as safe to consume. Food companies have until the summer of 2018 to reformulate their products without PHOs.[12] The FDA estimates that removing *trans* fats from food products could prevent thousands of heart attacks and deaths each year.[12]

Many processed foods, such as margarines, frozen meals, and baked goods, still contain PHOs. Until 2018, you can avoid them by reading food labels: Foods containing half a gram of *trans* fat or less per serving can claim to be "*trans* fat free," so look for the words "hydrogenated" or "vegetable shortening" in the ingredients list. If they're present, the food contains *trans* fats.

Recommended Fat Intake

National nutritional guidelines do not recommend a low-fat diet. Instead, fats should make up between 20% and 35% of your total calories.[4] Try to avoid *trans* fats entirely and keep saturated fats to less than 10% of your total calories by replacing them with unsaturated fats.[10]

If you're like most other busy people, you don't have time to monitor your diet closely every day. So for some easy ways to choose healthful fats, see the **Practical Strategies** box at right.

protein An energy-yielding macronutrient that helps build biological compounds and body tissues, including muscle, bone, skin, and blood.

amino acids Nitrogen-containing compounds that are the building blocks of proteins.

Proteins

Dietary **protein** is a macronutrient available from both plant and animal sources. Although it's one of the energy nutrients, protein is used for fuel only if your body does not have adequate amounts of carbohydrate and fat to burn. Assuming that you're well nourished, your body uses the protein you eat to build biological compounds, cells, and tissues.

The Role of Amino Acids

Some misconceptions surround the roles of protein in the diet and in the body. For instance, people who associate meat with protein and protein with strength may eat lots of meat to build their muscles. This is unnecessary: Whenever you consume proteins, whether they come from meats or plants, your body breaks them apart into their component building blocks, which are nitrogen-containing compounds known as **amino acids.** Once absorbed through the intestinal tract, amino acids enter the bloodstream and become part of the amino acid pool. Just as you might go to an auto parts store to buy an air filter or some spark plugs for your car, your body cells draw from the amino acid pool the precise amino acids they need to build or repair a wide variety of body proteins. These include muscle and other body tissues as well as chemicals such as enzymes, which speed up metabolic reactions in your body. In short, you consume dietary protein primarily to maintain your stock of amino acids for your body cells to generate whatever proteins they need.

Complete and Incomplete Proteins

Although all of the 20 amino acids your body needs are available in foods, you don't have to consume them all. That's because your body can produce ample amounts of 11 of them independently. The other 9 are called *essential amino acids* because your body either cannot make them or cannot make sufficient quantities of them to maintain your health. Thus, you need to consume these amino acids in your diet.

Dietary proteins are considered *complete proteins* if they supply all nine essential amino acids in adequate amounts. In contrast, *incomplete proteins* are lacking one or more of the essential amino acids. Meat, fish, poultry, dairy products, soy, and quinoa provide complete proteins. Most plant sources provide incomplete proteins. However, combinations of plant proteins—peanut butter on whole grain bread, for instance, or brown rice with lentils—can complement each other in such a way that the essential amino acids missing from one are supplied by the other. The combination yields complete proteins. Incidentally, foods with complementary amino acids don't have to be consumed at the same meal. People following a plant-based diet simply need to consume a variety of plant proteins throughout the day.

✱ PRACTICAL Strategies
Choosing Healthful Fats

To choose healthful fats, start by sorting the good guys from the bad. Make it a standard practice to pick foods with zero *trans* fats and replace saturated fats with unsaturated fats. Here are some additional tips:

- Instead of spreading cream cheese or butter on your toast, try peanut, almond, cashew, or walnut butter.
- Unless you're a vegetarian, eat fatty fish such as salmon and tuna twice a week to meet your omega-3 fatty acid needs. Consume small amounts of vegetable oils, walnuts, flaxseed, and leafy green vegetables daily.
- For other protein foods with healthful fats, choose legumes and other vegetables served over whole grains, or a small serving of lean red meats (rump, round, loin, and flank) or skinless poultry.
- Trim all visible fat from red meat and poultry. Instead of choosing fried meats, poultry, or fish, choose baked or broiled. Remove the skin from poultry before eating it.
- Skip the French fries. Opt for a baked sweet potato or side salad instead.
- Instead of ice cream, which is high in saturated fat, choose low-fat frozen yogurt or Greek yogurt.
- When the munchies hit, go for air-popped popcorn; whole grain pretzels or rice cakes; or a handful of nuts, seeds, or dried fruit.
- Make sure that all foods you buy are *trans* fat free.

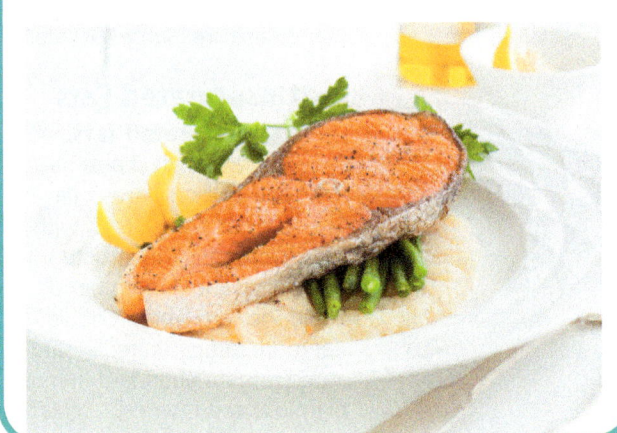

Recommended Protein Intake

For good health, experts recommend that adults consume between 10% and 35% of their calories as protein.[4] Staying within this range provides adequate protein for tissue maintenance and body functioning. Moreover, recent research suggests that an adequate ratio of protein to total calories may be important even within a single meal. The *protein-leverage hypothesis* proposes that protein intake signals the brain that we're full. Thus, when the protein content of a meal is "diluted," for example by bread or other refined grains, our drive to satisfy our protein need will cause us to consume too many total calories.[13]

How much protein *you* need largely depends on your body weight and level of activity. Healthy adults typically need 0.36 grams of protein per pound (0.8 grams per kilogram) of body weight—for example, 54 grams per day for a 150-pound person.[4] Runners and other athletes in aerobic sports can require one-and-a-half times as much protein, and strength athletes, such as bodybuilders, can require up to twice as much.[14] Few people in the United States suffer from protein deficiencies. Research indicates that even athletes, on average, consume protein well in excess of their needs.[15] Don't fall for the myth that consuming excessive protein—whether from foods or expensive supplements—will help you build muscle. Any protein you consume beyond your body's needs is stored as fat.

Unfortunately, many animal sources of protein are high in saturated fat. See the **Practical Strategies** box at right for ways to go lean with protein.

Vitamins

Vitamins are carbon-containing compounds required in small amounts to support human metabolism. For example, although they do not provide energy, vitamins do help your body break down carbohydrates, fats, and proteins for energy.

Humans need 13 vitamins. Four of these—vitamins A, D, E, and K—are *fat soluble*, meaning they dissolve in fat and can be stored in your body's fatty tissues. Because your body can store them, taking too much of these vitamins—typically in supplements—can be toxic. However, you don't have to consume the fat-soluble vitamins daily. Nine vitamins—vitamin C and the eight B-complex vitamins (thiamin, riboflavin, niacin, pantothenic acid, B_6, biotin, folic acid, and B_{12})—are *water soluble*. They dissolve in water, and excesses are generally excreted from the body in urine. Your body can store vitamin B_{12} in the liver, but you cannot store any of the other water-soluble vitamins. Thus, toxicity is unlikely unless you're taking a high-potency supplement. On the other hand, it's important to consume adequate amounts nearly every day.

vitamins Compounds needed by the body in minute amounts for normal growth and function.

Sources of Vitamins

Table 5.1 shows the primary food sources for the 13 vitamins. As you can see, some are abundant in fruits, vegetables, and whole grains. Others are more plentiful in animal-based foods. Vitamin B_{12} is available naturally only from animal foods, so vegans (strict vegetarians) have to get it from supplements or from eating processed foods to which B_{12} has been added.

Vitamin D has many functions in your body but is best known for its role in bone health. Your body is able to manufacture vitamin D from a cholesterol compound in your skin if you have adequate exposure to sunlight. For most people, this means about 5 to 30 minutes of exposure between the hours of 10 a.m. and 3 p.m. twice a week, on bare arms and legs, without sunscreen.[16] People who cannot get this much average sun exposure each week—for instance, during the winter in a cold climate, or in an area with heavy smog—should consume enough vitamin D either in foods such as oily fish and fortified milks, or in supplements.

⚙ PRACTICAL Strategies
Go Lean with Protein

- Choose lean cuts of meats such as rump, round, loin, and flank. Better yet, choose poultry (remove the skin). Best of all, choose fish.
- Avoid fried meats, as this cooking method adds fat. Choose baked, broiled, or grilled.
- For a lunchtime sandwich, choose turkey, roast beef, canned tuna or salmon, or peanut butter. Avoid deli meats like bologna or salami, which are high in saturated fat and sodium.
- Vary your protein sources by consuming vegetarian meals several times a week. Choose legumes, soy products such as tofu dogs and burgers, nuts, and seeds.
- Don't forget eggs, which are a complete and easily digestible source of protein. In fact, a hard-boiled egg makes a great snack.
- Choose a small portion of nuts or seeds as a snack, on salads, or in main dishes to replace meat or poultry.

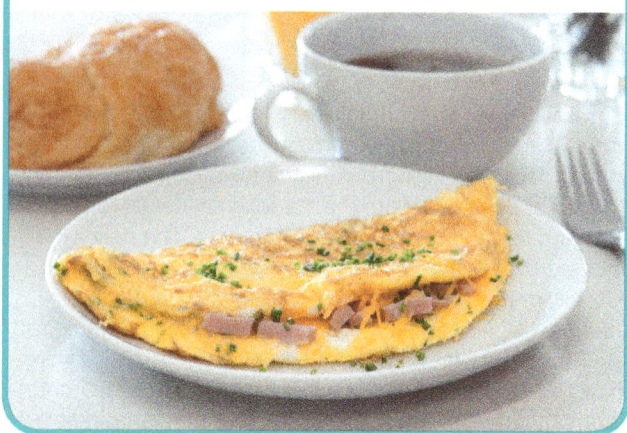

Vitamin Deficiencies

Because vitamins are readily available from the U.S. food supply, deficiencies among people in the United States are rare. However, there are exceptions. For example, people with dark skin need longer sun exposure to synthesize vitamin D and consistently have lower levels of vitamin D in their blood than people with light skin. As noted earlier, people who avoid all animal-based foods are at increased risk for vitamin B_{12} deficiency. Finally, a deficiency of folate may develop in people who don't consume dark green vegetables, legumes, or fortified commercial breads and breakfast cereals. Women who don't get adequate folate in their diet before and after becoming pregnant are at increased risk for giving birth to a newborn with a neural tube defect, a serious and sometimes fatal birth defect in which the spinal cord fails to close properly. The critical period for healthy development of the neural tube is the first four weeks after conception, typically before a woman even realizes she is pregnant. For this reason, all women of childbearing age, whether or not they intend to become pregnant, are advised to consume 400 micrograms of folic acid daily either from a supplement or from fortified foods.[17]

TABLE 5.1 Key Facts About Vitamins

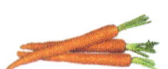 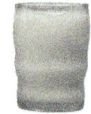 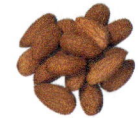 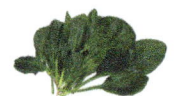 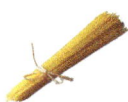 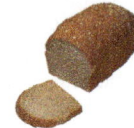 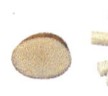 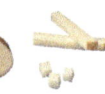

Fat Soluble				Water Soluble		
Vitamin A	**Vitamin D**	**Vitamin E**	**Vitamin K**	**Vitamin B$_1$ (Thiamin)**	**Vitamin B$_2$ (Riboflavin)**	**Vitamin B$_6$**
Functions: Required for vision, cell differentiation, reproduction; contributes to healthy bones and a healthy immune system	Functions: Regulates blood calcium levels; maintains bone health; assists in cell differentiation	Functions: Protects white blood cells, enhances immune function, improves absorption of vitamin A; protects cell membranes, fatty acids, and vitamin A from oxidation	Functions: Needed for the production of proteins that assist in blood clotting and maintenance of healthy bone	Functions: Needed for carbohydrate and amino acid metabolism	Functions: Needed for carbohydrate and fat metabolism	Functions: Needed for carbohydrate and amino acid metabolism; synthesis of blood cells
Food Sources: Beef, chicken liver, egg yolk, milk, spinach, carrots, mango, apricots, cantaloupe, pumpkin, yams	Food Sources: Canned salmon and mackerel, fortified milk or orange juice, fortified cereals	Food Sources: Sunflower seeds, almonds, vegetable oils, fortified cereals	Food Sources: Kale, spinach, turnip greens, Brussels sprouts	Food Sources: Pork, fortified cereals, enriched rice and pasta, peas, tuna, beans	Food Sources: Beef liver, shrimp, dairy products, fortified cereals, enriched breads and grains	Food Sources: Chickpeas (garbanzo beans), red meat/fish/poultry, fortified cereals, potatoes

Minerals

Minerals are elements that cannot be made or broken down. Minerals in your diet come from a wide variety of plant and animal foods, and even from the water you drink.

Your body needs more than a dozen minerals to function, and many minerals provide structure. The *major minerals* are those your body needs in amounts greater than 100 milligrams daily. These include sodium, potassium, chloride, calcium, phosphorus, sulfur, and magnesium. You need *trace minerals* in much smaller amounts, typically less than 10 milligrams daily. The trace minerals include iron, fluoride, iodine, selenium, zinc, copper, manganese, and chromium. **Table 5.2** provides more information about selected minerals.

A varied and balanced diet provides most people with all the minerals they need, and supplements are not generally recommended. However, physicians sometimes prescribe iron supplements for patients at risk for iron-deficiency anemia, or fluoride drops to promote healthy tooth development for infants and toddlers who do not drink fluoridated water. What about calcium supplements? Should you take them to maintain healthy bone? See the **Special Feature** on page 106 to find out.

One major mineral commonly found to excess in the American diet is sodium. Although the recommended intake is about one teaspoon of salt per day, most Americans consume much more, largely through processed foods. This is a concern because some Americans are sodium sensitive, and high blood pressure is more common in these people if they consume a high-sodium diet. (See Chapter 13 for more information on high blood pressure.)

▶▶ For more detailed information on specific vitamins and minerals, visit Oregon State University's Micronutrient Information Center at http://lpi.oregonstate.edu/infocenter/vitamins.html.

Water

You may be able to survive for weeks or even months without food, but you can live for only a few days without **water,** which is essential to most of your body's chemical reactions. It is vital, for instance, to digestion, absorption, circulation, body temperature regulation, and many other functions. Water also contributes to a feeling of fullness when consumed with a meal.

You have to drink water to replace what you lose in sweat, urine, feces, evaporation off your skin, and exhalation of breath from your lungs. When you're sick with a runny nose, fever, diarrhea, or vomiting, you lose even more water. Most adult women can maintain an adequate water intake by drinking 9 cups (2.2 liters) of beverages daily and men by drinking 13 cups (3 liters) of beverages daily.[18] If you are physically active or live in a very hot climate, you may require more total water.

Although beverages provide the greatest percentage of the water we consume, nearly all foods contain water as well. In addition, the body's metabolism of the energy-yielding nutrients generates metabolic water. Let's take a look at some commonly consumed beverages:[19]

- **Bottled water.** Plain drinking water hydrates your body and is calorie free. Although it may be convenient, bottled water is typically no safer or more healthful than plain tap water, and its bottling and packaging takes a greater toll on the environment than filling your own reusable bottle or cup from the faucet.
- **Sports beverages.** Traditional sports drinks provide water, some minerals, and a source of carbohydrate.

> **minerals** Elements needed by the body to regulate functions and provide structure.
>
> **water** A liquid composed of hydrogen and oxygen that is necessary for life.

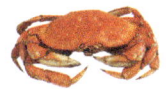 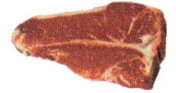 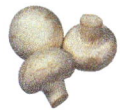 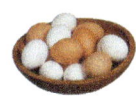 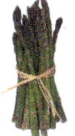 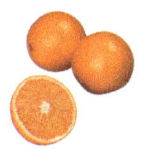

Water Soluble

Vitamin B₁₂	Niacin	Pantothenic Acid	Biotin	Folate (Folic Acid)	Vitamin C
Functions: Assists with formation of blood; required for healthy nervous system	**Functions:** Needed for carbohydrate and fat metabolism; assists in DNA replication and repair; assists in cell differentiation	**Functions:** Assists with fat metabolism	**Functions:** Involved in carbohydrate, fat, and protein metabolism	**Functions:** Needed for amino acid metabolism and DNA synthesis	**Functions:** Antioxidant; enhances immune function; assists in synthesis of important compounds; enhances iron absorption
Food Sources: Shellfish, red meat/fish/poultry, dairy products, fortified cereals	**Food Sources:** Beef liver, red meat/fish/poultry, fortified cereals, enriched breads and grains, canned tomato products	**Food Sources:** Red meat/fish/poultry, mushrooms, fortified cereals, egg yolk	**Food Sources:** Nuts, egg yolk	**Food Sources:** Fortified cereals, enriched breads and grains, legumes (lentils, chickpeas, pinto beans), spinach, romaine lettuce, asparagus, liver	**Food Sources:** Sweet peppers, citrus fruits and juices, broccoli, strawberries, kiwi fruit

Source: Adapted from Thompson, Janice, Melinda Manore, and Linda Vaughan, *The Science of Nutrition*, 4th ed., © 2017, pp. 294–295. Reprinted and electronically reproduced by permission of Pearson Education, Inc., Upper Saddle River, New Jersey.

They can help athletes and manual laborers avoid fluid imbalances during strenuous physical activity lasting an hour or longer; however, a typical 20-ounce bottle contains 34 grams (8.5 teaspoons!) of added sugars that most people don't need.

- **Milk and milk substitutes.** Soy milk and low-fat cow's milk are healthful beverage choices, providing protein, calcium, vitamin D, and several other vitamins and minerals.
- **Sugary drinks.** Many health experts believe that beverages loaded with added sugars, such as soft drinks, bottled teas, flavored milks, and juices, have contributed greatly to America's obesity problem. Whether in the form of high-fructose corn syrup, "pure cane sugar," honey, or "fruit juice concentrate," the added sugar provides the same 4 calories per gram, and as package sizes continue to increase, the calorie count for such beverages can be astronomical. Moreover, when you eat a certain amount of solid food, your brain gets the signal that you're full, but drinking the same number of calories as fluid doesn't trigger this "satisfaction" response in your brain, so you're still hungry. For these reasons, some weight-loss experts advise their overweight clients to entirely eliminate sugary drinks from their diet. Think this is a little extreme? Visit the **Consumer Corner** and check out the sugar and calorie contents of some popular beverages.
- **Beverages containing caffeine.** Coffee, tea, and hot cocoa all provide caffeine, a stimulant that can

TABLE 5.2 Key Facts About Selected Minerals

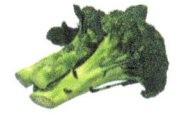 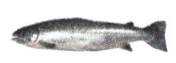 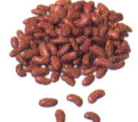 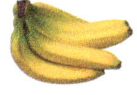 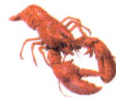

Calcium	Iron	Magnesium	Potassium	Zinc
Functions: Primary component of bone; needed for acid–base balance, transmission of nerve impulses, and muscle contraction	**Functions:** Helps transport oxygen in blood cells; assists many functional systems	**Functions:** Component of bone; aids in muscle contraction; assists many functional systems	**Functions:** Needed for fluid balance, transmission of nerve impulses, and muscle contraction	**Functions:** Assists many functional systems; aids in immunity, growth, sexual maturation, and gene regulation
Food Sources: Dairy products, fortified juices, fish with bones (such as sardines or salmon), broccoli, kale, collard greens	**Food Sources:** Clams, chicken, turkey, fish, ham	**Food Sources:** Oysters, beef, pork, chicken, turkey, tuna, lobster, shrimp, salmon, milk, yogurt, whole grain cereals, almonds, walnuts, sunflower seeds, beans	**Food Sources:** Fruits (bananas, oranges, grapefruit, plums), vegetables (spinach, beans)	**Food Sources:** Red meat, poultry, seafood (oysters, tuna, lobster)

Source: Adapted from Thompson, Janice, Melinda Manore, and Linda Vaughan, *Science of Nutrition*, 4th ed., ©2017, pp. 297–298. Reprinted and electronically reproduced by permission of Pearson Education, Inc., Upper Saddle River, New Jersey.

SPECIAL FEATURE

Feeding Your Bones

Calcium is the main component of the mineral crystals that make up healthy bone. As you age from childhood to adulthood, your bones are not only lengthening, they're also increasing in density. They do this by depositing calcium-containing crystals on a protein "scaffold" in the bone interior. If you don't eat a nourishing diet during these critical years, your bones may not be able to reach optimal density. As you age, you may be at increased risk for *osteoporosis*, a disease characterized by brittle bones that fracture easily.

- So what nutrients are important for bone health? If you're aged 19 to 50, you should consume at least 1,000 milligrams of calcium a day. If you consider that an 8-ounce glass of milk or soy milk contains about 300 milligrams of calcium, and a cup of cooked kale about 100, you can see that meeting this level of daily calcium intake can be challenging. Calcium is also available in cheese and yogurt, many legumes and certain other vegetables, and in fortified foods. What about supplements? They used to be commonly recommended, but research doesn't support their effectiveness in preventing osteoporosis, and they have many troubling side effects.[1,2] So your best bet is to obtain calcium from an overall healthful diet.

- Vitamin D is another important nutrient for bone health because it regulates your body's absorption of calcium. You also need vitamin K and the minerals phosphorus, magnesium, and fluoride. Finally, adequate protein intake is essential to healthy bone.

- What else can you do to keep your bones strong? Stay active. Any weight-bearing activity, from jumping rope to jogging to carrying textbooks up a flight of stairs, places positive stress on your skeleton and encourages your bones to increase or maintain their density.

Sources: **1.** Reid, I. R. (2014). Should we prescribe calcium supplements for osteoporosis prevention? *Journal of Bone Metabolism, 21*(1), 21–28. doi: 10.11005/jbm.2014.21.1.21. **2.** Tai, V., Leung, W., Grey, A., Reid, I. R., & Bolland, M. J. (2015). Calcium intake and bone mineral density: Systematic review and meta-analysis. *British Medical Journal, 351*, h4183.

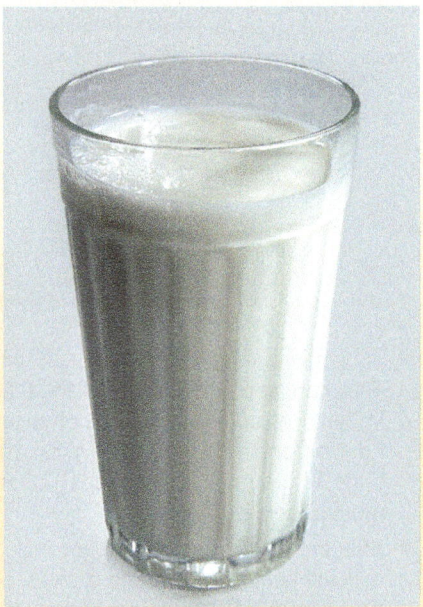

---

interfere with sleep. However, they can be healthful beverage choices if consumed in moderation, earlier in the day. Energy drinks vary greatly in their caffeine content, from a few milligrams to as much as 250 milligrams per serving. An average 8-ounce cup of brewed coffee contains about 100 milligrams, but you sip it slowly, whereas you can chug an energy drink, dumping a load of caffeine into your bloodstream. In 2012, the FDA released a warning linking the consumption of energy drinks to thousands of emergency room visits and at least five deaths.[20]

LO 5.1 QUICK CHECK

By definition, complete proteins
a. provide all 20 amino acids.
b. provide all 9 essential amino acids.
c. are derived from meat, fish, poultry, and eggs.
d. are completely digestible.

What About Functional Foods and Dietary Supplements?

LO 5.2 Discuss the potential benefits and concerns related to consumption of functional foods and dietary supplements.

Today, people are increasingly interested in consuming **functional foods**—that is, foods that confer some kind of health benefit in addition to the benefits provided by their basic nutrients. For example, researchers are studying non-nutrient substances in food that may improve your digestion, boost your immunity, delay aging, or prevent heart disease or cancer. Although many such non-nutrient substances are currently under investigation, we'll limit our discussion to those you're most likely to hear about—phytochemicals, probiotics, and prebiotics.

> **functional foods** Foods thought to confer health benefits beyond those provided by their basic nutrients.

106 CHAPTER 5 ■ Nutrition

CONSUMER CORNER
Drinking Calories: What's in Your Bottle?

When you choose a beverage, whether from a vending machine or at the dining hall or deli, do you ever stop and read the Nutrition Facts panel on the bottle? If you do, you might be shocked to learn what's inside. Here are the sugar and calorie counts of 16-ounce servings of some popular beverages:

Beverage	Sugar	Calories
Snapple Lemon Iced Tea	11½ teaspoons of sugar	200 calories
Pepsi Cola	13 teaspoons of sugar	200 calories
Minute Maid Orange Juice	12 teaspoons of sugar	220 calories
Rockstar Energy Drink	15½ teaspoons of sugar	248 calories
Ocean Spray Cran-Apple Drink	16 teaspoons of sugar	260 calories
Nesquik Chocolate Milk	14½ teaspoons of sugar	400 calories

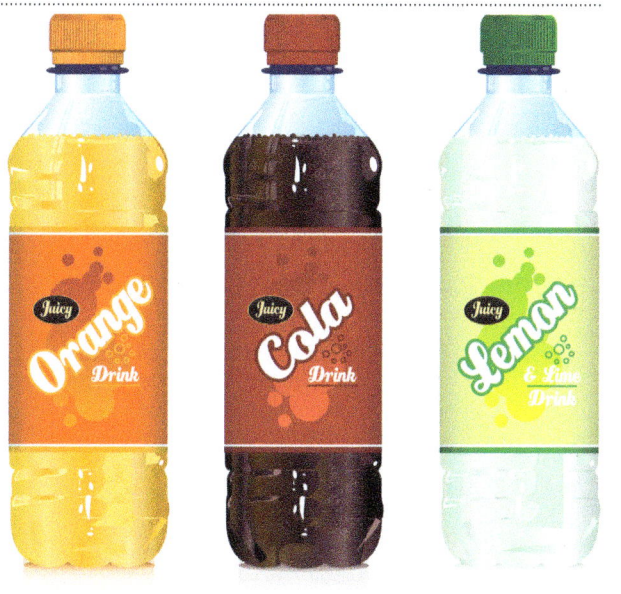

Phytochemicals

Phytochemicals are compounds that occur naturally in plants (*phyto-* means "plant") and are thought to support our health but are not nutrients. Sources of phytochemicals include not only whole plant foods but also many processed foods—from tomato sauce to tea—made from plants.

Many phytochemicals act as **antioxidants**. You've probably heard this term before but may wonder precisely what it means. As part of your normal day-to-day functioning, chemical reactions called *oxidation reactions* continually occur, producing *free radicals*, chemicals that can damage cells. Environmental factors such as pollution also contribute to free radical production. Damage from free radicals has been linked to cancer, cardiovascular disease, Alzheimer's dementia, and other disorders. Antioxidants stabilize free radicals, so they're not able to harm your cells. Some antioxidants are micronutrients: The most important of these are vitamins C and E and the mineral selenium. Many other antioxidants are phytochemicals.[21] In addition to their antioxidant activities, phytochemicals are thought to exert a wide range of healthful effects in the body, including, for example, opposing mechanisms that contribute to diabetes[22] and promoting mechanisms that may act to reduce the storage of body fat.[23]

You might have heard about three groups of antioxidant phytochemicals:

phytochemicals Naturally occurring plant substances thought to have health-promoting properties.

antioxidants In nutrition, compounds (mainly nutrients and phytochemicals) that help protect the body from harmful chemicals called free radicals.

- **Carotenoids.** These phytochemicals, such as beta-carotene and lutein, are found in red, orange, and deep-green foods such as tomatoes, carrots, and kale.
- **Flavonoids.** These phytochemicals are found in berries, black and green tea, chocolate, whole grains, and soy products.
- **Organosulfur compounds.** These phytochemicals are found in foods like garlic, onions, broccoli, cauliflower, and cabbage.

Researchers agree that the health benefits of phytochemicals result from their interactions with other substances in

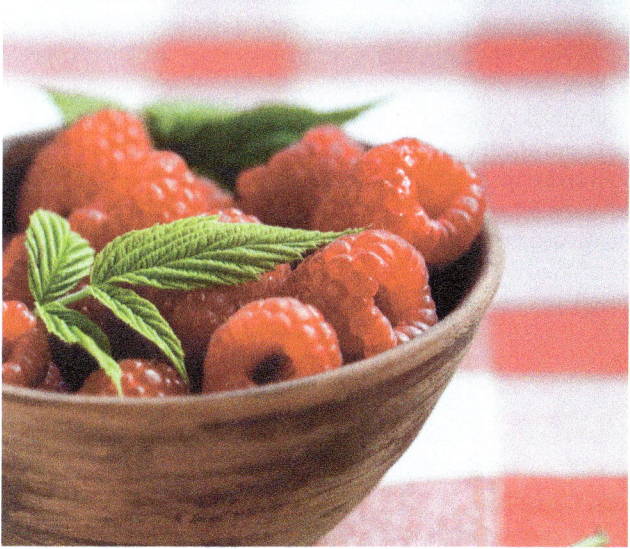

Raspberries are a rich source of antioxidant phytochemicals.

STUDENT STORY

What Should I Do?

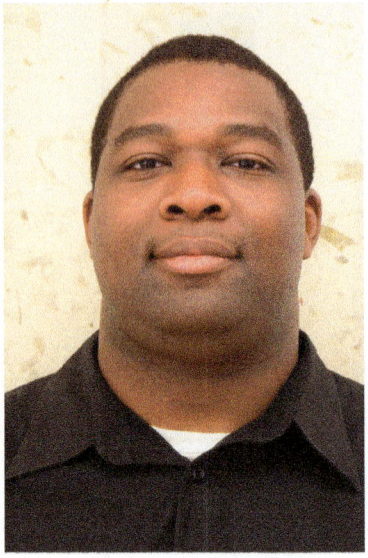

"HI, I'M PETER. I was raised on Wonder Bread, soda, and a lot of fast food. I didn't think much about what I ate; everyone I knew ate the same way. Now that I'm in college, I have some friends who are super health-conscious. One is a vegetarian, and another will only eat organic food from crazy expensive supermarkets. I like meat too much to ever become vegetarian, and I don't have the money to buy fancy food. But my doctor recently told me I am at risk of becoming diabetic because of my diet and my weight. I want to change my diet, but I need it to work for me. What's a realistic solution?"

What Do You Think?

1. List several nutrient-dense foods that you would encourage Peter to eat.
2. What four items should be limited in a healthful eating pattern? List several examples of foods and beverages you'd encourage Peter to avoid or minimize in his diet. Why are those foods poor choices?
3. Eating on a budget is an issue for most college students. How can Peter eat nutritiously without spending a fortune?

foods.[21,24] Phytochemical supplements (that is, those found in pill form) can't begin to imitate the qualities of natural foods, have not been shown to be beneficial, and may even be dangerous.

In addition to their nutrients and phytochemicals, of course, fruits and vegetables are a great source of dietary fiber. So it's no wonder that many nutrition experts recommend that you consume 5 to 9 servings of fruits and vegetables a day. How many college students actually do that? In a 2015 survey, fewer than 6% of college students said that they usually eat at least 5 servings of fruits and vegetables a day.[25]

▶▶ Want to find out how many fruits and veggies you should eat each day, in cups? Or find recipes to help you increase your fruit and veggie intake? Check out the activities on Fruits & Veggies: More Matters, at **www.fruitsandveggiesmorematters.org**.

Probiotics and Prebiotics

Probiotics are living, beneficial microbes that develop naturally in fermented dairy foods such as yogurt, buttermilk, and kefir, as well as in fermented vegetable foods such as sauerkraut, miso, kimchi, and tempeh (fermented tofu). The most common are types of bacteria. If deliberately consuming foods full of live bacteria sounds less than appealing to you, consider that your body already contains about as many bacteria as body cells, trillions of which reside in your large intestine, where they support your digestion and make other important contributions to your health. In fact, *probiotic* means "pro-life."

Research into our body's resident bacteria indicates that they promote good health by crowding out harmful bacteria, viruses, and yeasts; producing nutrients, including certain vitamins; promoting bowel regularity; assisting your immune system; degrading potential carcinogens (cancer-causing agents); and helping the body use energy and avoid building up body fat.[26,27] The bacteria you consume in probiotic foods are thought to exert similar beneficial effects.

When you consume a probiotic food, beverage, or supplement, the bacteria adhere to the lining of your large intestine for only a few days, so it is important to consume them regularly.

Another way to increase your population of beneficial bacteria is to consume foods containing **prebiotics.** These are nondigestible food ingredients (typically carbohydrates) that stimulate the growth and/or activity of beneficial bacteria in the large intestine.[28] Prebiotics don't feed you because they pass through the GI tract without being digested or absorbed. Rather, when they reach the large intestine, they "feed" the helpful bacteria there. An example is inulin, a carbohydrate found in a few fruits, onions, green vegetables, and whole grains, and added to some processed foods. In fact, inulin is often added to yogurt, producing a *synbiotic*—that is, a food, beverage, or supplement providing both pro- and prebiotics.

> **probiotics** Living microbes present in fermented foods, the consumption of which improves the microbial balance in the large intestine.
>
> **prebiotics** Nondigestible food ingredients that benefit human health by stimulating the growth and/or activity of beneficial bacteria in the large intestine.
>
> **dietary supplements** Products taken by mouth that include ingredients such as vitamins, minerals, amino acids, or herbs intended to supplement the diet.

Dietary Supplements

Do you regularly take dietary supplements? According to a recent survey of students at five U.S. universities, about 66% use a dietary supplement at least once a week, and 12% consume five or more supplements a week.[29] Although supplements are popular, they are not without risk.

Dietary supplements are products taken by mouth that include ingredients such as vitamins, minerals, amino acids, herbs, or other substances that are intended to supplement the diet. They are sometimes prescribed by an M.D.; for example, physicians commonly prescribe prenatal supplements to pregnant women. "Holistic" physicians such as osteopaths and naturopaths are more likely to prescribe a wider variety of dietary supplements, including herbs. Many consumers, however, decide to take supplements without consulting a health-care provider.

Types of Supplements

Certainly the most popular class of dietary supplements among Americans is multivitamin/mineral supplements

(MVMs). More than one out of three Americans takes at least one MVM, and many people take more than one.[30] As shown in the **Student Stats** at right, vitamins and minerals are the most popular supplement used by college students.

Botanical supplements, commonly referred to as *herbs,* are also popular. These are plants or plant parts used for their therapeutic properties. Some botanicals, such as ginger, chamomile, and peppermint taken as teas to aid digestion, are considered mild and generally safe. Others can be toxic. The fact that a product is manufactured from a plant does not necessarily mean it is "natural" or safe to consume.

>> The National Center for Complementary and Integrative Health (NCCIH) provides fact sheets on the most commonly used herbs. Find them at **https://nccih.nih.gov**.

Another popular class of supplements is known as *ergogenic aids*. These are substances used to enhance exercise and athletic performance. A few appear to be effective but most are not. Carnitine, chromium, and ribose, for example, are popular supplements claimed to increase energy during training and competition, but research indicates that none of the three have any benefit.[19] Steroids, another class of ergogenic aids, increase the risk of cardiovascular disease, cancer, liver damage, and other disorders and can lead to masculinization in women and feminization in men.[19] (To learn more about steroids and other performance-enhancing drugs, see Chapter 6.)

Supplement Safety

If you're considering using dietary supplements, consult with your physician before investing your money. Most are ineffective, and some are even dangerous. In 2015, an investigation in New York State found that four out of five supplements for sale in stores like Walmart and GNC did not contain the ingredient identified on the label; moreover, many were contaminated by potential allergens such as wheat even though they were labeled as wheat and gluten free.

How could this happen? Doesn't the FDA regulate supplements? The short answer is no. Whereas the FDA requires extensive research supporting the efficacy and safety of a prescription drug or an over-the-counter (OTC) medication before it can be sold, supplements do not get this same scrutiny. In addition, although federal laws bar supplement advertisements from making specific claims about improving health or curing disease, a quick glance at supplements' websites reveals that they routinely make such promises. The FDA does, however, have the authority to investigate such sites and to remove a supplement from the market if it has evidence that the supplement is unsafe. Manufacturers of fraudulent supplements can even be prosecuted: In 2015, the U.S. Justice Department, working with the FDA, brought criminal and civil suits against 117 individuals and companies marketing fraudulent supplements, some of which had caused serious disease and even deaths.

Before taking any dietary supplements, consider these guidelines:

- **Talk with your doctor first.** Some supplements may simply be a waste of money, whereas others are harmful. Caution is especially advised for pregnant women, people with chronic diseases, and people using prescription or OTC drugs.

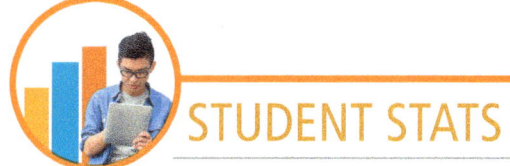

STUDENT STATS

Top Supplements Used by Students

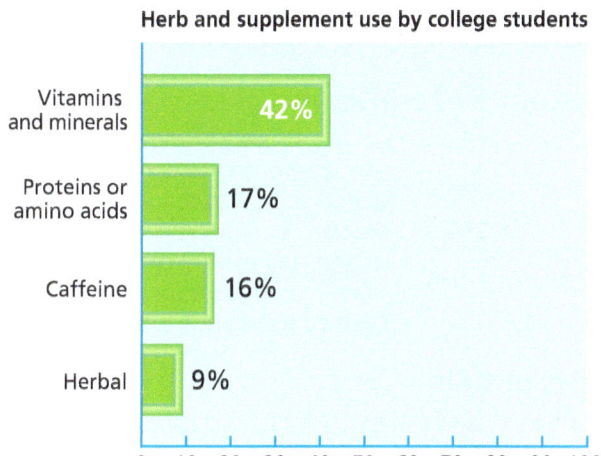

Herb and supplement use by college students

- Vitamins and minerals: 42%
- Proteins or amino acids: 17%
- Caffeine: 16%
- Herbal: 9%

Percent of students reporting use of herbs and supplements in a given week

Data from "Patterns of dietary supplement use among college students" by H. R. Lieberman, B. P. Marriott, C. Williams, et al., 2015, *Clinical Nutrition, 34*(5), 976–985. doi: 10.1016/j.clnu.2014.10.010.

- **Look for the USP verification mark.** This symbol on the label doesn't guarantee that the supplement has any particular therapeutic action, but it does indicate that the product meets minimum safety and purity standards as set forth by U.S. Pharmacopeia, a nonprofit organization.
- **Avoid supplements that contain high doses of a single vitamin or mineral, unless prescribed.** Some products containing such "mega-doses" may be toxic. This is especially true for the fat-soluble vitamins A and D. Vitamin A is especially toxic: Excessive intakes can cause organ damage and, during pregnancy, can result in birth defects or spontaneous abortion.

>> For additional tips on evaluating dietary supplements, visit the FDA's website at **www.fda.gov** and type "fraudulent dietary supplements" in the Search bar.

LO 5.2 QUICK CHECK

Prebiotics are

a. helpful bacteria found in yogurt and certain other fermented foods.
b. indigestible food components that stimulate the growth of bacteria in the large intestine.
c. naturally occurring plant chemicals thought to have antioxidant and other health-enhancing properties.
d. substances used to enhance exercise and athletic performance.

What Tools Can Help You Eat Right?

LO 5.3 Demonstrate how to use the DRIs, MyPlate, and other resources to design a healthful diet.

You've learned how nutrients and other health-promoting substances function in your body. But how do you choose real foods to get the amounts you need? In this section, you'll learn how to use four tools to help you eat right.

Dietary Reference Intakes (DRIs)

For more than 50 years, scientists have provided consumers with a set of energy and nutrient standards to protect against nutrient deficiencies, support healthy functioning, and prevent chronic diseases. These recommendations are called the **Dietary Reference Intakes (DRIs)**.

> **Dietary Reference Intakes (DRIs)** A set of energy and nutrient recommendations for supporting good health.

Types of DRIs

The DRIs include six types of recommendations **(Figure 5.3)**:[4]

- **Estimated Average Requirement (EAR).** The amount of a nutrient that meets the needs of half the people of a given age and gender. EARs are not very useful for consumers, but food scientists use them to calculate the RDAs.
- **Recommended Dietary Allowance (RDA).** The intake of a nutrient that is proposed to meet the needs of 98% of all healthy people of similar age and gender.
- **Adequate Intake (AI).** The amount of a nutrient that appears to be sufficient to maintain health. The AI is used as a guide to nutrient intake when an RDA cannot be determined. In other words, a nutrient has either an RDA or an AI but not both.
- **Tolerable Upper Intake Level (UL).** The maximum amount of a nutrient that appears to be safe for most healthy people to consume daily. This level is not, however, the recommended intake.
- **Estimated Energy Requirement (EER).** The average number of calories needed per day to maintain health and neither gain nor lose weight. Obviously, this will vary according to your gender, age, height, weight, and level of physical activity.
- **Acceptable Macronutrient Distribution Range (AMDR).** This DRI is specific to the energy-yielding nutrients. It defines a healthful range of carbohydrate, fat, or protein intake expressed as a percentage of your total daily calories **(Table 5.3)**. As an example, the AMDR for fat is 20%–35%, so if you typically consume 2,000 calories per day, a healthful fat intake would range between 400 and 700 calories.

>> You can access DRI tables online at the USDA's Food and Nutrition Information Center at **http://fnic.nal.usda.gov**. In the Search bar on the home page, type "DRI."

The DRIs Vary for Different Groups

Because of our age, gender, level of physical activity, or diet preferences, we all have unique nutrition needs. Here, we discuss a few of the key differences.

At different ages, people need different amounts of nutrients. For example, to promote bone density, children and teens aged 9 to 18 actually need more calcium (1,300 mg/day) than adults do (1,000 mg/day). In fact, calcium needs are never higher than in this period, even during pregnancy.

Because of structural and functional differences, men and women, on average, also have somewhat different needs for total calories, many vitamins and minerals, and fluids.

Athletes and others who engage in regular, vigorous exercise require much the same diet as non-athletes but need to make sure they meet their needs for total energy and fluids.[31] In addition, athletes may need more protein per pound (or kilogram) of body weight.

People who follow a vegetarian diet may also have unique nutrition needs. See the **Diversity & Health** box on page 111 for more details.

TABLE 5.3 Acceptable Macronutrient Distribution Range (AMDR)

Nutrient	AMDR*
Carbohydrate	45–65%
Fat	20–35%
Protein	10–35%

*AMDR values are expressed as percentages of total energy or as percentages of total calories.

Source: Data from *2005 Dietary Reference Intakes for energy, carbohydrates, fiber, fat, fatty acids, cholesterol, protein, and amino acids (macronutrients),* by the Institute of Medicine, Food and Nutrition Board, 2005, Washington, DC: National Academies Press.

FIGURE 5.3 Dietary Reference Intakes (DRIs). Most of the DRIs recommend specific amounts to consume, but the AMDR recommends a percentage of your daily calories that should be consumed as carbohydrate, fat, or protein.

Dietary Reference Intakes (DRIs)	
DRIs for most nutrients	DRIs for energy and macronutrients
Estimated Average Requirement (EAR)	Estimated Energy Requirement (EER)
Recommended Dietary Allowance (RDA)	Acceptable Macronutrient Distribution Range (AMDR)
Adequate Intake (AI)	
Tolerable Upper Intake Level (UL)	

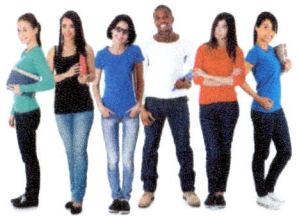

DIVERSITY & HEALTH

Vegetarian Diets

Broadly speaking, being a vegetarian means avoiding foods from animal sources. But the term has many subcategories:

- *Vegans* consume nothing derived from an animal—no meat, poultry, seafood, eggs, milk, cheese, or other dairy products, and typically no gelatin or honey. Many vegans also avoid wearing or using products made from or tested on animals.
- *Lacto-ovo-vegetarians* avoid meat, poultry, and seafood but will consume dairy products and eggs.
- *Pesco-vegetarians* avoid red meat and poultry but will eat seafood (*pesce* means "fish"), dairy products, and eggs.
- *Semivegetarians* (also called *flexitarians*) may avoid only red meat, or may eat animal-based foods only once or twice a week.

Except for fruit, every edible plant contains protein, so well-planned vegan and vegetarian diets do provide enough. When meals and snacks contain a variety of plant-based foods and caloric intake is sufficient to meet energy needs, protein needs can be met easily.

Vegetarians who consume dairy products and eggs don't have different micronutrient needs from their nonvegetarian counterparts. But vegans may not get enough vitamin B_{12}, which is available only from animal sources or fortified foods or supplements. Other micronutrients of concern include riboflavin, vitamin D, vitamin A, calcium, iron, and zinc. Even so, planned wisely, a vegan diet can provide adequate nutrients for overall good health.

Although health experts don't necessarily recommend that everyone become a vegetarian, many suggest that you increase the number of vegetarian meals you consume each week. Why? Plant-based diets tend to be lower in saturated fat and higher in unsaturated fats, many vitamins and minerals, fiber, and phytochemicals than the typical American diet. Studies show that such diets can reduce your risk for obesity and cardiovascular diseases.[1] Plant-based diets are also better for the environment because calorie-for-calorie, they use fewer natural resources and release less pollution, including greenhouse gases that contribute to climate change.[2]

What steps can you take to move toward a plant-based diet? Build your meals around legumes or other vegetables and whole grains. Think lentil soup with barley, a bean burrito on a whole grain tortilla, or mixed vegetables over quinoa pasta. Switch to veggie versions of your favorite foods, from pizza to tacos to burgers to chili. Most importantly, have confidence that nonmeat meals will provide you with all the nutrition that your body needs.

What Do You Think?

1. Let's say you weigh 145 pounds (about 68 kilograms) and are not an athlete. How much protein do you need each day? Would the following vegetarian foods provide enough protein for one day? Whole grain breakfast cereal with 1 cup soy milk: 12 grams; peanut butter sandwich on whole grain bread: 18 grams; snack of pumpkin seeds: 10 grams; and vegan black bean enchiladas: 13 grams.
2. Why do vegans have to consume vitamin B_{12} in fortified foods or supplements?
3. What other reasons, besides concerns for their health and/or for the environment, might prompt people to adopt a vegetarian diet? Discuss.

Sources: **1.** Academy of Nutrition and Dietetics. (2016, January 7). *Vegetarianism: The basic facts.* www.eatright.org. **2.** Eshel, G., Shepon, A., Makov, T., & Milo, R. (2014). Land, irrigation water, greenhouse gas, and reactive nitrogen burdens of meat, eggs, and dairy production in the United States. *Proceedings of the National Academy of Sciences, 111*(33), 11996–12001. doi: 10.1073/pnas.1402183111.

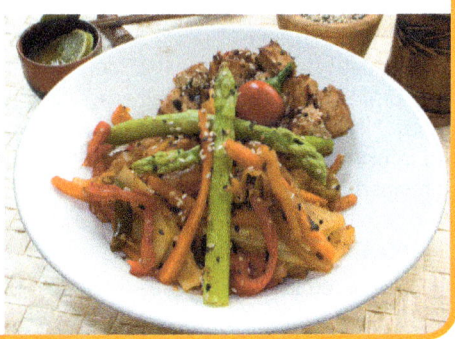

Do the DRIs seem confusing? For most people, they are. That's why many government agencies have developed tools that present the DRIs in more meaningful ways. One such tool is the food label found on nearly all packaged foods sold in the United States.

Food Labels

Food labels provide a lot of helpful information—if you read them! In addition to identifying the product and manufacturer, they include a list of all ingredients in the food in descending order by weight. So if you're considering buying a carton of yogurt and notice that sugar is the second ingredient on the list, you might want to choose another brand.

Nutrition Facts Panel

An especially helpful part of food labels is the *Nutrition Facts* panel, which provides nutrient information required by the FDA (**Figure 5.4**, next page). On the panel you'll find the recommended serving size for this food, as well as the number of servings per package, and the calories per serving. Changes because of new FDA NF panel, May, 2016. If you're watching your calorie intake, you should know that a food that has about 40 or fewer

STUDENT STORY

Why I'm Vegetarian

"**HI, I'M NIDYA.** I am a vegetarian, and I decided to become one basically because of my cousin. She's also a vegetarian and she showed me a PETA video that showed how they treated animals when they kill them for food. So I guess ever since then I've been kind of traumatized and I stopped eating meat. That was about two years ago.

In my household, since my family is Mexican, there's meat every day. So instead I eat a lot of beans and rice and fish and also vegetables, fruits, and salads, so I usually get all my nutrients."

What Do You Think?

1. What type of vegetarian is Nidya, as her diet includes fish?
2. Is Nidya eating any foods providing complementary amino acids? If so, what are they?
3. What are the benefits and drawbacks of Nidya's diet?

calories per serving is considered low in calories, and 400 or more is high.[32]

Beneath this line, the panel identifies the macronutrients, sodium, added sugars, and fiber found in a serving of the food. Notice that both saturated fat and *trans* fat are listed to inform you of the quantities of these unhealthful fats provided by this food.

Percent Daily Value

If you wanted to compare the amount of fiber in two different breakfast cereals you were considering buying, all you'd need to consider is the number of grams of fiber per serving on each label. But let's say you wanted to make sure that you meet your need for fiber each day and would like to find out what *percentage* a serving of your favorite breakfast cereal would contribute toward your daily need. For that, you'd look at the right-hand column of the Nutrition Facts panel to find the **Percent Daily Value (% DV)**. The percentages in this column give you a rough estimate of how much a serving of the food contributes to the overall intake of nutrients in a "typical" 2,000-calorie diet. So if you usually eat about 2,000 calories a day, and your favorite brand of corn flakes provided just 4% of your % DV for fiber, another cereal might be a better choice.

> **Percent Daily Value (% DV)** Nutrient standards that estimate how much a serving of a given food contributes to the overall intake of nutrients in a typical 2,000-calorie diet.

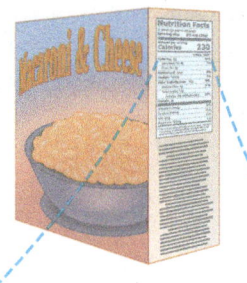

Nutrition Facts	
8 servings per container	
Serving size	2/3 cup (55g)

Amount per serving	
Calories	**230**

	% Daily Value*
Total Fat 8g	10%
Saturated Fat 1g	5%
Trans Fat 0g	
Cholesterol 0mg	0%
Sodium 160mg	7%
Total Carbohydrate 37g	13%
Dietary Fiber 4g	14%
Total Sugars 12g	
Includes 10g Added Sugars	20%
Protein 3g	
Vitamin D 2mcg	10%
Calcium 260mg	20%
Iron 8mg	45%
Potassium 235mg	6%

* The % Daily Value (DV) tells you how much a nutrient in a serving of food contributes to a daily diet. 2,000 calories a day is used for general nutrition advice.

FIGURE 5.4 Read Food Labels Wisely. When reading a Nutrition Facts panel, note the serving size, calories per serving, and nutrients per serving.

Even if your daily calorie needs are higher or lower than 2,000, you can still use the % DV to help judge the nutritional quality of a food: 5% DV or less is a low level for that nutrient, whereas 20% or more is high. So a frozen veggie burger that provided 5% of the DV for saturated fat, 0% for cholesterol, and 24% for protein would be a nutritious choice.

The bottom of the Nutrition Facts panel identifies the amount per serving and the %DV of four nutrients of concern in the U.S. diet: vitamin D, calcium, iron, and potassium. These are nutrients many Americans don't consume in adequate amounts, and poor intake is associated with an increased risk for chronic disease.

Use the % DV whenever possible. Consider not only the serving size but also how many servings you will actually consume. If you double the serving size listed on the package, then you must also double the calories, nutrients, and % DV. To help you interpret the serving sizes listed on food labels, see **Figure 5.5**.

Label Claims

Milk is milk, right? So how come one carton just identifies the name of the farm, whereas another claims, "Excellent source of calcium!" And would that claim influence you to choose that brand of milk, even if a comparison of the Nutrition Facts panels showed that both brands provide the identical 30% DV for calcium? Food marketers are hoping it would. Are such ploys legal? Actually, they are.

The FDA allows food companies to put two types of regulated claims on food labels:

- **Nutrient claims.** These draw your attention to the amount of a given nutrient in the food. For instance, a brand of soup may boast that it's "low sodium" and "a good source of fiber." Nutrient claims must be supported by the DV identified on the Nutrition Facts panel. For example, a juice cannot claim "Excellent source of calcium!" unless it provides 20% or more of the DV for calcium.
- **Health claims.** The FDA also allows food labels to include a small number of strictly worded claims related to dietary influences on human health. These claims cannot, however, suggest that eating the given product will improve the consumer's health. For example, an approved health claim on a low-fat, high-fiber, whole oat cereal might state: "Three grams of soluble fiber from oatmeal daily in a diet low in saturated fat and cholesterol may reduce the risk of heart disease. This cereal has 2 grams per serving."[33]

The FDA allows, but does not regulate, a third type of claim related to a product's contribution to human structure or function. Examples of such structure/function claims are "Builds stronger bones" and "Immune system support." When you see such claims on food labels, bear in mind that there's no guarantee they're true.

Dietary Guidelines for Americans

The *Dietary Guidelines for Americans* has been published jointly every five years since 1980 by the U.S. Department of Health and Human Services (HHS) and the U.S. Department of Agriculture (USDA). The *2015–2020 Dietary Guidelines* provide expert advice for achieving and maintaining a healthful weight and reducing your risk for chronic disease. See page 114 for the key messages.

MyPlate

In May 2011, the USDA released an interactive, personalized guide to healthful eating called MyPlate. It was updated with the *2015–2020 Dietary Guidelines*. When you log onto **www.choosemyplate.gov**, you can

- Learn about different foods and food groups
- Analyze your current diet and physical activity level
- Get a personalized daily food plan
- Find tips for healthful eating and for increasing physical activity
- Learn how to plan healthful menus
- Get information on how to lose weight

MyPlate also includes a simple but vibrant graphic representing the recommended types and amounts of foods you should eat at each meal. The relative portion sizes of each of the five food groups—vegetables, fruits, grains, protein foods, and dairy—are indicated in the plate graphic with segments of five different sizes and colors (**Figure 5.6**).

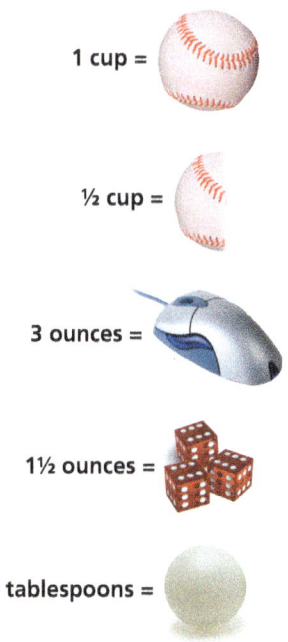

FIGURE 5.5 **Estimating Serving Sizes.** Comparing food amounts to common household items can help you estimate the serving sizes of your foods.

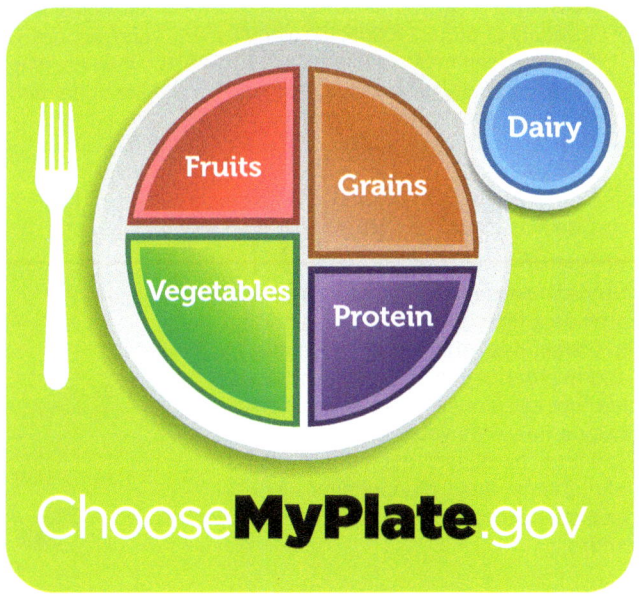

FIGURE 5.6 **The USDA's MyPlate.** To generate your personalized MyPlate plan, visit **www.choosemyplate.gov**.

Source: U.S. Department of Agriculture, 2011. www.choosemyplate.gov.

SPECIAL FEATURE

Dietary Guidelines
A Blueprint for Better Nutrition

The *2015–2020 Dietary Guidelines for Americans* are intended to help Americans achieve and maintain a healthful weight and to focus on consuming foods and beverages high in nutrients and low in empty calories. By following the *Dietary Guidelines,* you can reduce your risk of obesity, cardiovascular disease, and diabetes and promote overall health.

1. Follow a healthful eating pattern across the life span.

Instead of focusing on a single food or nutrient, focus on the quality of your whole diet over time. Recognize that every food and beverage choice you make contributes to your total intake of nutrients—and calories. Eat a wide range of healthful foods, including:

- A variety of vegetables from all subgroups—legumes, leafy green, orange, etc.
- Fruits, especially whole fruits
- Grains, at least half of which are whole grains
- Fat-free or low-fat milk, cheese, and yogurt and/or fortified soy beverages
- A variety of protein foods, including seafood, lean meats and poultry, eggs, legumes, nuts, seeds, and soy products
- Oils

2. Choose a variety of nutrient-dense foods in recommended amounts.

Nutrient-dense foods and beverages provide a high level of fiber-rich carbohydrates, healthful fats, amino acids, and micronutrients for a relatively low number of calories. Think of your daily calorie needs as your "budget" and use it to "purchase" the highest level of nutrients, fiber, phytochemicals, and pro- and prebiotics you can afford.

3. Limit calories from added sugars and saturated fats and reduce sodium intake.

A healthful eating pattern limits:
- Added sugars to less than 10% of total daily calories
- Saturated fats to less than 10% of total daily calories
- Sodium to less than 2,300 milligrams per day
- Alcohol to no more than one drink per day for women and two drinks per day for men

4. Shift to healthful food and beverage choices.

Choose nutrient-dense foods and beverages across and within all food groups in place of less healthful choices.

5. Support healthful eating patterns for everyone.

Support healthful eating patterns at home, on campus, at work, and in your community.

How can you follow a healthful eating pattern?

- Make major sources of saturated fats—such as cookies, ice cream, pizza, sausages, and hot dogs—occasional choices, not everyday foods.
- When cooking, switch from solid fats like butter and lard to plant oils.
- Drink water instead of sugary drinks. A 12-ounce cola contains about 140–150 empty calories.
- Select fruit for dessert. Eat sweets less often.
- Choose low-sodium versions of soup, bread, and frozen meals.
- Add spices or herbs to season food without adding salt.
- To help avoid oversized portions, use a smaller plate or bowl and stop eating when you are satisfied, not when you are full.
- If you have access to a kitchen, use it! When you cook your own food, you're in control of what's in it.
- When eating out, choose dishes that include legumes and other vegetables and avoid fried foods. Order a meal and a salad or vegetable side and share it with a friend.

Get plenty of physical activity.

Pick activities that you like and start by doing what you can, at least 10 minutes at a time. Every bit adds up, and the health benefits increase as you spend more time being active.

>> To view the full set of *2015–2020 Dietary Guidelines for Americans,* visit **www.health.gov**.

Source: Adapted from the *2015–2020 Dietary Guidelines for Americans,* by the U.S. Department of Health and Human Services and the U.S. Department of Agriculture, January 2016. www.health.gov.

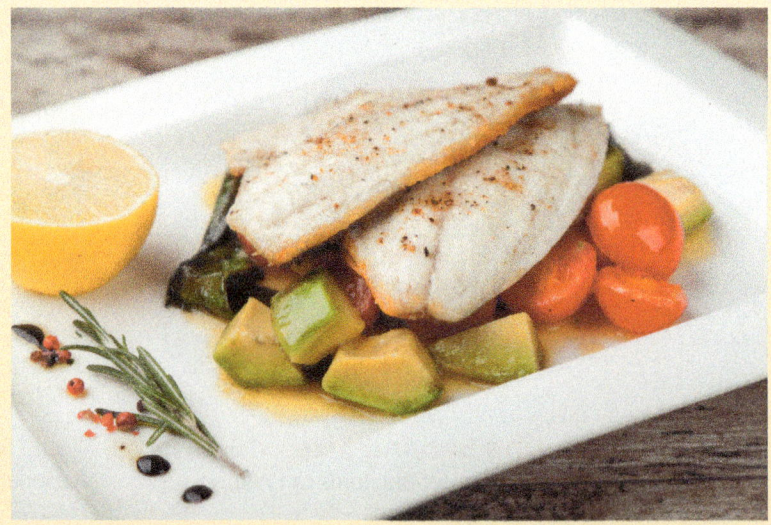

Food Groups in MyPlate

What foods are in each of the five groups? Let's take a look.[34]

Vegetables. As you can see in Figure 5.6, the vegetable group is the largest of the five. In fact, fruits and vegetables together should make up half your plate! Any vegetable or 100% vegetable juice counts as a member of the vegetable group. Vegetables may be raw or cooked, fresh, frozen, canned, or dried.

An important subset of the vegetables group is legumes, which include beans, peas, and lentils. Legumes are in the vegetable group because they're excellent sources of the dietary fiber and micronutrients available from other vegetables. However, they're also included in the protein foods group because they provide abundant plant protein as well as two minerals—iron and zinc—that we normally associate with meat. In fact, many people consider legumes the vegetarian alternative for meat. In recognition of their abundant protein, micronutrients, and fiber—not to mention the fact that they're naturally low in fat—the USDA recommends that everyone, including meat eaters, consume legumes at least a few times a week, if not every day.

> **nutrient-dense foods** Any food in which the proportion of healthful nutrients is high relative to the number of calories.
>
> **empty calories** Calories from solid fats or added sugars.

Fruits. Both whole fruit and 100% fruit juice count as fruit choices. Fruit can be canned (in water, not syrup), frozen, puréed, or dried. Berries, citrus fruits, apples, bananas, grapes, raisins, and fruit cocktail are common choices.

Grains. Any food made from wheat, rice, oats, cornmeal, barley, or another cereal grain is a grain product. Bread, pasta, oatmeal, breakfast cereals, tortillas, and grits are examples. The USDA recommends that you make at least half of your daily grain choices whole grains.

Protein Foods. Meats, poultry, seafood, eggs, legumes, processed soy products, nuts, and seeds are considered part of the protein foods group. Meat should be lean, and you should avoid eating the skin of poultry. Include at least 8 ounces of seafood a week (typically two servings). Everyone, not just vegetarians, should choose legumes at least a few times a week in place of animal-based proteins.

Dairy. Both cow's milk and calcium-fortified soy milk are dairy choices, as are cheeses and yogurt. The USDA recommends low-fat or skim dairy choices. Calcium-rich choices for people who do not consume dairy products include kale, bok choy, collard greens, and turnip greens; many legumes; calcium-fortified cereals, juices, and other products; and soy products such as tofu made with calcium sulfate.

What About Oils? Although they are not one of the five food groups, oils—fats that are liquid at room temperature—provide healthful unsaturated fatty acids, and you should consume them daily. If you eat nuts (including peanut butter), fish, and/or salad dressings, or cook with oils, you are probably already meeting your needs.

Empty Calories

Recall that the *Dietary Guidelines* recommend that you consume **nutrient-dense foods.** Peanut butter on whole grain bread is a nutrient-dense snack because it provides abundant plant protein, plant oils, fiber-rich carbohydrates, and micronutrients (not to mention antioxidant phytochemicals) for a relatively low number of calories.

Notice that a peanut butter sandwich is also very low in saturated fat, and except for highly processed brands, peanut butter contains no added sugars. In other words, a peanut butter sandwich is free of **empty calories**—that is, calories from solid fats or added sugars. The USDA recommends that you limit the empty calories you eat. Examples of foods loaded with empty calories are candies, cookies, cakes, doughnuts, ice cream, alcohol, soft drinks, fruit drinks, pizza, cheese, sausages, hot dogs, bacon, and ribs.

How Much of Each Group Do You Need?

Now that you know what the five food groups are, you might be wondering *how much* of each food group you should eat. There's no one-size-fits-all answer: The amounts you need reflect your age, gender, height, current weight, and activity level. To create a personalized eating plan, go to **www.supertracker.usda.gov** and choose "Create a Profile." Fill in the information requested, and in seconds, you'll learn how much of each food group you need.

When your plan appears, you'll notice that the recommended daily intakes of vegetables, fruits, and dairy are given in cups; for example, 1 cup of carrot juice or 1 cup of sliced carrots. In a few cases, however, a cup is not a cup! Lettuce and other leafy green vegetables are high-volume items: 2 cups is equivalent to a 1-cup serving. In contrast, dried fruits are dense, so ½ cup counts as a 1-cup serving. And what about dairy foods? A cup of milk, a cup of calcium-fortified soy milk, and a cup of yogurt are all 1-cup servings, as are 1½ ounces of hard cheese, and ⅓ cup of shredded cheese.

Recommended amounts of grains and protein foods are given in ounces and *ounce-equivalents*, which, as their name implies, are serving sizes that are equivalent to an ounce. For instance, an egg, ½ cup of cooked pasta, and ½ ounce of sunflower seeds all qualify as ounce-equivalents. For more examples, see **Figure 5.7**.

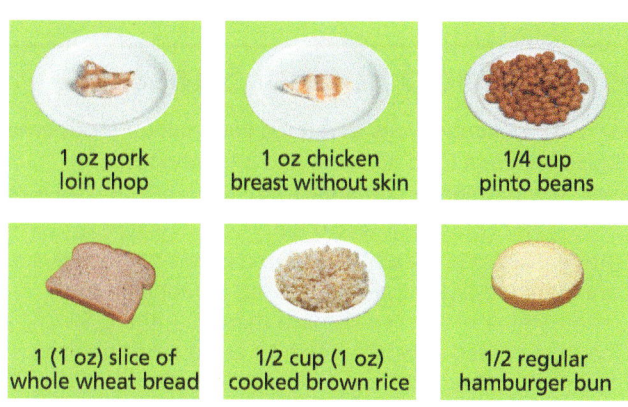

FIGURE 5.7 What's an "ounce-equivalent"? Here are sample 1-"ounce-equivalent" servings of various meats, beans, and grains.

When you're **hungry**, nutrition may not be the first thing on your mind, but making healthful choices is still important. To eat right:

CHOOSE THIS. NOT THAT.

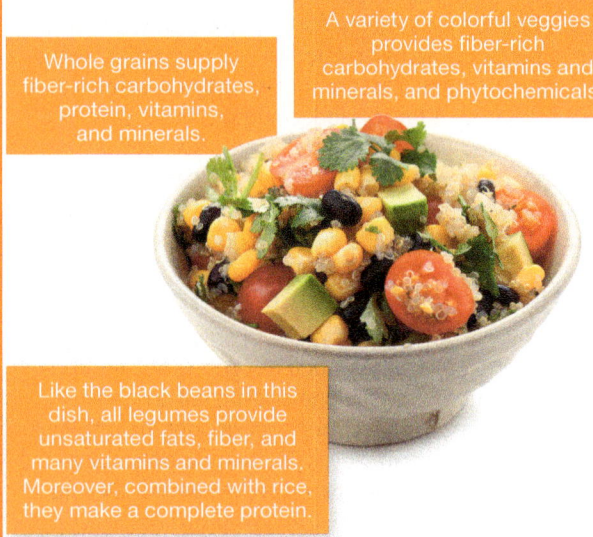

Whole grains supply fiber-rich carbohydrates, protein, vitamins, and minerals.

A variety of colorful veggies provides fiber-rich carbohydrates, vitamins and minerals, and phytochemicals.

Like the black beans in this dish, all legumes provide unsaturated fats, fiber, and many vitamins and minerals. Moreover, combined with rice, they make a complete protein.

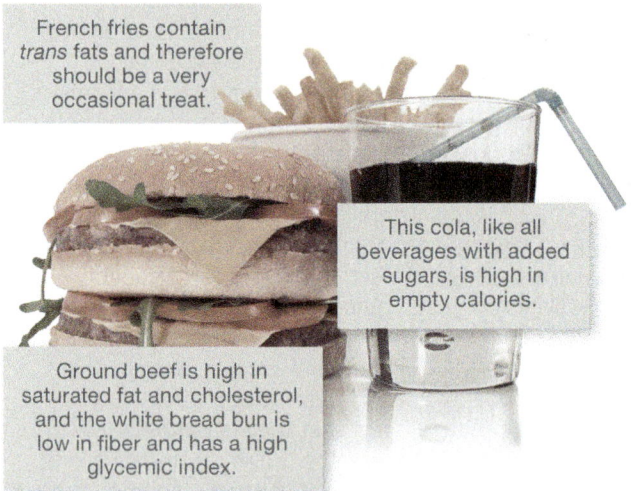

French fries contain *trans* fats and therefore should be a very occasional treat.

This cola, like all beverages with added sugars, is high in empty calories.

Ground beef is high in saturated fat and cholesterol, and the white bread bun is low in fiber and has a high glycemic index.

A Healthful Lunch:
Plant-based meals are naturally rich in healthful unsaturated fats, fiber, and micronutrients. They provide plenty of protein and have a low glycemic index. And they're delicious!

An Empty-Calorie Lunch:
The foods in this meal are full of empty calories and provide very few healthful nutrients and little fiber.

LO 5.3 QUICK CHECK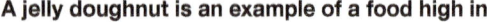

A jelly doughnut is an example of a food high in
a. empty calories.
b. nutrient density.
c. fiber-rich carbohydrates.
d. natural sugars.

Is Our Food Supply Safe?

LO 5.4 Describe ways to reduce your risk for foodborne illness, manage food allergies and intolerances, and avoid environmental contaminants.

After a 2009 outbreak of foodborne illness caused by contaminated peanut products killed 9 people in the United States and sickened more than 700, the U.S. Congress passed new legislation to safeguard America's food supply. The 2011 legislation increased inspections of food processing plants and gave the FDA greater authority to order the recall of tainted food. Moreover, a new national website, **www.foodsafety.gov,** was launched to provide Americans with a "gateway" to food safety tips and recall alerts. Unfortunately, the most recent data from the U.S. Centers for Disease Control and Prevention (CDC) indicate that these measures have done little to reduce the estimated 48 million cases of foodborne illness—including an estimated 3,000 deaths—that occur in the United States each year.[35,36]

Foodborne Illness

Foodborne illness, which most people call **food poisoning,** generally refers to illnesses caused by microbes consumed in food or beverages or by the toxins that certain microbes secrete into food that has not been properly preserved or stored. In otherwise healthy adults, foodborne illness often resolves in a few days without treatment. However, infants and toddlers, pregnant women and their fetuses, the elderly, and those with weakened immune systems, such as people

foodborne illness (food poisoning) Illness caused by ingesting foods or beverages contaminated by pathogenic microorganisms or their toxins.

with HIV infection, cancer, or diabetes, are at increased risk for severe complications and death.

Pathogens Involved in Foodborne Illness

Pathogens are disease-causing agents (*patho-* indicates "disease"). Viruses and bacteria are the two types of microbial pathogens most commonly responsible for foodborne illness. The culprit responsible for the most cases, by far, is norovirus, which causes abdominal cramps, vomiting, and diarrhea.[37] This highly contagious virus is transmitted from person to person, most commonly in places like restaurants and hotels where food is served to the public. In 2015, for example, nearly 350 customers in California and Massachusetts were sickened with norovirus after eating at Chipotle Mexican Grill. Inspections revealed several violations of food safety regulations; for example, employees had come to work sick, and food had been stored at a temperature that allowed the virus to reproduce.

danger zone Range of temperatures between 40° and 140° Fahrenheit at which bacteria responsible for foodborne illness thrive.

food allergy An adverse reaction of the body's immune system to a food or food component.

The species of bacteria most commonly implicated in foodborne illnesses is *Salmonella*. Infection with *Salmonella*, called *salmonellosis*, causes fever, diarrhea, abdominal cramps, nausea, and vomiting. Any raw food of animal origin, such as meat, poultry, and eggs, can harbor *Salmonella* bacteria, as can some fruits and vegetables.[38] Other species of bacteria that commonly cause foodborne illness are *Campylobacter*, *Listeria*, and *Escherichia coli* (*E. coli*). Although responsible for fewer cases of foodborne illness, the *Clostridium botulinum* bacterium produces a nerve toxin that is one of the most deadly substances known. A potentially fatal poisoning, called *botulism*, can develop after a person ingests even a microscopic amount of contaminated food. Botulism is commonly linked to improperly canned foods. If you're shopping for groceries and see a dented or bulging can, bring it to the store manager.

Microscopic worms and other parasites can also contaminate food or water and cause serious illness. In contrast, threads of mold on stale bread or old strawberries make the food look so unappealing that you're not likely to eat it; thus, molds are not commonly implicated in foodborne illness.

Reducing Your Risk for Foodborne Illness

Generally, pathogenic microbes spread easily and rapidly, requiring only nourishment, moisture, a favorable temperature, and time to multiply. Almost any food can harbor microbes. So, of course, can unwashed hands, as well as sponges, dish towels, cutting boards, and kitchen utensils.

So what can you do to keep food safe? Check out these steps:[39]

1. **Clean.** Wash your hands, kitchen items, and fruits and veggies. Here's how:

   - Wash your hands for at least 20 seconds with soap under warm or cold running water. Do it before you eat any meal or snack, as well as before, during, and after preparing food.
   - Wash utensils and small cutting boards with hot soapy water after each use. To clean surfaces and larger cutting boards that won't fit in the sink, mix 1 tablespoon of bleach with 1 gallon of water, flood the surface, and let it sit for 10 minutes before rinsing with clean water and allowing to air dry.
   - Use paper towels or clean cloths to wipe up spills. Wash kitchen cloths in hot water.
   - Before you cut or peel them, wash fruits and vegetables. If they're delicate, rinse them under running water.

2. **Separate.** Use different cutting boards for bread, produce, and raw meats, poultry, and seafood. At the grocery store, keep meats, poultry, and seafood separate from all other foods in your shopping cart. Keep them wrapped in your fridge, or if you don't plan to use them for a few days, freeze them. Keep eggs in their packaging and put them in the main compartment of the fridge where they'll stay cooler, not in the door.

3. **Cook.** The bacteria that cause food poisoning multiply quickest in the **danger zone** between 40°F and 140°F. Cook meats, poultry, seafood, and egg dishes until they are at or above 140°F. Use a food thermometer.

4. **Chill.** Notice that "room temperature" is right in the middle of the danger zone. In fact, bacteria can reproduce—and secrete their toxins—in foods left at room temperature within 2 hours. On a hot day, that time can be as short as an hour! So always refrigerate or freeze foods, including leftovers, promptly.

If you're not sure whether a food has been prepared, served, and/or stored safely, don't risk it. Heed the advice "When in doubt, throw it out!"

>> To find cooking temperatures, storage tips, video stories, and other help for reducing your risk of foodborne illness, visit **www.foodsafety.gov**.

Food Allergies and Intolerances

The FDA estimates that millions of Americans have allergic reactions to foods each year.[40] Broadly speaking, we can describe a **food allergy** as an adverse reaction of the body's immune system to a food or food component, usually a dietary protein. The body's immune system recognizes a food allergen as foreign and, in an attempt to combat the invasion, produces symptoms of inflammation. These may include swelling of the lips or throat, digestive upset, skin hives or rashes, or breathing problems. The most severe response, called *anaphylaxis*, includes most of these symptoms within minutes of exposure to the allergen. If not treated quickly, it can progress to anaphylactic shock, in which the cardiovascular and respiratory systems become overwhelmed. Without immediate treatment, anaphylactic shock is usually fatal.

Eight foods cause more than 90% of all food allergies: milk, eggs, peanuts, tree nuts (such as almonds, Brazil nuts, cashews, hazelnuts, pine nuts, and walnuts), soy, wheat, fish, and shellfish (such as lobster, crab, and shrimp).[40] The FDA requires that food labels clearly identify the presence of any of these eight allergens. The only known "treatment" for food allergies is avoidance of the offending food; however, some medical researchers have had success with a program of progressive introduction of the food into the patient's diet—under close supervision.

An adverse food reaction that doesn't involve the immune system is known as a **food intolerance.** This type of reaction typically develops within a half hour to two hours after eating the offending food. The most common example is *lactose intolerance*, which is caused by an inadequate level of a digestive chemical needed to properly break down the milk sugar lactose. Symptoms, which occur after consuming dairy products, include abdominal bloating and cramping, and diarrhea.

food intolerance An adverse food reaction that doesn't involve the immune system.

pesticides Chemicals used to kill pests; in agriculture, chemicals used to help protect crops from weeds, insects, fungus, slugs and snails, birds, and mammals.

Food intolerances have also been reported to wheat and to gluten, a protein present in wheat, rye, and barley. Gluten intolerance should not be confused with *celiac disease*, an immune system disorder in which consumption of gluten prompts inflammation and destruction of the lining of the small intestine and can lead to malabsorption and life-threatening weight loss. Many people who do not have celiac disease nevertheless report that avoiding gluten relieves digestive problems, joint pain, or other symptoms. These individuals may be diagnosed with *non-celiac gluten sensitivity* (*NCGS*), a disorder that is acknowledged but not currently well understood. Both celiac disease and NCGS are subjects of ongoing research.[41]

Food Residues

Food residues are chemicals that are not naturally part of food but remain in the food despite cleaning and processing. Two residues of concern to consumers are pollutants and pesticides.

Many different chemicals are released into the air, soil, and water as a result of industry, agriculture, automobile emissions, and improper waste disposal. Plants can absorb those pollutants and pass them on to the humans and food animals that eat the plants. Fish and land animals can also absorb pollutants directly into their tissues as well as ingest them when they eat other animals that are contaminated. Pollution residues have been found in virtually all categories of foods.

Pesticides are chemicals used in the field and in storage areas to help protect crops from weeds (herbicides), insects (insecticides), and other pests. When pesticide residues are not effectively removed, they can build up and damage body tissues. The health effects depend on the type of pesticide. Some are not toxic, whereas others can cause neurological disorders, affect glands, or increase the risk of cancer.

The U.S. Environmental Protection Agency (EPA) provides the following tips to reduce your exposure to pesticides:[42]

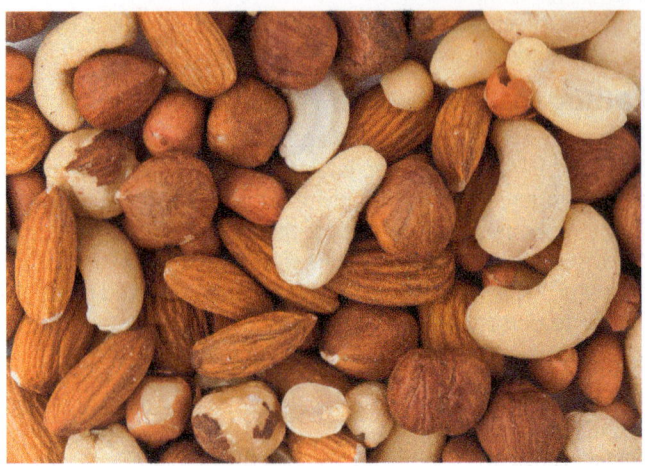

Nuts are a common source of food allergies.

- Scrub all fresh fruits and vegetables thoroughly under running water.
- Peel fruits and vegetables whenever possible and discard the outer leaves of leafy vegetables.
- Because pesticides tend to build up in an animal's fatty tissues, trim the fat from meat and the skin from poultry and fish.
- Eat a variety of foods from various sources.

Considering the harmful effects of pollution and pesticides, are organic foods better? What about foods labeled "non-GMO," "Local," or "Fair Trade"? To find out, visit the **Consumer Corner** on page 119.

LO 5.4 QUICK CHECK

Which of the following statements about pesticides is true?
a. Pesticide residues are a concern associated only with plant foods.
b. Herbicides protect crops from insects, rodents, and birds.
c. Although many people are concerned about the health effects of pesticides, pesticides are not known to be harmful.
d. To reduce your exposure to pesticides in lettuce, you should not only wash it but also discard the outer leaves.

Change Yourself, Change Your World

LO 5.5 Identify strategies for making nutritious, inexpensive choices when shopping, cooking, and eating out.

Armed with the information in this chapter, you're ready to improve your own diet and advocate for healthier food choices on campus. Improving your diet begins with an assessment of where you are right now. What food groups should you eat more of? What do you need to decrease? Are you eating too many calories overall, or too few? For answers, see the **Self-Assessment** on page 120.

Once you've identified your dietary drawbacks, use the **Choosing to Change Worksheet** at the end of this chapter to generate a plan for improving your food choices. But

CONSUMER CORNER
Organic, Non-GMO, Local, Fair Trade: What to Choose?

You're at the deli, waiting for your sandwich, and debating between several choices of beverage.

You could go with a carton of "certified organic" milk with "no GMOs!" Or what about a bottle of the "all natural" apple juice made from "Locally Grown!" apples? Then again, the "fair trade" coffee at the self-serve counter smells divine. Although you're not sure what these terms actually mean, they all sound good. So which should you buy?

Organic foods are grown without the use of toxic and persistent fertilizers or pesticides, genetic modification, or irradiation (exposing a food to radiation as a means of preservation). Red meat, poultry, eggs, and dairy products that are certified organic come from animals fed only organic feed and not given growth hormones or antibiotics. To earn the USDA organic seal, a food must contain 95% organically produced ingredients by weight, excluding water and salt. Farms must be certified organic by the USDA, and any companies that handle the food after it leaves the farm must also be certified. In contrast, the claim "all natural" has no regulated definition, so it can mean pretty much anything the food producer, including the maker of the apple juice, wants it to mean.

Are organic foods safer choices than foods grown with pesticides? That depends. If a conventionally grown fruit or vegetable can be thoroughly scrubbed or peeled, or if it tends to have a low pesticide residue anyway, then its safety is probably comparable to that of organically grown versions. Foods that don't tend to absorb pesticides include onions, corn, peas, pineapples, grapefruit, and several others. Foods that tend to show a high level of pesticides include apples, celery, sweet bell peppers, grapes, peaches, and strawberries, among others.[1]

Do organic foods provide more nutrients than conventional foods? To date, research has been inconclusive.[2,3] Thus, it's up to you to weigh the pros and cons of organic versus conventional foods.

Because the milk is certified organic, it's also "non-GMO," whether or not the carton specifically says so. GMOs are *genetically modified organisms*—that is, animals or plants derived from parent organisms whose DNA has been manipulated. Non-GMO milk is from dairy cows fed only with non-GMO crops; moreover, the cows themselves are not GMOs. In the United States, genetic modification is most often employed to produce crops that can tolerate conventional herbicides.[4] Although less common, genetic modification of animals is used to increase resistance to disease or produce meat or poultry products lower in saturated fat.

Supporters of genetically modified foods say that their use has increased agricultural productivity and enabled the world to feed its growing population. They also point to reduced use of energy and acreage for planting, water for irrigation, and pesticides for crop protection.[5] Opponents point out that the widespread use of genetically identical seeds has reduced food diversity and created "monocultures" that are highly vulnerable to plant diseases and climate events. Moreover, creating herbicide-tolerant crops has allowed farmers to apply even *more* herbicides. One result has been the evolution of herbicide-resistant *superweeds* that grow faster and tougher than traditional weeds, requiring the application of even more toxic herbicides.[6] Genetically modified seeds are also protected by patents, and farmers are not allowed to save seeds from their genetically modified crops to plant the following year. This means that they must continually purchase seed, the price of which has risen by half since widespread adoption of genetically modified crops.[4]

At this point, you may be thinking that the organic, non-GMO carton of milk is your best bet. But dairy production generates far more pollution than production of plant-based foods and beverages.[7] And although the apple juice isn't organic, it *is* locally grown. Why is that important? A common definition of a "local food" is a food produced within a 100-mile radius of the consumer. Transporting foods long distances in the conventional market system in the United States requires huge refrigerated trucks or railway cars

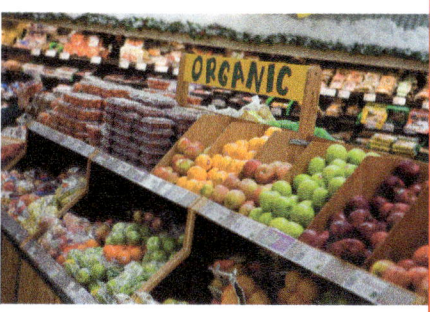

to haul the food, using energy for transportation and refrigeration and emitting pollution all along the way.

So how about that coffee? It was shipped to a local distributor from Columbia, so it's far from locally grown, but it does claim to be "fair trade." Fair-trade coffees (and other goods) are produced and sold in international partnerships between growers and buyers that promote sustainability and secure the rights of marginalized farmers and laborers.[8] These rights include safe and humane working conditions, as well as reasonable prices for crops and living wages for labor, which reduces farm families' reliance on child labor.

So which beverage should you buy? There's no right answer, of course. Each has merit and costs in terms of its nutritional quality, safety, environmental effects, and impact on the lives of others.

References: **1.** Environmental Working Group. (n.d.) *EWG's 2015 shopper's guide to pesticides.* www.ewg.org. **2.** Smith-Spangler, C., Brandeau, M. L., Hunter, G. E., Bavinger, J. C., Pearson, M., et al. (2012). Are organic foods safer or healthier than conventional alternatives? A systematic review. *Annals of Internal Medicine, 157*(5), 348–366. **3.** Baranski, M., Srednicka-Tober, D., Volakakis, N., Seal, C., Sanderson, R., et al. (2014). Higher antioxidant and lower cadmium concentrations and lower incidence of pesticide residues in organically grown crops: A systemic literature review and meta-analysis. *British Journal of Nutrition, 26*, 1–18. **4.** U.S. Department of Agriculture Economic Research Service. (2014, July 14). *Adoption of genetically engineered crops in the US: Recent trends in GE adoption.* www.ers.usda.gov. **5.** Klumper, W., & Qaim, M. (2014). A meta-analysis of the impacts of genetically modified crops. *PLOS One*, e111629. doi:10.1371/journal.pone.0111629. **6.** Fernandez-Cornejo, J., Wechsler, S., Livingston, M., & Mitchell, L. (2014, February). *Genetically engineered crops in the United States.* U.S. Department of Agriculture Economic Research Service. www.ers.usda.gov. **7.** Tubiello, F. N., Salvatore, M., Condor Golec, R. D., Ferrara, A., Rossi, S., et al. (2014, March). *Agriculture, forestry, and other land use emissions by sources and removals by sinks.* Food and Agriculture Organization of the United Nations. www.fao.org. **8.** Fair Trade USA. (2016). *What is fair trade?* www.fairtradeusa.org.

SELF-ASSESSMENT
Do You Follow a Healthful Eating Pattern?

The following 10 healthful eating behaviors are based on the *2015–2020 Dietary Guidelines for Americans.* Below each statement, check how often each applies to you.

1. I eat a variety of vegetables each day, including dark green, red, and orange vegetables, and beans and peas.

   Always ☐   Sometimes ☐   Never ☐

2. I make half of each meal vegetables and fruits.

   Always ☐   Sometimes ☐   Never ☐

3. I consume at least half of all grain foods as whole grains.

   Always ☐   Sometimes ☐   Never ☐

4. I choose lower-fat milk, yogurt, and cheese, or I drink fortified soy beverages.

   Always ☐   Sometimes ☐   Never ☐

5. I choose a variety of protein foods that are lower in saturated fat and higher in unsaturated fats, including omega-3 fatty acids. These choices may include seafood, lean meat, poultry, eggs, beans and peas, soy products, and nuts and seeds.

   Always ☐   Sometimes ☐   Never ☐

6. I use oils instead of solid fats when possible.

   Always ☐   Sometimes ☐   Never ☐

7. I choose and prepare foods with little salt and consume less than 2,300 milligrams of sodium per day.

   Always ☐   Sometimes ☐   Never ☐

8. I strictly limit my intake of foods and beverages with added sugars.

   Always ☐   Sometimes ☐   Never ☐

9. Whenever I can, I choose nutrient-dense foods and beverages in place of less healthful choices.

   Always ☐   Sometimes ☐   Never ☐

10. If I consume alcohol, I consume it in moderation—up to one drink per day for women and two drinks per day for men—and only because I am of legal drinking age.

    Always ☐   Sometimes ☐   Never ☐

HOW TO INTERPRET YOUR SCORE The more "Always" responses, the better. Focus on improving the eating behaviors for which you selected "Never" or "Sometimes." The *Choosing to Change Worksheet* at the end of the chapter will assist you in improving these areas.

To complete this Self-Assessment online, visit MasteringHealth™

---

even with a plan in place, how do you put it into action? Follow the suggestions provided here.

Think Smart When Making Choices

You understand the reasons why it's better to choose a black bean burger over a hamburger, but will you do it when you're in the dining hall—today? By adopting a smart thinking style, you'll find it easier not just to understand nutrition guidelines but to embrace them. Here are some strategies:

- **Be realistic.** Make small changes consistently over time. If your fruit intake is low, try adding a serving to one of your meals each day or as a snack. Or if you need to increase your calcium intake, start having a cup of yogurt every day as your afternoon snack.
- **Be sensible.** Pay attention to portion sizes and try to minimize your intake of empty calories.
- **Be adventurous.** Choose a fruit, vegetable, or whole grain you've never tried before.
- **Be flexible.** If you happen to overeat for one meal, let it go. Get back on track the next meal.
- **Be active.** You don't need to run 10 miles a day. You just need to be physically active. Consistently choose the stairs instead of the elevator. Walk over to your friends' dorm rather than calling them on your cell phone. Every step counts, so just get moving. (For more tips, see Chapter 6.)

Eat Smart When Eating Out

If you're like most other college students, you get a lot of your meals from the campus dining hall, food kiosks, and fast food outlets. But you can still make smart choices. For instance, compare these two fast food meals:

- A McDonald's Big Mac, large fries, and small iced mocha contain about 1,340 calories, 13% of which are from saturated fat.
- A McDonald's Artisan Grilled Chicken Sandwich, side salad with Italian dressing, and black coffee contains 425 calories, about 3% of which are from saturated fat.

As you can see, small choices you make every day can make a big difference in your nutrition, weight, and health. For some tips for eating at fast food restaurants, see the **Practical Strategies** box on page 121.

>> This site compares serving sizes, calories, saturated fat, *trans* fat, and sodium content for several popular fast foods: **www.acaloriecounter.com/fast-food.php**.

Shop Smart When Money's Tight

You might believe that it costs more to eat right, but in fact, some of the cheapest foods in your supermarket are also among the most healthful. Here are some smart choices:

- **Legumes.** Dried beans, peas, and lentils are a must-have staple. If you don't have the time to cook them, stock up on canned beans. They cost less than 50 cents per serving and provide 7 grams of protein, 6 grams of fiber, folate, calcium, and iron.
- **Canned tuna.** A small can provides two servings, each of which should cost you less than 75 cents, while

✲ PRACTICAL Strategies
Finding Nutrient-Dense Fast Foods

Fast food isn't, by definition, junk. Even at national chains, nutrient-dense choices are available. Here are some tips for how to find them:

- Order a "garden" burger, a bean burrito, or a slice of veggie pizza.
- When ordering meat, choose lean meats, poultry, or fish.
- Skip the cheese.
- Don't super-size it! Instead, order the size of burger or sandwich that will satisfy you without leaving you uncomfortably full.
- Order a side salad with vinaigrette instead of fries.
- If you crave fries, order the smallest serving size.
- Avoid sugary drinks. They won't help you feel full and are loaded with empty calories. Ask for a carton of low-fat milk or a glass of water instead.
- Skip dessert or order a piece of fruit instead. Watch out for those "yogurt parfaits" offered at many fast food restaurants. They're typically loaded with empty calories.
- Monitor your sensations of fullness as you eat and stop as soon as you're satisfied.

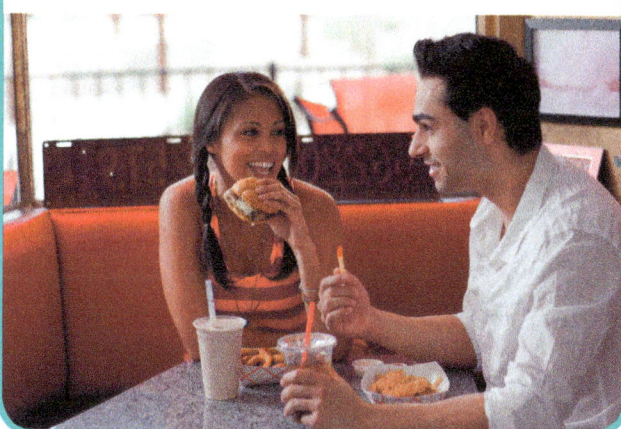

providing 12 grams of protein and about 250 milligrams of omega-3 fatty acids.

- **Lean meats, poultry, and fish.** Fill most of your plate with veggies and grains, accompanied by a small portion of high-quality lean meat, poultry, or fish. You'll save money and reduce your intake of saturated fat, not to mention calories.
- **Whole grains.** Choose brown rice, whole oats, and whole wheat bread. These foods are all inexpensive and are loaded with nutrients and fiber.
- **Frozen vegetables.** These are just as nutritious as fresh vegetables, less expensive, and quick to prepare: Pour the amount you want into a bowl with a tablespoon of water and microwave.
- **Fresh and frozen fruits.** Buy fruits in season or buy frozen fruit.

The bottom line? Make smarter food choices every day. Over time, they'll become a natural part of your healthful eating pattern.

Campus Advocacy

The *Dietary Guidelines* encourage Americans to support healthful eating for everyone. Whenever you choose a healthful food, you're doing just that. Whether you're buying frozen blueberries in your supermarket or ordering the bean burrito at your favorite Mexican hangout, you're sending the message that consumers value healthful foods and that it's profitable to offer them. At the same time, avoiding foods with empty calories limits their profitability and discourages their production.

On campus, make friends with the staff at your dining hall. Provide feedback—positive and negative—about the nutritional quality of the selections offered and ask for more plant-based meals. Find out where the food they serve comes from. Is produce locally grown when possible, and what food safety measures are in place? Check out the vending machines on campus, too. Do they offer nutritious snacks and beverages—or only junk? Who decides what's sold, and how can you improve the choices?

>> The USDA created the MyPlate on Campus program to empower college students to work with their campuses to promote healthful lifestyles. Visit the site to sign up as a MyPlate on Campus Ambassador, find a MyPlate on Campus Toolkit, and access other resources designed specifically for college students: **www.choosemyplate.gov/college**.

And while you're advocating for more healthful food choices, don't forget those less fortunate, including students on your campus. A recent study of more than 4,000 undergraduates at 10 U.S. community colleges found that, in the previous 30 days, 22% had gone hungry and another 26% had eaten less than they felt they should because of lack of money.[43] One way to help is to advocate for an on-campus food bank. Contact the College and University Food Bank Alliance for more information, at **www.cufba.org**. To help those less fortunate both on and off campus, consider joining a branch of the National Student Campaign Against Hunger and Homelessness. For more than 25 years, this organization has trained college students to fight hunger and homelessness directly and to advocate for long-term solutions. To find out more, go to **www.studentsagainsthunger.org**.

LO 5.5 QUICK CHECK

Which of the following actions best exemplifies the *Dietary Guidelines* urging us to support healthful eating patterns for everyone?
a. Log onto www.choosemyplate.gov and develop a personalized diet plan.
b. Offer your friends unlimited pizza and soft drinks if they'll help you repaint your apartment.
c. Provide positive feedback to the dining hall manager about the healthful choices offered.
d. Demand that your neighborhood grocer stop selling alcohol.

>> Watch videos of real students discussing their nutrition at **Mastering**Health™

Choosing to Change Worksheet

To complete this worksheet online, visit MasteringHealth

To conduct a self-assessment of your diet, log on to www.supertracker.usda.gov and select the interactive tool **Food Tracker.** To use the Food Tracker, you must keep track of everything you eat and drink for at least one *typical* day and enter the information into the website. For more accurate results, enter your food and drink information for three days—two typical weekdays and one typical weekend day. After you have completed entering all food and drink, under the My Reports drop-down menu, select Food Groups & Calories and print your report. You are ready to evaluate the quality of your current diet based on the daily food group targets.

Directions: Fill in your stage of behavior change in step 1 and complete the rest of the worksheet with your stage of change in mind.

Step 1: Assess your stage of behavior change. Please check one of the following statements that best describes your readiness to improve your diet.

_____ I do not intend to improve my diet in the next six months. (Precontemplation)

_____ I might improve my diet in the next six months. (Contemplation)

_____ I am prepared to improve my diet in the next month. (Preparation)

_____ I have been improving my diet for less than six months. (Action)

_____ I have been improving my diet for more than six months. (Maintenance)

Step 2: Analyze your diet. Review your Food Groups & Calories Report from the Food Tracker. Let's start with a comparison of your intake with MyPlate recommendations. Below, list the food groups for which your intake did and did not meet the target.

Food groups that met target intake: _____

Food groups that didn't meet target intake: _____

Next, look at the section on the bottom called "Limits." How does your intake of empty calories from solid fats and added sugars compare with the Allowance listed? What contributed most to your empty calorie intake (solid fats or added sugars)?

_____

Step 3: Plan to improve your diet. Jot down a plan for *increasing* your intake of the food groups that didn't meet your target intake and for *decreasing* your intake of the less healthful items. An example is provided.

Food Group	Plan for Change
Dairy	*By the end of this semester, I'll be consuming at least three servings of calcium-rich foods or beverages every day.*

Step 4: Anticipate obstacles. Write about any obstacles that might interfere with your ability to meet your goals. For instance, are you concerned that you won't have enough money to purchase fresh fruits and vegetables? Or that your lunch break is so short that you have no time for anything but fast food? For each obstacle, jot down a strategy to get around it.

_____

_____

_____

Step 5: Work within your stage of change. Given your stage of change, how likely do you think it is that you will implement the plan in step 3? What might encourage you to complete your plan?

_____

_____

_____

CHAPTER 5 STUDY PLAN

CHAPTER SUMMARY

LO 5.1
- The science of nutrition explores how the foods and beverages you consume affect your body and health. Nutrients in food are essential for the body's survival. The six major classes of nutrients are carbohydrates, proteins, fats, vitamins, minerals, and water.
- Carbohydrates provide 4 calories per gram. Glucose derived from the breakdown of carbohydrates is a key energy source during physical activity. Fiber is a non-nutrient, nondigestible carbohydrate that helps maintain health.
- Fats, at 9 calories per gram, are the most concentrated energy source in foods. Unsaturated fats are more healthful than saturated fats.
- Proteins contain 4 calories per gram. They are made up of combinations of amino acids. Proteins can be used for fuel, but their primary role is in building body tissues and functional compounds.
- Vitamins, minerals, and water are calorie free. Vitamins are compounds that support many body functions, from growth to metabolism. Minerals are discrete elements that regulate body processes and contribute to body structures. Water is vital to digestion and nutrient transport, serves as a lubricant, regulates body temperature, and is the medium in which the body's chemical reactions take place.

LO 5.2
- Functional foods provide health benefits beyond those of their basic nutrients. These benefits may be conferred by their phytochemicals, probiotics, or other non-nutrients.
- Phytochemicals are naturally occurring plant chemicals thought to enhance human health. Many have antioxidant properties; that is, they stabilize the free radicals that are a byproduct of metabolism.
- Probiotic bacteria present in yogurt and other fermented foods and beverages help to replenish the healthful bacteria that reside in our large intestine. Prebiotics are indigestible carbohydrates that support the growth of these healthful bacteria.
- Multivitamin/mineral supplements, herbs, and ergogenic aids are all popular among college students, but the FDA doesn't regulate the safety and effectiveness of dietary supplements. Therefore, you should check with your health-care provider before using them.

LO 5.3
- The Dietary Reference Intakes are six groups of energy and nutrient intake levels recommended for good health.

MasteringHealth™
Build your knowledge—and health!—in the Study Area of **MasteringHealth™** with a variety of study tools.

- The U.S. Food and Drug Administration regulates the information on food labels, including on the Nutrition Facts panel. Read the panel when food shopping, compare products, and choose those with the highest nutrient density.
- The *2015–2020 Dietary Guidelines for Americans* provide expert advice on designing and maintaining a healthful diet, which can help you maintain a healthful weight and reduce your risk for chronic disease.
- MyPlate is an interactive website developed and revised along with the *Dietary Guidelines*. Log onto **www.choosemyplate.gov** for help evaluating your current diet and developing and following a diet that's right for you.

LO 5.4
- Foodborne illness occurs when microbes, such as viruses and bacteria, or their toxins contaminate foods. The microbe most commonly implicated in foodborne illness is norovirus.
- You can reduce your risk of foodborne illness by following four steps: clean, separate, cook, and chill. The "danger zone" at which food microbes readily multiply is between 40°F and 140°F.
- A food allergy is an adverse reaction of the immune system to a component—usually a protein—in a food. Food intolerances such as lactose intolerance are digestive disorders and do not involve the immune system.
- Food residues of concern include pollutants and pesticides. All produce should be washed thoroughly before consumption.

LO 5.5
- Follow a healthful eating pattern: Assess your current eating behaviors and then create a personalized nutrition plan that includes more nutrient-dense foods and fewer foods with empty calories.
- Eat well on a budget by focusing your purchases on inexpensive versions of nutrient-dense foods, such as legumes, canned tuna, and frozen vegetables.
- Follow the *Dietary Guidelines* to support healthful eating patterns for everyone. Make healthful food purchases, and choose and provide positive feedback about healthful meal items wherever you dine.

GET CONNECTED

>> Visit the following websites for further information about the topics in this chapter:

- MyPlate
  www.choosemyplate.gov
- Foodsafety.gov
  www.foodsafety.gov
- *Dietary Guidelines for Americans*
  www.health.gov/dietaryguidelines
- Food and Drug Administration: For Consumers
  www.fda.gov/ForConsumers/default.htm
- Academy of Nutrition and Dietetics
  www.eatright.org
- The Center for Science in the Public Interest
  www.cspinet.org

MOBILE TIPS!
Scan this QR code with your mobile device to access additional nutrition tips. Or, via your mobile device, go to **http://chmobile.pearsoncmg.com** and choose by topic: nutrition.

Website links are subject to change. To access updated web links, please visit MasteringHealth™

TEST YOUR KNOWLEDGE

LO 5.1

1. Which of the following substances contributes the most calories?
   a. alcohol
   b. proteins
   c. carbohydrates
   d. vitamins

2. Which of the following is characteristic of a nutrient?
   a. It is low in added sugars, saturated fats, and calories.
   b. It cannot be degraded by the body.
   c. The body cannot make it in sufficient quantities to support healthy functioning.
   d. After digestion, it can be converted to energy.

3. Proteins are
   a. made up of long chains of fatty acids.
   b. made up of units known as essential amino acids.
   c. classified as an energy-yielding macronutrient.
   d. available only from animal-based foods, soy, and quinoa.

LO 5.2

4. Dietary supplements
   a. do not need FDA approval before they are marketed.
   b. cannot be removed from the market by the FDA.
   c. are generally safe if the label identifies the product as "all natural."
   d. are safe and effective if the product label shows the USP mark.

5. Which of the following statements about phytochemicals is true?
   a. Phytochemicals are not found in processed foods.
   b. Phytochemicals are found in all types of foods, from meats, eggs, and dairy products to fruits, vegetables, and grains.
   c. All antioxidants are phytochemicals, and all phytochemicals are antioxidants.
   d. Phytochemicals are not nutrients.

LO 5.3

6. Which of the following statements about the DRIs is true?
   a. The AMDR identifies the amount of protein, fat, and carbohydrate that an average adult should consume each day.
   b. The AI designates a nutrient intake level when an RDA cannot be determined.
   c. The DRIs include the RDA, the AI, and the % DV.
   d. The UL is the ideal intake recommended to promote health.

7. The *2015–2020 Dietary Guidelines for Americans*
   a. recommend that you consume no more than 2,000 calories a day.
   b. recommend that you consume a low-fat diet.
   c. recommend that you limit your intake of added sugars.
   d. recommend that you adopt a vegetarian diet.

LO 5.4

8. The species of bacteria most commonly implicated in foodborne illness is
   a. norovirus.
   b. *Salmonella*
   c. *Clostridium botulinum*.
   d. mold.

9. Most foodborne illnesses
   a. are deadly.
   b. are due to overcooking meat.
   c. can be prevented by using safe food-handling practices.
   d. can be prevented by choosing organic foods.

LO 5.5

10. Which of the following is a smart strategy for improving your nutrition?
    a. Shop for, cook with, and order menu items containing legumes.
    b. Maximize your intake of foods with empty calories because they are less likely to cause you to gain weight.
    c. Avoid all genetically modified foods.
    d. If your food budget is tight, purchase a variety of dietary supplements to make sure you get the nutrition you need.

WHAT DO YOU THINK?

LO 5.1
1. Identify three reasons that whole grain bread is more healthful than bread made with refined flour.

LO 5.2
2. Andy, a carpenter, cut his hand and developed a bacterial infection in the wound. His doctor prescribed an antibiotic to kill the bacteria and also suggested that Andy begin eating a serving of yogurt each day. Why?

LO 5.3
3. You're comparing two breakfast cereals that have similar micronutrients and calories per ¾-cup serving. Cereal A provides 4 grams of protein and 5 grams of dietary fiber, and it has no added sugars and no saturated fat. Cereal B provides 4 grams of protein and 1 gram of dietary fiber, and it has 16 grams of added sugars and no saturated fat. Which cereal should you choose, and why?

LO 5.4
4. You've brought homemade potato salad to an outdoor barbecue on a hot July day. Identify the greatest amount of time that the salad can safely be left without refrigeration and, using the concept of the "danger zone," explain why.

LO 5.5
5. Identify one food from each of the five food groups that is both nutrient dense and affordable, even on a tight budget.

6

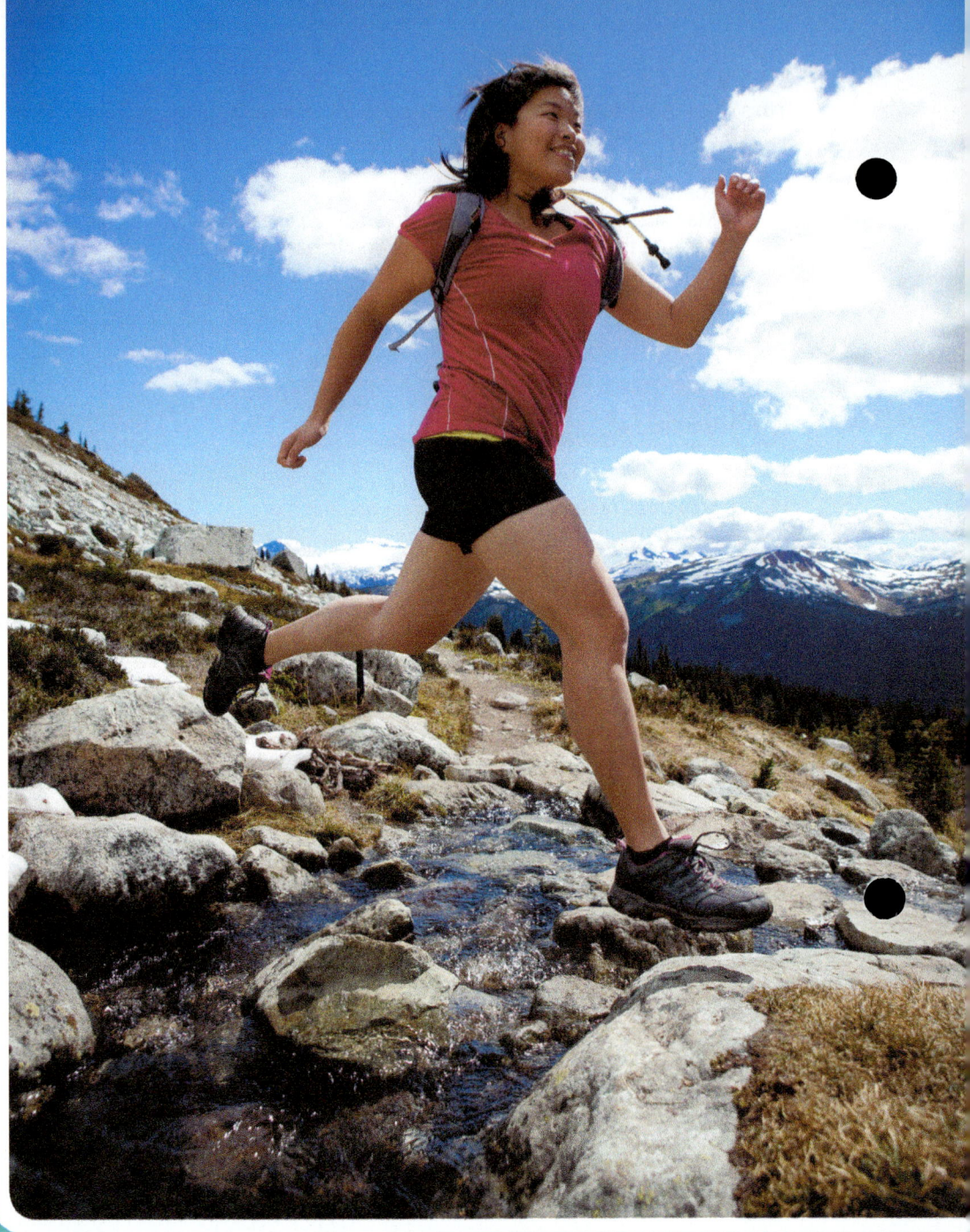

> People who are physically active for about 7 hours a week have a 40% lower risk of dying early than those who are active for less than 30 minutes a week.[i]

> Young adults with low cardiovascular fitness levels are two to three times more likely to develop diabetes in 20 years than those who are fit.[ii]

> In a recent study, women who performed 1 year of strength training significantly improved their ability to maintain mental focus and resolve conflicts.[iii]

PHYSICAL ACTIVITY FOR FITNESS AND HEALTH

LEARNING OUTCOMES

LO 6.1 Identify the five components of health-related physical fitness.

LO 6.2 Explain the health benefits of physical activity.

LO 6.3 Identify the principles of fitness training.

LO 6.4 Consider different types of physical activity for your fitness plan.

LO 6.5 Assess how much physical activity you need.

LO 6.6 Discuss how to exercise safely.

LO 6.7 Design an effective personalized fitness program.

As a society, we are out of shape.

Many of our daily activities no longer require significant physical effort, and busy schedules cut into our time for exercise—an especially critical problem for students, who often see their physical activity levels decline in college. Even when we do have time for recreation, hours that could be spent getting exercise or playing sports are instead dedicated to TV or a digital device. The result: Americans are experiencing more long-term health problems, such as overweight and obesity, diabetes, cardiovascular disease, and mental illness.

The good news is that in recent years, the percentage of people in the United States who report getting at least some regular physical activity has grown somewhat, with about 49% of those 18 years or older meeting guidelines for cardiorespiratory activity and about 21% meeting guidelines for both cardiorespiratory and strength-training activity.[1] If given the chance to be more active, our bodies thrive. Even small changes in physical activity levels can make a significant difference in your fitness and health, both in school now and in the years ahead.

What Is Physical Fitness?

LO 6.1 Identify the five components of health-related physical fitness.

Most of us equate fitness with appearance. We assume that people with trim builds are more fit, while those with flabby triceps are less fit. But physical fitness is not that simplistic. **Physical fitness** is the ability to perform moderate to vigorous levels of activity and to respond to physical demands without excessive fatigue. Physical fitness can be built up through physical activity or exercise. **Physical activity** is movement that substantially increases energy expenditure. Taking the stairs instead of the elevator and biking to class instead of driving count as types of physical activity. **Exercise** is physical activity that is carried out in a planned and structured format. Any type of activity will provide health benefits, but optimal physical fitness can only be achieved through regular exercise. Team sports, brisk walks, and working out at the gym all count as exercise.

There are two types of physical fitness: **skills-related fitness** and **health-related fitness.** In this chapter, we will focus on health-related fitness, specifically its five key components: cardiorespiratory fitness, muscular strength, muscular endurance, flexibility, and body composition.

> **physical fitness** The ability to perform moderate to vigorous levels of activity and to respond to physical demands without excessive fatigue.
>
> **physical activity** Bodily movement that substantially increases energy expenditure.
>
> **exercise** A type of physical activity that is planned and structured.
>
> **skills-related fitness** The capacity to perform specific physical skills related to a sport or other physically demanding activity.
>
> **health-related fitness** The ability to perform activities of daily living with vigor.
>
> **cardiorespiratory fitness** The ability of your heart and lungs to effectively deliver oxygen to your muscles during prolonged physical activity.
>
> **muscular strength** The maximum force your muscles can apply in a single maximum effort of lifting, pushing, or pressing.

Cardiorespiratory Fitness

Put together *cardio* for "heart" and *respiratory* for "breath," and you've got a good idea of what this component of fitness covers. **Cardiorespiratory fitness** refers to the ability of your heart and lungs to effectively deliver oxygen to your muscles during prolonged physical activity. Experts agree that cardiorespiratory fitness should be the foundation on which all the other areas of fitness are built. It is the component that is the best indicator of overall physical fitness, and it helps lower your risk of chronic disease and premature death.[2] In fact, the American Heart Association believes that cardiorespiratory fitness is one of the most important factors in overall health, and poor cardiorespiratory fitness is one of the strongest predictors of future risk for cardiovascular disease and other health problems—stronger, in fact, than other traditional risk factors like hypertension, smoking, obesity, elevated blood lipid levels, and type 2 diabetes.[3] You can boost your cardiorespiratory fitness by doing any continuous, rhythmic exercise that works your large muscle groups and increases your heart rate, such as brisk walking, swimming, or cycling, or programs such as CrossFit, which blends a rigorous cardiorespiratory workout with activities that build strength.

Muscular Strength

Muscular strength is the maximum force your muscles can apply in a single effort of lifting, pushing, or pressing. Building stronger muscles will help keep your skeleton properly aligned, aid balance, protect your back, boost your athletic performance, and increase your metabolic rate. Building muscular strength also results in much higher bone

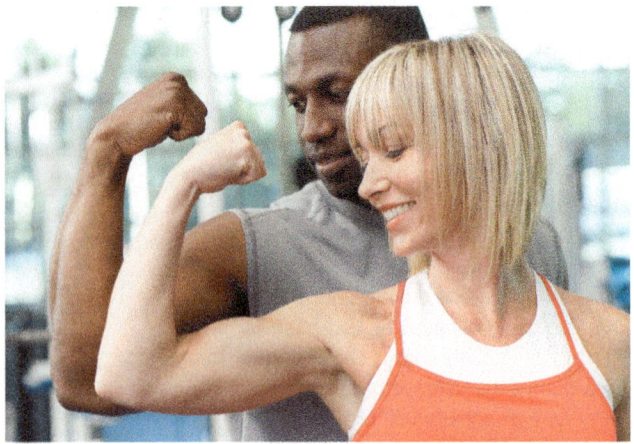

Men's and women's bodies react differently to resistance training.

mineral density and stronger bones.[4] You can build muscular strength by performing strength training exercises using machines, free weights, resistance bands, or simply the weight of your own body (as in push-ups, for example).

Muscular Endurance

Muscular endurance is the capacity of your muscles to repeatedly exert force, or to maintain force, over a period of time without tiring. Muscular endurance is measured in two ways: *static muscular endurance*, or how long you can hold a force that is motionless, and *dynamic muscular endurance*, or how long you can sustain a force in motion. A sustained sit-up, where you contract your abdominal muscles and do not move until they fatigue, is an example of static muscle endurance. Repeated sit-ups, done until you can't contract your abdominals any more, rely on dynamic muscle endurance. So do *plyometrics,* a type of fast-paced jumping exercise that focuses on building both speed and strength. Muscular endurance is important for posture and for performing extended activities. Muscular endurance can be improved by gradually increasing the duration that your muscles work in each bout of strength exercises, such as slowly increasing the number of push-ups you perform during exercise.

Flexibility

Flexibility refers to the ability of your joints to move through their full ranges of motion, such as how far you can rotate your neck from side to side or how far you can bend forward from the hips toward your toes. Flexibility depends on muscles as well as connective tissues such as the ligaments and tendons. Flexibility relieves muscle tension, reduces joint and back pain, and improves posture. Stretching exercises and activities such as yoga, Pilates, and tai chi can help improve flexibility.

Body Composition

Body composition refers to the relative proportions of fat tissue and lean tissue (such as muscle and connective tissues) in your body. A low ratio of fat to lean tissue is optimal. As we'll discuss in Chapter 7, many of us carry more body fat than is healthful. Excessive body fat, especially in the abdominal area, increases the risk of three of the four leading causes of death in the United States: heart disease, cancer, and stroke. It is also related to other serious conditions, including osteoarthritis, diabetes, hypertension (high blood pressure), and sleep apnea. Research indicates that even if you are healthy in other ways, having too much body fat will still negatively affect your health.[5]

Body composition affects your level of fitness, but the reverse is also true: As you become more physically fit, your body composition will usually improve. However, it's also important to note that each person's body may respond to exercise in different ways. For example, lifting weights will often yield different results in men and women. Men are more likely to see increased muscle bulk, while women may notice less bulk even while seeing increased muscle strength and tone.

Many factors, including your diet, body type, and genetics, play a role in how your body responds to pumping iron. But your sex is a key differentiator, largely because of hormones. Certain hormones, such as testosterone and androgens, are linked to muscle growth. Because men's bodies make more of these particular hormones, their muscles are more likely to increase in size under a resistance-training program.

> **muscular endurance** The capacity of muscles to repeatedly exert force, or to maintain a force, over a period of time.
>
> **flexibility** The ability of joints to move through their full ranges of motion.
>
> **body composition** The relative proportions of the body's lean tissue and fat tissue.

Differences in muscle size don't equal a difference in the benefits of strength training, however. Both men and women achieve valuable fitness and health gains from regular resistance workouts, including protection for our bones as we age. In women, for example, one study found a connection between muscle mass and bone health at locations where women are prone to fractures later in life, such as the hip.[6]

LO 6.1 QUICK CHECK

Which of the following is a prime example of dynamic muscular endurance?

a. a long continuous series of sit-ups
b. holding a hamstring stretch for 60 seconds
c. holding a heavy weight over your head for 60 seconds
d. a single sit-up held for as long as possible

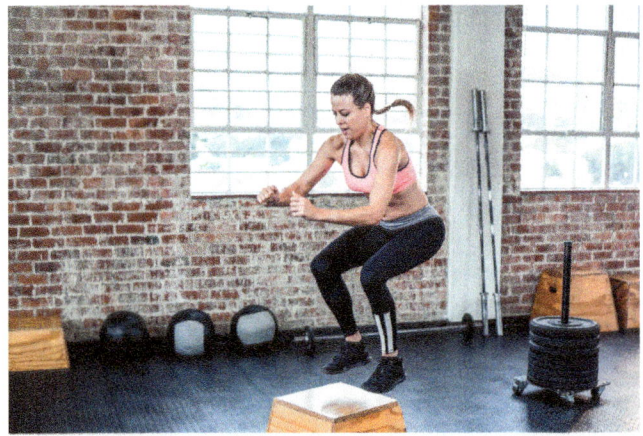

Pylometrics: A form of jumping-centered exercise that focuses on building speed and strength.

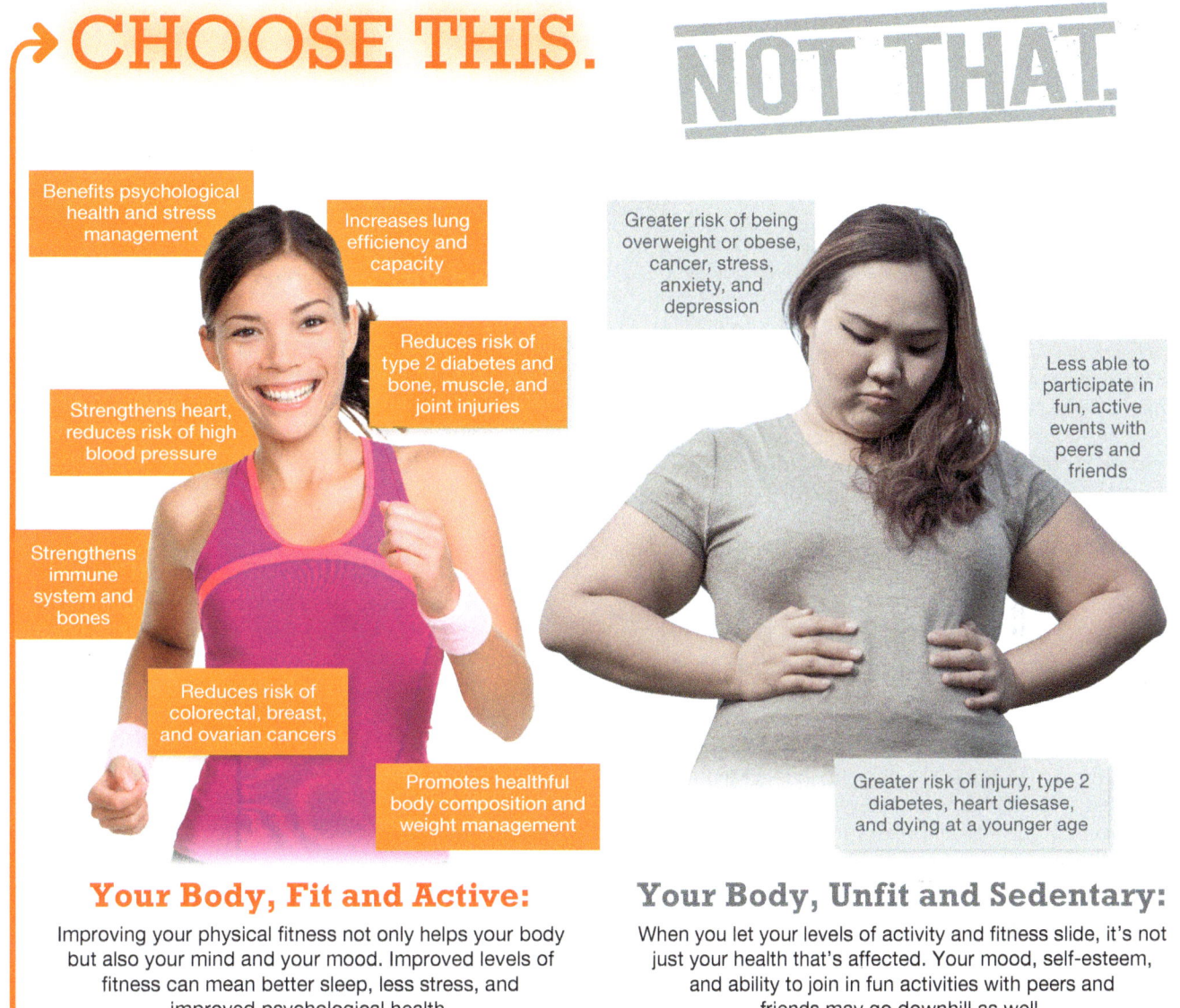

Get active, live better, live happier. To give yourself the overall lift that comes from being more fit:

CHOOSE THIS. NOT THAT.

Your Body, Fit and Active: Improving your physical fitness not only helps your body but also your mind and your mood. Improved levels of fitness can mean better sleep, less stress, and improved psychological health.

- Benefits psychological health and stress management
- Increases lung efficiency and capacity
- Reduces risk of type 2 diabetes and bone, muscle, and joint injuries
- Strengthens heart, reduces risk of high blood pressure
- Strengthens immune system and bones
- Reduces risk of colorectal, breast, and ovarian cancers
- Promotes healthful body composition and weight management

Your Body, Unfit and Sedentary: When you let your levels of activity and fitness slide, it's not just your health that's affected. Your mood, self-esteem, and ability to join in fun activities with peers and friends may go downhill as well.

- Greater risk of being overweight or obese, cancer, stress, anxiety, and depression
- Less able to participate in fun, active events with peers and friends
- Greater risk of injury, type 2 diabetes, heart diesase, and dying at a younger age

What Are the Benefits of Physical Activity?

LO 6.2 Explain the health benefits of physical activity.

Physical activity is one of the best things you can do for yourself. It benefits every aspect of your health, at every stage of your life. Some of these benefits are purely physical, such as a stronger heart and healthier lungs. But physical activity can also put you in a better mood and help you manage stress. As you age, it will help postpone physical decline and many of the diseases that can reduce quality of life in your later years.

Choose This, Not That summarizes the major benefits of physical activity; we'll discuss each one next.

Stronger Heart and Lungs

As the organs that pump your blood and deliver oxygen throughout your body, your heart, lungs, and entire circulatory system literally keep you going. By increasing your body's demand for oxygen, physical activity helps keep these systems strong and efficient, even as you age. Physical activity also appears to help stabilize the parts of your brain that control the function of these vital systems.[7]

Participating in physical activity and exercise can cut your risk of cardiovascular disease in half through its positive effects on several major risk factors: It lowers LDL (bad) cholesterol, raises HDL (good) cholesterol, helps prevent or control diabetes, and helps you lose excess weight.[8] In addition, because physical activity keeps your blood vessels healthier, it lowers your risk of high blood pressure.

The stronger your heart and lungs, the longer you're likely to live. One study followed more than 20,000 men who weren't overweight but had differing levels of cardiorespiratory fitness.[9] The researchers found that just being thin isn't enough to protect your health; fitness is also key. In the 8-year-long study, thin men with low rates of cardiorespiratory fitness were twice as likely to die from any cause as thin men with higher rates of cardiorespiratory fitness.

Management and Prevention of Type 2 Diabetes

Exercise can control your blood glucose level and blood pressure, help you lose weight and maintain weight loss, and improve your body's ability to use insulin, all of which help control or prevent type 2 diabetes. If you have type 2 diabetes, any daily physical activity is helpful. If you are at risk for the disease, even as little as 30 minutes of exercise a day 5 days a week can help lower your risk.[10] When combined with a healthful diet, exercise proves more powerful than prescription medication in lowering type 2 diabetes risk. A federal health study of people at high risk for diabetes showed that daily exercise and a healthful diet lowered risk by 58%, compared with a 31% reduction in risk for a common prescription diabetes drug.[11,12]

Reduced Risk of Some Cancers

Inactivity is one of the most significant risk factors for cancer that you can control. Physical activity lowers the long-term risks of developing colorectal cancer in men and women and breast and ovarian cancers in women.[13,14] One long-term study of more than 110,000 women found that those who performed at least 5 hours of moderate to strenuous exercise a week cut their risk of breast cancer by at least half.[14] Activity appears to help in part by controlling weight, a risk factor for certain cancers. It may also help by regulating certain hormones that are factors in some types of cancers and by encouraging your body to process and remove substances—including potential toxins that might cause cancer—more quickly.

Increased Immune Function

Do you want to lower your risk of getting sick during the next cold and flu season? Physical activity can help you fend off common illnesses by boosting your immune system. In one study, 60% to 90% of active individuals felt that they experienced fewer colds than their nonactive counterparts.[15] Scientists aren't entirely sure how physical activity helps build immunity, but exercise's role in flushing impurities from the body, along with regulating hormones related to immune function and stress may play a part.[16]

Stronger Bones

Physical activity builds and protects your bones.[17] Weight-bearing exercise such as walking, running, or lifting weights makes your bones denser and stronger. Non–weight-bearing exercise, such as swimming, is healthful in other ways but does not strengthen bones. Bone strength helps protect your skeleton from injury, so it is important for everyone, but it is especially important for those at risk for **osteoporosis,** a serious condition that mostly affects older adults, in which reduced bone mineral density causes the bones to become weak and brittle. Although many college-aged students don't think they need to worry about osteoporosis, bone density peaks during early adulthood, so this is precisely the time to build the bone strength that could prevent the onset of the disease later.

> **osteoporosis** A condition in which reduced bone mineral density causes the bones to become weak and brittle.

Reduced Risk of Injury

The stronger bones, muscles, tendons, and ligaments that result from physical activity can help protect you from injury. A strong back, for example, is much less likely to get strained and sore the next time you lift boxes while moving to a new dorm or apartment. Strong muscles can help you keep your balance and avoid falls, and strong joint-supporting muscles can help reduce the risk of a variety of injuries, including sprains, tendinitis, runner's knee, and shin splints.

Healthful Weight Management

Physical activity helps you lose and control weight in more ways than one. Not only does it burn calories, it also boosts your metabolism, so your body uses more calories. This boost in metabolism occurs both during and after workouts. Consistent exercise can slowly lower your overall percentage of body fat and help build and maintain muscle, whereas if you try to lose weight by dieting alone, you risk burning muscle mass along with body fat. Having more muscle also increases your metabolism and helps you maintain your weight long term.

Benefits to Psychological Health, Stress Management, and Sleep

When people say they work out to "blow off steam," they are describing the effect physical activity has on their stress levels. Physical activity reduces stress and anxiety, and it also helps boost concentration. These benefits appear to hold true no matter what type of physical activity you enjoy.

Certain studies have shown that exercise can be just as effective in relieving depression as antidepressant medication.[18] And the latest research concludes that exercise can prevent depression in the first place.[19] Any type of physical activity is considered helpful, but in one study of college women with signs of depression, vigorous-intensity exercise classes led to the most significant decrease in symptoms.[20]

In addition, active lifestyles may help you be more focused during the day and more tranquil at night. Physical activity may be associated with higher levels of alertness and mental ability, including the ability to learn and achieve academically.[5,21] Cardiorespiratory fitness, in particular, can promote academic achievement and job productivity.[3] A physically active lifestyle may also be beneficial when bedtime rolls around: A daily routine that includes at least moderate levels of exercise has been associated with improved sleep quality.[22]

LO 6.2 QUICK CHECK

Weight-bearing exercise is especially protective against which of the following conditions?
a. muscle strain
b. diabetes
c. osteoporosis
d. asthma

Principles of Fitness Training

LO 6.3 Identify the principles of fitness training.

You'll receive the greatest health benefits if you approach your exercise routine in a systematic way. In order to design an effective fitness program, you should first understand the basic principles of fitness training: *overload, specificity, reversibility, individuality,* and *diminishing returns*.

Overload

Whatever your fitness capabilities, improving means pushing yourself to the next level. The **overload** principle requires that you increase the stress placed on your body, creating a greater demand than your body is accustomed to meeting. This forces your body to adapt and become more fit. In other words, you improve by exercising beyond your comfort zone.

For overload to work effectively, new stresses should be steady and gradual. This requires **progressive overload,** or increasing the demands on your body gradually and safely over time to avoid injury. You can achieve progressive overload safely by modifying and personalizing one or more of the exercise variables collectively known as **FITT,** which stands for

- *Frequency,* or the number of times you engage in a particular physical activity each week.
- *Intensity,* or the level of effort at which you exercise. For cardiorespiratory fitness, intensity is usually measured in terms of how fast you get your heart beating (your heart rate). For muscular strength and endurance training, intensity depends on the amount of resistance and number of repetitions. For flexibility, intensity is measured by the depth of the stretch.
- *Time* (duration), or the amount of time you spend on a particular exercise.
- *Type,* or the sorts of exercise you choose to engage in.

Exercise type is closely linked to the principle of specificity, which we'll look at next. (To see the FITT principle applied to various types of workouts, see **Table 6.1**.)

Specificity

According to the **specificity** principle, in order to improve a specific component of fitness, you must perform exercises designed to address that component in a deliberate, targeted way. Many exercises improve some components of fitness but not others. Cycling, for example, is great for cardiorespiratory fitness, but it doesn't build upper body strength or increase your flexibility. You should take into account the principle of specificity when deciding which activities you choose to perform.

Reversibility

Your personal level of fitness can easily go up—or down. The **reversibility** principle states that your fitness level will decline if you don't maintain your physical activity. Fitness declines can happen quickly, sometimes in as little as 10 days.[23] Therefore, it is important to maintain a consistent exercise routine to avoid reversing your fitness gains. Even if you can't take on a new round of progressive overload and increased physical stress at a particular time, maintaining your current workout will help keep your level of fitness from declining.

---

overload Increasing the stress placed on your body through exercise, which results in an improved fitness level.

progressive overload Gradual overloading of the body over time in order to avoid injury.

FITT Exercise variables that can be modified in order to accomplish progressive overload: frequency, intensity, time, and type.

specificity The principle that a fitness component is improved only by exercises that address that specific component.

reversibility The principle that fitness levels decline when the demand placed on the body is decreased.

TABLE 6.1 The FITT Principle in Action

FITT Dimensions	Cardiorespiratory Exercise	Strength Training	Flexibility
Frequency	3–5 times per week	2–3 times per week	At least 2–3 days per week, preferably more
Intensity	60–85% of personal maximum heart rate	8–12 repetitions, or until the point of muscle fatigue	Tension (not pain), followed by feeling of release of tension
Time	At least 20 minutes or more (continuous)	As needed to work out safely	30–60 seconds
Type	Running, hiking, walking, swimming, rowing, stair climbing, vigorous dancing	Weight machines, free weights, resistance bands	Stretching

Source: Data from Haskell, W. L., Lee, I. M., Pate, R. R., Powell, K. E., Blair, S. N., et al. (2007). Physical activity and public health: Updated recommendation for adults from the American College of Sports Medicine and the American Heart Association. *Medicine & Science in Sports & Exercise*, 39(8), 1423–1434.

STUDENT STORY

Cardiorespiratory Fitness

"HI, I'M SEAN. I've been lifting weights for the past 2 years. I've gained about 12 pounds of muscle since I started lifting, yet I get tired very easily doing any cardiorespiratory exercises like jogging. I feel like I'm pretty fit as far as my muscular strength goes, but what can I do to improve my cardiorespiratory health?"

What Do You Think?

1. Why wasn't Sean seeing any cardiorespiratory benefits from lifting weights? What fitness training principle applies to his situation?
2. What types of exercises could Sean do to build cardiorespiratory fitness?
3. What other important component of fitness does Sean appear to be missing entirely?

Individuality

The principle of **individuality** says that you will respond to the demands you place on your body in your own unique way. We each react differently to specific exercises, with some people gaining more benefit from a particular exercise than others. Identifying the exercises best suited to you is a key part of designing an effective fitness program. Whatever your individual needs and responses, however, one overarching principle applies to all of us: We can all benefit from exercise.

Diminishing Returns

According to the principle of **diminishing returns,** if you maintain a constant level and type of physical activity, your body will gradually adjust to the required level of activity and benefit less, receiving less of a "return" on your exercise investment. To continue to improve your levels of fitness, vary the types and intensity of your physical activity so that you are always challenged. In strength training, for example, some fitness experts recommend a practice called *muscle confusion,* or regularly changing the weight-lifting exercises in your routine, to give your body a new strength stimulus.

LO 6.3 QUICK CHECK

The reversibility principle states that
a. when weightlifting, you need to exercise both sides of your body equally.
b. you need to vary the types of exercise that you do to build overall fitness.
c. backward motion is as important as forward motion for building muscle endurance and balance.
d. your fitness level will decline if you don't maintain your physical activity.

What Types of Physical Activity Should You Consider?

LO 6.4 Consider different types of physical activity for your fitness plan.

Any type of regular, sustained physical activity is beneficial, especially if you have been inactive for a while. However, in order to increase your overall health and fitness, you should look into activities that increase your cardiorespiratory fitness, muscular strength and endurance, and flexibility.

Aerobic Exercise

You can build cardiorespiratory fitness through **aerobic exercise,** which is any prolonged physical activity that raises your heart rate and works the large muscle groups. Aerobic exercise makes your heart, lungs, and entire circulatory system stronger by requiring them to work harder to deliver adequate oxygen to your muscles.

> **individuality** The principle that individuals respond to fitness training in their own unique ways.
>
> **diminishing returns** The principle that individuals adapt to a constant, static fitness routine and receive fewer benefits as a result.
>
> **aerobic exercise** Prolonged physical activity that raises the heart rate and works the large muscle groups.
>
> **target heart rate range** The heart rate range to aim for during exercise. A target heart rate range of 64% to 91% of your maximum heart rate is recommended.

Types of Aerobic Exercise

There are numerous forms of popular aerobic exercise, including the following:

- Running and jogging
- Hiking or brisk walking for extended periods of time
- Cycling and "spinning" (a structured workout on a stationary bicycle)
- Swimming
- Fast-paced running-based games, such as basketball or soccer
- Cardio classes, including aerobic dance videos and step aerobics training
- Vigorous martial arts, such as karate or cardio kickboxing

The types of aerobic exercise you choose, however, represent just one step toward improved fitness. Based on the FITT principle discussed earlier, you also need to consider other factors—including just how hard you work out.

Intensity of Aerobic Exercise

Aerobic intensity is usually measured by heart rate because increased heart rate indicates that your cardiorespiratory system is working harder. In order to achieve the maximum cardiorespiratory benefit, you should aim to raise your heart rate so that it falls within your **target heart rate range.** For healthy adults who are not entirely sedentary or exceptionally active, the American College of Sports Medicine (ACSM) recommends a target heart rate range of anywhere from 64% to 91% of your maximum heart rate.[24] See the **Self-Assessment** on page 133 for two ways to determine these indicators.

SELF-ASSESSMENT
Determining Your Maximum Heart Rate And Target Heart Rate Range

During aerobic exercise, the rate at which your heart is working lets you know if you are exercising effectively. You will gain the most cardiorespiratory benefit if you exercise within your target heart rate range. Two formulas are commonly used to determine target heart rate: one focused on "maximum heart rate" and another, known as the Karvonen Formula, which uses both resting and maximum heart rates to calculate your target heart rate.

Maximum Heart Rate Formula

To start, you need to know your maximum heart rate. The American College of Sports Medicine (ACSM) has found the most accurate way to determine your maximum heart rate is through the following equation:[1]

$206.9 - (0.67 \times \text{age}) = \text{maximum heart rate}$

Step 1: _____ × 0.67 = _____
         (your age)

Step 2: 206.9 − _____ = _____ = maximum heart rate
                (answer from Step 1)

Target Heart Rate Range

In the "maximum heart rate" calculation, the ACSM suggests a target heart rate range of 64%–91% of your maximum heart rate, based on your current activity level. You can narrow down that number by adding an "intensity" number tied to your current level of fitness.[1]

- If you perform only minimal physical activity right now, aim for a target heart rate of about 64%–74% of your maximum heart rate. Use the following formulas to determine your target heart rate range:
  Low end of target heart rate range:
  _____ × 0.64 = _____
  (maximum heart rate)
  High end of target heart rate range:
  _____ × 0.74 = _____
  (maximum heart rate)

- If you perform sporadic physical activity right now, aim for a target heart rate of about 74%–84% of your maximum heart rate. Use the following formulas to determine your target heart rate range:
  Low end of target heart rate range:
  _____ × 0.74 = _____
  (maximum heart rate)
  High end of target heart rate range:
  _____ × 0.84 = _____
  (maximum heart rate)

- If you perform regular physical activity right now, aim for a target heart rate of about 80%–91% of your maximum heart rate. Use the following formulas to determine your target heart rate range:
  Low end of target heart rate range:
  _____ × 0.80 = _____
  (maximum heart rate)
  High end of target heart rate range:
  _____ × 0.91 = _____
  (maximum heart rate)

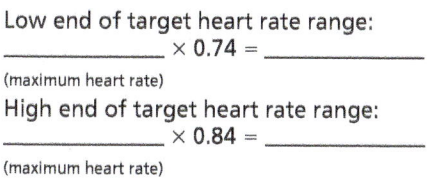

Karvonen Formula

Since this method includes resting heart rate, start with this measurement by finding the pulse in the carotid artery in your neck. Place your first two fingers (not your thumb) on the side of your neck next to your windpipe. Using a clock or watch, take your pulse for 6 seconds and then multiply that number by 10. The result will be your number of heart beats per minute, which is your resting heart rate.

From there, your target heart rate is calculated as follows:[2]

(Max HR − Resting HR × Intensity) + Resting HR
For example, the calculation and results for a 20-year-old who exercises regularly might look like this:

- Max HR = 200 (220 − 20), resting HR = 60, intensity = 0.80
- 200 − 60 = 140
- 140 × 0.80 = 112
- 112 + 60 = 172 beats per minute (target heart rate)

Measuring Your Heart Rate During Exercise

While you exercise, you can measure your heart rate by taking your pulse in your carotid artery, as described above. You may also choose to use an app that measures heart rate via your smart phone or other personal device.

HOW TO INTERPRET YOUR SCORE Some cardiorespiratory equipment in gyms, such as stair climbers, offer real-time heart rate calculators. But you can easily track your heart rate using the measurement method above.

If your heart rate is below your target heart rate range, increase your intensity until you are in your target range; if your heart rate is above your target heart rate range, reduce your intensity.

There are several methods for calculating maximum heart rate and target heart rate ranges. The formula presented above is the ACSM's most accurate method; some organizations or online calculators may calculate your target heart rate range differently.

To complete this Self-Assessment online, visit MasteringHealth™

References: **1.** American College of Sports Medicine. (2010). *ACSM's guidelines for exercise testing and prescription*, 8th ed. Baltimore, MD: Wolters Kluwer/Lippincott Williams & Wilkins. **2.** Karvonen, J., & Vuorimaa, T. (1988). Heart rate and exercise intensity during sports activities. Practical application. *Sports Medicine*, 5, 303–311.

Aerobic exercises are often categorized as lifestyle/light-intensity, moderate-intensity, or vigorous-intensity activities. According to the Centers for Disease Control and Prevention (CDC), light-intensity activity gets you moving but raises your heart rate to less than 50% of your maximum heart rate, moderate-intensity activities raises your heart rate to 50% to 70% of your maximum heart rate, and vigorous-intensity activities raise your heart rate to 70% to 85% of your maximum heart rate.[25] **Table 6.2** shows examples and benefits of these three categories of aerobic activities.

The best way to begin an aerobic exercise program is to start by performing exercises at intensities near the low end of your target heart rate range, especially if you have not exercised in a while. Start with a minimum of 10 minutes of activity at a time, more if you are able. Slowly increase the duration of your exercise by 5 to 10 minutes every 1 or 2 weeks for the first 4 to 6 weeks of your program.[24] After that, you can build fitness by gradually increasing the duration, frequency, or intensity of exercises. To help gauge the intensity of your workout, you may want to use a tool called the Rating of Perceived Exertion (RPE). This numerical scale, which ranges from 0 to 10, assesses how easy or difficult you find a particular activity. For details, see **Figure 6.1**.

Always be sure to warm up before and cool down after an aerobic session and to follow other safety precautions for exercise. See pages 145–148 for more about warming up, cooling down, and safety.

Incorporating Aerobic Exercise into Your Daily Life

Dedicated time for aerobic exercise is important but doesn't hinge on time at the gym. Even engaging in activity for as little as 10 minutes can be an effective way to get more exercise into your life. Simple changes, such as doing some errands on foot instead of in the car, can quickly add up to significant aerobic exercise.

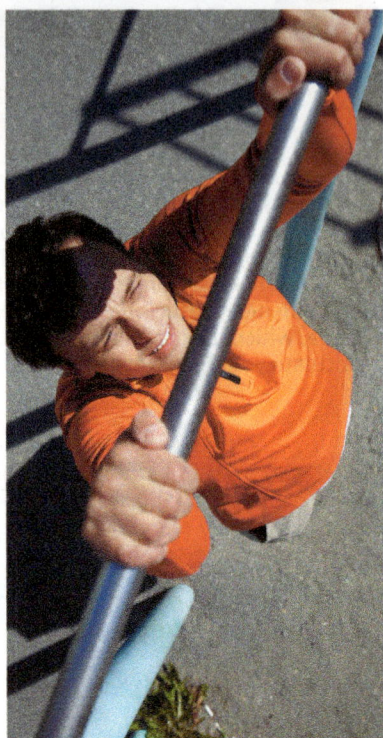

Rating of Perceived Exertion (RPE) Scale

10	Very, very heavy
9	
8	
7	Very heavy
6	
5	Heavy
4	Somewhat heavy
3	Moderate
2	Light
1	Very light
0.5	Just noticeable
0	Nothing at all

FIGURE 6.1 **Rating of Perceived Exertion.** The RPE scale, used to measure the intensity of your exercise, runs from 0 to 10. The numbers are associated with how easy or difficult you find an activity. For example, 0 (nothing) would represent the perceived ease of sitting still; 10 (very, very heavy) is how you would perceive doing a very difficult, tiring activity. In most cases, you should exercise at a level that feels 3 (moderate) to 4 (somewhat heavy).

Source: Cleveland Clinic. (2016). *Rated Perceived Exertion (RPE) scale*. http://my.clevelandclinic.org.

TABLE 6.2 Physical Activity Intensities

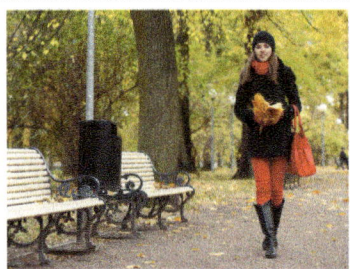	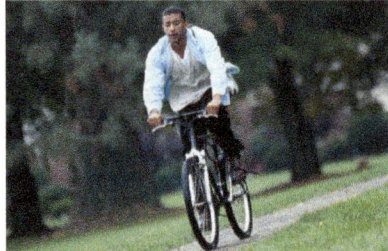	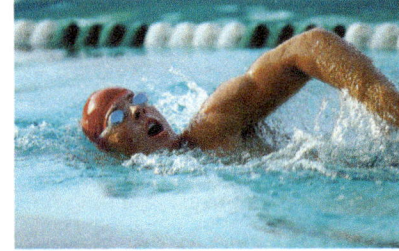
Activity Intensity Level: Lifestyle/light	**Activity Intensity Level:** Moderate	**Activity Intensity Level:** Vigorous
Heart Rate Range: Less than 50% maximum heart rate	**Heart Rate Range:** 50%–70% maximum heart rate	**Heart Rate Range:** 70%–85% maximum heart rate
Examples: Light yard work and housework, leisurely walking, self-care and bathing, light stretching, light occupational activity	**Examples:** Walking 3–4.5 miles per hour on a level surface, resistance training, hiking, climbing stairs, dancing, doubles tennis, using a manual wheelchair, recreational swimming, water aerobics, moderate yard work and housework	**Examples:** Jogging, running, basketball, soccer, circuit training, backpacking, aerobic classes, competitive sports, swimming laps, martial arts, singles tennis, heavy yard work or housework, hard physical labor/construction, bicycling 10 miles per hour or faster up steep terrain
Health Benefits: A moderate increase in health and wellness in those who are completely sedentary; reduced risk of some chronic diseases	**Health Benefits:** Increased cardiorespiratory endurance, lower body fat levels, improved blood cholesterol and pressure, better blood sugar management, decreased risk of disease, increased overall physical fitness	**Health Benefits:** Increased overall physical fitness, decreased risk of disease, further improvements in overall strength and muscular endurance

Source: Adapted from Centers for Disease Control and Prevention, Physical activity for everyone: Target heart rate and estimated maximum heart rate, www.cdc.gov; and Hopson, J., Donatelle, R., & Littrell, T. (2012). Get fit, stay well!, brief ed. Reprinted and Electronically reproduced by permission of Pearson Education, Inc., Upper Saddle River, New Jersey.

SPECIAL FEATURE

Core Concerns: Why You Should Strengthen Your Core

Your core muscles run the entire length of your torso, stabilizing the spine, pelvis, and shoulders. They also provide a solid foundation for movement of the arms and legs and make it possible for you to stand upright, move on two feet, balance, and shift movement in any direction. Standing upright and walking around on two feet is not easy on your body. A strong core distributes the stresses of bearing your weight and protects the back.

Weak core muscles can compromise the appropriate curvature of your spine, often resulting in low back pain and other injuries. The greatest benefit of core strength is increased functional fitness—the fitness that is essential to both daily living and regular activities. Core strength can be built through exercises such as abdominal curls, planks, back extensions, Pilates, and any other exercises that work core muscles.

▶▶ Watch a video about core training at www.youtube.com/watch?v=Lj0q_L2U7EQ.

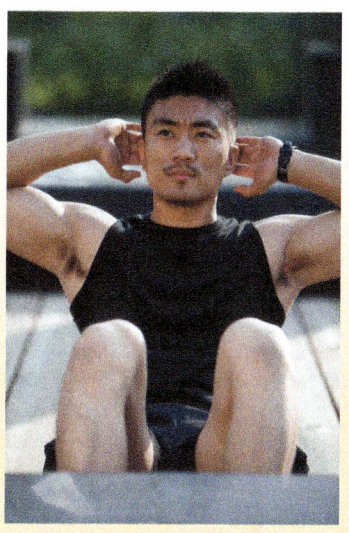

If you don't have time for a long walk, try breaking your time on foot into shorter stretches that fit into your daily routine. One study found that people who met physical activity guidelines but did so through bouts of exercise that lasted less than 10 minutes still saw some health improvements.[26] In another study of young men, ten 3-minute brisk walks per day were as effective as one longer walk at lowering resting blood pressure and levels of fats in the blood after meals.[27]

There are lots of other ways to get moving. Ride your bike instead of driving. Take the stairs. If you like being outside, try hiking, swimming, or playing sports like Ultimate Frisbee or soccer. If you prefer indoor exercise, consider using an elliptical trainer, taking a Zumba or CrossFit class, or following along with an aerobic workout DVD at home. It's easy to make aerobic exercise fun if you find activities that are so enjoyable that the time—and your workout—flies by.

Exercise for Muscular Strength and Endurance

Not all full-body exercises increase cardiorespiratory fitness. Short, intense activities—such as sprint running, sprint swimming, or heavy weight lifting—usually require more oxygen than the body can take in and deliver quickly. As a result, the muscles develop an oxygen deficit, and you tire in a short amount of time. However, these **anaerobic exercises** increase your body's ability to deliver short bursts of energy and build muscular strength.

Many people think building muscle means increasing the amount of weight you can lift—in other words, building strength. But endurance is also an important component of muscular fitness. Strength allows you to lift that heavy box when you move to your next apartment, but muscular endurance lets you carry it all the way out to the moving truck.

In order to build muscle, the muscle must work against some form of resistance—this is called *resistance training* or *strength training*. You can create resistance for your muscles to work against using free weights (such as dumbbells or barbells), weight machines, resistance bands, or even your own body weight. Free weights, resistance bands, and your own body weight give you flexibility, allowing you to do many different exercises. Weight machines are usually designed to be used for only one or two specific exercises. On the other hand, machines promote correct movement and safe lifting and allow you to easily change the amount of resistance and pinpoint specific muscles.

anaerobic exercise Short, intense exercise that causes an oxygen deficit in the muscles.

isometric exercise Exercise in which the muscle contracts but the body does not move.

isotonic exercise Exercise in which the muscle contraction causes body movement.

Isometric Versus Isotonic

Resistance exercises can be isometric or isotonic. In **isometric exercise,** the muscle contracts, but there is no visible movement. This is accomplished by working against some immovable form of resistance, such as your body's own muscle (pressing the palms together) or a structural item (pushing against the floor when performing a "plank" exercise). It is most helpful to hold isometric contractions for six to eight seconds and to perform each exercise 5 to 10 times. During **isotonic exercise,** muscle force is able to cause movement. The tension in the muscle remains unchanged, but the muscle length changes. Performing a biceps curl with a free weight, walking up stairs, and doing a push-up are examples of isotonic exercises.

Repetitions and Sets

When developing a resistance training program, you should decide on the numbers of repetitions and sets you will do for each exercise. **Repetitions** are the number of times you perform the exercise continuously. **Sets** are separate groups of repetitions. The numbers of sets and repetitions to do depends on whether you are trying to build strength or endurance. Doing a few repetitions (approximately 8–12) with heavier weights or more resistance develops strength. Doing more repetitions (approximately 15–25) with lighter weights or less resistance develops endurance. Increase the amount of resistance once you can easily perform the desired number of repetitions.

repetitions The number of times you perform an exercise repeatedly.

sets Separate groups of repetitions.

recovery The period necessary for the body to recover from exercise demands and adapt to higher levels of fitness.

static flexibility The ability to reach and hold a stretch at one endpoint of a joint's range of motion.

dynamic flexibility The ability to move quickly and fluidly through a joint's entire range of motion with little resistance.

Training Tips

When participating in a resistance training program, be sure to follow these guidelines:

- Use proper technique when performing weight-lifting exercises. See **Practical Strategies: Safe Weight Lifting**.
- Because resistance exercises are specific to the particular muscles they are designed for, be sure to include exercises for all the major muscle groups.
- Rest for 2 to 3 minutes between sets. If you are building muscular endurance, you can slightly shorten the time between sets.[24]
- Vary your resistance training routine from time to time to reduce the risk of injury and keep your workouts from getting dull. Revisit your program as you get stronger. You may also need different levels or types of resistance training to preserve fitness and muscle mass as you get older.

Figure 6.2 on pages 137–138 shows examples of some simple resistance exercises you can perform.

Recovery

Once you've begun a resistance program, be sure to allow overloaded muscle at least 48 hours for repair and **recovery** before another exercise bout. However, because muscles begin to atrophy after about 96 hours, don't let too much time pass without another training session. You can do resistance training on consecutive days if you work different muscle groups on different days (for example, lower body versus upper body), as long as each muscle group receives the recommended 48 hours of recovery time.

▶▶ Keep a log of your workouts so you can be sure to allow each muscle group adequate recovery time. Try these online logs:

PRACTICAL Strategies
Safe Weight Lifting

- If you are just beginning to use weights, make an appointment with a fitness specialist who can teach you the proper techniques that reduce your risk of injury and maximize strengthening.
- Always warm up before lifting weights.
- Take your time and lift mindfully.
- Breathe out as you lift the weight and in as you release the weight. Don't hold your breath as doing so can cause dangerous increases in blood pressure.
- Focus on the muscle you're trying to work. Feel the effort in the muscle, not in the joint.
- Equally train opposing muscle groups, such as the lower back and abdomen or the biceps and triceps.
- Use only the amount of weights that your body can handle without having to cheat by using other muscles or momentum.
- When using free weights, always have a partner who can check your form and "spot" for you.
- Pain does not equal a great workout. Muscle pain or soreness during or after your workout may mean that the muscle you are trying to strengthen has been damaged, and injury will delay further strengthening. Increase the weight you lift and number of reps gradually, to give your muscles time to adapt without injury.
- If you do feel post-lifting soreness, massage the affected area or apply alternating hot and cold therapy. These remedies often help damaged muscle fibers by increasing circulation and fluid flow in the injured area.

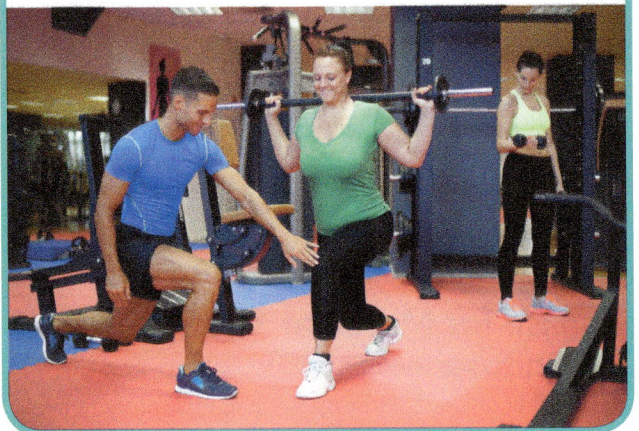

www.sparkpeople.com and www.supertracker.usda.gov/physicalactivitytracker.aspx.

Exercises for Improving Flexibility

There are two major types of flexibility. **Static flexibility** is the ability to reach and hold a stretch at one endpoint of a joint's range of motion. **Dynamic flexibility** is the

(a) Squat

 Stand with feet shoulder-width apart, toes pointing forward, hips and shoulders aligned, abdominals pulled in. Bend your knees and lower until you have between a 45- and 90-degree angle. Keep your knees behind the front of your toes. Contract your abdominals while coming up.

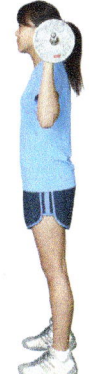 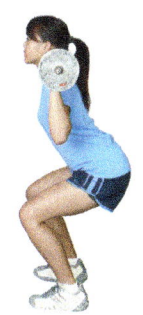

(b) Lunge

 Stand with feet shoulder-width apart. As you step forward, keep your front knee in line with your ankle; make sure the front knee does not extend over your toes. Distribute your weight evenly between the front and back leg.

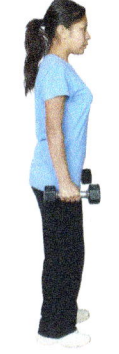 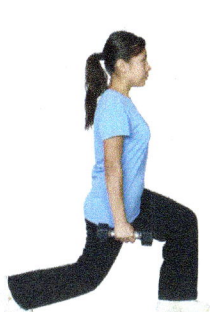

(c) Leg Abduction

 Connect a resistance band to a stable object and loop around your outside leg. Stand with good posture and hold onto something stable. Slowly extend your leg out and return.

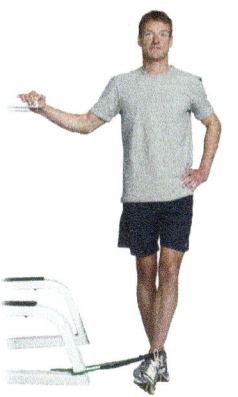 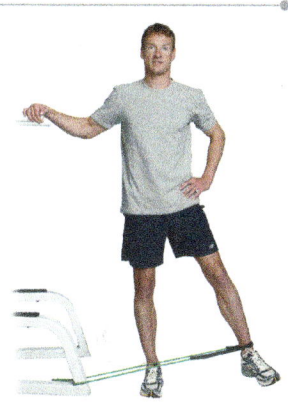

(d) Biceps Curl

 Sit on a bench or chair with a dumbbell in each hand. Sit with good posture (ears and shoulders over hips and abdominals contracted) and your feet planted on the ground for balance. Lift one dumbbell up to your shoulder, turning your palm toward your shoulder as you lift. Slowly lower the dumbbell to the starting position as you lift the dumbbell in your other hand.

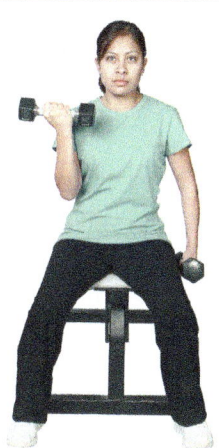

FIGURE 6.2 **Simple Resistance Exercises.** Be sure to perform exercises equally on both sides.
Source: Text from Hopson, J., Donatelle, R., & Littrell, T., *Get fit, stay well!* 4th ed. © 2018. Reprinted and electronically reproduced by permission of Pearson Education, Inc., Upper Saddle River, New Jersey.

(e) Curl-Up

Lie on a mat with your arms by your sides, palms down, elbows straight, and fingers extended. Bend your knees at about a 90-degree angle. Curl your head and upper back upward, reaching your arms forward, then curl back down so that your upper back and shoulders touch the mat. During the entire curl-up, your feet and buttocks should stay on the mat.

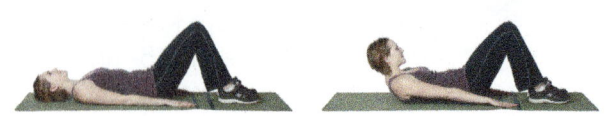

(f) Reverse Curl

 Lie on your back and place your hands near your hips. Lift your legs to 90 degrees from the floor. Your knees may be bent or straight. Contract your abdominals, pulling them in, while you lift your hips off the floor. Slowly return hips to the floor. Be careful not to rock back and forth.

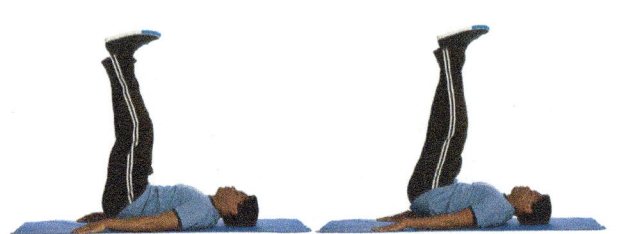

(g) Back Extension

 Start lying on your stomach with your arms and legs extended, forehead on the mat. Lift and further extend your arms and legs using your back muscles. Hold for 3–5 seconds and slowly lower back down.

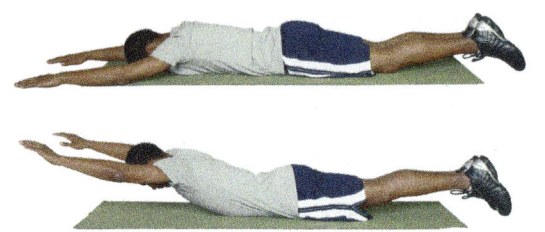

(h) Plank

 Support yourself in plank position (from the forearms or hands) by contracting your trunk muscles so that your neck, back, and hips are completely straight. Hold for 5–60 seconds, increasing time as you become stronger. Your forearms should be slightly wider than your shoulders.

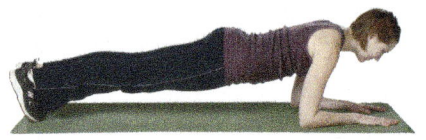

(i) Modified Push-Ups

 Support yourself in push-up position as shown by contracting your trunk muscles. Place hands slightly wider than your shoulders. Keep your neck, back, and hips completely straight; do not let your trunk sag in the middle or raise your hips. Slowly lower your body down toward the floor, being careful to keep a straight body position. Your elbows will press out and back as you lower to a 90-degree elbow joint. Press yourself back up to start position.

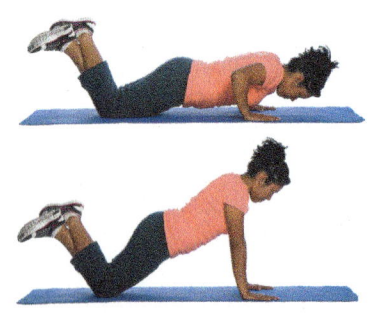

FIGURE 6.2

ability to move quickly and fluidly through a joint's entire range of motion with little resistance. Static flexibility determines whether a martial artist can reach her leg as high as her opponent's head; dynamic flexibility enables her to kick her leg that high in one fast, fluid motion. Flexibility can vary a lot among individuals, but everyone can increase flexibility through consistent stretching exercises.

Stretching

Stretching applies gentle, elongating force to both a muscle and its connective tissue. **Static stretching,** the most common form of stretching, involves a gradual stretch and then hold of the stretched position for a certain amount of time. Static stretching can be either active or passive. In **active stretching,** you apply the force for the stretch. **Passive stretching,** on the other hand, is performed with a partner who gently applies the force to the stretch. Passive stretching may provide a more intense flexibility workout but also increases the risk of injury because you are not controlling the stretch yourself. **Ballistic stretching** focuses on the use of dynamic repetitive bouncing movements to stretch a muscle beyond its normal range of motion. If performed improperly, though, ballistic stretching can increase the risk of injury, so recreational exercisers should avoid this form of stretching.[28] **Dynamic stretching,** or slow movement stretching, incorporates controlled movements that mimic a specific sport or exercise. Dynamic stretches are often included during the warm-up before a sports event. An example in soccer would be gently swinging a leg back and forth as if to kick an imaginary ball.

static stretching Gradually lengthening a muscle to an elongated position and sustaining that position.

active stretching A type of static stretching in which you gently apply force to your body to create a stretch.

passive stretching Stretching performed with a partner who increases the intensity of the stretch by gently applying pressure to your body as it stretches.

ballistic stretching Performing rhythmic bouncing movements in a stretch to increase the intensity of the stretch.

dynamic stretching A type of slow movement stretching in which activities from a workout or sport are mimicked in a controlled manner, often to help "warm up" for a game or an event.

Flexibility varies for each part of the body, and flexibility exercises are specific to the body area they're designed for, so when creating a flexibility program, be sure to stretch all the major muscle and joint areas of the body (neck, shoulders, upper and lower back, pelvis, hips, and legs). Don't stretch cold muscles. Instead, warm up by walking or jogging or doing some other low-intensity activity for at least 5 minutes prior to stretching or stretch at the end of your workout. The following tips will help you create a flexibility program:[29]

- Hold static stretches for 10–30 seconds.
- Perform two to four repetitions of each stretch, accumulating 60 seconds per stretch.
- Stretch at least 2 or 3 days per week.
- Stretch until your muscle feels tight or until you feel slight discomfort.
- Do not hold your breath while stretching. Try to relax and breathe deeply.
- Do not lock your joints while stretching.

Holistic Flexibility Programs

In addition to regular stretching exercises, there are several other types of mind- and whole body–centered activities that increase flexibility. These types of activities are also sometimes referred to as *neuromotor exercise,* or workouts designed to improve balance and agility. Three of the most popular are yoga, Pilates, and tai chi:

- *Yoga* moves you through a set of carefully constructed poses designed to increase flexibility and strength. Yoga also addresses mood and thought, using techniques such as breathing exercises to reduce stress and anxiety.
- *Pilates* combines stretching and resistance exercises to create a sequence of precise, controlled movements that focuses on flexibility, joint mobility, and core strength. Because Pilates movements are so precise, it is best to begin Pilates in a group or private class.
- *Tai chi* is a Chinese practice designed to work the entire body gently through a series of quiet, fluid motions. The discipline also focuses on your energy, referred to in Chinese as "chi" (sometimes spelled "qi"), or life force. The practice aims to keep a participant's body and chi in balance, requiring a focus on mood and thought.

Limits of Stretching

Many people like to stretch because they believe it prevents injuries. But a series of research studies indicates otherwise.[30] Researchers have found that stretching is ineffective at preventing injuries unless it is in preparation for an activity that demands a wide range of flexibility, such as gymnastics. Stretching also seems to be ineffective at preventing muscle soreness.[31] Static stretching may even be linked to decreased muscle strength and endurance, although other types of stretching may not have this effect.[32] If you are performing an activity in which there is a high demand for muscle strength or endurance, stretch *after* the activity rather than before.

While it's important to know the limits and best uses of stretching, it's also critical not to forgo this important fitness component. Flexibility can't prevent some types of injury, but it is essential for daily wellness and also provides a full range of motion for activities such as swinging, throwing, reaching, or swimming.

Figure 6.3 on pages 140–141 shows simple flexibility exercises you can easily perform on your own.

>> Wherever you download apps, search for podcasts on topics like running, action sports, yoga, or activities in the great outdoors.

LO 6.4 QUICK CHECK

Which of the following is not an example of isotonic exercise?
a. performing a biceps curl with a free weight
b. an extended shoulder stretch held for 60 seconds
c. walking up stairs
d. punching a punching bag

(a) Neck Stretches

Head turn: Gently turn your head to look over one shoulder, keeping both of your shoulders down. Head tilt: Keeping your chin level and your shoulders down, tilt your head to one side.

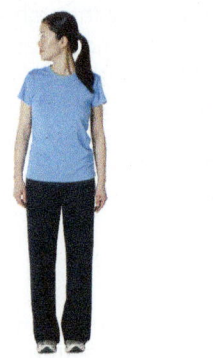
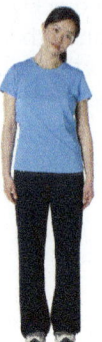

(b) Upper-Back Stretch

Reach your arms in front of you and clasp your hands while rounding your back and lowering your head.

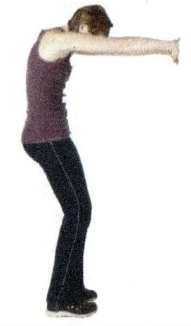

(c) Shoulder Stretch

Reach one arm across your chest and hold it above or below the elbow with the other hand.

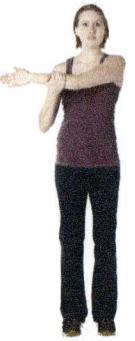

(d) Tricep Stretch

Lift your arm overhead, reaching the elbow toward the ceiling. Press the arm back from the front or reach your other arm over your head and gently pull the elbow toward your head.

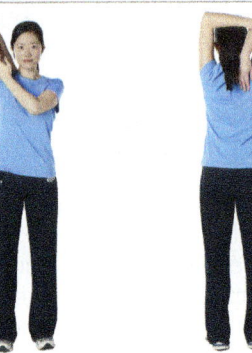

(e) Torso Twist

Sit with your legs straight out in front of you. Bend one knee and cross it over your other leg. Turn your body toward the bent knee and twist to look behind you. Place the opposite arm on the bent leg to gently press the stretch further.

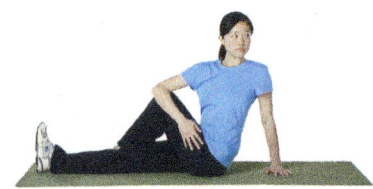

FIGURE 6.3 **Simple Stretching Exercises.** Be sure to perform exercises equally on both sides for at least 30 to 60 seconds each.

Source: Text from Hopson, J., Donatelle, R., & Littrell, T., *Get fit, stay well*! 4th ed. © 2018. Reprinted and electronically reproduced by permission of Pearson Education, Inc., Upper Saddle River, New Jersey.

(f) Hip Stretch

While lying on your back, bend one knee and hip 90-degrees and keep the other leg straight. Slowly move the bent leg across your body toward the floor. Keep your arms wide and both shoulders down.

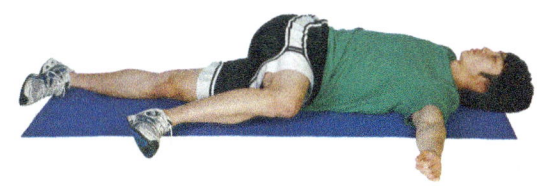

(g) Inner-Thigh Butterfly Stretch

 Bring the bottoms of your feet together and pull your feet gently toward you. Actively contract your hip muscles to lower your knees closer to the ground.

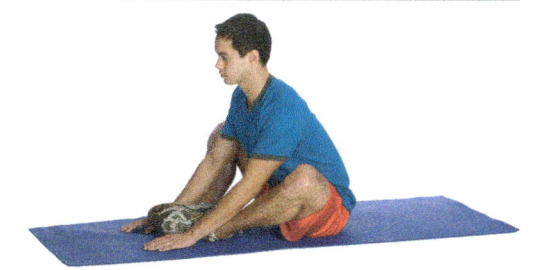

(h1) Hip Flexor Stretch

 Stand tall with one foot forward and one foot back in a lunge position. Lift up the heel of the back leg and press your hips forward.

(h2) Quadriceps Stretch

 Grab your foot from behind and pull it back toward your rear until you feel a stretch in the front of your thighs. Maintain straight body alignment and keep your thighs parallel. Assist your balance by holding onto a stable object.

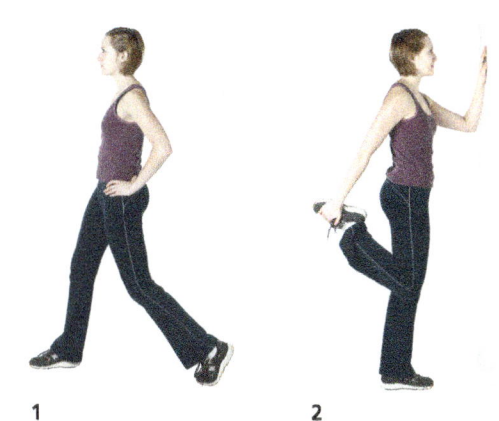

1   2

(i) Hamstrings Stretch

 Sit with one leg extended and the other leg bent with the knee facing sideways. Keeping your back as straight as possible, lean your body forward, moving your chest closer to your extended leg. If you are moderately flexible, you can reach for and hold your foot but only if this does not cause pain.

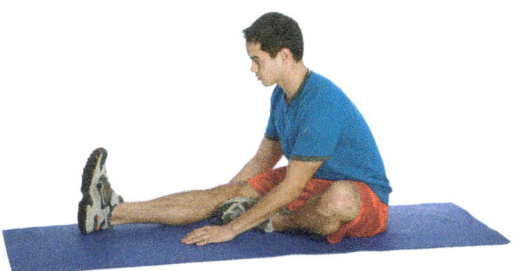

(j) Gluteal Stretch

 Lie on your back with one leg bent and the foot on the floor. Place the ankle of the other leg on your thigh just above the knee (toward the hip). Lift both legs toward the chest and support them with your hands clasped behind your thigh.

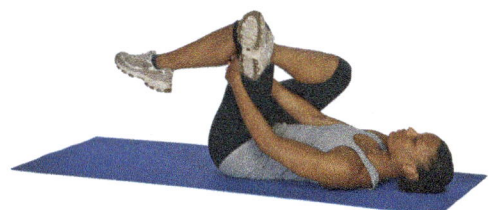

(k) IT (iliotibial band) Stretch

Place one hand on a piece of sturdy exercise equipment or a wall for support, or on your hip. Cross the leg that is on the same side as the equipment/wall/hip over the other leg at the ankle. Extend the outside arm over your head, reaching toward the equipment/wall/hip where your hand is placed.

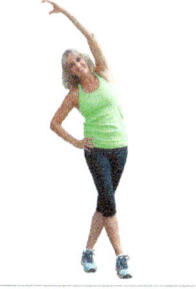

FIGURE 6.3

How Much Physical Activity Do You Need?

LO 6.5 Assess how much physical activity you need.

Creating a fitness program involves more than determining what types of exercise to do; you also need to decide how often to be active so that you can move from overload to recovery and back again in an effective, consistent way.

Guidelines for Health Maintenance

The *Physical Activity Guidelines for Americans* from the U.S. Department of Health and Human Services recommends the following activity levels for the creation and maintenance of health-related fitness in healthy adults:[33]

- At least 2 hours and 30 minutes (150 minutes) of moderate-intensity aerobic activity each week

OR

- At least 1 hour and 15 minutes (75 minutes) of vigorous-intensity aerobic activity each week

OR

- An equivalent mix of moderate- and vigorous-intensity aerobic activity each week

AND

- Resistance exercise 2 days a week or more, for all major muscle groups, in sets of at least 8–12 repetitions

> *"A good way to meet the aerobic guidelines is to perform 30 minutes of moderate-intensity activity 5 days a week."*

More detailed guidelines from the American College of Sports Medicine build on the government fitness recommendations and include specific suggestions for flexibility and neuromotor exercise. **Table 6.3** and **Figure 6.4** summarize this set of exercise recommendations.

A good way to meet the aerobic guidelines is to perform 30 minutes of moderate-intensity activity 5 days a week. For greater health benefits, increase your weekly aerobic activity to 300 minutes (5 hours) of moderate-intensity activity or 150 minutes (2 hours and 30 minutes) of high-intensity activity.[33] If weight loss or maintenance of weight loss is one of your fitness goals, aim for at least 60–90 minutes of moderate-intensity physical activity a day.[34] How much physical activity is typical on college campuses? See **Student Stats** on page 144 for a snapshot.

TABLE 6.3 Exercise Guidelines from the ACSM

Exercise Type	ACSM Guidelines
Cardiorespiratory	Adults should get at least 150 minutes of moderate-intensity exercise per week or 75 minutes of vigorous-intensity exercise per week, or an equivalent mix of both.
	Exercise recommendations can be met through 30–60 minutes of moderate-intensity exercise (5 days per week) or 20–60 minutes of vigorous-intensity exercise (3 days per week), or an equivalent mix of both.
	One continuous session and multiple shorter sessions (of at least 10 minutes) are both acceptable to accumulate the desired amount of daily exercise.
	Gradual progression of exercise time, frequency, and intensity is recommended for best adherence and least injury risk.
	People unable to meet these minimums can still benefit from some activity.
Resistance	Adults should train each major muscle group 2–3 days each week using a variety of exercises and equipment.
	Two to four sets of each exercise will help adults improve strength and power.
	For each exercise, 8–12 repetitions improve strength and power, 10–15 repetitions improve strength in middle-aged and older persons starting exercise, and 15–20 repetitions improve muscular endurance.
	Adults should wait at least 48 hours between resistance training sessions.
	Very light or light intensity is best for older persons or previously sedentary adults starting exercise.
	A gradual progression of greater resistance, and/or more repetitions per set, and/or increasing frequency is recommended.
Flexibility	Adults should do flexibility exercises at least 2–3 days each week to improve range of motion.
	Each stretch should be held for 10–30 seconds to the point of tightness or slight discomfort.
	Repeat each stretch two to four times, accumulating 60 seconds per stretch.
	Static, dynamic, ballistic, and PNF stretches are all effective.
	Flexibility exercise is most effective when the muscle is warm. Try light aerobic activity or a hot bath to warm the muscles before stretching.
Neuromotor	Neuromotor exercise (sometimes called "functional fitness training") is recommended for 2–3 days per week.
	20–30 minutes per day is appropriate for neuromotor exercise.
	Exercises should involve motor skills (balance, agility, coordination, and gait), proprioceptive exercise training, and multifaceted activities (tai chi and yoga) to improve physical function and prevent falls in older adults.

Data from Garber, C., Blissmer, B., Deschenes, M., Franklin, B., Lamonte, M., et al. (2011). Quantity and quality of exercise for developing and maintaining cardiorespiratory, musculoskeletal, and neuromotor fitness in apparently healthy adults: guidance for prescribing exercise. *Medicine & Science in Sports & Exercise*, 43(7), 1334–1359.

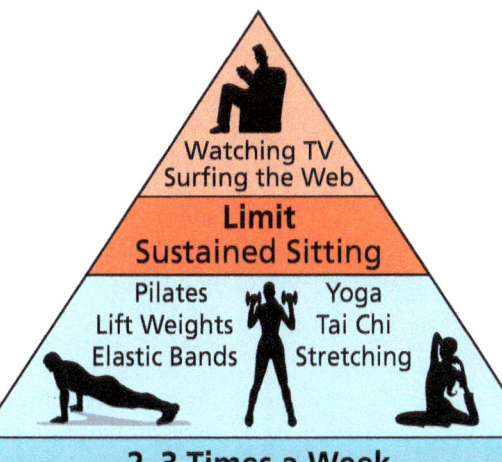

My Physical Activity & Exercise Pyramid

Lifestyle Physical Activity	Cardiorespiratory Exercise	Resistance, Flexibility, and Neuromotor Exercise	Sedentary Behavior
Engage in daily physical activity at home or work or by commute. Some activity is better than none.	Plan aerobic exercise that elevates your training heart rate to a moderate or vigorous intensity.	Strengthen major muscle groups. Perform 8 to 12 reps per set, and do 2 to 4 sets per exercise.	Too much sustained sitting is not the same as too little exercise or physical activity.
Engage in intermittent light- or moderate-intensity physical activity anytime, anywhere.	Plan 5 moderate sessions of ≥ 30 min or 3 vigorous sessions of ≥ 20 min or a combination of both weekly.	Stretch major muscle groups. Hold each stretch 10–30 seconds, repeat to accumulate 60 seconds.	Trim total daily sitting time to prevent subsequent multiple adverse health outcomes.
Engage in ≥ 30 min daily, preferably ≥ 10 min at a time. Accumulate ≥ 150 min per week. More minutes = more health benefits.	Plan sporting or recreational activities that involve moderate or vigorous bursts of aerobic activity with brief rest periods.	Select functional fitness exercises that simultaneously use multiple muscles and joints to improve strength, balance, and agility.	Take regular activity breaks to interrupt sustained sitting. Stand up and walk around for 2 minutes every 30 minutes.

FIGURE 6.4 **My Physical Activity and Exercise Pyramid.** This pyramid summarizes the different types of activities, each with unique benefits, recommended for adults to improve and maintain physical fitness and health. The recommendations link activities of daily living with a comprehensive exercise program.

Source: Dr. Jerome Kotecki, Ball State University. Reprinted with permission of Ball State University © 2015.

metabolic equivalent of task (MET) A unit of measurement that describes the energy expenditure of a particular activity.

Another way to measure and track your activity level is to think about your METs. A **MET, or metabolic equivalent of task,** is a unit of measurement that describes the energy expenditure of a specific task. One single MET represents the rate of energy expended while a person is at rest. From there, METs increase as activity levels rise. A four-MET activity, for example, expends four times the energy used when the body is at rest.[35]

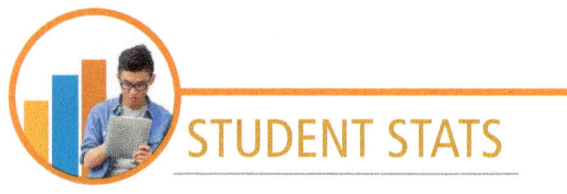

STUDENT STATS

Physical Activity on College Campuses

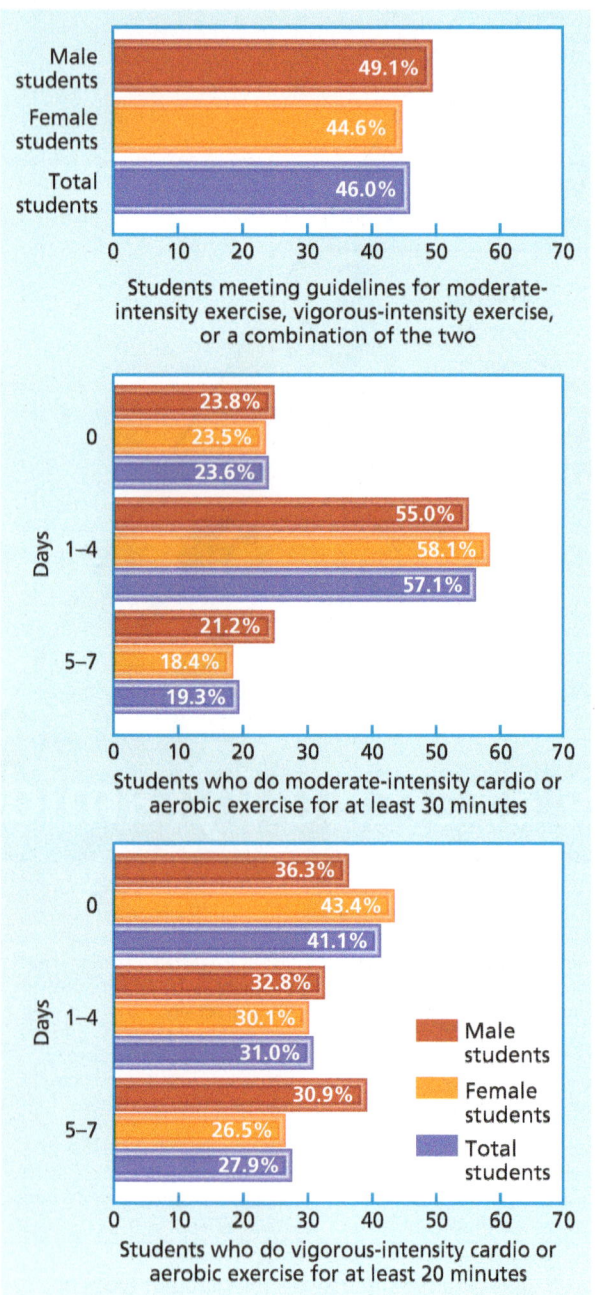

Data from *ACHA-NCHA II: Undergraduate reference group executive summary, spring 2015*, by the American College Health Association, 2015.

If you do a 4-MET activity for 30 minutes, you can multiply those numbers to get your *MET minutes*—a useful measure of your activity level. A 4-MET activity done for 30 minutes equals 120 MET minutes (4 × 30 = 120). Federal health experts recommend that each of us aim for 500 to 1,000 MET minutes per week. See **Table 6.4** for a list of common activities and their corresponding MET levels.[35]

Avoid Sustained Sitting

"Sustained sitting," or sedentary behaviors, should be minimized as much as possible. Sedentary behavior is typically defined as any behavior with exceedingly low energy expenditure. These behaviors include seated "couch potato activities," such as watching television, playing video games, and staring at a computer screen. In one study, researchers found that the amount of leisure time spent sitting is linked to increased risk of death, even if you work out.[36] The researchers found that sitting 6 or more hours a day outside work or class, compared to less than 3 hours, was significantly associated with a greater risk of death. Try to limit the overall quantity of daily sustained sitting, as well as take frequent breaks to interrupt and intersperse sustained sitting by standing up and moving about briefly every 30 minutes.

Increase Your Level of Activity

The following tips can help you increase your activity levels and meet—or even go beyond—the physical activity recommendations.

If You Aren't Active Now

If you usually get little or no regular physical activity, start by doing what you can and then look for ways to add more. If you tire easily, you can work out in as little as 10-minute intervals.[37] Below are a few easy ways you can add activity into your life:

- Park your car at the far end of the parking lot.
- Walk briskly or ride your bike to class.
- Begin an active new social hobby like tennis, yoga, or dance classes.
- To make sure your new activities encompass all the types of fitness you need, don't forget to include resistance and flexibility exercises at least 2 days per week.

If You Get Some Physical Activity Now

If you engage in some physical activity on a regular basis, focus on increasing your activity level:[37]

- Increase the intensity of your aerobic exercise by replacing moderate- with vigorous-intensity activities.
- Be active for longer; instead of walking for 30 minutes, try walking for 50 minutes.
- Be active more often; if you work out 2 days a week, try building up to 4 days a week.
- If you already meet the minimum recommendations for activity, strive for the elevated recommendations of 300 minutes of moderate-intensity or 150 minutes of vigorous-intensity activity per week.

If You Are Overweight

Many people who are overweight or obese feel that they can't start an activity program, but that isn't true. To get started with an activity program, try the following:

- If your current weight puts stress on your joints, choose non–weight-bearing exercise. Swimming and water-based exercise classes can get you moving without stressing your joints.

TABLE 6.4 Common Activities and Their METs

Moderate Activity (3.0 to 6.0 METs)	Vigorous Activity (more than 6.0 METs)
Walking at a moderate to brisk pace of 3–4.5 mph	Jogging and running
Bicycling at a pace of 5–9 mph or stationary bicycling at moderate effort	Bicycling at a pace of more than 10 mph or up a steep incline
Aerobics high-impact	Teaching an aerobics class
Yoga	Martial arts, jumping rope
Weight training, using free weights or weight machines	Circuit weight training, rowing machine used with vigorous effort

Source: Adapted from Centers for Disease Control and Prevention. (n.d.) *General physical activities defined by level of intensity.* www.cdc.gov.

- Remember that everyday activities, such as housework, walking the dog, or washing the car, can get you moving. Any activity that puts your body in motion helps. Try increasing your physical activity slightly each day.
- If you haven't worked out in a while, begin with light-intensity (40%–50% of your maximum heart rate) aerobic activity that gets your whole body moving. This will provide health benefits, expend energy to help with weight loss, and set the foundation for progression to higher intensities.

▶▶ Watch videos about the Physical Activity Guidelines for Americans at **www.cdc.gov/physicalactivity/everyone/videos/index.html**.

LO 6.5 QUICK CHECK

What are the basic recommendations for strength training?
a. Resistance exercise 2 days a week or more, for all major muscle groups, in sets of at least 8–12 repetitions.
b. Resistance exercise daily for all major muscle groups.
c. Resistance exercise 2 days a week, focusing on weight machines for optimal form.
d. Resistance exercise 4 days a week or more, for all major muscle groups, in sets of at least 8–12 repetitions.

Exercise Safe, Exercise Smart

LO 6.6 Discuss how to exercise safely.

Exercising safely is not difficult if you keep a few basic guidelines in mind.

Get Medical Clearance and Be Prepared

Before you begin any exercise program, make an appointment with a doctor to make sure you do not have any health conditions that should be taken into account. Plan to wear a helmet, pads, and other protective gear when cycling, skateboarding, or participating in any other activities where a fall is possible. See the **Consumer Corner** box on page 146 for more information on how to pick a proper shoe for exercise.

Warm Up and Cool Down

Before you start any moderate- to vigorous-intensity exercise, give yourself about 15 minutes to warm up. Warming up is not the same as stretching; effective warm-up involves gentle overall motion or a slowed-down version of the activity you are about to pursue, to increase your heart rate and blood flow to the muscles needed for exercise. When you are finished with your workout, give yourself another 15 minutes to cool down by performing slower and less intense movements, slowly returning your body to a less active state.

Get Training

Learning proper workout techniques from a qualified instructor will help prevent injury and increase your success at the activity. When you are choosing a trainer or fitness instructor, look for certifications from nonprofit organizations like the American College of Sports Medicine and training in CPR and first aid; your trainer should also undergo ongoing professional training on new techniques. Choose someone who makes you feel comfortable and provides helpful feedback to you during your workout.

Eat Right

What food should you eat when you exercise? Consider these suggestions, adapted from the Mayo Clinic:[38]

- **Eat breakfast.** Your body needs fuel before exercise. If you plan to eat within an hour of your workout, reach for something light, such as whole grain cereal.
- **Need a snack before your workout?** Think small and healthful. Good options include fresh fruit, yogurt, and crackers with peanut butter.
- **After your workout, eat within 2 hours.** Smart snacks include yogurt and fruit, nuts, and string cheese and crackers. If it's time for a meal, be sure it includes protein, carbs, and fiber.

Stay Hydrated

Adequate water consumption is a critical part of any workout. Studies show that dehydration limits strength, power, and endurance.[39] It is most effective to keep drinking water before, during, and after exercise as opposed to gulping down water all at once at the end of your workout. If you find yourself feeling thirsty, fatigued, with weak muscles and a minor headache, you may need to rehydrate.

To stay hydrated, fitness specialists say that water is your best choice. If, however, activity is prolonged and performed at a high intensity level, you may consider commercial sports drinks. These beverages combine water with flavorings, sugars that provide energy, and *electrolytes,* salts that help your body function properly. For everyday workouts, however, sports drinks are often unnecessary. These beverages are

CONSUMER CORNER
Choosing Athletic Shoes

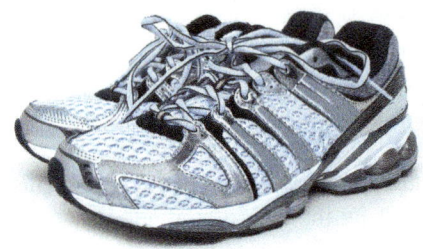

When shopping for athletic shoes, it's important to choose shoes that are made for the particular activity you are participating in because while athletic shoes look similar on the outside, each kind is constructed differently. The following tips will help you pick the best shoe:[1]

- Always go to a store that specializes in athletic shoes to find the best selection and the most knowledgeable salespeople.
- Shop for shoes at the end of the day, when your feet are at their largest.
- Wear the type of socks you plan on wearing with the shoes, in order to get the best fit.
- Watch for width. If the sides of the heel, toes, or arch feel tight, the shoe is not wide enough.
- If you have high arches, make sure to purchase a shoe or separate insoles with lots of arch support and cushioning.
- Purchase shoes made specifically for your sex. However, women with wide feet may consider trying men's or boy's shoes, which are made a bit larger throughout the heel.
- Bring your old shoes with you. Shoe professionals can give you tips based on the wear pattern on your old shoes.
- Try on both shoes, and walk, run, or perform the types of movements you will use the shoe for. The shoes should feel immediately comfortable, and your heel should fit snugly in each shoe and not slip as you walk.
- Don't assume that you wear the same shoe size in athletic shoes as you do in regular shoes.
- Running shoes should be replaced every 300–500 miles, cross-training shoes after 5–7 months, and aerobic shoes after 100–120 hours of use.[2] If your shoes are wearing through, it's time to replace them regardless of how long you've had them.
- This interactive graphic can help you select the best walking shoes: www.mayoclinic.com/health/medical/FS00001.

References: **1.** Mayo Clinic. (2014). *Walking shoes: Features and fit that keep you moving.* www.mayoclinic.com. **2.** Mahoney, S. (2015). *The differences between track and running shoes.* www.livestrong.com.

---

often expensive, provide little essential nutrition, and contain unnecessary levels of sugar. If you prefer the taste of sports drinks to plain water but aren't performing vigorous-intensity, prolonged exercise, try mixing just a little sports drink, juice, or a few slices of lemon or lime into a bottle of water.

Prepare for Hot or Cold Weather

If you exercise outside in cold weather, wear layered clothing that keeps you warm and wicks sweat away from your body but lets you move at the same time. Wear a hat because much of your body heat is lost through your head and protect your fingers and toes from the cold. If you start shivering, stop your workout, add more layers of clothing, and head inside. Constant shivering is an early sign of **hypothermia,** a potentially fatal condition in which your core body temperature dips too low. If your core temperature isn't raised, you will become uncoordinated, drowsy, and confused and will have difficulty speaking. If anyone you work out with develops these symptoms, he or she should be warmed up and taken to a hospital.

If you are working out in a hot climate, try to exercise in early morning or evening, when the weather tends to be cooler and less humid. If you get too dehydrated in hot weather, you put yourself at risk for **heat exhaustion,** a mild form of heat-related illness. Symptoms of heat exhaustion include nausea, headache, fatigue, and faintness; they indicate that you need to slow down, drink water, and head for a cooler spot.

If your overheating worsens, you face the possibility of **heatstroke,** a potentially fatal condition in which the body's core temperature reaches or exceeds 105°F. In heatstroke, your overheated core temperature overwhelms your body's cooling capabilities, causing dry, hot skin and rapid heart rate. Brain damage and death can follow. If you or a companion experience any of the symptoms, seek emergency medical attention by calling 911 immediately. In the meantime, a person experiencing heatstroke needs rest, a cooler location, ice packs applied to the body—especially the neck, armpits and groin area—and lots of cool fluids to drink immediately. Outdoor sports that require heavy pads, such as football, make it tough for your body to regulate its temperature effectively on hot days and put you at higher risk for heatstroke. If you participate in gear-heavy sports that leave you feeling overheated, talk to your coach about taking steps to make everyone cooler.

hypothermia A potentially fatal condition in which your core body temperature drops too low.

heat exhaustion A mild form of heat-related illness that usually occurs as a result of exercising in hot weather without adequate hydration.

heatstroke A life-threatening heat-related illness that occurs when your core temperature rises above 105°F.

Start Slowly and Watch Out for Red Flags

To avoid injuries, it's important to start slowly when you begin an exercise program. If you are just starting your fitness plan, for example, give yourself time before trying an intense workout such as CrossFit or training for a 10K run.

MEDIA AND Fitness
Do Fitness Apps Work?

When working out, more and more people bring a new piece of gear along with their towel and water bottle: their phone. In one recent survey of smart phone users, 38% of those who had downloaded a health-related app had included at least one fitness app in their selections.[1] But mobile apps are a relatively new part of fitness, and at least so far, they appear to offer mixed results in improving your workout.

Apps can be fun, give you new workout suggestions, and provide connections to others who have similar fitness goals and challenges. One recent study found more than 100,000 fitness apps available for download. But many aren't grounded on sound fitness science. In one key study, researchers looked at 30 popular fitness apps and found that most aren't based on exercise guidelines established by the American College of Sports Medicine. Only 1 of the 30 apps—the Sworkit Lite Personal Workout Trainer—met more than half the criteria from the guidelines.[2]

Other studies have found that many fitness apps aren't based on the scientific theories and guidelines proven to motivate real health behavior change.[3] One common shortcoming is the limited ability for users to customize an app to important personal factors such as height, weight, or age.[3] When choosing an app, consider only apps based on established fitness guidelines and that allow you to personalize your experience.

Another study found that health-related apps with slightly higher costs (more than the popular $0.99 price for many apps) were more likely to be based on factors important to lasting behavior change.[3] In other words, it may be worth paying a little bit for an app to get help achieving long-term results. Fee-based apps that have received positive feedback for quality include the fee-base versions of C25K (Couch to 5k), iTreadmill, iFitness, and FitnessBuilder.[4]

What Do You Think?

1. Have you used a fitness-related app to help with a workout? Why or why not?
2. What are some of the benefits of social connection and support in using fitness apps? What might be some of the drawbacks?
3. Based on what you've learned about behavior change, what are two or three important factors that would form the basis of a fitness app more likely to help you achieve long-term results?

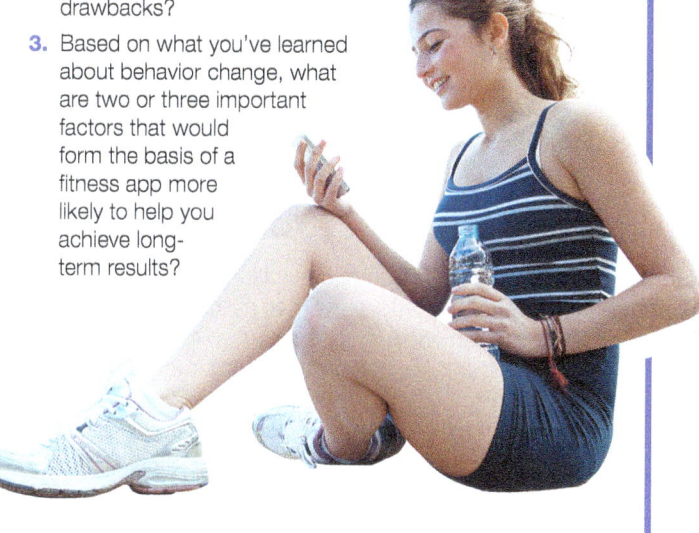

References: 1. Pew Internet and American Life Project. (2012). *Mobile health 2012*. www.pewinternet.org. 2. Modave, F., Bian, J., Leavitt, T., Bronwell, J., Harris, C., & Vincent, H. (2015). Low quality of free coaching apps with respect to the american college of sports medicine guidelines: review of current mobile apps. *Journal of Medical Internet Research, 3*, e77. 3. Cowan, L., Van Wagenen, S., Brown, B., Hedin, R., Seino-Stephan, Y., et al. (2012). Apps of steel: Are exercise apps providing consumers with realistic expectations? A content analysis of exercise apps for presence of behavior change theory. *Health Education & Behavior, 40*(2), 133–139. 4. West, J., Hall, C., Hanson, C., Barnes, M., Giraud-Carrier, C., & Barrett, J. (2012). There's an app for that: Content analysis of paid health and fitness apps. *Journal of Medical Internet Research, 14*(3), e72.

If you experience any of the following symptoms while exercising, stop immediately, no matter your level of fitness. Talk with your doctor or campus health service about any of these symptoms:

- Pain, tightness, or pressure in your chest, neck, arm, or shoulder
- Dizziness or nausea
- Cold sweats
- Severe muscle cramps
- Extreme shortness of breath
- Pain in your joints, feet, ankles, or legs

Care for Injuries

Injuries occasionally do happen with exercise. Common complaints include contusions (bruises), joint sprains, muscle strains, shin splints, and tendinitis. These injuries most often cause pain, swelling, or skin discoloration.

Another common complaint during exercise is **cramps.** These severe muscle contractions are your body's way of telling you to take a break. If you get a cramp, stop your activity. Drink some water and massage or apply pressure to the cramped muscle. You can also try taking a few deep breaths to give your body—and your cramped muscles—extra oxygen.

cramp An involuntary contracted muscle that does not relax, resulting in localized intense pain.

Minor injuries to the muscles and joints should be treated with the *RICE protocol*:

- **Rest.** Stop exercising as soon as you feel pain and rest the injured area.
- **Ice.** Apply an ice pack to the injured area for no more than 20 minutes at a time intermittently for the first 24–48 hours. The cold of the ice helps to decrease the swelling. After 48 hours you can apply a heating pad to the area, which improves blood flow and promotes healing.

- **Compression.** Compressing the area with an elastic bandage both holds the ice pack in place and decreases the swelling.
- **Elevation.** If possible, elevate the injured area above your heart. Doing so will minimize swelling and discomfort.

Be Wary of Performance-Enhancing Drugs

Prominent athletes, including well-known Olympic athletes, cyclists, and players in Major League Baseball, have made headlines after investigators discovered their use of performance-enhancing drugs. But use of these substances isn't confined to the top tiers of sports. According to health estimates, up to 3 million Americans have used performance-enhancing drugs, including an estimated 4.7% of males and 1.2% of females.[40] In a national survey, about 20% of U.S. teenagers described these substances as easy to get, and anywhere from 7% to 11% reported using a potentially dangerous substance, without a prescription, for its perceived performance-enhancing benefits.[41] Some performance-enhancing drugs carry dangerous side effects, and a few are even illegal for use or sale in the United States. The following are some of the common types of performance-enhancing drugs:

- **Anabolic steroids.** Sometimes called "roids" or "juice," these synthetic derivatives of the male hormone testosterone can encourage muscle growth and build lean body tissue. Using anabolic steroids to improve athletic performance is illegal, and these drugs pose serious health risks, including liver cancer, fluid retention, high blood pressure, and severe acne. In men, anabolic steroids may shrink testicles and lower sperm counts. In women, steroid use can cause cessation of the menstrual cycle, growth of facial and body hair, and deepening of the voice. Anabolic steroids can also lead to dangerous psychological side effects, including aggression, extreme mood swings, rage, and even violent behavior.
- **Creatine.** Sometimes referred to as "muscle candy," creatine is a substance naturally produced by the body and stored in skeletal muscles. Creatine is thought to help muscles during short, high-intensity activity, but research on creatine has been inconclusive. Taking creatine may cause dehydration, reduce blood volume, and produce imbalances in blood chemistry. Federal health officials warn that creatine supplements should be used only under a doctor's care.[42]
- **Human growth hormone.** Also known as HGH, human growth hormone is a naturally occurring compound made by the body to fuel cell growth and regeneration. Its use as an athletic supplement has been widespread because HGH is difficult to detect during drug testing. Scientists warn that the long-term effects of using HGH are unknown, and researchers have found no significant athletic benefits tied to use of the hormone. Use of HGH in athletes, for example, did not improve strength and actually appeared to worsen athletic performance. HGH users also experienced more soft tissue swelling and fatigue.[43]

- **Androstenedione.** Also called "andro," this steroid precursor is thought to enhance athletic performance and boost testosterone and has been linked to many high-profile controversies among professional athletes. Androstenedione is illegal for sale or use in the United States, and its side effects include breast development and impotence in men, abnormal periods and facial hair in women, and liver disease and blood clots.
- **Ephedra.** Also referred to as "ephedrine" or by its Chinese name "Ma Huang," ephedra is typically used to boost energy and promote weight loss. Ephedra has such serious adverse effects that the U.S. Food and Drug Administration has banned its sale. Research has not shown ephedra to be effective in boosting energy or athletic performance, but it has shown side effects such as high blood pressure, irregular heartbeat, stroke, gastrointestinal distress, and psychological problems.[44]
- **Dehydroepiandrosterone.** Often known as DHEA, this hormone, made in the body, helps lead to the production of male and female sex hormones and is sometimes taken in synthetic form to try to improve athletic performance or weight-lifting capability. But it carries many of the same side effects and risks seen with steroid use, and DHEA use is banned by the National Collegiate Athletic Association (NCAA).
- **Chromium picolinate.** Often referred to simply as "chromium," this mineral is sometimes taken to try to build muscle tissue or boost energy, even though researchers have found it be ineffective.[45] Side effects include liver and kidney damage.

LO 6.6 QUICK CHECK

For everyday workouts, sports drinks are
a. ideal for hydration.
b. ideal for electrolyte balance.
c. better than water.
d. often unnecessary.

Change Yourself, Change Your World

LO 6.7 Design an effective personalized fitness program.

Improved fitness is as much a public health goal as it is a personal one. Some of the factors that contribute to one's level of fitness reflect individual choice—whether to drive or cycle, watch TV or go outside, spend time online or spend time at the gym. But the communities in which we live also play a key role. Getting fit starts with you, but through the choices you make, you also have the potential to help improve the lives of others.

Personal Choices

In the busy life of a student, scheduling regular exercise may seem daunting. But if you set goals, find activities you enjoy, and periodically reassess your progress, you'll be able to stay motivated, have fun, and enjoy the benefits of fitness.

DIVERSITY & HEALTH

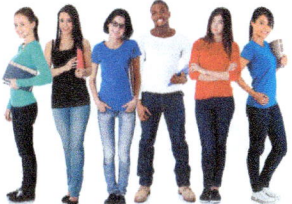

Safe Exercise for Special Populations

Exercise can do everyone good. If you have health concerns, the key is to modify your fitness program to reduce risk and maximize the benefits you receive. The following measures can help you have a safe and effective workout.

Asthma

- If prescribed, use pre-exercise asthma inhalers before beginning exercise.
- Extend your warm-up and cool-down to help your lungs prepare for and recover from exercise.
- Check for environmental irritants that could promote an asthma attack, such as a recently mowed lawn, high pollen counts, or high levels of air pollution, and consider exercising indoors at those times. If exercising in cold weather, cover your mouth and nose with a scarf or mask.
- Try swimming. The warm, moist environment is soothing, and swimming helps build cardiorespiratory endurance.
- If you begin to cough, wheeze, have difficulty breathing, or have tightness in your chest, halt exercise and use your inhaler or other prescribed medication.

Pregnancy

- Avoid contact sports or activities that may cause trauma or a fall. Walking and swimming are great low-impact options, but you can also dance, run, or hike.
- You can still perform resistance exercises. Focus on muscular endurance exercises rather than strengthening exercises.
- Halt exercise if you experience vaginal bleeding, dizziness, headache, chest pain, calf pain or swelling, pre-term labor, or decreased fetal movement.
- After the first trimester, avoid exercises in which you lie on your back; they can reduce blood flow to the uterus.

Diabetes

- Monitor your blood glucose before and after exercise, especially when beginning or modifying your exercise program.
- Wear a diabetes ID bracelet during exercise.
- Carry a snack if you will be active for a few hours.
- If you begin to feel shaky, anxious, or suddenly begin to sweat more, halt exercise and consume a fast-acting carbohydrate.
- Make sure to wear well-fitting shoes and check your feet for blisters or sores before and after exercise.

What Do You Think?

1. Does your campus athletic center or fitness center make efforts to accommodate the needs of those with special safety concerns? If not, what other options are available on your campus?
2. Have you ever had a teammate or fitness partner who has asthma? How can you help them work out or play a sport safely and comfortably?
3. Given how exercise works alongside insulin in regulating blood sugar, why might people with diabetes need to be especially careful when exercising?

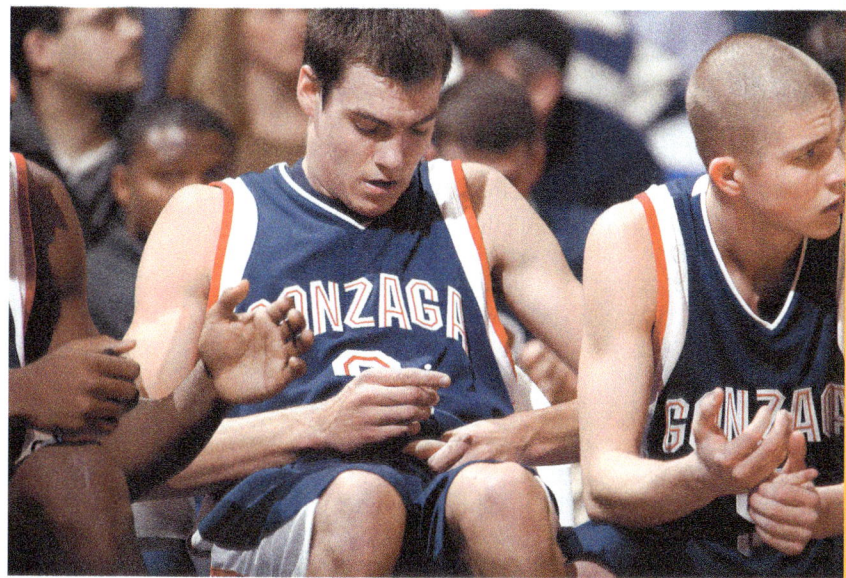

This college basketball player with diabetes is preparing an insulin injection for himself.

Set Realistic Goals

One of the most important aspects of a fitness program is working at an intensity and rate that make sense for you as you are. It is important to realistically assess your current fitness level in order to set fitness goals that are appropriate. Fitness goals can be based on a specific activity-related improvement you want to make, such as cycling 40% farther than you currently can; a health-related goal, such as reducing your blood pressure; or a social or lifestyle desire, like preparing for a backpacking trip with your friends. Make sure your goals are easily measurable so you can clearly tell when you've met one. If you don't make a particular goal you have set, don't get discouraged. Take the chance to reevaluate your goal and possibly break it down into smaller subgoals.

>> Take this self-assessment for a quick idea of how fit you are: www.nhs.uk/Tools/Pages/Fitness.aspx.

Find Activities You Enjoy

To exercise on a regular basis, focus on physical activities you naturally enjoy. Ask yourself which of those activities will help you reach your fitness goals, which ones you are most likely to stick with, and which ones you can afford. Don't be afraid to mix it up; a wide range of activities can bring you all the benefits of fitness and will stave off boredom. If you can afford to take tennis lessons only twice a month, combine that with free aerobics classes at school and resistance exercises you can perform at home.

Schedule Time

One key to sticking with exercise is to schedule in exercise as you would a job or a class. If you have a set time devoted to exercise, you will be more likely to stick with it. See step 3 of the **Choosing to Change Worksheet** at the end of this chapter for a schedule where you can plan activity.

Team Up!

Find a friend or family member with similar fitness goals and make plans to work out together regularly. You'll not only enjoy the company and extra motivation to stay on track but may achieve greater health benefits. One study found that people with regular workout partners, especially workout partners who'd received a significant amount of fitness training and coaching, lost more weight compared with those who trained alone.[46]

Overcome Obstacles

You can probably come up with a long list of reasons why you do not exercise regularly. Here are some common obstacles and solutions for overcoming them:

- **I don't have time.** Remember that only 30 minutes of moderate exercise a day can improve or maintain your fitness and that amount can be broken down into 10-minute sessions. Substituting exercise for TV or computer time is a good place to start. If you don't have time for the gym, exercise at home. If you have children, actively play with them. Some gyms also offer free or inexpensive child care.
- **I don't know how.** If you don't know how to play a particular sport, take a class. Consider working with a personal trainer, who will build your skills with lots of one-on-one attention. Many campus wellness centers offer low-cost personal training and classes.
- **I don't like the gym.** If working out on the machines isn't your thing, try alternative exercises, like rock climbing, Ultimate Frisbee, or video games designed for fitness, like the Wii Fit.
- **I'm embarrassed about how I look.** If you aren't ready to hit the campus pool in a bathing suit, start with activities where you'll be comfortable in sweat pants and a T-shirt. Also, seek out exercise environments in which you feel comfortable (for example, a women-only fitness center).
- **I don't have the money.** If you can't afford a gym membership, choose exercises that require no more than a good pair of shoes, such as walking or running. Or purchase low-cost equipment like exercise bands, exercise balls, or dumbbells. Your campus or community recreation center may have free or low-cost gyms or classes.

Assess Your Progress

Every 4 to 6 weeks, get motivated by assessing how far you've come. Look back on all the exercise you've done, think about the positive effects on how you feel or how fit you are becoming, and evaluate how close you are to the goals you set. At the beginning of an exercise program, you may want to assess your progress even more often.

▶▶ Watch videos of real students discussing physical activity and fitness at **Mastering**Health™.

LO 6.7 QUICK CHECK

You are more likely to get regular exercise if you
- a. work out whenever you have a little spare time.
- b. schedule workouts as you would a class or job.
- c. use a tracking app.
- d. None of the above.

STUDENT STORY

Adapting Exercise to My Needs

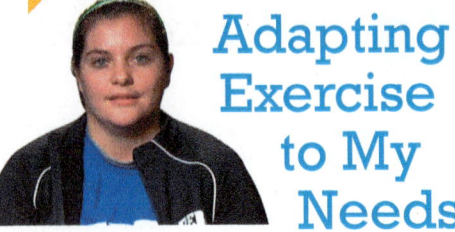

"HI, I'M MOLLY. I have hip dysplasia so some of the movements that other people can do, I can't do as well. I don't have as good flexibility and mobility and sometimes when I run or I do other things for a long time, things hurt. So I've had to adapt the way that I exercise so that I can still get that activity, but do it in a way that doesn't hurt me. And one of those ways is that I swim. I'll do laps or go swimming with my friends and that is something that doesn't put pressure on my hips but it's still a great way to exercise. And I also like to ride my bike. I reach my target heart rate and it's something that I can do just as well as anyone else."

What Do You Think?

1. Do you have any needs—physical or otherwise—that you want to structure your exercise around? How will you go about doing that?
2. Exercising with friends and varying your exercise activities, as Molly does, can help you stay motivated. What else will help you stay motivated with your fitness program?
3. What are some of your own self-created justifications for not exercising? How can you draw inspiration from people with physical limitations who still find ways to exercise?

# Choosing to **Change** Worksheet

To complete this worksheet online, visit MasteringHealth

In this chapter you have learned about the importance of physical fitness. To improve your overall fitness, follow the steps below.

Directions: Fill in your stage of behavior change in step 1 and complete the rest of the worksheet with your stage of change in mind.

Step 1: Assess your stage of behavior change. Please check one of the following statements that best describes your readiness to improve your overall fitness.

_____ I do not intend to improve my overall fitness in the next six months. (Precontemplation)

_____ I might improve my overall fitness in the next six months. (Contemplation)

_____ I am prepared to improve my overall fitness in the next month. (Preparation)

_____ I have been improving my overall fitness for less than six months. (Action)

_____ I have been improving my overall fitness for more than six months. (Maintenance)

In order to create and maintain a fitness program, you should set goals, find activities you enjoy, schedule time, overcome obstacles, and assess your progress.

Step 2: Set a fitness goal.

1. What is your SMART goal for fitness? Do you want to run 5 miles? Touch your toes? Bench press a specific weight? Something else? Make sure the goal is specific, focused, and easily measurable and set a realistic timeline for your goal. If your goal is large, break it down into smaller subgoals.

Goal: _____   Timeline: _____

Subgoal 1: _____   Timeline: _____

Subgoal 2: _____   Timeline: _____

Subgoal 3: _____   Timeline: _____

2. What activities do you enjoy that could help you meet your fitness goals? Think about activities that you honestly like, that you have relatively easy access to, and that you can afford. Write down all the activities that meet these criteria. Remember, participating in more than one type of activity will help you combat boredom.

_____

_____

Step 3: Schedule time for fitness. How do you find time to get enough exercise? One of the best ways is to write it down in a schedule as you would for any other commitment. Fill out the table below to create an exercise schedule for yourself.

Type of Activity	Monday	Tuesday	Wednesday	Thursday	Friday	Saturday	Sunday	Recommended Minimum Amount
Aerobic exercise								150 minutes moderate-intensity OR 75 minutes vigorous-intensity OR equivalent combination of both
Resistance training								2 nonconsecutive days per week in sets of 8–12 reps
Flexibility exercise								2–3 days per week for at least 60 seconds per stretch

Step 4: Overcome obstacles. What obstacles might you face in adhering to a fitness program, and what could you do to combat them? See page 150 for tips.

Obstacle	How to Overcome
_____	_____
_____	_____
_____	_____
_____	_____

CHAPTER 6 STUDY PLAN

CHAPTER SUMMARY

LO 6.1
- Physical fitness is the ability to perform moderate- to vigorous-intensity physical activity and to be able to respond to physical demands without excessive fatigue.
- The five key components of health-related fitness are cardiorespiratory fitness, muscular strength, muscular endurance, flexibility, and body composition.

LO 6.2
- Physical activity builds the health of your heart and lungs. It also lowers your risk of certain diseases, increases immunity, helps your bones stay strong, helps you manage your weight, and helps you cope with stress.

LO 6.3
- The principles of fitness training are overload, specificity, reversibility, individuality, and diminishing returns.

LO 6.4
- A well-rounded fitness program should include a mix of activities that build your cardiorespiratory fitness, work your muscles, and increase your flexibility.

LO 6.5
- You need at least 150 minutes of moderate-intensity or 75 minutes of vigorous-intensity aerobic activity each week, or an equivalent mix of the two. You also need 2 to 3 days of resistance training and flexibility exercise per week.
- In addition to engaging in regular physical activity, limit sustained sitting. If you find yourself sitting for extended periods of time, get up and move around at least every 30 minutes.
- If you haven't exercised for a while, you can meet activity recommendations by starting slowly and building up. If you already work out, you can try exercising longer, more often, or at a greater intensity. If you are overweight or obese, it is especially important to add activity to your life, focusing first on regular low-intensity aerobic activities.

LO 6.6
- You can avoid injury while you exercise by taking some simple precautions, such as getting medical clearance, warming up and cooling down, getting training, wearing suitable clothes, eating right, staying hydrated, caring for injuries, and avoiding performance-enhancing drugs.

LO 6.7
- To maintain fitness habits, remember to set measurable goals, focus on activities you enjoy, schedule time, find ways around obstacles, and assess your progress.
- Your workouts may be more successful and enjoyable with others. Team up with a friend to exercise or help start a fitness program on campus or in your community.

MasteringHealth™
Build your knowledge—and health!—in the Study Area of MasteringHealth™ with a variety of study tools.

GET CONNECTED

Visit the following websites for further information about the topics in this chapter:

- American College of Sports Medicine Public Resources
  www.acsm.org
- American Council on Exercise
  www.acefitness.org
- President's Challenge Program: The Active Lifestyle Activity Log
  www.presidentschallenge.org

MOBILE TIPS!
Scan this QR code with your mobile device to access additional tips about physical activity for fitness and health. Or, via your mobile device, go to **http://chmobile.pearsoncmg.com** and choose by topic: fitness and health.

Website links are subject to change. To access updated web links, please visit MasteringHealth™

TEST YOUR KNOWLEDGE

LO 6.1
1. Which one of the following is not a component of physical fitness?
   a. cardiorespiratory fitness
   b. muscular strength
   c. flexibility
   d. balance

LO 6.1, 6.2
2. Muscular strength
   a. does not help your bones.
   b. is the same thing as muscular endurance.
   c. is important for performing extended activities.
   d. is the maximum force your muscles can apply in a single effort.

LO 6.1
3. Body composition
   a. refers to your ratio of muscle to lean tissue.
   b. only matters in weight loss.
   c. can be changed by physical activity.
   d. None of these answers are correct.

LO 6.4
4. Aerobic exercise includes
   a. isometric and isotonic exercises.
   b. static and dynamic exercises.
   c. prolonged activity that raises the heart rate.
   d. short, intense activities that create an oxygen deficit.

LO 6.2, 6.5
5. Students under a lot of stress
   a. shouldn't exercise because it will just take time they don't have.
   b. can get stress relief from working out.
   c. are better off in the gym than working out on their own.
   d. won't be able to stick to an exercise program.

LO 6.3
6. The principle of individuality means that
   a. you should only do one type of exercise during each workout.
   b. you need to do exercises in different orders each day.
   c. you can improve only one component of fitness at a time.
   d. each individual adapts to exercise differently.

LO 6.5
7. The CDC recommendations for exercise for health maintenance include
   a. resistance exercise 1 day a week or more.
   b. 150 minutes of moderate-intensity aerobic activity or 75 minutes of vigorous-intensity activity each week.
   c. 250 minutes of moderate-intensity aerobic activity or 150 minutes of vigorous-intensity activity each week.
   d. weekly resistance exercise or aerobic activity but not both.

LO 6.6
8. If you find yourself getting really hot, nauseated, and faint during a workout, you should
   a. stop, find a cool spot, and drink water.
   b. keep going—this means you are getting a good workout.
   c. keep going if your friends or teammates are.
   d. stop and dial 9-1-1.
9. Sports drinks
   a. should be used only with light exercise.
   b. provide the vitamins you need to keep exercising.
   c. can be used during prolonged exercise.
   d. are always a good idea when working out.

LO 6.7
10. To make exercise a habit, you should
    a. focus on physical activities that make you happy.
    b. do activities you don't like because you need work in those areas.
    c. buy a lot of expensive equipment; it will motivate you to work out.
    d. work out at the highest possible intensity so you get fit quickly.

WHAT DO YOU THINK?

LO 6.1
1. What is the key difference between exercise and physical activity? How can you get more physical activity into your daily routine, even if you aren't exercising that day?

LO 6.2
2. Why isn't just being thin as protective to your health as being physically fit?

LO 6.3
3. How does the principle of specificity apply to your own types of physical activity and exercise? Does your own routine include activities specific to all the various types of fitness you need?

LO 6.4
4. How much emphasis does your own daily activity routine or exercise regime place on flexibility? If you've been neglecting this aspect of fitness, what are three things you can start doing to improve your flexibility?

LO 6.6
5. How can we as a society discourage use of performance-enhancing drugs? When a sports star admits to using performance-enhancing drugs, does that turn people off to illegal doping or just make the problem worse through greater publicity?

7

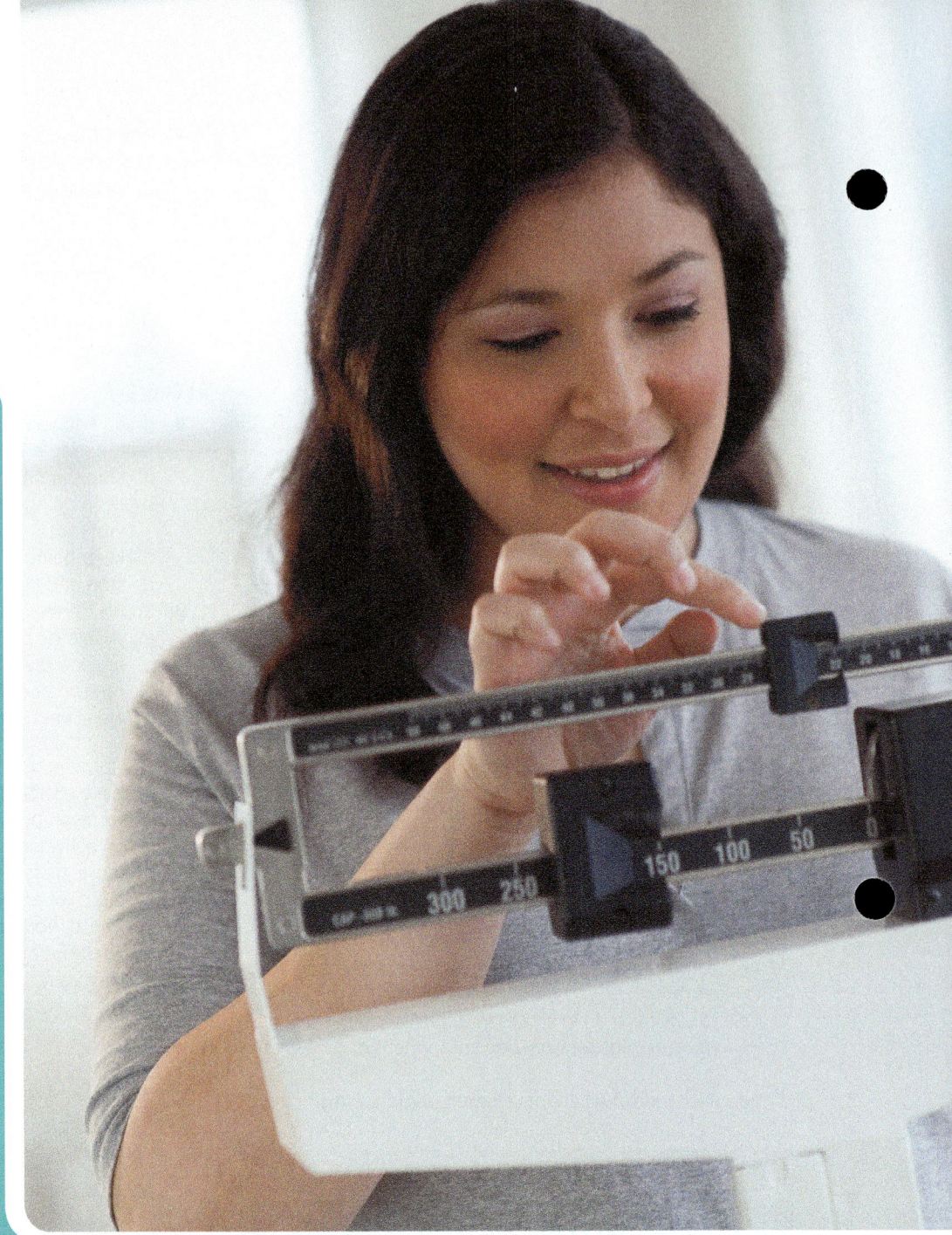

> An estimated 68.5% of American adults age 20 and older are overweight or obese.[i]

> Obesity-related health-care costs in the United States add up to more than $270 billion per year.[ii]

> Obesity is now responsible for more than 3 million deaths worldwide each year—triple the number of deaths due to malnutrition.[iii]

> In the United States, 4.3% of college students report being underweight.[iv]

BODY IMAGE, BODY WEIGHT

LEARNING OUTCOMES

LO 7.1 Identify important factors in body image and body weight.

LO 7.2 Describe alarming trends in weight gain.

LO 7.3 Explain the risks and costs of obesity.

LO 7.4 Identify factors that contribute to weight gain.

LO 7.5 Explain how to reduce excess body weight.

LO 7.6 Describe strategies for maintaining a healthy weight at college.

LO 7.7 Describe common body image and eating disorders.

Excess body weight is one of our society's most serious health concerns—

so much so that the Centers for Disease Control and Prevention has declared obesity a national epidemic. An estimated 68.5% of American adults over age 20 and 31.8% of those 19 and under are **overweight** or **obese.**[1] The problem is also spreading globally in both industrialized and developing nations—in 2014, 39% of the world's adult population was overweight.[2]

Amid this pressing public health concern, others face difficult issues at the other end of the weight spectrum. In the United States, 1.7% of adults[3] and 4.3% of college students are **underweight.**[4] Some of these individuals may need nutritional or medical help to reach a healthful weight, while others may be suffering from potentially dangerous eating disorders such as bulimia or anorexia nervosa.

Why should you care about your body weight? It affects your risk of disease and, in serious cases, may lead to an early death. Your body weight also influences your self-confidence and self-image, which in turn affects your relationships, goals, and activities—essentially all aspects of your life.

Body Image and Body Weight

LO 7.1 Identify important factors in body image and body weight.

When was the last time you looked at your body in a mirror and thought it could be more attractive? When did you last criticize yourself for your body shape or size? Did you use harsh terms that you'd never use to describe a friend? If you are like many other people, those self-criticisms come easily and all too often.

The way you view, critique, and feel about your own body is called **body image.** Whether positive or negative, how you view your body can shape the way you feel, the way you treat yourself, and the way you eat—all of which have important health implications. Body image concerns affect males and females of all ages:

- Numerous studies have found that children absorb adult ideas about thinness and ideal body type, often from media images, and then use those ideas to judge themselves.[5]
- Men often share women's self-criticisms of size and shape, although they may experience them more sharply at different points in their lives. One 20-year-long study found that men's dissatisfaction with their bodies went up with time and age. Women, while persistently displeased with their bodies, were often more critical when they were younger and become more self-accepting as they grew older.[6]
- College is prime time for harsh self-judgment. In a study of college students, about 70% of female students and 35% of male students were dissatisfied with their bodies.[7] About 70% of female students considered themselves unattractive to the opposite sex, as did about 45% of male students.

overweight The condition of having a body weight that exceeds what is generally considered healthful for a particular height. A weight resulting in a BMI of 25 to 29.9.

obese A weight disorder in which excess accumulations of nonessential body fat result in increased risk of health problems. A weight resulting in a BMI of 30 or higher.

underweight A weight resulting in a BMI below 18.5.

body image A person's perceptions, feelings, and critiques of his or her own body.

>> Beauty-product manufacturer Dove has created a series of videos called Real Beauty Sketches, which explore women's body images. Watch the videos here: www.dove.com/us/en/stories/campaigns/real-beauty-sketches.html.

Many Factors Influence Body Image

For the vast majority of us, external influences shape our body image. Every day we see hundreds of images of women who appear to be effortlessly fit and thin and of men who seem to have been born buff. The opinions of friends and family members also contribute to our perceptions of our bodies.

Girls and women are often under the most pressure to conform to societal ideals of the "beautiful body." Magazines and fashion-oriented websites geared toward young women are packed with images that associate extreme thinness with beauty, desirability, and success. Numerous research studies have linked viewing such images to the development of negative self-perceptions. In one study in which college women were shown either neutral images or "thin-ideal" images from magazines, exposure to the skinny imagery was directly linked to an increasingly negative view of one's own body, regardless of the person's actual size.[8]

Our obsession with social media is also affecting body image. For example, a recent survey of female college students found that those who were regularly on Facebook had negative feelings about their own bodies after looking at others' posted photos. The researchers concluded that comparisons to social media might have an even more negative effect on a woman's body image than comparisons to traditional media images because comparisons to our friends are much more relevant. However, these posted images can be just as unrealistic as ones in traditional media because most have been edited and enhanced.[9]

Defining a Healthful Body Weight

If media images and social pressures are poor guides for assessing one's weight, where should each of us look to determine our most healthful weight and shape? Some of the answers lie in numbers—measurements that indicate everything from weight to percentage of body fat. Others depend on more personal factors. We'll look at the numbers first.

Health-care professionals commonly use body mass index (BMI) and waist circumference measures because these assessments are easy and inexpensive to perform. Together, these measures can be valuable in assessing some of a person's weight-related health risks, such as heart disease risk, and monitoring changes over time.[10]

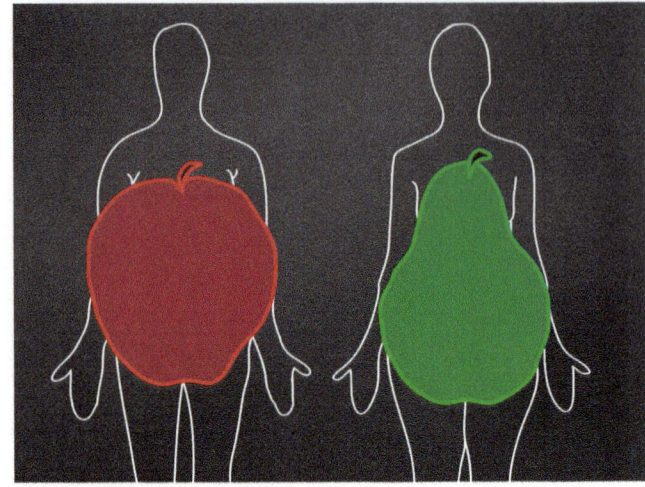

(a) Apple-shaped fat patterning   (b) Pear-shaped fat patterning

Those with apple type bodies carry more fat around their waists, which can put them at higher risk for certain diseases than those with pear type bodies.

Body Mass Index (BMI)

Body mass index (BMI) is one of the most common measures for assessing weight, as well as for defining *overweight* and *obese*. A ratio between your height and your weight, BMI is one of several indicators used to predict risk factors for health problems later in life. A BMI between 18.5 and 24.9 indicates a **healthful weight,** and people within this category generally have fewer weight-related health risks. Risks increase as BMI falls below or rises above this range; both underweight and overweight can impair health.[11] To determine your own BMI and related weight category, see **Figure 7.1** on page 157 and the **Self-Assessment** on page 158.

BMI, however, is not always an accurate health indicator. Athletes with large amounts of lean muscle mass, for example, may have BMIs that classify them as overweight, even though they are at a healthful weight for their build. BMI also sometimes underestimates total body fat in older people who have lost muscle. In addition, one large recent scientific analysis of many weight-related studies found that, especially for older people, having a BMI that equaled being overweight—but not obese—lowered the risk of death compared with people of normal weight.[12] Based on such findings, many experts increasingly say that many factors, such as cholesterol levels or blood pressure, need to be considered along with BMI and that BMI should not be used as the sole indicator of weight-related health.

body mass index (BMI) A numerical measurement, calculated from height and weight measurements, that provides an indicator of health risk categories.

healthful weight The weight at which health risks are lowest for an individual; usually a weight that results in a BMI between 18.5 and 24.9.

Body Measurements

Beyond BMI, two waist measurements are used to predict weight-related health problems: *waist circumference* and *waist-to-hip ratio*. Waist circumference is an indicator of how much body fat you carry. In general, a waist measuring more than 35 inches in a woman or 40 inches in a man points to increased health risks. As waist circumference increases, disease risks increase.

Body shape may also influence disease risk. Individuals who carry fat mainly around the waist (so called *apple-shaped* fat patterning) are more likely to develop certain health problems, such as heart disease or diabetes, than those who carry fat mainly in the hips and thighs (also called *pear-shaped* fat patterning). Waist-to-hip ratio (waist circumference divided by hip circumferences) separates the apples from the pears. Excess fat around the waist is a risk factor for heart disease, even in those with normal BMIs.[13]

> ❝ *A BMI between 18.5 and 24.9 indicates a healthful weight, and people within this category generally have fewer weight-related health risks. Risks increase as BMI falls below or rises above this range; both underweight and overweight can impair health.* ❞

▶▶ You can skip the math and use the online calculators at http://www.health-calc.com.

Personal Factors

Personal factors, such as your age, genetics, and body type, should influence your assessment of your body weight. Consider the following questions:

	Underweight		Healthful weight							Overweight					Obese					Extremely obese			
BMI	17	18	18.5	19	20	21	22	23	24	25	26	27	28	29	30	31	32	33	34	35	36	37	39	≥40
Height										**Weight in pounds**														
4'10"	81	86	89	91	96	100	105	110	115	119	124	129	134	138	143	148	153	158	162	167	172	177	186	191
4'11"	84	89	92	94	99	104	109	114	119	124	128	133	138	143	148	153	158	163	168	173	178	183	193	198
5'	87	92	95	97	102	107	112	118	123	128	133	138	143	148	153	158	163	158	174	179	184	189	199	204
5'1"	90	95	98	100	106	111	116	122	127	132	137	143	148	153	158	164	169	174	180	185	190	195	206	211
5'2"	93	98	101	104	109	115	120	126	131	136	142	147	153	158	164	169	175	180	186	191	196	202	213	218
5'3"	96	102	104	107	113	118	124	130	135	141	146	152	158	163	169	175	180	186	191	197	203	208	220	225
5'4"	99	105	108	110	116	122	128	134	140	145	151	157	163	169	174	180	186	192	197	204	209	215	227	232
5'5"	102	108	111	114	120	126	132	138	144	150	156	162	168	174	180	186	192	198	204	210	216	222	234	240
5'6"	105	112	115	118	124	130	136	142	148	155	161	167	173	179	186	192	198	204	210	216	223	229	241	247
5'7"	109	115	118	121	127	134	140	146	153	159	166	172	178	185	191	198	204	211	217	223	230	236	249	255
5'8"	112	118	122	125	131	138	144	151	158	164	171	177	184	190	197	203	210	216	223	230	236	243	256	262
5'9"	115	122	125	128	135	142	149	155	162	169	176	182	189	196	203	209	216	223	230	236	243	250	263	270
5'10"	119	126	129	132	139	146	153	160	167	174	181	188	195	202	209	216	222	229	236	243	250	257	271	278
5'11"	122	129	133	136	143	150	157	165	172	179	186	193	200	208	215	222	229	236	243	250	257	265	279	286
6'	125	133	136	140	147	154	162	169	177	184	191	199	206	213	221	228	235	242	250	258	265	272	287	294
6'1"	129	137	140	144	151	159	166	174	182	189	197	204	212	219	227	235	242	250	257	265	272	280	295	302
6'2"	132	140	144	148	155	163	171	179	186	194	202	210	218	225	233	241	249	256	264	272	280	287	303	311
6'3"	136	144	148	152	160	168	176	184	193	200	208	216	224	232	240	248	256	264	272	279	287	295	311	319
6'4"	140	148	152	156	164	172	180	189	197	205	213	221	230	238	246	254	263	271	279	287	295	304	320	328

FIGURE 7.1 **Body Mass Index (BMI).** BMI is often used to predict risk factors for health problems later in life. To determine your BMI, find your height and then scan across to find your weight. Then scan up to find your BMI.

- **What is a healthful *range* of weight for you?** There is no single ideal weight that is right for all of us. Identifying a healthful range of weight and accepting that it's normal for your weight to fluctuate within that range is a much more practical approach. The following section discusses several methods for determining the range of weight that's most healthful for you.
- **What's your body composition?** Your *body composition*, or the percentage of fat compared to muscle and other tissues that we just discussed, matters more than the number on your bathroom scale. Although it varies with age, healthful amounts of total body fat range from 8% to 24% for adult men; adult women should have a body fat range between 21% and 35%.[14]
- **How old are you?** Most of us gain weight as we age. It's not realistic to expect that you will always weigh what you did in high school.

- **What's going on in your life?** Extremely busy periods in our lives often make it tougher to stay at the lower range of a healthy weight.
- **How does gender factor in?** As we discuss on page 162, men and women tend to gain and store weight in different ways.
- **What's your body type?** Some of us are naturally willowy, others stocky, and others curvy. Aim to look and feel like a healthy version of yourself, not someone else.

LO 7.1 QUICK CHECK

Which of the following is true about individuals who have a tendency to store weight primarily in the hips and thighs?
  a. They are considered to have apple-shaped fat patterning.
  b. They are at increased risk for heart disease.
  c. They are at increased risk of diabetes.
  d. They are considered to have health-protective pear-shaped fat patterning.

SELF-ASSESSMENT
Assessing Your Weight-Related Health Risks

To assess your health risks related to weight, use these three key measures: BMI, waist circumference, and waist-to-hip ratio.

Determine your BMI

The formula for computing BMI is (your weight in pounds × 703)/your height in inches^2

Classification of Overweight and Obesity by BMI

	BMI	Obesity Class
Underweight	< 18.5	
Normal	18.5–24.9	
Overweight	25.0–29.9	
Obesity	30.0–34.9	I
	35.0–39.9	II
Extreme Obesity	≥ 40.0	III

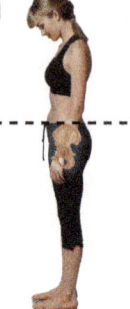

Measure your waist circumference

1. Place a tape measure around your bare abdomen, just above your hip bones (see photo).
2. Be sure that the tape is snug but not pushing into your skin.
3. Breathe out and measure the girth of your abdomen.

Calculate your waist-to-hip ratio

4. Measure your waist as described.
5. Use the same technique to measure your hips at the widest part.
6. Divide your waist measurement by your hip measurement.

Waist-to-Hip Ratio and Associated Health Risk Levels

Classification	Men	Women
Lower Risk	< 0.90	< 0.80
Moderately High Risk	0.90–1.0	0.80–0.85
High Risk	> 1.0	> 0.85

How To Interpret Your Score

- **BMI:** Calculate your BMI and check it against the BMI table. Underweight, overweight, obesity, and extreme obesity are all associated with increased health risks.
- **Waist circumference:** A waist measuring more than 35 inches in a woman or 40 inches in a man points to greater health risks.
- **Waist-to-hip ratio:** Calculate your waist-to-hip ratio and check it against the waist-to-hip ratio table. This ratio is an indicator of where you carry your excess fat. A higher ratio may mean you carry excess fat in your abdomen; a lower ratio indicates you carry more fat in your lower body.

To complete this Self-Assessment online, visit MasteringHealth™

Alarming Trends in Body Weight

LO 7.2 Describe alarming trends in weight gain.

With 2 in 3 American adults qualifying as overweight or obese, weight concerns are a major personal and public health problem. But this wasn't always the case. Rates of overweight and obesity began trending upward in the late 1980s.

Weight Trends in the United States

Over the past 35 years, adult obesity rates in the United States have doubled, and today more than two-thirds of American adults are overweight or obese. In 1990, no U.S. state had an obesity rate above 15%; today, 45 states have adult obesity rates above 25%.[15] (See **Figure 7.2**.) On average, American adults weigh 24 pounds more today than they did in 1960. Child obesity rates more than tripled between 1980 and 2002, and currently almost a third of children are overweight or obese. In the past few years, obesity rates have leveled off among all girls, but they continue to rise among men and boys of all ethnicities, as well as among African American and Mexican American women. Black women have the highest rate of obesity, at 56.6%, compared to a national average of 34.9%.[16]

>> A coproduction of HBO and the National Institutes of Health, the documentary *Weight of the Nation* goes in-depth into America's obesity epidemic. Stream it for free at **http://theweightofthenation.hbo.com/films**.

Weight Trends Around the World

Weight concerns are hardly confined to the United States. Globalization has spread Western eating and lifestyle habits—especially an affinity for high-fat, high-sugar foods and a decline in physical activity—worldwide. International health experts are now tackling overweight and obesity as global problems.

Worldwide rates of obesity and overweight have increased alarmingly, rising from 857 million in 1980 to 2.1 billion in 2013. This represents a 28% increase among adults and a startling 47% increase among children since 1980.[17] Obesity rates have grown threefold since 1980 in parts of Europe, the Middle East, the Pacific Islands, Australia, New Zealand, and China.[2] In 2013, more than 60% of the world's obese people lived in developing countries.[17] Ironically, problems of obesity and malnutrition often coexist in some developing countries, with richer residents seeing rapid weight gains even as some of their fellow citizens suffer from a lack of adequate nutrition.

As in the United States, an increase in chronic disease is following this rise in weight. Countries such as India and China, which once had relatively low rates of heart disease and diabetes, are already seeing significant increases in these conditions. In 2010, heart disease emerged as the top cause of death and disability worldwide; just 20 years earlier, it was the fourth-leading cause.[18]

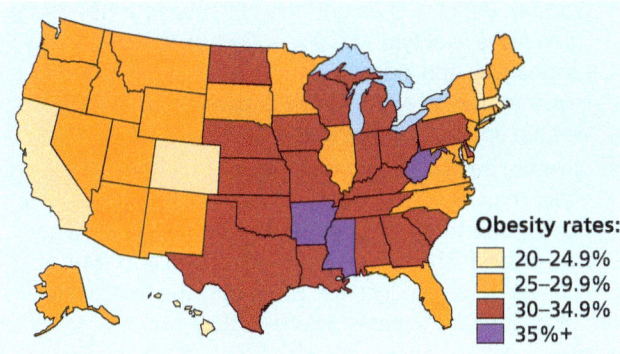

FIGURE 7.2 **Obesity in the United States, 2014.**
Source: Data from Levi, J., Segal, L. M., Rayburn, J., & Martin, A. (2015). *The state of obesity 2015.* http://stateofobesity.org.

Weight Trends on Campus

Most first-year students gain some weight once they start college—usually about 7 to 8 pounds[19] rather than the "freshman 15" you've probably heard about. This weight often doesn't disappear once the first year is over. Instead, many students gain a few more pounds each year of college. In one study that tracked a group of male and female students over their four years in college, about 70% gained weight (almost 12 pounds on average) between freshman year and graduation, and the percentage qualifying as overweight or obese climbed from 18% to 31%.[20] Male students experienced weight gain more often: About 42.9% of them qualified as overweight/obese, compared with about 37.9% of female students. About 50% of college students said they were trying to lose weight.[4]

What's the big culprit behind campus weight gain? While excess calories clearly contribute, a decline in physical activity also appears to be a major factor. Female students, for example, often find that their level of physical activity drops substantially in college.[21] For all students, larger amounts of time spent watching television and smaller amounts of physical activity have been closely linked with excess weight.[20]

The problem is compounded by the fact that more students are starting college at heavier weights than ever before. Approximately 20.5% of American adolescents between the ages of 12 and 19 are obese, compared with a teen obesity rate of 4.6% in 1970.[1] For many, these problems start during early childhood, with 8.4% of preschoolers between ages 2 and 5 qualifying as obese.[1] Overweight children are far more likely to carry extra pounds into adulthood.[11]

LO 7.2 QUICK CHECK

Approximately how many American adults are overweight or obese?

a. 1 in 3 (33%)   c. 1 in 5 (20%)
b. 2 in 3 (66%)   d. 1 in 10 (10%)

Risks and Costs of Obesity

LO 7.3 Explain the risks and costs of obesity.

You could be tempted to think: How bad can a few extra pounds be, when so many people you know carry some? But just because weight concerns are common doesn't make them any less serious.

Health Risks

Extreme obesity shortens life expectancy by about 14 years,[22] and being overweight or obese is associated with many health problems, including:

- **Type 2 diabetes.** Type 2 diabetes is strongly associated with increased body weight. More than 85% of people with type 2 diabetes are overweight or obese.[23] Excess fat makes your cells resistant to insulin, a hormone that allows glucose to be transported out of the bloodstream and into cells. When *insulin resistance* develops, glucose stays in the bloodstream, leaving cells depleted of energy and causing damage to blood vessels throughout the body.

- **Abnormal levels of blood lipids.** Obesity is associated with low blood levels of HDL cholesterol ("good" cholesterol) and high levels of LDL cholesterol ("bad" cholesterol) and triglycerides. Over time, abnormal blood lipids can contribute to *atherosclerosis*—an accumulation of deposits on the lining of blood vessels that narrows them and impedes blood flow. Atherosclerosis puts a person at risk for coronary heart disease and stroke. With increasing weight, there is a 9% to 18% increase in the prevalence of abnormal blood lipids.[24]

- **Coronary heart disease (also called coronary artery disease).** This disease results from atherosclerosis in arteries that supply the heart. The narrowed arteries reduce the amount of blood that flows to the heart. Diminished blood flow to the heart can cause chest pain (*angina*). Complete blockage can lead to a heart attack.

- **Stroke.** Atherosclerosis occurs in arteries throughout the body, including those that feed the brain. A stroke occurs when an artery supplying a region of the brain either becomes completely blocked or ruptures. In either case, brain tissue in that region is deprived of blood, and the functions controlled by it cease. Being obese raises your risk for having a stroke.

- **High blood pressure (hypertension).** High blood pressure is twice as common in obese adults because

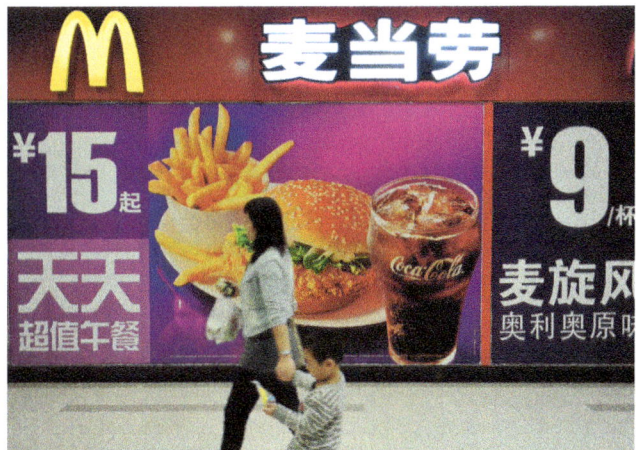

As developing countries adopt more Westernized diets, their **rates of overweight and obesity** are increasing.

CHAPTER 7 ■ Body Image, Body Weight

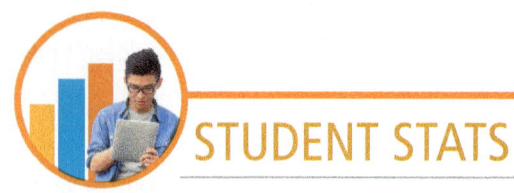

STUDENT STATS

Overweight, Obesity, and Dieting on Campus

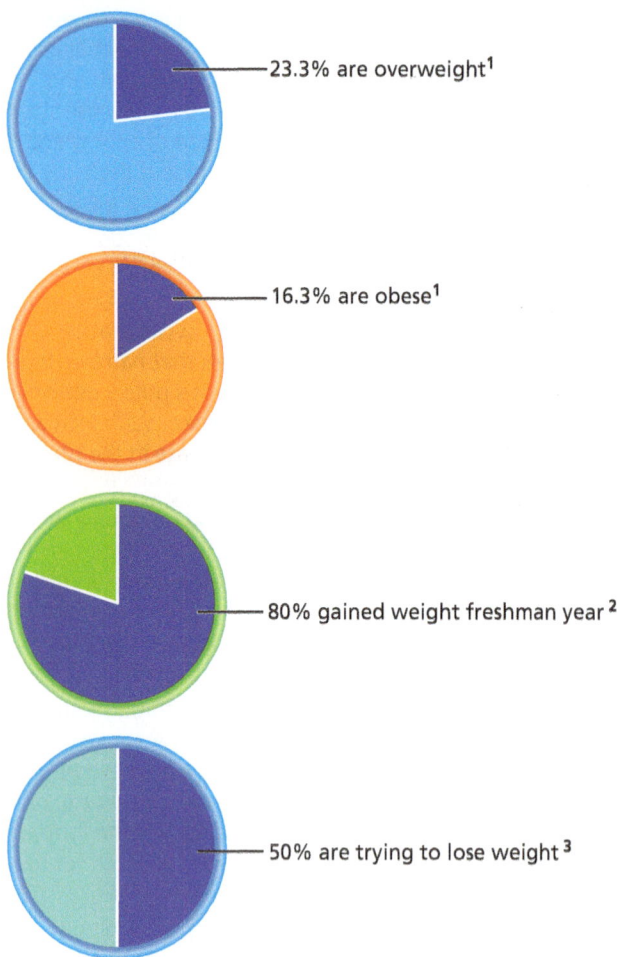

- 23.3% are overweight[1]
- 16.3% are obese[1]
- 80% gained weight freshman year[2]
- 50% are trying to lose weight[3]

References: **1.** American College Health Association. (2015). *ACHA-NCHA II: Undergraduate reference group executive summary, fall 2015.* www.acha-ncha.org. **2.** Bondenlos, J. S., Gengarelly, K., & Smith, R. (2015). Gender differences in freshmen weight gain. *Eating Behaviors, 19,* 1–4.

metabolic syndrome A group of obesity-related factors that increase the risk of cardiovascular disease and diabetes, including large waistline, high triglycerides, low HDL cholesterol, high blood pressure, and high fasting blood glucose.

they have increased blood volume, higher heart rates, and blood vessels with a reduced capacity to transport blood.

- **Metabolic syndrome and increased cardiometabolic risk.** A group of obesity-related risk factors for cardiovascular disease and diabetes is referred to as **metabolic syndrome,** and an expanded group of risk factors is referred to as *cardiometabolic risk.* They include, for example, a waist measurement of 40 inches or more for men and 35 inches or more for women. (We discuss metabolic syndrome and cardiometabolic risk in Chapter 13.)

- **Cancer.** Being overweight may increase your risk for developing several types of cancer, including colon, rectal, esophageal, and kidney cancers. Excess weight is also linked to uterine and postmenopausal breast cancer in women and prostate cancer in men.
- **Osteoarthritis.** This joint disorder most often affects the knees, hips, and lower back. Excess weight places extra pressure on these joints and wears away the cartilage that protects them, resulting in joint pain and stiffness. For every 2-pound increase in weight, the risk for developing arthritis increases 9% to 13%.
- **Sleep apnea.** Sleep apnea causes a person to stop breathing for short periods during sleep. A person who has sleep apnea may suffer from daytime sleepiness, difficulty concentrating, and even heart failure. The risk for sleep apnea is higher for people who are overweight.
- **Gallbladder disease.** The gallbladder is a small sac that stores bile from the liver and secretes it into the small intestine to break apart dietary fats. Gallbladder disease includes inflammation or infection as well as the formation of gallstones (solid clusters formed mostly of cholesterol). Overweight people may produce excessive cholesterol and/or may have an enlarged gallbladder that may not work properly.
- **Fatty liver disease.** The level of stored fat often increases in the livers of overweight and obese people. When fat builds up in liver cells, it can cause injury and inflammation, leading to severe liver damage, *cirrhosis* (scar tissue that blocks proper blood flow to the liver), or even liver failure.
- **Pregnancy complications.** Pregnant women who are overweight or obese raise their risk of pregnancy complications for both themselves and their child. These women are more likely to develop insulin resistance, high blood glucose, and high blood pressure. The risks associated with surgery, anesthesia, and blood loss also are increased in obese pregnant women.

Excess weight is also linked to physical discomfort, social and emotional troubles, and (in the case of obesity) lower overall life expectancy. A long-term study conducted by Oxford University found that life expectancy of severely obese individuals may be reduced by 3 to 10 years.[25] **Figure 7.3** summarizes some of the major health risks associated with overweight and obesity.

Financial Burden of Obesity

Experts estimate that overweight and obesity cost the United States about $270 billion a year in health-care costs and lost productivity.[26] Annual costs for obesity-related illnesses are an estimated $190.2 billion, which is 21% of annual medical spending in the United States.[27]

The individual costs are high as well—especially for women. In a study of the personal costs of obesity, researchers found that it costs an obese woman about $4,870 more per year to live in the United States compared with a woman of healthy weight, and it costs an obese man about $2,646 more per year than a healthy-weight man.[28] Some of these costs are medical, such as for doctor's visits and medications. Others are work related, pertaining to wages and missed work days. And

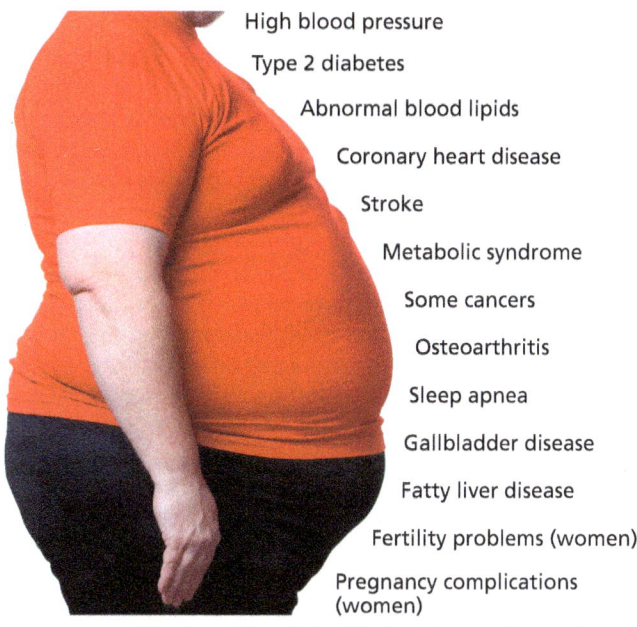

FIGURE 7.3 **Major Health Risks Associated with Overweight and Obesity.**

some are personal, such as for transportation and life insurance premiums.

LO 7.3 QUICK CHECK

All of the following except _____ are diseases associated with overweight/obesity.
a. coronary heart disease
b. stroke
c. cancer
d. Parkinson's disease

Factors that Contribute to Weight Gain

LO 7.4 Identify factors that contribute to weight gain.

The number on the bathroom scale rises or falls because of a simple concept: **energy balance.** The calories in the foods and beverages you consume are a form of "energy in." Your body uses this energy to perform all of its activities, from breathing and circulation to studying and exercising. Think of these activities as "energy out." If, over time, the calories you consume match the calories you expend, then you are in energy balance, and your weight will not change. If you take in fewer calories than you use, you'll lose weight. Take in more calories than you use, and you'll gain weight **(Figure 7.4).**

energy balance The state achieved when energy consumed from food is equal to energy expended, maintaining body weight.

basal metabolic rate (BMR) The rate at which the body expends energy for only the basic functioning of vital organs.

But while excess weight ultimately results from an energy intake in excess of energy used, many factors influence how that equation plays out in each of us. We discuss these factors next, starting with those that are less controllable.

Biology and Genetics

Why does it seem as if some people can eat whatever they want all day long and not gain a pound, while others who monitor every mouthful just keep watching the scale go up? This is partly due to misperceptions; for instance, some people fail to count snacks that add up during the day. But it also occurs because factors unique to us as individuals affect our energy needs.

Differences in Basal Metabolism

About two-thirds of the energy a person needs each day goes toward *basal metabolism*—that is, the body's maintenance of basic physiological processes (like keeping vital organs functioning) when at complete digestive, physical, and emotional rest. The remainder of energy a person uses is for food digestion, adjusting to environmental changes (such as temperature changes), stress, and physical activity.

The rate at which basal metabolism occurs in an individual is his or her **basal metabolic rate (BMR).** A similar

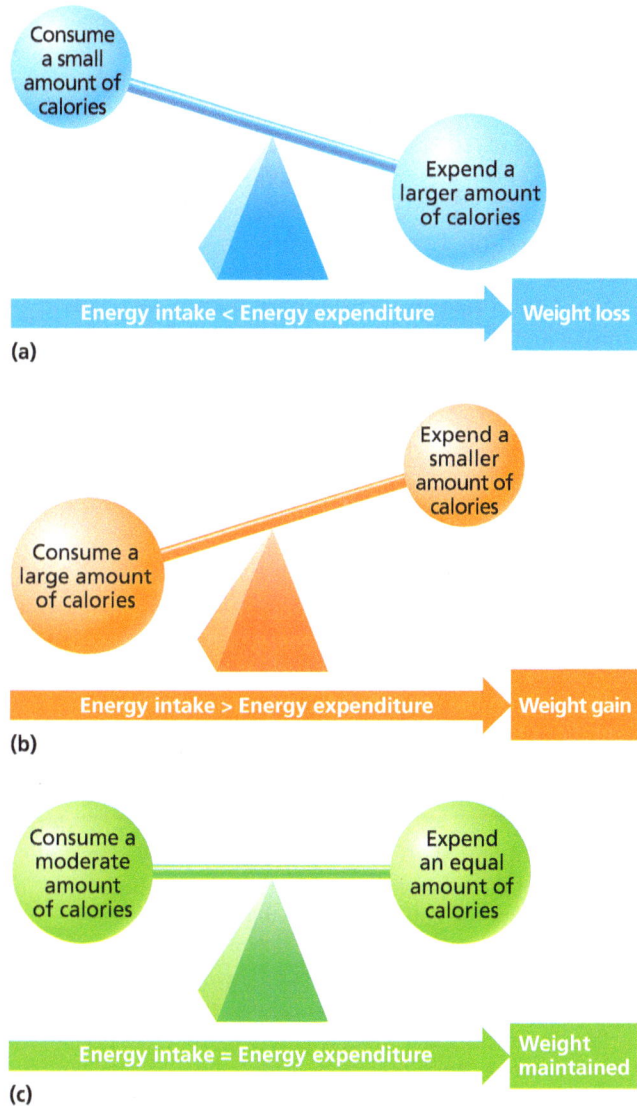

FIGURE 7.4 **Energy Balance.** Energy balance is attained when the calories you consume equal the calories you expend.

Source: Thompson, J., & Manore, M. (2014). *Nutrition: An applied approach*, 4th ed. Reprinted and electronically reproduced by permission of Pearson Education, Inc., Upper Saddle River, New Jersey.

measure of energy output, called *resting metabolic rate* (*RMR*), is measured when a person is awake and resting quietly. BMR and RMR may vary greatly from person to person and may vary for the same person with a change in circumstance or physical condition. In general, BMR and RMR are highest in people who are growing (children, adolescents, pregnant women), are tall (greater surface area = more heat loss = more calories burned), and have more lean body mass (physically fit people and males).

Regular physical activity can build your muscles, a component of your lean body mass. If you increase your physical activity from light to moderate or heavy, you will burn more energy through exercise while increasing your BMR; together these factors can contribute greatly to weight loss.

Age

As people age, they tend to become less active and lose muscle mass. Because of this, BMR declines about 2% for each decade.[29] This reduced energy expenditure in turn reduces calorie needs. However, older adults who remain active can avoid gaining weight as they age. Aerobics, strength training, and flexibility exercises are all recommended.

Sex and Gender Differences

Men and women each have unique factors that contribute to weight gain. Men may be more likely than women to consume high-calorie diets in response to social expectations. "Real men," according to the stereotype, eat ribs, not salad. In one study of college students, male students were less interested in making careful food choices because healthy eating was more a female concern.[30] Furthermore, in a study of more than 300,000 adults, men were more likely to underestimate their weight than women. When asked to predict which of five weight categories they would fall into, 23% of the men (compared to 8% of women) guessed their weight range as being one category healthier than it actually was.[31] So men may be underestimating their weight and minimizing their obesity risk. However, preventing weight gain is just as important in men as in women, if not more so; men are more likely to store fat in their abdomens, which, as discussed earlier, confers greater health risks, such as heart disease.[32,33]

Women, on the other hand, have unique health considerations that increase their risk of excess weight. Female hormones play an important role in fat storage.[34] Women's bodies need adequate fat for the production of female reproductive hormones, and women naturally keep body fat stores in reserve for pregnancy and breast-feeding. As evidence of this, it is not uncommon for women with inadequate body fat to cease menstruating. Because women are typically smaller and tend to have a higher percentage of body fat than men, and body fat burns less energy than lean tissue, women, on average, need fewer calories than men do.

Life cycle factors also affect women's weight more drastically than men's. While pregnancy leads to necessary weight gain, many women find that the extra pounds are difficult to lose afterward. In addition, between puberty and menopause, women are more likely to store body fat in their hips and thighs, but after menopause, fat storage patterns begin to more closely resemble men's, with fat storage shifting to the abdominal area, increasing the risk of conditions such as heart disease.

Genetics

Overweight and obesity often run in families. If one or both of your parents are overweight or obese, your chances of being overweight increase. Some of this influence may be due more to habits than genes since families tend to share eating and exercise patterns (whether the habits are healthful or unhealthful). However, studies have shown that genes, too, can affect the tendency to gain weight, how much fat a person stores, and where he or she carries excess weight. Scientists are studying specific genes, such as a certain variation of a gene that is related to fat mass and obesity, known as FTO. FTO appears to increase a person's risk of obesity by 30% to 70%, depending on the specific variety of FTO and how many copies of that obesity-linked variation a person carries.[35] Most experts agree that the most significant role genes play in obesity is in programming an individual to respond to our current environment of excess food consumption coupled with inactivity. Some individuals respond by storing more energy as fat in an environment of excess, while others lose less fat in an environment of scarcity (such as when dieting). Genetic variation between individuals appears to be what influence these different responses.[36]

Race and Ethnicity

Overweight and obesity disproportionately affect certain racial and ethnic groups. Overweight and obesity are problems for[16]

- 76.2% of African Americans
- 81% of Native Americans/Alaskan Natives
- 78% of Hispanic Americans
- 67.2% of Caucasian Americans
- 48.6% of Asian Americans

The reasons for these disparities are complex. Factors may include cultural differences in diet and exercise, socioeconomic differences in patterns of food consumption, inequalities in access to nutritious food, inequalities in access to education about nutrition and fitness, and genetic differences.

The disparities occur in more than just body weight. One study of *central obesity*, or excessive fat concentrated in the abdomen, found that while levels of abdominal fat have increased for Caucasian Americans, African Americans, and Mexican Americans since 1900, African American women have seen the largest shifts.[37] If patterns of central obesity increases continue, the researchers estimate that by 2020, about 71% of African American women would qualify as having central obesity and would be likely to face the increased health risks it confers.

Health History

Certain health issues or medications may trigger weight gain. In some cases, weight gain may reflect hormonal imbalances triggered by an underactive thyroid. In this condition, called hypothyroidism, the thyroid gland fails to make enough thyroid hormone, which leads to a variety of symptoms, including excess weight, fatigue, and being more sensitive to cold. If you have concerns about your thyroid, your doctor can check your thyroid hormone levels with a simple blood test.

Recent studies suggest that antibiotics received in infancy[38] as well as long-term exposure to antibiotics from meat products[39] can contribute to weight gain in adults by causing a long-term increase in a type of bacteria in the gut that extract additional calories from food. These additional extracted calories that aren't used are stored as fat.

Individual Behaviors

Although factors such as biology and genetics are important considerations in an individual's weight, they cannot alone explain the dramatic surge in weight gain seen worldwide in recent decades. Personal choices related to diet and physical activity clearly have had a major effect.

Increased Calorie Consumption

The average American today consumes about 570 more calories per day than in 1977.[40] Many of these increased calories are in the form of fats and sugar: By 2005, total added fats and oils available for consumption in the U.S. diet reached 86 pounds per person, compared with 53 pounds per person in 1970, and total sugars and sweeteners reached 142 pounds per person, compared with about 120 pounds in 1970.[41] Our diets are especially high in saturated fats (fried foods, fatty meats, cheeses), added sugars (especially in soft drinks, many breakfast cereals, and desserts), and refined grains (pasta, white bread, flour tortillas).

Did you grab a snack before sitting down to study this chapter? If so, what did you choose? Even seemingly small decisions about what and how much you eat can significantly increase your calorie consumption over time. The **Practical Strategies** box on page 169 lists several helpful choices to try.

Large portion sizes and dining away from home also increase calorie intake. Across the board, portion sizes have ballooned. Servings of fast foods and soft drinks, for example, often are two to five times larger now than when they were introduced.[42] For example, in 1954, a serving of McDonald's French fries weighed 2.4 ounces and contained 210 calories. By 2015 the fries had reached 5.9 ounces and 510 calories.[42,43]

>> Take the Portion Distortion Quiz to see how increasing portion sizes piles on the calories at **www.nhlbi.nih.gov**. (Search for "portion distortion.")

Lack of Physical Activity

Fewer than 1 in 3 Americans gets the recommended minimum of 30 minutes of moderate activity a day most days of the week. In fact, one-third of Americans over the age of 18 do not engage in any leisure-time physical activity at all, and that percentage climbs steadily with age.[44] About 25% of those between the ages of 18 and 24 get no leisure-time physical activity, and among those 65 or older, that number jumps to 49%.[45]

Many people now earn their living while sitting for hours. In 1860, the average workweek was 70 hours of heavy physical labor, compared with 40 hours of sedentary work today. The least physically active groups are older adolescents and adults over 60 years old who spend about 60% of their waking time in sedentary pursuits.[45] Americans also spend approximately 60 hours per week on average in front of a screen (television, computer, tablet, video, smart phone).[46]

Coupled with the fact that Americans typically spend almost an hour a day commuting to and from work, little time is left in the day for physical activity.[47] With less physical activity, lean body mass decreases, and fat takes its place.

STUDENT STORY

Active Loser

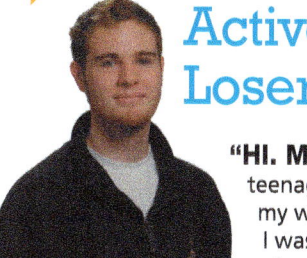

"**HI. MY NAME IS JOSH.** As a teenager, I often struggled with my weight. When I was 14 or 15 I was overweight, and I felt really down about myself and had low self-esteem. So, in an effort to lose weight and to get more healthy, I started looking for activities that I enjoyed and I found basketball and I found running. And through these activities, I started gradually losing weight, and I stuck to it. And so, if I could suggest anything for losing weight, I'd say find an activity that you like and which you can motivate yourself to do."

What Do You Think?

1. What side of the energy balance equation did Josh change to lose weight: energy in or energy out?
2. Do you think it really matters that Josh likes the activities he's doing, or will any activity work to lose weight?
3. What activities do you like that you could use to lose weight?

Social Factors

Many social factors in our everyday lives encourage behaviors that run counter to healthful weight management:

- Long work and school days, combined with commuting, leave many people little time for staying healthy. A study of college students found that those with a drive time of 16 minutes or more were 64% more likely than those with a shorter commute to be overweight or obese.[48]
- Some people reach for food as comfort in times of stress. One study found that the stresses of everyday life often trigger the urge to eat, and many people favor less healthful food options.[49]
- The fast food so many of us go for could be more aptly named "fat food." Most popular fast food choices are stuffed with calories and saturated fat.[43]

While these social factors affect all aspects of American society, they play an especially acute role for those facing the greatest economic challenges. In what researchers sometimes call the "food insecurity–obesity paradox," individuals and families of lower socioeconomic status are often at the greatest risk for obesity. A complex web of factors appears to underlie this paradox, including limited ability to access and purchase healthful foods, fewer opportunities for physical activity, and high levels of stress. Also influential are cycles of food deprivation and overeating, in which lack of food at some points leads to overeating and weight gain at others.[50] Many nutrition experts now push for food assistance programs that provide healthy nutrition choices and promote physical activity rather than simply providing adequate calories.[51]

Physical Factors

Look at the built environment, and you'll likely see examples of how we have literally helped construct the obesity epidemic. Health experts now describe many of our built areas as "obesogenic environments," meaning that they are spaces that promote obesity. Here are just a few examples:

- Many neighborhoods lack sidewalks, resulting in more driving and less walking. Protected bike routes are rare in many communities.
- In some neighborhoods, supermarkets are scarce, leaving residents to rely on smaller stores that rarely carry healthful choices such as fresh fruits and vegetables. In many such neighborhoods, fast food is often the most available restaurant option.
- Many people don't have ready access to gyms or other opportunities for physical activity and recreation. Paradoxically, those at greatest risk for obesity often have the least access. One group of researchers found that when they built a playground and a walking path in a lower-income neighborhood, the proportion of residents observed being active increased significantly, indicating that even relatively simple improvements to the built environment can carry important benefits.[52]

Public Policy

Laws, regulations, and federally sponsored promotional programs around food also affect our nutritional environment, perhaps not always for the better. While public health officials now pour substantial money and attention into understanding and addressing the obesity epidemic, critics argue that other agencies create policies that make obesity more likely, sometimes by promoting the consumption of foods higher in fat and calories over those that are less calorie dense. According to one group's research, more than 60% of recent agricultural subsidies have directly and indirectly supported meat and dairy production, while less than 1% have gone to fruits and vegetables.[53]

Congress recently passed the Healthy Hunger-Free Kids Act, which requires schools to include more fruits, vegetables, and whole grains in meals. Unfortunately, while students may be eating better at school, they are moving less. The CDC recommends that children and adolescents participate in 60 minutes of daily physical activity, with a substantial percentage being provided by school physical education class. However, nearly half of students across the nation reported that they had no PE classes in an average week.[54]

LO 7.4 QUICK CHECK ✓

According to the "energy equation," when the calories you consume equal the calories you use, you

a. gain weight.
b. lose weight.
c. achieve an obesogenic environment.
d. achieve energy balance.

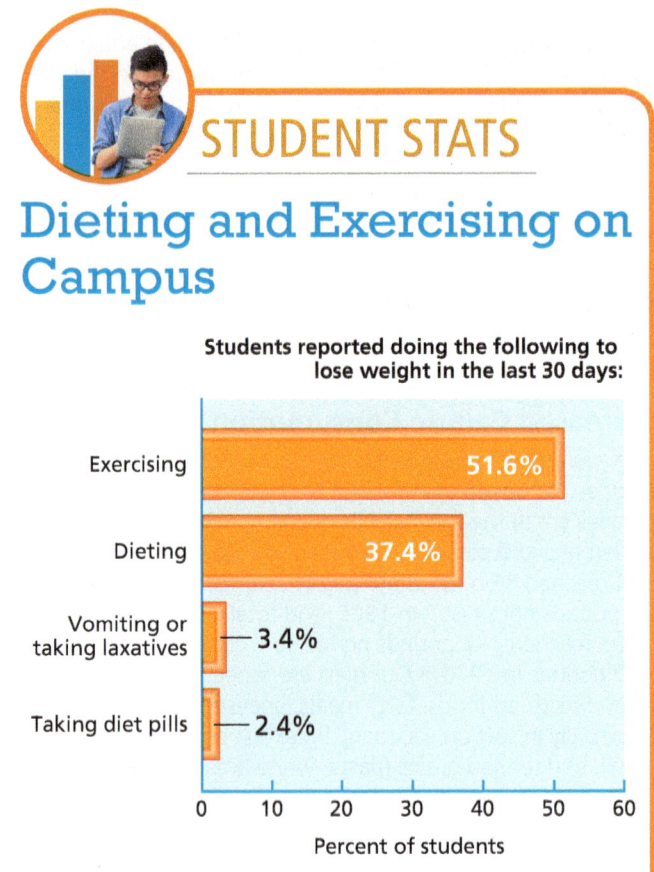

STUDENT STATS

Dieting and Exercising on Campus

Students reported doing the following to lose weight in the last 30 days:

- Exercising: 51.6%
- Dieting: 37.4%
- Vomiting or taking laxatives: 3.4%
- Taking diet pills: 2.4%

Source: 2015 data from American College Health Association. (2015). *ACHA-NCHA II: Undergraduate reference group executive summary, fall 2015.* www.acha-ncha.org.

Reducing Excess Body Weight

LO 7.5 Explain how to reduce excess body weight.

For most people, the key to healthful weight management lies in the ability to ensure that less energy is coming in and more energy is going out. This requires consistent work. Losing weight doesn't have to mean depriving yourself. But it does mean eating wisely and changing your lifestyle to be as physically active as possible.

Some of us practice successful weight management on our own. But many of us benefit from some support, whether that help comes from a friend, a trainer, a counselor, a formal program, or a doctor.

Can Dieting Work?

Hunger is the physiological sensation caused by a lack of food. Hunger is triggered in our brains, as a response to signals sent by the digestive tract and hormones circulating in our blood. Hunger is different from **appetite,** the psychological response to the sight, smell, thought, or taste of food that prompts or postpones eating. Appetite can prove helpful, stimulating you to eat before you get too hungry. It can also

> **hunger** The physiological sensation caused by the lack of food.
>
> **appetite** The psychological response to the sight, smell, thought, or taste of food that prompts or postpones eating.

satiety Physical fullness; the state in which there is no longer the desire to eat.

satiety helps turn off the desire to eat more.

Given that both hunger and appetite compel us to eat, can dieting work? Weight-loss diets can be helpful for some people, especially those who like the support of a structured plan or program. However, dieting is a slow, steady process. You can't achieve healthful or permanent weight loss by starving yourself for a week. Diets also work best prove harmful, steering you toward too much food or toward tempting but unhealthful food choices. When we've eaten and relieved or prevented hunger, a feeling called if they are accompanied by regular exercise. To keep the weight off, successful dieters must work to make their new eating and exercise habits into a way of life that they can sustain long term.

Millions of Americans follow weight-loss diets **(Table 7.1)**. In a year-long study that compared four popular diets—Atkins, Ornish, The Zone, and Weight Watchers—roughly half the participants lost an average of 7 pounds and improved some of their health indicators, such as heart disease risk.[55] But in a pattern familiar to many dieters, the other half of the study's participants dropped out.

TABLE 7.1 Popular Diets

Name	Description	Foods to Eat	Foods to Avoid	Practicality	Analysis
Atkins Diet	Claims that eating too many carbohydrates causes obesity and other health problems. Emphasizes the consumption of protein and fat over carbohydrates.	Meat, fish, poultry, eggs, cheese, low-carb vegetables, butter, oil	Carbohydrates, specifically bread, pasta, most fruits and vegetables, milk, alcohol	Difficult to eat in restaurants because only plain protein sources and limited vegetables or salads are allowed. Difficult to maintain long term because of limited food choices. Focus on meat and dairy can get expensive.	The composition of a sample menu is 8% carbohydrate, 56% fat, and 35% protein. Initial weight loss is mostly water. Does not promote a positive attitude toward food groups. Eliminates virtually all carbohydrate foods. May encourage overly high fat consumption.
Eat Right for Your Type	Claims that blood type is the key to your immune system, which determines your diet and supplementation.	Varies based on blood type	Varies based on blood type	Promotes some foods, such as dairy and wheat, even if individuals experience intolerances for those foods, potentially leading to gastrointestinal discomfort and other health problems.	This diet has no scientific basis. People may use this diet to attempt to fight cancer, asthma, infections, diabetes, arthritis, hypertension, and infertility, but there is no evidence that it is effective.
Jenny Craig	This program's philosophy for successful weight loss is (1) a healthful relationship with food, (2) an active lifestyle, and (3) a balanced approach to living. Dieters are required to have a 15-minute personal consultation weekly with Jenny Craig "counselors" (who lack formal nutrition/behavior training). A variety of online support tools are also available to strengthen dieters' motivation.	Promotes Jenny Craig–brand packaged meals, snacks, and supplements. Fruits, vegetables, and nonfat dairy foods are limited per Jenny Craig's 28-day menu planner. Vegetarian choices are available.	"Homemade" meals, commercial items (except those carrying the Jenny Craig label), sweets, and other foods that are not listed on Jenny Craig's 28-day menu planner	Eating packaged meals long term may be difficult and not realistic.	The targeted composition of the 1,200- to 1,500-calorie menus is 60% carbohydrate, 20% fat, and 20% protein. Packaged meals are not conducive to teaching dieters how to shop, cook, and eat their own healthful, calorie-controlled meals. Many meal options contain more than recommended levels of sodium. The cost of purchasing required ready-made meals can be expensive.
Slim-Fast	This program promotes Slim-Fast products as staples of breakfast and noon meals; evening meal is 500 calories and nutritionally balanced. Portion control, avoidance of sugary and fatty foods, and frequent water consumption are encouraged. Dieters are expected to track food intake, physical activity, and weight changes via online Slim-Fast tools.	Promotes 3–5 servings of fruits and vegetables daily. Promotes Slim-Fast products, vegetables, fruits, whole grains, salad, lean proteins, low-fat cheese, water, and other non-calorie beverages. Snacks of 120 calories or fewer are allowed.	Regular candy, cookies, and other sweets, fried or other high-fat foods, some dairy products and snack items	Buying meal-replacement bars and shakes for breakfast and lunch meal replacement becomes expensive over time.	The targeted composition of the 1,200- to 1,800-calorie menus is 63% carbohydrate, 15% fat, and 22% protein. The "sensible" evening meal is the most educational component of the plan because it teaches dieters about appropriate portions of a moderate-calorie meal. Dieters are expected to purchase Slim-Fast products for their breakfast and lunch meals. This requirement leads to dieters' "burnout" and limits individuals' ability to select healthful, traditional foods.

(continued)

TABLE 7.1 Popular Diets (continued)

Name	Description	Foods to Eat	Foods to Avoid	Practicality	Analysis
South Beach Diet	This diet advocates the intake of "good" fats and "good" carbohydrates for cardiac protection, improved nutrition, and the management of hunger, insulin resistance, and weight control. The diet is divided into three phases. Three meals plus two snacks are the eating pattern for all phases of the diet.	Mostly healthful foods are consumed. Lean proteins, some fruits, vegetables, and oils are the staples of this diet. Initially: seafood, chicken breast, lean meat, low-fat cheese, most vegetables, nuts, and oils are promoted. Later: whole grains, most fruits, low-fat milk or yogurt, and beans are promoted.	Refined carbohydrates and added sugars, fatty meats, full-fat cheese, refined grains, sweets, juice, potatoes	Phase I of the diet is restrictive and may be difficult to complete. Phase II includes more foods, and Phase III is maintenance. While the diet includes many recommended recipes, the focus on meat and cheese can make the diet's recipes costly to follow.	The composition of a sample menu from Phase I of the plan is 42% carbohydrate, 43% fat, and 15% protein. Research to support this diet and its long-term effectiveness is very limited. The two short-term studies that were completed had a small sample size and were funded by South Beach Diet affiliates.
Volumetrics	The Volumetrics eating plan focuses on enhancing the feeling of fullness while simultaneously consuming fewer calories. The diet aims to maximize the amount of food available per calorie. Foods are assigned to one of four categories based on their energy (calorie) density. Category 1 foods can be enjoyed on a daily basis; Category 4 foods are portion controlled and consumed on an occasional basis.	Focuses on fiber-rich foods with high moisture content. Fruits, vegetables, whole grain pasta, rice, breads and cereals, soups, salads, low-fat poultry, seafood, meats, and dairy are promoted. Moderate amounts of sugar and alcohol are permitted, too.	No foods are forbidden, but limiting fatty foods like deep-fat-fried items, sweets, and fats added at the table is recommended. Limited amount of dry foods (crackers, popcorn, pretzels, etc.) due to their high caloric value and low satiety index.	The large amount of fiber-rich foods recommended for meals and snacks may cause gastrointestinal distress for some dieters. The diet also requires that substantial amounts of time be dedicated to food preparation, which may not work for all dieters.	The composition of the diet is ≥ 55% carbohydrate, 20% to 30% fat, and 15% to 35% protein. Fiber intake is 25 to 38 grams/day. This is a sensible and nutritionally balanced eating plan developed by a nutrition researcher.
Weight Watchers	A program that uses weekly meetings, weigh-ins, and online tracking for motivation and behavioral support for diet and exercise changes. Clients follow a point system that they can track either manually or online.	Theoretically, all foods are allowed. Fruits, vegetables, whole grains, lean protein, low-fat or nonfat dairy, and 2 teaspoons of healthful oils are staples of the program.	Although there are no "forbidden" foods, limiting intake of foods high in saturated and *trans* fats, sugar, and alcohol is emphasized.	Weekly Weight Watchers meetings have been shown to significantly strengthen participants' weight-loss successes. If a dieter is unable to attend weekly meetings, his or her results could be impacted. When clients reach and maintain their target weights, they are allowed to attend meetings for free.	The composition of the diet plan is 50% to 60% carbohydrate, 25% fat, and 15% to 25% protein. No research supports the program's effectiveness, but its sensible advice is used and supported by millions, including nutrition experts.

Source: Based on "Best Diets Overall," by *U.S. News and World Report*, January 2013; "Nutrition Fact Sheets: Fad Diets," by the Northwestern University Feinberg School of Medicine website, January 2007; and "Top Diets Reviewed," by Consumer Reports website, June 2007.

Comparing Diets

Three common dieting approaches are low-calorie diets, low-fat diets, and low-carbohydrate diets.

Low-Calorie Diets

Cutting 500 to 1,000 calories a day typically leads to a loss of 1 or 2 pounds a week. (**Figure 7.5** shows a healthful way to reduce the calories in a daily diet.) But a low-calorie diet is rarely a simple matter of food math. Without a healthful eating plan in place, abruptly restricting one's daily calorie intake below recommended levels can be dangerous and deprive you of the energy you need for daily activities. You may find yourself withholding calories all day, only to lunge for a double cheeseburger at night.

>> *Frontline: Diet Wars* investigates popular diets and America's obesity problem. Search for "Frontline diet wars" at www.pbs.org.

Low-Fat Diets

Diets that focus on reducing daily fat intake are also common. Most diets aim to cut total fat intake to about 25% of calories or less. Long-term weight loss is a challenge with low-fat diets because dieters find them difficult to follow and to maintain. That said, we can all benefit from following these general fat intake guidelines:

- **Cut *trans* fats from your diet.** *Trans* fats occur naturally in meat and dairy products and are artificially created when manufacturers add hydrogen to vegetable oil—a process called hydrogenation. Consumption of *trans* fats reduces your "good cholesterol" (HDL) and raises your "bad cholesterol" (LDL), thereby increasing your risk of cardiovascular disease. Prepackaged snack and dessert foods (crackers, chips, cookies, cakes, pies, etc.) that contain partially hydrogenated oil are a significant source of *trans* fat. Food manufacturers are required to list *trans* fat content on food labels; be aware, however, that labeling regulations allow any food product with 0.5 gram of *trans* fats or less *per serving* to claim 0 grams of *trans* fats on the label. If you eat multiple servings of such foods, you may wind up consuming significant amounts of *trans* fats after all. Restaurant foods, such as French fries, may also contain *trans* fats and do not carry labeling requirements.[56] However, in 2015 the U.S. Food and Drug Administration (FDA) determined that partially

Higher-Calorie Diet (about 3,300 calories/day)		Lower-Calorie Diet (about 1,700 calories/day)	
Breakfast: 1½ C. Fruit Loops cereal 1 C. 2% milk 1 C. orange juice 2 slices white toast 1 Tbsp. butter (on toast)	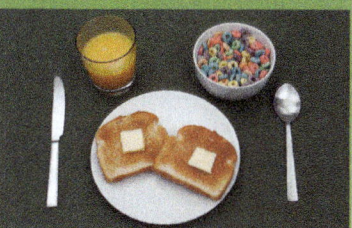	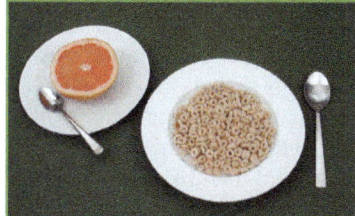	**Breakfast:** 1½ C. Cheerios cereal 1 C. skim milk ½ fresh pink grapefruit
Lunch: McDonald's Big Mac hamburger French fries, extra-large 3 Tbsp. ketchup Apple pie	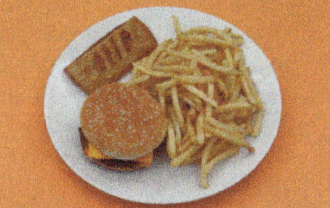	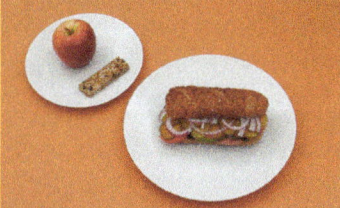	**Lunch:** Subway cold cut trio 6-inch sandwich Granola bar, hard, with chocolate chips (24 g) 1 fresh medium apple
Dinner: 4½ oz. ground beef (80% lean, crumbled), cooked 2 medium taco shells 2 oz. Cheddar cheese 2 Tbsp. sour cream 4 Tbsp. store-bought salsa 1 C. shredded lettuce ½ C. refried beans 6 Oreos	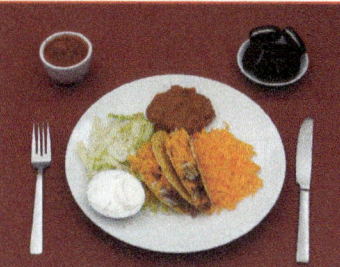	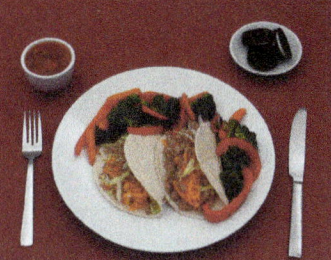	**Dinner:** 5 oz. ground turkey, cooked 2 soft corn tortillas 3 oz. low-fat Cheddar cheese 4 Tbsp. store-bought salsa 1 C. shredded lettuce 1 C. cooked mixed veggies 3 Oreos

FIGURE 7.5 **How to Cut Calories While Maintaining a Balanced Diet.** The meals on the right show healthful alternatives to the higher-calorie meals on the left.

Source: Thompson, J., & Manore, M. (2014). *Nutrition: An applied approach*, 4th ed. Reprinted and electronically reproduced by permission of Pearson Education, Inc., Upper Saddle River, New Jersey.

hydrogenated oils that contain artificially produced *trans* fat are not safe and should not be used as food additives.[57] This determination will further reduce the availability, and therefore the consumption, of *trans* fats in the U.S.

- **Consume more "good" fats.** Fats found in plant oils, nuts, seeds, and fish should make up the majority of fats in your diet.

Low-Carbohydrate Diets

First popularized by Dr. Robert Atkins, low-carbohydrate diets propose greatly reducing sugar and starch intake and increasing intake of lean protein. Recent studies have supported the earlier claims that low-carbohydrate diets may be effective for weight loss. This may be due in part to the fact that dieters expend less energy metabolizing high-carbohydrate foods than when eating exactly the same number of calories in fats or proteins.[58] Furthermore, certain high-glycemic carbohydrates (such as sugar, bread, and white potatoes) spike blood sugar levels, causing hunger, cravings, and, ultimately, overeating.

Most nutrition experts agree that Americans eat too many refined carbohydrates, especially from added sugars. But fiber-rich carbohydrates—including fruits, legumes and other vegetables, and whole grains—are nutritious foods that your body needs. Try these guidelines:

- **Choose fiber-rich carbohydrates.** Choose carbohydrates found in whole grains, fruits, and vegetables and avoid refined carbohydrates found in commercial baked goods, soft drinks, and candy.
- **Watch your total calories.** To lose weight, you need to consume fewer calories than you expend, regardless of whether those calories are carbohydrates, fats, or proteins.
- **When choosing protein-rich foods, look for leaner options.** Fish, skinless chicken breasts, or rump, round, flank, and loin cuts of meat are choices lower in saturated fats. Better yet, choose plant proteins, which provide healthful unsaturated fats and are high in fiber and micronutrients.

Diet "Aids"?

Walk into most grocery or health food stores, and you'll find a variety of foods, drinks, and pills claiming to help you lose weight. It's worth considering these products carefully before getting out your wallet.

It's easy, for example, to find numerous high-protein energy bars or protein drinks that claim to help with weight loss. But many of these products are high in empty calories from added sugars. In addition, high-protein food items are not necessary for weight loss; maintaining energy balance, rather than high levels of a particular nutrient, is the most important factor over the long term.

Diet pills claim to help with weight loss in a variety of ways, from tricking your body into thinking it's full to regulating hormones that affect your desire to eat. Although many diet pills have never been proven to work, manufacturers of these products do a booming business. In 2010, Americans spent $2.69 billion on over-the-counter diet aids, including pills and meal replacements such as low-calorie energy bars.[59] One study of college students found that female students who perceived themselves to have a higher BMI than they actually had were more than twice as likely to have used a diet drug.[60]

Most over-the-counter diet pills are considered dietary supplements, a category that the FDA only minimally regulates.[61] They do not need to be proven safe by the manufacturer unless they include a new ingredient, and they are not tested by the FDA until they have already gone on the market and problems have been reported. In addition, because labeling requirements remain less strict for supplements, many supplement firms downplay the risk of side effects in packaging and advertising. However, the FDA has recently reported that some over-the-counter diet aids advertised as supplements have been removed from the market for containing laxatives and unreported prescription diet, hypertension, and seizure medications or other potentially harmful drugs not approved in the United States.[62] Buyer, beware.

Only one diet aid has received full clearance from the FDA for sale as an over-the-counter weight-loss medication. Alli, a lower dose of the prescription weight-loss medication orlistat, was released to the public in 2007. This drug works by causing your body to excrete some of the fat that passes through your digestive tract, and it is intended to help you lose about 5% of your body weight over time. But its side effects, such as digestive discomfort and gas with oily spotting, can be unpleasant. Alli is also expensive, costing about $50 for a one-month supply of the pills.

>> Visit *Medline Plus* for reliable information about drugs and supplements: **www.nlm.nih.gov**. (Search for "medline plus supplements.")

Clinical Options for Obesity

In 2015, 16.3% of college students had BMIs in the obese category.[4] Because obesity is a significant health risk, your health care provider may recommend medical treatment if your BMI is 30 or higher. Options range from psychotherapy to prescription drugs to weight-loss surgery.

Psychotherapy

Psychotherapy can be a vital component of both weight-loss and weight-management programs. This is especially true for people who turn to food to reduce stress or assuage depression. Others may have significant body image issues that are most effectively addressed with the help of a therapist. Psychologists have found that both individual and group therapy can be helpful in treating obesity and related issues such as shame or a distorted view of one's own body.[63]

Prescription Drugs

The only prescription weight-loss medications approved by the FDA for short-term use are diethylpropion, phendimetrazine, and phentermine. These three medications are classified as controlled substances because they have the potential to be abused. Common side effects include headache, increased blood pressure and heart rate, nervousness, insomnia, dry mouth, and constipation.

Three prescription medications are FDA approved for long-term use by people who are significantly overweight:

- Orlistat (Xenical) stops about a third of the fat from the food you eat from being digested. On average, patients lose a modest 5 to 7 pounds after taking the drug for a year. As discussed previously, a lower-dose version, Alli, is available over the counter. Common side effects, which worsen if you eat more that 30% of you calories from fat, include stomach pain, gas, diarrhea, and leakage of oily stool. Rare cases of severe liver injury have also been reported.
- Lorcaserin (Belviq) is one of the two weight-loss drugs approved by the FDA in 2013. Phentermine-topirate (Qsymia) is the other. Belviq works by affecting the chemicals in your brain that make you feel full. Common side effects include headaches, dizziness, fatigue, dry mouth, cough, and constipation. You should not take it if you are pregnant or taking certain antidepressants.
- Phentermine-topiramate (Qsymia) is a combination of two FDA-approved drugs, phentermine and topiramate. Phentermine is an appetite suppressant similar to an amphetamine, and topiramate is an anti-seizure medication that makes you feel full. Although phentermine as a weight-loss drug has historically been approved only for 12 weeks of use, the doses in Qsymia are much lower, and patients can take the drug for an extended period. Qsymia can cause birth defects and should not be taken by those who may be pregnant, those who have glaucoma or thyroid problems, or those who are taking certain medications. Side effects are similar to those of Belviq.

Surgery

A growing number of obese people—about 200,000 each year in the United States alone—are opting for surgery to alter the sizes of their stomachs and reduce the amount of food they can ingest.[64] This type of surgery, called **bariatric surgery,** comprises several different types of procedures. One subset of procedures, known as *gastric banding,* involves partitioning off part of the stomach with a removable band. The other subset, *gastric bypass,* involves permanently reducing the size of the stomach. After either type of procedure, the reshaped stomach can hold only a limited amount of food—sometimes as little as an ounce—resulting in greatly reduced calorie intake. In more extreme types of surgery, other portions of the digestive tract are also altered to limit calorie absorption. In early 2011, the FDA approved the use of a relatively less invasive weight-loss procedure, called LAP-BAND, for those with a BMI of 30 or higher and at least one obesity-related condition.

> **bariatric surgery** Weight-loss surgery using various procedures to modify the stomach or other sections of the gastrointestinal tract in order to reduce calorie intake or absorption.

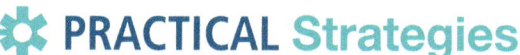

Cutting Calories, Not Nutrition

You can reduce the total number of calories you eat while boosting your intake of healthful nutrients by following these basic guidelines:

- **Shop smart.** Never shop on an empty stomach and avoid buying high-calorie foods that you'll have difficulty eating in moderate amounts.
- **Track your food intake.** Research shows that people who keep track of what they eat are more successful at losing weight. You can use a free online tracker, like the MyPlate SuperTracker (www.supertracker.usda.gov) or www.sparkpeople.com or try one of the many smart phone apps, such as *MyFitnessPal* or *Lose It*.
- **Fill your plate will lower-calorie foods.** If you fill most of your plate with vegetables alongside smaller portions of foods higher in calories, you can still have a filling, nutritious meal without busting your calorie count for the day.
- **Eat whole foods as close to their natural state as possible.** Highly processed foods are more likely to contain empty calories and less fiber.
- **Don't skip meals.** Skipping meals will only leave you overwhelmingly hungry later on and consequently more likely to overeat.
- **Avoid drastic measures.** Drastic calorie cutting causes your BMR to drop. At the same time, your feelings of hunger and deprivation make you crave food even more strongly. Sustained weight loss requires steady, gradual lifestyle change. Aiming to lose 10% of your body weight over a six-month period is a reasonable goal.
- **Drink water instead of sugary drinks filled with calories.** Approximately 20% of our total calorie consumption comes from what we drink.[1] Juices, "vitamin waters," soft drinks, and energy drinks are all extra sources of calories.
- **Use artificial sweeteners in moderation.** Artificial sweeteners are low- or no-calorie sugar substitutes. Artificial sweeteners containing aspartame (for example, Equal and NutraSweet) have been found to be safe in moderation; however, they may affect blood sugar levels and increase diabetes risk.[2] People with phenylketonuria (PKU) should avoid aspartame because it contains phenylalanine, which their bodies cannot process.
- **Change one habit at a time.** Instead of trying to overhaul all of your eating habits at once, choose one meal or snack and make small changes little by little.

References: **1.** Vartanian, L. R., Schwartz, M. B., & Brownell, K. D. (2007). Effects of soft drink consumption on nutrition and health: A systematic review and meta-analysis. *American Journal of Public Health, 97*, 667–675. **2.** Fagherazzi, G., Vilier, A., Saes Sartorelli, D., Lajous, M., Balkau, B., & Clavel-Chapelon, F. (2013). Consumption of artificially and sugar-sweetened beverages and incident type 2 diabetes in the *Etude Epidemiologique aupres des Femmes de la Mutuelle Generale de l'Education Nationale*—European Prospective Investigation into Cancer and Nutrition Cohort. *American Journal of Clinical Nutrition, 97*(3), 517–523.

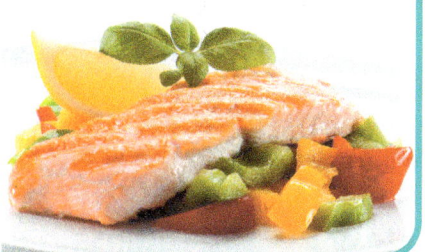

Some patients see significant weight loss and other health improvements after undergoing these procedures, such as a significant reduction in blood glucose. But others eventually regain the weight they lost, find they can no longer absorb certain nutrients properly, or experience chronic diarrhea or vomiting or other problems. Also, any major surgery involving an obese patient carries an unusually high risk for complications, such as infection and the formation of blood clots. Overall, about 1 in 200 patients dies within 90 days following the surgery.[65]

The Importance of Physical Activity

Physical activity does more than burn off calories and reduce body fat. While a particularly strenuous workout might leave you reaching for a snack, regular exercise over time appears to help reduce feelings of hunger and mediate appetite.[66] It also builds muscle, which burns more calories than fat tissue. Choose an activity you like. If you make exercise fun, weight loss will be more enjoyable!

Keep in mind the basic exercise guidelines we discussed in Chapter 6. If you are trying to maintain weight loss or lose weight, aim for 60–90 minutes of exercise each day. At least two to three times a week, some of that exercise should focus on building muscle. If you have time for nothing else, try to build a little more walking into your routine each day. It can make a significant difference in the long term.

>> Lots of free online programs that can track your diet and physical activity, such as **www.supertracker.usda.gov**, **www.sparkpeople.com**, and **www.fitday.com**.

What If You Want to Gain Weight?

If you want or need to gain weight for optimal health, you should consume more calories than you expend. Consider the following approaches:

- **Boost your calories but in healthful ways. Table 7.2** lists a healthful 3,000-calorie-per-day diet that can be used to gain weight.
- Eat smaller meals more frequently throughout the day. If you don't have much of an appetite, try eating four or five smaller meals throughout the day rather than two or three big ones.
- Add calories to your favorite meals. If you enjoy salad, for example, choose an olive oil dressing instead of a fat-free version. Add in some protein as well, such as diced chicken, cheese, avocado, or tofu.

TABLE 7.2 Healthful Weight Gain: A Sample 3,000-Calorie Diet

Meal	Food
Breakfast	1 cup Grape Nuts
	2 cup 2% milk
	1 cup cranberry juice
Snack	6 Tbsp. raisins
	1 cup orange juice
Lunch	8 oz. 2% milk
	3 oz. tuna
	2 tsp. mayonnaise
	1 bun
	Lettuce, tomatoes, sprouts
	2 oz. chips/snack food
	1 cup whole baby carrots
Snack	Met-Rx fudge brownie bar
	1 cup orange juice
Dinner	5 oz. chicken
	1 cup instant mashed potatoes with 1/3 cup 2% dry milk powder
	1 cup 2% milk
	1 Tbsp. *trans* fat-free margarine
	1 cup green beans
	Lettuce salad with vegetables
	2 Tbsp. salad dressing
Snack	16 oz. water
	16 animal crackers

- Get regular exercise to build both appetite and muscle. Participate in activities such as weight lifting to increase muscle mass and swimming to improve cardiovascular fitness.

How Do You Maintain a Healthful Weight?

Reaching or being at a healthful weight is only one piece of the puzzle. Once you've achieved your target weight, you have to maintain it.

Long-term weight management doesn't have to mean endless days of dull meals or counting calories. Instead, look at your food habits, your level of physical activity, and your feelings about eating and choose options that make it easy and fun to keep your weight in balance. Keep the following in mind:

- Your healthful weight is a range, not a fixed number.
- Aim to be more active in your everyday life.
- When choosing physical activity, aim for consistency over intensity.
- Snack smarter by replacing higher-calorie snacks such as chips and energy bars with fruits and vegetables.
- Don't be too hard on yourself when you do overeat; just get back on track as soon as possible.

LO 7.5 QUICK CHECK

What is the psychological response to the sight, smell, thought, or taste of food that prompts or postpones eating?

a. hunger
b. appetite
c. satiety
d. BMR

Change Yourself, Change Your World

LO 7.6 Describe strategies for maintaining a healthy weight at college.

College doesn't have to mean scary food in the dining hall and worrying about the "freshman 15." However, if you've tried to lose weight, you may have discovered how difficult it can be to do it on your own. People and organizations are available to give you support.

Start by visiting your campus health and fitness centers. Many offer a variety of services and programs related to achieving a healthy weight. If you are a student, these services are often less expensive than you'll find elsewhere.

You can also consider joining a community-based or commercial weight-loss program. Nonprofit groups such as Overeaters Anonymous and TOPS (Take Off Pounds Sensibly) provide supportive help in understanding and rethinking emotional responses to food and are either free or relatively low cost. Commercial groups, such as Weight Watchers or Jenny Craig, are also readily available, although at a higher price. Some base their weight-loss plans around purchasing prepared meals from the program, which can get expensive, especially on a student budget.

When deciding whether any weight-loss program is right for you, federal health experts suggest looking for these elements:[67]

- Healthy eating plans that reduce calories but do not forbid specific foods.
- Tips to increase moderate-intensity physical activity.
- Tips on healthy habits that also keep your cultural needs in mind, such as lower-fat versions of your favorite foods.

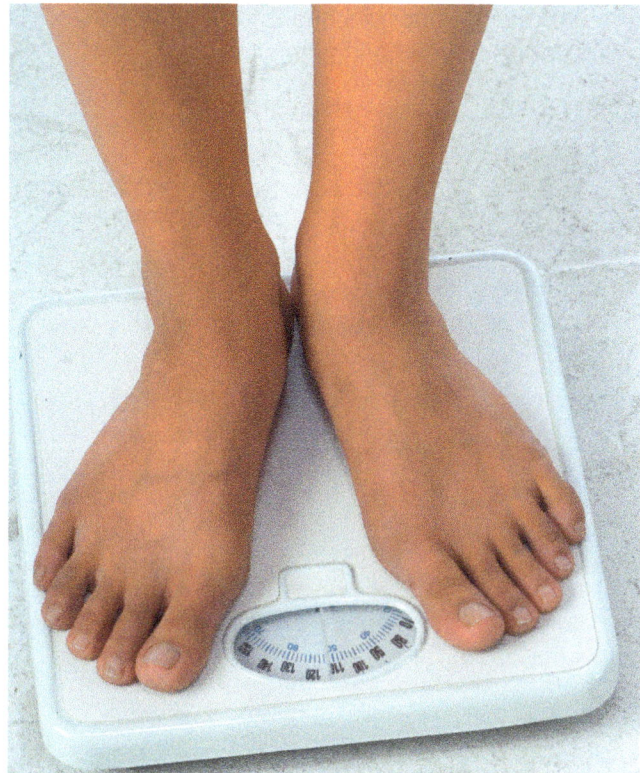

Talking to someone at your campus health center or joining a weight-loss program can be a first step to **losing weight.**

- Slow and steady weight loss. Depending on your starting weight, experts recommend losing weight at a rate of 1/2 to 2 pounds per week.
- Medical care if you are planning to lose weight by following a special formula diet, such as a very low-calorie diet (a program that requires careful monitoring from a doctor).
- A plan to keep the weight off after you have lost it.

>> If you're interested in joining a commercial weight-loss program or trying a new product, check out the Federal Trade Commission's resources to help you assess them: **www.consumer.ftc.gov**. (Search for "weight-loss-fitness.")

Campus Resources for Maintaining a Healthy Weight

The Real Food Challenge (**www.realfoodchallenge.org**) is a network of students working to bring better options to campuses. This group, which has chapters at about 300 colleges and universities so far, aims to "shift $1 billion of annual college food purchases away from industrial agriculture towards local, sustainable, and fair sources." That's an ambitious goal, but the group provides support and training for campus chapters and also has ways to start smaller, such as getting just one real food item into the menu at your dining hall. If your school doesn't have a chapter, start one, and if it does, get involved. Groups such as these show that students don't have to be at the mercy of the campus food service.

Maybe you make most of your own meals. If so, consider starting a cooking club with like-minded friends, where you share the planning, shopping, cooking—and mealtime.

If your campus doesn't offer safe walking and biking options, work with other students to lobby the administration and make these changes happen. In addition to working toward a healthful campus environment, it's also essential to avoid judging others because of weight. Many colleges and universities now offer courses in so-called fat studies, which prompt students to research issues such as how weight is perceived in different countries and what our media obsession with thinness reveals about our values as a society. Or check out National Association to Advance Fat Acceptance (NAAFA), at **www.naafaonline.com**.

LO 7.6 QUICK CHECK

Which of the following is true about weight control in college?
a. Most people don't have to worry about gaining weight in college.
b. It can be difficult to lose weight on your own.
c. Most colleges do not have programs/services to help with weight control.
d. College-sponsored weight management services are typically expensive.

Body Image and Eating Disorders

LO 7.7 Describe common body image and eating disorders.

Have you ever thought about the fact that ads for junk foods like chips or cheeseburgers are funding videos and programs featuring actors so thin they look like they've never had a bite of either? For some people, contradictions like this contribute to the development of a distorted view of their body or a dangerous relationship with food.[68]

Body Image Disorders

While many of us have concerns about our bodies and our appearance from time to time, some people experience worries about body image to such a strong degree that their thoughts and perceptions interfere with their happiness and daily life.

Body Dysmorphic Disorder

In **body dysmorphic disorder (BDD),** a person can't stop thinking about a perceived flaw with his or her appearance, even though the flaw is typically minor or imagined. Though BDD can apply to any physical feature, it often centers on weight and body shape, and it often starts during the teen years. Men and women experience the disorder in equal numbers.[69]

> **body dysmorphic disorder (BDD)** A mental disorder characterized by obsessive thoughts about a perceived flaw in appearance.

This condition can have serious effects, including depression, anxiety, social isolation, eating disorders, seeking out unnecessary cosmetic

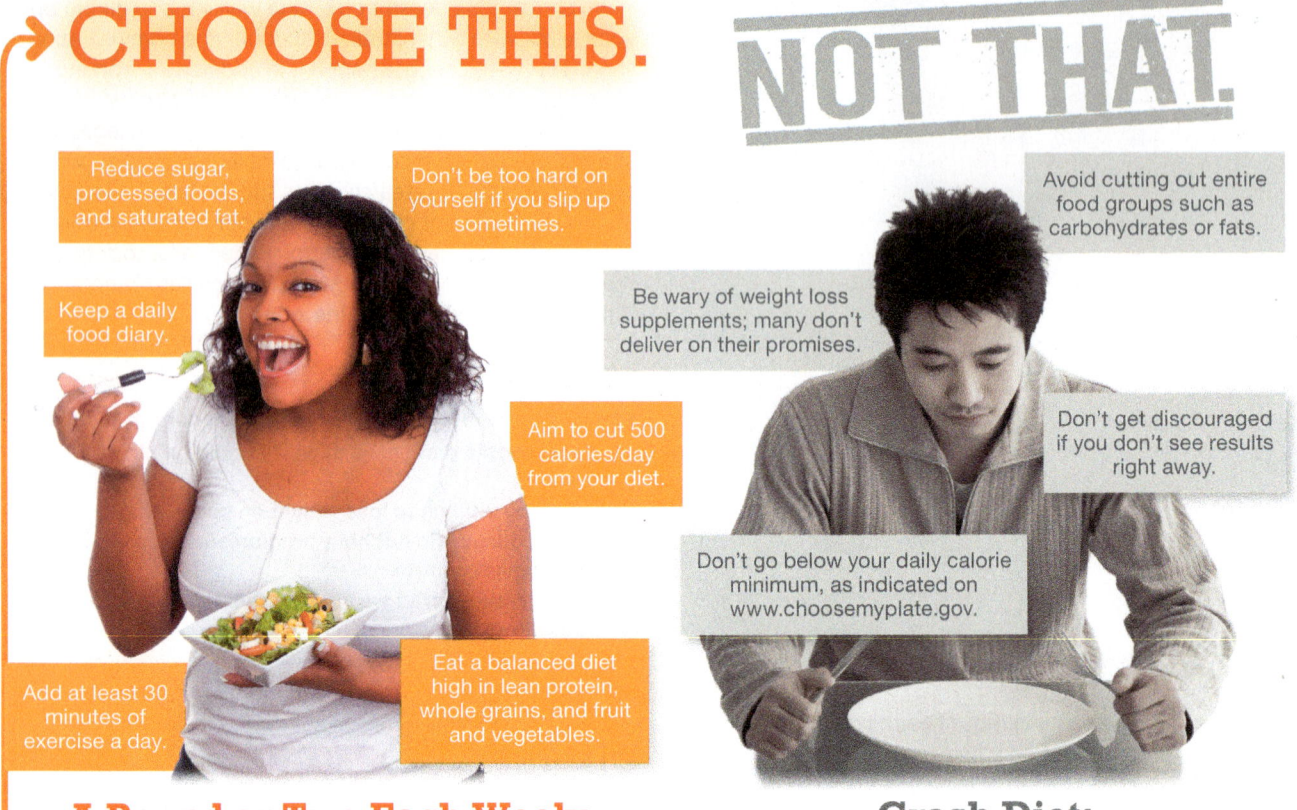

When you want to lose some weight, you can reach your goal healthfully or set yourself up for frustration. To drop pounds in a healthy way:

CHOOSE THIS.
- Reduce sugar, processed foods, and saturated fat.
- Don't be too hard on yourself if you slip up sometimes.
- Keep a daily food diary.
- Aim to cut 500 calories/day from your diet.
- Add at least 30 minutes of exercise a day.
- Eat a balanced diet high in lean protein, whole grains, and fruit and vegetables.

A Pound or Two Each Week: When you want to lose weight, you want the pounds gone NOW. But a slower, steadier pace will be more manageable and bring longer-lasting results.

NOT THAT.
- Avoid cutting out entire food groups such as carbohydrates or fats.
- Be wary of weight loss supplements; many don't deliver on their promises.
- Don't get discouraged if you don't see results right away.
- Don't go below your daily calorie minimum, as indicated on www.choosemyplate.gov.

Crash Diet: Trendy diets may sound like a path to getting skinny fast, but they are often not balanced and will leave you feeling depleted. They also don't help keep weight off later.

procedures or surgeries, and even suicidal thoughts. Treatment often centers on psychotherapy, although in some cases antidepressant medications may also be recommended.

Social Physique Anxiety

Many of us get a little uncomfortable at the thought of appearing before others in shorts or a bathing suit, but for those with **social physique anxiety,** this concern is amplified to a degree that makes them extremely nervous and fearful of having their bodies judged by others. Those with this disorder are likely to experience consequences such as social isolation or extreme self-criticism.[70] While males and females may both experience this disorder, women and girls are more likely to have higher levels of social physique anxiety and lower levels of physical self-esteem than males.[71]

Eating Disorders

Sometimes people let negative body image or other psychological factors steer them toward unhealthful eating behaviors. When these behaviors produce drastic weight changes and put health and even life at risk, they are called **eating disorders.** Teenage girls are at highest risk for most eating disorders, especially if they are preoccupied with being thin, experience social or family pressure to be thin, come from more affluent families, and have tendencies toward extreme self-control and perfectionism. But young men and athletes under pressure to adhere to a particular body shape are also vulnerable. According to national estimates, about 2.7% of 13- to 18-year-olds, including 3.8% of girls and 1.5% of boys, suffer from an eating disorder.[72]

Three dangerous eating disorders are anorexia nervosa, bulimia nervosa, and binge eating disorder. Other eating and weight-related behaviors, while not yet classified by medical experts as full-blown eating disorders, can also have serious health effects; these include night-eating syndrome, the female athlete triad, and orthorexia nervosa.

Anorexia Nervosa

People with **anorexia nervosa** see food as an enemy that must

social physique anxiety A mental disorder characterized by extreme fear of having one's body judged by others.

eating disorders A group of mental disorders, including anorexia nervosa, bulimia nervosa, and binge eating disorder, that is characterized by physiological and psychological disturbances in appetite or food intake.

anorexia nervosa A mental disorder characterized by extremely low body weight, body image distortion, severe calorie restriction, and an obsessive fear of gaining weight.

172 CHAPTER 7 Body Image, Body Weight

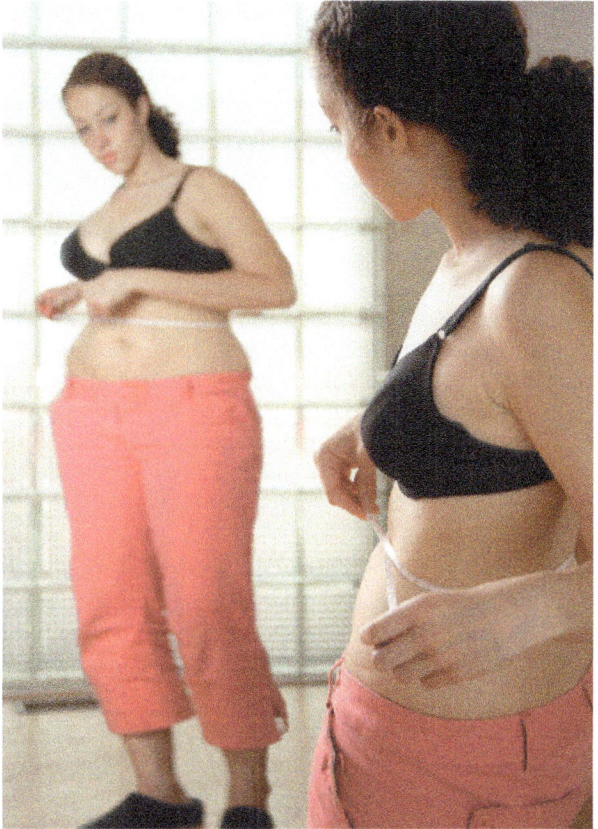

Being overly critical of your body can interfere with your happiness.

be controlled. They eat as little as possible, often setting up elaborate rituals and practices to control food intake. They have an extremely unhealthful body image, seeing themselves as fat even when they are dangerously underweight. In the United States, experts estimate that about 0.6% of the population suffers from anorexia, including about 0.9% of women and 0.3% of men.[73] About 0.3% of teenagers develop the condition.[74]

Although the exact cause of anorexia nervosa is unknown, a variety of factors play a role in many cases. Psychological factors, such as a tendency toward obsessive-compulsive personality traits, may make it more possible for some people to focus intently on their weight and forgo food even when hungry. Environmental factors, such as the body image concerns and media influences discussed earlier, often play a part.

Signs and symptoms of anorexia nervosa include the following:

- An intense fear of gaining weight or being overweight
- A highly distorted body image that continues to see fat where none exists
- An inability to maintain a normal body weight
- A refusal to eat or eating patterns that tightly restrict food intake

Anorexia nervosa is classified as a serious mental disorder. Starvation leads to wasting: A body deprived of calories will begin to break down the proteins in muscle and other body tissues to use for energy. This can cause serious and sometimes irreparable damage throughout the body, especially to the heart muscle, and can prompt sudden death. People suffering from anorexia nervosa are 18 times more likely to die early than people in the same age group in the general population.[75] Other physical consequences of anorexia nervosa are illustrated in **Figure 7.6.**

Treatment for the disorder is key, although experts estimate that only about 34% of those with the disorder receive care.[76] The good news, though, is that once treatment is accessed, most patients do respond. In one survey of teenagers diagnosed with anorexia, more than 65% followed their treatment plan closely, and the vast majority showed healthful, positive outcomes in the years following their care.[77] The type and duration of treatment varies according to the severity of the illness. Patients with less severe cases often receive a blend of treatment and support services, such as psychiatric care, medications, and nutritional counseling in outpatient settings that allow them to continue to live at home. Patients with more severe cases, especially those whose life is at risk, may receive treatment in the hospital, where patient care, including nutritional support in the form of supervised feedings, can be more closely monitored.[78]

During and after treatment for anorexia nervosa, support from family and friends is key. Many treatment plans include family therapy to help loved ones find new ways

Brain and Nerves
Can't think right, fear of gaining weight, sad, moody, irritable, bad memory, fainting, changes in brain chemistry

Hair
Hair thins and gets brittle

Heart
Low blood pressure, slow heart rate, fluttering of the heart, palpitations, heart failure

Blood
Anemia and other blood problems

Muscles, Joints, and Bones
Weak muscles, swollen joints, bone loss, fractures, osteoporosis

Kidneys
Kidney stones, kidney failure

Body Fluids
Low potassium, magnesium, and sodium

Intestines
Constipation, bloating

Hormones
Periods stop, growth problems, trouble getting pregnant. If pregnant, higher risk for miscarriage, having a C-section baby with low birth weight, and postpartum depression.

Skin
Bruise easily, dry skin, growth of fine hair all over body, get cold easily, yellow skin, nails get brittle

FIGURE 7.6 **Major Physical and Health Effects Associated with Anorexia.**
Source: Adapted from National Institute of Mental Health. (2014). *Eating disorders: About more than food.*

to support the patient and each other and avoid prior patterns of behavior that may have contributed to the condition. Patients also benefit from finding new ways to manage stress and reduce anxiety, helping themselves acquire a more healthful body image and relationship with food. Patients are also helped by disengaging from "pro-anorexia" websites and online forums where those with untreated anorexia nervosa discuss how they sustain their disorder or hide it from friends and family. To help, several large blogging and social media platforms have removed posts and websites that could promote anorexia and other eating disorders.[79]

Bulimia Nervosa

Bulimia nervosa is a disorder marked by an ongoing cycle of seeking large amounts of food and then trying to get rid of the calories consumed. People who have this disorder have elaborate food rituals that typically start with **binge eating,** the consumption of a large amount of food in a short amount of time. After a binge, bulimics then try to remove these calories from their bodies by **purging** through self-induced vomiting, heavy laxative use, fasting, or excessive exercise.

> **bulimia nervosa** A mental disorder characterized by episodes of binge eating followed by a purge behavior such as vomiting, laxative abuse, or extreme exercise.
>
> **binge eating** The rapid consumption of an excessive amount of food.
>
> **purging** Behaviors such as vomiting, laxative abuse, or overexercising that are intended to reduce the calories absorbed by the body.

An estimated 0.6% of American adults develop bulimia nervosa in their lifetime, including about 0.5% of women and 0.1% of men.[80] About 0.9% of teenagers develop the condition.[71] Unlike with anorexia nervosa, those suffering from bulimia nervosa often maintain a healthy or normal weight, but as in anorexia nervosa, bulimics are often intensely anxious about gaining weight and extremely critical of their own bodies. Many conduct bulimic behavior in secret, sometimes as often as several times each day.[81]

Bulimia nervosa carries serious health risks, including dental problems such as cavities and tooth enamel erosion, dehydration from vomiting and other forms of forced purging, stomach problems such as ulcers and even stomach rupture, and cardiac risks, including irregular heartbeat and heart failure. Signs of bulimia nervosa include the following:

- Regular binge eating episodes, at a rate of at least once per week for several months
- Binges followed by purging, strict dieting, or excessive exercise to prevent weight gain
- Using self-induced vomiting or laxatives as part of purging
- An obsession with weight and body shape
- Calluses on the knuckles or backs of the hands due to repeated self-induced vomiting

As with anorexia nervosa, treatment for bulimia nervosa can be extremely effective. Bulimia treatments usually focus on a combination of medical, psychiatric, and psychosocial care tailored to the needs of the individual patient. Some patients also benefit from antidepressant medications such as fluoxetine (Prozac), which is the only prescription drug approved by the FDA as a treatment for bulimia. These medications help some patients reduce depression and anxiety, as well as reduce binge-purge behavior and the chance of relapse.[82]

Binge Eating Disorder

Binge eaters may periodically consume thousands of calories in a matter of hours, do little to burn off those calories afterward, and then repeat a session of binge eating within a few days. As more binges lead to weight gain, many binge eaters say they begin to feel depressed, worried, and concerned about their ability to control their appetite. Those feelings lead many binge eaters to eat in private or try to hide their eating from others. About 2.8% of U.S. adults, including 3.5% of women and 2% of men, suffer from binge eating disorder.[83] About 1.6% of teenagers develop the condition.[74]

Signs of binge eating disorder include the following:

- Recurring episodes of eating large amounts of food in a short period of time while having feelings of being out of control. Behavior occurs at least once a week over three months.
- Eating too quickly and even when not hungry.
- Having feelings of guilt, embarrassment, or disgust because of the binging behavior.
- Binge eating alone to hide the behavior.[84]

Treatment options for binge eating disorder are similar to those used to treat bulimia nervosa and may include nutritional counseling, behavior therapy, and antidepressant medication.

Other Unhealthful Eating Behaviors

Other unhealthful eating behaviors do not qualify as full-blown eating disorders but still have serious effects on weight, mental health, and well-being. These behaviors are classified as **disordered eating,** a range of unhealthful eating habits in which food is used primarily to deal with emotional issues. Disordered eating is common on college campuses; in one study, about 17% of students said they had experienced some kind of disordered eating.[85]

> **disordered eating** A range of unhealthful eating behaviors used to deal with emotional issues that does not warrant a diagnosis of a specific eating disorder.

Night-Eating Syndrome

While it's common for many of us to occasionally visit the fridge after dinner, some people suffer from a regular pattern of night-time eating, disrupted sleep, and mood disorders that can add up to depression and weight gain. Those with night-eating syndrome often skip breakfast and eat little during the first part of the day. Then, beginning in the evening, food intake increases dramatically, often focusing on starchy or sugary foods. People with this syndrome may eat before going to bed and then wake up several times during the night for more food.

This syndrome isn't yet fully understood. Researchers suspect that a range of sleep and health difficulties may play a role, leading the body to seek food in an effort to better produce and regulate sleep-related hormones.

SELF-ASSESSMENT
Could I Have an Eating Disorder?

To help find out, a doctor would ask you the following questions:

- Do you regularly eat large quantities of food and continue eating long after you're full?
- Do you worry that you have lost control over how much you eat?
- Do you regularly avoid food, even when you're hungry?
- Do you have obsessive negative feelings about how your body looks?
- Do you feel extremely anxious about gaining weight?

HOW TO INTERPRET YOUR SCORE Score 1 point for every "yes" answer. If you score 2 points or more, talk with a health professional.

TTo complete this Self-Assessment online, visit MasteringHealth™

Estimates of its prevalence vary widely; while experts estimate that about 1.5% of the general population suffers from the condition, a study of a group of college students found that about 5.7% experienced some form of the disorder.[86,87] Night-eating syndrome can be difficult to treat but is sometimes addressed with hormonal supplements such as melatonin or antidepressant medications.[83]

Female Athlete Triad

The multifaceted disorder **female athlete triad** is most prevalent in female athletes participating in sports or activities that require a lower body weight, such as gymnastics, diving, distance running, or dance. Women and girls with this syndrome experience a trio of disorders: disordered eating (focusing on weight control and calorie restriction), amenorrhea (irregular or absent menstrual period), and osteoporosis (low bone density).[88] The combination of disordered eating and frequent high-intensity exercise leaves the body with inadequate energy to maintain fat stores and reproductive functioning. Low blood levels of the female reproductive hormone estrogen lead to cessation of menstrual periods and loss of bone density. This in turn increases the athlete's risk for fractures. Depending on the athlete's age, the loss of bone density may be irreversible, resulting in a lifelong increased risk for fractures. Because this disorder is difficult to treat, medical experts stress prevention, urging coaches, friends, and parents of female athletes to avoid excessive focus on an athlete's weight, watch for signs of the triad, and seek professional help if they suspect that the disorder is present.[89]

A related disorder is **anorexia athletica,** in which excessive exercise is used as a type of purge. Those with this disorder work out much more frequently and with more intensity than is recommended or even healthy. Failure to exercise at such high levels leads to overwhelming guilt and anxiety. The excessive exercising often interferes with professional obligations and personal relationships.

Orthorexia Nervosa

While they may not obsess over calories or being thin, those suffering from **orthorexia nervosa** have an unhealthy obsession with healthy eating. This behavior usually starts out with an attempt to eat more healthfully and eventually becomes a fixation on food quality and purity. Sufferers adopt a very rigid diet. Experts believe that orthorexia is motivated less by health than by the need to feel in control and body image issues. The condition can become all-consuming and may result in social isolation. Counseling with an eating disorder professional is the recommended treatment.

Getting Help for a Body Image or Eating Disorder

If you struggle with a negative body image or unhealthful eating behaviors, seek support and treatment from trained professionals. Many people who experience eating disorders and disordered eating also get a great deal of help from guided support groups. In these groups, you'll not only receive help in shifting your self-perceptions and habits but get valuable advice from others who have been in your shoes. If you have a serious eating disorder, you may first need medical treatment to stabilize your body and stop your health from deteriorating.

Try the following if you think someone you know has an unhealthful eating or weight-control behavior:

- Locate support and treatment resources on campus or in your community.
- Once you know where to find help, have a compassionate, open conversation with the person you are concerned about.
- Try not to talk with your friend or loved one about dieting, body size, or weight. Instead, focus on behaviors that worry you and how they might be unhealthful.
- Offer to direct the person to the treatment resources you've found and offer to go along for support if desired.
- Know that one conversation may not go far. Keep trying. If you let your friend or loved one know that you are concerned, that person will know where to turn when he or she is ready to seek help.

---

female athlete triad A multifaceted disorder typically seen in female athletes and characterized by disordered eating, amenorrhea and osteoporosis

anorexia athletica A mental disorder that involves using compulsive and excessive exercising as a purge.

orthorexia nervosa Disordered eating characterized by a fixation with obsessively healthy eating.

> "*Remember that your worth is not defined by your appearance, and your health is not defined by the number on the scale.*"

Personal Choices: Develop a More Positive Body Image

While energy balance—calories in versus calories burned—is important, it's also critical to understand how you view your body and your health. Here are a few strategies for building a more positive body image to help yourself achieve and maintain a healthy weight and shape:

- Accept yourself for who you are. Beauty comes in many shapes and sizes.
- Pay attention to your fitness rather than your appearance. Build healthy habits that benefit both your mind and your body.
- Be kind to yourself. No one can look their healthiest or eat wisely all the time. Accept your setbacks as temporary obstacles rather than as personal failures.
- Know that the beauty and fitness industries are businesses designed to make money, not be health-care providers. Take corporate and mass media beauty and fitness advice with a large grain of salt.
- Remember that your worth is not defined by your appearance, and your health is not defined by the number on the scale.

>> Watch videos of real students discussing weight management and body image at **Mastering**Health™

LO 7.7 QUICK CHECK

Which group is at highest risk of developing most eating disorders?

a. middle-aged women　　c. older adults
b. young boys　　　　　　d. teenage girls

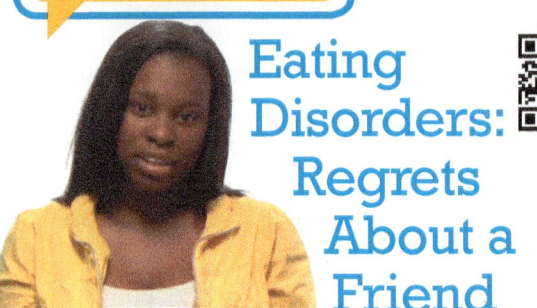

STUDENT STORY
Eating Disorders: Regrets About a Friend

"HI, MY NAME IS VIEGE. My freshman year in college I had a friend named Lisa, who suffered from an eating disorder. She would always starve herself to try to look like other people or starve herself to get a guy. To be honest with you, I really didn't take it seriously. I just told her that it's just a phase she was going through and everything will be all right. And then, as I saw her getting skinnier and skinnier, I was like, 'Hey, maybe you do need to get some help.' And all she would say is, 'I'm not crazy. I just want to be beautiful.' So I just let it go. And that was the biggest mistake I've ever made because a couple months later, Lisa was rushed to the hospital because she had something wrong with her heart.

So, if you do have a friend that's struggling with eating disorders, you should probably talk to them. You may not think of it as serious but it can be, even if they're young."

What Do You Think?

1. What do you think was wrong with Viege's friend's heart? What could have caused her to be hospitalized?
2. Early on, why do you think Verge failed to take her friend's problem seriously? Do you think this is a common reaction to early signs of an eating disorder?
3. What would prompt you to talk to a friend about a possible eating disorder? Do you think it's your place to convince a friend to get help?

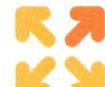 ## Choosing to **Change** Worksheet

To complete this worksheet online, visit Mastering Health™

What can you do to manage your weight? What is an appropriate goal for weight management? Follow the steps below to develop a weight-management plan.

Directions: Fill in your stage of behavior change in step 1 and complete the rest of the worksheet with your stage of change in mind.

Step 1: **Assess your stage of behavior change.** Please check one of the following statements that best describes your readiness to manage your weight.

_____I do not intend to change my body weight in the next six months. (Precontemplation)

_____I might change my body weight in the next six months. (Contemplation)

_____I am prepared to change my body weight in the next month. (Preparation)

_____I have been changing my body weight for less than six months. (Action)

_____I have been changing my body weight for more than six months. (Maintenance)

Step 2: Create a weight-management plan

1. What can BMI and waist-to-hip ratio tell a person about the effect of weight on health? How do you feel about your weight when you look in the mirror? Do you want to maintain your current weight? Gain weight? Lose weight? How many pounds? Write down exactly what you want to accomplish with your weight-management plan.

BMI and waist-to-hip ratio: _____

Effect on health: _____

Weight-management goal: _____

_____

2. Given your current stage of behavior change, what can you do next to accomplish your weight-management goal? Which side of the energy balance equation do you want to change: energy in or energy out? Or do you want to modify both? Include a realistic timeline for your next step and list a reward for yourself once you have accomplished your next step.

Next step: _____

_____

Timeline: _____

Reward: _____

3. Consider that a healthful prescription for weight loss is cutting 500 to 1,000 calories a day, through reduced calorie intake or increased exercise. This typically leads to a weight loss of 1 or 2 pounds a week. To gain weight, you add a similar amount of calories daily. Now, consider the weight-management techniques introduced in this chapter. Which techniques can you try to better manage your weight? Keep in mind that you should not cut calories below your recommended MyPlate levels, which you can find at www.choosemyplate.gov.

_____

_____

_____

4. If you want to simply maintain your current weight, what will you do to ensure that your energy expenditure meets the energy you consume? Think about extended amounts of time when you might consistently consume more food (such as holiday breaks) or where you might be less active than usual (such as during finals). What steps can you take during those times to make sure you stay in energy balance?

_____

_____

_____

Step 3: Promote a healthful body image.

1. What are your current feelings about your body? When you think about your body, are you usually thinking about how it looks? How it feels? What it does for you? Write down your general thoughts.

_____

_____

2. What do you like about your body? Write down *at least* three things.

_____
_____
_____

3. Are there factors that lead you to think negatively about your body (for example, images you see in the media, opinions of friends or family members, the presence of scars or injury, etc.)? If so, how could you combat those factors and improve your body image?

_____
_____
_____

CHAPTER 7 STUDY PLAN

CHAPTER SUMMARY

LO 7.1
- Weight affects your health, not just your appearance. Many, however, become preoccupied with body image when thinking about weight.
- BMI, together with other factors such as waist circumference and waist-to-hip ratio, can help indicate whether your weight will increase your risk for certain health conditions and diseases.

LO 7.2
- Overweight and obesity are serious and common health problems not just in the United States but around the world.
- Excess body weight is a critical issue for college students. Decline in physical activity is often a major contributor to college weight gain.

LO 7.3
- Health risks of excess weight include high blood pressure, type 2 diabetes, abnormal blood fats, coronary heart disease, stroke, cancer, osteoarthritis, sleep apnea, gallbladder disease, fatty liver disease, and fertility and pregnancy complications.
- To understand your weight and its effects on your health, you need to know your body composition, blood chemistry, and other factors, not just how much you weigh.

LO 7.4
- Your weight is shaped by your energy balance, physical activity, basic energy needs, age, genes, gender, and environment.
- Ultimately, excess weight results from an imbalance of calories consumed and calories used.

MasteringHealth™
Build your knowledge—and health!—in the Study Area of **MasteringHealth**™ with a variety of study tools.

LO 7.5
- Reaching a healthful lower weight requires consistent, long-term work on both eating habits and increasing physical activity. Short-term diets are often of limited help. Diet aids can be expensive, may not work, and may be harmful.
- Medical options, including prescription drugs and bariatric surgery, may be beneficial for people who are extremely obese.
- To gain weight, boost your calories in healthful ways by eating nutritious foods. Also, eat more often and exercise to stimulate your appetite.

LO 7.6
- Access campus resources to help you achieve your weight goals.
- Maintaining a healthful weight is most effective when you establish and consistently follow eating and exercise habits you enjoy and use them to keep your weight within a healthful range.

LO 7.7
- Societal contradictions that encourage weight gain while glorifying thinness can lead to negative views of our own bodies. These body image issues contribute to disordered eating and eating disorders.
- Eating disorders are complicated psychiatric conditions affected by family, social dynamics, and feelings of self-worth. Eating disorders that carry significant health risks

- include anorexia nervosa, bulimia nervosa, and binge eating disorder.
- Disordered eating behaviors, while not qualifying as psychiatric disorders, are also unhealthy. Eating disorders and disordered eating can significantly harm a person's health, or even lead to death in some cases. Effective treatments are available.
- If you know someone who you think might have an eating-related disorder, help them find resources on campus for support and treatment

GET CONNECTED

»» Visit the following websites for further information about the topics in this chapter:

- American College of Sports Medicine Exercise Guidelines
  www.acsm.org
- Academy of Nutrition and Dietetics
  www.eatright.org
- Centers for Disease Control and Prevention: Overweight and Obesity
  www.cdc.gov (Search for "obesity")
- National Institute of Mental Health: Eating Disorders
  www.nimh.nih.gov (Search the health publications section for "eating disorders")

MOBILE TIPS!
Scan this QR code with your mobile device to access additional tips about weight management and body image. Or, via your mobile device, go to **http://chmobile.pearsoncmg.com** and choose by topic: weight management and body image.

- USDA Nutritional Database
  http://ndb.nal.usda.gov
- World Health Organization: Obesity
  www.who.org (Search for "health topics obesity")

Website links are subject to change. To access updated web links, please visit Mastering Health™

TEST YOUR KNOWLEDGE

LO 7.1

1. What is BMI?
   a. a ratio between your height and your weight, used to help assess health risks
   b. a measurement of how much fat you have
   c. a measurement of how much muscle you have
   d. a 100% reliable indicator of how healthy you are

2. What is the healthful weight range for someone who is 5 feet 11 inches tall?
   a. 133 to 172 pounds
   b. 140 to 171 pounds
   c. 149 to 183 pounds
   d. 164 to 196 pounds

LO 7.2

3. Between 1980 and 2002, childhood obesity rates _____.
   a. remained the same
   b. increased by 10%
   c. doubled
   d. tripled

4. When most students start college, how many pounds do they gain?
   a. 1 to 4
   b. 7 to 8
   c. 9 to 12
   d. 13 to 16

LO 7.3

5. Which of the following conditions is not related to being overweight?
   a. sleep apnea
   b. high blood pressure
   c. fatty liver disease
   d. low LDL levels

LO 7.4

6. What percentage of 18- to 24-year-olds engage in no leisure-time physical activity?
   a. 75%
   b. 50%
   c. 25%
   d. 10%

LO 7.5

7. What is the best approach to weight loss?
   a. Eat more protein and drink more water.
   b. Take in fewer calories and exercise more.
   c. Avoid foods containing carbohydrates.
   d. Take in more energy and eat less fat.

8. In order to maintain weight loss, you should
   a. eat as little as possible.
   b. stop working out; it makes you hungry.
   c. never allow yourself to have a high-calorie day.
   d. focus on eating fruits and vegetables.

LO 7.7

9. Which of the following statements about body image is true?
   a. In body dysmorphic disorder, a person focuses on a perceived physical flaw.
   b. Among college students, about 10% of males and 35% of females are dissatisfied with their body.
   c. Men and boys are more likely to have higher levels of social physique anxiety than women and girls.
   d. Women become less self-accepting of their bodies with age.

10. The risk for fractures is increased in women with
    a. bulimia nervosa.
    b. night-eating syndrome.
    c. the female athlete triad.
    d. compulsive overeating.

WHAT DO YOU THINK?

LO 7.1
1. What are the most important factors to consider when determining your own most healthful weight?

LO 7.2
2. Over the past 35 years, obesity rates in the United States have more than doubled. Why do you think this has occurred?

LO 7.3
3. Why should a healthy college student be concerned about weight management? What steps should he/she take now to ensure a healthier future?

LO 7.5
4. Of all the weight management/loss strategies discussed in this chapter, which do you think would work for you? Why?

LO 7.7
5. How would you help a friend who exhibits unhealthful eating or weight-control behaviors?

8

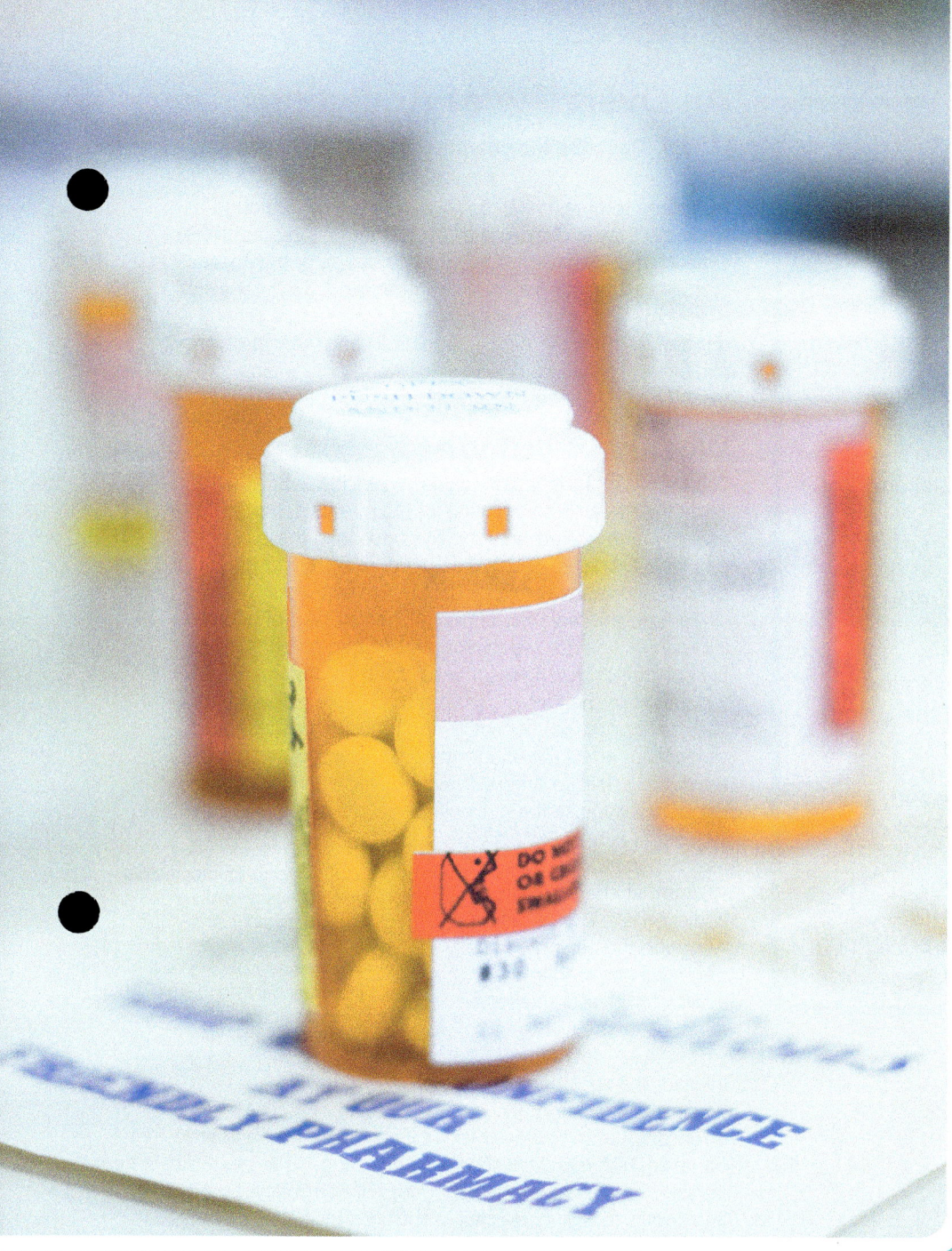

> More than 27 million Americans age 12 and up currently use illicit drugs.[i]

> Drug overdose deaths, escalating for the past decade, have reached "epidemic" levels, claiming more than 125 American lives every day.[ii]

> Despite the dangers of "drugged driving," driving after marijuana use is more common among college students than driving after drinking.[iii]

ADDICTIONS AND DRUG USE

LEARNING OUTCOMES

LO 8.1 Describe the characteristics of addiction.

LO 8.2 Identify four common behavioral addictions.

LO 8.3 Compare the prevalence of drug use among college students and in the general population.

LO 8.4 Discuss the physical and psychological effects of initial and chronic drug use.

LO 8.5 Identify commonly abused drugs and describe their mechanisms, effects, and health risks.

LO 8.6 Discuss common drug-prevention strategies used throughout the United States.

LO 8.7 List community, campus-based, and clinical options for treatment of drug abuse.

LO 8.8 Outline personal strategies for overcoming addictions and preventing drug abuse.

Singer's death linked to lethal drug cocktail.

Actor's spending out of control! When addiction or abuse involves a celebrity, you hear about it. But what about the untold stories—the more than 47,000 drug-overdose deaths in the United States each year, the 27 million Americans who use illicit drugs, or the 2 million Americans whose lives are ruined by a gambling addiction?[1–4] Chances are, you've witnessed some form of addiction among your own family members or friends—or maybe the untold story is your own.

Even if your life hasn't been directly touched by addiction, you share the costs. These costs include the economic burden of increased health care, social services, and law enforcement, as well as the costs of broken families, death by overdose, and ravaged communities.

What can you do about addictions and drug abuse? Change starts with knowledge—about the nature of addictions, how to avoid them, how to recover, and how to help yourself or a friend.

An Overview of Addiction

LO 8.1 Describe the characteristics of addiction.

From time to time, we all do things for fun even though we know they might cause us trouble in the long term: We cut classes, eat that extra bowl of ice cream, or buy those concert tickets that we "really can't afford." Such behavior is normal—and reflects the power of the pleasure centers in our brains. But some people repeatedly engage in problematic behaviors that have long since stopped providing any real pleasure. In short, they develop an addiction.

What Is Addiction?

The American Society of Addiction Medicine defines **addiction** as a chronic disease of brain reward, motivation, memory, and related circuitry. Dysfunction in these brain circuits is characterized by the pursuit of reward and/or relief by substance abuse or other destructive behavior.[5]

Perhaps the most fundamental characteristic of addiction is *craving*.[5] An addicted person experiences an uncontrollable compulsion to engage in a particular behavior and seeks it out even in the face of significant negative consequences, such as poor grades, loss of relationships or employment, violence, or arrest. Although these negative consequences are entirely clear to others, the addict has a diminished capacity to recognize them. Denial of both the negative consequences and the addiction itself is common.[5]

Another characteristic of addiction is *loss of pleasure*. Although the person originally may have engaged in the activity for pleasurable recreation, he or she now derives very little satisfaction from it. Instead, the addict's motivation becomes an increasingly powerful compulsion to relieve the physical discomfort and emotional anguish experienced when abstaining. As a result, the person experiences an *escalating loss of control* over the act and comes to feel increasingly controlled by it.[5] At the same time, the person has an increased sensitivity to stressors as well as increased anxiety and emotional pain.

Without treatment, addiction is progressive; that is, the behavior becomes more frequent and/or severe.[5] Recovery is often preceded by one or more cycles in which the person abstains from the behavior then relapses, but with treatment, full recovery is possible.

How can you tell if you or someone you care about has an addiction? See the **Practical Strategies** box for a list of signs.

> **addiction** A chronic, progressive disease of brain reward, motivation, memory, and related circuitry characterized by uncontrollable craving for a substance or behavior despite both negative consequences and diminishment or loss of pleasure associated with the activity.

LO 8.1 QUICK CHECK

Which of the following is an example of a brain circuit involved in addiction?

a. laziness
b. excuse-making
c. reward
d. none of the above

182 CHAPTER 8 • Addictions and Drug Use

⚙ PRACTICAL Strategies
Warning Signs of Addiction

How can you tell if you or someone you care about has an addiction? Look for the following signs:

- **Craving.** Does the person seem compelled to engage in a particular behavior, such as gambling or doing drugs and getting high?
- **Loss of control.** Does the person seem to be engaging in the behavior less because of the pleasure it brings and more because he or she can't stop?
- **Negative consequences.** Is the behavior becoming increasingly reckless, such as a pattern of skipping class and missing exams? Does the person continue the destructive behavior despite serious negative consequences such as academic failure, financial ruin, injury or illness, arrest, or loss of relationships with others?
- **Denial.** Does the person fail to recognize or acknowledge that the addiction is causing problems?

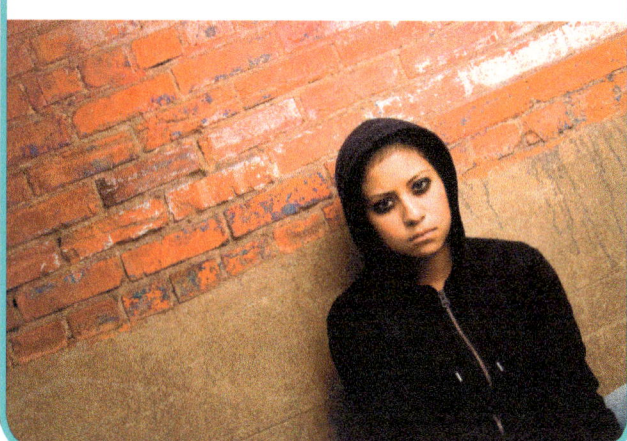

What Are Behavioral Addictions?

LO 8.2 Identify four common behavioral addictions.

The American Psychiatric Association (APA) recognizes a diagnosis category called **behavioral addictions.** This category applies to patients who are addicted to an activity such as gambling.[6] The patient's subjective experience, the brain networks involved, the progression of the disorder, and the effective treatment are equivalent to those for substance addictions.

Pathological Gambling

About 85% of U.S. adults have gambled at least once in their life.[4] For most of us, a night at the casino doesn't pose a problem. However, for an estimated 2 million people in the United States, roughly 1% of adults, gambling is an addiction.[4] Although gambling is illegal for anyone under age 21 in many states, most addicted gamblers get their start in high school, and young adults are especially vulnerable. Studies estimate that 6% of American college students have a serious gambling problem that can result in psychological difficulties, unmanageable debt, and failing grades.[7]

The APA considers a gambling habit *pathological* (harmful) when players experience destructive traits such as the following:

- Being preoccupied with thoughts and plans related to gambling
- Needing to gamble with increasing amounts of money to achieve the desired excitement
- Feeling restless or irritable when attempting to cut back or stop gambling, or being unable to do so
- Using gambling to escape feelings of helplessness, guilt, anxiety, or depression

Other telltale signs include lying to friends and family to hide the extent of the problem and borrowing or stealing to finance the habit.

Hypersexual Disorder

A variety of sources estimate that between 3% and 6% of the U.S. population could meet the criteria for sexual addiction, which the APA refers to as *hypersexual disorder*.[8] Characteristics include recurrent and intense sexual fantasies, urges, and behavior that consume excessive time and cannot be controlled, despite negative consequences such as sexually transmitted infections, unintended pregnancy, broken relationships, and financial problems. The person typically gains little satisfaction from sexual activity and in fact may experience feelings of deep guilt and shame.

Compulsive Spending

Compulsive spending (also referred to as compulsive buying or shopping) is thought to affect more than 1 in 20 U.S. adults overall, including about 8% of university students.[9] Most compulsive spenders are young—typically of traditional university age, according to researchers and have incomes below $50,000. When a compulsive spender buys something, the act triggers the release of chemicals in the brain that cause a rush of euphoria. Compulsive spenders are also more likely than ordinary shoppers to experience uncontrollable buying binges, make senseless and impulsive purchases, and feel depressed after shopping.[9]

> **behavioral addiction** A form of addiction involving a compulsion to engage in an activity such as gambling, sex, or shopping rather than a compulsion to use a substance.

Technology Addiction

A growing number of studies worldwide suggest that as many as 18% of regular Internet users become addicted; that is, their Internet use interferes with their academic success, work, relationships, hours of sleep, or exercising.[10] Moreover, the addict turns to Internet use to alter his or her mood, especially to escape from depression or anxiety.

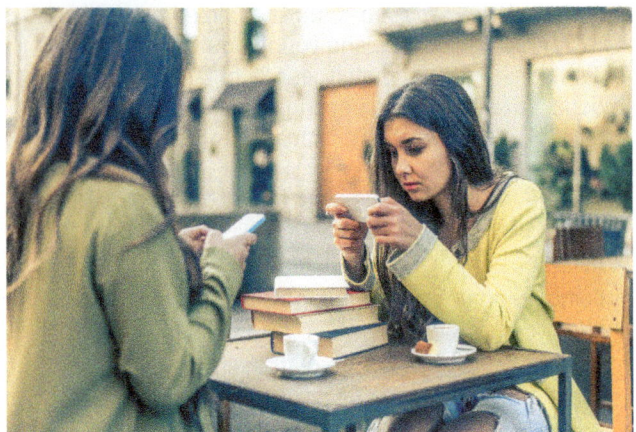

Technology addictions are a growing concern in this device-driven age.

Another use of technology that's increasingly getting media attention is "addiction" to texting. Undoubtedly, Americans love to text: We send or receive about 5 billion text messages per day.[11] Many of these messages are sent by people of college age; a national survey found that young adults between the ages of 18 to 24 years old send about 50 messages a day.[12] Does this level of texting constitute an addiction? Those who say it does point to research showing that texting triggers a reaction in the brain's "reward system," which we'll discuss next, and theorize that texting feeds it. Moreover, many people continue to text excessively despite serious negative consequences—including damage to the tendons in their hands or traffic accidents caused by texting while driving. Other addiction experts say that, although frequent texting is a bad habit, before we can classify it as an addiction, more research is needed.[13]

>> View the complete results of the 2014 National Survey on Drug Use and Health at www.samhsa.gov. (Search for "survey on drug use.")

LO 8.2 QUICK CHECK

Which of the following is a characteristic of compulsive spenders?
a. wealthy, making more than $250,000 a year
b. 35 to 44 years old
c. middle class, typically making more than $50,000 a year
d. young, tending to be of traditional university age

Patterns of Drug Use

LO 8.3 Compare the prevalence of drug use among college students and in the general population.

Do you use drugs? Many of us quickly say no, but the answer to this question is not simple. A **drug** is any chemical that is taken in order to alter the body physically or mentally for a non-nutritional purpose. Drugs that alter feelings, mood, perception, or psychological functioning are considered **psychoactive**.

> **" Although you may not realize it, you might routinely use one or more psychoactive drugs."**

If you drink caffeinated beverages or take certain pain relievers, sleeping pills, or allergy medicines, you are using psychoactive drugs. Of course, some are much more harmful than others: There is a big difference between having a daily cup of coffee and being addicted to cocaine.

In 2014, about 10% of Americans age 12 and older used **illicit drugs**—that is, drugs that are regulated by the U.S. Drug Enforcement Agency (DEA) as unlawful substances, including prescription medications used unlawfully.[3,14] Among Americans age 18 to 25, that figure was more than double—about 22%.[3]

drug A chemical substance that alters the body physically or mentally for a non-nutritional purpose.

psychoactive Capable of altering feelings, mood, perceptions, or psychological functioning.

illicit drugs Drugs regulated by the U.S. Drug Enforcement Agency as unlawful substances, including prescription medications used unlawfully.

Much of this drug use is far from "recreational," with dangerous consequences that federal health experts say add up to a growing public health emergency. More Americans died from drug overdoses in 2014 than during any previous year on record.[1] In addition, that year, more Americans died from drug overdose than lost their lives in motor vehicle crashes.[1]

Which illicit drugs do young adults most commonly use? To compare, check out the **Student Stats** graph.

Despite these pressing public health concerns, it's important to note that drug use can sometimes seem more pervasive than it actually is. College students, for example, tend to vastly overestimate the percentage of their peers who use drugs. In a national survey conducted in 2015, students reported believing that over 80% of their peers use marijuana, when only 17% of students reported actually using it.[15] The number of students who report using other illicit drugs was even lower—about 11%. Even if some drug use goes unreported, those numbers still add up to less than one-third of students using illicit drugs—meaning that plenty of other students have found more positive ways of coping with stress and having fun.

>> View a video of young adults telling personal stories about their drug addictions at http://pact360.org (Click on "Youth360.")

LO 8.3 QUICK CHECK

In 2014, how many Americans died from illicit drug overdose?
a. more than 30,000
b. more than 45,000
c. more than 65,000
d. more than 100,000

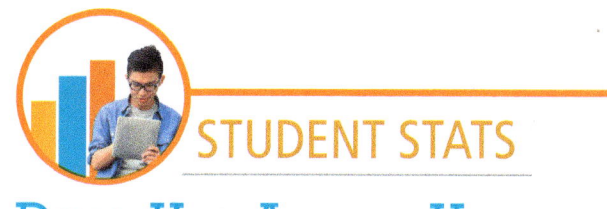

STUDENT STATS

Drug Use Among Young Adults

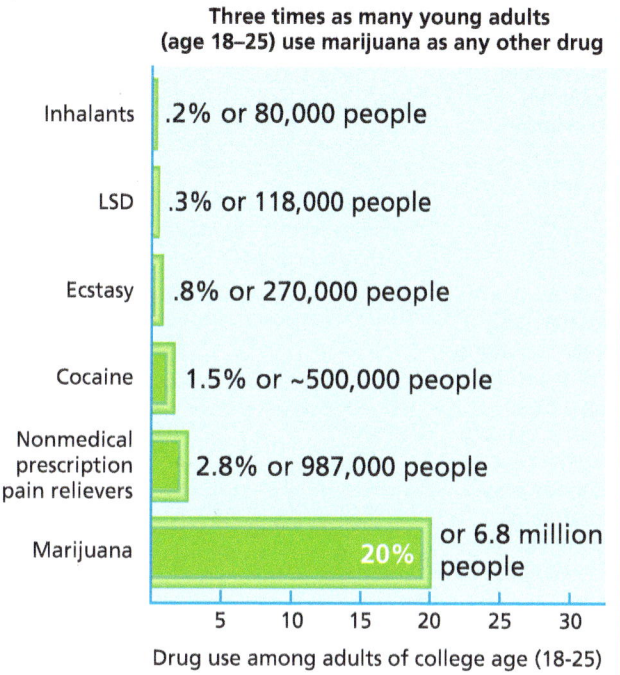

Three times as many young adults (age 18–25) use marijuana as any other drug

- Inhalants: .2% or 80,000 people
- LSD: .3% or 118,000 people
- Ecstasy: .8% or 270,000 people
- Cocaine: 1.5% or ~500,000 people
- Nonmedical prescription pain relievers: 2.8% or 987,000 people
- Marijuana: 20% or 6.8 million people

Drug use among adults of college age (18-25)

Data from Substance Abuse and Mental Health Services Administration. (2015). *Behavioral health trends in the United States: Results from the 2014 National Survey on Drug Use and Health* (HHS Publication No. SMA 15-4927, NSDUH Series H-50). www.samhsa.gov.

How the Body Responds to Drugs

LO 8.4 Discuss the physical and psychological effects of initial and chronic drug use.

By definition, all psychoactive drugs intoxicate the brain, producing characteristic physical, psychological, and behavioral changes. Before we explore the chemistry behind these changes, let's define some terms.

Drug Misuse and Abuse

Drug misuse is the inappropriate use of a legal drug, either for a reason for which it was not medically intended or by a person without a prescription. Using your roommate's prescription antibiotic because you think you have a sinus infection is an example of drug misuse.

In contrast, **drug abuse** is the use (most often the excessive use) of any legal or illegal drug in a way that is detrimental to your health. If, for example, you take prescription painkillers to get high or use street amphetamines to lose weight, you are abusing drugs. All drug use involves some level of health risk, but the risks are significantly increased if you misuse or abuse drugs.

Initial Effects on the Brain

People self-administer drugs in a variety of ways, from ingestion to inhalation (**Table 8.1**). But no matter how they get into the body, once they enter the bloodstream, drugs interfere with the brain's communication system, altering how nerve cells send, receive, and process information. The most addictive substances trigger a rush of the neurotransmitter *dopamine*. Dopamine is the brain's "feel-good" neurotransmitter, a chemical messenger that produces feelings of pleasure and satisfaction. When the brain is overstimulated chemically, users experience a sense of euphoria that primes their bodies to repeat the stimulation. Eventually the brain adapts to the drug by producing less of its own neurotransmitters. As a result, when the drug is no longer externally supplied, users may feel "flat" or depressed.

> **drug misuse** The inappropriate use of a legal drug, either for a reason for which it was not medically intended or by a person without a prescription.
>
> **drug abuse** The use (most often the excessive use) of any legal or illegal drug in a way that is detrimental to your health.
>
> **tolerance** Reduced sensitivity to a drug so that increased amounts are needed to achieve the usual effect.

Effects of Chronic Use

Prolonged or repeated use of chemical substances can actually alter the brain's structure and how it works. The body can eventually develop **tolerance,** meaning that the brain has grown so accustomed to the drug that more of the drug is required to achieve the same effect that a smaller amount used to produce. Tolerance may also cause users to keep using a drug just to feel "normal."

TABLE 8.1 Common Methods of Drug Administration

Method	Description	Typical Drugs
Ingestion	Swallowing a drug and absorbing it through the digestive system	Alcoholic beverages, pills, LSD
Injection	Using a syringe to inject a drug directly into the skin, muscle, or bloodstream	Cocaine, methamphetamine, heroin
Inhalation	Breathing a drug into the lungs through the mouth or nostrils (snorting or smoking)	Marijuana, tobacco, cocaine (crack), inhalants such as paint thinner or glue
Mucosal absorption	Absorbing a drug through the mucous membranes	Chewing tobacco (absorbed through the membranes in the mouth); snorted cocaine (absorbed through the membranes in the nose)
Topical administration	Applying a drug directly onto a body surface, like the skin	Nicotine patch

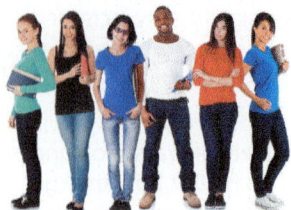

DIVERSITY & HEALTH

Drug Use and Overdose

Recent national surveys and studies of drug use in the United States reveal the following specifics about what health officials term an "epidemic" of drug overdose deaths.

Overall
- About 10% of the U.S. population (27 million individuals age 12 or older) currently use illicit drugs.[1] Prescription drugs used nonmedically, including opioids, are the second most commonly used group of illicit drugs, with more than 4 million users.[1]
- In 2014, more than 47,000 Americans died of a drug overdose. Illicit use of opioids (prescription forms and heroin) was involved in more than 60% of those deaths.[2]

Race and Ethnicity
- Caucasians experience the highest rate of drug overdose deaths, with the overdose death rate almost doubling between 2002 and 2014 among this group. Caucasians' rate of drug overdose deaths in 2014 (12.3 per 100,000 people) was almost three times higher than that of Hispanics (4.3) and almost four times higher than that of African Americans (3.2).[3] Among young adults age 25 to 34, drug overdoses are driving up the death rate to levels not seen since the end of the AIDS epidemic more than two decades ago.[4]

Gender
- Males have a far higher death rate from overdose than females. The drug overdose death rate for males of all races and ethnicities in 2014 climbed to 18.3 per 100,000 people, compared to 11.1 for females of all races and ethnicities.

For Caucasian men and boys, that rate spiraled to 23.2.[3]

Geography
- Death rates from overdoses in rural areas now outpace the overdose death rates in large urban areas. In 2014, West Virginia, New Mexico, New Hampshire, Kentucky, and Ohio saw the highest rates of drug overdose deaths, often in rural counties. The overdose problem is a relatively new one for rural counties in such states, according to a federal analysis of overdose data. Because drug overdose was historically more of a big-city issue, some health researchers believe that these counties may not have adequate treatment programs to address the surge in drug abuse related to opioids.[2]

What Do You Think?

1. What factors might account for the higher rates of drug overdose deaths among males?
2. What aspects of the medical system might be contributing to the opioid overdose problem?
3. What particular challenges might rural areas face in helping residents with drug addiction?

Sources: **1.** Substance Abuse and Mental Health Services Administration. (2015). *Behavioral health trends in the United States: Results from the 2014 National Survey on Drug Use and Health* (HHS Publication No. SMA 15-4927, NSDUH Series H-50). www.samhsa.gov. **2.** Rudd, R., Aleshire, N., Zibbell, J., & Gladden, M. (2016). Increases in drug and opioid overdose deaths—United States, 2000–2014. *Morbidity and Mortality Weekly Report, 64*(50), 1378–1382. **3.** National Center for Health Statistics. (2016). *Drug poisoning mortality: United States, 2002–2014.* http://blogs.cdc.gov. **4.** Kolata, G., & Cohen, S. (2016, January 16). Drug overdoses propel rise in mortality rates of young whites. www.nytimes.com.

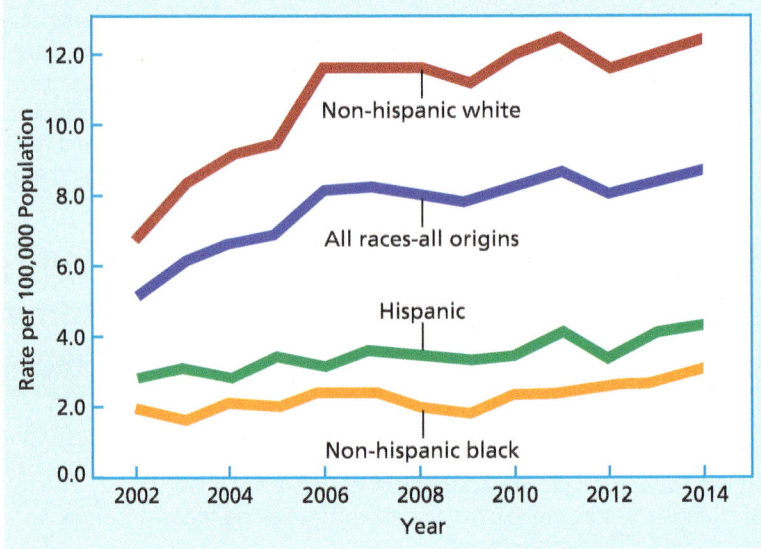

Rates of death by drug overdose have climbed dramatically in the past decade.

Source: CDC/NCHS, National Vital Statistics System, 2016.

This cycle of drug use and tolerance feeds drug addiction. Like other forms of addiction, drug addiction is a complex condition characterized by uncontrollable craving and use—despite negative consequences. In the past, people believed that drug addiction was due to moral failure, laziness, or lack of willpower. Today, addiction to drugs is typically described in terms of **dependence,** which has both psychological and physical roots.

Psychological dependence ("psychological addiction") means a mental attachment to a drug—the belief that a drug is needed to relieve stress, anxiety, or other uncomfortable feelings. With *physical dependence,* the body requires the regular use of a substance in order to function. A physically dependent person also develops tolerance; therefore, larger and larger doses are needed to achieve a high, or to even feel normal. Both psychological dependence and physical dependence are characterized by intense cravings for the drug.

> **dependence** The state of being mentally attached to and/or physically needing a drug.
>
> **withdrawal** The process in which, and symptoms that develop when, a person stops using a drug.
>
> **toxicity** The dosage level at which a drug becomes poisonous to the body.

The APA defines *substance use disorder* as a pattern of substance use that ranges from mild to severe and that is characterized by two to three of the following within a one-year period:[16]

- Developing tolerance to the substance.
- Using the substance in larger quantities or over a longer period than intended.
- Becoming unable to cut down or control one's use of the substance.
- Spending an inordinate amount of time on activities aimed at obtaining the substance, using it, or recovering from its effects.
- Sacrificing important social, occupational, or recreational activities due to the substance use.
- Continuing to use the substance despite knowledge that the substance has either caused or is exacerbating a physical or psychological problem.
- Experiencing withdrawal symptoms. **Withdrawal** refers to the process and experience of ceasing to take a drug that has created a physical dependence. Withdrawal can make some drugs extremely difficult to quit; symptoms include craving, headaches, nausea, and vomiting.

How Drugs Leave the Body

Both the extent and the duration of a drug's effect on the body depend on several factors, from body size to ethnicity. For example, a heavyset person will be less affected by the same dose of the same drug than a slender person, and Caucasians generally clear psychoactive drugs from the body more quickly than do Asian Americans. Moreover, drugs differ in their *distribution half-life,* the amount of time it takes a drug to move from the bloodstream to body tissues such as muscle and fat. The liver is responsible for metabolizing (breaking down) all kinds of toxins, from environmental pollutants to psychoactive drugs, into chemicals that can be excreted by the bowels in feces and by the kidneys in urine. Some substances can also be eliminated through exhaled breath, sweat, saliva, or in the breast milk of nursing mothers.

A drug's physiological effect on the body can also be altered when two or more drugs are combined. In *additive interactions,* the effect of one drug is combined with the effect of another. In *antagonistic interactions,* the effect of one drug is diminished when combined with another drug. The dosage level at which a drug becomes poisonous to the body and can cause temporary or permanent damage is referred to as its **toxicity.**

LO 8.4 QUICK CHECK

Dopamine is
a. a hormone that causes addiction.
b. a chemical compound in many narcotics that increases their addictive properties.
c. the brain's "feel-good" neurotransmitter.
d. a synthetic substance used to treat addiction.

Commonly Abused Drugs

LO 8.5 Identify commonly abused drugs and describe their mechanisms, effects, and health risks.

As noted earlier, illicit drug use includes unlawful use of prescription drugs, which is a growing problem in the United States. The following section discusses these and other commonly abused drugs.

Prescription and Over-the-Counter Medications

Taken as directed, medications can improve health and boost quality of life, but all carry risks, including unwanted side effects. These risks increase when medications are not taken properly. These are the four most common types of misuse:

- Taking the incorrect dose
- Taking the medicine at the wrong time
- Forgetting to take a dose
- Failing to take all the medicine

These behaviors can slow healing, promote complications, or, in the case of antibiotics, lead to the reproduction of "super bugs" that are resistant to the drug.

In addition to problems of misuse, experts now consider the abuse of prescription drugs to be an epidemic, spreading at a rate that mirrors the spread of HIV/AIDS in the United States.[1] About 6.5 million Americans reported abusing prescription drugs in 2014,[3] and a national survey conducted by the American College Health Association found that almost 14% of college students reported using prescription drugs that were not prescribed to them.[15]

Over-the-Counter Drugs

Over-the-counter (OTC) drugs are medications that can be purchased without a prescription. They include pain relievers and medications used to reduce allergy symptoms and to treat coughs and colds. There are now more than 700 OTC products available that contain ingredients that were available only by prescription three decades ago—some at greater dosage strength.[17]

OTC drugs pose many of the same challenges as prescription drugs. They are not meant to be taken in higher doses or for longer periods than indicated on the label. If symptoms do not go away after a few days of using an OTC drug, it is time to see your health-care provider. Some OTC medications can interact with other medicines, herbal and other dietary supplements, foods, and alcohol. Some OTC drugs are hazardous for people with certain medical conditions, such as asthma. Pregnant women should always check with a doctor before taking any OTC drug.

The U.S. Food and Drug Administration (FDA) cautions against the misuse of several common OTC pain relievers.[18] For example, taking too much acetaminophen can lead to serious liver damage. If ingested with alcohol—as little as three drinks per day—the risk of liver damage increases. The anti-inflammatory drug ibuprofen also has serious adverse effects if taken to excess or with alcohol. These include diarrhea, nausea, and vomiting, ulcers, internal bleeding, and kidney damage.

Cough and cold formulations can also be dangerous, especially when given to children. The FDA has withdrawn some of these medications for children younger than age 2 and advises that caregivers always consult the child's pediatrician before using OTC remedies.[19]

Prescription Drug Abuse

The second most commonly abused class of prescription drugs is stimulants, including drugs traditionally prescribed for attention deficit/hyperactivity disorder (ADHD), such as Ritalin and Adderall. In 2014, about 1 million Americans abused prescription stimulants.[3] Abuse typically starts among young adults age 18 to 25, and the problem is increasing on campus. (See the **Special Feature**.)

Other commonly abused prescription drugs include sedatives, antidepressants, and erectile dysfunction drugs. Again, many prescription drugs, including opioids and stimulants, have a high potential for addiction. And prescription drug abuse—especially when it involves combinations of drugs—can be fatal.

>> View a PBS Newshour segment on the increasing misuse and abuse of prescription drugs at **http://video.pbs.org/**. (Search for "too much pain medication.")

Opioid Abuse

In 2014, more than 4.3 million Americans reported abusing prescription pain medications in the past year.[3] The most commonly abused pain medications are prescription *narcotics* (from the Greek word meaning "numbing"), pain relievers that were originally derived from opium, a milky fluid found in the unripe seedpods of the opium poppy. Today, most narcotics are synthetic versions called **opioids**. They include morphine, which is often given to patients before or after surgery to alleviate severe pain, and codeine, which is used for milder analgesia (pain relief) or severe coughs. Other prescription opioids include hydrocodone (Vicodin) and oxycodone (marketed under the brand names OxyContin, Percodan, and Percocet).

Narcotics attach to special receptors on cells and block the transmission of pain signals to the brain. When taken as directed, they can effectively manage pain. Common side effects include nausea and constipation, and in too large a dose, they can cause respiratory depression, coma, and death. Abuse of prescription narcotics is implicated in hundreds of thousands of emergency department visits annually in the United States and is now the primary cause of overdose deaths, including more than 28,700 in 2014.[1,20]

In addition to being dangerous and addictive on their own, prescription narcotics are increasingly linked to heroin, a morphine derivative classified as an illicit drug.

Heroin

Fast-acting and highly addictive, **heroin** is typically sold as a white or brown powder, or as a sticky black substance known as "black tar heroin." Known on the street as "smack," "H," and "junk," heroin is usually injected directly into a vein, although it can also be smoked. In a 2014 study, about 435,000 people in the United States reported heroin use in the past year.[3]

Heroin is particularly addictive because it crosses into the brain quickly, producing an intense "rush" of pleasure accompanied by a sensation of heaviness. Withdrawal symptoms may begin within a few hours and include drug craving, restlessness, muscle and bone pain, diarrhea, and vomiting. Although these symptoms typically subside after about a week, they persist in some people for many months. Nearly a quarter of people who use heroin become dependent.[21]

> **opioids** Drugs derived from opium or synthetic drugs that have similar sleep-inducing, pain-reducing effects.
>
> **heroin** An illicit, highly addictive opioid.

Recent studies suggest that people who abuse prescription opioids are also at increased risk for heroin use. While many opioid abusers do not appear to transition to heroin, the majority of recent heroin users told researchers that they started with prescription opioids before they turned

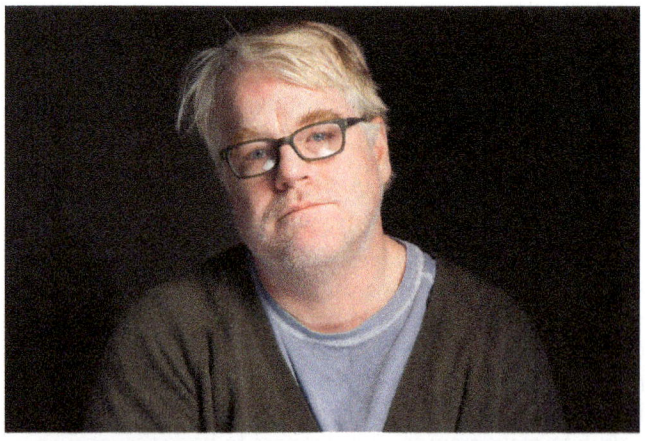

Mixing drugs is especially dangerous.
A lethal combination of drugs caused the death of actor Philip Seymour Hoffman.

SPECIAL FEATURE

Are "Study Drugs" Smart—or Safe?

In recent years, there has been an increase in college students' misuse of prescription stimulants, such as Adderall, Ritalin, and Concerta, which are intended for the treatment of attention deficit/hyperactivity disorder (ADHD). Evidence suggests that between 6% and 34% of college students have used a prescription stimulant (PS) without a valid prescription.[1,2]

The drugs work by increasing blood flow and levels of neurotransmitters in a region of the brain involved in decision making and impulse regulation. Users believe that the drugs help keep them alert and focused for extended periods of study or work time. But does PS use translate into academic success?

It would seem logical that drugs that improve attention and concentration should also promote learning and academic achievement. But studies have found a correlation between PS use and improvement in rote memory, not complex memory, and complex memory is more likely to be required for college exams.[3] Moreover, because the drugs cause students to think more narrowly, they can stifle creativity. So students may be better able to process data but less able to make meaningful connections.

In addition, modest improvements in academic skills with PS use were limited to subjects who had lower levels of ability to begin with, indicating that PS drugs are more effective at correcting deficits than in enhancing performance.[3] Smart, creative students actually derive little benefit from using these drugs.

Interestingly, the placebo effect may contribute to students' perceptions of PS use improving their performance. In one study, subjective feelings of being stimulated were produced solely by *expecting* to receive a PS.[3]

While benefits of PS use are minimal, the academic risks are significant. First, these drugs are controlled substances; thus, their unauthorized use (without a prescription) is a violation of most campus drug policies (and a federal crime). Corrective actions may range from mandatory participation in drug treatment to suspension or dismissal. For example, Duke University prohibits the nonmedical use of prescription stimulants for any academic purposes. Such use has been added to the university's formal definition of cheating.[3]

PS misuse also poses significant health risks.[2,3] Large doses can lead to psychosis, seizures, and an increased or erratic heart rate that can result in heart attack, stroke, and sudden death. Even at small doses, the drugs disrupt normal sleep patterns and cause nervousness, headaches, decreased appetite, and fever. Many of the drugs have a high potential for abuse and are highly addictive; withdrawal symptoms can include exhaustion, depression, anxiety, insomnia, and thoughts of suicide.

Cases of suicide among students using prescription stimulants are increasingly in the news. In 2013, for example, the parents of student John Edwards filed a medical-malpractice lawsuit against Harvard University. A sophomore, Edwards committed suicide six months after a psychiatric clinical nurse specialist at the campus health services center prescribed Adderall following a single consultation. Edwards' parents contend that their son never had ADHD.[4]

As a result of such cases, dozens of colleges are tightening the rules under which health services staff are allowed to prescribe ADHD medications. Many require students to sign contracts in which they promise to visit a mental health professional monthly, submit to regular blood testing, and not share or sell the pills.[5]

References: **1.** Dodge, T., Williams, K. J., Marzell, M., & Turrisi, R. (2012). Judging cheaters: Is substance misuse viewed similarly in the athletic and academic domains? *Psychology of Addictive Behaviors, 26*(3), 678–682. **2.** Arria, A., & DuPont, R. (2010). Nonmedical prescription stimulant use among college students: Why we need to do something and what we need to do. *Journal of Addiction Discovery, 29*(4), 417–426. **3.** Lakhan, S. E., & Kirchgessner, A. (2012). Prescription stimulants in individuals with and without attention deficit hyperactivity disorder: Misuse, cognitive impact, and adverse effects. *Brain and Behavior, 2*(5), 661–677. **4.** Schwartz, A. (2013, May 3). *Harvard student's suicide as case study* www.nytimes.com. **5.** Schwartz, A. (2013, April 30). *Attention-deficit drugs face new campus rules.* www.nytimes.com.

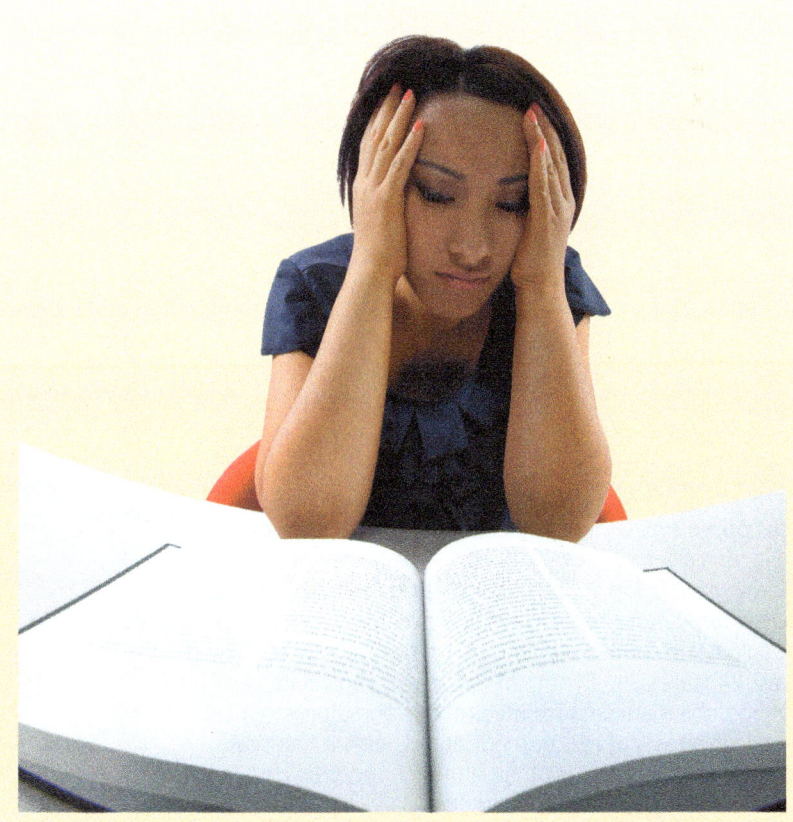

to heroin. Health researchers are now studying the possible connections more closely to better understand how addressing the two types of drug abuse together might lead to better treatments for the opioid epidemic.[22]

Marijuana

Of all well-known drugs, **marijuana** has received the most recent widespread legal attention—and perhaps the most public debate.

As of mid-2016, the District of Columbia and 4 states—Alaska, Colorado, Oregon, and Washington—allowed recreational use of marijuana, and at least 14 more were considering legalizing the drug. By that time, at least 20 states had also decriminalized small amounts of marijuana for personal use, meaning that the legal penalties associated with such use of the drug were generally not severe and typically did not include jail sentences.[23]

Yet these recent changes do not equal widespread acceptance of marijuana. Ohio's state legislature has rejected legalization. And at the federal level, marijuana is still classified as an illicit drug. While groups who support legalization claim that small amounts are relatively harmless, critics question that claim, pointing to documented short- and long-term health effects.

Marijuana is the most commonly used illicit drug in the United States.[3] In the most recent National Survey on Drug Use and Health, about 22 million Americans reported having used marijuana in the previous 30 days, representing about 8% of the population over the age of 12.[3]

Marijuana (the plant *Cannabis sativa*) grows wild and is farmed in many parts of the world. "Pot" is a dry, shredded mix of flowers, stems, seeds, and leaves of the plant that is usually rolled and smoked as a cigarette (joint) or by using a water pipe (bong) that passes the smoke through water to cool it. It is also sometimes mixed in food such as brownies, or brewed as a tea.

Short-Term Effects

Over the years, marijuana growers have bred the plant to contain increasingly higher percentages of its psychoactive ingredient, tetrahydrocannabinol (THC). When a person inhales THC in marijuana smoke, it takes just a few minutes to move from the lungs to the bloodstream to the brain. Ingesting marijuana from food moves THC to the brain more slowly. In the brain, THC binds to cannabinoid receptors, initiating a series of cellular reactions that ultimately result in a dopamine surge, which causes users to experience a high. The heart beats faster (sometimes double the normal rate), the bronchi (large air passages in the lungs) become enlarged, and blood vessels in the eyes expand, reddening the whites of the eye. Other manifestations include dry mouth, hunger, and sleepiness.

Some users report that the drug makes them feel relaxed and that time seems to slow, while others feel euphoric, with colors and sounds seeming more intense. Physicians in at least 24 states, the District of Columbia, and Guam can now prescribe marijuana for medical use, sometimes to help relieve side effects of cancer medications, such as nausea or severe pain. Patients report that, although the drug does not relieve pain, it helps them tolerate it.

Other short-term effects are less pleasant. They include impaired coordination, confusion, reduced reaction time, and difficulty thinking, solving problems, learning, and remembering. These effects can last for days or weeks in chronic users[24] and can also lead to "drugged driving," a dangerous condition similar to driving under the influence of alcohol. Public awareness of the risks of driving after marijuana use hasn't kept pace with the drug's popularity. In one survey, only about 7% of college students reported driving after they drank, but about 30% of marijuana users reported driving after using the drug.[25]

> **marijuana** One of the most commonly used drugs in the United States; derived from the plant *Cannabis sativa*.

Moreover, because marijuana raises the heart rate, the risk for a heart attack in the hour after its use increases more than fourfold.[26] Finally, THC is well documented for producing "the munchies," and weight gain is not uncommon with frequent use.

Long-Term Effects

Chronic marijuana use can have serious effects on mental and physical health **(Figure 8.1)**. Indeed, opponents of medical marijuana use often cite these adverse effects in explaining their opposition.

A number of studies have shown an association between chronic use and increased rates of anxiety, depression, psychosis, and personality disturbances; however, it is not clear whether marijuana use causes these disorders, exacerbates them, or reflects an attempt to self-medicate symptoms already present.[24] Long-term attention, learning, and memory have all been shown to be impaired in heavy, chronic marijuana users.

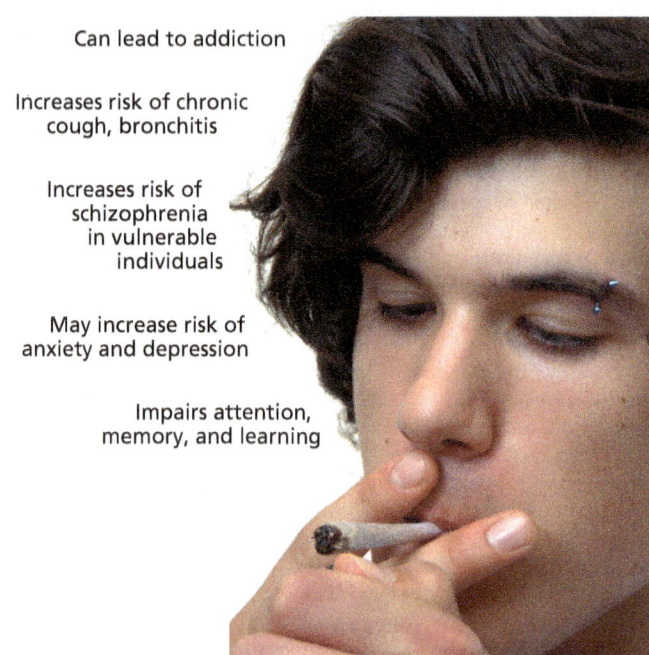

FIGURE 8.1 **Long-Term Effects of Marijuana Use.** Smoking marijuana can cause health problems throughout the body.

Marijuana smoke contains more cancer-causing chemicals than tobacco smoke and is similarly irritating to lung tissues. Thus, people who smoke marijuana can end up with many of the same respiratory problems associated with tobacco smokers, including daily cough and phlegm production and lung infections. Frequent and/or long-term marijuana use may also increase a man's risk of developing the most aggressive type of testicular cancer.[27]

Increasingly, research is finding that marijuana can be a hard habit to kick. Addiction develops in about 9% of all users but in 25% to 50% of daily users.[24]

>> For more information on the health effects of marijuana, visit **www.drugabuse.gov**.

Stimulants

Stimulants are a class of drugs that stimulate the function of the central nervous system, resulting in increased heart rate, blood pressure, and alertness. Commonly referred to as "uppers," stimulants also elevate mood. Legal stimulants include nicotine, caffeine, and prescription stimulants lawfully used. Illegal stimulants include cocaine, amphetamines, methamphetamine, and "bath salts" as well as prescription stimulants used nonmedically.

Caffeine

Caffeine is a white crystalline powder that, in its pure form, tastes very bitter. However, as a component in coffee, tea, soft drinks, energy drinks, and chocolate, it is the most popular psychoactive drug in the world. **Table 8.2** lists the caffeine content in selected foods, beverages, and OTC medications.

TABLE 8.2 Caffeine Content of Selected Foods and Beverages

Food/Beverage/Pill	Caffeine (milligrams)
Generic brewed coffee, 8 oz.	95–200
NoDoz, maximum strength, 1 tablet	200
Excedrin, extra strength, 2 tablets	130
Rockstar, 8 oz.	79–80
Red Bull, 8.4 oz.	76–80
Restaurant-style espresso, 1 oz.	40–75
Black tea, 8 oz.	14–61
Mountain Dew, 12 oz.	46–55
Coca-Cola Classic, 12 oz.	30–35
Generic decaffeinated brewed coffee, 8 oz.	2–12
Arizona iced tea, lemon flavored, 8 oz.	11
Hershey's kisses, 9 pieces	9

Source: Data from Mayo Clinic. (2012). *Caffeine content for coffee, tea, soda and more.* www.mayoclinic.com.

The effects of caffeine start less than an hour after consumption. As the drug stimulates the body's central nervous system, users feel more alert and energetic. Heart rate and blood pressure increase, and concentration and athletic performance can improve. While most people can safely drink two to four cups of coffee a day, excessive caffeine consumption can cause restlessness, anxiety, dehydration, and irritability. Caffeine can also trigger headaches and insomnia and lead to abnormal heart rhythms. Pregnant women who drink a cup and a half of coffee a day may double their risk of having a miscarriage.[28]

Caffeine is physically addictive, and regular users can suffer withdrawal symptoms if they suddenly go "cold turkey." Withdrawal usually lasts two to nine days and may include headaches, anxiety, fatigue, drowsiness, and depression.

Cocaine

Cocaine is derived from South American coca leaves, which people have ingested for thousands of years. "Coke" refers to cocaine in its fine white powder form. It is inhaled (snorted) or dissolved in water and injected intravenously. *Freebase cocaine* is a form of the drug that has been purified and converted into a crystalized substance that can be smoked. Freebase cocaine can also be further processed into small rock-like pellets known as *crack*, which refers to the crackling sound that the drug makes when heated.

Cocaine is a strong central nervous system stimulant that triggers the release of dopamine. Almost immediately, its use causes a rush of euphoria. These effects typically disappear within a few minutes or a few hours. To maintain a state of euphoria, users must continue taking the drug.

Taken in small amounts, cocaine usually makes the user feel energetic and mentally alert. It can also temporarily reduce appetite. Some people find that it helps them perform simple physical and mental tasks more quickly, while others experience confusion. Paranoia is also common.

Common side effects include increased heart rate, blood pressure, and respiration, chest pain, blurred vision, fever, and muscle spasms. Cocaine use can also cause abnormal heart rhythms, heart damage, strokes, abdominal pain and nausea, seizures, coma, and death.

Continued use commonly leads to tolerance. Repeated snorting of cocaine can lead to nosebleeds, a reduced sense of smell, and a chronically runny nose. Injection can trigger allergic reactions and put users at risk for infection with bloodborne diseases such as HIV and hepatitis. A hazard of the powder is that dealers often cut it with additives such as cornstarch, talcum powder, sugar, or other stimulants such as amphetamines.

Mixing cocaine and alcohol is especially dangerous. Taken together, the two drugs are converted by the body into cocaethylene, which is more toxic than either drug alone and can cause death.

stimulants A class of drugs that stimulate the central nervous system, causing acceleration of mental and physical processes in the body.

caffeine A widely used stimulant found in coffee, tea, soft drinks, chocolate, and some medicines.

cocaine A potent and addictive stimulant derived from leaves of the coca shrub.

>> Learn more about cocaine abuse at **www.drugabuse.gov**.

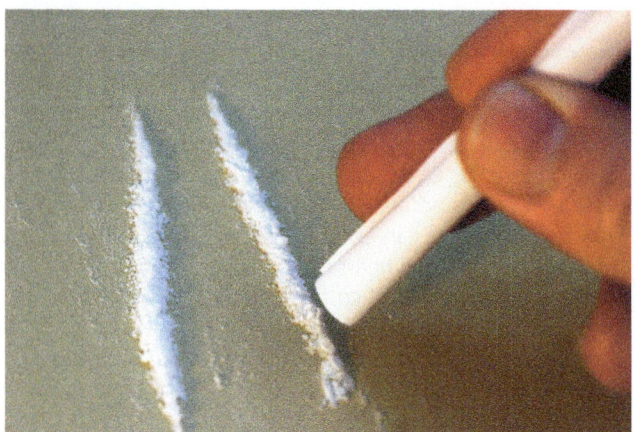

Cocaine use can result in heart damage, stroke, and sudden death.

Amphetamines

Amphetamines exert their stimulant effects by increasing the concentration of neurotransmitters in different regions of the brain. This increases the user's sense of alertness, decreases appetite and the need for sleep, and enhances physical performance. Amphetamines also induce feelings of well-being and euphoria.

The effects and risks associated with amphetamines are similar to those of cocaine. Even healthy young adults have suffered heart attacks after using them. Addiction is especially common because their effect causes users to take them repeatedly to avoid the "down" they begin to feel as soon as the drug wears off.

Amphetamines are legally classified as Schedule II drugs, meaning that they have a high potential for abuse and addiction but also have a recognized medical use. They are found in prescription drugs used to treat ADHD and in drugs used for certain rare sleep disorders and for chronic fatigue syndrome.

Methamphetamine

The highly addictive **methamphetamine** is a chemical similar to amphetamines, but it is much more potent, longer lasting, and more harmful to the central nervous system. Despite serious side effects, users often find themselves hooked by intense craving for the drug. The addiction is very difficult to treat. Methamphetamine is prescribed medically for ADHD and extreme obesity; however, because of its high potential for abuse, it is legal only by a one-time, nonrefillable prescription. Most methamphetamine sold on the street is made by small illegal labs. It can be ingested, injected, smoked, or snorted. "Crystal meth" refers to methamphetamine in its clear crystal form.

Short-Term Effects. Like amphetamines, methamphetamine exerts its effects by causing the brain to flood with neurotransmitters. However, its added methyl group of atoms allows it to cross into the brain more efficiently and to degrade more slowly. Even small amounts of methamphetamine can cause a rapid or irregular heartbeat, boost blood pressure, and reduce appetite. Other side effects include irritability, anxiety, insomnia, confusion, and tremors. Users quickly develop tolerance, needing more of the drug to get the same high. But increasing the dose can cause convulsions, cardiovascular collapse, and death.

Long-Term Effects. Chronic methamphetamine use may alter areas of the brain associated with emotion and memory, which could account for many of the emotional and cognitive problems that have been observed in abusers.[29] It may also result in aggressiveness, anorexia, hallucinations, and a paranoia that sometimes causes homicidal or suicidal thoughts. Some users hallucinate that bugs are crawling all over them and therefore scratch themselves repeatedly.

> **amphetamines** Central nervous system stimulants that are chemically similar to the natural stimulants adrenaline and noradrenaline.
>
> **methamphetamine** A highly addictive and dangerous stimulant that is chemically similar to amphetamine but more potent and harmful.
>
> **bath salts** Any of a group of drugs containing a synthetic compound similar to cathinone, an amphetamine-like stimulant.

Over time, some methamphetamine users begin to develop what is known as "meth mouth"—severely stained teeth that appear to be rotting away or falling out. Methamphetamine can also damage tissues and blood vessels, promote acne, and slow down the healing of sores. Open sores, in fact, are a hallmark of methamphetamine use (**Figure 8.2**).

>> View "before" and "after" images of people who became addicted to methamphetamine at **www.facesofmeth.us**.

Bath Salts

The term **bath salts** refers to drugs containing one or more chemicals related to the stimulant cathinone.[30] They are typically sold in small packets marketed as bath salts, plant food, or jewelry cleaner. Users ingest, inhale, or inject them.

The stimulant effect of these drugs is said to be as much as 10 times more potent than that of cocaine, but they also induce hallucinations. Together, the combination can produce extreme agitation, panic attacks, paranoia, delirium, suicidal thoughts, and violent behavior. Heart attack, stroke, seizures, and kidney failure have also been reported. Criminal assaults and emergency department visits are common consequences of use, and numerous deaths have been reported. Moreover, the drugs produce intense cravings and are highly addictive.[30]

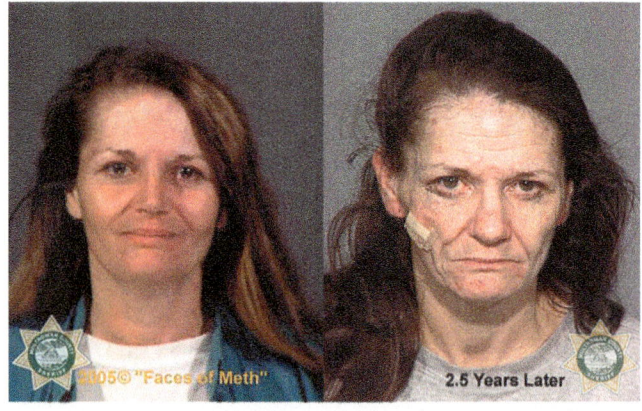

FIGURE 8.2 **Methamphetamine.** Methamphetamine use can take a dramatic physical toll.

Hallucinogens

Hallucinogens are so named because, in addition to altering perceptions, thoughts, and mood, they cause hallucinations, which are sensory impressions (e.g., sights, sounds, smells) that are not based in reality. Some hallucinogens come from plants, like the button-shaped top of the mescal cactus that produces mescaline, and certain types of mushrooms. Manufactured hallucinogens can be even more potent.

LSD

Lysergic acid diethylamide, commonly called **LSD,** is one of the strongest mood-altering chemicals. Commonly known as "acid," it is derived from lysergic acid, found in a fungus that grows on rye and other grains. Its hallucinogenic effects were discovered in 1943 when the scientist who first synthesized it accidentally swallowed some. LSD "trips" were promoted in the 1960s as a means of enhancing creativity or experiencing spiritual insight, and the fad emerged again among teens in the 1990s.

The effects of LSD are unpredictable. First effects are experienced within 30 to 90 minutes. The user swings from one emotional state to another or feels several emotions simultaneously. A large dose can cause delusions and visual hallucinations. Physical changes include dilated pupils, sweating, sleeplessness, tremors, and increased temperature, heart rate, and blood pressure.

LSD is not addictive, but some users grow tolerant. Sometimes users have "bad trips" that are extremely disturbing, or experience "flashbacks," reliving parts of a previous LSD experience long after the drug has worn off. Flashbacks may occur a few days or even a few years after use.

PCP

The street names for **phencyclidine (PCP)** include "angel dust," "killer weed," "embalming fluid," and "rocket fuel." As these names suggest, the drug can have volatile and even fatal effects. Originally developed in the 1950s as an anesthetic, its medical use was discontinued because of its adverse effects. Today, street PCP is produced in illegal labs. Users typically apply it to a smokable, leafy material such as mint or marijuana. Many people take in PCP unknowingly when someone else adds it to marijuana, LSD, or methamphetamine.

PCP is a **dissociative drug,** meaning that it produces feelings of detachment from a person's surroundings. Some users say PCP gives them the perception of strength and invulnerability, but others have very bad reactions, including confusion, agitation, and delirium. No one knows why reactions vary so much. Other effects include shallow breathing, flushing, sweating, numbness of the extremities, and poor muscular coordination.

At high doses, the effects can range from nausea and vomiting to blurred vision, seizures, coma, and death. PCP is known for triggering violent behavior, and suicides have been associated with the drug. Some symptoms, such as memory loss, speech difficulties, and depression, can last for up to a year after taking PCP.

Psilocybin (Magic Mushrooms)

Psilocybin, also known as "magic mushrooms," is a hallucinogen present in certain mushrooms grown in South America, Mexico, and parts of the United States. The mushrooms are often brewed as a tea or eaten with foods that mask their bitter flavor.

Within 20 minutes of ingestion, users begin to notice changes, usually hallucinations and an inability to separate fantasy from reality. Panic attacks can also occur. The effects usually fade after 6 hours. Psilocybin is not known to be addictive, and there seem to be no withdrawal effects. But serious risks include the onset of psychosis in susceptible users, and poisoning if another, deadlier mushroom has been confused with the psilocybin mushroom.

Club Drugs

The National Institute on Drug Abuse uses the term **club drugs** to refer to methamphetamine, LSD, MDMA (Ecstasy) and several other psychoactive substances that tend to be used at bars, nightclubs, and parties.[31] A few of these are discussed here.

MDMA (Ecstasy)

Methylenedioxymethamphetamine (MDMA), commonly known as ecstasy, is a synthetic drug chemically

---

hallucinogens Drugs that alter perception and are capable of causing auditory and visual hallucinations.

lysergic acid diethylamide (LSD) A powerful hallucinogen manufactured from lysergic acid, a substance found in a fungus that grows on rye and other grains.

phencyclidine (PCP) A dangerous synthetic hallucinogen that reduces and distorts sensory input and can unpredictably cause both euphoria and dysphoria.

dissociative drug A medication that distorts perceptions of sight and sound and produces feelings of detachment from the environment and self.

psilocybin A hallucinogenic substance obtained from certain types of mushrooms that are indigenous to tropical regions of South America.

club drugs Illicit substances, including MDMA (ecstasy), GHB, and many others that are commonly used at nightclubs and parties.

methylenedioxymethamphetamine (MDMA) A synthetic drug, commonly called "ecstasy," that works as both a stimulant and a hallucinogen.

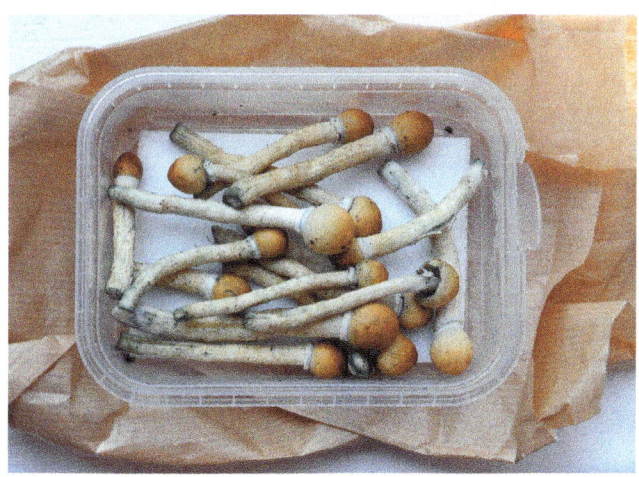

Psilocybin, also called "magic mushrooms," induces hallucinations and can cause psychosis in some users.

similar to methamphetamine. It was used by 0.8% of young adults in 2014.[3] Ecstasy comes in tablets, often as colorful pills imprinted with smiley faces, peace signs, or hearts. It is also known as "E," "X," and "XTC."

After ingesting a tablet, it takes about 15 minutes for the drug to enter the bloodstream and reach the brain. Its positive effects can include feelings of self-confidence, peacefulness, empathy, and increased energy. About 45 minutes later, the user feels the peak of the high, which can last for 3 to 6 hours.

>> View a segment about the dangers of Molly, a new formulation of MDMA www.today.com. (Search for "Molly drug.")

Ecstasy's negative effects—including confusion, anxiety, and paranoia—are similar to those of stimulants.[32] Physical effects can include nausea, blurred vision, chills, sweating, muscle tension, rapid eye movement, involuntary teeth clenching, faintness, and increases in heart rate and blood pressure. Because the stimulant effects enable users to dance for long periods, some have suffered dehydration and heatstroke. Heatstroke can lead to kidney, liver, or cardiovascular failure, and is nearly always fatal when untreated.

Regular use of ecstasy can cause depression, anxiety, insomnia, and memory problems that last up to several weeks. Studies have shown that some regular MDMA users have significant memory loss and attention deficits.[32]

Date-Rape Drugs

Less commonly used club drugs include GHB and Rohypnol. These are referred to as "date-rape drugs" because perpetrators commonly slip them into drinks to make victims drowsy or unconscious. The Drug-Induced Rape Prevention and Punishment Act of 1996 increased the federal penalties for using any controlled substance to aid in a sexual assault.

Gamma-hydroxybutyric acid (GHB) is used for its euphoric effects and for the perception of increased libido and sociability. High doses are associated with seizures, respiratory distress, and comas. GHB is addictive, and withdrawal symptoms include insomnia, anxiety, tremors, and sweating.

Rohypnol is a sedative that can cause drowsiness, visual disturbances, dizziness, and confusion. It can also cause partial amnesia, rendering users unable to remember certain events that they experienced while under the influence of the drug, including sexual assault.

Inhalants

Psychoactive **inhalants** include more than 1,000 common household items, such as paint, glue, and felt-tip markers, which people sniff to get high. In 2014, 0.2% of young adults reported having abused an inhalant in the past year.[3] Common household chemicals are often used as inhalants.[33] These include solvents such as paint thinner, aerosols such as hair spray, gases such as refrigerant gases, and nitrites such as fragrance sprays. Inhalants typically cause a feeling of intoxication similar to that of alcohol, usually for just a few minutes.[33] By repeated sniffing, users extend the high for several hours.

Health risks vary by type of inhalant but include permanent hearing loss, bone marrow damage, and brain damage.[33] Butane, propane, and the chemicals in aerosols have all been linked to what is known as "sudden sniffing death"—fatal heart failure within minutes of repeated inhalations. Some users cover their heads with a paper or plastic bag to inhale a higher concentration of chemical. This can cause suffocation. Chronic abuse of solvents can cause severe liver and kidney damage.

> **gamma-hydroxybutyric acid (GHB)** A central nervous system depressant known as a "date rape drug" because of its use to impair potential victims of sexual assault.
>
> **Rohypnol** A powerful sedative known as a "date rape drug" because of its use to impair potential victims of sexual assault.
>
> **inhalants** Chemical vapors that, when inhaled, produce mind-altering effects.
>
> **depressants** Substances that depress the activity of the central nervous system and include barbiturates, benzodiazepines, and alcohol.
>
> **barbiturates** Types of central nervous system depressants prescribed to induce sleep or sedation.
>
> **benzodiazepines** Medications commonly prescribed to treat anxiety and panic attacks.

Depressants

Depressants (also known as "downers") include alcohol, barbiturates, and benzodiazepines. All are substances that depress the central nervous system and slow the brain's activity. The effect is a drowsy or calm feeling that can reduce feelings of anxiety or pain and help induce sleep. Misuse of depressants can result in addiction, health problems, and even death.

Barbiturates and Benzodiazepines

Barbiturates are a type of central nervous system depressant typically prescribed to induce sleep and reduce anxiety. Barbiturate sedation can range from mild and short term to severe and long term (inducing coma). The drugs were popular in the early 20th century, but because of their side effects, potential for abuse, and safety concerns, fewer than 10% of current depressant prescriptions in the United States are for barbiturates.

Benzodiazepines are commonly prescribed to induce sleep, relieve anxiety and panic attacks, and help

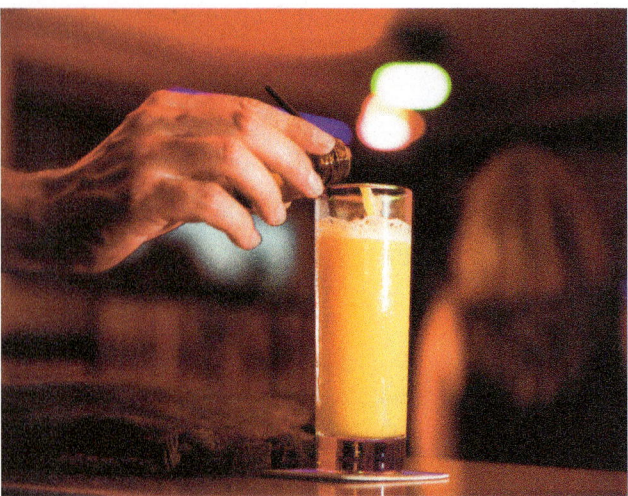

Date-rape drugs, such as GHB or Rohypnol, can be slipped into drinks when you're not looking.

prevent seizures. They were first marketed in the 1960s and, because they're considered safer and less addictive than barbiturates, they have become the depressant of choice in many medical practices. More than a dozen benzodiazepines are approved for use in the United States, including lorazepam (Ativan), alprazolam (Xanax), and diazepam (Valium).

Effects

In small doses, depressants reduce inhibition, induce calmness and muscle relaxation, and impair judgment. Excessive doses can cause slurred speech and loss of motor coordination. Very high doses can lead to respiratory depression, coma, and death. Veterinarians routinely use barbiturates to euthanize animals, and 1 in 10 humans who overdose on barbiturates do not survive.[34]

Depressants are not usually prescribed for long-term use, because such use can result in memory loss, irritability, amnesia, hostility, and disturbing dreams. Long-term users can develop tolerance and physical dependence, and withdrawal can be dangerous. Because depressants work by slowing the brain's activity, abruptly ending long-term use can cause the brain to race out of control. Insomnia and anxiety—the same symptoms that may have prompted a person to use these drugs in the first place—are common. More severe withdrawal can include fever, delirium, seizures, and cardiovascular collapse. Hospitalization may be required for those seeking to end their dependence on these drugs.

Table 8.3 (next page) provides a summary of commonly abused drugs, their intoxication effects, and the associated health risks.

LO 8.5 QUICK CHECK

Oxycodone is an example of which type of drug?
a. inhalant
b. opioid
c. stimulant
d. OTC medication

Preventing Drug Abuse

LO 8.6 Discuss common drug-prevention strategies used throughout the United States.

The aim of prevention programs is to reduce the factors that contribute to drug abuse while simultaneously promoting protective factors. Parental involvement, for example, is a known protective factor: Communicating the risks of drug abuse to children and teens cuts their risk of engaging in the behavior in half.[35] When valid substance abuse prevention programs are properly implemented, they can be effective.[36]

The following prevention strategies are in use throughout the United States:

- **Public awareness campaigns.** The federal government has spent millions of dollars on public awareness campaigns meant to discourage drug use. Although the effectiveness of these campaigns is subject to debate, the National Institute on Drug Abuse reports that rates of abuse go down when perceptions of harm go up, which typically happens with public awareness campaigns. Moreover, two research studies found that young people who reported exposure to a public awareness campaign on the risks of marijuana were less likely to begin use.[37]
- **Drug testing.** In an effort to discourage drug use—and to catch those who are users—some schools, athletics organizations, the U.S. military, and many workplaces conduct *random drug testing*. The process usually involves taking a urine sample and testing for traces of common drugs. Drug-free results on such tests may be required as part of the hiring process or as a condition of continued employment or membership. The Occupational Safety and Health Administration (OSHA) recommends a strategy in which companies that perform random drug testing also offer employees drug education and assistance programs.[38]
- **Federal policies.** In 2016, the Obama administration announced a new set of policies, backed by $1.1 billion in federal funding, to try to reduce the epidemic of prescription drug and heroin abuse. Some of its key initiatives include increased public awareness campaigns, increased monitoring of prescription drugs, including narcotics, increased availability of drug treatment medications and programs, and increased access to medical treatment for these addictions.[39]

LO 8.6 QUICK CHECK

Workplace drug testing is often conducted
a. at random.
b. on an annual basis.
c. in conjunction with employee evaluations.
d. jointly with local police.

Getting Help for a Drug Problem

LO 8.7 List community, campus-based, and clinical options for treatment of drug abuse.

Historically, drug abuse in the United States was seen as more of a moral problem than as a public health problem. The legacy of that stance is that arrest and punishment took precedence over placing drug users into treatment programs. However, courts now often try to strike a balance between punishment and the goal of recovery. And many people enter drug treatment without ever coming into contact with the legal system.

In 2014, about 21.6 million Americans were classified by the U.S. Department of Health and Human Services as having a *substance abuse disorder*, a recurring drug or alcohol problem significant enough to cause health problems, disability, and/or failure to meet major responsibilities at work, school, or home. About 7 million of these cases were drug related.[3]

Yet many people who need treatment may never receive it due to lack of health insurance or inability to afford treatment. In 2014, about 22.5 million people age 12 or older needed treatment for an illicit drug or alcohol use problem. But only 4.2 million (about 18%) received any treatment in the same year.[40]

TABLE 8.3 Commonly Abused Drugs

Category	Representative Drugs	Method of Administration	Intoxication Effects and Health Risks
Cannabis	Marijuana (street names: pot, dope, weed, grass, joint, reefer)	Inhaled or ingested	Effects: Psychoactive agent THC causes a sense of euphoria. Heart rate increases, bronchi enlarge, blood vessels expand. Risks: Addiction, impaired cognition, lung damage, increased cancer risk
Stimulants	Cocaine (street names: crack, rock, blow, C, coke, snow)	Inhaled or injected	Effects: Derived from coca leaves, this drug first produces feelings of increased energy and euphoria. Heart rate and blood pressure increase, appetite drops. Risks: Addiction, irritability, anxiety, paranoid or violent behavior, damage to heart, brain, and other vital organs
	Amphetamines (street names: speed, uppers, crank)	Inhaled, ingested, injected	Effects: This large, varied group of synthetic drugs improves mood and alertness. Heart rate and blood pressure increase. Risks: Addiction, restlessness, appetite suppression, hallucinations, erratic or violent behavior
	Methamphetamines (street names: meth, crystal, ice, glass, tina)	Inhaled, ingested, injected	Effects: A common form of amphetamine, this highly addictive drug quickly produces a sense of euphoria followed by a dramatic drop in emotion and energy as the drug wears off. Risks: Addiction, appetite suppression, dental damage, brain damage, psychosis, paranoia, aggression
Hallucinogens	LSD (street names: acid, blotter)	Ingested	Effects: Effective even at very low doses, this drug is known for producing powerful hallucinations. Other effects include nausea, increased heart rate, tremors, and headaches. Risks: Shortened attention span, miscarriage and preterm labor in pregnant women, paranoia, disordered thinking
	PCP (street name: angel dust)	Inhaled, ingested, injected	Effects: This synthetic drug can lead to both euphoria and extreme unhappiness and can also produce hallucinations. Risks: Slurred speech, poor coordination, loss of sensitivity to pain, nausea, vomiting, violent behavior, coma, and even death
	Psilocybin (street names: shrooms, magic mushrooms)	Ingested	Effects: This group of mushrooms, if ingested, has effects similar to those of LSD. Effects last for up to 6 hours. Risks: Paranoia, disordered thinking, nausea, erratic behavior
Club Drugs	MDMA (street names: ecstasy, E, X, XTC, Molly)	Ingested	Effects: This synthetic drug creates feelings of warmth and friendliness and also increases heart rate and blood pressure. Risks: Hallucinations, brain damage, disordered thinking, disturbed sleep; extremely dangerous if mixed with alcohol
	GHB (street name: G)	Ingested	Effects: This is a central nervous system depressant that disrupts memory and can lead to unconsciousness. Risks: Temporary amnesia, nausea, vomiting, seizures, memory loss, hallucinations, coma
	Rohypnol (street name: roofies)	Ingested	Effects: This drug is a powerful tranquilizer that slows physical and mental responses and is the best known of the daterape drugs. Risks: Temporary amnesia, slowed physical and mental reactions, semiconsciousness, unconsciousness
Inhalants	Solvents (e.g., paint thinner), aerosols (e.g., spray paint), gases (e.g., nitrous oxide), nitrites (e.g., leather cleaner)	Inhaled	Effects: Found in ordinary household products, these substances can produce a feeling of being "high" or drunk. Risks: Dizziness, impaired speech, impaired physical coordination, vomiting, hallucinations, loss of consciousness, death
Depressants	Barbiturates (street names: barbs, downers)	Ingested or injected	Effects: This group of drugs slows the functions of the central nervous system and is legally prescribed for anxiety and insomnia. Risks: Slowed pulse and breathing, slurred speech, impaired memory, addiction, sleep problems, impaired coordination
	Benzodiazepines (street names: downers, benzos)	Ingested or injected	Effects: This group of depressants functions as tranquilizers and includes common medications such as Valium. Risks: Drowsiness, dizziness, loss of libido, confusion, depression; less addictive than barbiturates
Opioids	Heroin (street names: smack, H, brown sugar, junk, horse)	Injected or inhaled	Effects: This opioid produces a feeling of drowsiness, dreaminess, and euphoria and can also lead to dramatic mood swings. Risks: Addiction, cardiovascular damage, respiratory illnesses, internal infections, death
	Prescription opioids (street names: Oxy, Captain Cody)	Ingested	Effects: This group of drugs produces feelings of sleepiness, dreaminess, and a reduced sensitivity to pain. Risks: Addiction, dangerous interactions with other drugs, nausea, vomiting, lack of physical coordination, death

Campus and Community-Based Options

Twelve Step programs, such as Narcotics Anonymous (NA), are free of charge and help many people struggling with substance abuse. Men and women come together to share their problems with drugs, to talk about their strategies for maintaining sobriety, and to support others facing the same challenges. The 12 steps take addicts through a process of personal growth, which includes making amends to all the people they have harmed. NA members have an average of nine years drug free.[41]

Twelve Step programs Addiction recovery self-help programs based on the principles of Alcoholics Anonymous.

Your campus health services center may offer assistance for students struggling with substance abuse. These services may include drug treatment, weekly support group meetings, substance-free housing, and opportunities to participate in community service projects. These services can be highly effective: Records from one Midwestern college show that, of an average of 60 students per year served in the previous decade, only 8 per year relapsed.[42]

>> View personal stories of hope and recovery from drug addiction at www.youtube.com. (Search for "You are not alone stories of hope.")

Clinical Options

The long-term goal of clinical drug treatment programs is, of course, to get people off harmful drugs for good. Many outpatient programs are available, but residential treatment is often necessary for persistent and severe addictions. In residential programs, patients live at the treatment center for weeks or months at a time. This removes them from environments and people who could tempt them to relapse, making it easier to develop new healthier habits.

Programs typically move through stages, beginning with *detoxification*, a process by which the person is therapeutically supported (with medications and other interventions)

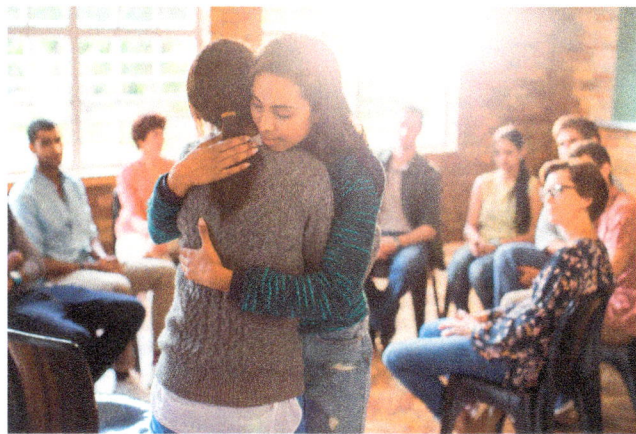

Support groups, usually available free of charge, help many people struggling with substance abuse.

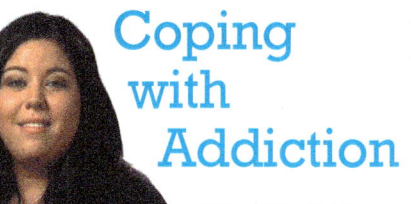

STUDENT STORY

Coping with Addiction

"HI, I'M ANA. I come from a background of alcoholism and addiction in my family. I've also struggled with it myself since I was 14. My dad was hardly ever around, and when he was, he struggled with addiction. I grew up thinking that was normal, despite what was taught at school. About a year ago, I heard about Alcoholics Anonymous and Narcotics Anonymous, and I've been with the program for a year. My dad's also with the program, and it's been great to have each other for support.

I used to drink a lot—binge drink with my friends—because that's what everybody did. And being around party drugs, designer drugs, was really kinda hard. Seeing everyone else use them, you really fall into the peer pressure of it all.

Now I definitely don't hang out with the same crowd. Back then, my friends and I pulled each other down. Not being around those kinds of people has really helped me a lot because I'm not around drugs or alcohol anymore, so I don't have the temptation there. I don't have the drugs to turn to.

AA and NA have helped because they're about getting over the fear of being judged and speaking about it. We feel like we're going to be ostracized from society and from our family if we admit to having a problem with addiction. But it's really important to speak out about it and ask for help, especially at a young age before all the other problems develop."

What Do You Think?

1. What factors put Ana at increased risk for addiction?
2. Ana talks about the fear of being judged for having an addiction. Why else might people avoid admitting that they have a problem? What might cause someone to finally admit to an addiction?
3. Ana mentions other problems that could develop due to addictions. What do you think she means? What types of problems does addiction cause in people's lives?

while the body clears itself of the drug and its byproducts and undergoes withdrawal. This is followed by treatment, which may include medications and psychotherapy.

Medications commonly used for opioid addiction include methadone and buprenorphine, which act on the same receptors as heroin and morphine, suppressing withdrawal symptoms and relieving cravings. All medications help patients disengage from drug seeking and become more receptive to behavioral treatments.[40]

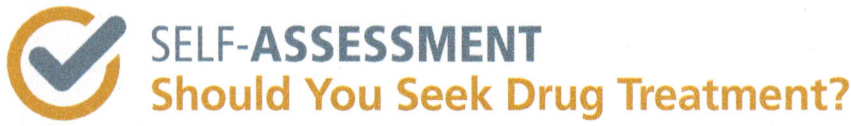
SELF-ASSESSMENT
Should You Seek Drug Treatment?

Answer Yes or No to the following 20 questions.

1. Have you used drugs other than those required for medical reasons?
2. Have you abused prescription drugs?
3. Do you abuse more than one drug at a time?
4. Do you use drugs more than once a week?
5. Have you tried to stop using drugs and not been able to do so?
6. Have you had blackouts or flashbacks as a result of drug use?
7. Do you ever feel bad or guilty about your drug use?
8. Do your spouse or parents ever complain about your involvement with drugs?
9. Has drug abuse created problems between you and your spouse or your parents?
10. Have you lost friends because of your use of drugs?
11. Have you neglected your family because of your use of drugs?
12. Have you been in trouble at work because of your use of drugs?
13. Have you lost a job because of drug abuse?
14. Have you gotten into fights when under the influence of drugs?
15. Have you engaged in illegal activities in order to obtain drugs?
16. Have you been arrested for possession of illegal drugs?
17. Have you ever experienced withdrawal symptoms (felt sick) when you stopped taking drugs?
18. Have you had medical problems as a result of your drug use, such as memory loss, hepatitis, convulsions, bleeding, etc.?
19. Have you gone to anyone for help for a drug problem?
20. Have you been involved in a treatment program especially related to drug use?

HOW TO INTERPRET YOUR SCORE The more "Yes" answers you have, the more likely it is that you should seek treatment for your drug use.

To complete this Self-Assessment online, visit MasteringHealth™

Source: DAST-20 Drug Abuse Screening Test, reproduced by permission of Dr. Harvey A. Skinner. ©Copyright 1982 by Harvey A. Skinner, PhD and the Centre for Addiction and Mental Health, Toronto, Canada. Reprinted by permission.

Recovery from addiction is often more complicated for a **polyabuser**—a person who abuses multiple drugs, often including alcohol. Polyabuse is frequently a factor in drug overdose incidents and deaths; in fact, a significant majority of U.S. emergency department visits for drug overdose involve polyabuse.[43] The behavior is particularly dangerous because of the collective toxicity of the drugs.

Should you seek drug treatment? Find out by completing the **Self-Assessment**.

LO 8.7 QUICK CHECK

Which of the following is a top reason people needing drug treatment don't receive it?

a. lack of personal responsibility
b. insurance and affordability issues
c. nationwide shortage of methadone
d. lack of interest from family and friends

Change Yourself, Change Your World

LO 8.8 Outline personal strategies for overcoming addictions and preventing drug abuse.

If you currently abuse drugs—or find yourself strongly tempted to do so—seek help now. If you're concerned about peer pressure, academic stress, or other issues pulling you toward drug abuse in the future, then your best strategy may be to think of yourself as your own personal advocate. Just as you surely have been advised to "think before you drink," health experts encourage you to *think before you act* when it comes to drugs and consider all the ramifications before you light up, shoot up, or pop a pill. Do you understand the short- and long-term health risks involved? Is a temporary high worth the risk of addiction and other health problems, family and relationship conflict, academic problems, financial trouble, a car accident—maybe even arrest—or death?

Personal Choices

By now you're familiar with the process of behavior change. But overcoming drug abuse can be more challenging than other types of behavior change because of the chemical effects that psychoactive drugs have on your brain. Employing the strategies discussed here can help.

Value Your Values

What are your values? Are honesty, integrity, and respect and kindness toward others important to you? What about your goals? Do you want to pursue an advanced degree, get hired for your dream job, or land a role on Broadway? Challenging yourself to identify how your choices about drugs reflect and support—or deny and derail—your values and goals can be an enlightening exercise. The next step is identifying specific steps you need to take to live in closer alignment with your values and to achieve your goals.

polyabuser A person who abuses more than one drug.

Make Some Trade-offs

If you're tempted to abuse drugs, or to continue to abuse them, you may believe that they'll provide a quick fix for your current problems. Although it's true that, for a few minutes or hours, you'll escape, what about those short- and long-term consequences? Make a better trade-off. **Endorphins** are your body's own "feel-good" chemicals. When they bind to opiate receptors in the brain, they increase pleasure and decrease pain. There are many healthful ways to prompt your brain to produce this "natural high," including exercise, meditation, creative writing, volunteer work, and spending time with people you love. Many people find that challenging themselves to overcome fears (by getting involved in public speaking or rock climbing, for example) boosts their endorphins.

> **endorphins** Hormones that act as neurotransmitters and bind to opiate receptors, stimulating pleasure and relieving pain.
>
> **intervention** A technique used by family and friends of an addict to encourage the addict to seek help for a drug problem.

Another important trade-off you might have to make is in your circle of friends. Tell them in unambiguous language that you're drug free. True friends will not only accept but respect your decision. Those who ridicule you or try to change your mind still deserve your care and concern, but not your time. Let them know you have no hard feelings but won't be able to hang out with them anymore. Recognize your vulnerable times, such as Friday and Saturday nights, and schedule drug-free activities in advance to make sure your calendar is filled. That way, you can honestly say, "Sorry, I'm busy," if someone invites you to a party where drugs will be available.

Build a Healthier Lifestyle

If you're in recovery, the experience will go more smoothly if you take care of yourself. Although withdrawal often disturbs sleep patterns, go to bed at a reasonable hour and try to get seven to eight hours of sleep. If your mind races, try repeating a positive affirmation or sending loving thoughts to any friends who are also struggling with abuse and addiction.

Don't ignore your diet. Depending on the drug you used, you may have lost significant weight. Withdrawal from certain drugs can promote gastrointestinal problems such as diarrhea, vomiting, and nausea at a time when you need nutrients, including fluids, to support your recovery. Guidelines from the National Institutes of Health recommend the following dietary practices for recovery:[44]

- Stick to regular mealtimes.
- Drink plenty of water and stay hydrated.
- Eat a diet that is relatively low in fat and has adequate protein and complex carbohydrates (including plenty of vegetables and whole grains).
- Take a multivitamin and mineral supplement.
- Don't mistake hunger or thirst for a drug craving. If a craving hits, eat a healthy meal or snack or drink a glass of water or a cup of caffeine-free herbal tea.

Finally, exercise. The endorphins released during physical activity will help decrease cravings and elevate your mood.

Ask for Help

If you're trying to quit drugs, but a craving hits you in the middle of the night, who is the one person you can call on for help? Maybe it's your mom or dad, a sibling, your best

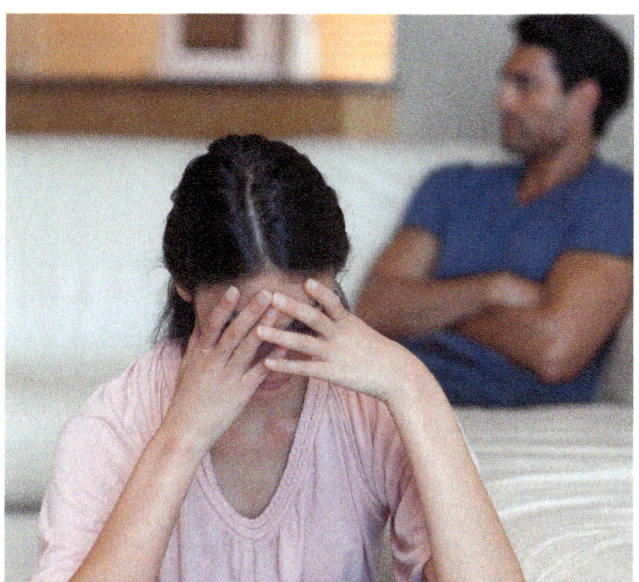

Don't be afraid to talk to someone if you're suffering with addiction.

friend, your sponsor, or another member of your Twelve Step program or support group. Whoever it is, tell him or her what you are going through and ask that they be "on call" for you. Remember, you don't have to "tough it out"; medications and clinical counseling are a phone call away. The Substance Abuse and Mental Health Services Administration's nationwide treatment referral help line is available 24 hours a day, at 1-800-662-HELP.

▶▶ You can also locate treatment centers in your area by clicking on the map at http://findtreatment.samhsa.gov.

Deal with Relapse

Even with help, more than half of patients in drug treatment may experience relapse.[36] Often, relapse occurs during times of stress. But some people are tempted to abuse again when they are well into their recovery, feeling healthy and strong. At these times, people can begin to feel nostalgic for their "early days" of drug use, when they felt they were in control. They may believe that they can return to this casual level of use, not realizing that the chemical changes prompted by their addiction don't make this possible.[45, 46]

Experts stress that "falling off the wagon" does not mean treatment doesn't work or that a user will never be free of the drug. Relapse can, however, be extremely demoralizing. It is better to look at relapse as practice than as failure. As with every other challenge in life, you may need to try several times before finally getting sobriety right.

Helping a Friend

As drug dependence progresses, it changes brain functioning significantly enough that users do not realize they have a problem or that it is interfering with their lives. In such cases, friends and family may stage what is called an **intervention,** an organized attempt to encourage a loved one to get professional help. Interventions usually involve direct, face-to-face demonstrations of love, support, and encouragement to enter treatment. Before you consider an intervention for a family member or friend, meet with a substance abuse counselor for guidance and for information about available treatment options.

>> An excellent resource for helping a loved one with a drug addiction is the Partnership at www.drugfree.org.

How can you promote a campus environment where drug abuse and addiction are recognized as serious health problems? Here are some ways to get involved:

- Recognize that every time you say no to drugs, you're challenging the idea that drug use is normal. Still, it's hard to "just say no." Be prepared with a "reply" such as: "No thanks, I've got a paper due tomorrow." Or, "I'm dealing with a health challenge right now, and that would only make it worse." Or try humor: "Sorry, but I need to preserve all the brain cells I have!"
- Spread the word. Although information alone usually isn't enough to stop drug abuse, when combined with other prevention and treatment efforts, it does make a difference, especially when the information comes from peers. For instance, let's say you know that a friend is abusing a prescription drug but mistakenly thinks that, because it was prescribed for a family member, it's safe and legal. Take the opportunity to ask some questions: *Do you know about the health risks of using this drug? Do you know that what you're doing is illegal?* Let your friend know you're concerned and offer to help.
- Volunteer to become a peer mentor. Many colleges have peer mentoring associations whose volunteers help their peers overcome substance abuse and other challenges.

>> Watch videos of real students discussing drug use and abuse at MasteringHealth™

LO 8.8 QUICK CHECK

Which of the following is a healthful way to boost endorphins?
a. Use only OTC drugs.
b. Limit yourself to recreational drug use only.
c. Choose alcohol over drugs.
d. Pursue activities that help you overcome your fears.

Choosing to Change Worksheet

To complete this worksheet online, visit MasteringHealth™

Although you may not realize it, you might routinely use one or more psychoactive drugs. If you drink caffeinated beverages like coffee, tea, cola, or energy drinks, or drink alcohol or smoke cigarettes, or take pain relievers, sleeping pills, or allergy medicine, you are using a psychoactive drug. Monitor your drug use for a week.

PART I   Keep a Drug Diary

List the drugs you consumed daily over the course of a week. Did you drink coffee? List the number of cups. How about energy drinks or caffeinated sodas? Tea? Did you smoke cigarettes? How many? Drink alcohol? Did you take prescription medications? Over-the-counter medications? Also make note of your stress level and mood at the time you used the drug.

Example:

Day	Substance	Amount	Drug	What Did It Do for You?	Stress Level 1= low stress 2 = moderate stress 3 = high stress	Mood (angry, happy, depressed, bored, frustrated, etc.)
1	Coffee	3 cups	Caffeine	Helped me wake up	3	Frustrated

Your Turn:

Day	Substance	Amount	Drug	What Did It Do for You?	Stress Level 1 = low stress 2 = moderate stress 3 = high stress	Mood (angry, happy, depressed, bored, frustrated, etc.)
1						
2						
3						
4						
5						
6						
7						

Review and Reflect on Your Drug Diary

1. Were you surprised about anything in your drug diary? _____ If yes, what surprised you?
   _____

2. Did you notice any patterns in your use of drugs? _____ If yes, what patterns were apparent?
   _____

3. Are you using any drugs as a coping mechanism to deal with your stress levels or moods? _____ If yes, which drugs?
   _____

4. Looking at your drug diary, are there any substances you would like to reduce or eliminate?
   _____

PART II Reducing or Eliminating Drug Use

Directions: Fill out your stage of change in step 1 and complete the remaining steps depending on which one applies to your stage of change.

Step 1: Assess your stage of behavior change. Please check one of the statements on the next page that best describes your readiness when it comes to reducing or eliminating the drug listed in question 4, above.

_____ I do not intend to eliminate or reduce use of this drug in the next six months. (Precontemplation)

_____ I might eliminate or reduce the use of this drug in the next six months. (Contemplation)

_____ I am prepared to eliminate or reduce the use of this drug in the next month. (Preparation)

_____ I eliminated or reduced use of this drug less than six months ago. (Action)

_____ I have eliminated or reduced use of this drug for more than six months and want to maintain it. (Maintenance)

Step 2: Working the precontemplation, contemplation, and preparation stages. Write down a healthier behavior you could put in place of your drug use. If you are in the preparation stage, create a SMART goal for your behavior change.

_____
_____
_____

Tell someone what you plan to do. Being accountable to others motivates you and also offers you the support and encouragement of others. Who did you tell?

_____

Step 3: Working the action and maintenance stages. Track your progress. For three days after you start reducing or eliminating your drug use, keep track of the results. Evaluate your progress and explain whether you intend to modify your plan.

_____
_____
_____

If you still have trouble cutting back on your drug use, see a health professional for help. Reread pages 197–199 of the chapter for information on where to find professional help. List the professional resources that will help you achieve your goal:

_____
_____

Step 4: Helping someone else who uses drugs. Ask yourself the following questions about your friend or loved one's drug use.

1. Are you concerned with the amount of drugs your friend or loved one uses? Yes No
2. Does trying to talk about your friend or loved one's drug or alcohol use cause a fight? Yes No
3. Do you worry about how much money and time your friend or loved one devotes to alcohol or drugs? Yes No
4. Do you make excuses or lie to cover up your friend or loved one's behavior when he or she is using? Yes No
5. Has he or she ever hurt or embarrassed you because he or she was drunk or high? Yes No
6. Does his or her behavior when he or she is drinking or using ever scare you or make you nervous? Yes No
7. Have you ever thought of calling the police on your friend or loved one while he or she is drunk or high? Yes No
8. Does his or her using make you feel stressed out? Yes No
9. Are you forced to take on his or her responsibilities because he or she is drunk, high, or hung over? Yes No

Source: Adapted from National Council on Alcoholism and Drug Dependence, Inc. (n.d.). *Concerned About Someone?* www.ncadd.org. Reprinted with permission from NCADD.

If you answered "Yes" to any of the nine questions, you may want to talk to your friend or loved one right away. Also, reread pages 197–199 for information on professional resources that may help and reread the information on pages 199–200 about how to help a friend with addiction.

CHAPTER 8 STUDY PLAN

CHAPTER SUMMARY

LO 8.1
- *Addiction* is a chronic disease of reward, motivation, memory, and related brain circuitry. One of its most fundamental characteristics is craving.

LO 8.2
- Behavioral addiction is a type of addiction that involves a compulsion to engage in a particular activity, usually with negative consequences.
- Recognized behavioral addictions include pathological gambling, hypersexual disorder, compulsive spending, and technology addiction.

LO 8.3
- Deaths from drug overdose have reached epidemic levels, driven largely by abuse of prescription and illegal opioids.
- College students greatly overestimate how many of their peers are using illicit drugs. Self-reported marijuana use among college students is about 17%.

LO 8.4
- *Drug misuse* is the inappropriate use of a legal drug. *Drug abuse* is the use of any drug that harms your health.
- Chemicals called neurotransmitters (such as dopamine) facilitate the transport of messages throughout the nervous system. Psychoactive drugs typically trigger a surge of "feel-good" chemicals, resulting in a sense of euphoria.

MasteringHealth™
Build your knowledge—and health!—in the Study Area of **MasteringHealth**™ with a variety of study tools.

- With regular use, the body develops tolerance to drugs, so progressively larger amounts are needed to achieve an effect. Psychological dependence is a mental attachment to a drug. Physical dependence occurs when the body requires the regular use of a drug in order to function. Withdrawal from a drug provokes a variety of symptoms, including nausea, vomiting, insomnia, and panic attacks.

LO 8.5
- Commonly abused drugs include prescription and over-the-counter medications, marijuana, stimulants (e.g., caffeine, cocaine, amphetamines, and methamphetamine), hallucinogens (e.g., LSD, PCP, psilocybin), club drugs (e.g., MDMA, GHB, Rohypnol), inhalants, depressants (e.g., barbiturates, benzodiazepines), and opioids, including certain prescription pain relievers and heroin.

LO 8.6
- Prevention efforts include public awareness campaigns, random drug testing in the workplace and on sports teams, and federal policies, such as those mandating increased monitoring of prescription drugs.

- Prevention efforts are especially effective when combined with treatment for those who need it.

LO 8.7
- Most people who need drug treatment do not receive it. Community-based programs such as Narcotics Anonymous can help.
- A growing number of colleges offer on-campus support services for students attempting to overcome substance abuse.
- Clinical drug treatment includes outpatient clinics and residential programs; both offer medications and counseling.

LO 8.8
- To prevent or stop drug abuse or addiction, you will most likely need change how you manage stress, the people you hang out with, and the activities you engage in. Practice good sleep habits, eat a nourishing diet, get exercise, and talk to a friend.
- An intervention is an organized attempt by an individual, a family, or another group to encourage a loved one to get professional help to overcome addiction.

GET CONNECTED

>> Visit the following websites for further information about the topics in this chapter:

- The Science of Addiction
  www.drugabuse.gov/publications/science-addiction
- Drugs of Abuse Information
  www.drugabuse.gov
- Narcotics Anonymous
  www.na.org

MOBILE TIPS!
Scan this QR code with your mobile device to access additional tips about avoiding substance abuse. Or, via your mobile device, go to http://chmobile.pearsoncmg.com and choose by topic: substance abuse.

- National Center on Addiction and Substance Abuse at Columbia University
  www.centeronaddiction.org.

Website links are subject to change. To access updated web links, please visit MasteringHealth™

TEST YOUR KNOWLEDGE

LO 8.1
1. One of the most fundamental characteristics of addiction is
   a. recognition that the behavior is causing significant harm.
   b. intense craving.
   c. sleep disturbances.
   d. euphoria.

LO 8.2
2. Which of the following is a behavioral addiction?
   a. pathological gambling
   b. hypersexual disorder
   c. addiction to video games
   d. all of the above

LO 8.3
3. The rate of drug abuse among full-time college students is
   a. significantly higher than the rate among college-age adults in general.
   b. significantly lower than the rate among college-age adults in general.
   c. about the same as the rate among college-age adults in general.
   d. somewhat higher than most college students believe it is.

LO 8.4
4. A person who must use more of a drug to experience an effect that a smaller dose used to produce has developed
   a. tolerance.
   b. psychological dependence.
   c. hypersensitivity to the drug.
   d. signs of withdrawal.

LO 8.5
5. Which of the following is responsible for the greatest percentage of overdose deaths?
   a. heroin
   b. cocaine
   c. methamphetamine
   d. prescription opioids

6. Adderall is grouped within the same class of drugs as
   a. methamphetamine.
   b. barbiturates.
   c. LSD.
   d. OxyContin.

7. Impaired memory is a potential adverse effect of use of
   a. marijuana.
   b. methamphetamine.
   c. MDMA.
   d. all of these drugs.

LO 8.6

8. The Occupational Safety and Health Administration recommends which of the following drug-abuse prevention strategies?
   a. mandatory random drug testing for all American workers
   b. termination of employees who test positive for drug abuse
   c. federal tax incentives for companies that perform regular random drug testing
   d. employee drug education and assistance programs for companies that perform random drug testing

LO 8.7, 8.8

9. Which of the following statements about drug treatment options is true?
   a. Membership fees for participation in Narcotics Anonymous are usually covered by health insurance providers.
   b. The most common reason people give for not entering treatment for drug abuse is lack of health insurance coverage and an inability to afford treatment.
   c. Community support groups and outpatient therapy are usually effective treatment options even for people with persistent and severe addictions.
   d. All are true.

LO 8.1, 8.8

10. The return to drug abuse after a period of drug abstinence is called
    a. persistence.
    b. remediation.
    c. relapse.
    d. codependency.

WHAT DO YOU THINK?

LO 8.1, 8.7

1. Do you know any families experiencing problems with addiction that pass from one generation to the next? What are some of the reasons this occurs? What could help these families break the cycle of addiction?

LO 8.5

2. What do you think about the effects of legalizing marijuana in some states. Does legalization reduce the potential for crime? Why or why not? Or does legalization just encourage more people to use marijuana, thereby magnifying the health and social problems it can cause?

LO 8.5

3. Buying, selling, giving away, or accepting even one Adderall pill is a federal crime. Do you see this behavior among your peers? Do you participate? If so, are you concerned about the health and legal risks? Why or why not?

LO 8.5, 8.7

4. What is your campus doing to prevent the use of date-rape drugs? Are those efforts effective? Why or why not?

LO 8.8

5. If you saw someone "spike" another student's drink at a party or bar, or offer someone marijuana that you knew to be laced with a stronger drug, what would you do? How can students work together to keep each other safe in social situations?

9

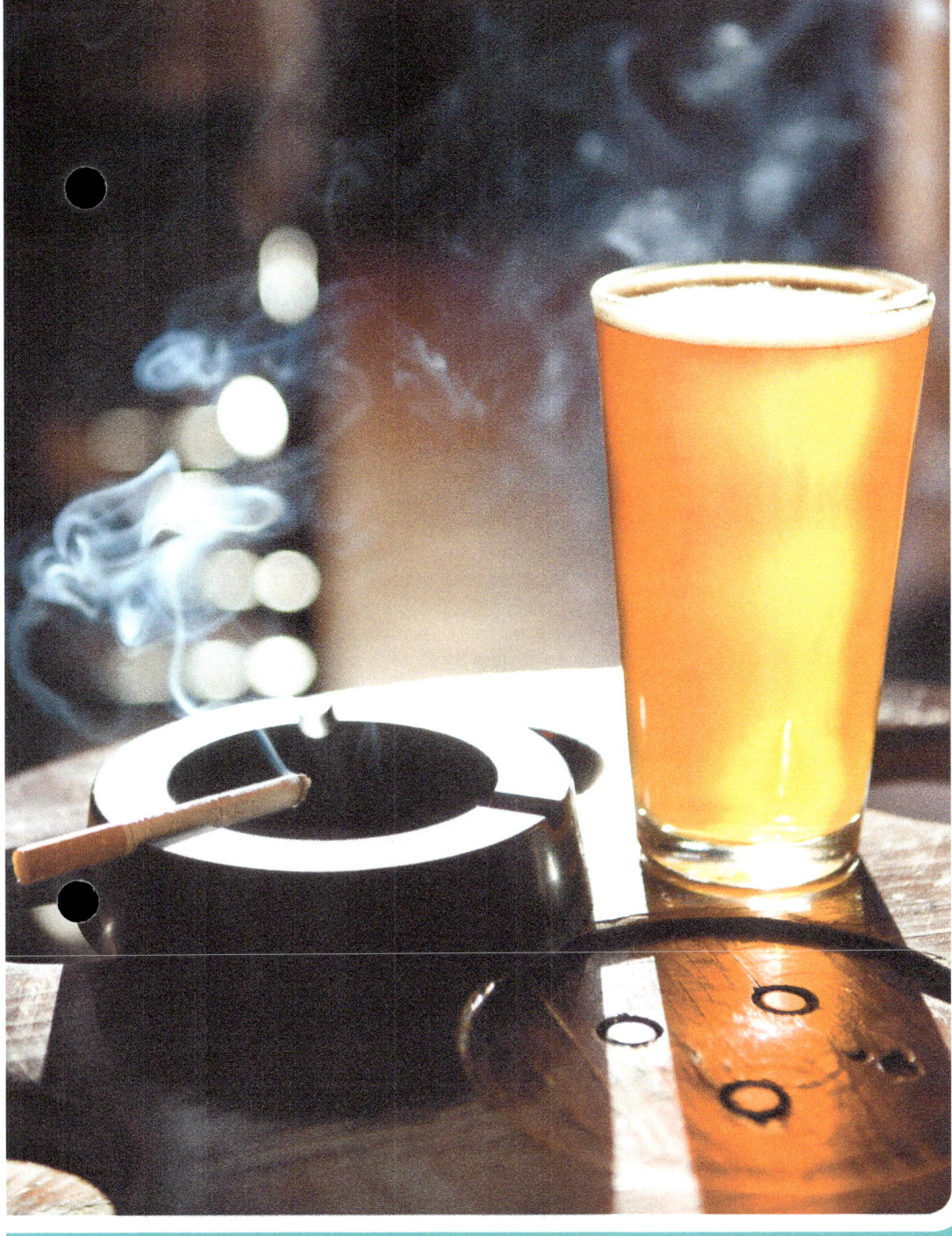

ALCOHOL AND TOBACCO USE AND ABUSE

> Alcohol is a factor in about 60% of fatal burn injuries, drownings, and homicides; 50% of severe trauma injuries and sexual assaults; and 40% of fatal motor vehicle crashes, suicides, and fatal falls.[i]

> About 25% of U.S. college students have never had a drink at all.[ii]

> 1 out of every 5 deaths in the United States is caused by a smoking-related illness.[iii]

> Secondhand smoke, laden with toxic chemicals, is responsible for almost 50,000 smoking-related deaths each year.[iii]

LEARNING OUTCOMES

LO 9.1 Discuss alcohol use in the United States.

LO 9.2 Describe how the body absorbs and metabolizes alcohol.

LO 9.3 Describe the short-term and long-term health effects of alcohol use.

LO 9.4 Explain how alcohol affects behavior.

LO 9.5 Recognize the types and signs of alcohol abuse.

LO 9.6 Identify alcohol abuse treatment options and prevention strategies.

LO 9.7 Discuss tobacco use in the United States.

LO 9.8 List the short-term and long-term health effects of tobacco use.

LO 9.9 Identify a range of tobacco products.

LO 9.10 Outline strategies for quitting smoking.

LO 9.11 Describe how to promote a smoke-free environment on campus.

There will be many times in college when you are exposed to two of the most popular drugs

in the United States: alcohol and tobacco. Both are easily accessible on college campuses, and students often feel pressure to try them. Although experimenting with these drugs may seem like a harmless rite of passage, their use can carry serious consequences. Just one drunken night can result in a fatal vehicle accident or make you vulnerable to sexual assault. Alcohol and tobacco are also both highly addictive. Many alcoholics trace the roots of their alcoholism to their college years, and smoking is notoriously hard to quit. The long-term health consequences of heavy drinking and smoking can be devastating and include diseases like cirrhosis (scarring of the liver), cancer, and heart disease.

Students tend to underestimate how easy it is to develop a drinking or smoking problem and how difficult it is to overcome one. By setting limits—or by abstaining from alcohol and tobacco altogether—you can reduce the likelihood that these addictive drugs might one day control you.

Alcohol Use in the United States

LO 9.1 Discuss alcohol use in the United States.

According to national surveys, slightly more than half of Americans drink alcohol—about 139.9 million people.[1] Among males, about 57.1% report being current drinkers compared to 47.5% of females. However, among those aged 12 to 17, the percentages of male and female drinkers are very similar (both about 13%). Among Caucasian adults of either sex, about 57.7% drink alcohol—a higher percentage than reported by any other racial or ethnic group.[1] See the **Diversity & Health** box on page 207 for a more detailed snapshot of drinking in the United States.

The 1984 Federal Uniform Drinking Age Act (FUDAA) financially penalizes any state that fails to prohibit the purchase or public possession of any alcoholic beverage by a person under 21. Because all states ultimately complied, the act effectively raised the national minimum legal drinking age to 21. Research shows that the FUDAA has had positive effects on health and safety, primarily in decreasing traffic crashes and fatalities, suicide, and consumption by those under age 21.[2-5]

Alcohol Use and Binge Drinking on Campus

An estimated 74.5% of college students nationwide have tried alcohol, and 29.9% report **binge drinking** in the last two weeks.[6] Binge drinking, or *heavy episodic drinking*, is defined by the National Institute on Alcohol Abuse and Alcoholism as a pattern of drinking alcohol that results in a blood alcohol concentration (BAC) of 0.08% or above.[7] (We will discuss BAC in more detail shortly.) For a typical adult, this corresponds to consuming five or more drinks (for men), or four or more drinks (for women) in about two hours. Note that some organizations define binge drinking even more narrowly—as consuming four or more drinks (for men) and three or more drinks (for women) within two hours.

The incidence of binge drinking is highest among young adults aged 18 to 24, whether they are in college, the military, or the workforce. In fact, the highest prevalence of alcohol dependence occurs in this age group.[7] Studies indicate that high school seniors heading to college are consistently less likely than their non–college-bound counterparts to report binge drinking.[8] However, once at college, these same students report more binge drinking than their peers who entered the workforce.

> **binge drinking** A pattern of drinking alcohol that results in a blood alcohol concentration of 0.08 or above (about five or more alcoholic drinks within two hours for men or four or more alcoholic drinks within two hours for women).

Binge drinking is arguably the most significant health risk behavior among college students today. If you consider the consequences—and just how widespread binge drinking

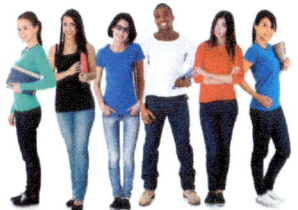

DIVERSITY & HEALTH

Alcohol and Tobacco Use: Breaking It Down

A recent national survey conducted by the Substance Abuse and Mental Health Services Administration revealed the following:

Overall

Alcohol	Tobacco
Among people aged 12 or older, 52.7% reported being current drinkers: about 139.7 million people.	Approximately 1 in 4 (25.2%) of those aged 12 or older (about 66.9 million people) use a tobacco product.
Among people aged 12 or older, 43.6% reported binge drinking (having five or more drinks on one occasion, on at least one day over the course of the previous month).	While the number of cigarette smokers has decreased significantly since 2002, the number of smokeless tobacco users and cigar smokers has remained about the same.
Among people aged 12 or older, 11.7% reported heavy drinking (having five or more drinks on one occasion, on at least five days over the course of the previous month).	Of smokers aged 12 or older, approximately, 1 in 5 (20.8%) smoke cigarettes, compared to 1 in 4 (24%) in 2002; 4.5% smoke cigars; 3.3% use smokeless tobacco.

Gender

Alcohol	Tobacco
Of males aged 12 or older, 57.3% reported being current drinkers, compared to 48.4% of females in the same age group.	Men are more likely to use a tobacco product than women. Of males aged 12 or older, 31.1% use a tobacco product compared to 19.7% of females.
Among those aged 12 to 17, 12.3% of females were current drinkers compared to 10.8% of males.	In the 12 to 17 age category, there is considerably less difference between the percentage of males (5.1%) and females (4.6%) who smoke compared to males (33.6%) and females (23.1%) in the 18 to 25 age category

Race/Ethnicity

Alcohol	Tobacco
Among Caucasians, 57.7% report being current drinkers, the highest rate of any racial/ethnic group. ■ Among mixed-race individuals, 49.5% report being current drinkers. ■ Among Native Americans, 42.3% report being current drinkers. ■ Among Hispanics, 44.4% report being current drinkers. ■ Among African Americans, 44.2% report being current drinkers. ■ Among Asian Americans, 38.7% report being current drinkers.	Among Native Americans, 37.8% report current tobacco use, the highest of any racial/ethnic group; ■ Among people of mixed-race background, 29.5% report current tobacco use. ■ Among Caucasians, 27.6% report current tobacco use. ■ Among African Americans, 26.6% report current tobacco use. ■ Among Hispanics, 18.8% report current tobacco use ■ Asians Americans report the lowest rate of current tobacco use at 10.2%
Rates of binge drinking (five or more drinks on at least one occasion over the previous month) were highest among Native Americans (27.7%), Hispanics (24.7%), Caucasians (23.5%), African Americans (21.6%), those of mixed race (21.0%), and Asian Americans (14.5%).	Native American/Alaskan Natives have the highest rate of current cigarette smoking (29.2%), followed by those of mixed race (27.9%), Caucasians (18.2%), African Americans (17.5%), Hispanics (11.2%) and Asian Americans (9.5%).

Age

Alcohol	Tobacco
Among individuals aged 18–25, 59.6% reported being current drinkers, the highest rate of any age group.	People aged 18–25 report a higher rate of current tobacco use (35.0%) than any other age group.

Education

Alcohol	Tobacco
Among individuals aged 26 and older, the rates of binge drinking or heavy drinking were lower among college graduates than among those who had attended some college but not yet obtained a degree. For heavy drinking, 4.8% of college graduates reported doing so, compared to 6.3% of those without a degree.	Only 15.1% of adults with college degrees are current tobacco users compared to 35.8% of adults who don't finish high school.
For binge drinking, 20.1% of college graduates reported engaging in that behavior, compared to 23.6% of non-college graduates.	Cigarette smoking is highest among persons with a GED (43.0%), followed by those with less than 12 years of school (22.9%). It is lowest among those with a graduate degree (5.4%), followed by those with an undergraduate degree (7.9%).

Geography

Alcohol	Tobacco
The rates of alcohol use are lowest in the South (48.7%), followed by the West (52.4%), Midwest (55.1%), and Northeast (58.3%).	Rates of smoking are highest in the Midwest (23.5%), followed by the South (22.4%), Northeast (19.8%), and West (16.7%).

What Do You Think?

1. These figures on alcohol and tobacco use include people as young as 12 years. What, if any, drinking and alcohol use did you notice among your peers in high school? How is it different from what you are experiencing in college?

2. What are some possible reasons behind varying rates of alcohol and tobacco use in different parts of the country?

3. Why do you think drinking and smoking rates are similar for both male and female teens but diverge as people get older?

Source: Center for Behavioral Health Statistics and Quality. (2015). *Behavioral health trends in the United States: Results from the 2014 National Survey on Drug Use and Health* (HHS Publication No. SMA 15-4927, NSDUH Series H-50).

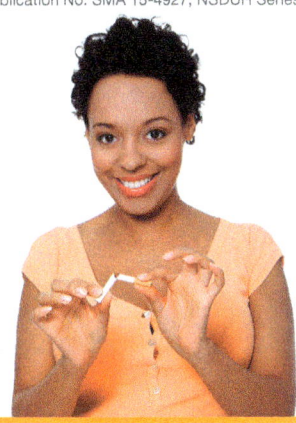

is—it is easy to see why. Alcohol is a factor in about 60% of fatal burn injuries, drownings, and homicides; 50% of severe trauma injuries and sexual assaults; and 40% of fatal motor vehicle crashes, suicides, and fatal falls.[9] In addition, binge drinking can lead to drunk driving, violence, vandalism, risky sex, forced sex, and poor academic performance.[10] Binge drinkers not only place themselves in harm's way but also raise risks for those around them. Those who live with or near heavy drinkers are exposed to more property damage, fights, and noise disturbances than those who do not.[11] Non-drinking students also report experiencing verbal abuse, drunk driving, and harassment of minority and international students at the hands of peers who have had too much to drink.[12] Of even more concern is the fact that each year, more than 696,000 students between the ages of 18 and 24 are assaulted by another student who has been drinking, and more than 97,000 students between the ages of 18 and 24 are victims of alcohol-related sexual assault or date rape.[13]

Although college students of all types may binge drink, it is most common among athletes, sports fans, fraternity and sorority members, and extremely social students. Women and minorities and religious, married, and older students tend to drink less.[14] The **Student Stats** feature provides a snapshot of overall drinking patterns on campus, based on a recent nationwide survey of college students.

▶▶ Listen to a Centers for Disease Control and Prevention (CDC) podcast on the dangers of binge drinking at **www.cdc.gov**. (Search for "podcast binge dangerous.")

Why Students Drink

Students cite many reasons for reaching for a drink. Researchers have classified the motivations into four different categories: coping (to avoid problems), conformity (to gain peer acceptance), enhancement (to induce a positive mood), and social (to make parties and outings more enjoyable).[15]

Peer pressure is often a major factor. When students are frequently offered alcoholic beverages at parties or goaded into consuming multiple drinks at a time by their friends, they may come to think that heavy drinking is normal behavior. Aware of the impact of social norms on students' drinking behaviors, alcohol abuse prevention experts try to counter student perceptions of their peers' drinking behaviors with the fact that the overwhelming majority of students drink responsibly. In fact, in a recent national survey, 15% of U.S. college students who had tried alcohol reported that they had not had a single alcoholic beverage within the past 30 days, and 25.5% of college students in this survey reported that they had never tried alcohol at all. However, students mistakenly believed that 92.1% of their peers had used alcohol in the past 30 days.[6]

Parents are also a major influence on the drinking patterns of college students. Parents who allow their children to drink alcohol in high school are not protecting their children from abusing alcohol when they leave the home for college. On the contrary, students whose parents allowed alcohol consumption in high school were significantly more at risk for alcohol misuse and its consequences in college.[16] Meanwhile, parental disapproval of drinking in high school does seem to have a protective effect against alcohol misuse in college.[16]

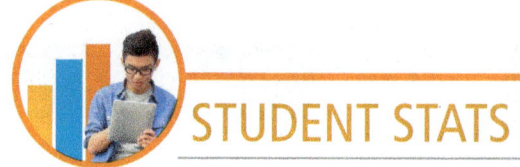

STUDENT STATS

Alcohol Use on Campus

A recent national survey of college students revealed that:

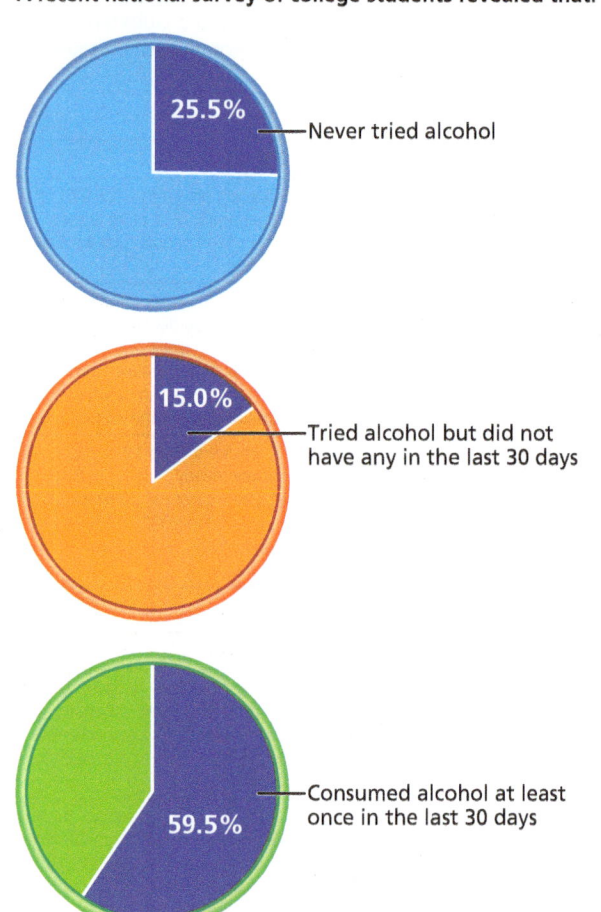

- 25.5% — Never tried alcohol
- 15.0% — Tried alcohol but did not have any in the last 30 days
- 59.5% — Consumed alcohol at least once in the last 30 days

Data from *ACHA-NCHA II: Undergraduate reference group executive summary, fall 2015*, by the American College Health Association, 2016.

▶▶ Is your drinking pattern risky? Assess yourself at **http://rethinkingdrinking.niaaa.nih.gov**. (Search for "pattern.")

The Makeup of Alcohol

Alcohol is a chemical substance that is toxic to the body. The key ingredient in every can of beer, glass of wine, and shot of tequila is **ethyl alcohol, or ethanol.** This intoxicating substance is produced through a process called *fermentation,* in which natural sugars are converted into alcohol and carbon dioxide with the help of yeast. To produce beer and wine, manufacturers add other ingredients, such as water, that dilute the drinks. To create hard liquor, they put the ethyl alcohol through another process, known as *distillation.* Distillation involves heating and then cooling the fermented liquid so that it ends up with a higher alcoholic

> **ethyl alcohol (ethanol)** The intoxicating ingredient in beer, wine, and distilled liquor.

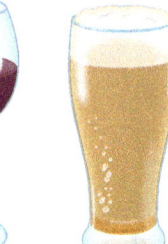
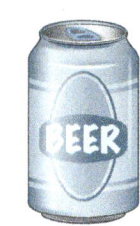

1.5 fl oz shot of 80-proof distilled spirits (gin, rum, tequila, vodka, whiskey, etc.) = 5 fl oz of table wine = 8–9 fl oz of malt liquor = 12 fl oz of regular beer

40% alcohol · about 12% alcohol · about 7% alcohol · about 5% alcohol

FIGURE 9.1 **"Standard" Serving Sizes.** A 1.5-ounce shot of liquor, 5-ounce glass of wine, 8- to 9-ounce malt liquor, and 12-ounce can of beer are all considered "standard" servings because they contain approximately the same amount of alcohol: 14 grams (½ ounce). Remember that not all beers, wines, and liquors are created equal. Some contain higher concentrations of alcohol than others.

proof value A measurement of alcoholic strength, corresponding to twice the alcohol percentage (e.g., 13% alcohol equals 26 proof).

standard drink A drink containing about 14 grams of pure alcohol (one 12-oz. can of beer, one 5-oz. glass of wine, or 1.5 oz. of 80-proof liquor).

absorption The process by which alcohol passes from the stomach or small intestine into the bloodstream.

metabolism The breakdown of food and beverages in the body to transform them into energy.

blood alcohol concentration (BAC) The amount of alcohol present in blood, measured in grams of alcohol per deciliter of blood.

concentration than before. These stronger beverages are often referred to by their **proof value,** a measure of their ethyl alcohol content. A proof is double the actual alcohol percentage; for example, 100-proof bourbon contains 50% alcohol by volume. Many red wines have an alcohol percentage of around 13%, or a proof value of 26.

>> For more information on what constitutes a "standard drink," visit http://rethinkingdrinking.niaaa.nih.gov and search for "standard."

Because different beverages have such varying levels of alcohol, a "standard" serving size also varies by drink type. A **standard drink** contains about 14 grams (or ½ ounce) of pure alcohol. That is the equivalent of a 12-ounce can of beer or 8 to 9 ounces of malt liquor. A 5-ounce glass of table wine is considered standard, as is 1.5 ounces of 80-proof liquor—roughly one shot glass **(Figure 9.1)**. Although these amounts may seem intuitive enough, researchers at the University of California at Berkeley found that when people were asked to serve themselves a standard drink at home, they poured considerably more alcohol than they should have.[17]

LO 9.1 QUICK CHECK ✓

Binge drinking is defined as
  a. consuming five or more drinks within two hours for men or four or more drinks within two hours for women
  b. drinking once a day every day
  c. consuming five or more drinks over the course of a week for both men and women
  d. drinking hard liquor

How the Body Absorbs and Metabolizes Alcohol

LO 9.2 Describe how the body absorbs and metabolizes alcohol.

When you consume an alcoholic beverage, the alcohol passes from your stomach and small intestine into your bloodstream, a process known as **absorption.** The alcohol then travels to your liver, where it is broken down by enzymes in a process known as **metabolism** (**Figure 9.2,** next page). (A small amount of alcohol is metabolized in the stomach as well, but 80% of alcohol metabolism takes place in the liver.) One enzyme in particular, *alcohol dehydrogenase* (ADH), converts alcohol into a byproduct called *acetaldehyde.* The acetaldehyde is then quickly transformed into acetate by other enzymes and is eventually metabolized to carbon dioxide and water. Some alcohol, however, is not metabolized by the body and is excreted in urine, sweat, and breath. It can be detected in breath and urine tests that gauge blood alcohol levels.

The liver can metabolize only a small amount of alcohol at a time, roughly one standard drink per hour, although metabolism varies among individuals. Alcohol that is not immediately metabolized by the liver continues to circulate in the bloodstream to other parts of the body, including the brain. If a person consumes alcohol at a faster rate than the liver can break it down, the person becomes intoxicated.

Blood Alcohol Concentration

The amount of alcohol contained in a person's blood is known as **blood alcohol concentration (BAC).** BAC is measured in grams of alcohol per deciliter of blood and is usually expressed in percentage terms. Having a BAC of 0.08% means that a person has 8 parts alcohol per 10,000 parts blood in the body. Also referred to as *blood alcohol level,* BAC can be affected by several factors, including:

- **How much and how quickly you drink.** Binge drinking causes a large amount of alcohol to enter your body in a very short period. Because your body cannot process alcohol at a fast pace, this results in a higher BAC.
- **What you drink.** All drinks are not created equal. The water in beer and wine acts as a buffer for alcohol so that people feel the effects of these beverages a little less than if they were to down a straight shot of hard liquor. Champagne and beer contain carbon dioxide, which increases the rate of alcohol absorption and causes more rapid intoxication. The type of mixer you choose can also make a big difference. Water and fruit juices mixed with alcohol may slow the absorption and intoxication process, whereas soda and other carbonated beverages speed it up. The temperature of the alcohol also affects absorption; a hot toddy moves into the bloodstream more quickly than a frosty margarita.

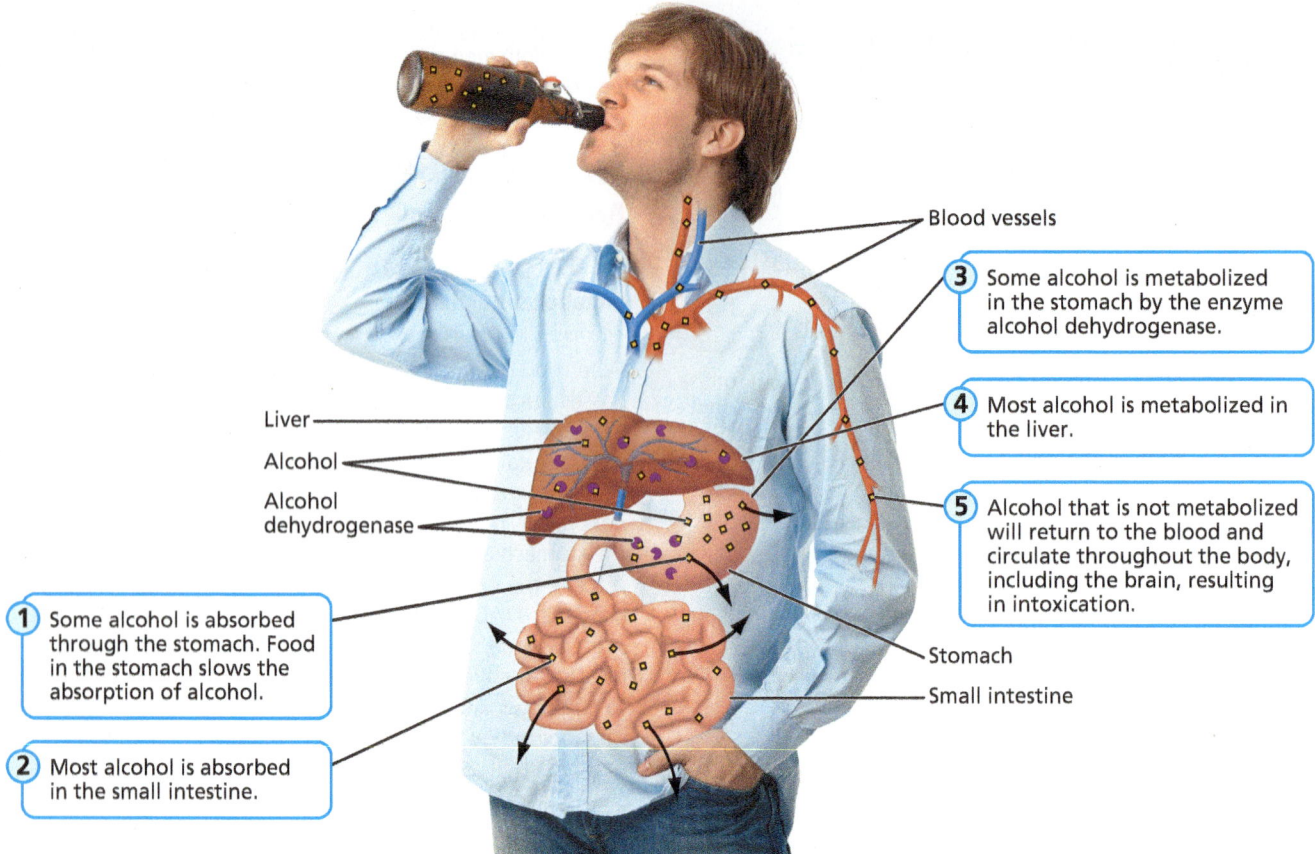

FIGURE 9.2 **Alcohol Absorption and Metabolism.** Alcohol is absorbed into the bloodstream through the stomach and small intestine. Metabolism takes place in the stomach and in the liver.

Source: Adapted from Blake, Joan Salge, *Nutrition and You*, 2nd ed., ©2012. Reprinted and electronically reproduced by permission of Pearson Education, Inc., Upper Saddle River, New Jersey.

- **Your sex.** Women are more vulnerable to alcohol than men and have a higher BAC after drinking the same amount of alcohol. This occurs for several reasons. First, women typically are smaller and consequently have less blood volume than men. They also have a higher percentage of body fat. Because alcohol is not easily stored in fat, it enters the bloodstream more quickly in women. Men have significantly more muscle and consequently have a higher percentage of water in their bodies. The added water helps dilute the alcohol men consume. Women absorb about 30% more alcohol into the bloodstream than men do. This is primarily because women produce less alcohol dehydrogenase, the enzyme responsible for the breakdown of alcohol in the stomach. **Figure 9.3** shows how BAC levels differ between men and women of similar weights.
- **Your age.** Research indicates that as people age, they become more sensitive to alcohol's effects.[18] The same amount of alcohol can have a greater effect on an older person than on a younger one.
- **Your weight.** The less you weigh, the less blood and water you have in your body to dilute alcohol. As a result, a lighter person will have a higher BAC than a heavier person who drinks the same amount.
- **Your physical condition.** People who are fatigued or stressed out tend to be more affected by moderate amounts of alcohol.

- **Your food intake.** Eating a meal before drinking, especially one high in protein and fat, helps slow the absorption of alcohol into the bloodstream. Conversely, drinking on an empty stomach speeds absorption. BAC rises more rapidly when you have not eaten because there is no food in your stomach in which to dilute the alcohol.
- **Medications.** Aspirin and other medications, including many sold over the counter, prevent the enzyme ADH from breaking down alcohol. This causes alcohol to accumulate in the blood faster (resulting in a higher BAC) and have longer-lasting effects. Women on birth control pills process alcohol more slowly than do other women, and they remain drunk longer.

>> Use this calculator to estimate your blood alcohol concentration: **http://bloodalcoholcalculator.org**.

LO 9.2 QUICK CHECK

Approximately how much alcohol can the liver metabolize in an hour?

a. The amount in one standard drink
b. It depends on the type of alcohol
c. The amount has never been approximated
d. The liver is flexible and will adjust its rate of metabolism to accommodate a person's speed of alcohol absorption

For Women

Drinks per hour	Body weight in pounds					
	100	120	140	160	180	200
1	0.05	0.04	0.03	0.03	0.03	0.02
2	0.09	0.08	0.07	0.06	0.05	0.05
3	0.14	0.11	0.10	0.09	0.08	0.07
4	0.18	0.15	0.13	0.11	0.10	0.09
5	0.23	0.19	0.16	0.14	0.13	0.11
6	0.27	0.23	0.19	0.17	0.15	0.14
7	0.32	0.27	0.23	0.20	0.18	0.16
8	0.36	0.30	0.26	0.23	0.20	0.18
9	0.41	0.34	0.29	0.26	0.23	0.20
10	0.45	0.38	0.32	0.28	0.25	0.23

For Men

Drinks per hour	Body weight in pounds					
	100	120	140	160	180	200
1	0.04	0.03	0.03	0.02	0.02	0.02
2	0.08	0.06	0.05	0.05	0.04	0.04
3	0.11	0.09	0.08	0.07	0.06	0.06
4	0.15	0.12	0.11	0.09	0.08	0.08
5	0.19	0.16	0.13	0.12	0.11	0.09
6	0.23	0.19	0.16	0.14	0.13	0.11
7	0.26	0.22	0.19	0.16	0.15	0.13
8	0.30	0.25	0.21	0.19	0.17	0.15
9	0.34	0.28	0.24	0.21	0.19	0.17
10	0.38	0.31	0.27	0.23	0.21	0.19

FIGURE 9.3 Blood Alcohol Concentration (BAC) Tables. The orange areas indicate legal intoxication.
Source: Data from P. E. Watson, I. D. Watson, and R. D. Batt, 1981, "Prediction of Blood Alcohol Concentrations in Human Subjects: Updating the Widmark Equation," *Journal of Studies on Alcohol*, Vol. 42, No. 7.

The Effects of Alcohol on the Body

LO 9.3 Describe the short-term and long-term health effects of alcohol use.

Excess alcohol consumption negatively affects the health of the drinker on many levels. Not only do heavy drinkers put themselves at higher risk of accidental injury and violence, they also increase their risks of developing lasting neurological problems and serious diseases, such as cancer, heart disease, and liver disease.

Intoxication

In the most basic sense, **alcohol intoxication** is just another term for being drunk. In a legal sense, it means having a BAC of 0.08% or greater. Intoxication levels vary, but generally a person weighing 150 pounds can expect the following symptoms:[19]

- At a BAC of 0.03% (after about one drink), you feel relaxed and slightly exhilarated.
- At a BAC of 0.06% (after two drinks), you feel warm and relaxed as well as experience decreased fine-motor skills.
- At a BAC of 0.09% (after three drinks), you notice a slowed reaction time, poor muscle control, slurred speech, and wobbly legs.
- At a BAC of 0.12% (after four drinks), you have clouded judgment, a loss of self-restraint, and an impaired ability to reason and make logical decisions.
- At a BAC of 0.15% (after five drinks), you have blurred vision, unclear speech, an unsteady gait, and impaired coordination.
- At a BAC of 0.18% (after six drinks), you find it difficult to stay awake.
- At a BAC of 0.30% (after 10 to 12 drinks), you are in a stupor or deep sleep.
- At a BAC of 0.50%, you are in a deep coma and in danger of death.

Immediate Effects of Alcohol on the Body

Within moments of ingestion, alcohol begins to cause changes in the body. As BAC increases, the drinker experiences the immediate symptoms mentioned previously and also these additional short-term effects (see **Figure 9.4**, next page):

- **Dehydration.** Alcohol is a diuretic, triggering more frequent urination. This can lead to dehydration and an electrolyte imbalance. Symptoms of mild to moderate dehydration include thirst, weakness, dryness of mucous membranes, dizziness, and lightheadedness.
- **Gastrointestinal problems.** Alcohol irritates the stomach and intestines, causing inflammation and indigestion. This is especially true when a person drinks a beverage with an alcohol concentration greater than 15%.[20]
- **Sleep disturbances.** Although alcohol has sedative effects that can make people feel sleepy, it actually tends to *disrupt* sleep and throw off the biological rhythms of the body. As a result, alcohol-induced sleep is often shorter in duration and poorer in quality. In addition, alcohol relaxes the throat muscles, facilitating snoring.
- **Alterations in the metabolic state of the liver and other organs.** These changes result in low blood sugar levels.

The effect many drinkers fear most, however, is a **hangover,** which begins within several hours after drinking has stopped and can last for up to 24 hours. A hangover is the constellation of unpleasant physical and mental symptoms that accompany a bout of heavy drinking. They include fatigue, headache, increased sensitivity to light and sound, redness of the eyes, dry mouth, muscle aches, thirst, vomiting, diarrhea, dizziness, vertigo, depression, and irritability.

alcohol intoxication The state of physical and/or mental impairment brought on by excessive alcohol consumption (in legal terms, a BAC of 0.08% or greater).

hangover Alcohol withdrawal symptoms, including headache and nausea, caused by an earlier bout of heavy drinking.

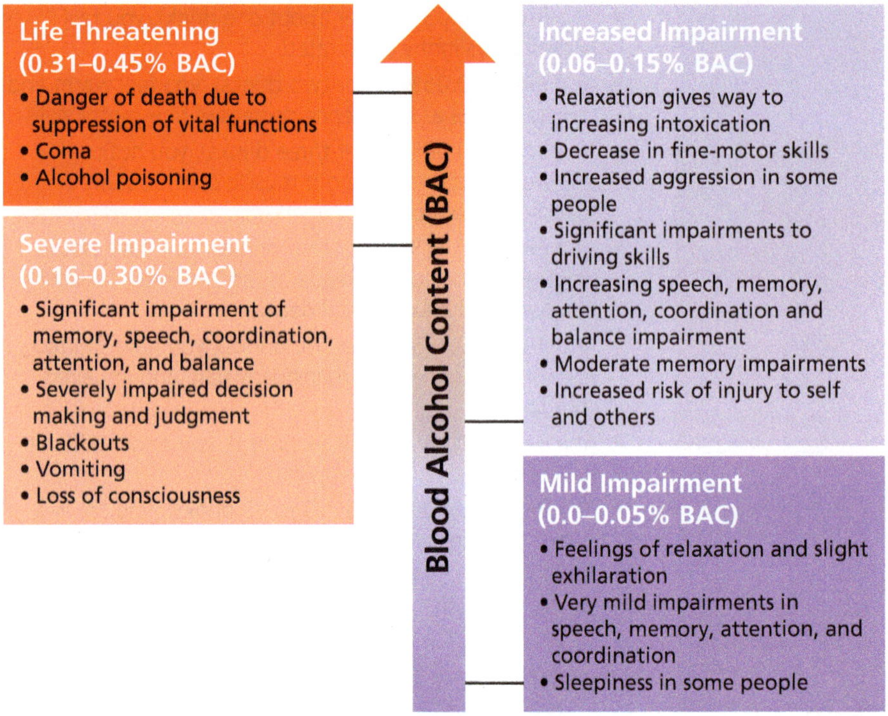

Life Threatening (0.31–0.45% BAC)
- Danger of death due to suppression of vital functions
- Coma
- Alcohol poisoning

Severe Impairment (0.16–0.30% BAC)
- Significant impairment of memory, speech, coordination, attention, and balance
- Severely impaired decision making and judgment
- Blackouts
- Vomiting
- Loss of consciousness

Increased Impairment (0.06–0.15% BAC)
- Relaxation gives way to increasing intoxication
- Decrease in fine-motor skills
- Increased aggression in some people
- Significant impairments to driving skills
- Increasing speech, memory, attention, coordination and balance impairment
- Moderate memory impairments
- Increased risk of injury to self and others

Mild Impairment (0.0–0.05% BAC)
- Feelings of relaxation and slight exhilaration
- Very mild impairments in speech, memory, attention, and coordination
- Sleepiness in some people

Blood Alcohol Content (BAC)

FIGURE 9.4 Impairment Increases with BAC Level.

Researchers believe that key contributors to hangovers are compounds found in alcoholic beverages known as *congeners*.[21] Congeners contribute to the taste, smell, and appearance of alcoholic drinks, but the body metabolizes them very slowly, and they are more toxic than ethanol. Research has shown that beverages containing a large number of congeners, such as whiskey, brandy, and red wine, cause greater hangover effects than beverages composed of more pure ethanol, such as gin and vodka.[22]

Alcohol Poisoning

Every year, dozens of students from universities and colleges across the country die from **alcohol poisoning** as a result of a dangerously high level of alcohol consumption and the toxic by-products that result when alcohol is metabolized by the body. Absorbing too much alcohol can depress the body's central nervous system, slowing breathing, heart rate, and the gag reflex that is needed to prevent choking. Inebriated students can lose consciousness, choke on their own vomit, and die from asphyxiation. In addition, victims can experience *hypothermia* (low body temperature) and *hypoglycemia* (too little blood sugar), which can lead to seizures. Vomiting can also cause seizures, which in turn can result in permanent brain damage.

Signs of alcohol poisoning include mental confusion, vomiting, seizures, slow or irregular breathing, low body temperature, and skin that is pale or bluish in color. If a person cannot be roused, that is another indication that emergency medical care is needed.

Alcohol poisoning should be taken as seriously as any other kind of poisoning. Giving a grossly intoxicated person a cup of coffee or a cold shower will not help. Neither will having him or her sleep or "walk it off." A person's blood alcohol concentration can continue to rise even while he or she is passed out. It is dangerous to assume that the person will be fine if left alone to sleep.

If you encounter someone who you suspect may have alcohol poisoning, call 911 immediately if the person:

- Is unconscious and you can't rouse him or her even by shaking.
- Has consumed other drugs.
- Is experiencing seizures.
- Is injured.
- Has a respiration rate of fewer than 8 breaths per minute.
- Is experiencing shallow or irregular breathing (10 seconds or more between breaths).

alcohol poisoning Dangerously high level of alcohol consumption, resulting in depression of the central nervous system, slowed breathing and heart rate, and compromised gag reflex.

Long-Term Effects of Alcohol on the Body

It is difficult to find a part of the body that alcohol does not damage if it is abused for long periods. Chronic, heavy use of alcohol has been linked to cancer, heart disease, liver problems, neurological ailments, and stomach disorders.

Cancer

Study after study has linked cancer and excessive alcohol use.[23,24] Cancers of the liver, breast, esophagus, mouth, larynx, throat, and pancreas have all been associated with chronic drinking patterns.[23] Among women assessed in one important study, breast cancer was responsible for the majority of alcohol-related cancer deaths. Importantly, even small amounts of alcohol can increase the risk of breast cancer, and the risk is cumulative. Compared to nondrinkers, a woman increases her breast cancer risk 4% to 7% with each drink consumed per day.

> *"A person's blood alcohol concentration can continue to rise even while he or she is passed out. It is dangerous to assume that the person will be fine if left alone to sleep."*

MYTH OR FACT?

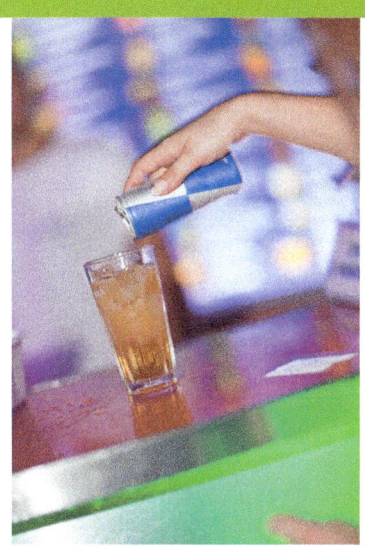

Is It Safe to Mix Alcohol and Caffeine?

Caffeinated alcoholic beverages (CABs), premixed drinks that combine alcohol, caffeine, and often other stimulants, first hit the market in the early 2000s. Marketed heavily to teens and young adults, they often had a higher alcohol content than beer. The FDA challenged CAB manufacturers' claims that these beverages were safe and, in November 2010, demanded that the seven largest CAB producers remove the caffeine from their products. What about the CABs you mix yourself by combining alcohol with highly caffeinated energy drinks? Are they safe?

Alcohol is a depressant. At high levels, it can actually cause death by depressing vital functions such as heart rate and respiration. The danger of combining alcohol with energy drinks is that the caffeine in these beverages can mask the depressant effects of alcohol. At the same time, caffeine has no effect on the metabolism of alcohol by the liver and thus does not reduce breath alcohol concentrations or reduce alcohol-related risks.

Also, consider these statistics from the CDC:

- Drinkers who consume alcohol mixed with energy drinks are three times more likely to binge drink than those who don't.

- Drinkers who mix alcohol and energy drinks are about twice as likely as those who don't to report negative events associated with drinking, such as being taken advantage of sexually, taking advantage of someone else sexually, or riding with a driver who was under the influence of alcohol.

Data from Centers for Disease Control and Prevention. (2015). *Fact sheets—Caffeine and alcohol.* **www.cdc.gov**.

Among men, cancers of the esophagus and upper airway were especially notable.[24] Drinkers who consumed more than 20 grams of alcohol (about 1.5 drinks) per day made up more than one-quarter of all alcohol-related cancer deaths.[24]

Scientists aren't sure exactly why alcohol consumption increases the risk of cancer. There is evidence that acetaldehyde, the toxic chemical produced when the body metabolizes alcohol, damages DNA, and this plays a role in certain cancers (e.g., head, neck, and esophagus). The increased circulating estrogens caused by alcohol consumption could play a role in the development of breast cancer. In regard to colon cancer, alcohol may block the metabolism of nutrients that play an important role in reducing cancer risks.

Cardiovascular Disease

Although there is some evidence that *moderate* alcohol use may lower the risk of some types of heart disease, excessive chronic alcohol use can raise the blood levels of triglycerides, a type of fat. It can also lead to high blood pressure, heart failure, and, in some chronic drinkers, stroke. Excessive use of alcohol can also have a direct toxic effect on the heart muscle cells, causing *cardiomyopathy*. Cardiomyopathy is a serious disease in which the heart muscle becomes inflamed and weakened. As a result, it cannot pump blood efficiently. The lack of blood flow affects all parts of the body, resulting in damage to multiple tissues and organ systems.

Liver Disease

Alcohol can cause three kinds of liver disease:

- **Fatty liver.** A buildup of fat cells in the liver that can cause abdominal discomfort.
- **Alcoholic hepatitis.** Also called inflammation of the liver. About one-third of heavy drinkers will develop alcoholic hepatitis, which causes progressive liver damage and is marked by nausea, vomiting, fever, and jaundice.
- **Alcoholic cirrhosis.** The most serious type of alcohol-related liver disease. An estimated 48.2% of the 31,500 deaths from cirrhosis each year are alcohol related, according to a national study.[25] With cirrhosis, normal liver tissue is replaced with scar tissue, causing life-threatening damage.

Neurological Effects

Alcohol can cause severe and possibly lasting brain damage in people under age 21, according to the American Medical Association. The brain grows and changes during adolescence and into the college years, and alcohol can negatively affect two brain areas involved in learning and behavior. Moderate drinking impairs learning and memory far more in youths than adults, with adolescents needing to drink only half as much to suffer the same negative brain effects.[26]

Alcohol and Pregnancy

A pregnant woman is not only "eating for two," she is also "drinking for two." The ingestion of high levels of alcohol during the first trimester of a pregnancy can cause a miscarriage. Alcohol ingested at other points in the pregnancy can lead to health problems and even brain damage in the fetus. Scientists coined the term **fetal alcohol syndrome** more than three decades ago to describe a pattern of birth defects that appeared in children of mothers who drank while pregnant. The telltale signs of the condition include facial abnormalities, retarded growth, and permanent intellectual and behavioral problems.

Today, drinking while pregnant is recognized as the leading cause of birth defects, developmental disabilities, and intellectual disability. The prevalence of fetal alcohol syndrome is estimated to be between 0.2 and 1.5 for every 1,000 births, and approximately 40,000 newborns are affected by an alcohol-related disorder each year.[27] Despite the known risks, an estimated 9.4% of pregnant women reported consuming alcohol while pregnant in a recent national survey.[28]

The greatest risk is to babies whose mothers are heavy drinkers, but scientists are unsure whether there is any safe level of alcohol use during pregnancy. In 2005, the U.S. surgeon general issued an advisory to pregnant women, urging them to abstain from alcohol altogether. Stating that it is "in the child's best interest for a pregnant woman to simply not drink alcohol," Dr. Richard Carmona said studies also indicate that babies can be affected by alcohol just after conception, before a woman even knows she is pregnant. For that reason, the federal government has begun recommending that women who may possibly be pregnant avoid alcohol.

fetal alcohol syndrome A pattern of mental and physical birth defects found in some children of mothers who drank excessively during pregnancy.

Health Benefits of Alcohol?

There is some evidence that people who regularly consume *small* amounts of alcohol may have a decreased risk of coronary heart disease, high blood pressure, and stroke compared with people who do not drink at all.[29] Other studies have shown that moderate drinkers (defined as people who regularly have one or two drinks per day) have the lowest mortality rate, whereas heavy drinkers have the highest, and teetotalers (those who don't drink) and light drinkers have rates that fall somewhere in the middle.[30]

However, another analysis looked broadly at studies supporting the health benefits of alcohol in heart disease and found fundamental problems with almost all of them, raising questions about how accurate the health claims for alcohol might truly be.[31] Women should also be aware that alcohol use—even moderate use—has been linked to an increased risk of breast cancer.[32] Among young people in particular, alcohol use is associated with *increased* risk of premature death from accidents or injuries. College students should not take up drinking or drink more frequently with the goal of improving their health.

LO 9.3 QUICK CHECK

If you encounter someone you think may have alcohol poisoning, which of the following should you do?
a. Give him or her coffee or other caffeinated beverage
b. Get him or her up and walking around
c. Get him or her into a cold shower
d. Call 911

The Effects of Alcohol on Behavior

LO 9.4 Explain how alcohol affects behavior.

Alcohol does not just have physical effects on the body; it is also associated with poor decision making and risky behavior. Among the most serious risks associated with alcohol use are drunk driving and alcohol-related sexual activity.

Drinking and Driving

In 2013, 10,076 people died in alcohol-related car crashes in the United States—about 31% of total traffic fatalities for the year, or about 1 every 52 minutes. Young adult drivers (aged 21 to 24) involved in fatal crashes were above the legal alcohol limit 32% of the time, significantly more than all other drivers (21%).[33]

College students are disproportionately affected by drunk driving. One study found that more than 1,825 students aged 18 to 24 died from alcohol-related car crashes and unintentional injuries in a single year.[13] More than one-fourth

STUDENT STORY

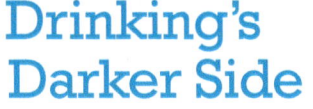

"HI, I'M COURTNEY. Out of my friends, most of us drink. There have been a lot of negative effects from drinking. This year alone, one of my sorority sisters fell and broke her hand. Another one has fallen and chipped a tooth. A lot of us spend way too much money when we go out. There's lots of negative effects.

A lot of people drink because it loosens them up to be able to socially interact. But I would tell someone who doesn't want to drink to definitely join organizations on campus. There are a lot of things you can do to meet people that have nothing to do with drinking."

What Do You Think?

1. Courtney lists injuries and financial impacts as negative effects from drinking. What other negative effects can you think of?
2. What factors make Courtney vulnerable to high-risk drinking?
3. Courtney suggests that students who don't want to drink join organizations to meet new people. What other alternatives for alcohol-free socializing can you think of?

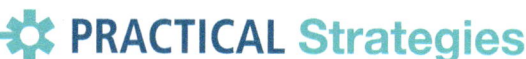

PRACTICAL Strategies

How to Protect Yourself from Risky Alcohol-Related Behavior

Accidents or injuries resulting from alcohol-related behavior are all too common on college campuses. The following guidelines can help keep you safe:

- **Don't drink to get drunk.** Alcohol-related risks increase dramatically with intoxication, so if you drink, drink moderately. Eat before you start consuming any alcohol and keep eating while you drink. During the evening, take breaks between drinks by alternating alcoholic beverages with non-alcoholic ones. Avoid drinking games that can cause you to drink alcohol more quickly than your body can handle.
- **Pair up with a friend.** If you are drinking away from home, don't do it alone. Always pair up with a friend and make a pact to stick together.
- **Make arrangements for getting home safely.** If you are heading to a drinking event, arrange for a sober driver or contact a cab company ahead of time. Most colleges have "safe ride" systems that provide safe late-night transportation services from popular night spots.
- **Don't accept drinks from strangers.** While at a party, club, or bar, don't give anyone the opportunity to slip drugs like Rohypnol or GHB into your drink. Never put your drink down. If your drink is out of sight, even for a few minutes, don't finish it. Get yourself a new one. Don't accept an open drink from anyone. If you order a drink in a bar, make sure you watch the bartender open the bottle or mix your drink.
- **Know the signs of alcohol poisoning.** Be prepared so that you can help a friend if the situation arises. If the person is unconscious, cannot be roused, has consumed other drugs, is experiencing seizures, is injured, and/or is exhibiting shallow or irregular breathing, call 911 immediately. Remember that other signs of alcohol poisoning include mental confusion, vomiting, low body temperature, and skin that is pale or bluish in color.

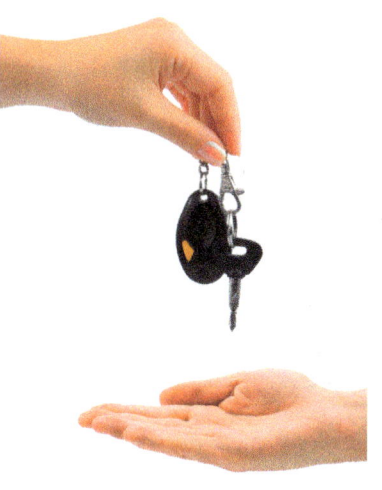

of college students in the United States have driven under the influence of alcohol.[13]

How does alcohol affect driving skills? The following are only some of the common impairments:

- **Judgment.** Alcohol reduces reason and caution, so you're more likely to take risks, from speeding to failing to stop at a light that's changing to red. Research has shown that as few as one or two drinks can impair mental and motor skills necessary for safe driving.[19]
- **Vision and hearing.** Alcohol reduces the acuity of hearing and vision, including depth perception, which helps you relate the position of your vehicle to others on the road.
- **Reaction time.** Impairments in focusing your attention, understanding your situation, and coordinating your response all contribute to significantly slowed reaction time.

Having a BAC of 0.08% or greater will qualify you for a DWI (driving while intoxicated) arrest in all 50 states if you are 21 years of age or older. Under zero-tolerance laws, it is illegal to have any alcohol in your system if you are underage and driving a vehicle. Drivers caught doing so could be charged in civil or criminal courts with a DWI or similar charge and, if convicted, could have their license suspended—in some states for one year or until they reach age 21, whichever is longer.

>> The Mothers Against Drunk Driving (MADD) website includes statistics on drunk driving, victim services, and opportunities to help eliminate drunk driving: **www.madd.org**.

Although penalties vary by state, a first conviction for DWI may result in jail time, a fine ranging from several hundred to several thousand dollars, and/or community service. The offender's driver's license will be suspended for a period, and he or she will be required to enroll in an alcohol rehabilitation program. In some states, a DWI conviction—even if a first offense—may remain on the person's criminal record for life. A second offense may involve mandatory prison time and a much higher fine. In addition, in at least 22 states, repeat offenders must have their cars outfitted with an ignition-interlock system, which detects alcohol use and prevents people from starting their vehicle if they have been drinking.[34]

Alcohol and Sexual Activity

Engaging in sexual intercourse while inebriated can be just as dangerous as riding in a speeding car after the driver has had too many drinks. In one study, 21.3% of college students reported participating in unplanned sexual activities after having too much to drink.[35] Drinking may also make it less likely that partners use protection while having sex under the influence, possibly exposing themselves to sexually transmitted diseases, such as AIDS or hepatitis B, as well as unplanned pregnancy.

For women, the risks can be even greater. Heavy drinking increases the odds that a woman will become a victim of violence or rape. One survey of college students between the ages of 18 and 24 years found that in a single year, about 97,000 were victims of alcohol-related sexual assault or date rape.[13]

Alcohol and Other Problems

Students who engage in heavy drinking also increase their risks of other problems. One of the most common consequences of high-risk drinking among college students is difficulty keeping up with academic responsibilities. In one survey, 25% of college students said they had missed class, fallen behind, flunked exams, or received lower grades as a result of their drinking.[36] Alcohol use is also closely associated with depression and can increase the risk that a depressed person will attempt suicide. Alcohol intoxication increases suicide risk up to 90 times, as compared with abstinence.[37]

A common refrain on T-shirts states, "I don't have a drinking problem. I drink, I get drunk. I fall down. No problem!" Health experts, however, are not laughing. One study found that in a single year, more than 1 million college students were injured or assaulted in drinking-related incidents.[13]

LO 9.4 QUICK CHECK

Laws that make it illegal for those under 21 to drive after consuming any alcohol are referred to as
a. DWI laws.
b. zero-tolerance laws.
c. DUI laws.
d. drunk-driving laws.

Alcohol Abuse

LO 9.5 Recognize the types and signs of alcohol abuse.

Excessive drinking is a pervasive problem in American society. In the United States, 17.6 million adults meet the criteria for either alcohol abuse or alcohol dependence.[38] **Alcohol abuse** refers to drinking that gets in the way of work, school, or home life and causes interpersonal, social, or legal problems. **Alcoholism,** technically known as **alcohol dependence,** is problem drinking taken a step further; alcoholics do not just enjoy drinks but crave them and experience withdrawal symptoms whenever they stop drinking.

Alcoholism

Alcoholism is defined as exhibiting at least three of the following symptoms during a one-year period:

- **Tolerance.** Needing to drink more and more alcohol to get drunk.
- **Withdrawal symptoms.** Having a physical dependence on alcohol to the extent that nausea, sweating, shakiness, tremors, seizures, and anxiety are experienced after stopping drinking.
- **Loss of control.** Drinking more or longer than intended.
- **Desire or an inability to quit.** Having a persistent desire to cut down on drinking or attempting unsuccessfully to do so.
- **Overwhelming time commitment.** Spending an excessive amount of time buying alcohol, drinking it, and recovering from its effects.

- **Interference with life.** Experiencing a reduction in social, recreational, or work activities due to alcohol use.
- **Continued use.** Drinking despite the knowledge that it is causing physical or psychological problems.

Risk Factors for Alcoholism

Genetic, physiological, psychological, and social factors all play a role in determining a person's susceptibility to alcoholism. To what extent each factor influences a person's susceptibility depends on the individual. The risk of alcoholism is higher for people who have a parent who abused alcohol, for instance, but not all children of alcoholics become alcoholics themselves. Other factors that increase a person's risk for abusing alcohol include low self-esteem, impulsiveness, a need for approval, peer pressure, poverty, and being a victim of physical or sexual abuse. Individuals who are under a great deal of chronic stress are also vulnerable. They may turn to alcohol to cope with their problems and try to make themselves feel better, a potentially destructive behavior that is called **self-medicating.**

The age at which a person begins drinking can also raise his or her risk for alcohol abuse. People who begin drinking as teenagers are more likely to develop problems with alcohol. Gender is another risk factor; statistics show that men are much more likely to become dependent on alcohol than are women.[1]

> **alcohol abuse** Drinking alcohol to excess, either regularly or on individual occasions, resulting in disruption of work, school, or home life and causing interpersonal, social, or legal problems.
>
> **alcoholism (alcohol dependence)** A physical dependence on alcohol to the extent that stopping drinking brings on withdrawal symptoms.
>
> **self-medicating** Using alcohol or drugs to cope with sadness, grief, pain, or mental health problems.

No matter what the cause, once people begin abusing alcohol, the problem often perpetuates itself. Heavy drinking can deplete or increase the levels of some chemicals in the body, causing it to crave or need alcohol to feel good again. Some people keep drinking simply to avoid the uncomfortable withdrawal symptoms.

Common Profiles of Alcoholics

Alcoholism knows no demographic boundaries. It can affect men and women of any race, class, age, and social group. That said, researchers have identified five subtypes of alcoholics that are the most prevalent in our society:

- **The young adult subtype.** Usually alcoholics by their 21st birthday, these young adult drinkers typically do not abuse other drugs and are free of mental disorders. They usually lack a family history of alcoholism and rarely seek help for their drinking problem. They may drink less often than other alcoholics but tend to binge drink when they do. They account for 31.5% of alcoholics in the United States.[39]
- **The young antisocial subtype.** These drinkers start at an earlier age than the young adult subtype and tend to come from families suffering from alcoholism. About half could be considered antisocial, and many have major depression, bipolar disorder, or anxiety problems. They are

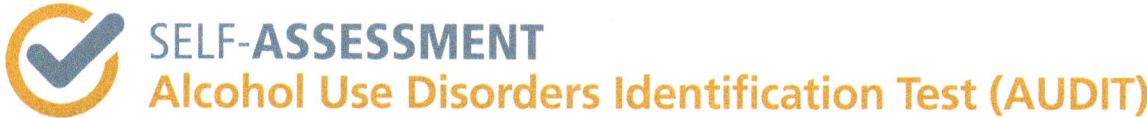

SELF-ASSESSMENT
Alcohol Use Disorders Identification Test (AUDIT)

Is the way or amount you drink harming your health? Should you cut down on your drinking? Taking the following Self-Assessment will help you answer these questions.

Please mark the answer that is correct for you.

1. How often do you have a drink alcohol?
   ☐ Never ☐ Monthly or less ☐ 2 to 4 times a month ☐ 2 to 3 times per week ☐ 4 or more times per week
2. How many drinks containing alcohol do you have on a typical day when you are drinking?
   ☐ 1 or 2 ☐ 3 or 4 ☐ 5 or 6 ☐ 7 to 9 ☐ 10 or more
3. How often do you have six or more drinks on one occasion?
   ☐ Never ☐ Less than monthly ☐ Monthly ☐ 2 to 3 times per week ☐ 4 or more times a week
4. How often during the last year have you found that you were not able to stop drinking once you had started?
   ☐ Never ☐ Less than monthly ☐ Monthly ☐ 2 to 3 times per week ☐ 4 or more times a week
5. How often during the last year have you failed to do what was normally expected from you because of drinking?
   ☐ Never ☐ Less than monthly ☐ Monthly ☐ 2 to 3 times per week ☐ 4 or more times a week
6. How often during the last year have you needed a first drink in the morning to get yourself going after a heavy drinking session?
   ☐ Never ☐ Less than monthly ☐ Monthly ☐ 2 to 3 times per week ☐ 4 or more times a week
7. How often during the last year have you had a feeling of guilt or remorse after drinking?
   ☐ Never ☐ Less than monthly ☐ Monthly ☐ 2 to 4 times per week ☐ 4 or more times a week
8. How often during the last year have you been unable to remember what happened the night before because you had been drinking?
   ☐ Never ☐ Less than monthly ☐ Monthly ☐ 2 to 3 times per week ☐ 4 or more times a week
9. Have you or someone else been injured as a result of your drinking?
   ☐ No ☐ Yes, but not in the last year ☐ Yes, during the last year
10. Has a relative or friend or a doctor or other health worker been concerned about your drinking or suggested you cut down?
    ☐ No ☐ Yes, but not in the last year ☐ Yes, during the last year

HOW TO INTERPRET YOUR SCORE The Alcohol Use Disorders Identification Test (AUDIT) can detect alcohol problems experienced in the last year. Questions 1–8 are scored as 0, 1, 2, 3, or 4 points from first to last option. Questions 9 and 10 are scored 0, 2, or 4 only. A score of 8 or above on the AUDIT generally indicates harmful or hazardous drinking.

To complete this Self-Assessment online, visit MasteringHealth™

Source: The Alcohol Use Disorders Identification Test: Interview Version from AUDIT Manual, box 4, p. 17, World Health Organization, Division of Mental Health and Prevention of Substance Abuse. Copyright ©2001 by World Health Organization. Reprinted with permission.

more likely to smoke cigarettes and marijuana as well as use cocaine. They account for 21% of all alcoholics.[40]

- **The functional subtype.** Typically middle-aged, well-educated, and smokers, these drinkers have stable jobs, good incomes, and families. About one-third have a family history of alcoholism, and about one-fourth have had a major bout of depression. They make up 19.5% of the alcoholic population.[40]
- **The intermediate familial subtype.** These middle-aged drinkers tend to have alcoholic parents. About half have been depressed. Most smoke cigarettes, and nearly 1 in 5 have had problems with cocaine and marijuana use. They account for 19% of alcoholics.[40]
- **The chronic severe subtype.** Chronic severe drinkers typically start drinking early in life and develop alcohol problems at a young age, too. They tend to be middle aged, antisocial, and prone to psychiatric disorders, including depression. They exhibit high rates of smoking, marijuana use, and cocaine dependence. Although they account for only 9% of U.S. alcoholics, about two-thirds of chronic severe drinkers seek help for their drinking problems, making them the most prevalent type of alcoholic in treatment.[40]

Although 22 is the average age when alcohol dependence begins, the onset varies from the mid-teens to middle age.[40]

Are you at risk for developing alcoholism or alcohol abuse? Take the **Self-Assessment** above.

LO 9.5 QUICK CHECK

John is a middle-aged, well-educated man with a stable job, good income, and a family. He is most likely which type of alcoholic?

a. young adult subtype
b. functional subtype
c. intermediate familial subtype
d. chronic severe subtype

Alcohol Abuse: Treatment and Prevention

LO 9.6 Identify alcohol abuse treatment options and prevention strategies.

Few people who abuse alcohol acknowledge that they have a drinking problem. Fewer still seek treatment or counseling for it. It can take a major health problem, accident, or hitting "rock bottom" to motivate a problem drinker to change his or her behavior. Even when drinkers decide that they want to quit, they may not know how to do so on their own. An estimated 21.6 million people in the United States need treatment for an alcohol use problem (about 8.4% of the population aged 12 or older), but only 2.3 million receive treatment at a specialized facility.[1]

Treatment Options

Advances in alcoholism treatment in recent years have provided more choices than ever before for patients and health professionals. They include:

- **Medications.** Newer medications (naltrexone, topiramate, and acamprosate) can make it easier to quit drinking by offsetting changes in the brain caused by alcoholism and reducing the craving for alcohol. They don't make you sick if you drink, unlike an older medication (disulfiram). None of these medications are addictive. They can also be used together with support groups or alcohol counseling.
- **Alcohol counseling, or "talk therapy."** Several counseling approaches are about equally effective—12 Step, cognitive-behavioral, motivational enhancement, or a combination of these. Getting help in itself appears to be more important than the particular approach used, as long as it offers empathy, avoids heavy confrontation, strengthens motivation, and provides concrete ways to change drinking behavior. These programs usually focus on abstinence from alcohol. They may offer individual or group therapy, connect patients with alcoholism support groups, provide informational lectures, or involve activity therapy sessions. Specialized counseling may focus on the individual or family and may involve months of sessions or just occasional appearances. Short, one-on-one counseling sessions known as "brief interventions" have been increasing in popularity in recent years. Unlike traditional alcoholism treatments that emphasize complete abstinence from alcohol, interventions encourage sensible drinking at healthy levels. They require minimal follow-up and can be very effective.[41]
- **Self-help groups.** Mutual help organizations include the 12 Step program Alcoholics Anonymous. People in these groups attend general meetings and support each other by sharing advice and their personal experiences with alcohol abuse and recovery.
- **Intensive treatment programs.** These programs include 14- to 28-day residential programs that typically employ a 12 Step approach combined with individual and group therapy in a strictly scheduled abstinence environment. They also include longer-term (three- to four-month) programs and halfway houses that offer life skill and job training as well as treatment for substance dependence and mental health problems.

>> Looking for an alcohol treatment center? To find a treatment program near you, go to **http://samhsa.gov** and search for "find treatment."

>> This site provides self-help strategies for cutting back on or quitting drinking: **http://rethinkingdrinking.niaaa.nih.gov** and search for "approach."

Dealing with Relapse

Once an alcoholic has decided to curb or stop drinking altogether, he or she must confront the possibility of *relapse*. **Relapse**—resuming the behavior of drinking to excess, or "falling off the wagon"—is experienced by up to 90% of drinkers when they first try to quit.[42] With hard work and commitment, however, it can be overcome. Research from the National Institute on Alcohol Abuse and Alcoholism reveals that 20 years after the onset of alcohol dependence, about three-fourths of individuals were fully recovered.[41] Even more surprising, more than half of these individuals were able to drink at low levels without showing symptoms of alcohol dependence.[41] That said, many alcoholics find that abstinence is ultimately the only way to keep alcohol use from disrupting their lives.

> **relapse** Returning to drinking after a period of sobriety.

Beating any addiction requires both patience and practice. The body has to be weaned off a substance it has been dependent on, and the mind has to give up a long-used emotional crutch. Recovering alcoholics often have to change their social patterns and entire lifestyle. If you relapse while trying to quit drinking, don't give up. Learn from what happened and decide what to do next.

Prevention Strategies

Reducing alcohol-related risks happens one drink at a time. Some simple choices can keep drinking under control, reduce your risk of becoming a victim of others' drinking, and help your peers make more healthful choices, too.

Reducing Your Risk of Problem Drinking

If your drinking is getting out of hand, what can you do to take control? Step one: Make sure you haven't given someone else—for instance, your peer group—the power to control your decisions about drinking. Check out the **Special Feature** box on page 219 for tips on resisting peer pressure. In addition, here are other personal choices you can make to cut down on your drinking and reduce your risks.

Start by respecting your limits. Remember that your liver can break down the amount of alcohol in just one standard drink per hour, on average. So if you're at a party, try to stay within that limit:[43]

- **Pace and space.** Sip slowly. Make every other drink totally alcohol free.
- **Include food.** Don't drink on an empty stomach.
- **Shuffle things up.** Don't just drink. Get out on the dance floor, join the group watching a movie, or talk with friends outside.

❝ *Make sure you haven't given someone else—for instance, your peer group—the power to control your decisions about drinking.* **❞**

SPECIAL FEATURE

Peer Pressure
Resisting the Pitch

When was the last time you did something against your better judgment? Maybe last Saturday night? Did you give in to peer pressure and do something you really did not want to do? How can you stand your ground next time?

The National Institute on Alcohol Abuse and Alcoholism identifies a few of the most common reasons people give in to peer pressure.[1] Do any of these sound familiar?

- Desire to be liked, to be popular, and to not lose friends
- Desire to appear sophisticated, hip, cool, one of the "in" crowd
- Fear of being rejected, put down, teased, or ridiculed
- Worry about hurting a friend's feelings
- Uncertainty about what you really want
- Unawareness of how to get out of a bad situation

If you find yourself giving in to peer pressure for any of these reasons—or others—realize that although such feelings may be uncomfortable, they can motivate you to change. Here's how:[1]

Take a reality check. A friend may say to you, "Everybody else is okay with it. Why aren't you?" But how many students are really going to that pregame party, or mixing shots with their beer, or taking part in the drinking game in the lounge? If necessary, broaden your view: Remind yourself of students you like to hang out with who don't engage in high-risk drinking and who aren't participating in the behavior you're being pressured to join.

Remind yourself of the risks. Do you really want to end the night on the floor, in an ambulance, or sobering up in campus security or the city jail?

Just say no. Don't say it smugly or aggressively but don't mumble or apologize either. Say no assertively, standing up straight and looking directly at the person or group who is pressuring you. Speaking firmly and politely, state that you don't want to join the behavior. Make it clear that this is your choice but don't offer to explain your reasons. If the challenge continues, try countering: Repeat that you don't want to participate and point out that real friends respect one another's choices.

Walk away. If necessary, be prepared to walk away from the situation.

Saying no when the pressure is on takes self-confidence. If yours is lacking, check out some resources for building self-esteem and assertiveness skills at your campus counseling center.

Source: 1. "Peer pressure," by the National Institute on Alcohol Abuse and Alcoholism, 2010, www.thecoolspot.gov/pressures.asp.

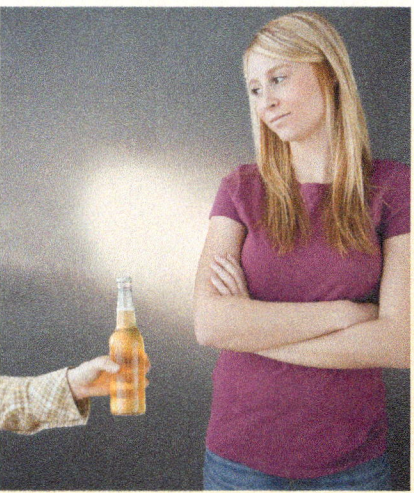

What if you're planning to go to a club or an off-campus party where you know alcohol will be served? Offer to be the designated driver or take a cab. If at all possible, attend the party with a trusted friend. Make a pact with each other not to engage in high-risk drinking and help each other stick to it.

Another potentially life-saving precaution is to avoid consuming alcohol during swimming, boating, or other water activities. Alcohol is involved in over 60% of fatal drownings.[9] Moreover, the American Boating Association reports that alcohol is involved in 31% of boating fatalities.[44]

Also avoid using other potentially dangerous machinery and equipment if you've been drinking. The truth is, when you're intoxicated, anything from a candle flame to a flight of stairs could become a life-threatening hazard.

Helping a Friend

What if you suspect that someone you care about is engaging in high-risk drinking? Trust your feelings. Confronting your friend now might save his or her academic career, health, or life. Here are some guidelines from the University of Texas at Dallas for talking to your friend about getting help for his or her high-risk drinking:[45]

- **Be informed.** Know before your talk where help is available, just in case your friend is ready to seek it.
- **Use I statements.** Say things like, "I'm afraid you'll get kicked out" or "I worry that you'll be charged with a DWI, or even worse—that you'll get killed . . . or kill somebody else." Pointing the finger or using the word *you* too much, as in "You've got to change," will only back your friend into a corner.
- **Don't judge and don't interrupt.** If your friend starts talking about the problem, don't break in. Sometimes just verbalizing about a situation can lead to a huge revelation.
- **Don't expect your friend to seek help after just one discussion.** It's difficult to predict how any individual person will react when confronted with his or her drinking problem. But it's still important to begin the process.

Reducing High-Risk Drinking on Campus

Students nationwide are helping to reduce high-risk drinking on their campuses. If you'd like to get involved, seek out one of the two national programs that may be active on your campus—and looking for student volunteers:

- **The BACCHUS Network.** Since 1975, the mission of the BACCHUS Network has been to actively promote student leadership on health and safety issues such as alcohol abuse. One of its goals is to train a network of peer educators who in turn empower other students. For information on starting a chapter or getting involved on your campus, visit www.bacchusnetwork.org.
- **Students Against Destructive Decisions.** Founded in Massachusetts, in response to the impaired driving deaths of local teens, SADD's original mission was to help young people say "no" to drinking and driving. Today, its broader mission is to provide students with the best prevention tools to deal with issues of underage drinking, other drug use, impaired driving, and other destructive decisions.[46] To get involved, check out **www.sadd.org**.

LO 9.6 QUICK CHECK

All of the following are guidelines for talking to a friend about getting help for high-risk drinking except
 a. be informed.
 b. use I statements.
 c. expect your friend to seek help immediately.
 d. don't judge or interrupt.

Smoking in the United States

LO 9.7 Discuss tobacco use in the United States.

Smoking remains the world's most preventable cause of death, each year killing 6 million people worldwide and 480,000 Americans. That translates to 1 of every 5 deaths in the United States. The good news is that in the decades since the 1964 landmark surgeon general's report *Smoking and Health*, the adult smoking rate in the United States has decreased from 43% to 18%.[47]

Certain population groups have higher smoking rates than others. For example, smoking is most common among the least educated. While 32% of adults with 9 to 11 years of education smoke, only 6% of those with graduate degrees do.[48]

The **Diversity & Health** box on page 207 provides a closer look at the prevalence of alcohol and tobacco use among various demographic groups.

Smoking on Campus

Of all tobacco users, people between 18 and 25 years old have the highest rate of use; 35% of people in that age range use tobacco.[49] About 25.5% of college students have tried smoking cigarettes at least once, although only 9.7% report smoking in the previous 30 days and just 2.7% report smoking daily.[6] If you thought the rates of smoking on your campus were higher, you're not alone: The **Student Stats** box examines actual versus perceived use of cigarettes among college students.

Why Do Some Students Smoke?

It would be difficult to find a student who has not heard that smoking can kill you. Why, then, do some students smoke? There are as many factors and reasons as there are individuals.

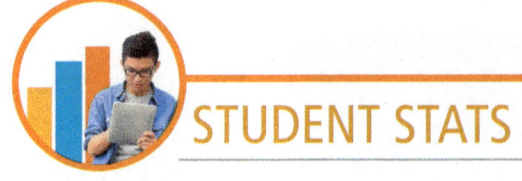

STUDENT STATS
Smoking on Campus

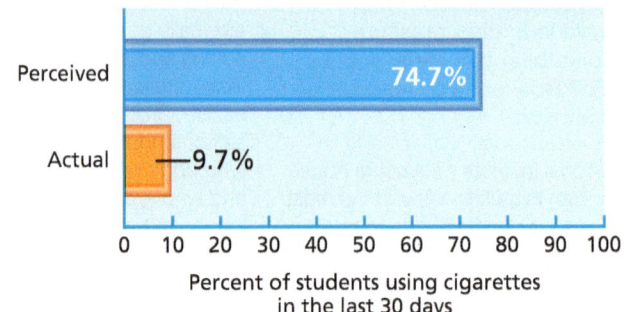

Students often greatly overestimate how many of their peers regularly smoke cigarettes.

Perceived: 74.7%
Actual: 9.7%

Percent of students using cigarettes in the last 30 days

Data from *ACHA-NCHA II: Undergraduate reference group executive summary, fall 2015*, by the American College Health Association, 2016.

Genetics. Substantial evidence from a number of twin and adoption studies suggests that persistent smoking is significantly influenced by hereditary factors.[50] In addition, molecular studies suggest that genetic variations account for at least some of the susceptibility to become addicted to **nicotine**, the key psychoactive and addictive ingredient in tobacco.[51] Still, no specific genes have been reliably identified, and many researchers emphasize that persistent smoking and addiction to nicotine develop as a result of complex genetic–environmental interactions.[52]

> **nicotine** An alkaloid derived from the tobacco plant that is responsible for smoking's psychoactive and addictive effects.

Family and Peer Exposure. One environmental factor is family exposure. Research shows that if children have a parent who smokes, they are at significant risk of becoming smokers themselves, and the risk goes up further if both parents smoke.[53] Moreover, students whose friends smoke may begin smoking so that they can maintain acceptance from their peer group, or they may begin smoking simply because they are more often in environments in which smoking is the norm. In one study, nonsmoking young adults who frequented bars, clubs, and similar establishments where smoking was unrestricted were at significantly higher risk for becoming smokers themselves.[54]

Age at Initiating Smoking. The younger people are when they start smoking, the more likely they are to become adult smokers. Research findings conclude that approximately 90% of adults who are regular smokers began at or before age 19.[55]

Psychosocial Factors. Stress is certainly a factor in tobacco use. Schoolwork, family tensions, and complicated social relationships with classmates have all been cited as reasons students smoke.

Young people experiencing interpersonal stress may rebel by experimenting with substances that their parents—and other authority figures in their lives—would not approve of. The fact that smoking is "bad" can actually make it more appealing to a teen wishing to challenge authority. In addition, some teens curious to experiment with a variety of recreational drugs may begin with smoking.

Behind such experimentation, there's often a failure to appreciate the real risks of tobacco use. Young adults sometimes have poor decision-making and risk-judging skills, and they believe they're invulnerable to harm. In one study, adolescents who had the lowest appreciation for the long-term health risks of smoking were more than three times as likely to start smoking as adolescents with the highest appreciation of the risks.[56] In another study, Florida community college students who smoked rated the health risks of smoking to be less significant than did their nonsmoking peers. Moreover, the smokers viewed their personal risk as lower than the risk to other smokers.[57]

Desire to Lose Weight. For decades, public health researchers have speculated that concerns about body weight were important factors in initiation of tobacco use among adolescents, particularly females. A 2008 study supports this theory. It found that, in general, females who perceived themselves to be overweight in grades 8 and 11 were more likely to be smokers as young adults.[58] Although it is true that nicotine can suppress appetite, taking up smoking to lose weight is one of the worst decisions anyone can make. The damage to health caused by smoking far outweighs any benefits in weight management.

Role of Media and Advertising. Media and advertising, including films, music videos, and expensive promotional campaigns, play a significant part in glamorizing smoking and making it acceptable. Characters in movies are commonly shown smoking, for example, even though the majority of Americans don't share the habit. Overall, the total weight of evidence from multiple types of studies worldwide demonstrates not just an association but a causal relationship between tobacco promotion and increased tobacco use.[59]

For a deeper look at how entertainment and ads contribute to smoking and alcohol use, see the **Media and Alcohol and Tobacco Use** box on page 222.

What's in a Cigarette?

Smoking cigarettes is by far the most common form of tobacco use. A typical cigarette in the United States contains 50% shredded tobacco leaf, 30% reconstituted tobacco (made from other parts of the tobacco plant, such as the stem), and 20% expanded tobacco (tobacco that has been "puffed up" like popcorn and functions as "filler").[60] It also contains nearly 600 additives with a wide range of functions. Cocoa, licorice, and vanilla, for example, are among the additives that help hide the harsh taste of tobacco. Meanwhile, ammonia—a chemical commonly used for household cleaning—boosts the delivery of *nicotine* (the key psychoactive ingredient in tobacco) into the lungs and bloodstream.

When a cigarette is lit and smoked, the burning tobacco produces a complex chemical mixture of more than 7,000 compounds, more than 60 of which are **carcinogenic,** meaning they cause cancer. These carcinogens include arsenic (a poison), formaldehyde (used in embalming fluid), polonium-210 (a radioactive substance), and **tar.** Tar is a sticky, thick brown residue that forms when tobacco is burned and its chemical particles condense. Other harmful chemicals in cigarette smoke include hydrogen cyanide, benzene (found in gasoline), and **carbon monoxide,** an especially dangerous gas that inhibits delivery of oxygen to the body's vital organs.

>> View video clips about the effects of tobacco advertising and more at http://www.tobaccofree.org/clips/.

LO 9.7 QUICK CHECK

What is the key psychoactive and addictive ingredient in cigarettes?
a. arsenic
b. nicotine
c. tar
d. carbon monoxide

Effects of Smoking on Health

LO 9.8 List the short-term and long-term health effects of tobacco use.

Smoking harms nearly every organ of the body, including the lungs, kidneys, bladder, heart, pancreas, stomach, and esophagus. It weakens the immune system and reduces life expectancy. Adults who smoke have a life expectancy more than 10 years shorter than those who don't smoke.[61] About half of long-term smokers will die because of their habit, according to the American Cancer Society.[62]

Short-Term Health Effects

From the moment a person takes the first puff of a cigarette, physiological changes take place in the body. Within 8 seconds of entering the body, nicotine is absorbed by the lungs and quickly moved into the bloodstream, where it is circulated throughout the brain. There, it triggers the release of large amounts of **dopamine,** a neurotransmitter that stimulates feelings of pleasure. Once smokers develop a tolerance to nicotine, they need more and more of it to achieve the same effects they experienced when they first began smoking. Eventually, smokers need to keep smoking just to feel "normal," as the body becomes addicted to nicotine. Stopping smoking can cause withdrawal symptoms such as cravings, irritability, insomnia, headache, inability to concentrate, and dry mouth.

---

carcinogenic Cancer-causing.

tar A sticky, thick brown residue that forms when tobacco is burned and its chemical particles condense.

carbon monoxide A gas that inhibits the delivery of oxygen to the body's vital organs.

dopamine A neurotransmitter that stimulates feelings of pleasure.

MEDIA AND Alcohol and Tobacco Use
How Entertainment and Ads Drive Drinking and Smoking

The media play a crucial role in shaping perceptions and habits related to drinking and smoking. Unfortunately, the message that's usually portrayed to viewers is that alcohol or tobacco use is fun, sophisticated, or cool.

Studies have found that frequent exposure to television and video portrayals of alcohol consumption as desirable can trigger new or increased drinking, with one study noting that "alcohol advertising and promotion increases the likelihood that adolescents will start to use alcohol, and to drink more if they are already using alcohol."[1] Take, for example, a period in our recent history: the 1990s. During that time, researchers linked increases in alcohol use to a decline in public service announcements cautioning against alcohol use and a corresponding increase in pro-use messages from the entertainment industry. In 1997, for example, alcohol appeared in 93% of the 200 most popular movie rentals, and the same year, the alcohol industry spent more than $1 billion on television, radio, print, and outdoor advertising.[2]

You might think the amount spent on alcohol advertising is high, but the tobacco industry leaves it in the dust. The major cigarette manufacturers spend more than $27.2 million *every day* to promote their products in the United States, and many of their efforts directly reach young adults.[3] Those efforts are also often apparently successful in both popularizing and triggering smoking; one large research analysis found that "nonsmoking adolescents who were more aware of tobacco advertising or receptive to it, were more likely to have experimented with cigarettes or become smokers" later.[4]

The depiction of smoking is pervasive in films, occurring in three-quarters or more of contemporary box-office hits.[5] Perhaps no form of media is more powerful in influencing smoking initiation: A 2008 report from the National Cancer Institute reached "the government's strongest conclusion to date" that smoking in films encourages smoking in youth.[5]

What Do You Think?

1. How often do you see ads and images glamorizing alcohol use as compared to ads or messages about its health risks, such as drunk driving?
2. How often are the depictions of smoking you see on film realistic in terms of everyday hassles (bad breath, smelly clothes) and health risks?
3. Why do you think smoking is so commonly shown in movies when the majority of the U.S. population doesn't smoke?

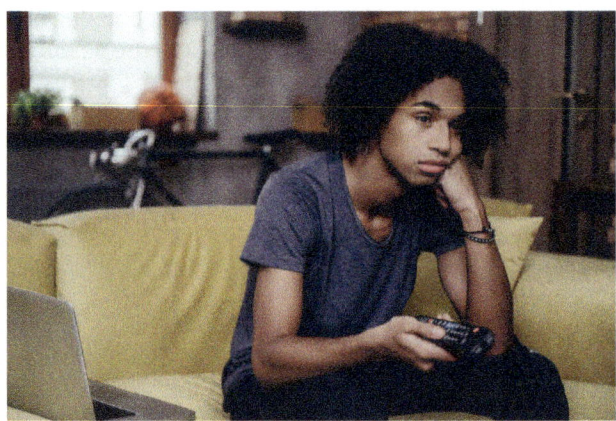

Watching movies and TV that depict tobacco use or excessive alcohol use can promote these behaviors.

References: **1.** "Impact of alcohol advertising and media exposure on adolescent alcohol use: A systematic review of longitudinal studies," by P. Anderson, A. Bruijn, K. Angus, R. Gordon, & G. Hastings, 2009, *Alcohol & Alcoholism*, 44(3), 229–243. **2.** "Substance abuse: The nation's number one health problem," by U.S. Department of Justice, 2001, OJJDP Fact Sheet, #17, www.ncjrs.gov. **3.** "Cigarette report for 2007 and 2008," by the U.S. Federal Trade Commission, 2011, www.ftc.gov. **4.** "Impact of tobacco advertising and promotion on increasing adolescent smoking behaviours," by C. Lovato, A. Watts, & L. Stead, 2011, *The Cochrane Collaboration*, Issue 10. Art. No.: CD003439. doi: 10.1002/14651858. **5.** "The role of the media in promoting and reducing tobacco use. NCI tobacco control monograph series," by the National Cancer Institute, 2008, http://cancercontrol.cancer.gov.

Other short-term health effects of smoking include:

- **Increased heart rate and blood pressure.** Nicotine causes the heart to beat faster. It also raises blood pressure.
- **Shortness of breath and reduction in stamina.** The carbon monoxide in cigarette smoke binds to a protein in red blood cells, disrupting these cells' ability to effectively deliver oxygen to the rest of the body.
- **Coughing.** Cigarette smoke damages the respiratory passageways, increasing the production of mucus and triggering the need to cough.
- **Heightened alertness.**
- **Decreased skin temperature.** Nicotine constricts blood vessels, resulting in less blood flow to the skin (reducing its temperature) and to the legs and feet.
- **Increased blood sugar.**
- **Dulled sense of smell and taste.**
- **Bad breath.**
- **Smelling like smoke.**
- **Decreased urine production.**
- **Risks to a developing fetus.**

Long-Term Health Effects

Cigarette smoking is so harmful that the surgeon general has called it "the leading preventable cause of disease and deaths in the United States." Since the surgeon general's 1964 report warning of the dangers of smoking, more than 20 million premature deaths have been attributed to cigarettes. Smoking is responsible for more than 87% of lung cancer deaths, 61% of pulmonary disease deaths, and 32% of all deaths from heart disease. Plus, research continues to identify associated diseases not previously thought to be caused by smoking, such as diabetes, rheumatoid arthritis, and colorectal cancer. Smoking also has many other adverse health effects, such as causing inflammation and impairing immune function.[47]

chronic obstructive pulmonary disease (COPD) A category of diseases that includes emphysema, chronic bronchitis, and asthma.

emphysema A chronic disease in which the air sacs in the lung become damaged, making breathing difficult.

chronic bronchitis Inflammation of the main airways in the lungs that continues for at least three months.

asthma A chronic pulmonary disease in which the air passages become inflamed, making breathing difficult.

Cancer

In the United States, smoking is responsible for 90% of lung cancer deaths in men and nearly 80% of those in women.[63] Smoking also increases the risk for cancers of the mouth, throat, larynx, stomach, kidney, bladder, pancreas, stomach, esophagus, colon/rectum, ovary, cervix, and blood.[64] A smoker's risk of developing these cancers increases with the number of cigarettes and the number of years he or she smokes. The odds of getting lung cancer are more than 25 times higher among smokers than among nonsmokers.[63] The risk, however, does begin to drop over time in those who quit for good.

Cardiovascular Disease

Smoking is a key risk factor for three major types of cardiovascular disease:

- **Coronary heart disease.** The leading cause of death in the United States, coronary heart disease often stems from the development of *atherosclerosis,* a progressive hardening of the coronary arteries. Smoking contributes to the development of atherosclerosis, which can result in a heart attack. Indeed, you are four times more likely to die of coronary heart disease if you smoke than if you don't.[47]
- **Stroke.** A stroke occurs when a blood vessel carrying oxygen and nutrients to the brain either bursts or is blocked by a clot. When that happens, part of the brain cannot get the blood and oxygen it needs and starts to die. It can cause speech problems, vision problems, memory loss, and paralysis on one side of the body. It can also be fatal. Cigarette smoking doubles a person's odds of having a stroke. The risk, however, steadily decreases after quitting smoking, with former smokers having roughly the same stroke risk as nonsmokers do 5 to 15 years after quitting.[47]
- **Abdominal aortic aneurysm.** An aortic aneurysm is a dangerously weakened and bulging area in the aorta, the major blood vessel that supplies blood to the body. A ruptured aortic aneurysm can cause life-threatening bleeding. Smoking is clearly associated with the condition. Several studies show that the risk of death from abdominal aortic aneurysm more than quadruples in smokers and doubles in former smokers.[47]

Respiratory Disease

Smoking damages the airways and alveoli of the lungs and can lead to **chronic obstructive pulmonary disease (COPD),** a category of diseases that includes emphysema, chronic bronchitis, and asthma.

In **emphysema,** the walls of the lungs' air sacs lose their elasticity and are destroyed. It becomes difficult for the lungs to transfer oxygen to the bloodstream, causing shortness of breath. Emphysema sufferers often have trouble performing simple physical activities such as shopping or climbing stairs. As the disease progresses, many emphysema patients must rely on an oxygen tank to help them breathe.

Chronic bronchitis is an inflammation of the main airways in the lungs that continues for at least three months. Symptoms include a chronic cough that produces mucus, shortness of breath, wheezing, and frequent respiratory infections.

Asthma is a chronic pulmonary disease in which the air passages become inflamed. The inflammation causes a narrowing of the airways, making breathing very difficult. Asthma symptoms include wheezing, coughing, shortness of breath, and chest tightness.

In 2014, COPD was the third leading cause of death in the United States.[65] Smoking is considered the "primary causative factor" in 80% of COPD deaths.[66]

Other Health Effects

Aside from the increased risks for cancer, cardiovascular disease, and respiratory disease, smoking can have additional health consequences:

- Greatly increased risk of developing diabetes and higher risk for complications such as kidney disease, blindness, and circulation problems that lead to amputations[47]
- Impaired immune function, resulting in a higher risk for diseases like tuberculosis and certain autoimmune disorders such as rheumatoid arthritis
- Adverse reproductive effects, such as erectile dysfunction in men and decreased fertility and ectopic pregnancy in women
- Loss of bone density in women following menopause
- Periodontitis, a gum infection that can lead to tooth loss
- Increased risk of developing macular degeneration and cataracts, leading causes of blindness
- Poorer general health
- Premature aging, wrinkling of skin, and stained teeth

Figure 9.5 summarizes the short- and long-term health effects of smoking.

Smoking and Pregnancy

When a pregnant woman smokes, so does her unborn baby. The nicotine, carbon monoxide, benzene, and other cancer-causing chemicals that enter her bloodstream are

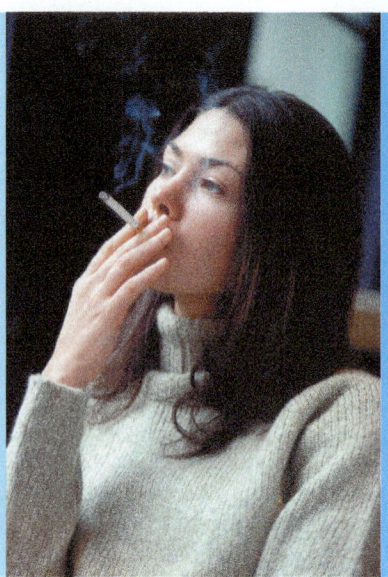

Short-term effects:
- Increased heart rate
- Increased blood pressure
- Shortness of breath
- Reduction in stamina
- Coughing
- Heightened alertness
- Decreased skin temperature
- Increased blood glucose
- Dulled sense of smell and taste
- Bad breath
- Smelling like smoke
- Health risks to developing fetus

Long-term effects:
- Greatly increased risk of cancer
- Greatly increased risk of cardiovascular disease
- Reduced lung function
- Periodontal disease
- Increased risk of gastroesophageal reflux
- Increased risk of peptic ulcers
- Reduced liver function
- Increased risk of type 2 diabetes
- Erectile dysfunction
- Decreased fertility
- Loss of bone density
- Vision impairment
- Premature aging and wrinkling of skin
- Stained teeth
- Nicotine addiction

FIGURE 9.5 **Short- and Long-Term Health Effects of Smoking.**

passed on to her fetus. Nicotine also reduces the amount of oxygen that reaches the fetus, negatively affecting its growth. Nicotine exposure during pregnancy has lasting negative consequences for fetal brain development.

Smoking while pregnant is like gambling—with the baby's life. Babies born to women who smoke are two to three times more likely to die of *sudden infant death syndrome* than babies born to women who did not smoke.[67] They also have 30% higher odds of being born prematurely and are more likely to weigh less than 5.5 pounds when they are born, increasing their risk for illness or death.[67] Smoking during pregnancy has also been linked to miscarriages and stillbirths. Up to 5% of infant deaths would be prevented if women did not smoke during pregnancy.[68]

Secondhand Smoke

Secondhand smoke is a mixture of **sidestream smoke**—the smoke emanating from the burning end of a cigarette or pipe—and **mainstream smoke,** which is exhaled from the lungs of smokers. Also called **environmental tobacco smoke,** it contains more than 250 chemicals known to be toxic or capable of causing cancer, including arsenic, ammonia, formaldehyde, and benzene.[69]

The smoke that nonsmokers are exposed to actually has higher concentrations of some harmful chemicals than the smoke inhaled by the smoker, according to the American Lung Association. This is because sidestream smoke is not filtered through a cigarette filter or a smoker's lungs. As a result, secondhand smoke has at least twice the amount of nicotine and tar as mainstream smoke. It also has five times the amount of carbon monoxide and has higher levels of ammonia and cadmium (chemicals found in glass cleaner and batteries, respectively).

Millions of people in the United States are essentially *passive smokers:* people who breathe in secondhand smoke from their environment. In national surveys, 43% of passive smokers have been found to have detectable levels of *cotinine*—the major breakdown product of nicotine—in their blood.[69]

The health risks to passive smokers are no less serious than if they were the ones lighting up a cigarette or puffing on a cigar. The U.S. surgeon general has concluded that "the scientific evidence indicates that there is no risk-free level of exposure to secondhand smoke." In fact, secondhand smoke can kill.

Health Effects of Secondhand Smoke

Secondhand smoke, which can linger in the air for hours after cigarettes have been extinguished, can exacerbate—or cause—a number of health conditions, including cancer, respiratory infections, and asthma. On a basic level, it can irritate the eyes, nose, throat, and lungs. It can also cause chest pain, coughing, and production of excessive phlegm. In a report spanning more than 700 pages, the U.S. surgeon general concluded that secondhand smoke can also cause:

- Premature death and disease in children and adults who do not smoke
- A 25% to 30% increase in a nonsmoker's heart disease risk
- Lung cancer in people who have never smoked
- Respiratory illnesses, including asthma, in children
- Ear infections in children
- Sudden infant death syndrome in some babies[69]

"The health effects of secondhand smoke exposure are more pervasive than we previously thought," the report summarized. "The scientific evidence is now indisputable:

> **secondhand smoke (environmental tobacco smoke)** The smoke nonsmokers are exposed to when someone has been smoking nearby; a combination of sidestream smoke and mainstream smoke.
>
> **sidestream smoke** Smoke emanating from the burning end of a cigarette or pipe.
>
> **mainstream smoke** Smoke exhaled from the lungs of smokers.

CONSUMER CORNER
Are "Light" Cigarettes Safer to Use?

You have probably seen advertisements for cigarettes that are "low-tar," "mild," "light," or "lite."

Some even purport to be "ultra-light." But are such cigarettes really any less dangerous than other cigarettes?

Although it's true that some cigarettes deliver less tar or nicotine than regular cigarettes in machine-based tests, health experts say there is no convincing evidence that they are less harmful to a person's health. On the contrary, studies have shown that when smokers switch to low-tar cigarettes, they often change the way they smoke, smoking more cigarettes, taking bigger puffs, and holding smoke in their lungs longer.[1]

- The U.S. surgeon general has concluded that "light" cigarettes do not actually decrease the health risks of smoking, primarily because these changes did not reduce smokers' actual exposure to tobacco toxicants.[1]
- The National Cancer Institute has determined that people who switch to light cigarettes are likely to inhale the same amount of hazardous chemicals as those smoking regular, or "full-flavored," cigarettes. They also remain at high risk for developing smoking-related cancers and other diseases.[2]
- There is no evidence that switching to light cigarettes actually helps smokers kick their habit.

The bottom line: "Light" cigarettes are still harmful to a person's health.

References: **1.** *How tobacco smoke causes disease: The Biology and behavioral basis for smoking-attributable disease, a report of the surgeon general,* by the U.S. Department of Health and Human Services, 2012. **2.** *Risks associated with smoking cigarettes with low machine-measured yields of tar and nicotine* [Monograph 13], October 2001, by the National Cancer Institute, http://cancercontrol.cancer.gov.

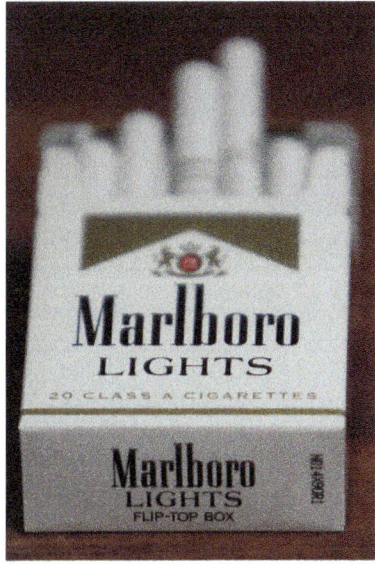

---

secondhand smoke is not a mere annoyance. It is a serious health hazard that can lead to disease and premature death in children and nonsmoking adults."[69]

Health experts estimate that secondhand smoke causes 3,400 lung cancer deaths and between 22,700 and 69,600 heart disease deaths in adult nonsmokers in the United States each year.[70]

Because their bodies are growing and developing, infants and children are particularly vulnerable to the effects of secondhand smoke. Secondhand smoke causes more than 750,000 middle-ear infections in children and increases the number and severity of asthma attacks in more than 200,000 asthmatic children.[70] It also reduces lung function in children and promotes the development of persistent wheezing.

LO 9.8 QUICK CHECK

Which of the following is the best definition of *carcinogenic*?
a. any substance containing tar
b. a cancer-causing substance
c. of or relating to a cigarette
d. any byproduct produced when something is burned

Other Forms of Tobacco

LO 9.9 Identify a range of tobacco products.

Cigars, clove cigarettes, bidis, pipes, and smokeless "spit" tobacco are other commonly used tobacco products. Like cigarettes, they are also associated with numerous health problems.

Cigars

Cigars contain many of the same addictive, toxic, cancer-causing substances as cigarettes. The smoke from cigars also contains many of the toxins found in cigarette smoke, including ammonia, carbon monoxide, and benzene, but in much higher concentrations. A single cigar can contain as much tobacco as an entire pack of cigarettes.[71]

Because most cigar smokers do not inhale, their risk of developing lung cancer is lower than it is for cigarette smokers. However, cigar smokers still have higher rates of lung cancer, heart disease, and COPD than do nonsmokers.[72]

Clove Cigarettes

Clove cigarettes, which have a distinctly sweet, pungent odor, are shaped like traditional cigarettes and are imported from Indonesia or other Southeast Asian countries. Also called *kreteks,* they usually contain tobacco, cloves, and other additives. Although they may smell and taste different from conventional cigarettes, there is no evidence that they are any safer. Clove cigarette smokers have higher rates of asthma and up to 20 times the risk for abnormal lung function, compared with nonsmokers.[73]

Recent federal laws ban the sale of flavored cigarettes, including clove cigarettes. It is not illegal to smoke them, but it is illegal to sell them.

Bidis

Bidis (pronounced bee-dees) are thin, hand-rolled cigarettes that come in a variety of flavors, including cherry, chocolate, grape, and mango. Imported from India and other Southeast

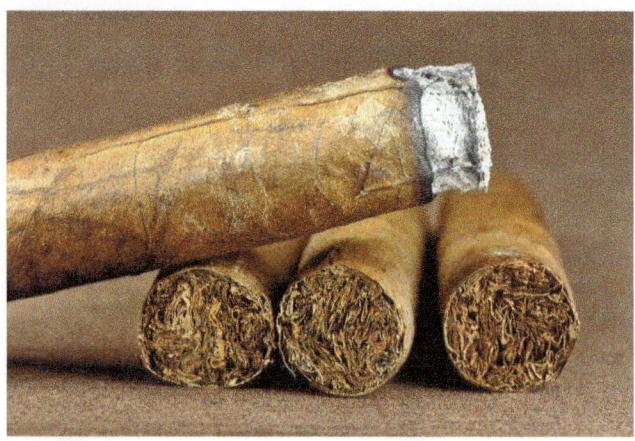

Cigars, clove cigarettes, bidis, and smokeless tobacco all increase the risk of cancer and heart disease.

Asian countries, they are packed with tobacco and wrapped in leaf, sometimes tied at the ends with colorful string.

Contrary to a popular misconception, bidis are *not* safer than cigarettes. A bidi contains approximately three to five times more nicotine than a regular cigarette.[73] Bidi smokers are at increased risk for several types of cancer, including oral, lung, stomach, and esophageal cancer, as well as coronary heart disease, emphysema, and chronic bronchitis.[73]

Hookahs

A hookah is a type of water pipe used for vaporizing and smoking flavored tobacco. Unlike a typical tobacco pipe, a hookah allows the smoke to pass through water before being inhaled by the smoker. Hookah use is gaining in popularity in the United States, and approximately 21% of college students report having tried a hookah.[6] While hookah smokers may think this is a safer method of tobacco smoking, the CDC warns that it has many of the same health risks as traditional smoking. In addition to exposure to the nicotine, tar, and other toxins in tobacco smoke, hookah users are also exposed to fellow smokers' germs, since the pipe is usually passed from person to person.

Smokeless ("Spit") Tobacco

For some young people, especially young men, the use of smokeless tobacco is almost a rite of passage, even though it carries dangerous health risks. Baseball fans are used to seeing their heroes use smokeless tobacco, also known as "spit" or "chew." Indeed, one in three major league baseball players uses smokeless tobacco.[74] In some communities, especially rural areas and small towns, younger men may pick up a tradition of using smokeless tobacco from fathers and older brothers.[75] No wonder, then, that many boys and young men have followed in the footsteps of their role models, using smokeless tobacco at alarming rates. Nationwide, about 11% of male high school students use smokeless tobacco, and 2% of adult men report having used smokeless tobacco products.[76]

Smokeless tobacco comes in several forms. *Snuff* is a fine-grain tobacco often sold in powered form, either loose or in teabag-like pouches that users "pinch" or "dip" between their lower lip and gum. Snus is a similar product that is usually packaged in small pouches; it requires the user to spit less often. *Chewing tobacco* comes in wads of shredded or "bricked" tobacco leaves that are placed between the cheek and gum. No matter the type, smokeless tobacco is meant to stew in the mouth for minutes at a time. Users suck on the tobacco juices and then spit to get rid of the saliva that builds up, hence the nickname "spit."

Although they don't emit harmful plumes of smoke like cigarettes and cigars do, smokeless tobacco products contain plenty of addictive nicotine. It is absorbed into the bloodstream through the mucous membranes that line the mouth, and users can become physically hooked without ever swallowing the tobacco soup that builds up in their mouths. The average dose of smokeless tobacco, in fact, contains up to four times the amount of nicotine in the average cigarette. One can of snuff is equivalent, nicotine-wise, to about four packs of cigarettes.

Regular use of smokeless tobacco increases a person's risk for cancers of the lip, tongue, cheeks, gums, and mouth. The products stain and wear down the teeth, cause gums to recede, and can cause a condition called **leukoplakia,** characterized by whitish lesions in the mouth. These lesions may become cancerous and are frequently found in snuff and chew users in their 20s.

> **leukoplakia** White spots on the mucous membranes in the mouth that may become cancerous.

Electronic Cigarettes

A newer nicotine product often advertised as a smoking cessation aid is the electronic cigarette (or e-cigarette), a battery-powered device that delivers a dose of nicotine in vapor form. According to the Food and Drug Administration (FDA), e-cigarettes have not been adequately studied and, therefore, consumers don't know what quantities of nicotine or other harmful substances are being inhaled during use. Consequently, in 2016 the FDA extended its authority to cover the regulation of e-cigarettes. These regulations prohibit the sale of e-cigarettes, hookah and all tobacco products to those under the age of 18 and also implement rigorous scientific review of tobacco product safety and claims.[77]

While proponents of e-cigarettes claim that they are a safer alternative to tobacco products, public health advocates insist that for teens, they are a gateway to tobacco cigarettes. Also, poison control centers have reported numerous nicotine poisoning cases among very young children caused by e-cigarettes.[78] Experts contend that this occurs because the nicotine in e-cigarettes is in liquid form, it comes in flavors kids like, and the products are not sold in childproof packaging.

LO 9.9 QUICK CHECK

Which of the following is a condition of the mouth characterized by whitish, often precancerous, lesions sometimes seen in those who use smokeless tobacco products?

a. melanoma
b. kreteks
c. periodontitis
d. leukoplakia

Getting Help to Quit Smoking

LO 9.10 Outline strategies for quitting smoking.

If you smoke, odds are you have thought about quitting. The majority of Americans who have ever smoked have now quit (55%),[79] and more than half of all smokers make a determined effort to quit each year.[77] And for good reason. Smokers are estimated to lose more than a decade of life. Researchers recently determined that if smokers quit before age 40, they can reduce that loss by 90%.[47]

Stopping smoking is not a simple matter. Nicotine activates the pleasure and reward centers of the brain and raises levels of the "feel good" neurotransmitter dopamine. Consequently, nicotine can be as addictive as heroin or cocaine. Those attempting to quit often must deal with withdrawal symptoms such as restlessness, depression, hunger, insomnia, and headaches. A smoker's brain develops an abundance of nicotine-binding receptors to accommodate the large doses of nicotine. Research findings conclude that for up to 6 weeks after people stop smoking, these receptors still exist.[80] Unfortunately, these nicotine-receptor brain cells contribute to the cravings and other discomforts of smoking withdrawal and probably explain why the first months of smoking cessation are very difficult for many people. The good news is that after 6 to 12 weeks of abstinence, the former smoker's nicotine receptor levels match those of a nonsmoker, and consequently relapse is less likely.

The health benefits of quitting smoking begin almost immediately. **Figure 9.6** illustrates the short- and long-term benefits of quitting.

Treatment Options

Studies show that effective cessation treatments can double or triple a smoker's chances of long-term abstinence.[81] Several types of products are available to aid smokers who wish to quit. Most of them, including nicotine gum, inhalers, lozenges,

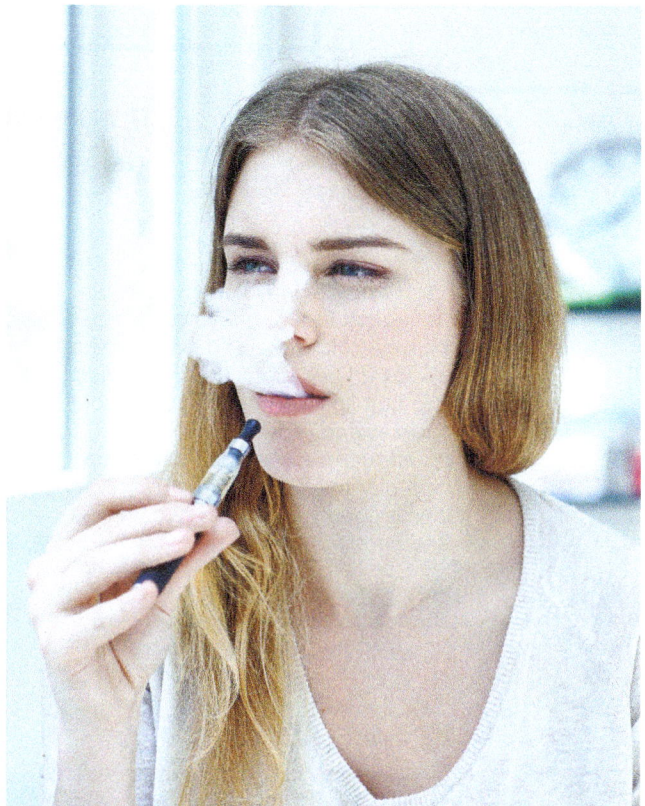

E-cigarettes are promoted as a safer alternative to smoking, but public health experts warn that they may be a gateway for teens to tobacco products.

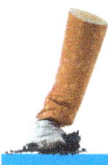

QUIT SMOKING

First 48 hours:

20 minutes	8 hours	24 hours	48 hours
• Blood pressure drops to normal. • Pulse rate drops to normal. • Body temperature of hands and feet increases to normal.	• Carbon monoxide level in blood drops to normal. • Oxygen level in blood increases to normal.	• Chance of heart attack decreases.	• Nerve endings start regrowing. • Ability to smell and taste is enhanced.

First year:

2 weeks to 3 months	1 to 9 months	1 year
• Circulation improves. • Walking becomes easier. • Lung function increases up to 30%.	• Coughing, sinus congestion, fatigue, and shortness of breath decrease. • Cilia regrow in lungs, increasing ability to handle mucus, clean the lungs, and reduce infection. • Overall energy level increases.	• Excess risk of coronary heart disease is half that of a smoker.

Future years:

5 years	10 years	15 years
• Lung cancer death rate for average former smoker (one pack a day) decreases by almost half.	• Lung cancer death rate similar to that of nonsmokers. • Precancerous cells are replaced. • Risk of cancer of the mouth, throat, esophagus, bladder, kidney, and pancreas decreases.	• Risk of coronary heart disease is that of a nonsmoker.

FIGURE 9.6 Benefits of Quitting Smoking. The health benefits of quitting smoking begin the moment you stop.

nasal sprays, and patches, are *nicotine replacement therapies* designed to help smokers gradually reduce their dependence on nicotine and reduce the severity of nicotine withdrawal symptoms. Others, such as bupropion (Zyban) and varenicline (Chantix), do not contain nicotine at all but reduce the smoker's craving for tobacco and ease withdrawal symptoms. (Note that serious safety concerns have recently arisen about both of these drugs.) You should talk with your doctor or a pharmacist before taking any smoking cessation products, especially if you have any allergies, have health problems, are taking any medications, or are pregnant or planning to become pregnant.

Note that nicotine replacement therapies are available only to those aged 18 and older. You should not continue smoking while taking a smoking cessation product. You should also avoid taking more than one smoking cessation product at the same time without consulting a doctor because improper use can result in nicotine overdose.

In addition to nicotine replacement therapies, smoking cessation programs are effective for approximately 20% to 40% of smokers.[81] There are several types of treatment options, including residential, individual and group therapy, and education and support groups.

Dealing with Relapse

Smokers commonly experience withdrawal symptoms when they first quit smoking, including difficulty concentrating, a negative mood, and the urge to smoke. These symptoms usually peak within one or two weeks. Not surprisingly, smokers are most likely to relapse early in the quitting process, although sometimes relapse can occur months or even years after quitting. Any smoking—even taking one single puff—increases the likelihood of a full relapse.

LO 9.10 QUICK CHECK

Which of the following statements is true about smoking cessation treatments?

a. Effective cessation treatments can triple a smoker's chances of long-term abstinence
b. Most smoking cessation treatments don't work
c. Nicotine replacement therapies are designed to flood the smoker's system with nicotine to make them sick and therefore no longer crave it
d. People of any age can obtain various types of nicotine replacement therapies

Change Yourself, Change Your World

LO 9.11 Describe how to promote a smoke-free environment on campus.

Smoking injures and kills. Whether you're a smoker and want to quit or want to reduce the threat of secondhand smoke, there are powerful choices you can make to reach your goal.

Personal Choices

If your goal is to quit smoking and avoid relapse, you need to follow a plan that works. The plan described here, adapted from the National Cancer Institute (NCI), is one you can trust.[82]

STUDENT STORY

Quitting Cold Turkey

"HI, I'M ADDISON. When I first started smoking I was 16 years old. I've tried to quit numerous times—always cold turkey. I'd last maybe a week if I was lucky. Recently I tried to quit again. This time I went cold turkey *and* I started working out, too. I tried to replace a bad habit with a healthier habit. I go to the gym every day, I haven't smoked in two weeks, and I hope to keep it that way."

What Do You Think?

1. What stage of behavior change is Addison in? (Review Chapter 1 if you can't remember the stages of behavior change.)
2. What do you think of Addison's plan to "replace" smoking with working out?
3. How can Addison improve his chances of quitting smoking for good?

Quitting is more likely to succeed if you're prepared. Start by thinking about why you want to quit. Write down your reasons and keep them with you. Make sure the reasons you list are meaningful to you. For instance:

- I'll have more stamina on the basketball court.
- I won't have to be embarrassed about bad breath and smelly clothes.
- I'll know that I'm the one in control of my life.

Next, take a good, hard look at how strong your addiction to nicotine really is. For instance, do you smoke only socially or by yourself as well? When you wake up in the morning, do you crave your first cigarette? How many cigarettes do you typically smoke in a day? Your honest answers may help you to decide whether you need professional support to quit. Going "cold turkey" usually works for only a very small percentage of smokers who have a low level of nicotine dependency.[82] Others need support.

Identify your triggers—the activities, feelings, and other factors that make you want to smoke. Is it coffee? Being around other smokers? Feeling bored, unhappy, or depressed? List a strategy for avoiding each trigger entirely or for substituting a behavior other than smoking. For example, if you typically smoke when you drive, replace cigarettes in your car with a stash of chewing gum. If a craving still hits, take a long, deep breath and remind yourself that it will go away, usually in just a few minutes.

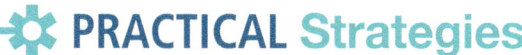

PRACTICAL Strategies

Quitting Smoking

The National Institutes of Health promotes the START method as an effective smoking cessation strategy.

S = Set a quit date.
Choose a date within the next two weeks as your official quit date. Smoking cessation experts suggest that you pick a special date as your quit date. Consider your birthday, a special anniversary, New Year's Day, July 4, "World No-Tobacco Day" (May 31), or the "Great American Smokeout" (the third Thursday in November).

T = Tell family, friends, and coworkers that you plan to quit.
If you are going to be successful in your attempt to quit, you need the help and support of others. So inform the important people in your life and let them know exactly how they can help you in your efforts.

A = Anticipate and plan for the challenges you'll face while quitting.
Studies show that most people who return to smoking do so within the first three months. Make plans ahead of time for dealing with cravings and withdrawal symptoms when they hit.

R = Remove cigarettes and other tobacco products from your home, car, and work.
Get rid of everything you can that reminds you of smoking. Change your routine, so that certain events and places don't prompt a cigarette craving. Throw away all cigarettes and smoking paraphernalia such as lighters, matches, and ashtrays.

T = Talk to your doctor about getting help to quit.
Your health-care provider can prescribe medication that can help you quit. There are also effective over-the-counter products that are helpful in dealing with nicotine withdrawal. These products include:

- Nicotine gum
- Nicotine inhaler
- Nicotine lozenge
- Nicotine nasal spray
- Nicotine patch
- Bupropion SR pills (prescription only)
- Varenicline pills (prescription only)

For more help, call 1-877-44U-QUIT (1-877-448-7848) to talk to a smoking cessation counselor from the National Cancer Institute. For help within your own state, call 1-800-QUITNOW (1-800-784-8669) or visit www.smokefree.gov.

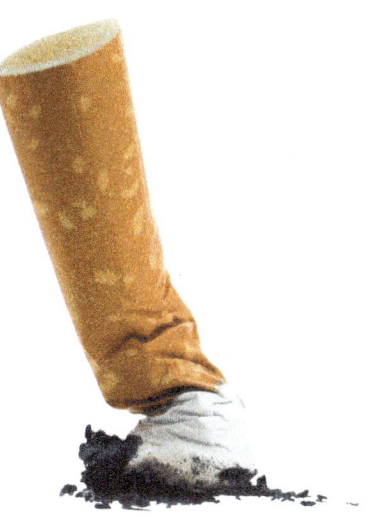

Finally, learn your options. Earlier in this chapter, we discussed campus and community-based support as well as medications and clinical smoking cessation programs. Stay open to the option of combining two or more of these methods. **Practical Strategies: Quitting Smoking** also summarizes a step-by-step strategy for taking the plunge to quit, prepared by the National Cancer Institute.

>> Ready to quit smoking today? Visit the National Cancer Institute's www.smokefree.gov.

Campus Advocacy

Many national public health organizations, from the U.S. Centers for Disease Control and Prevention to the American College Health Association, support not only indoor smoking bans on college and university campuses but outdoor bans as well. This is in part because indoor smoking bans may encourage smokers to cluster just outside buildings, saturating these areas with tobacco smoke, which can then drift back into the building.[83]

If you'd like to advocate for a smoke-free campus, the American College Health Association recommends a policy that includes the following provisions:[84]

- Prohibit smoking and all forms of tobacco on all campus grounds and in all campus-related facilities, including residence halls and fraternities and sororities, as well as at all indoor and outdoor campus events.
- Prohibit the sale, advertising, and free distribution of tobacco products and tobacco-related merchandise on campus and at sporting events.
- Provide accessible tobacco treatment on campus and promote it.
- Prohibit campus organizations, including athletic organizations, from accepting money or other forms of sponsorship from tobacco companies.
- Prohibit the university from holding stock in or accepting donations from the tobacco industry.

>> Watch videos of real students discussing their experiences with alcohol and tobacco at **Mastering**Health™

LO 9.11 QUICK CHECK

For those wanting to advocate for a smoke-free campus, the American College Health Association recommends a policy that includes which of the following?

a. a designated area for smoking
b. a campus-wide ban that prohibits indoor and outdoor smoking
c. the sale of tobacco products on campus to generate funds to support smoking-cessation programs
d. tobacco company sponsorship of anti-smoking campaigns on campus

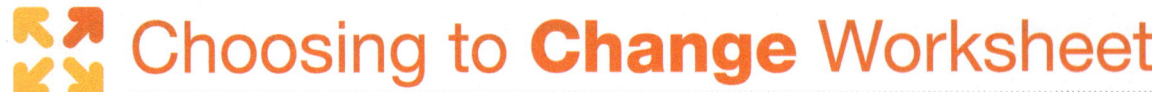

Choosing to Change Worksheet

To complete this worksheet online, visit MasteringHealth

Alcohol and tobacco are highly addictive drugs that can be very difficult to curb or eliminate from your daily life. The following worksheet can help you work toward a healthier lifestyle. If you are one of the many college students who do not use tobacco and do not drink alcohol or drink only moderately and infrequently, then use this worksheet to interview a friend who struggles with his or her alcohol or tobacco use.

Directions: Fill in your stage of change in step 1 and complete steps 2 or 3, depending on which one applies to your stage of change. Step 4 provides information for finding help with a drinking problem.

Step 1: Assess your stage of behavior change. Check one of the following statements that best describes your feelings about your drinking or smoking habits.

_____ I do not intend to quit or cut back on my drinking or tobacco use in the next six months. (Precontemplation)

_____ I might quit or cut back on my drinking or tobacco use in the next six months. (Contemplation)

_____ I am prepared to quit or cut back on my drinking or tobacco use in the next month. (Preparation)

_____ I have cut back on my drinking or tobacco use less than six months ago. (Action)

_____ I do not drink or use tobacco, or I cut back on my drinking or tobacco use more than six months ago. (Maintenance)

Step 2: Work within the precontemplation or contemplation stage of change. Reread the sections on the physical and behavioral effects of alcohol use or the effects of smoking on health on pages 211–215 or 221–225 and consider how you benefit from continuing your behavior or changing it.

Perceived Benefit of Continuing Excessive Drinking or Tobacco Use	Perceived Benefit of Stopping or Modifying Excessive Drinking or Tobacco Use
What do I give up if I change?	How will this help me?
1.	1.
2.	2.
3.	3.
4.	4.
5.	5.
6.	6.

Now, add up your totals:

_____ reasons to change _____ reasons to stay the same

What one benefit do you think will motivate you the most?

_____

What one barrier do you think will present the biggest obstacle for you?

_____

Step 3: Work within the preparation, action, or maintenance stage of change. If you are ready to quit or cut back on your drinking or smoking, or have already started, complete the following.

1. What is your SMART goal? If you are in the preparation stage, create a SMART goal for your change and write it down. If you are in the action or maintenance stages, write down the SMART goal you are working with.

_____

_____

2. Identify emotional or situational triggers. What situations or emotions make you most want to drink or use tobacco? Common triggers include anxiety, boredom, meals, peer pressure, and socializing with friends.

_____

_____

3. Target one of the triggers and substitute an alternate healthier behavior instead of drinking or using tobacco. For example, if you know that you are more likely to drink at the end of a stressful day, instead decide to take a walk or go work out at the gym.

Target trigger: _____

Alternative healthy behavior response: _____

Step 4: Find help. If alcohol or tobacco is seriously disrupting your life, seek help. The following websites are two great places to start: http://findtreatment.samhsa.gov and www.smokefree.gov. Also, keep in mind that most college campuses have student health centers staffed with counselors who can help support you in breaking an alcohol or smoking habit.

_____

_____

CHAPTER 9 STUDY PLAN

CHAPTER SUMMARY

LO 9.1
- Alcohol and tobacco are the most commonly used drugs in the United States and on college campuses.
- People of traditional college age are among the heaviest users of both of these addictive substances.

LO 9.2
- Alcohol is absorbed into the bloodstream from the stomach and small intestine. It is metabolized by the liver. If a person consumes alcohol at a faster rate than the liver can break it down, intoxication occurs.
- Blood alcohol concentration (BAC) is affected by numerous factors, including how much and how quickly alcohol is consumed, type of alcohol, sex, age, weight, physical condition, food intake, and medications.

LO 9.3
- The short-term effects of alcohol use include lightheadedness, loss of inhibition, compromised motor coordination, slowed reaction times, slurred speech, dulled senses, dehydration, and hangover.
- Long-term effects include increased risk of cancer, cardiovascular disease, liver disease, and neurological problems.

LO 9.4
- Alcohol impairs judgment and can lead to high-risk behaviors, including impaired driving, unprotected sex, and assault.

MasteringHealth™

Build your knowledge—and health!—in the Study Area of **MasteringHealth™** with a variety of study tools.

LO 9.5
- Alcohol dependence is characterized by a tolerance to and craving for alcohol.
- Overcoming addiction can be challenging, but many people recover eventually.

LO 9.6
- Residential treatment programs, medications, Internet resources, and counseling can help problem drinkers quit drinking and avoid relapse.

LO 9.7
- Students smoke for a variety of reasons. Both heredity and the environment are factors, including family and peer exposure, stress, and promotion of smoking in films and other media and advertising.

LO 9.8
- The short-term effects of smoking include increased heart rate and blood pressure, shortness of breath, coughing, alertness, decreased skin temperature, increased blood sugar, dulled senses, bad breath, smelling like smoke, and decreased urine production.

- The long-term effects of smoking include increased risk of cancer, cardiovascular disease, respiratory disease, and other health problems.
- Secondhand smoke contains higher concentrations of some harmful chemicals than the smoke inhaled by smokers. People, especially children and infants, who inhale secondhand smoke can suffer from the same health problems as smokers.

LO 9.9
- Cigars, clove cigarettes, bidis, pipes, and smokeless tobacco are commonly used tobacco products. Like cigarettes, these are also associated with health problems.

- Marketed as a smoking cessation aid, e-cigarettes are battery-powered devices that deliver nicotine in vapor form.

LO 9.10
- Quitting smoking has numerous immediate and long-term health benefits.
- Nicotine replacement therapies (such as nicotine gums, inhalers, and patches) are designed to help smokers gradually reduce their dependence on nicotine and reduce the severity of withdrawal symptoms.

LO 9.11
- Many former smokers have found assistance with quitting through campus resources.

GET CONNECTED

>> Visit the following websites for further information about the topics in this chapter:

- Rethinking Drinking: Alcohol and Your Health
  http://rethinkingdrinking.niaaa.nih.gov
- Alcoholics Anonymous
  www.aa.org
- Al-Anon and Alateen
  www.al-anon.alateen.org
- American Lung Association's Freedom from Smoking Online
  www.ffsonline.org

MOBILE TIPS!
Scan this QR code with your mobile device to access additional tips about avoiding alcohol and tobacco abuse. Or, via your mobile device, go to **http://chmobile.pearsoncmg.com** and choose by topic: alcohol and tobacco abuse.

- Centers for Disease Control and Prevention: Tobacco
  Search for "tobacco" at www.cdc.gov
- National Cancer Institute
  www.smokefree.gov

Website links are subject to change. To access updated web links, please visit **MasteringHealth™**

TEST YOUR KNOWLEDGE

LO 9.1
1. A standard drink is equivalent to
   a. 1.5 ounces of 80-proof liquor.
   b. 5 ounces of table wine.
   c. 12 ounces of beer.
   d. all of the above.

LO 9.2
2. Blood alcohol concentration can be affected by all of the following except
   a. how expensive the alcohol is.
   b. how much a person drinks.
   c. how fast a person drinks.
   d. how much a person has eaten prior to drinking.

LO 9.3
3. Long-term effects of alcohol on the body include
   a. increased risk of cancer.
   b. increased risk of cardiovascular disease.
   c. increased risk of liver disease.
   d. all of the above.

LO 9.4
4. A college student who drinks heavily is at increased risk of
   a. participating in unplanned sexual activity.
   b. contracting an STI.
   c. being involved in a sexual assault.
   d. all of the above.

LO 9.5
5. Factors associated with an increased risk for alcohol dependence include
   a. female gender.
   b. poverty.
   c. Asian ethnicity.
   d. initiating drinking at age 21 or over.

LO 9.6
6. What percentage of alcoholics relapse during their first attempt to quit drinking?
   a. 25%
   b. 40%
   c. 75%
   d. 90%

LO 9.7
7. What is the key psychoactive ingredient in cigarettes?
   a. ammonia
   b. carbon monoxide
   c. nicotine
   d. formaldehyde

LO 9.8
8. The immediate physical effects of smoking include all of the following *except*
   a. increased heart rate and blood pressure.
   b. increased skin temperature.
   c. increased level of blood sugar.
   d. shortness of breath.

LO 9.9
9. Smokeless tobacco is
   a. thought to be less addictive than cigarettes.
   b. used by about 18% of high school seniors.
   c. associated with an increased risk of cancer.
   d. all of the above.

LO 9.10
10. Quitting smoking
    a. is helped by the fact that nicotine lowers the "feel good" neurotransmitter dopamine.
    b. will provide health benefits within as little as 6 to 12 weeks.
    c. is difficult in part because excess nicotine-binding receptors in the brain promote craving.
    d. can be aided by beginning a nicotine replacement therapy before you quit.

WHAT DO YOU THINK?

LO 9.1
1. While college-bound high school seniors are less likely than their non-college-bound counterparts to binge drink, once at college, these same students report more binge drinking than their peers who entered the workforce. Why do you think this occurs?

LO 9.5
2. If you suspect that a friend has a problem with alcohol, what signs would confirm your suspicions?

LO 9.6
3. Why are college students particularly susceptible to alcohol-related problems? What is one change that could be made on your campus that would reduce problem drinking?

LO 9.7
4. Most students who smoke know that smoking can kill, and yet they continue their habit. Why?

LO 9.9
5. Are e-cigarettes a safer alternative to tobacco products? Should manufacturers of e-cigarettes be allowed to promote them as being safer?

10

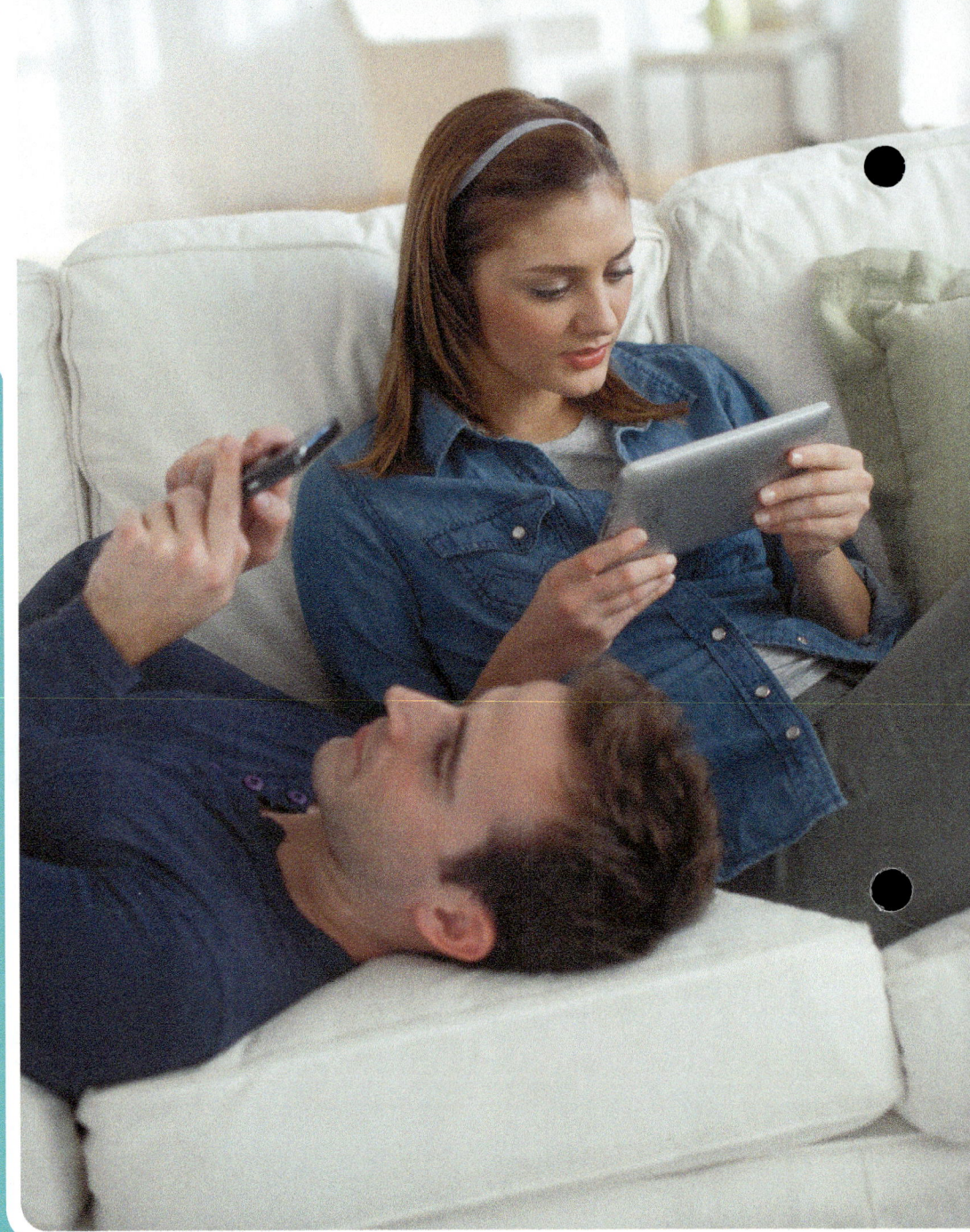

> More than 1 billion people use Facebook every day.[i]

> More than 50% of unmarried Americans aged 15 to 24 have lived with a partner outside marriage. About 40% of those couples tie the knot within three years.[ii]

> More than 20% of American adults over age 25 have never been married, more than double the number in 1960.[iii]

SOCIAL RELATIONSHIPS AND COMMUNICATION

LEARNING OUTCOMES

LO 10.1 Identify the characteristics of effective communication.

LO 10.2 Understand how self-perception, early relationships, and gender roles influence relationships.

LO 10.3 Identify the benefits of healthy long-term friendships.

LO 10.4 Discuss different forms of intimate relationships and Sternberg's Triangular Theory of Love.

LO 10.5 Describe at least three different types of committed relationships.

LO 10.6 Explain the factors that should be considered before starting a family.

LO 10.7 Discuss strategies for building and maintaining healthy relationships.

We are social beings, craving connections with others and the support, love,

and sense of contentment they give us. Our families teach us and guide us through the highs and lows of life. Our friends listen to us, laugh with us, and share in our successes and failures. Our lovers provide us with intimacy, companionship, and comfort. Our relationships with others fulfill us, define us, nurture us, and make us feel safe. Good relationships can relieve stress and, indeed, help keep us healthy.

Maintaining relationships, however, takes effort. Being able to speak up, listen well, and resolve conflicts are critical skills to develop for all personal relationships. In this chapter, we discuss the characteristics of effective communication, examine what constitutes a healthy relationship, identify signs of dysfunctional relationships, and explore various categories of committed relationships. Along the way, we will introduce methods of building relationship skills that strengthen healthy ties to friends, colleagues, family members, and partners. We will emphasize that although there is no such thing as a perfect relationship or a perfect family, strong unions are based on mutual affection, respect, commitment, companionship, and honesty.

Communication in Relationships

LO 10.1 Identify the characteristics of effective communication.

The cornerstone of every successful relationship is effective communication. That idea seems straightforward enough, but in real life, true communication can be challenging. All of us, at times, experience difficulty in communicating our thoughts, feelings, and needs. In addition, understanding the intentions and concerns of others isn't always easy. Effective communication is a skill that can be developed and continually improved. Without it, many relationships fail.

Communicating Feelings

True communication entails much more than just making smalltalk. It involves sharing honest feelings and other personal information—our hopes, our dreams, our secrets, our fears. This kind of sharing, called **self-disclosure,** was first described in 1971 by psychologist Sidney M. Jourard, in his foundational work, *The Transparent Self*. "If we want to be loved, we must disclose ourselves. If we want to love someone, he must permit us to know him," he wrote. "This would seem to be obvious. Yet most of us spend a great part of our lives thinking up ways to avoid becoming known."[1]

> **self-disclosure** The sharing of honest feelings and personal information about yourself with another person.

It is not always comfortable to share one's feelings. To do so can leave a person feeling vulnerable and exposed. If you think back through your own life, odds are you have known someone who had difficulty saying "I love you" or telling you what he or she was feeling or thinking. In order to be truly close to another person, however, we need to occasionally let down our guard and speak freely and honestly about what is on our minds.

Communication Skills

Especially when dealing with disagreements or other uncomfortable situations, certain communication strategies are helpful:

- **Stay focused.** Focus on the current issue, your feelings about it, and finding a solution.
- **Take responsibility.** Own what is yours and admit when you've made mistakes.
- **Use "I" messages.** Begin the discussion with an "I feel" statement. Making the discussion about the other person may make him or her feel attacked and trigger defensiveness.
- **Listen effectively.** A big part of being a good communicator is being a careful listener.
- **Be solution focused.** Try to look for a win–win compromise. Effective communication requires that you find a resolution that both parties can be happy with.
- **Step away if necessary.** Sometimes the timing isn't right for resolving a relationship conflict. If tempers flare and the conversation is headed toward an unproductive verbal fight, take a break. But don't just forget about it. Problems don't disappear just because you don't talk

about them. Return to the issue when it can be approached with a more constructive attitude.

- **Avoid jumping to conclusions or making quick judgments.** Let the other person complete his or her thought before forming an opinion. If you have a question about what another person means, ask for a clarification.
- **Resist antagonizing the other person.** For example, resist correcting grammatical errors or nitpicking at other details that do not matter to the real issue at hand.
- **Seek help if you need it.** If you or your partner continues to have difficulty communicating about relationship issues in a constructive way, it may be a good idea to seek help from a counselor or other professional who can help.

Nonverbal Communication

Sometimes you can get a message across without saying a single word. Imagine a teenager who has been out way past her curfew. When she arrives home, she unlocks the front door and tiptoes inside, hoping to make it to her bedroom unnoticed. But in the living room, she sees her father, still awake in his easy chair, tapping his feet, arms crossed, face scowling. Message received.

Savvy communicators know that it isn't just what you say but *how* you say it that matters. Nonverbal cues such as posture, gestures, eye contact, and even touch help us broadcast our thoughts, whether we realize it or not. This is known as **nonverbal communication,** sometimes called *body language*. If a friend has a glazed-over look in her eyes or is yawning while you are talking, that body language can communicate that she is bored. A person with upright posture and good eye contact conveys confidence, whereas someone who is hunched over and whose eyes dart back and forth communicates nervousness and discomfort. Crossed arms can convey defensiveness—or simply that someone is cold. The ability to ensure that your body language is in tune with what you intend to say is a key characteristic of an effective communicator.

> *"In order to be truly close to another person, however, we need to occasionally let down our guard and speak freely and honestly about what is on our minds."*

Being a Good Listener

Listening is an integral part of successful communication. Although it might seem like a simple skill, good listening actually requires concentration, focus, and attentiveness. Some strategies for effective listening include:

- **Be silent while another person is sharing his or her feelings or concerns.** Speak up only when you have a question or want to summarize what you have heard.
- **Empathize with what the other person is saying.** If you put yourself in the other person's shoes, you will gain a better idea of his or her viewpoint.
- **Try to set aside any anger or resentment you may be feeling.** These emotions can interfere with your ability to truly listen.
- **Make other people feel comfortable speaking to you.** This can be done by maintaining eye contact, keeping a relaxed posture, and nodding and smiling so that others know you are listening.
- **Give the speaker your undivided attention.** Get rid of any distractions. Close the door and turn off your cell phone.

Resolving Conflicts

Put any relationship under a microscope, and you will see conflicts arise. Conflict is a normal part of relationships because people have different needs, viewpoints, interests, and backgrounds. However, not everyone handles conflicts in the same way. Some people actively avoid discussing their concerns or annoyances, believing that it is better to keep the peace than start what could become an ongoing feud. This communication style is commonly referred to as **conflict avoidance.** Others prefer to be more direct and confrontational and have no problem making it clear when they are unhappy with a situation.

The most effective way to resolve conflict is for two people to voice their concerns maturely and engage in constructive criticism rather than resort to name calling and finger pointing. Settling disagreements, of course, is not always easy. **Conflict resolution** is an acquired skill. To avoid **conflict escalation,** the opposing parties should agree to fight

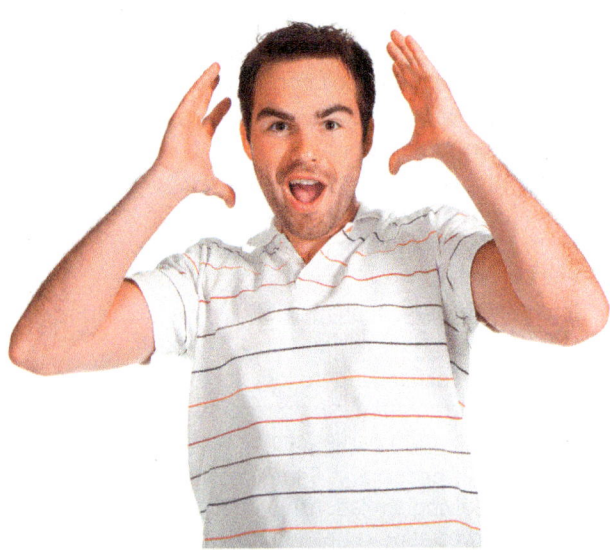

Body language can communicate a lot of information. Do you think this person is relaxed or surprised?

> **nonverbal communication** Communication that is conveyed by body language.
>
> **conflict avoidance** The active avoidance of discussing concerns, annoyances, and conflict with another person.
>
> **conflict resolution** Resolving a conflict in a manner that both people can accept and that minimizes future occurrences of the conflict.
>
> **conflict escalation** Increasing conflict to a more confrontational, painful, or otherwise less comfortable level.

236 CHAPTER 10 ■ Social Relationships and Communication

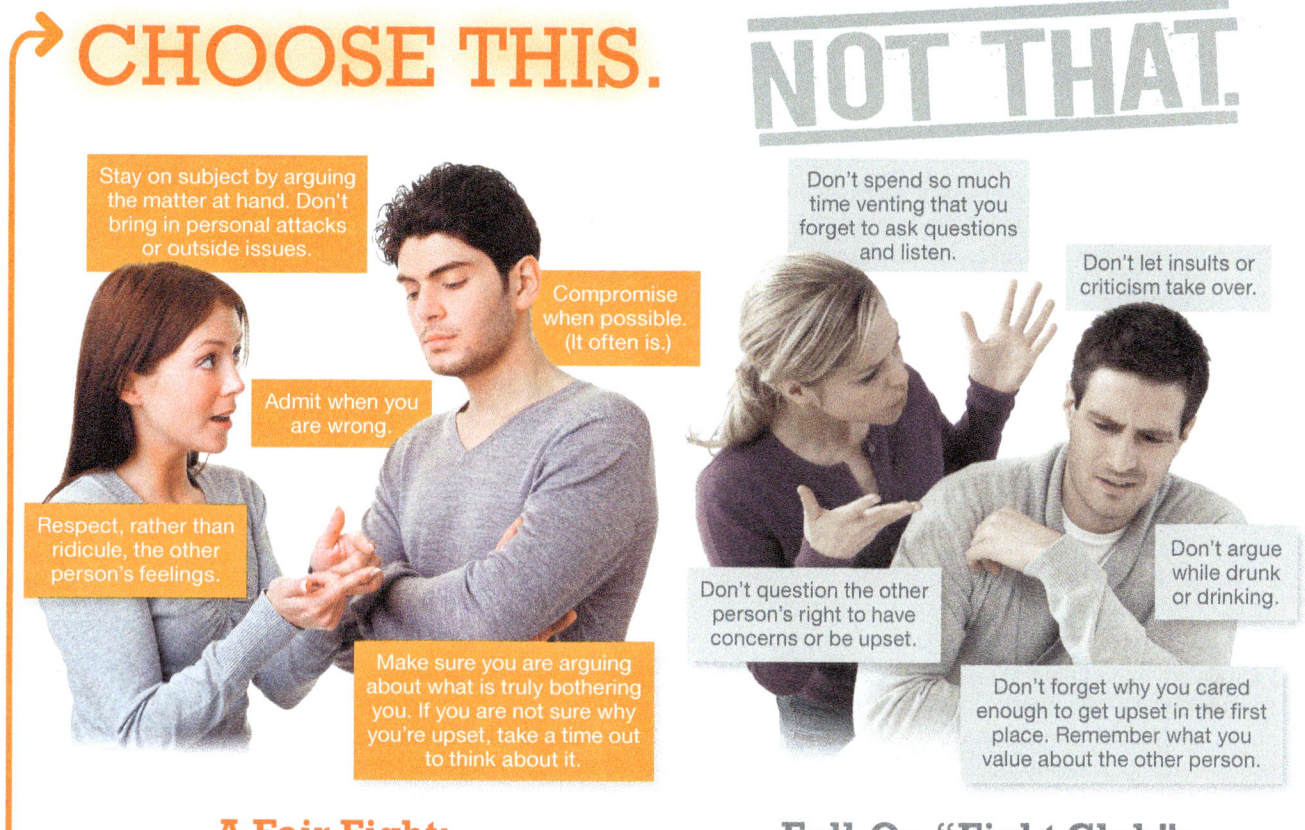

When you want to resolve a conflict, you can find common ground productively or make the problem worse. To settle conflicts in a healthy way:

CHOOSE THIS.

- Stay on subject by arguing the matter at hand. Don't bring in personal attacks or outside issues.
- Compromise when possible. (It often is.)
- Admit when you are wrong.
- Respect, rather than ridicule, the other person's feelings.
- Make sure you are arguing about what is truly bothering you. If you are not sure why you're upset, take a time out to think about it.

A Fair Fight:
When you are feeling frustrated or angry with someone, it's easy to go on the offensive. But doing so will just breed more anger. Instead, try these tactics.

NOT THAT.

- Don't spend so much time venting that you forget to ask questions and listen.
- Don't let insults or criticism take over.
- Don't question the other person's right to have concerns or be upset.
- Don't argue while drunk or drinking.
- Don't forget why you cared enough to get upset in the first place. Remember what you value about the other person.

Full-On "Fight Club":
Do you argue to improve your relationships or to prove you are right? Set some ground rules when you fight and don't use fights as an excuse to be mean or hurtful.

---

fair, be respectful, and stay away from personal attacks and put-downs.

Strategies for effective conflict resolution include:[2]

- Acknowledge that a conflict exists. Don't ignore the problem, even if it feels hard to address it.
- Strive to resolve conflict rather than to "win."
- Voice your frustrations as soon as possible rather than allowing them to build up.
- Approach the conflict as you would any other problem that needs to be solved: Define the problem, express the facts (and your feelings) regarding the problem, identify what needs to be resolved, and listen to possible solutions. You should evaluate each possible solution, agree on one, and make specific plans on how and when to implement it. After a solution is adopted, evaluate it. Is everyone satisfied with the outcome, or would another solution work better?
- Communicate your concerns and opinions clearly, honestly, and directly instead of expecting the other person to read your mind.
- Listen to the other person's feedback and summarize what you think he or she has said.
- Postpone a discussion to an agreed-upon time if one person is tired or not ready to work on the problem.
- Strive to "fight fair" rather than seeking a quick win by embarrassing the other person. For suggestions, see the **Choose This, Not That** feature above.
- Decide how you'll evaluate the outcome of the conflict and whether all sides agree that the initial solution is working. If the initial solution isn't working, discuss what steps can be taken to resolve the conflict.

Gender Roles and Communication

Although both men and women share a common need to communicate information, thoughts, and feelings, research reveals that there are often differences in how they go about it. One of the most fundamental differences is the motivation, or driving force, behind a man's communication and a woman's communication. Men are more likely to communicate in order to perform tasks and seek social status; women are more likely to communicate to build personal connections and seek social interactions.[3] Although individuals vary, researchers have found that in general:

- Women seek to connect to others in conversation; men want to be independent information givers.
- Women often want to build consensus before making a decision; men prefer to make decisions expediently on their own.
- Women attempt to minimize differences; men may prefer giving orders and pointing out areas of superiority.[4]

There are also gender differences in overall communication style. In general, these include the following:

- Men speak significantly fewer words each day than women, probably because men like to get to the bottom line and women like to build connections and share details.
- Women process their problems out loud. They often use conversation to think through a problem and work toward a solution. In contrast, men often think through a problem silently and then verbalize their solution.
- Men are more likely to speak bluntly and state requests directly. Women are more likely to be tactful, use indirect speech, listen, and offer feedback or make requests.
- Women are more likely to use "circular" speech and may change the topic in the middle of a conversation, returning to it later to weave multiple topics together. Men are more likely to be linear communicators and thinkers; they want to finish one topic before going on to another.[5]
- Women are more frequent users of digital communication tools and prefer directly interactive media that more immediately build connections and relationships, such as text messaging or online video calls, to technologies that are less immediately interactive, such as leaving a post in an online forum.[3]

Neither communication style is better or worse; they're just different. And understanding the differences can improve male–female communication and relationships.

LO 10.1 QUICK CHECK

Which of the following is an example of nonverbal communication?

a. communicating by texting with a friend
b. crossing arms and gazing at the floor during a conversation
c. holding a business discussion using video conferencing
d. none of the above

Developing Relationships

LO 10.2 Understand how self-perception, early relationships, and gender roles influence relationships.

Most of us are social creatures from the time we are born, craving closeness and connections to others. And whether we are at home, school, or work, we spend much of our time in the presence of other people. Several personal factors influence how we develop relationships with others, including our self-perception, our early relationships, and cultural gender roles.

Self-Perception

How we relate to others depends, in part, on how good we feel about ourselves—our self-concept. As discussed in Chapter 2, self-esteem is a sense of positive self-regard that results in elevated levels of self-respect, self-worth, self-confidence, and self-satisfaction. People with low self-esteem are more likely to feel lonely and socially isolated. They tend to be preoccupied with the thought of rejection and often behave agreeably toward others because they want to be liked.[6] One psychology professor found that college students with low self-esteem often blame themselves for a boyfriend's or girlfriend's unhappiness, even when other factors are clearly responsible.[6] The finding is true not only of young lovers but of couples in long-term relationships. Researchers have found that even after a decade of marriage, people with low self-esteem misread subtle cues and believe their partners love them far less than they actually do.[7]

Early Relationships

The first relationship we ever experience is the family relationship. Early experiences with our families are important because they help form the template for all subsequent relationships we experience in our lives. Some experts theorize that our relationships with others are patterned after the attachment we had with parents and other caregivers when we were children, a concept known as **attachment theory**.[8] These early interactions may shape our expectations of adult relationships and be responsible for the individual differences in relationship behaviors and needs.[9]

> **attachment theory** The theory that the patterns of attachment in our earliest relationships with others form the template for attachment in later relationships.
>
> **gender roles** Behaviors and tasks society considers appropriate for men and for women.

Exactly what constitutes a "family" changes over time, but it is generally defined as a domestic group of people with some degree of kinship, be it through marriage, blood, or adoption. Families today take many different forms, including households headed by single parents, blended families with stepparents and stepsiblings, extended family households with relatives or family friends all living under the same roof, foster families, and gay and lesbian partnerships, to name just a few. There is no perfect or "right" kind of family, but in a healthy family environment, children are respected and nurtured and learn how to have strong relationships of their own.

Gender Roles

Gender roles are the behaviors and tasks society considers appropriate for men and for women. Just as many girls are trained at an early age to play with dolls and stuffed animals, boys are encouraged to appreciate cars and trains and to emulate seemingly all-powerful "superheroes." As we grow up, some experts think that beginning in adolescence, girls' tendencies to place greater value on interpersonal connections than boys do can leave girls more vulnerable to depression and lower self-esteem.[10] In other words, while relationships are important, keeping them in perspective provides a more healthful balance.

Gender roles often extend into adulthood. However, we live in a time of changing gender roles. A generation ago, men were traditionally expected to work and support the family, while women were encouraged to stay home to raise the children. Today, many women opt to juggle both family and career, whereas some men make the decision to be stay-at-home fathers. Yet attitudes and stereotypes about gender roles remain. In addition, some research has shown that traditional gender roles become more pronounced in married couples after the birth of a child.[11]

LO 10.2 QUICK CHECK

Attachment theory relates to which of the following?
a. attachments people have to material possessions
b. connections to friends made online and the strengths of these connections
c. attachments to parents and other caregivers during childhood
d. none of the above

Friendships

LO 10.3 Identify the benefits of healthy long-term friendships.

Do you have a BFF? If so, being a "best friend forever" benefits you both in many ways. Besides providing someone to hang out with and confide in, friendships can be important for good health.[12] For example, a study of teenagers found that those who had a circle of friends in high school, rather than just one or two friends, enjoyed better health and lower health-care costs over the next five years after graduation.[13] The quality of that social support matters: It must provide a sense of belonging and also help people to be more competent and feel more capable.

Friendships may be more complex and less immediate today. One landmark study found that between 1985 and 2004, the number of Americans who felt that they have someone to discuss important matters with dropped by almost one-third. The study also found that the percentage of people who spoke about important matters only with family members jumped from 57% to 80%.[14] Other research, however, adds perspective to those findings, saying that friendships are shifting under the influences of technology, with weaker virtual friendships sometimes becoming more accessible than in-person contact.

In one recent survey, more than half of American teens said that they had made at least one new friend entirely online.[15] The changing nature of friendship doesn't make it any less important; however, loneliness can harm your health. One study showed that college students with lower levels of social support were more likely to experience mental health problems, including a sixfold risk of depressive symptoms.[16] Loneliness is also associated with stress and poor life satisfaction (see Chapter 2).[14]

Maintaining Old Friendships

Friendships can be some of the longest, most fulfilling relationships in your life, outlasting romantic relationships and even marriages. But the demands of being a student can make it hard to keep up with older friendships. If you are

---

STUDENT STORY

A New BFF

"HI, I'M BRITTANY, AND THIS IS MY FRIEND SANDY. We're both freshmen and we've been friends for about a semester now, ever since we became neighbors in our dorm. We started eating dinner together occasionally and then began hanging out more and more often. We like the same music, we study together, go to the gym, and just hang out and have fun. Recently both of my parents were laid off, and Sandy has been really great in helping me deal with it; she listens to me talk, and I feel like she's really there for me. In a few weeks, a group of us are going to Florida for spring break, and next year, we're even going to get an apartment together. I thought it was going to be difficult making friends in college but I'm so glad I've found such a good one already!"

What Do You Think?

1. What are the benefits of Brittany and Sandy's friendship? What personal and environmental factors helped make them friends?
2. Why do you think Brittany confided in Sandy about her parents being laid off? How did Sandy help?
3. What can Brittany and Sandy do to make sure that they have a good living situation when they move in together next year?

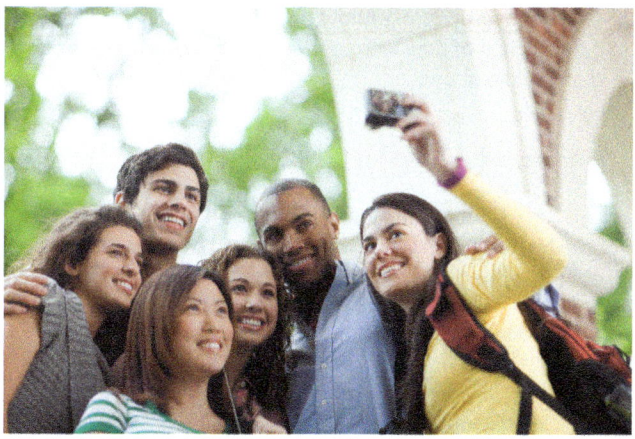

Friendships can boost emotional and physical health.

> *"Friendships can be some of the longest, most fulfilling relationships in your life, outlasting romantic relationships and even marriages."*

struggling with maintaining your tried-and-true relationships now that you're in college, consider these tips:

- **Understand that you and your friends are changing.** Don't be afraid to show how you're changing and don't expect your friends to stay exactly the same, either.
- **Don't overwhelm old friends with information about your college life.** It's exciting to fill in your friends with what you are doing now but be sure to listen to their stories as well.
- **Keep in touch.** Phone, email, video chat services like Skype, instant messaging, and social networking applications like Facebook and Twitter are all great ways to update your friends about what you're doing and to hear about them. However, if you really want to maintain a friendship with someone, take the time to send him or her a personal message or pick up the phone.
- **Don't be afraid to reconnect.** If you've lost touch with an old friend, research indicates that you can still rekindle the friendship even after years without contact.[17]

›› Listen to this National Public Radio story on college friendships: www.npr.org/templates/story/story.php?storyId=112330125.

›› These videos explore the effects of social networking: www.pbs.org/wgbh/pages/frontline/digitalnation/relationships/socializing.

LO 10.3 QUICK CHECK

Strong friendships can outlast which of the following?
a. romantic relationships—even marriage
b. extended periods without any contact
c. stretches of time with only online or phone contact
d. all of the above

Intimate Relationships

LO 10.4 Discuss different forms of intimate relationships and Sternberg's Triangular Theory of Love.

intimacy A sense of closeness with another person formed by being emotionally open and caring.

Intimacy is the emotionally open and caring way of relating to another person. An intimate relationship is usually one that is deep and has evolved over time, in which two people feel safe and comfortable sharing their innermost thoughts and secrets.

Sternberg's Triangular Theory of Love

Psychologist Robert Sternberg theorized that there are three primary components of healthy, loving relationships:

- **Intimacy.** The emotional component, intimacy is the feeling of closeness and connectedness experienced in loving relationships.
- **Passion.** The motivational component, passion is the intensity that fuels romance, physical attraction, and sex.
- **Commitment.** The cognitive component, commitment is the short-term decision to love another person and the long-term decision to stay committed to maintaining that love.[18]

Sternberg used the shape of a triangle to illustrate his theory, which he called the Triangular Theory of Love **(Figure 10.1)**. Sternberg postulated that the type and intensity of love a couple experiences depends on the strength of each of the three components in their relationship. The factors can be combined to characterize seven different types of love:

- **Liking.** Liking is intimacy alone. It is a closeness to another person, without passionate feelings or a long-term commitment.
- **Infatuation.** Infatuation is passion alone, also known as "love at first sight."
- **Empty love.** Empty love is commitment alone. The passion is not there, and neither is the intimacy. Empty love is present in some stagnant relationships or just before a couple breaks up.
- **Romantic love.** Romantic love is passion and intimacy without commitment, physical attraction with an emotional bond.
- **Companionate love.** Companionate love is commitment and intimacy without passion. It is essentially a

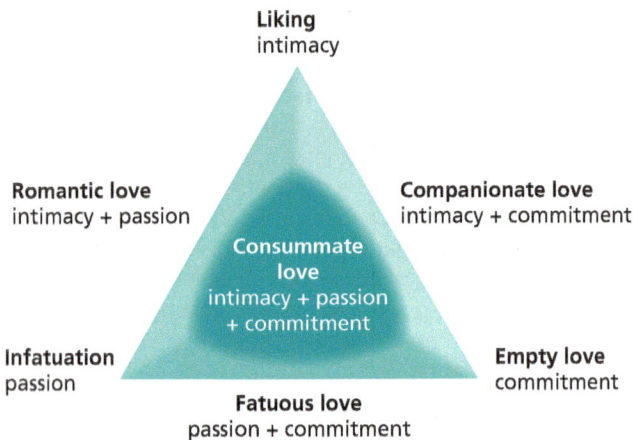

FIGURE 10.1 Sternberg's Triangular Theory of Love.
Source: Sternberg, R. J. (1986). "A Triangular Theory of Love." *Psychological Review, 93*(2), 119–135. Reprinted with permission.

SPECIAL FEATURE

Social Media, Communication, and Cyber-Bullies

On February 4, 2004, Harvard computer science student Mark Zuckerberg launched "Thefacebook" and forever changed the world of social connections—and sometimes, unfortunately, social torment.[1]

Originally used only by Harvard students, Facebook and other social networking sites and apps have become almost essential tools for socializing in our modern world. Despite lots of competition from Twitter, Google Plus, YouTube, and Pinterest, Facebook (together with its subsidiary Instagram) is still the leading social networking site, with more than 1 billion active users throughout the world every day.[2] One study of college students found that Facebook made a meaningful difference in maintaining connections in a geographically mobile world, such as letting students stay close to friends from high school who are now going to school elsewhere.[3]

Despite the popularity of Facebook and other social media, they are not without critics. Privacy proponents worry that members' information is too easily accessed by those with both personal and business motives. Social critics say that real-world connections are being neglected for less meaningful ones online. On campuses, professors complain that students are wasting a tremendous amount of time on digital interactions and that they are distracted in class. Professors at some U.S. colleges have even banned laptops and mobile devices from classrooms because of social media such as Facebook.[4]

Using Social Media in a Healthy Way

Regardless of criticisms, social media such as Facebook is here to stay. You can communicate through social media in a healthy way by following a few tips:[5]

- **Limit your number of friends.** Limit your friends list to those you really care about or use available tools to create a circle of truly close contacts with whom you can maintain meaningful connections.
- **Don't tag friends in unflattering photos.** If you aren't sure, don't tag it.
- **Manage your profile and privacy settings.** You may not want your boss or professor seeing your photos from last weekend. So if you have both personal and professional "friends," make sure you know how to use the custom settings to control what specific people can see. Policies in regard to profile and privacy settings often change, so stay on top of how your information can be used and shared.
- **Think before you post.** Don't post anything you wouldn't say in real life or don't want the entire Internet to read.
- **Don't list personal info.** Never post your address, phone number, class schedule, or any other personal information that you don't want thousands of people to know.
- **Limit the amount of time you spend on social media.** Because information is updated constantly on social media, it can become addicting. Try ignoring your virtual friends for a while and spending some face-to-face time with your real live friends.

Confronting Cyber-Bullying

Sometimes, unfortunately, social media is far from friendly. Outlets such as Facebook, along with technologies like texting, have been used to facilitate *cyber-bullying*. This type of harassment, defined as repeated, deliberate harm inflicted through digital platforms and electronic devices, is meant to inflict embarrassment and emotional pain, sometimes with tragic results. About 20% of 11- to 18-year-olds admit to harassing others in this manner.[6] One study of college students found that about 22% said they had been victims of cyber-bullying.[7] In high-profile cases around the country, teens and young adults have been victims of assaults related to cyber-bullying, and some victims have even committed suicide.[8,9]

If cyber-bullying is affecting you or someone you know, a few quick actions can help confront the problem:[10]

- **Call out the bullying for what it is.** Don't ignore the problem, which only encourages further harassment. Acknowledge the issue as something serious and harmful and take it seriously.
- **Don't be a bystander.** Whether in person or online, bullies often seek an audience. Don't stand by and watch. Let the bully know that the harassment is not acceptable and take steps to help the victim feel supported and safe.
- **Think before you post.** Online situations can easily escalate with a simple click. Rather than going for an easy laugh at someone else's expense, think about what you are about to say. Would you want someone to say it about you or post a similar photo of you?
- **Model how to treat others with respect.** By avoiding bullying behavior and calling out others who engage in it, you help create online spaces that are safer—and more fun—for everyone.

▶▶ Visit Facebook's anti-bullying page at the Facebook Help Center: **www.facebook.com/help** and searching for "Bullying."

References: **1.** Tabak, A. (2004, February). Hundreds register for new Facebook website. *Harvard Crimson*. www.thecrimson.com. **2.** Facebook Newsroom. (2016). *Company info: Stats*. http://newsroom.fb.com. **3.** Luther, J. (2012, January 26). Laptop bans in classes receive mixed reaction. *The Chronicle*. www.dukechronicle.com. **4.** Manago, A., Taylor, T., & Greenfield, P. M. (2012). Me and my 400 friends: The anatomy of college students' Facebook networks, their communication patterns, and well-being. *Developmental Psychology, 48*(2), 369–380. **5.** O'Halloran, D. (2015, March 11). *The complete guide to Facebook privacy settings*. www.techlicious.com. **6.** Patchin, J. W., & Hinduja, S. (2012). School-based efforts to prevent cyberbullying. *The Prevention Researcher, 19*(1), 7–9. **7.** Indiana State University. (2011). *Bullying still occurs in college, professors find*. www.indstate.edu. **8.** Oppel, R. (2013, March 17). *Ohio teenagers guilty in rape that social media brought to light*. www.nytimes.com. **9.** Hughes, M. (2012, May 21). Rutgers suicide: Man who filmed gay roommate sentenced to 30 days. *The Guardian*, www.telegraph.co.uk. **10.** U.S. Department of Health and Human Services. (n.d.). *Respond to bullying*. www.stopbullying.gov.

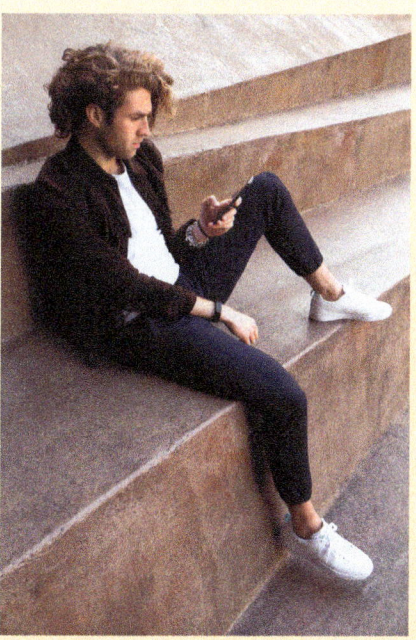

STUDENT STORY

Talk it Out

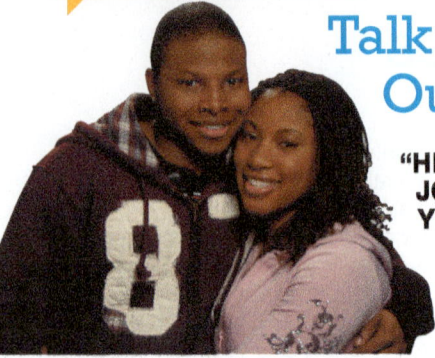

"HI, WE'RE JONATHAN AND YEANI, and we've been a couple for six months. There are a lot of obstacles that we face in our relationship, especially when it comes to juggling our schoolwork in addition to all the other aspects of our lives. At times, things seem hard. We each get stressed out by school and we can get on each other's nerves, but it's nice to have someone to lean on, and to know that you don't have to go through all your problems alone. For us, communication and trust have really helped make our relationship successful. Our best advice to new couples trying to make things work in college is to be open with one another and don't be afraid to express your concerns, doubts, fears, or any other emotions with your partner."

What Do You Think?
1. Do you think juggling a relationship with school is a common source of stress for college couples? What can you do to help balance school and relationship time?
2. Why do you think Jonathan and Yeani chose to be in a relationship rather than just hook up?
3. Do you agree with their advice for new couples in college? What else do you think college couples should do to keep their relationship healthy?

---

committed friendship in which the passion has died down, as sometimes occurs in people who have been married a long time.
- **Fatuous love.** Fatuous love is commitment and passion without intimacy, a whirlwind romance that often does not last very long.
- **Consummate love.** Consummate love is the whole package: intimacy, passion, and commitment. It is the kind of love many of us strive for.[18]

Sternberg also identified an eighth category—nonlove—which is the absence of intimacy, passion, and commitment. This type of casual interaction makes up the majority of our relationships with other people.

What Causes Attraction?

You have probably heard the saying "opposites attract," but scientists have found this to be untrue. Studying the factors that bring two people together for a romantic relationship reveals that we tend to pick partners who are a lot like ourselves—who are of similar economic class, educational level, religion, and racial or ethnic group and who share the same interests or values. This tendency to be attracted to people who share some of our characteristics is known as **assortative mating.** Some studies have also found that we look for people who share a similar level of physical attractiveness to us, with more attractive people being more particular about the physical attractiveness of their potential partners.[19]

> **assortative mating** The tendency to be attracted to people who are similar to ourselves.

Beauty, of course, is more than skin deep. Who we are and how we behave also influence whether others are attracted to us. One study found that men and women who were honest or helpful were perceived as better looking. Those who were rude or unfair or displayed other negative traits were generally considered to be less attractive.[20]

Although similarities in physique may bring us together, it is similarity in personality—and a generous attitude toward one's partner—that appears to be most indicative of whether the relationship will be a happy and lasting one.[21] Why? In one study, researchers found that when they asked members of couples to both describe their own personality traits and their partner's, it was those couples who described each other more generously than they described themselves who also had the highest levels of marital satisfaction.[21] In other words, not only sharing personality traits but seeing those positive traits magnified in one's partner appears to build enduring bonds.

Dating

Dating—that is, spending time with another person one-on-one to determine whether there is an attraction or a desire to see more of one another—has evolved over the years. In earlier generations, men would typically ask women out on a formal date, and steady dating would be considered a "courtship" intended to lead to marriage. But that linear path has been replaced by a less direct one, in which couples often meet through friends and get to know each other in groups or by spending time together more casually. If the relationship progresses, many young couples often live together before marriage.[22] A formal date is often now viewed as "the old way," or an event saved for special occasions.

Hooking Up

On campus, the concept of dating has largely been replaced with *hooking up*—casual, noncommittal physical encounters that may range from "making out" to oral sex or intercourse. "Hooking up on college campuses has become more frequent than dating in heterosexual sexual interaction," noted one study.[23] However, while hooking up may be common, it does not mean that it is popular with everyone. The same study found that men prefer this type of interaction, but women tend to prefer dating. Another study found that hooking up is more common in the first two years of college and then appears to become less common, especially among female students.[24]

Many students have had negative experiences. Because hooking up is often fueled by alcohol, your judgment during such an encounter can be impaired. Some of the negative effects from hooking up include negative impact on psychological well-being and social status; regrets; decreased relationship skills; and sexual risk taking, including an increased likelihood of sexually transmitted infections (STIs) and unplanned pregnancy.[25,26] Some relationship and mental health experts are also concerned that hooking up doesn't help today's singles learn the skills needed to build intimacy and test out whether someone would be a good long-term or marriage partner.

Online Dating

Online dating is now a dating mainstay, especially in the years after college, when life off-campus makes it harder to meet potential partners. Dating services are a booming business. Popular sites such as eHarmony, Match, Tinder, and OkCupid report millions of users each month. These services assist members in finding suitable partners by providing a place where they can both advertise themselves online with a personal profile and view the profiles of others looking for partners. Members search profiles using criteria such as sex, age, location, and interests. Online dating easily and effectively increases the pool of potential partners. Also, because face-to-face meetings are not immediate, potential partners have the opportunity to build their relationships via phone calls, texting, email, and other technology before having a face-to-face encounter.

It's important to remember that online dates are basically strangers. So in order to stay safe while using an online dating service, keep these precautions in mind:

- Never give out your full name, address, or other personal information until you have met the person and are sure he or she is trustworthy.
- Make sure to meet your date in a public place, like a restaurant or café. Avoid going to isolated places with a new date and don't arrange to meet at your home. Always tell a friend beforehand what you are doing and where you are going.
- If something doesn't feel right when you meet the person, don't be afraid to cut your date short.

Same-Sex Relationships

As many as 9 million people in the United States identify as lesbian, gay, bisexual, transgender, queer or questioning, or intersex (LGBTQI).[27] Researchers estimate that about 3% of college students are gay or lesbian, although they caution that obtaining exact numbers is difficult because some students may not feel comfortable sharing information about their sexual orientation.[28] Some LGBT students may prefer not to disclose their sexual orientation until they are a few years into their college experience. One survey of LGBT Americans found that the median age for "coming out" to friends and/or family is 20 years old.[29]

In many ways, committed **homosexual** couples are similar to committed **heterosexual,** or straight, couples.[30] Studies conclude that long-term same-sex couples are just as committed and satisfied in their relationships as heterosexual married couples.[30,31] In at least one study, same-sex couples reported more positive feelings toward their partners and less conflict than married straight couples.[31] Indeed, same-sex couples often have more egalitarian or equal relationships because they do not subscribe to traditional gender roles. If there is a major difference, it is seen in lesbian couples, whom scientists have found are "especially effective at working together harmoniously."[31]

>> Online support for students seeking to better understand and communicate their sexual identity can be found by going to www.hrc.org and searching for "Coming Out," or by going to www.glsen.org.

One striking difference for LGBTQI couples is the disapproval and discrimination that same-sex couples often face from society and sometimes even from family members. Prior to a 2015 U.S. Supreme Court ruling, in some states, homosexual couples could not legally marry or adopt children, and some religions frown upon homosexuality. Such discrimination lead homosexual couples to feel stigmatized, isolated, and powerless. Societal attitudes and pressures against homosexuality, including **homonegativity**—unfavorable views of a person because he or she is, or is perceived to be, homosexual—or **homophobia**—a fear and hatred of homosexuality—can also discourage intimacy between same-sex friends if it makes them fear being labeled gay or lesbian.[32] Chapter 11 discusses issues related to homosexuality in more detail.

> **homosexual** A person who is sexually attracted to someone of the same sex.
>
> **heterosexual** A person who is sexually attracted to someone of the opposite sex.
>
> **homonegativity** Unfavorable views of those who are or are perceived to be homosexual.
>
> **homophobia** Fear and hatred of homosexuality.

Healthy Relationships

Successful relationships are built on trust, respect, and communication. They enable each individual to retain his or her own identity and foster personal growth rather than smother it.

Some people have an idealized view of healthy relationships, believing that they are free of conflict and require little effort to maintain. However, no deep, intimate relationship is without challenges. Well-adjusted couples learn how to steer clear of avoidable problems and to be respectful, supportive, and sensitive to each other's feelings. With cooperation and compromise, as well as a commitment to work together, couples can help each other through some of the most trying times of life—the loss of a job, the death of a parent or child, or the onset of a chronic, debilitating disease. The **Practical Strategies** box on page 244 provides tips for maintaining a strong and healthy relationship.

How do you know if your intimate relationship is a healthy one? Are you at a point in your relationship where the negatives are outweighing the positives? Taking a step back and assessing the strength of your relationship with a boyfriend, girlfriend, or partner can be illuminating (see the **Self-Assessment**).

⚙ PRACTICAL Strategies

Tips for Maintaining a Strong Relationship

Although there is no simple recipe for success, the following strategies can help you maintain a strong, healthy relationship with your boyfriend, girlfriend, spouse, or partner:

- **Be honest with the other person.** Strive to maintain a warm, comfortable relationship in which you can confide in each other about virtually anything.
- **Trust and respect each other.** Be able to disagree without using put-downs or threats. Try to understand the other person's feelings, even if you don't share his or her ideas.
- **Communicate effectively.** Ask how your loved one thinks and feels rather than expecting him or her to be a mind reader. Share your own thoughts and offer empathy when needed.
- **Give your loved one freedom and encouragement.** Recognize that each person has the right to his or her own opinions, feelings, friends, and dreams. Encourage each other's enjoyment and success in life.
- **Encourage common interests and shared activities.** Engage in activities and hobbies you both like, including new ones. Discovering and learning new things together builds bonds and helps keep your relationship fresh.
- **Be kind to one another.** Help each other out and show care through consistent respect rather than abuse followed by apologies.
- **Be appreciative.** Remind yourself of all the good things that you admire about your loved one.
- **Be attentive, every day.** Each morning, try asking yourself, "What can I do for five minutes today to make my partner's life better?"
- **Share decision making.** Make decisions together rather than tell each other what to do.[1,2]

References: **1.** Employee Assistance. (n.d.). *Characteristics of a healthy and enjoyable friendship or dating relationship.* www.eap.partners.org. (Originally from Liz Claiborne, Inc.) **2.** Brody, J. (2013, January 14). *That loving feeling takes a lot of work.* http://well.blogs.nytimes.com.

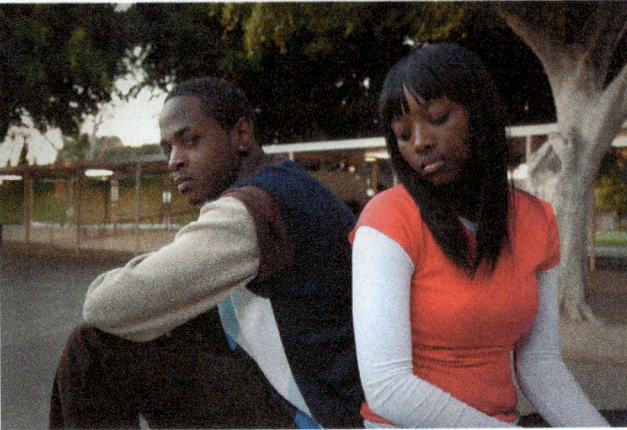

Addressing problems in relationships can help you fix them.

Dysfunctional Relationships

While some relationships are uplifting, others are toxic, becoming more of a burden than a joy. Dysfunctional relationships can come in many forms, with one or both partners being manipulative, controlling, mean, disrespectful, or even verbally or physically abusive. This kind of negative behavior is often learned in the home at an early age. Children observe how their parents relate to each other and may think the hostile or unhealthy ways they interact are normal. Research has shown that adolescents who witnessed their parents' marital violence were more likely to be physically aggressive toward romantic partners themselves.[33] Similarly, adolescents exposed to marital discord may later show symptoms of posttraumatic stress disorder (PTSD) and tend to have conflict in their own marriages many years later.[34]

Often, the signs that a relationship is dysfunctional or somehow amiss are subtle:[35]

- You focus on the other person at the expense of yourself.
- You feel pressured to change to meet your partner's ideals.
- Your partner expects you to justify what you do and whom you see, or you expect your partner to do so.
- One of you makes all the decisions without listening to the other's input.
- You are afraid to disagree, and your ideas are criticized.
- You lie to each other.
- You feel stifled and trapped, unable to escape the pressures of the relationship.
- You or your partner is addicted to drugs or alcohol, and it impacts your relationship.

If you have noticed any of these signs in your relationship, it may be time to think about whether it is indeed a good match for you.

Another problem that can damage relationships is **jealousy**, a response to a threat to a relationship from an actual or imagined rival for a partner's attention.[36] Although it is natural to feel jealous once in a while, jealousy becomes serious when it is a precursor to domestic violence or interferes with

jealousy A response to a threat to a relationship from an actual or imagined rival for a partner's attention.

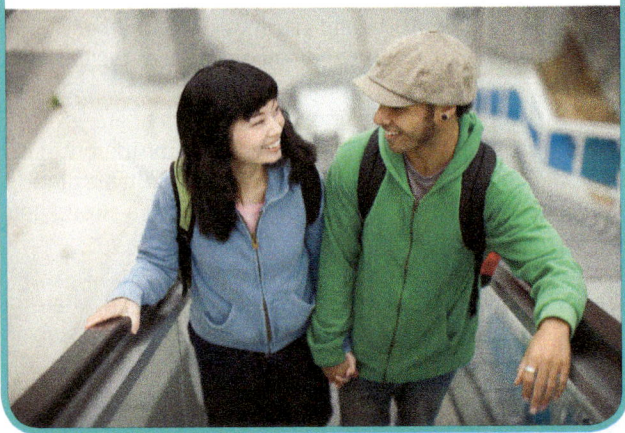

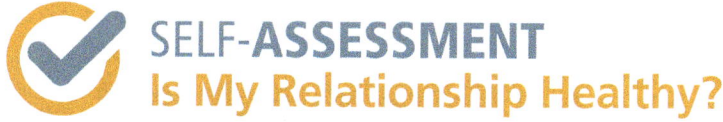

SELF-ASSESSMENT
Is My Relationship Healthy?

Check "Yes" or "No" in response to each of the following questions.

1. I am very satisfied with how we talk to each other. _____ Yes _____ No
2. We are creative in how we handle our differences. _____ Yes _____ No
3. We feel very close to each other. _____ Yes _____ No
4. My partner is seldom too controlling. _____ Yes _____ No
5. When discussing problems, my partner understands my opinions and ideas. _____ Yes _____ No
6. I am completely satisfied with the amount of affection from my partner. _____ Yes _____ No
7. We have a good balance of leisure time spent together and separately. _____ Yes _____ No
8. My partner's friends or family members rarely interfere with our relationship. _____ Yes _____ No
9. We agree on how to spend money. _____ Yes _____ No
10. I am satisfied with how we express spiritual values and beliefs. _____ Yes _____ No

HOW TO INTERPRET YOUR SCORE The more "Yes" answers you checked, the more likely you are to be part of a happy couple.

To complete this Self-Assessment online, visit **MasteringHealth**™

Source: Adapted from Olson, D. H., & Olson, A. K. (2000). *Empowering couples: Building on your strengths.* Copyright © 2000 by Prepare-Enrich/Life Innovations, Inc., Minneapolis, MN. Reprinted with permission.

---

the relationship in other ways. Jealousy is associated with low self-esteem, irrational thinking, depression, divorce, and physical violence. It is not a marker of true love but rather of insecurity, immaturity, and a need to be in control. An underlying cause of extreme jealousy is a fear of abandonment. Ironically, the behavior of extremely jealous partners often causes these fears to come true.

Experts suggest that couples deal with jealousy directly and attempt to talk about the feelings underlying it. Often, talking about what sparks the jealousy may be enough to reduce it. A jealous partner can benefit from remembering that uncertainty is part of any relationship; no one can control how another person thinks or feels. If you are suffering from jealousy yourself, work on building your self-esteem because low self-esteem is one of the sources of jealousy. If your partner is jealous, be available and respond to his or her concerns, offer reassurance, and keep in mind that changes do not happen immediately and sometimes counseling may even be needed to help you and your partner move forward.[37]

One situation demands that you immediately leave a relationship: physical abuse. If a partner is threatening you physically or is being physically abusive to you or your children, remove yourself and your children from the relationship as soon as possible. Chapter 15 discusses physical abuse and domestic violence in more detail.

When Relationships End

Despite our best efforts, many relationships eventually end. Those that lead to marriage are still vulnerable to the problems that can eventually result in a split: infidelity, jealousy, competitiveness, illness, money problems, and growing apart.

Breaking up, however, can be difficult, especially if you did not initiate the split. Recovering from a failed relationship takes time and effort. The follow are some strategies that can facilitate the recovery process:[38]

- **Talk about it.** Share your feelings with a good friend or family member.
- **Focus on what is good about you.** Resist the urge to blame yourself and exaggerate your faults while mending a broken heart.
- **Take care of yourself.** Exercise, eat well, and get plenty of sleep.
- **Let your emotions out.** Do not be afraid to cry.
- **Do things you normally enjoy.** Have some fun.
- **Keep yourself busy.** Get your mind off your pain for a while.
- **Give yourself time to recover.** Recognize that your hurt will not go away overnight.

LO 10.4 QUICK CHECK

According to Sternberg's Triangular Theory of Love, passion is which of the following components?
a. motivational
b. cognitive
c. sexual
d. emotional

Committed Relationships

LO 10.5 Describe at least three different types of committed relationships.

Most adults value having a committed relationship with another person. Nationwide surveys reveal that the majority of unmarried adults say they would like to be in a long-term committed relationship such as marriage.[39] Committed relationships come in various forms, including cohabitation, marriage, and domestic partnership.

Cohabitation

One of the greatest transformations in family life in the United States during the past century has been the significant increase in **cohabitation**—unmarried couples living together under the same roof. Many couples today opt to live together before getting engaged or married. Some continue in long-term, committed relationships without ever tying the knot. Cohabitation is now so common and accepted in our society that researchers estimate that more than 60% of couples in the United States now live together before getting married.[40] For some, cohabitation represents a chance to get to know each other better before taking marriage vows. Others choose to cohabit to benefit from the companionship, intimacy, and shared living costs cohabitation allows.

cohabitation Living together in the same household; usually refers to unmarried couples.

There is also a downside to cohabitation. Most cohabiting couples are denied the legal and financial benefits afforded to married couples. These include family leave, Social Security benefits after the death of a partner, and access to a partner's pension, health insurance coverage, and untaxed retirement savings.[41] In addition, cohabiting couples in the United States report the lowest levels of wealth among household types. Their relationships may also be less stable than those of married partners. One study found that nearly 40% of unmarried, cohabiting parents in their 20s who had a baby between 2000 and 2005 split up by the time their child was 5, which is a separation rate three times higher than that for parents in their 20s who were married when they had a child.[42] One theory for these differences is that marriage fosters certain behavior changes by the couple and those around them that cohabitation just doesn't encourage.[43] Recent research is hopeful, however, indicating that these trends may be changing as cohabitation becomes more common and accepted in society. It also shows that cohabiting couples who are engaged before they move in together may be more successful than couples who live together but have no plans to marry.[44]

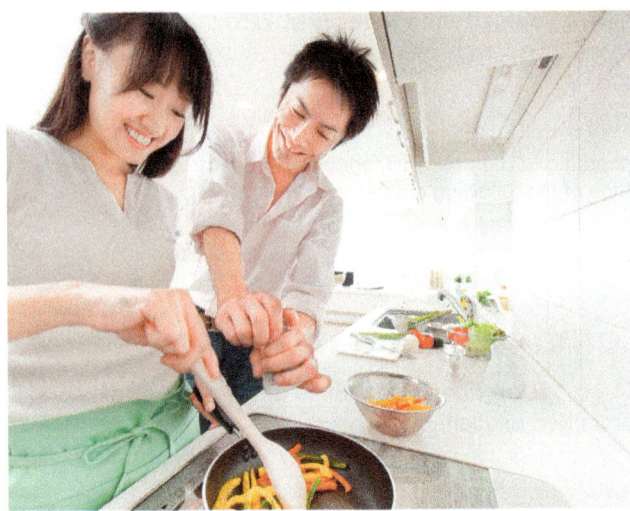

Cohabitation can have benefits, but it also has drawbacks.

> **"** *Study after study has shown that marriages in general—and good marriages in particular—provide a wealth of physical, psychological, and financial benefits.*"

Marriage

About 80% of Americans will marry by age 40.[22] Despite the increasingly casual nature of many of our romantic relationships, marriage remains so valued that it is the focus of a major social struggle: Same-sex couples have waged an intense legal and political battle to have their unions recognized and legalized nationwide, resulting in a significant 2015 decision from the U.S. Supreme Court that overturned state-level bans on same-sex marriage. See the **Diversity & Health** box for more information.

Aside from its romantic associations, marriage has practical implications, benefits, and obligations. It is a legally binding contract, giving a sense of legitimacy to the relationship in the eyes of society and the law.[45] It signals to others that each spouse has entered into a long-term commitment that carries with it expectations of fidelity, mutual support, and lifetime partnership.

Benefits of Marriage

Study after study has shown that marriages in general—and good marriages in particular—provide a wealth of physical, psychological, and financial benefits. The longer a person stays married, in fact, the more the benefits accrue.[45] The benefits include:

- **Better mental health.** Married people tend to be happier and more satisfied with their lives, on average, than unmarried people, according to an analysis of 22 studies.[46]
- **Better physical health and longer life expectancies.** Being married is linked to fewer sick days, less use of hospital facilities, and less likelihood of having chronic health conditions.[46] Married men can expect to live, on average, at least seven years longer than never-married men, whereas married women tend to live at least three years longer than their never-married counterparts.[46]
- **Better financial health.** Married couples tend to have higher household incomes than unmarried people.[41]

Are married people healthier because they are married? Or is it that healthier people are somehow more likely to get married? Although researchers suspect that both could be at play, there is evidence that marriage fosters healthful and helpful behaviors. For example, a study of 3.5 million Americans found that married people have a lower risk of heart disease than those who are single, widowed, or divorced.[47]

DIVERSITY & HEALTH

Same-Sex Marriage: The State of Our Current Debate

In 2015, when the U.S. Supreme Court ruled that no state could ban same-sex marriage, same-sex couples earned the right to marry throughout the country.[1] But as often happens when the law addresses social issues, a legal ruling doesn't mean an end to the debate.

The issue of same-sex marriage can be socially polarizing. Perhaps that's because it exposes differences in our interpretation of certain doctrines we hold "sacred"—from the American ethic of fairness to religious and cultural teachings. For instance, some proponents of same-sex marriage have long argued that the guarantees of equal protection and due process in the U.S. Constitution require that same-sex couples be treated no differently from heterosexual couples. At the same time, opponents argue that marriage is an institution founded to promote and protect the need to procreate and, therefore, should only occur between a male and a female.

What's at stake? Although the debate is certainly fueled by a clash of values, far more significant are the rights that marriage brings. In 2004, a federal report identified a total of 1,138 federal statutory provisions in which marital status is a factor in determining or receiving benefits, rights, and privileges.[2] A couple's status can affect whether they are entitled to certain tax advantages, health-care benefits, community property rights, and rights to surviving children. Moreover, homosexual couples have been denied the right to become foster parents and adoptive parents, to petition for their partners to immigrate, and to become residents in the same nursing home. Until 2011, same-sex partners could even be denied the right to visit each other in the hospital.[3]

Legal protections for same-sex marriages at the federal level are slowly being matched by gradual increases in social acceptance. Dozens of polls conducted over the past decade show that the percentage of Americans who favor legal marriage between homosexual partners is inching upward. Despite generational, political, and regional differences, America's overall support for same-sex marriage is growing.

What Do You Think?

1. Do you think same-sex couples should have the legal right to marry? Why or why not?
2. Prior to the 2015 Supreme Court decision, what were the practical implications for same-sex couples if such marriages were not recognized in their state of residence?
3. Why do you think younger Americans tend to be more supportive of same-sex marriage than older generations?

Sources: **1.** National Conference of State Legislatures. (2015, June 26). Same-sex marriage laws. www.ncsl.org. **2.** U.S. General Accounting Office. (2004, January 23). Defense of Marriage Act: Update to Prior report. GAO-04-353R, Washington, DC. **3.** Smith, A. M. (2010, August 18). Same-sex marriage: Legal issues. Congressional Research Service. http://assets.opencrs.com.

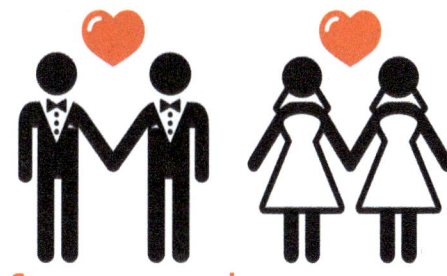

Same-sex marriage continues to be a topic of social debate in the United States.

Separation and Divorce

"Till death do us part" is a phrase that is often included in marriage vows. For about half the couples getting married for the first time, however, the marriage will end not when one person passes away but when one decides to file for divorce.[22] Divorce has become an increasingly common and accepted practice in the United States, as the moral and social stigmas surrounding it have greatly diminished. Divorce rates actually peaked in the early 1980s, and the rate of divorces and annulments has gone down slightly since then; over the past several years they have stabilized at just under 50%.[48]

Researchers attribute the divorce rate to a number of factors, including society's increasingly high expectations for marriage. During the 1950s and early 1960s, surveys of college students demonstrated that marriage was sought after because of the opportunities it afforded couples—namely, the chance to own a home, live a stable lifestyle, and have children. Today, college students say they value marriage because they believe it will provide them with emotional fulfillment.[49]

Risk factors for divorce include a pattern of negative interactions between spouses, having parents who are divorced, marrying younger than age 21, having less education, having lower income, and reacting strongly or defensively to problems and disappointments.[50] For those in really bad marriages, divorce can represent a relief, an end to seemingly never-ending marital woes.[51] For most people, though, divorce results in a crisis that causes severe emotional pain and distress to the entire family. Whereas adults often experience temporary stress and sadness, their children may develop long-term emotional problems that can get worse as they grow older.[52] Children of divorced parents are 50% more likely to get a divorce themselves one day.[53]

There are factors that decrease your risk of divorce. Divorce rates are lowest for people with at least some college education, who have annual incomes over $50,000, who are religious, who have parents who are married, and who wait until age 25 to marry and have children.[41]

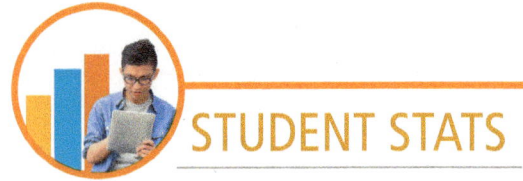

STUDENT STATS
Students and Relationships

Percentage of undergraduates, age 19–23, who are considered someone else's dependent: 85.3%

Percentage of undergraduates, age 19–23, who are considered independent: 14.7%

Among independent students*:

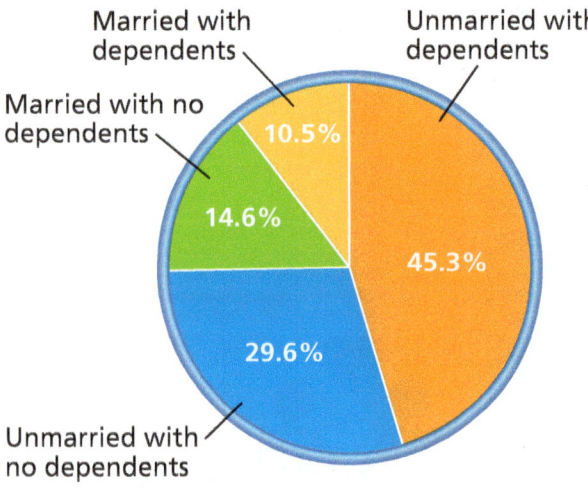

- Married with dependents: 10.5%
- Unmarried with dependents: 45.3%
- Married with no dependents: 14.6%
- Unmarried with no dependents: 29.6%

*Independent students are age 24 or over and students under 24 who are married, have dependents, are veterans or on active duty, are orphans or wards of the courts, are homeless or at risk of homelessness, or were determined to be independent by a financial aid officer using professional judgment. Other undergraduates under age 24 are considered to be dependent.

Data from U.S. Department of Education. (2014). *Profile of undergraduate students, 2011–2012.* http://nces.ed.gov.

Domestic Partnerships

Domestic partnerships, permitted in many states, offer some couples an alternative to marriage. In a domestic partnership, a couple lives together, stays in a long-term committed relationship, and legally registers as domestic partners. In return, they often have access to their partner's employer-sponsored benefits such as health insurance and bereavement leave. Domestic partnerships are also recognized by some states, counties, and cities, in which case they give couples access to other privileges, including the ability to visit a partner in the hospital. Yet the benefits vary widely by location and fall far short of those provided through marriage. In many states, domestic partnerships are open to committed couples—homosexual or heterosexual—who have lived together usually for more than one year.

domestic partnership A legal arrangement in which a couple lives together in a long-term committed relationship and receives some, but not all, of the rights of married couples.

Staying Single

In 1980, the median age at marriage was 22 years for women and 24.7 years for men. Fast-forward 30 years, and the age rose to 25.8 years for women and 28.3 years for men—the oldest in U.S. history.[54] In 2013, one national survey found that about 65% of Americans aged 18 to 34 had never been married.[39] The trend to stay single is occurring in all racial groups in the United States but is most pronounced among younger people who are not Caucasian.[54]

Why are Americans waiting longer to marry or avoiding marriage entirely? Some opt to focus on their education and career. Rising cohabitation rates have also meant that many adults enjoy intimacy and companionship while remaining legally single. Women today are also much more financially independent and less pressured to marry in order to attain economic stability. Attitudes about marriage and childrearing have also changed, with far more couples having children out of wedlock. According to one study, 48% of first births now occur outside marriage.[42]

Singles can, and do, lead very fulfilling lives, enjoying successful careers, close personal friendships, and strong family ties. Some date frequently, others rarely. Some choose to live with a partner long term. Singles are often stereotyped as being alone and lonely, but in reality, they are likely to have networks of important people and friendships that have lasted years beyond many marriages.[55]

LO 10.5 QUICK CHECK

Which of the following describes marriage?
a. a romantic partnership
b. a legally binding contract
c. an emotional partnership
d. all of the above

Starting a Family

LO 10.6 Explain the factors that should be considered before starting a family.

Most young adults in the United States anticipate that they will be parents one day. For some, raising children is one of the life achievements they most look forward to, and three-quarters of Americans say that their family is the most important element in their life.[41] The American family, however, has undergone a dramatic transformation in recent decades. Women are waiting longer to have children, spacing births further apart, and ending their fertility at earlier ages than ever before. In addition, about 18% of women now say they would not mind at all if they never had children.[41] Consequently, the U.S. birth rate is at an all-time low.

Nontraditional families are also on the rise, with single-parent households increasing more than sixfold since 1950 and unmarried-couple households more than quadrupling.[56] In 2015, only 70% of U.S. children lived with two married, biological parents.[57] These changes in the traditional organization of the American family don't necessarily signal the decline of our social structure. They do, however, point to how flexible and complex American family arrangements have become and remind us that there is no such thing as a "typical" family.

Choosing to Have Children

Having a baby can be one of the most rewarding experiences in life. It can also be one of the most difficult, trying a new parent's patience and testing a couple's relationship.

If you are considering parenthood, ask yourself whether you are ready for the following dramatic changes:

- **Relationship changes.** Caring nonstop for a newborn baby can leave little time for couples to focus on their own relationship. Especially during the child's first year, parents are likely to fight more and be intimate less. Married couples often experience a decrease in their overall satisfaction with their marriage.[58]
- **Changes in your relationships with family members and friends.** Your parents may have ideas about what your priorities should be, and they may differ from yours. Your friendships could also change because new babies leave much less time for socializing with friends.
- **Less time for yourself.** Having little time to sleep or take good care of yourself is a complaint of many new parents. The amount of work it takes to care for a newborn can be overwhelming.[58]

In addition, assess the following:

- **Your health.** If you are a prospective mother, you should evaluate how healthy you are and how to prepare your body for a pregnancy. If you smoke or drink, quit. Eat nutritious foods, get regular exercise, and begin taking prenatal vitamins right away. If you are a prospective father, you should also work at adopting a more healthful lifestyle, including avoiding tobacco, alcohol, and recreational drugs because using these substances before conception could affect your fertility or perhaps even contribute to poor fetal health.[59]
- **Your finances.** Consider your monthly budget and the added expenses that come with a baby, including food, diapers, clothing, furniture, and possibly a bigger place to live. Assess the decrease in income you will see if one of you takes time off work. Come up with a plan on how to cover the medical bills and the cost of child care, if you will need it.
- **Your child care arrangements.** Agree on who will care for your child. You? Your partner? A family member? A daycare center? Are any of these options affordable?
- **Parenting styles.** What values do you want to emphasize? Do you and your partner have similar beliefs on discipline?

Stepfamilies

About 40% of all American marriages are a remarriage for at least one of the spouses, and many of these families include children from prior relationships.[60] "Blended families" have become commonplace in modern society, as more parents have opted to divorce and later remarry. Indeed, about three-fourths of divorced adults do go on to remarry, many within the first few years of their original marriage's end.[61] In about 65% of these remarriages, one or both partners have children from a previous relationship, according to the National Stepfamily Resource Center.[62]

When a stepfamily is first coming together, life can be unpredictable and chaotic. It can take several years for members of previously distinct families to integrate, and they do not always succeed.[63] Members of a stepfamily need to form new roles and norms within their new family rather than try to re-create the original family. Setting realistic expectations and encouraging open communication can be extremely useful in fostering strong stepfamily relationships.

Single Parenthood

Even if you were not raised by a single parent, odds are you know someone who was. Of the 74.2 million children living in the United States in 2009, about 22% lived with only one parent.[57] This statistic reflects the high divorce rate, the small number of partners who are widowed, and the growing number of parents who have never been married. About 40% of children today are born to unmarried mothers.[64]

One of the greatest hurdles single mothers face is economic hardship. An estimated 30% of women who have a child born out of wedlock live in poverty, compared with just 8% of women who were married at the time of their child's birth.[65] Single mothers, on average, also have lower levels of education than other women, which can hurt their job prospects and lower their earnings potential.

Just how children fare growing up in a single-parent household varies and has been the source of some controversy. Experts recognize that a family's structure is not as important as how it functions. Yet children from single-parent families have a risk of difficult life outcomes that is two to three times higher than that of children from married, two-parent families.[66] Children born out of wedlock are more likely to experience a wide range of behavioral and emotional problems, reach adulthood with less education, and earn less income. They are more likely to be "idle"—out of school and out of work—in their late teens and early 20s. They experience more symptoms of depression and have more troubled marriages and higher rates of divorce.

But do these gloomy predictions hold for children born to women who deliberately choose single motherhood? A growing number of sociologists are saying no. Women who are financially independent and well-educated—lesbian or heterosexual—are increasingly choosing to have children without a partner. Sociologist Suzanne Bianchi of the University of Maryland explains that these women make sacrifices in their personal lives and careers to make single parenting work, putting their children first. Wellesley College sociologist Rosanna Hertz agrees: "The child really becomes the focal point of their lives."[67] One study of 1,500 U.S. multiethnic 12- and 13-year-olds supports these observations: Cornell professor Henry Riciutti found that, when income and level of education are factored in, there's "little or no difference" between the intellectual development, academic achievement, and behavior of children in single-parent and two-parent families. The study also suggests that any risks of single parenting can be greatly reduced with increased access to economic, social, educational, and parenting support.[68]

Characteristics of Happy Families

Researchers have devoted a great deal of time to looking at strong families, measuring their affection and communication, trying to decipher their secrets for success. What they have found is that a happy family is not one without trouble or weaknesses. Some have experienced financial difficulties, health problems, or other setbacks. But strong families learn how to adapt and endure; they take a constructive approach to dealing with crises, often because they have a shared agreement about what constitutes their own particular version of "success."[69]

Members of strong families value these traits:[70]

- **Commitment.** They are dedicated to the family and promoting each other's happiness. They are honest, faithful, and dependable.
- **Appreciation and affection.** They care for each other and are not afraid to express it. They give compliments and show their affection freely.
- **Positive communication.** They are good talkers and good listeners. They do argue but avoid blaming each other and are able to compromise.
- **Time together.** They spend quality time together as often as they can and arrange their schedules to ensure that this happens.
- **Spiritual well-being.** They have hope, faith, and compassion as well as shared ethical values.
- **The ability to manage stress and crises.** They see crises as both challenges and opportunities for growth. They pull together during tough times and give support to each other. They set their own definitions of success and work together to take steps both large and small to reach their goals.

LO 10.6 QUICK CHECK ✔

How does the current U.S. birth rate compare to historical rates?
a. about the same as in 1980
b. about the same as in 1990
c. at an all-time low
d. at an all-time high

Change Yourself, Change Your World

LO 10.7 Discuss strategies for building and maintaining healthy relationships.

Healthy relationships involve many challenges, from misunderstandings and hurt feelings to episodes of significant emotional pain. Still, failing to build healthy relationships simply is not an option! In the words of civil rights leader Martin Luther King, Jr., "We must learn to live together as brothers, or perish together as fools."[71] The rewards of healthy relationships are abundant.

Personal Choices

If you want to build and maintain healthy relationships, a smart first step is to practice the skills—including effective communication and conflict-resolution skills—described earlier. In addition, it's important to adopt the following behaviors:

- **Stay true to who you are.** Everyone wants to experiment with different beliefs, values, and behaviors. But when you adopt attitudes and behavior patterns that don't feel authentic, just because you think doing so will help you fit in or keep a relationship going, you're doomed to dishonest, superficial relationships. Be yourself—right from the start.
- **Respect others for who they are.** Have you ever found yourself thinking about breaking off a relationship because you're just "too different"? If so, it might be time to think again. If you can learn to value your differences—in beliefs, standards, experiences, skills, behaviors, style—you might find that you're able to forge a highly energetic relationship in which you and your partner become more productive and creative. Sociologist Mark Granovetter refers to this phenomenon as "the strength of weak ties," and it's a key reason to value diversity in your relationships.[72]
- **Learn to give and receive.** This doesn't mean the two of you have to be rich! The most meaningful gifts in lasting relationships are gifts of time, attention, listening, and emotional support. Give these gifts unselfishly and accept them from your partner with gratitude.
- **Lighten up.** Make room in your relationships for fun! Take a break from studying to take a bike ride or keep a Saturday free for a trip to the beach. Keep humor a part of your personal connections.

Campus Advocacy

College students come together from regions all over the world not only to acquire knowledge but to learn to respect and negotiate differences—including differences in culture, religion, language, ability, sexual orientation, and much more. What can you do to build bridges to others on your campus? Here are some simple ideas.

Keep the Lines of Communication Open

One international student described her two years of study at an American university as "a challenging experience."[73] She noted that students on her campus tended to associate only with those like themselves and often avoided even speaking to students from other countries. She offered this advice for keeping the lines of communication open:[73]

- **Initiate a conversation.** If the person has difficulty speaking English, give him or her some time to think through a translation or to take out the person's electronic dictionary and find the right words.
- **Remember that words are not the most important part of human communication.** Observe the person's facial expression and gestures; take a look!
- **During a conversation, empathize.** Try to see the world through the other person's perspective.

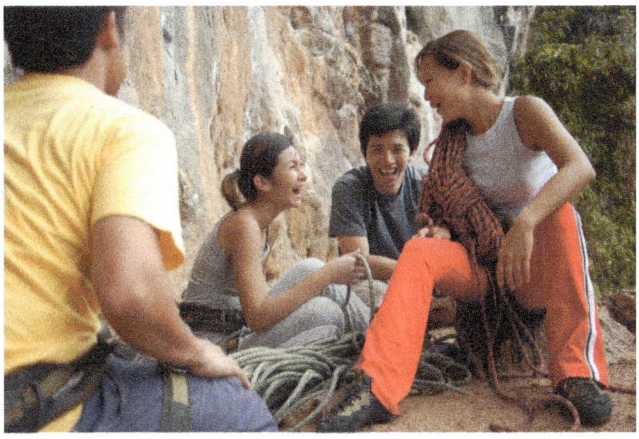

Taking the time to appreciate your friends and partners for who they are can **strengthen your relationships.**

Join a Campus Organization That Promotes Tolerance

Many different organizations provide training and tools to combat *bias*—unfair preferences—and promote an atmosphere of tolerance on campus. For example:

- **The National Educational Association of Disabled Students (NEADS)** has a network of 40 campus-based groups to support students with disabilities. Membership is open to all students, regardless of level of ability. For information about forming a group or becoming a member, go to **www.neads.ca** and search for "Campus Student Groups."
- **Campus Pride** is a national nonprofit group working to create a safer college environment for LGBT (lesbian, gay, bisexual, or transgender) students across the United States. Find out more about this organization at **www.campuspride.org.**

In addition to checking into these two examples, find out what's happening on your campus and get involved.

Explore New Options

You don't have to join an organization to build diverse relationships on campus. Try attending a few services of a campus religious organization that you're not familiar with. Volunteer to help plan a social or cultural event sponsored by an international students' organization. Advocate for a culture of respect on campus, both among students and in the rules set by the administration, that discourages bullying (in person or online) and states that such behavior is not tolerated at your school.[74] You might argue that you're only one person, but in reality, you're part of a vast network of relationships. By reaching out in simple ways like these, you challenge the belief that differences can keep us from building strong, meaningful relationships.

LO 10.7 QUICK CHECK

Which of the following is an important gift to give in any close relationship?
 a. time
 b. attention and being present
 c. emotional support
 d. all of the above

Watch videos of real students discussing communication and relationships at **MasteringHealth**

Choosing to **Change** Worksheet

To complete this worksheet online, visit MasteringHealth

Successful healthy relationships are built on trust, respect, and communication. They enable each individual to retain his or her own identity and foster personal growth rather than smother it. With this in mind, think about one relationship that is important to you and needs improvement. Write down this relationship in step 1.

Directions: Fill in your stage of change in step 1 and complete the remaining steps with your stage of change in mind.

Step 1: Assess your stage of behavior change. My relationship with _____ is important to me and needs improvement. Please check one of the following statements that best describes your readiness to improve this relationship.

_____ I do not intend to participate in building a healthy relationship in the next six months. (Precontemplation)

_____ I might participate in building a healthy relationship in the next six months. (Contemplation)

_____ I am prepared to participate in building a healthy relationship in the next month. (Preparation)

_____ I have been building a healthy relationship for less than six months but need to do more. (Action)

_____ I have built a healthy relationship for more than six months and want to maintain it. (Maintenance)

Step 2: Assess your communication skills. It is important to know how to communicate effectively with others. Think about the communication skills listed on pages 235–238. List the skills that you feel you have mastered in your own life. Then list one area in particular that you would like to improve.

Mastered: _____

_____

Needs improvement: _____

_____

Step 3: Get feedback on your communication style. Find someone close to you whom you trust and who you can have an open discussion with. Ask that person about your communication skills—that is, what your strengths are and what might need improvement. Try not to become offended if the person suggests areas for improvement; honest feedback is the hallmark of a true friend. What did that person say, and how do you feel about it?

_____

_____

_____

Step 4: Improve your listening. Listening is a major component of communication. Consider the good listening skills that were discussed on page 236. Which techniques can you try to become a better listener? Provide examples of how you will apply these skills in your chosen relationship.

Techniques: _____

_____

Examples: _____

_____

Step 5: Put yourself in someone else's shoes. Another way to improve a relationship is to try to see things through the other person's eyes. Take a moment to think about your chosen relationship and write down key factors in that person's life and situation. Answer the following questions: Who are the important people in his or her life and why? What other people is he or she having problems with and why? What are his or her current stressors? What is he or she looking forward to or worried about?

_____

_____

_____

Step 6: Write a note. Imagine that you are writing a note to the person with whom you want to improve your relationship. What would you say? Write it down.

_____

_____

_____

_____

Step 7: Determine the next step. Given your current stage of behavior change, what will be your next step in building the relationship you want to improve? If you are in the preparation stage of change, write down your SMART goal.

_____

_____

CHAPTER 10 STUDY PLAN

CHAPTER SUMMARY

LO 10.1
- Good communication includes being able to articulate your honest thoughts and feelings, being a good listener, and being aware of how body language can affect how others interpret what you are saying.
- Effective conflict resolution requires that both parties voice their concerns in a mature way and engage in constructive criticism rather than resorting to personal attacks and put-downs.

LO 10.2
- Self-perception, early relationships, and gender roles affect how we develop relationships throughout life.

LO 10.3
- Strong friendships and social ties contribute to our overall health.
- Online friendships are common and can be fun, but they often do not provide the same level of support and connection as in-person contact.

LO 10.4
- Sternberg's Triangular Theory of Love identifies intimacy, passion, and commitment as the three primary components of healthy, loving relationships.
- Healthy relationships are based on trust, respect, and communication. Dysfunctional relationships are characterized by physical or verbal abuse, manipulation, and disrespect.

MasteringHealth™
Build your knowledge—and health!—in the Study Area of **MasteringHealth**™ with a variety of study tools.

LO 10.5
- Cohabitation, marriage, and domestic partnerships are examples of different kinds of committed relationships.
- In the United States, same-sex couples now share the same right to marry that heterosexual couples enjoy.

LO 10.6
- Raising children can be rewarding as well as stressful. Couples should ask themselves if they are truly ready for the changes that parenting requires.
- Strong families are characterized by commitment, appreciation, affection, positive communication, time together, spiritual well-being, and the ability to adapt to changes.

LO 10.7
- To build and maintain healthy relationships, it is important to develop effective communication and conflict-resolution skills, to respect others, to pay attention to those you care for, and to rise above petty differences and annoyances.

GET CONNECTED

>> Visit the following websites for further information about the topics in this chapter:

- Conflict Resolution Information Source
  www.crinfo.org
- American Psychological Association
  www.apa.org
- Human Rights Campaign
  www.hrc.org
- Loveisrespect.org
  www.loveisrespect.org

MOBILE TIPS!
Scan this QR code with your mobile device to access additional tips for healthy, happy relationships. Or, via your mobile device, go to **http://chmobile.pearsoncmg.com** choose by topic: relationships.

- American Association for Marriage and Family Therapy
  www.aamft.org
- Go Ask Alice
  www.goaskalice.columbia.edu

Website links are subject to change. To access updated web links, please visit MasteringHealth™

TEST YOUR KNOWLEDGE

LO 10.1
1. Sharing your feelings and other personal information with another person is called
   a. self-assuredness.
   b. self-love.
   c. self-appreciation.
   d. self-disclosure.

2. All of the following are examples of nonverbal communication except
   a. eye contact.
   b. email.
   c. arm movements.
   d. facial expressions.

LO 10.4
3. In Sternberg's Triangular Theory of Love, which of the following is not a primary component of healthy relationships?
   a. passion
   b. contentment
   c. commitment
   d. intimacy

4. Assortative mating refers to the tendency of people to
   a. be attracted to people who have opposite interests to their own.
   b. fall in love at first sight.
   c. "hook up" instead of date.
   d. select romantic partners who are similar to themselves.

LO 10.2
5. Attachment theory states that
   a. becoming close to a romantic partner weakens existing friendships.
   b. close friends will grow to be more and more like one another.
   c. the more attached you become to someone, the more healthy the relationship becomes.
   d. early childhood relationships shape our expectations of adult relationships.

LO 10.3
6. Friendships are
   a. stronger today with modern technology.
   b. helpful in promoting health.
   c. difficult to rekindle if you have been out of touch.
   d. all of these answers are correct.

LO 10.1, 10.7
7. All of the following will help you maintain relationships except
   a. staying true to who you are.
   b. respecting others.
   c. avoiding conflict.
   d. being generous.

LO 10.5
8. In general, married people
   a. enjoy better mental and physical health than unmarried people.
   b. live longer than unmarried people.
   c. are financially better off than unmarried people.
   d. All of these answers are correct.

9. The divorce rate in the United States is
   a. just under 50%.
   b. just under 75%.
   c. around 33%.
   d. increasing.

LO 10.6
10. What percentage of remarriages in the United States include children from a prior relationship?
    a. 25%
    b. 45%
    c. 65%
    d. 85%

WHAT DO YOU THINK?

LO 10.5
1. Do you think health organizations should make statements about social issues?

LO 10.1, 10.3, 10.4
2. What are three ways that digital technology can help interpersonal relationships? What are three ways the same technology can harm them?

LO 10.4, 10.7
3. What steps should schools take, if any, to prevent online bullying?

LO 10.2, 10.5
4. Amid the hook-up culture, what are some ways to find and build committed relationships?

LO 10.6
5. What do you think are the most important factors in providing a secure, healthy environment for raising children?

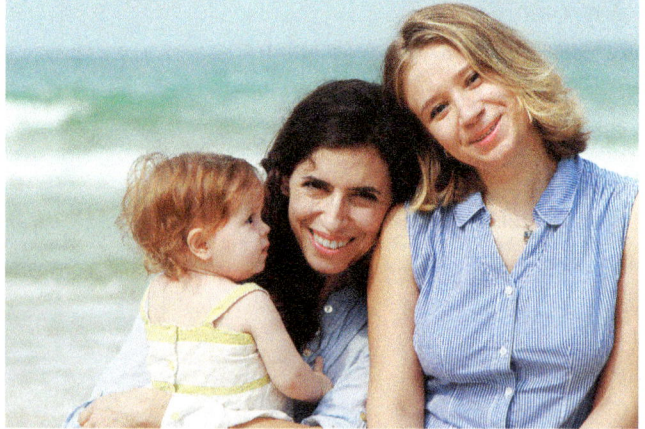

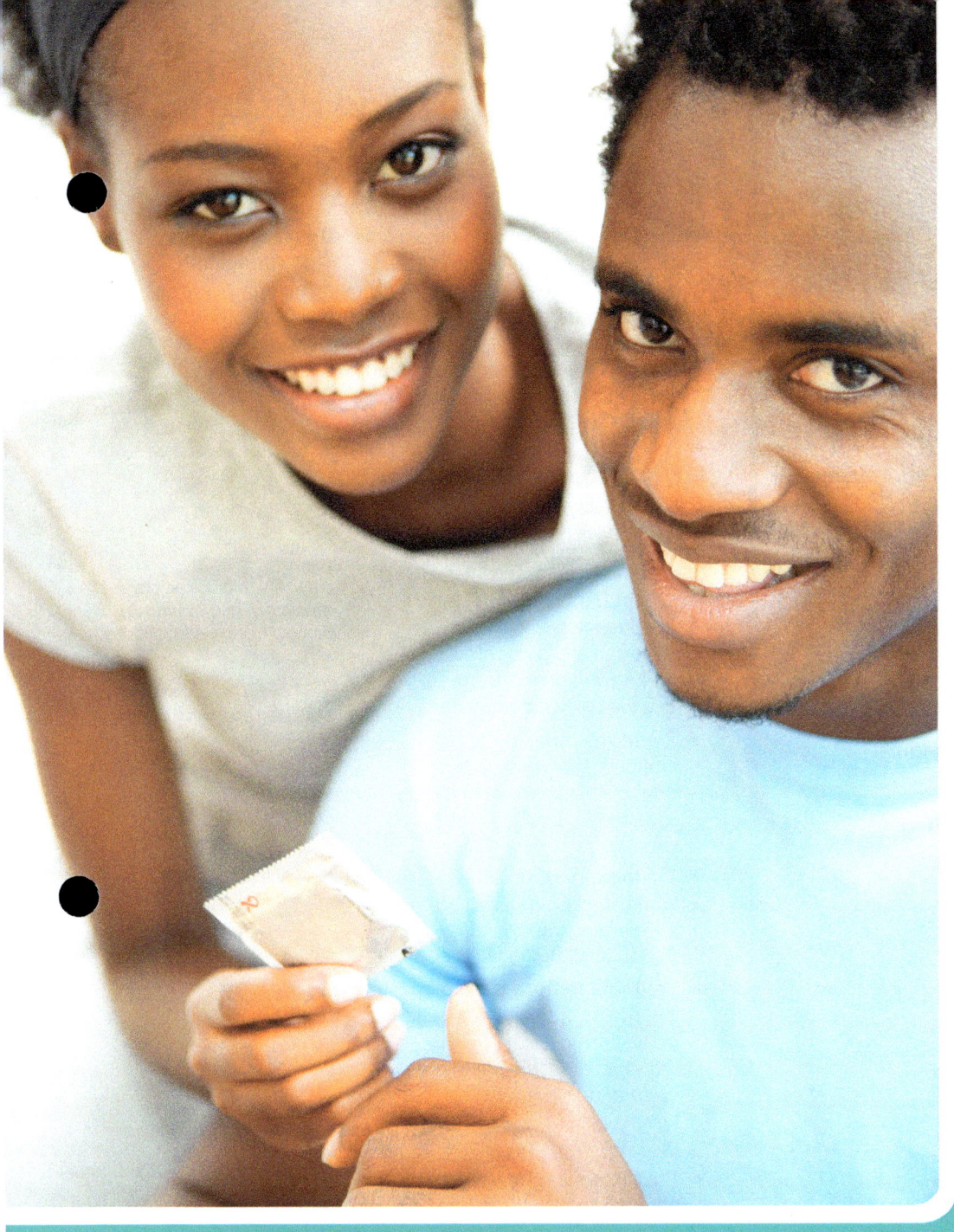

11

> About 37.2% of college students report that they have never engaged in vaginal intercourse.[i]

> Approximately 49.9% of college students report that they did not use contraception the last time they had vaginal intercourse.[i]

> In the United States, half of all pregnancies are unplanned—about 3 million each year.[ii]

SEXUALITY, CONTRACEPTION, AND REPRODUCTIVE CHOICES

LEARNING OUTCOMES

LO 11.1 Describe the primary structures in female and male sexual anatomy.

LO 11.2 Outline the key events of the female menstrual cycle.

LO 11.3 Identify the phases of the sexual response cycle and discuss common sexual dysfunctions.

LO 11.4 Define *abstinence*, *non-intercourse sexual activity*, and *sexual intercourse*.

LO 11.5 Discuss sexual orientation and gender identity.

LO 11.6 Compare and contrast different methods of contraception.

LO 11.7 Discuss surgical and medical abortion.

LO 11.8 Describe the key stages of pregnancy and childbirth.

LO 11.9 Discuss causes of and treatment for infertility.

LO 11.10 Consider ways of developing and promoting healthy sexuality.

Sex is something people rarely think about intellectually.

Sure, you may fantasize about it, but pondering the physiological and wellness aspects of sex is usually not high on a college student's list of priorities. Yet sex is worth deeper thought than we often give it. Our sexuality—including how we see ourselves and how we relate to others—affects our health, our sense of pleasure, our romantic relationships, and our decisions about whether and when to have a family. Understanding your **sexuality,** knowing your reproductive options, and making choices that best fit your values and goals are important elements of your overall health and well-being.

Sexual Anatomy And Health

LO 11.1 Describe the primary structures in female and male sexual anatomy.

Beginning at puberty, our bodies continually prepare for reproduction. A woman's ovaries release an egg each month, whereas a man's testes are constantly manufacturing new sperm. Given these biological realities, sexual decisions we make in a split second can alter the course of our lives dramatically, sometimes leading to an unplanned pregnancy or a sexually transmitted infection (STI) (see **Chapter 12**) that permanently affects fertility.

Female Sexual Anatomy and Sexual Health

A woman's sexual anatomy includes both external and internal sex organs **(Figure 11.1).** The term **vulva** refers to all of the female external organs collectively—also known as *genitals*. These include the following structures:

- The **mons pubis** is the fatty, rounded area of tissue in front of the pubic bone; it is covered in pubic hair after puberty.
- The **labia majora** is the fleshy, larger outer lips (*labia* means "lips") surrounding the labia minora.
- The **labia minora** is the thin, inner folds of skin, which rest protectively over the *clitoris*, the *vaginal opening*, and the *urethral opening*, through which urine is released from the body.
- The **clitoris** is an organ composed of spongy tissue with an abundance of nerve endings that make it very sensitive to sexual stimulation. During sexual arousal, the clitoris fills with blood and plays a key role in producing the female orgasm. In fact, the clitoris is the only organ in either sex with the sole purpose of sexual arousal and pleasure.

The internal organs include the following:

- The **vagina** is the tube that connects a woman's external sex organs with her *uterus*. It serves as the passageway through which menstrual flow leaves the body as well as the passageway through which sperm enters the body during heterosexual intercourse. During childbirth, it functions as the birth canal.
- The **uterus,** also known as the **womb,** is a pear-shaped organ, normally about the size of a fist. It is here that a

---

sexuality The biological, physical, emotional, and psychosocial aspects of sexual attraction and expression.

vulva All of the female external organs collectively. Also called *genitals*.

mons pubis The fatty, rounded areas of tissue in front of the pubic bone.

labia majora The fleshy, larger outer lips surrounding the labia minora.

labia minora The thin, inner folds of skin, which rest protectively over the *clitoris*, the *vaginal opening*, and the *urethral opening*, through which urine is released from the body.

clitoris An organ composed of spongy tissue and nerve endings that is very sensitive to sexual stimulation.

vagina A tube that connects a woman's external sex organs with her uterus.

uterus (womb) A pear-shaped organ where a growing fetus is nurtured.

growing fetus is nurtured. The innermost lining of the uterus is called the *endometrium*. It is shed monthly in non-pregnant women of **childbearing age,** a range often defined as being between 15 and 44 years of age.¹ The narrowed end of the uterus that projects into the top of the vagina is called the *cervix*. Sperm deposited into the vagina swim through the opening of the cervix into the body of the uterus.

- The **ovaries** are the two chambers, one on either side of the pelvic cavity, where a woman's eggs, or *ova*, are stored. Every month, at approximately midway through her **menstrual cycle,** a woman *ovulates*; that is, one of her ovaries releases an egg. The ovaries produce the hormone *estrogen*.

- The **fallopian tubes** are two tubes—one on either side of the uterus—that connect the uterus to the ovaries. After ovulation, the egg is swept into the nearby fallopian tube. It then travels through the tube to the uterus. If it encounters sperm within the tube, the egg may become fertilized. Whether fertilized or not, the egg then continues to be swept into the uterus.

Good sexual health includes preventive care. According to the American Congress of Obstetricians and Gynecologists (ACOG), girls should have their first gynecologic visit between the ages of 13 and 15. Unless a girl is sexually active or is experiencing problems, these first visits most likely will not include a pelvic exam.

New ACOG guidelines indicate that women should have their first pelvic exam and cervical cancer screening at age 21. Screening includes a Pap test and, for some women, testing for human papillomavirus (HPV). The frequency of subsequent screenings depends on a woman's age and

childbearing age The age range during which a woman can become pregnant.

ovaries The two female reproductive organs where ova (eggs) reside.

menstrual cycle The monthly physiological cycle marked by *menstruation*.

fallopian tubes The pair of tubes that connect the ovaries to the uterus.

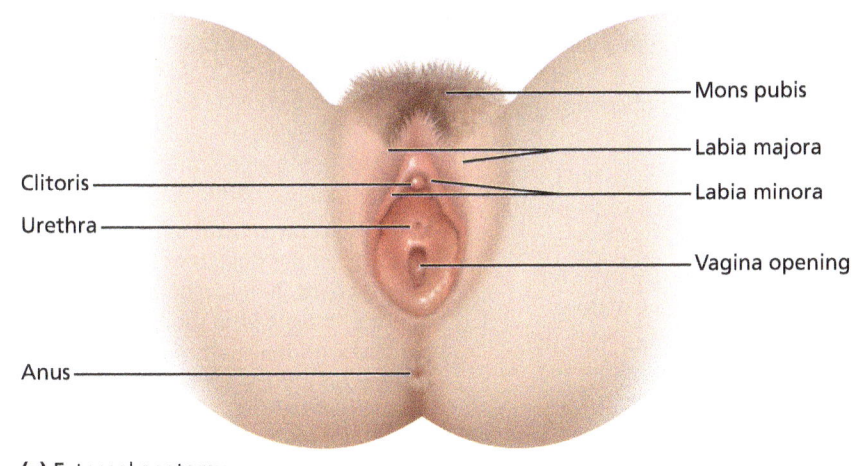

(a) External anatomy

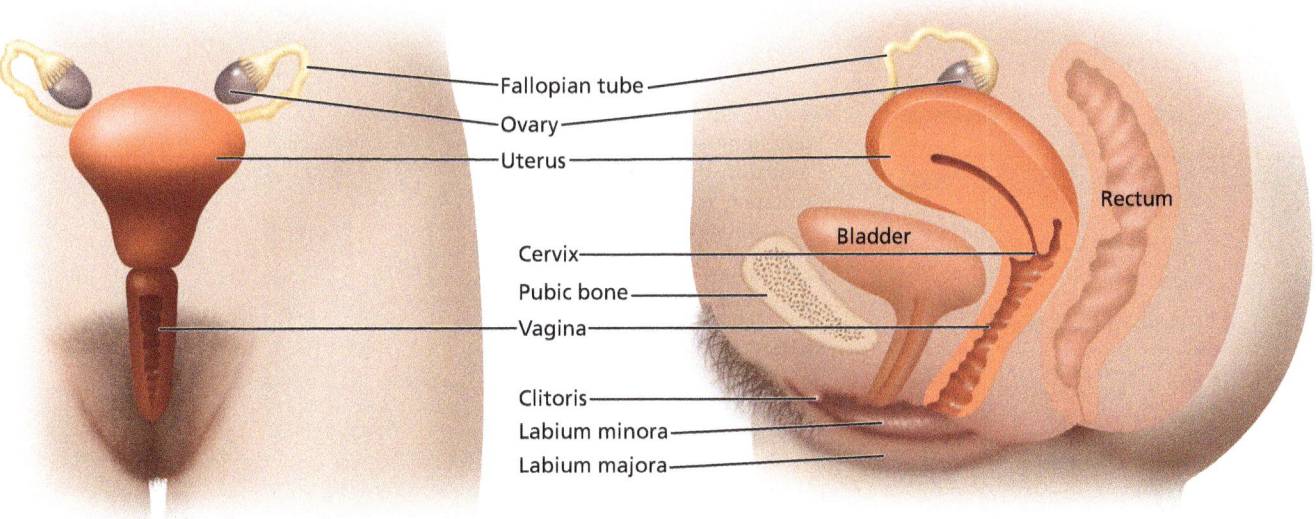

(b) Internal anatomy

FIGURE 11.1 **Female Sexual Anatomy.**

health history (see Chapter 12).[2] Unfortunately, about 42% of college-age women do not get screened regularly.[2] This reduces the odds of detecting medical problems early and also deprives women of the opportunity to discuss important sexual health issues and reproductive concerns with a health professional.

Male Sexual Anatomy and Sexual Health

A man's reproductive anatomy also includes both internal and external organs **(Figure 11.2)**. These are the external organs:

- The **penis** is the male sexual and reproductive organ, which consists of the shaft (body) and a slitted tip called the glans penis (head). Made up of soft, spongy tissue, the penis fills with blood during sexual arousal and becomes firm and enlarged, a state known as an **erection.** Boys are born with a hood of skin, known as the *foreskin,* covering the head of the penis. In more than half of boys born in the United States, parents opt to have the skin surgically removed through a procedure called **circumcision** (see **Myth or Fact?**).
- The **scrotum** is the skin sac at the base of the penis that contains the *testes* (testicles). The scrotum is responsible for regulating the temperature of the testes, which need to be kept cool to facilitate production of *sperm,* the male reproductive cells.

These are the internal male organs:

- The **testes (testicles)** are the reproductive glands that manufacture sperm.
- The **epididymis** are coiled tubes—one above each testicle—where sperm are held until they mature.
- The **vas deferens** is the tube that ascends from the epididymis—one on each side of the scrotum—and transports sperm into the *ejaculatory duct*.
- The **accessory glands** are a set of glands that lubricate the reproductive system and nourish the sperm. They include the *seminal vesicles,* small sacs that store *seminal fluid,* which provides sugars and other nutrients that feed and activate sperm. The seminal vesicles secrete seminal fluid into the ejaculatory duct, which also receives sperm from the vas deferens. This mixture of sperm and seminal fluid is called **semen.** Another accessory gland that contributes to semen is the *prostate gland,* a walnut-shaped structure below the bladder. It secretes into semen an alkaline fluid that helps protect sperm from the acidic environment of the vagina. Below the prostate are the *Cowper's glands,* pea-shaped glands on each side of the urethra that discharge a lubricating secretion into the urethra just before ejaculation.
- Within the prostate, the ejaculatory duct joins the **urethra,** a much longer duct that travels from the bladder through the shaft of the penis and carries fluids to the outside of the body. Both urine from the bladder and semen from the ejaculatory duct pass through the urethra, although not at the same time.

> **penis** The male sexual and reproductive organ.
>
> **erection** The process in which the penis fills up with blood as a result of sexual stimulation.
>
> **circumcision** Surgical removal of the foreskin of the penis.
>
> **scrotum** The skin sac at the base of the penis that contains the testes.
>
> **testes (testicles)** Two reproductive glands that manufacture sperm.
>
> **epididymis** The coiled tube on top of each testicle where sperm are held until they mature.
>
> **vas deferens** The tube ascending from the epididymis that transports sperm.
>
> **accessory glands** The glands (seminal vesicles, prostate gland, and Cowper's gland) that lubricate the reproductive system and nourish sperm.
>
> **semen** Male ejaculate, consisting of sperm and other fluids from the accessory glands.
>
> **urethra** The duct that travels from the bladder through the shaft of the penis, carrying fluids to the outside of the body.

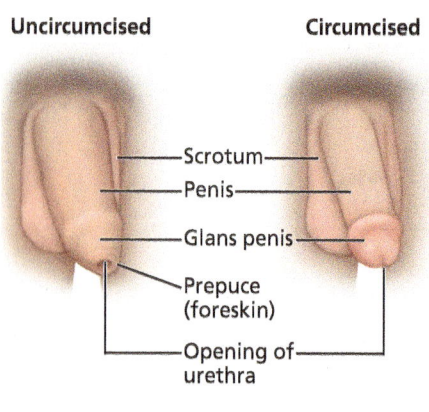

(a) External anatomy

(b) Internal anatomy

FIGURE 11.2 Male Sexual Anatomy.

MYTH OR FACT?

Should Boys Be Circumcised for Health Reasons?

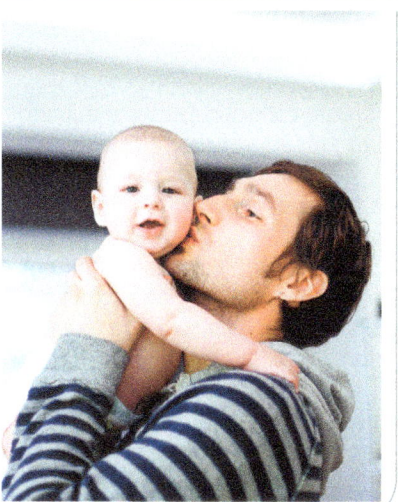

Infant boys are born with a hood of skin, known as the *foreskin,* covering the head of the penis. In more than half of boys born in the United States, parents opt to have the foreskin surgically removed through a procedure called *circumcision*.

Circumcision rates vary greatly across the country and throughout the world. The surgery was performed on 54.7% of newborn boys in the United States in 2010.[1] Circumcision is also widely performed in the Middle East and Canada, but in Europe, Latin America, China, and India, it is uncommon.

In some families, the decision to circumcise is primarily a religious one. In both the Jewish and Muslim faiths, circumcision is a common rite of passage. In others, it is more of a cultural determination: Boys are circumcised because their fathers were. What remains most controversial is circumcising for health-related reasons, although recent research is adding more weight to the procedure's potential health benefits.

These benefits start with cleanliness. Circumcision boosts personal hygiene, making it somewhat easier to wash the penis. It also reduces the risk of urinary tract infections in infancy. Men who have been circumcised have lower rates of penile cancer, and several types of research studies have documented a reduced risk of acquiring and transmitting some sexually transmitted infections, including HIV.[2] Safer sex practices, however, are much more important at stopping the spread of those diseases than circumcision is. Still, one economic study determined that circumcision provides enough health benefits that if U.S. circumcision rates were to fall to levels seen in Europe, the decline would add more than $4 billion to U.S. health-care costs.[3]

In 2012, the American Academy of Pediatrics revised its policy on circumcision, stating that the benefits of the surgery "justify access to the procedure for families who choose it."[4] Although the academy stopped short of recommending circumcision for all newborns, it stated that health insurance should cover the cost of the procedure. In 2014, the Centers for Disease Control and Prevention (CDC) released the first federal guidelines on circumcision, stating that "the scientific evidence is clear that the benefits outweigh the risks."[2]

Opponents of circumcision point out that the procedure can be painful. It also comes with risks, including the potential for infection and excessive bleeding. In rare cases, the penis may not heal properly or a second surgery may be needed. Some opponents argue that circumcision reduces penile sensation and sexual function; however, well-designed studies of these issues are few and inconclusive.

References **1.** Centers for Disease Control and Prevention. (2011). Trends in in-hospital newborn male circumcision—United States, 1999–2010. *Morbidity and Mortality Weekly Report, 60*(34), 1167–1168. **2.** Centers for Disease Control and Prevention. (2014). *Recommendations for providers counseling male patients and parents regarding male circumcision and the prevention of HIV infection, STIs, and other health outcomes.* www.regulations.gov. **3.** Johns Hopkins Medicine. (2012, August 20). *Declining rates of U.S. infant male circumcision could add billions to health care costs, experts warn.* www.hopkinsmedicine.org. **4.** American Academy of Pediatrics. (2012). Circumcision policy statement. *Pediatrics, 130*(3), 585–586.

Like women, men should take their sexual health seriously and get regular medical checkups. Sexually active men are also encouraged to perform genital self-exams, looking for any abnormalities that could indicate an STI or testicular cancer, which is most often diagnosed in young men (see Chapter 12).

LO 11.1 QUICK CHECK

What is the correct term for a female's external sexual organs collectively?

a. vagina
b. vulva
c. clitoris
d. mons pubis

The Menstrual Cycle

LO 11.2 Outline the key events of the female menstrual cycle.

A rite of passage for girls as they transition into womanhood is **menarche** (pronounced *me-NAR-kee*), the onset of **menstruation,** the discharge of blood and endometrial tissue from the vagina. Also called a *period* or *menstrual period,* menstruation usually lasts from 3 to 7 days. In the United States, the average age at menarche is 12, although it is considered normal to start as early as 8 or as late as 15.[4]

> **menarche** The first onset of menstruation.
>
> **menstruation** The cyclical discharge of blood and tissue from the vagina.

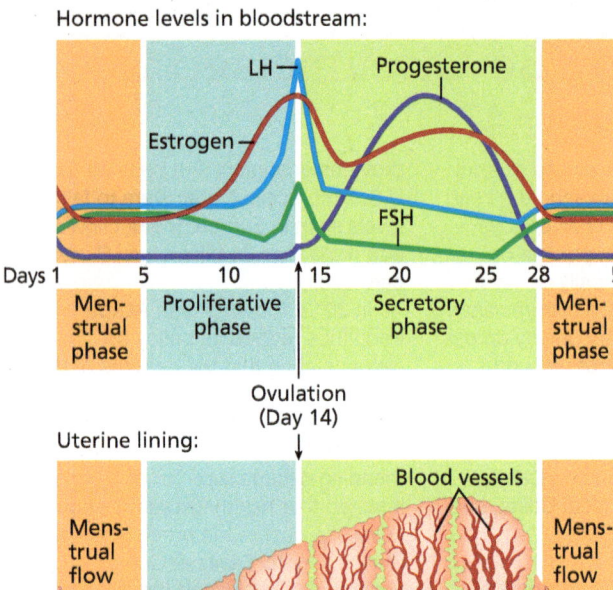

FIGURE 11.3 **Phases of the Menstrual Cycle.**
The menstrual cycle consists of a menstrual phase, a proliferative phase, and a secretory phase.

Menopause, the time at which women stop menstruating, usually occurs in a woman's early 50s.

Menstruation is just one of several physiological events in a woman's *menstrual cycle* **(Figure 11.3)**. Because it is controlled by hormones, the menstrual cycle can be interrupted by anything that affects hormone production—including illness, excessive dieting with or without excessive exercise, and breast-feeding. The menstrual cycle also ceases during pregnancy. Otherwise, in women of childbearing age, it repeats approximately every month, spanning from 21 to 35 days (average is 28 days).[4]

▶▶ View an animation of the menstrual cycle at **www.womenshealth.gov**. (Search for "menstrual cycle.")

Phases of the Menstrual Cycle

The menstrual cycle is characterized by a series of events involving the uterus and the ovaries. Fluctuations in the levels of four female reproductive hormones control these events, which are typically grouped into three phases: the **menstrual phase,** the **proliferative phase,** and the **secretory phase** (see Figure 11.3).

Menstrual Phase

The first day of a woman's menstrual flow is designated as day 1 of the menstrual cycle. Menstruation results from the breakdown of the endometrium after the body "recognizes" that a pregnancy has not occurred. During the menstrual phase, a hormone called *follicle-stimulating hormone (FSH)* is released from the pituitary gland in the brain. A woman's ovary contains thousands of egg sacs called *follicles*. FSH stimulates the maturation of the immature eggs within a few of these follicles. As the eggs develop, the follicles begin releasing an ovarian hormone, *estrogen,* into the bloodstream. As estrogen reaches the uterus, it causes menstruation to end (around day 6).

Proliferative Phase

During the proliferative phase, estrogen causes the lining of the uterus to thicken to prepare for the possibility of a fertilized egg. A woman may also notice a copious, slippery discharge of mucus from her vagina. This characteristic *cervical mucus* helps facilitate the mobility of sperm and protect them from the otherwise acidic environment of the vagina. Its presence also indicates that a woman is about to **ovulate**—that is, release a mature egg (*ovum*) from the ovary. Ovulation occurs around day 14 of a 28-day cycle and is caused by the release of *luteinizing hormone (LH)* from the pituitary gland. In some women, ovulation is accompanied by sharp pain on one side of the lower abdomen lasting for several minutes to several hours. This "mid-cycle pain" is entirely normal and can help a woman pinpoint more precisely the time when she is fertile.

Secretory Phase

Once the ovum has been ejected, the remaining follicle sac degenerates into a *corpus luteum,* a tiny gland that begins releasing a fourth reproductive hormone, progesterone. Rising levels of progesterone enter the bloodstream and travel to the uterus, further thickening the endometrial lining in preparation for the arrival of a fertilized egg.

If sperm are present in sufficient numbers in the fallopian tube when an ovum is also present, fertilization is likely to occur. The fertilized egg will then produce the hormone *human chorionic gonadotropin (hCG),* which is needed to sustain a pregnancy. In fact, over-the-counter pregnancy test kits work by detecting the presence or absence of hCG in a woman's urine. Within 3 to 4 days, the fertilized ovum reaches the uterus.

An unfertilized ovum is viable only for about 12 to 24 hours. If fertilization does not occur within this time period, it will quickly deteriorate and, around day 25, the endometrium will start to degenerate. Within 3 to 4 days, menstruation begins and the cycle repeats.

menopause The time when a woman stops having menstrual cycles.

menstrual phase The phase of the menstrual cycle characterized by menstrual flow, the release of follicle-stimulating hormone from the pituitary gland to the brain, and the release of estrogen into the bloodstream.

proliferative phase The phase of the menstrual cycle characterized by a thickening of the lining of the uterus and discharge of cervical mucus. This phase ends when luteinizing hormone triggers the release of a mature egg.

secretory phase The phase of the menstrual cycle characterized by the degeneration of the follicle sac, rising levels of progesterone in the bloodstream, and further increase of the endometrial lining.

ovulate To release an egg from the ovary.

Disorders Associated with the Menstrual Cycle

Although normal menstruation is a sign of health and maturity, in some women it's accompanied by pain, excessive bleeding, or other problems.

Premenstrual Syndrome

As many as 85% of women experience mildly disturbing emotional and physical symptoms just prior to menstruation.[5] These symptoms can include breast tenderness, fluid retention, headaches, backaches, uterine cramping, irritability, mood swings, appetite changes, depression, and anxiety. Approximately 15% of women experience a constellation of the symptoms at a "sufficient severity to interfere with some aspect of life" and, consequently, are considered to have **premenstrual syndrome (PMS).**[6] The symptoms of PMS typically appear in the week or two before the period begins and dissipate after menstrual bleeding starts.

Exactly what causes PMS isn't entirely clear. Some women may simply be more sensitive to the changes in female reproductive hormones that occur during the menstrual cycle. Chemical changes in the brain may also play a role. Stress and psychological problems do not cause the syndrome, although there is evidence that they can exacerbate it.[7]

Some lifestyle changes can reduce the symptoms of PMS. These include avoidance of smoking, alcohol, caffeine, salt, and sugary foods. A balanced diet rich in vegetables, fruits, and whole grains can be helpful, along with regular exercise and adequate, restful sleep. Some women find that a multivitamin and mineral supplement providing adequate levels of B vitamins, magnesium, and vitamin E is helpful, and women, especially those aged 19–50, should consume recommended amounts of calcium. Over-the-counter pain medications can be used to relieve symptoms. In more severe cases in women who do not want to become pregnant, birth control pills may be prescribed, which stop ovulation and reduce menstruation.[7]

premenstrual syndrome (PMS) A collection of emotional and physical symptoms that occur just prior to menstruation.

premenstrual dysphoric disorder (PMDD) Severe and debilitating psychological symptoms experienced just prior to menstruation.

dysmenorrhea Pain during menstruation that is severe enough to limit normal activities or require medication.

endometriosis A condition in which endometrial tissue grows in areas outside the uterus.

Premenstrual Dysphoric Disorder (PMDD)

Some women experience the psychological symptoms of PMS in a more severe and debilitating way. This condition, known as **premenstrual dysphoric disorder (PMDD),** can interfere with daily functioning and social relationships. (*Dysphoria* refers to a generalized feeling of sadness, anxiety, or discontent.) The 3%–8% of women who suffer from PMDD[8] experience at least five of the following symptoms, including at least one of the first four:

- Mood swings, suddenly sad or tearful episodes, or increased sensitivity to rejection
- Persistent irritability or anger
- Depressed mood, feelings of hopelessness, or self-deprecating thoughts
- Anxiety or tension
- Sense of being overwhelmed or out of control
- Sleep disturbances
- Food cravings or other significant changes in appetite
- Low energy or fatiguing easily
- Difficulty focusing
- A loss of interest in daily activities and relationships

The treatments recommended for PMS are also used for PMDD, and some women with the condition have found relief taking *selective serotonin reuptake inhibitor (SSRI)* antidepressants.

Dysmenorrhea

More than half of all menstruating women experience some pain for 1 to 2 days each month.[9] In most of these women, the pain is mild; however, sometimes the pain is severe enough to interfere with normal activities. This is called **dysmenorrhea,** or painful menstruation, and can include severe abdominal cramps, back or thigh pain, diarrhea, and even headaches in the days immediately preceding and during menstruation.[10] Dysmenorrhea is the leading cause of absenteeism from school in adolescent girls.[10]

The cramping pain of dysmenorrhea is due to *prostaglandins,* chemicals that regulate many body functions, including contraction of smooth muscle—like the muscle in a woman's uterus. Prostaglandins cause uterine muscle cells to contract, expelling the uterine lining. This is why over-the-counter prostaglandin inhibitors like ibuprofen and naproxen are usually effective in treating dysmenorrhea. The discomfort also usually wanes spontaneously with age and often disappears after pregnancy.

Endometriosis

Endometriosis is a condition in which endometrial tissue grows in areas outside the uterus, such as the fallopian tubes, ovaries, and other structures in the pelvic region.[11] This tissue responds to the same hormonal signals that

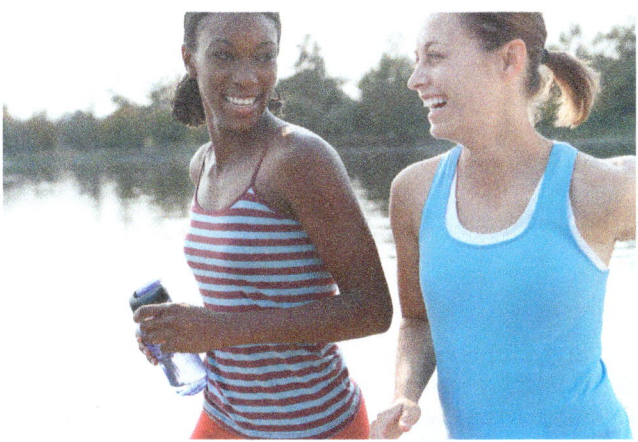

Exercise can help relieve the symptoms of **premenstrual syndrome.**

affect the uterus and so breaks down and bleeds monthly into the abdominopelvic cavity. The condition can cause severe pain in the pelvic region that may be associated with the menstrual cycle, as well as scarring that can result in infertility. Endometriosis occurs most commonly in women in their 30s and 40s but can occur at any time during the reproductive years. A physician can evaluate a woman for endometriosis during a physical examination, and it can be confirmed with laparoscopic surgery, in which a thin, lighted tube is inserted into the abdominopelvic cavity. If endometrial tissue is found, it can often be removed during the same procedure.[11]

Amenorrhea

Amenorrhea is clinically defined as having no periods for at least 3 consecutive months.[4] Missed periods are normal in women who are pregnant and throughout the first few months of breast-feeding. They can also signal a serious underlying disorder of the reproductive organs. However, amenorrhea can usually be traced to severe weight loss, often in athletes who train vigorously while restricting calorie intake to maintain a competitive weight. It is also a common consequence of eating disorders, certain hormonal imbalances, and significant stress. Some medications, including birth control pills, can also suppress menstruation.

Symptoms can include headaches and vaginal dryness, but doctors are most concerned about its long-term effects on bone health. Recall that it is during the normal menstrual cycle that the ovaries produce the reproductive hormone estrogen. Because estrogen plays a key role in building new bone tissue, amenorrhea puts women at significant risk for low bone density. Ultimately, women who experience long-term amenorrhea can suffer from osteoporosis and bone fractures at a relatively early age.

LO 11.2 QUICK CHECK ✔

Which of the following conditions involves the growth of endometrial tissue in areas outside the uterus?
a. PMDD
b. endometriosis
c. amenorrhea
d. dysmenorrhea

The Sexual Response Cycle

LO 11.3 Identify the phases of the sexual response cycle and discuss common sexual dysfunctions.

Famed sex researchers William H. Masters and Virginia E. Johnson were the first to scientifically study the body's physiological reaction to sexual stimulation. They described four distinct stages of the **human sexual response cycle:**

- **Excitement.** The first phase, **excitement,** occurs as a result of any erotic mental or physical stimulation that leads to arousal. In both sexes it is characterized by increased heart and respiration rate and also increased blood pressure. Nipple erection, especially as a result of direct stimulation, occurs in almost all females and in approximately 60% of males. Both may also experience a "sex flush," which is the reddening of the skin due to vasocongestion (blood vessel engorgement). In males, the penis becomes mostly erect and the testicles draw upward. In females, the labia increase in size and the clitoris swells. Lubrication occurs as a result of vasocongestion of the vaginal walls.

- **Plateau.** The second phase, **plateau,** is more intense excitement that takes partners to the edge of orgasm, leading hearts to beat rapidly and making genitals sensitive to touch. In males, the urethral sphincter, a valve at the base of the penis that prevents urination during ejaculation, closes. Muscles at the penis base also begin to contract rhythmically. Males also secrete a pre-ejaculatory fluid (that may contain small amounts of sperm) and the testicles rise closer to the body. In females, the outer third of the vagina swells and the pelvic muscle tightens, creating what Masters and Johnson refer to as the *orgasmic platform.*

- **Orgasm.** The plateau phase concludes with **orgasm,** the peak or climax of sexual response. It is accompanied by rhythmic muscle contractions of the genitals and surrounding areas. Most describe it as an intensely pleasurable feeling of release of sexual tension. In men, orgasm is accompanied by ejaculation.

- **Resolution.** In the **resolution** phase, the body returns to normal functioning. It often includes a sense of both well-being and fatigue.[12]

Men usually experience a *refractory period,* a period of time when they are not immediately able to respond to stimulation with an erection and may actually find continued stimulation unwelcome or even painful. Most women do not experience a refractory period and may be able to immediately return to the plateau stage, allowing for the possibility of multiple orgasms.

Sexual Dysfunctions

Sexual dysfunctions are problems that can occur during any stage of the sexual response cycle—curbing desire, interrupting arousal, reducing pleasure, or preventing orgasm. An estimated 43% of women and 31% of men report having had at least one symptom of sexual dysfunction at some point in their life.[13]

> **amenorrhea** Cessation of menstrual periods.
>
> **human sexual response cycle** Distinct phases extending from the first moment of sexual desire until the calm after orgasm.
>
> **excitement** The first phase of the sexual response cycle, marked by erection in men and lubrication and clitoral swelling in women.
>
> **plateau** The second phase of the sexual response cycle, characterized by intense excitement, rapid heartbeat, genital sensitivity, the secretion of pre-ejaculatory fluid in men, and vaginal swelling in women.
>
> **orgasm** The peak, or climax, of sexual response, characterized by rhythmic muscle contractions of the genitals and surrounding areas and ejaculation in men.
>
> **resolution** The stage of the sexual response cycle in which the body returns to normal functioning.
>
> **sexual dysfunctions** Problems occurring during any stage of the sexual response cycle.

Female Sexual Dysfunctions

A variety of problems, including the following, can keep a woman from enjoying sex:[14]

- **Painful intercourse.** Pain during intercourse is very common: Nearly 75% of adult women have experienced it at some time during their lives.[15] Often the pain is temporary and occurs only under certain circumstances, such as when the penis first enters the vagina or during vigorous thrusting. In other cases, the problem is long term. The causes vary with the type of pain reported, but some of the most common are insufficient vaginal lubrication, prior injury, inflammation, an allergic reaction to a birth control product (such as a spermicide or a latex condom), or an underlying problem such as an infection, ovarian cyst, or endometriosis. Lack of desire or arousal or emotional factors such as stress, low self-esteem, or a history of sexual abuse occasionally play a role. Often, simply a change in position or the use of a lubricant can correct the problem. If the pain is frequent or severe, a health-care provider should be consulted to rule out gynecologic conditions. In some cases, hormonal medications or therapy to address problems with sexual response can help.

- **Low level of sexual desire.** About 5%-15% of women experience a persistently low sex drive.[16] Common physical causes include fatigue, medication side effects, alcohol abuse, pregnancy, breast-feeding, and menopause. In addition, psychological problems and unresolved issues within the relationship can be factors. Lifestyle changes such as regular exercise and stress management can help, as can couples counseling. Hormonal therapy is also available. Finally, some women find that *Kegel exercises*—tightening the pelvic floor muscles as if stopping the flow of urine, holding for a few seconds, and releasing—can help put them back in touch with their sexual anatomy and their sex drive.

- **Inability to achieve orgasm.** About 1 in 5 women worldwide have difficulty experiencing orgasm.[17] The problem can occur as a side effect of prescription medications, including certain antidepressants. Medical problems, relationship problems, embarrassment, or a history of sexual abuse or rape can also prevent some women from reaching orgasm. However, one common factor is simply insufficient stimulation of the clitoris. Switching position can produce more clitoral stimulation during intercourse. Masturbation or use of a vibrator during sex can also help.[17]

Male Sexual Dysfunctions

Being unable to perform sexually can be damaging to a man's self-esteem and place stress on the relationship. Problems related to male sexual function include the following:

- **Erectile dysfunction (ED)** is the inability to get or maintain an erection firm enough for sexual intercourse.[18] Most prevalent among older men, ED most commonly results from injury or underlying disease, but it can stem from fatigue, stress, depression, use of certain medications, or excessive alcohol or tobacco use. As treatment, a physician may prescribe lifestyle modifications such as weight loss or quitting smoking. Oral medications can help by boosting the flow of blood to the penis, but they can have serious side effects and are not intended for men with certain underlying health conditions. Surgery may be recommended in cases of underlying injury, and counseling or sex therapy is also an option.

- **Premature ejaculation (PE)** is a condition in which a man ejaculates earlier than he would like to or earlier than his partner would like him to. Although in the past sex researchers and therapists attempted to define PE based on a quantitative time frame (how long it took to ejaculate), today most agree that a male has a problem when poor ejaculatory control interferes with the sexual satisfaction of one or both partners. PE can result from physical factors, but in most cases it is due to psychological factors such as anxiety. In college-aged men it frequently occurs because of lack of experience, intense arousal, and alcohol use.[19] However, hormonal imbalance, infection, nervous system disorders, and other physical causes should be ruled out if PE is chronic. Treatment of any underlying physical problem is important. In many cases, sexual counseling and incorporating a delaying tactic called the "squeeze technique" can resolve the problem.[20] Strengthening pelvic floor muscles with Kegel exercises can also help.

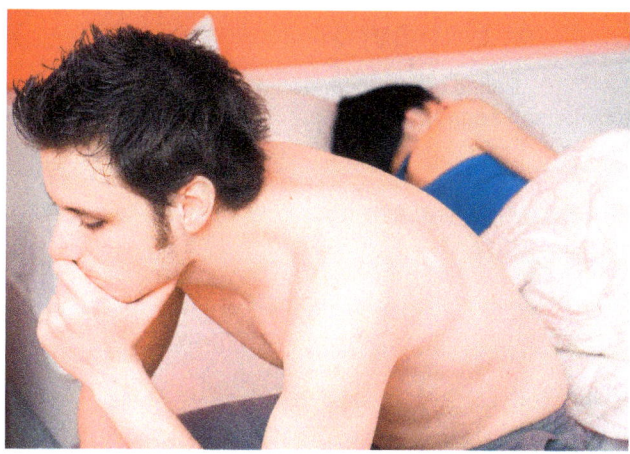

Sexual dysfunctions can occur in both men and women.

erectile dysfunction (ED) Inability of a male to obtain or maintain an erection.

premature ejaculation (PE) A condition in which a male ejaculates earlier than he would like to.

>> For more information on the "squeeze technique," visit the Mayo Clinic website at www.mayoclinic.com. (Search for "squeeze technique.")

LO 11.3 QUICK CHECK ✓

In college-aged men, premature ejaculation (PE) is often a result of all of the following *except*

a. testicular cancer.
b. alcohol use.
c. lack of experience.
d. intense arousal.

Sexual Behavior

LO 11.4 Define *abstinence, non-intercourse sexual activity,* and *sexual intercourse*.

A wide range of human sexual behaviors and interests are considered "normal." Biologist Alfred Kinsey's research in the late 1940s and early 1950s provided a basis for social comparison and helped answer a question many people wondered about: "Who's doing what with whom, and how often are they doing it?" Since Kinsey, many researchers have concluded that the continuum of "normal" sexual behavior in our society is broad and varied.

Abstinence and Celibacy

Abstinence refers to the avoidance of sexual intercourse. Whether it is by deliberate choice or due to circumstance, many people find themselves abstaining from sexual activity for extended periods. Long-term abstinence is referred to as *celibacy*. According to results from the annual National College Health Association annual survey, a significant number of college students are waiting to have sex. In a 2015, 37.2% of college students reported that they had never had vaginal intercourse compared to 28.8% in 2000.[3,21] Some choose celibacy for religious or moral reasons; others choose it out of a desire to avoid becoming pregnant or contracting an STI.[22]

Sexual Intercourse

Sexual intercourse, or *coitus,* is sexual union involving genital penetration. For many heterosexuals, the term is synonymous with **vaginal intercourse,** the insertion of the penis into the vagina. In a recent national survey, 62.6% of male and 67.7% of female college students reported that they have had vaginal intercourse.[3] The use of condoms is advised to avoid unintended pregnancy while reducing the risk for STIs; however, less than half (47.8%) of college students indicate that they use condoms during vaginal sex.[3]

The decision to have sexual intercourse is an important one. To review what should be considered when making this decision, complete the **Self-Assessment** on page 265.

Long considered a taboo in U.S. society, **anal intercourse** has increasingly become accepted, especially among younger generations. According to surveys from the Centers for Disease Control and Prevention (CDC), about 40% of men and 35% of women aged 25–44 have had anal sex with a partner of the opposite sex,[23] and 24.3% of college students report that they have had anal sex.[3] The CDC also reports that 6% of men aged 15–44 have had anal sex with another man at some point in their lives. The practice involves penile penetration of the anus and rectum. Because these tissues are much more fragile than those of the vagina, anal intercourse is one of the riskiest of sexual behaviors in terms of both injury and transmission of infectious disease. It represents one of the primary risk factors for acquiring HIV, the virus that causes AIDS, and is also associated with the spread of syphilis and gonorrhea. Condoms can be used, but they tend to break during anal sex. Sex educators advise couples engaging in anal sex to use a lubricant along with a condom.

abstinence Avoidance of sexual intercourse.

vaginal intercourse Intercourse characterized by the insertion of the penis into the vagina.

anal intercourse Intercourse characterized by the insertion of the penis into a partner's anus and rectum.

oral sex Stimulation of the genitals by the tongue or mouth.

fellatio Oral stimulation of the penis.

cunnilingus Oral stimulation of the vulva or clitoris.

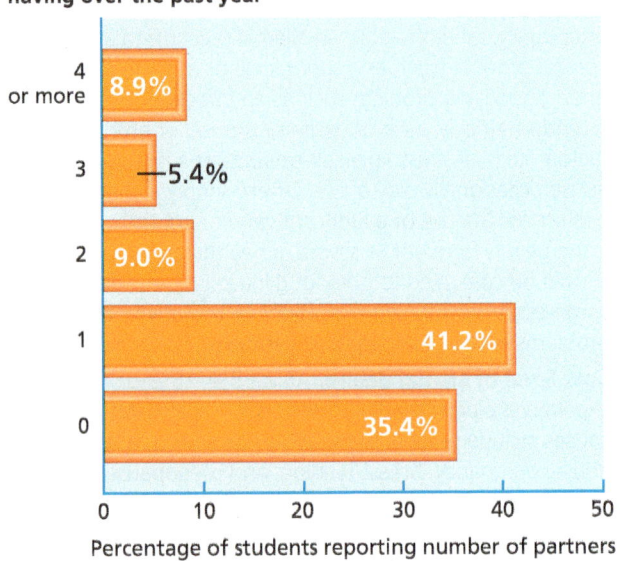

STUDENT STATS

Sex and the College Student

Number of sexual partners college students reported having over the past year

Number of partners	Percentage
4 or more	8.9%
3	5.4%
2	9.0%
1	41.2%
0	35.4%

Data from American College Health Association. (2015). *ACHA-NCHA II: Undergraduate reference group executive summary, fall 2015.* www.acha-ncha.org.

Oral Sex

Oral sex is the stimulation of the genitals by the tongue or mouth. **Fellatio** is oral stimulation of the penis, and **cunnilingus** is oral stimulation of the vulva, especially the clitoris. In a national survey, 65.9% of college students report having had oral sex.[3] Some couples use oral sex as *foreplay,* stimulation that is erotic and is intended to increase arousal prior to sexual intercourse. Some engage in oral sex in place of sexual intercourse, and others avoid the practice. Although oral sex does not result in pregnancy, it is not necessarily "safer" sex. Unprotected oral sex can leave a partner vulnerable to the transmission of herpes, syphilis, hepatitis B, HPV, and gonorrhea (see Chapter 12). Using a condom or dental dam can help prevent the spread of STIs; however, only 5.7% of sexually active college students report using a condom or dental dam when having oral sex.[3]

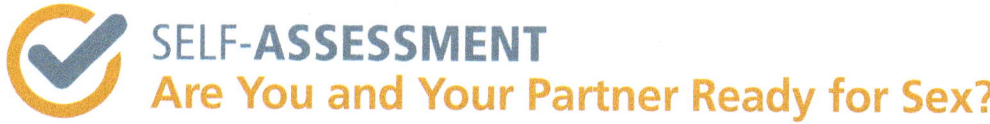

SELF-ASSESSMENT
Are You and Your Partner Ready for Sex?

Maybe you've only been on two dates. Maybe you've been "just friends" for 2 years. But sooner or later, the question is going to demand an answer: Are the two of you ready for your relationship to become sexual? Here are some questions that can help you decide.

1. Is your decision to have sex completely your own (that is, you feel no pressure from others, including your partner)? __Yes __No
2. Is your decision to have sex based on the right reasons? (The wrong reasons are peer pressure, a need to fit in or make your partner happy, or a belief that sex will make your relationship with your partner better or closer. If you decide to have sex, it should be because you feel emotionally and physically ready and your partner is someone you love, trust, and respect.) __Yes __No
3. Do you feel your partner would respect any decision you made about whether to have sex? __Yes __No
4. Do you trust and respect your partner? __Yes __No
5. Are you able to comfortably talk to your partner about sex and your partner's sexual history? __Yes __No
6. Do you know how to prevent pregnancy and STIs? __Yes __No
7. Are you and your partner willing to use contraception to prevent pregnancy and STIs? __Yes __No
8. Have you and your partner talked about what both of you would do in the event of pregnancy or if one of you were to develop an STI? __Yes __No
9. Do you feel completely comfortable with the idea of having sex with this partner? __Yes __No

HOW TO INTERPRET YOUR SCORE If you answered "No" to *any* of these questions, you are not really ready for sex with this partner. If you think you should have sexual intercourse because others want you to or everyone else is doing it, these are not the right reasons. You should only decide to have sex because you trust and respect your partner, you know the possible risks, you know how to protect yourself against the risks, and, most importantly, because you know that you are ready!

To complete this Self-Assessment online, visit MasteringHealth™

Source: "Quiz: Are You Ready for Sex?" © 2010 by the Center for Young Women's Health at Children's Hospital, Boston. All rights reserved. Used with permission.

> **"A wide range of human sexual behaviors and interests are considered 'normal.'"**

Communicating About Sex

Each year in the United States, more than 15 million cases of STIs are diagnosed and well over 1 million unplanned pregnancies are terminated.[24] Given these statistics, it seems obvious that practicing safer sex is crucial. But before you can practice it, you have to talk about it. It's also important to communicate what you're comfortable with in terms of sexual behaviors, frequency, and other potentially sensitive issues. So how do you get up the nerve to talk candidly about sex? See **Practical Strategies** on page 277.

Non-Intercourse Sexual Activity

There are a number of ways people experience sexual pleasure without actually engaging in sexual intercourse. Among them are masturbation, sexual fantasies, and outercourse. Pornography, another form of non-intercourse sexual activity, is discussed in the **Media and Sexuality** box on page 266.

Masturbation

Masturbation is the manipulation of one's own genitals for sexual pleasure. It is a healthy and common expression of sexuality. Research indicates that 92% of male college students and 68% of female college students have masturbated.[25]

Two other forms of non-intercourse sexual activity often accompany masturbation: sexual fantasy and viewing pornography. Sexual fantasies are sexual or romantic thoughts, daydreams, and imagined scenarios featuring fictional characters or actual people. They may reflect a person's unconscious desires, allowing the person to imagine sexual experiences that they may not feel comfortable acting out in real life. Pornography is viewed by 43% of college males at least once or twice a week.[26] For most, it causes no problems, but for some, excessive use can interfere with healthy sexual relationships.

Outercourse

Although the definition can vary, **outercourse** generally refers to sexual intimacy without penetration of the vagina or anus. Outercourse includes everything from kissing and "making out" to manual stimulation of the genitals and mutual masturbation. Because no semen enters the vagina during outercourse, there is no risk of pregnancy. The risk of STIs is also minimized, although infections like herpes and HPV can still spread via skin-to-skin genital contact.

masturbation Manipulation of one's own genitals for sexual pleasure.

outercourse Sexual intimacy without penetration of the vagina or anus.

sexting The use of cell phones or similar electronic devices to send sexually explicit text, photos, or videos.

Sexting

Sexting (the use of electronic devices to send sexually explicit text, photos, or videos) has become more mainstream

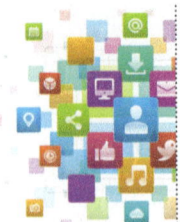

MEDIA AND Sexuality
Is Porn a Problem?

Pornography, explicit sexual material used for sexual excitement and erotic stimulation, has never been more available. Porn appears in a host of media, including books, magazines, photos, animation, film, sculpture, painting, and video games; however, the two top revenue generators are video sales and rentals and Internet sites. Of all websites, approximately 12% (4.2 million) are pornographic, and 25% of all search engine requests (68 million) are related to pornography. In the United States alone, pornography is estimated to be a $12 billion business.[1]

With porn so ubiquitous in our society, college campuses are far from exempt. A study conducted by East Carolina University found that 43% of college students reported looking at pornography at least once or twice a week. Almost 32% of college men reported viewing pornography three to five times per week, while fewer than 4% of college women reported doing so. The findings from this study also suggest that the Internet is the primary source of pornography for college students.[2] Interestingly, according to Pornhub, the world's biggest porn site, 63% of its traffic in 2015 was from mobile devices, up from 12% just 5 years ago.[3]

Along with commercial pornography websites, there has been an increase in noncommercial, free sites where visitors can post their own photos and videos. Some of these sites are devoted to college students and are referred to as "dorm porn." Some experts contend that such noncommercial pornographic websites reflect a larger trend toward digital self-exploitation.[4]

In the East Carolina University study, men expressed greater approval of pornography, and women reported feeling more threatened by it. Is there anything behind these concerns? Pamela Paul, a prominent researcher and author on the effects of pornography, cites several issues surrounding pornography that can be problematic.[5] Looking at porn wastes time: Studies are delayed or cut short, work is interrupted, and relationships are put on hold. It also wastes money: Once users become "acclimated" to free sites, they move to expensive services. Porn has addictive elements, claiming increasing amounts of time and money; interfering with activities of daily living, goals, and relationships; and involving a sense of compulsion. Particularly on the Internet, users find themselves turning more often to increasingly violent and shocking images, including those involving abuse, torture, or children. Many users report feeling increasingly debased by their porn use; images that once would have disgusted them come to seem "routine," and ever harder-core porn becomes a requirement for sexual arousal.

Porn has specific effects on romantic relationships as well. Porn is essentially a form of voyeurism, involving looking at but not interacting with the model or actor. As such, it elevates the physical—body parts and acts—while ignoring all other qualities that make us human. Viewers learn to relate to others as objects rather than to form and maintain relationships with them. Not surprisingly, porn reduces the viewer's ability to be close to others—including their current partner.

What Do You Think?

1. Do you agree that men and women often have different views about porn? If so, what do you think are some of the factors behind these differences?
2. What are some common stereotypes about men and women depicted in pornography?
3. How might these stereotypes be detrimental to a person's real-life relationships?

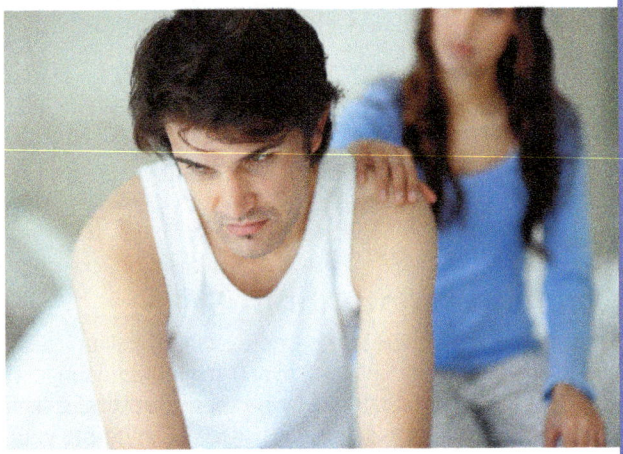

Excessive use of pornography can interfere with relationships in real life.

data. www.pornhub.com. 4. Jaishankar, K. (2009). Editorial: Sexting: A new form of victimless crime? *International Journal of Cyber Criminology*, 3(1), 21–25. 5. Paul, P. (2010, March 7). The cost of growing up on porn. www.washingtonpost.com.

References 1. Brigham Young University. (2010). *National pornography statistics.* https://wsr.byu.edu. 2. O'Reilly, S., Knox, D., & Zusman, M. E. (2007). College student attitudes toward pornography use. *College Student Journal, 41,* 402–404. 3. Pornhub Insights. (2015, September 30). Apple vs. Android. Pornhub

---

on college campuses. A recent study of college students found that most who engaged in this behavior did so in the context of a romantic relationship. While sexting seems to have become an acceptable form of sexual expression for today's young adults,[27] there are still risks associated with it.

Before sending any texts or images with sexual content, consider the following:

- **Make sure all participants are adults.** Some states have enacted specific laws against sexting involving minors, and it is a crime in all states for an adult to possess or distribute sexually explicit images of a minor or to coerce or solicit a minor to send these images.

- **Sexting under the influence can have unintended consequences.** Sexting can have consequences, so make sure you are in full control of your faculties before you make the decision to send what might later be an embarrassing photo or video.

- **Don't succumb to pressure from peers or a partner.** Anyone who pressures you about any type of sexual activity isn't the type of person you want to be involved with. Think very carefully about the potential future consequences of an explicit message, photo, or video.
- **Remember that a sext is forever.** Once something is launched into cyberspace, it is out there forever. There is no such thing as privacy online. Remember that an explicit photo or video that was originally intended for one person can surface later on and cause a great deal of harm to your reputation, career, and personal relationships.

>> Do you have questions about sex that you are afraid to ask? *Go Ask Alice* is a website sponsored by Columbia University that answers many frequently asked questions: www.goaskalice.columbia.edu.

LO 11.4 QUICK CHECK

Which of the following is the correct term for oral sex performed on a female?
a. outercourse
b. fellatio
c. coitus
d. cunnilingus

Sexual Orientation and Gender Identity

LO 11.5 Discuss sexual orientation and gender identity.

At a very early age, humans begin to develop their **sexual orientation,** their romantic and physical attraction toward others. Experts believe that our natural tendency to be attracted to men or women—or both—is shaped by a confluence of biological, environmental, and cognitive factors, with sexual orientation being neither a conscious choice nor something that can be readily changed.

Sex researcher Alfred Kinsey theorized that sexual orientation could be delineated on a continuum, divided into seven parts. At one end of the Kinsey Scale are **heterosexuals,** "straight" people who are solely attracted to the opposite gender. On the other end are **homosexuals,** *gays* or *lesbians* who are attracted to people of the same gender. In the middle are **bisexuals,** individuals who are attracted to members of their own sex as well as the opposite sex. In between these points on the scale are varying levels of bisexuality.

Heterosexuality

Worldwide, the majority of people describe themselves as heterosexual. In the United States, CDC survey found that 96.6% of adults aged 18–64 identified themselves as straight, 1.6% as gay or lesbian, 0.7% as bisexual, and 1.1% as "other."[28]

Heterosexuality is the only sexual orientation that receives full social and legal legitimacy in most countries. As a result of this and other cultural factors, homosexuals and bisexuals can be subjected to "heterosexism," which includes negative attitudes, bias, and discrimination in favor of heterosexual relationships. Those with a heterosexist view think that their orientation is the only "normal" one.

> "In the United States, the American Psychiatric Association removed homosexuality from its manual of psychiatric disorders in 1973."

Homosexuality

Homosexuality is deeply rooted in many world cultures, having been an accepted practice in some parts of the ancient world. In other regions it has been and is still shunned. For example, psychiatrists in some countries, including China, India, and Brazil, still consider it a mental illness.

In the United States, the American Psychiatric Association removed homosexuality from its manual of psychiatric disorders in 1973, in response to a growing understanding of homosexuality as a normal variant of sexual orientation. In 2015, the U.S. Supreme Court ruled that the Constitution guarantees a right to same-sex marriage.[29] Correspondingly, there has been an increasing acceptance of homosexuality in U.S. culture. For example, in a 1973 survey, 70% of people in the United States reported believing that homosexual relations are always sinful; but in 2009, only 49% expressed this belief.[30] As of 2015, the majority of Americans (55%) supported same-sex marriage, compared with 35% who supported it in 2001.[31]

Still, many homosexuals continue to face discrimination and harassment in the United States, a fact acknowledged by 64% of the population.[30] This discrimination can take many forms, including **homonegativity**—negative attitudes toward homosexuality—or **homophobia**—irrational fear of, aversion to, or discrimination against homosexuals or homosexuality. The harassment often begins at an early age. In one study, researchers found that homosexual and bisexual students "are at greater risk of suicidal thoughts, suicide attempts, victimization by peers, and elevated levels of unexcused absences from school," with 84.6% of such students reporting verbal abuse and 40.1% reporting having been physically assaulted because of their sexual orientation.[32] They were also twice as likely to have skipped school in the previous month out of a concern for their own safety. Homonegativity and homophobia sometimes erupt into criminal

sexual orientation Romantic and physical attraction toward others.

heterosexuals People who are sexually attracted to partners of the opposite sex.

homosexuals People who are sexually attracted to partners of the same sex.

bisexuals People who are attracted to partners of the same and the opposite sex.

homonegativity Negative attitudes toward homosexuality.

homophobia Irrational fear of, aversion to, or discrimination against homosexuals or homosexuality.

violence: In 2014, the FBI reported that 18.6% of all hate crimes were against homosexuals.[33]

Bisexuality

One common (and inaccurate) definition of bisexuality is having sexual relations with people of the same and opposite genders, often outside of a monogamous relationship. Yet, as the Kinsey Scale indicates, sexual orientation may be experienced as a continuum, rather than a set of rigid rules, and many bisexual people may find that their preference on this continuum can vary over time.[34] Some bisexuals may choose not to act on their innate impulses, whereas others have not had the opportunity to do so. Some may pursue a monogamous relationship with a man at one point in their lives and a committed relationship with a woman later. A better gauge of bisexuality is having an attraction to both men and women. The intensity of the attraction can change over time, but bisexuality should not be seen as a "phase" that a person is going through. In one long-term study of bisexual women, the subjects reported being attracted to both sexes throughout the 10-year study period.[35] Bisexuality, the experts wrote, is a "stable identity" rather than a "transitional stage."

Gender Identity

Whereas the term *sex* refers to an individual's biological status as male or female, *gender* is "one's innermost concept of self as male, female, a blend of both, or neither."[36] It includes how people perceive themselves and how they identify themselves. An infant's biological sex usually becomes a profound component of the growing child's gender identity. But for some people, their biological sex and the gender they identify with differ.

transgender A person whose gender identity or gender expression is different from his or her biological sex.

transsexual A person who has permanently changed or is transitioning to the opposite gender through clinical interventions such as hormone therapy and surgery.

Gender expression is the appearance of a person's *gender identity* (clothing, voice, hair, etc.), which may or may not conform to his or her biological sex. **Transgender** people have gender identities that are the opposite of their biological sex. Those who choose to express their own sense of gender identity rather than the one that corresponds to their biological sex are considered to be going through the process of *gender transition*. This process might include the use of new names and pronouns, dressing differently, and/or asking to be socially recognized as another gender. The transition process is complex and varies from person to person; it may or may not include medical treatments such as taking hormones or surgery. It is important to note that being a transgender person does not imply any specific sexual orientation.

The term **transsexual** originated in medical and psychological practice to describe people who have changed or are changing their bodies to another sex through clinical interventions such as hormone therapy and surgery. Many in today's lesbian, gay, bisexual, or transgender (LGBT) community prefer the term *transgender*.

Only those who experience clinically significant distress due to their biological sex differing from their gender identity

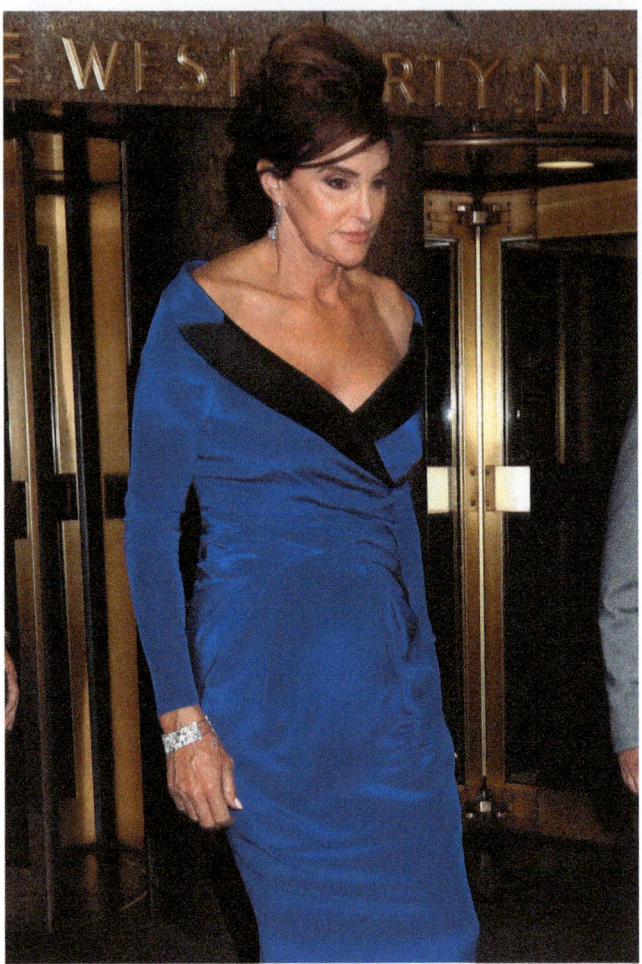

Until 2015, Caitlin Jenner was previously known as Bruce Jenner, a U.S. Olympian.

are considered to suffer from *gender dysphoria*. This diagnosis replaces the older term *gender identity disorder*; it emphasizes that many who identify with the opposite gender are not experiencing clinically significant distress and therefore do not have a mental illness. Despite the complexities of their lives, many transgender individuals report feeling comfortable with their gender identity and sexual orientation.[37]

LO 11.5 QUICK CHECK

John, who was born "Jane," now lives his life as a male instead of a female. Which of the following best describes John?
a. homosexual
b. heterosexual
c. transgender
d. homophobic

Conception and Contraception

LO 11.6 Compare and contrast different methods of contraception.

More than half of pregnancies in the United States are unintended.[38] The U.S. abortion rate, while lower than its all-time high, continues to be among the highest in the

STUDENT STORY

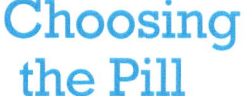

Choosing the Pill

"**HI, I'M BETTY.** When discussing contraceptives with my mom, she gave me so many options. She works in maternal health care, so she had this huge planner out and she was like 'this is a female condom and this is this and that'—and it was just like, I don't even want to know all the other stuff. I didn't want an IUD and I didn't want a female condom or anything like that. . . . I was like, let me go to the simplest form. That way if I decide 'OK, if I don't want to take this anymore, then I can get rid of it. I ended up deciding to get on the pill. The pros are that you always know when your period is going to arrive, it lessens PMS and cramping, and you won't get pregnant. The cons—you have to continuously stay on it. You have to keep it as a ritual: like, get in the shower, brush your teeth, and before you brush your teeth, take your pill. Sometimes it can make you nauseous. That's another con, but other than that, it's great."

What Do You Think?

1. Given what you've learned in this chapter, do you think birth control pills alone are enough to protect you (or your partner) against pregnancy? How about STIs? Explain your answer.
2. Betty was able to turn to her mom for contraceptive advice. Think about the resources available to you. How will you learn more about contraceptive options and decide which one is right for you?
3. Betty explained her "ritual" for taking the pill. Why is it important for women to incorporate oral contraceptives into their daily routine?

industrialized world. In addition, failure to use protective birth control options such as condoms exposes millions of people to STIs that can cause life-threatening disease and infertility. So whether or not you are planning to have children, it is important to understand your fertility, how to protect it, and the family planning methods available.

Conception

At birth, a female's ovaries are filled with more than 1 million ovarian follicles, each containing an immature egg. After puberty, a woman's body prepares itself for pregnancy each month by ovulating—releasing one egg. Meanwhile, a man's testes are constantly creating sperm, millions of which can be released into a woman's vagina during ejaculation. The vast majority of these sperm will never find their way to their target; millions will leak from the vagina or be destroyed in its acidic environment. The few thousand sperm that do reach the egg—typically while it is still within the fallopian tube—next face the difficult task of penetrating the egg's tough outer layer. After a sperm breaches this outer layer, the egg undergoes a chemical change that blocks any further sperm from penetrating its membrane. The "winning sperm" then travels to the egg's nucleus, and fertilization—or **conception,** the combination of the genetic material (DNA) of an egg and sperm cell—occurs.

Even then, pregnancy is not guaranteed. The fertilized egg, now called a **zygote,** must complete its journey through the fallopian tube and emerge into the uterus, where it can implant in the endometrium, in a process called **implantation.** Any scar tissue within the tube can "snag" the zygote so that it attaches to the wall of the tube, where it cannot grow. In some cases the zygote will make it into the uterus but fail to implant, and the entire process from menstruation to ovulation will begin all over again.

conception Fertilization of a female egg with male sperm.

zygote A fertilized egg.

implantation Lodging of a fertilized egg in the endometrium of the uterus.

contraception Any method used to prevent pregnancy.

Figure 11.4 summarizes the processes of conception through implantation.

Contraceptive Options

Contraception is any method used to prevent pregnancy. Approximately 70% of U.S. women between the ages of 25 and 44 use some form of contraception.[39] Contraceptive options differ in terms of method, price, effectiveness, and side effects, but all have the same goal of prevening pregnancy. They do this in a number of ways:

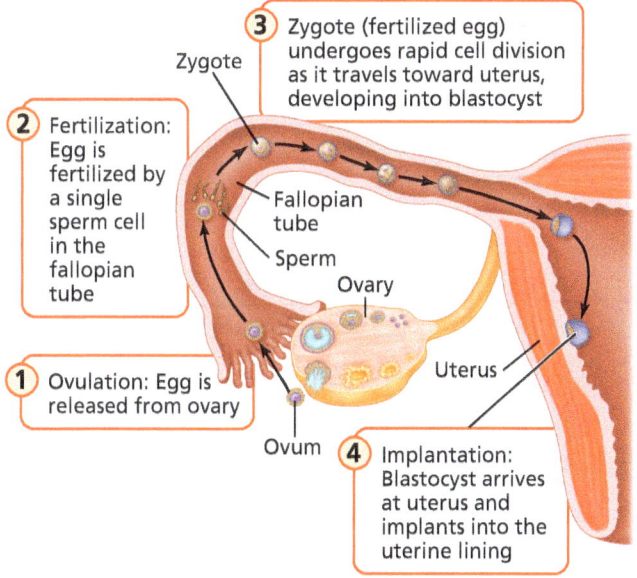

FIGURE 11.4 Events Involved in Conception. The process of conception includes ovulation, fertilization, and implantation.

Source: Thompson, J., Manore, M., & Vaughan, L. (2011). *The science of nutrition*, 3rd ed. Reprinted and electronically reproduced by permission of Pearson Education, Inc., Upper Saddle River, New Jersey.

- *Natural methods* involve no pills or devices and are therefore always available and cost-free.
- *Barrier methods* work to prevent sperm from reaching an egg.
- *Hormonal methods* deliver hormones to a woman that prevent ovulation. If no egg is released, fertilization cannot occur.
- *Surgical methods* are available for women and men and are the most permanent options.

Table 11.1 summarizes different forms of contraception, organized into four categories: cost-free methods, over-the-counter methods, those requiring a prescription, and surgical interventions. As we take a closer look at these methods, take note of differences in availability, cost, effectiveness, ease of use, and whether the method provides protection against STIs. The **Student Stats** box on page 273 illustrates the most popular forms of contraception reported by college students.

TABLE 11.1 A Summary of Contraceptive Options

Method	Description	Advantages	Disadvantages	Failure Rate*	Average Cost
Cost-Free Methods					
Intimacy without intercourse	Engaging in sexual or sensual behavior without vaginal penetration	Prevents pregnancy and STIs	Requires mutual commitment, trust, and self-control	No statistics available	No cost
Fertility awareness (rhythm or calendar method)	Understanding the monthly menstrual cycle and avoiding intercourse on fertile days	No cost	No protection against STIs; not as effective if cycle is irregular; high possibility of failure	1–25	No cost
Withdrawal	Withdrawing the penis before ejaculation	No cost	No protection against STIs; high risk of pregnancy; requires physical and psychological control and awareness	19	No cost
Over-the-Counter Methods					
Male condom (such as Durex, Lifestyles, Trojan)	Very thin sheath that fits over an erect penis to prevent semen from entering vagina	No medical exam required; side effects are uncommon; latex condoms protect against many STIs	Only about 80%–94% effective at preventing pregnancy; if not used correctly, unintended pregnancies can occur; requires planning	2–15	$0.50–$3.00 each use
Female condom (such as Reality, FC2)	A thin sheath with a soft outer ring and a pliable inner ring; the condom covers the inside of the entire vagina	Protects against STIs	Some users may have difficulty inserting the condom correctly	5–21	$0.50–$3.00 each use
Contraceptive sponge (such as Today Sponge)	A round, soft foam sponge containing spermicide with a nylon loop for removal	Easy to obtain, no medical exam required; easy to carry; can be left in place for up to 30 hours	No protection against STIs and increases risk of STIs and other infections; may cause irritation in some women	9–16	$9–$15 for a packet of three sponges
Spermicides (such as Encare, VCF, Gynol)	Chemical compounds that immobilize sperm	Easy to obtain, no medical exam required; variety of forms for convenience	May leak; high failure rate if used alone; doesn't protect against STIs; increases risk of some STIs	18–29 if used alone, but spermicides increase protection when used with other barrier methods	$0.50–$3.00 each use
Emergency contraception (EC) (Also known as the "morning-after pill," such as Plan B One-Step Next Choice One Dose, My Way, Take Action)	A single pill or two pills containing a synthetic form of progestin that can suppress ovulation and disrupt implantation	Effective when used within 72 hours after unprotected intercourse to prevent pregnancy, although most effective within the first 24 hours following intercourse	Not effective if woman has already ovulated prior to using; begins to lose effectiveness 24–72 hours after intercourse; does not protect against STIs	No statistics available	$35–$60

TABLE 11.1 A Summary of Contraceptive Options (continued)

Method	Description	Advantages	Disadvantages	Failure Rate*	Average Cost
Methods Requiring Prescriptions					
Diaphragm	A soft dome-shaped cup with a flexible rim that is filled with spermicide and fits inside the vagina, covering the cervix	Does not require the ingestion of hormones; may be left in place for up to 24 hours	No protection against STIs; cannot be used during menstruation; some women find insertion difficult; may become dislodged; requires an exam and fitting by a health-care provider; may cause urinary tract infection or vaginal irritation in some users	6–16	$100–$200 for device, fitting, and spermicide
Cervical cap	A pliable cup filled with spermicide that fits inside the vagina, covering the cervix	Does not require the ingestion of hormones; may be left in place for up to 48 hours	No protection against STIs; cannot be used during menstruation; some women find insertion difficult; may become dislodged; requires an exam and fitting by a health-care provider; may cause urinary tract infection or vaginal irritation in some users	6–16	$100–$200 for device, fitting, and spermicide
Intrauterine Device (IUD): ParaGard	A small T-shaped plastic device that releases copper	No action necessary before, during, or after sex; can be left in place for 10–12 years	No protection against STIs; in rare cases, may cause infections or the device may slip out	Less than 1	$200–$300
Intrauterine Device (IUD): Mirena Liletta Skyla	A small T-shaped plastic device that releases progestin	No action necessary before, during, or after sex; may lessen periods or cause them to cease; can be left in place for up to 5 years	No protection against STIs; in rare cases, may cause infections or the device may slip out	Less than 1	$200–$300
Birth control pills (*A variety of combination pills are available.*)	Pills containing the hormones estrogen and progestin, which prevent pregnancy; one pill should be taken at the same time each day	Convenient; helps protect against cancer of the ovaries and uterus; some women have lighter periods and milder cramps	No protection against STIs; requires taking a pill each day, which may be hard to remember; refills must be on hand; requires ingesting artificial hormones; adverse effects possible; consultation with health-care provider is essential	1–8	$20–$35 per month
Emergency contraception (EC)/*ella*	A "morning-after pill" that can be taken up to 5 days after sexual intercourse to suppress ovulation and prevent pregnancy	Unlike OTC EC, can be taken up to 5 days after sexual intercourse and still be effective	Not effective if woman has already ovulated prior to using; does not protect against STIs; requires a prescription	No statistics available	No information available at press time
"Mini-pill"	Pills containing the hormone progestin, which prevents pregnancy	Convenient; helps protect against cancer of the ovaries and uterus; some women have lighter periods and milder cramps; better choice for women who are at risk for developing blood clots	No protection against STIs; requires taking a pill each day, which may be hard to remember; refills must be on hand; requires ingesting artificial hormones; several adverse effects possible; consultation with health-care provider is essential	1–8	$20–$35 per month
Transdermal patch	A thin plastic patch that is placed on the skin, which releases the hormones estrogen and progestin slowly into the body	Convenient—woman does not have to remember to take a pill every day; may reduce risk of endometrial cancer and other cancers; relieves PMS and menstrual cramping and improves acne	No protection against STIs; may cause bleeding between periods, breast tenderness, or nausea and vomiting; may cause skin irritation at patch site; may alter a woman's sexual desire; may be less effective in women who weigh more than 198 pounds; several long-term adverse effects possible; consultation with health-care provider is essential	1–8	$25–$30 per month
Vaginal ring (NuvaRing)	A small flexible ring that slowly releases the hormones estrogen and progestin into the body	Convenient—woman does not have to remember to take a pill every day; may reduce risk of endometrial cancer and other cancers; relieves PMS and menstrual cramping and improves acne	No protection against STIs; may cause bleeding between periods, breast tenderness, or nausea and vomiting; may increase vaginal discharge and lead to irritation or infection; may alter a woman's sexual desire; several long-term adverse effects possible; consultation with health-care provider is essential	1–8	Cost of initial health-care appointment plus $15–$50 per month

TABLE 11.1 A Summary of Contraceptive Options (continued)

Method	Description	Advantages	Disadvantages	Failure Rate*	Average Cost
Monthly injections	An injection containing the hormones estrogen and progestin	Convenient, may help reduce risk of certain cancers and promote lighter, shorter periods	No protection against STIs; requires monthly visit to health-care provider; side effects may include bloating/weight gain, headaches, vaginal bleeding, and irregular periods; women over age 35 or who smoke or have certain health conditions are at risk for serious adverse effects	1–3	$30–$35 month
Quarterly injections	An injection containing the hormone progestin	Convenient; requires only one injection four times a year; helps protect against endometrial cancer; reduces monthly bleeding and anemia; in most cases, women stop having their periods	No protection against STIs; side effects may include amenorrhea, headaches, depression, loss of interest in sex, and bone loss; fertility may be delayed for many months after discontinuing; not advised for women who want less than a year of birth control	1–3	$60–$75 for 3 months
Implant	A thin plastic rod containing the hormone progestin	Convenient; lasts 5 years; helps protect women from endometrial cancer	No protection against STIs; insertion and removal of implants requires a small cut in the skin, and scarring may occur; if implants fail, there is a greater chance of ectopic pregnancy; side effects may include acne, headaches, weight gain	1	$450–$750 for 5 years
Surgical Methods					
Tubal ligation	The fallopian tubes are surgically tied or otherwise sealed	Convenient; no hormonal effect; permanent solution to birth control	No protection against STIs; invasive; permanent	Less than 1	$1,500–$6,000
Hysterectomy	Surgical removal of a woman's uterus, sometimes along with her ovaries and fallopian tubes	May be necessary to treat health conditions such as excessive menstrual bleeding or tumors	Irreversible	No statistics available	No information available
Vasectomy	A minor surgical procedure performed at a hospital or clinic in which the vas deferens is tied off and cut on both sides of the scrotum	Convenient; procedure does not affect sexual desire or hormone levels; male may resume sex as soon as it is comfortable; permanent solution to birth control	No protection against STIs; after the procedure the male will still have viable sperm for a period of time; sterilization is considered permanent	Less than 1	$350–$1,000, including sperm count test after procedure

*Number of women out of 100 likely to become pregnant during the first year of use. Number ranges indicate perfect versus typical use.

Source: Data from Planned Parenthood. (2013). Comparing effectiveness of birth control methods. www.plannedparenthood.org.

Cost-Free Methods

Three methods of contraception are always available and without cost. They are intimacy without intercourse, fertility awareness, and withdrawal. Note that none of these methods are 100% reliable.

Intimacy Without Intercourse. Some couples who desire a sexual relationship yet want to avoid the risks of pregnancy and STIs opt for non-intercourse sexual activities like kissing, "making out," manual stimulation of the genitals, and mutual masturbation. Because intercourse doesn't occur, the chance of pregnancy or STIs is theoretically zero. However, in reality, this method requires a high level of commitment, self-discipline, and mutual cooperation and trust.

Fertility Awareness (Rhythm or Calendar Method). With **fertility awareness (rhythm or calendar method),** a woman tracks on a calendar the day her period begins each month. Ideally, she also logs the days on which she had copious, slippery cervical mucus because its presence indicates that she is fertile (the mucus occurs as ovulation approaches). Finally, if possible, she makes a note of the day on which she experienced midcycle pain (indicating ovulation). **Figure 11.5** provides an example of fertility tracking. Because most women's cycles vary somewhat from month to month, it's essential that a woman using the fertility awareness method track her cycles for several months (a full year is ideal) before relying on this method. Also, keep in mind that this method is not fail-safe; women with irregular menstrual cycles should rely on other methods of contraception.

> **fertility awareness (rhythm or calendar method)** Tracking of a woman's monthly menstrual cycle; may be used as a method of preventing pregnancy if the woman tracks carefully and has regular periods, although it is not fail-safe.

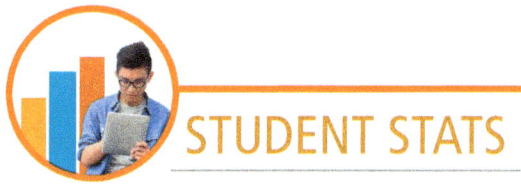

STUDENT STATS

Contraception and College Students

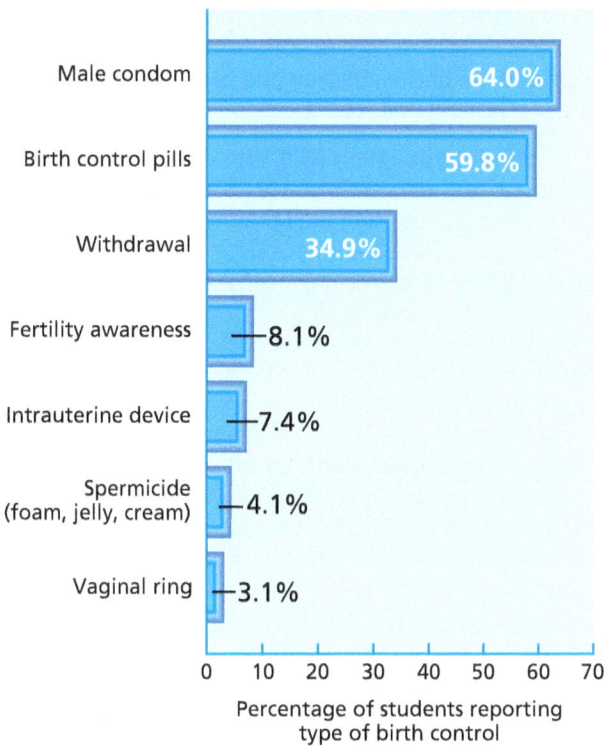

Top methods of contraception used by college students*

- Male condom — 64.0%
- Birth control pills — 59.8%
- Withdrawal — 34.9%
- Fertility awareness — 8.1%
- Intrauterine device — 7.4%
- Spermicide (foam, jelly, cream) — 4.1%
- Vaginal ring — 3.1%

Percentage of students reporting type of birth control

* Who engaged in vaginal intercourse and used contraception

Data from American College Health Association. (2015). *ACHA-NCHA II: Undergraduate reference group executive summary, fall 2015.* www.acha-ncha.org.

> "In addition to the careful planning required, the fertility awareness method requires couples to abstain from sexual intercourse for 11 days out of each cycle."

Using the data from several months, the woman next calculates her average cycle length (for example, 28 days, 32 days, etc.). Because sperm can survive for 5 days in the vagina—possibly more—and an egg is viable for up to 2 days, a woman is theoretically able to conceive as many as 5 days before she ovulates and as many as 2 days afterward. However, to be on the safe side, women should avoid intercourse for 7 days prior to ovulation and 4 days afterward.

Some women also track their body temperature, which typically rises slightly after ovulation. However, because the temperature increase is so slight—usually less than 1 degree—and must be recorded at the same time every morning before getting out of bed, many women do not have success with this method.

In addition to the careful planning required, the fertility awareness method requires couples to abstain from sexual intercourse for 11 days out of each cycle. If couples also abstain during the first few days the woman is having her period, this can eliminate half of all days each month. During that time, the couple can use other forms of contraception or engage in non-intercourse sexual activity. Also note that when the couple does engage in unprotected intercourse, both partners may be at risk for STIs.

Withdrawal. Also called *coitus interruptus*, the **withdrawal** method requires the man to withdraw his penis from his partner's vagina before he ejaculates. Often the man is unable to do this, and consequently the withdrawal method is associated with a very high failure rate (see Table 11.1). Even if the man can exert the required self-control, pregnancy can still occur because the pre-ejaculate fluid may contain sperm. This method also provides no protection against STIs and can be unsatisfying for both partners. Despite these disadvantages, almost one-third of females age 15 to 24 report having relied on withdrawal in the previous 3 years.[40]

> **withdrawal** Withdrawal of the penis from the vagina before ejaculation.

Over-the-Counter Methods

Over-the-counter methods are available without a prescription or physical examination. They include condoms, which may be available from campus health clinics and other sources free of charge; the contraceptive sponge; spermicides; and emergency contraceptives.

Start of period: ○   Avoid sex: ✗

FIGURE 11.5 Fertility Awareness Tracking. Jotting down key events in the menstrual and ovulatory cycles can help couples identify which dates to avoid intercourse.

Condoms. The **condom (male condom)** is a thin sheath, typically made of latex, polyurethane, or lambskin (those made of lambskin do not provide as much protection against infection as condoms made of latex or polyurethane). The condom is unrolled over the erect penis prior to vaginal penetration. If used correctly **(Figure 11.6)** and consistently, condoms offer excellent protection against pregnancy and STIs. Either can occur, however, if the condom breaks or comes off during sex. Most condoms are lubricated. It's important to check the expiration date on the condom packet and to discard a condom if the expiration date has passed.

Some men feel that wearing a condom decreases their level of stimulation and pleasure. Experimenting with different sizes, types, and brands, as well as using a water-based personal lubricant, may help.

The female condom is a lubricated latex or polyurethane sheath with flexible rings on either end **(Figure 11.7).** Using an applicator, the woman inserts it into the vagina until the inner ring rests against the cervix. The outer ring remains outside the body, partly covering the labia. The female condom can be inserted several hours before sex and provides protection against both pregnancy and STIs. However, some women find it awkward to insert, and it can cause some discomfort during sex. It can also get pushed upward into the vagina. Finally, it is associated with a higher pregnancy rate than the male condom.

Contraceptive Sponge. A flexible foam disk containing spermicide, the **contraceptive sponge** is moistened with water and inserted into the vagina until it rests against the cervix. The sponge can cause irritation and dryness. It does not protect against STIs; in fact, it slightly increases the risk of contracting one. It must be left in place for 6 hours after intercourse and is associated with an increased risk of urinary tract infections, vaginal infections, and toxic shock syndrome.

Spermicides. A **spermicide** is a substance containing nonoxynol-9, a chemical that kills or immobilizes sperm. Spermicides are available as foams, gels, film, and suppositories. They are not very effective in preventing pregnancy, don't protect against STIs, and have been associated with an increased risk of HIV infection and bacterial urinary tract infection in women (see Table 11.1).[41]

Emergency Contraception (EC). Also called the **"morning after" pill, emergency contraception (EC)** is a one-dose pill containing the hormone levonorgestrel, a progestin. It is available over-the-counter under the brand name Plan B One-Step and in generic forms (e.g., Take Action, Next Choice One-Dose, My Way). While EC is effective up to 72 hours after unprotected sex, it is most effective within the first 24 hours after intercourse.[42] EC works by tricking the body into believing that pregnancy has already occurred, preventing ovulation, fertilization, or implantation. If a woman is already pregnant, EC will do nothing to stop the pregnancy. EC should not be confused with *RU-486*, the so-called abortion pill. A prescription-only form of EC called *ella* is available (discussed in the following section).

Methods Available by Prescription

Many more sophisticated methods of contraception are available by prescription. Prescription barrier methods include the diaphragm, cervical cap, and IUD. Prescription hormonal products are available in various delivery methods. All of these options are for women. Research into such methods for males is ongoing.

> **condom (male condom)** A thin sheath typically made of latex, polyurethane, or lambskin that is unrolled over an erect penis prior to vaginal penetration.
>
> **contraceptive sponge** A flexible foam disk containing spermicide that is inserted in the vagina prior to sex.
>
> **spermicide** A substance containing chemicals that kill or immobilize sperm.
>
> **emergency contraception (EC; "morning after" pill)** A pill containing levonorgestrel, a synthetic hormone used to prevent pregnancy after unprotected sex.

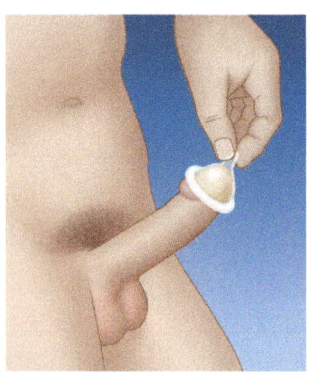 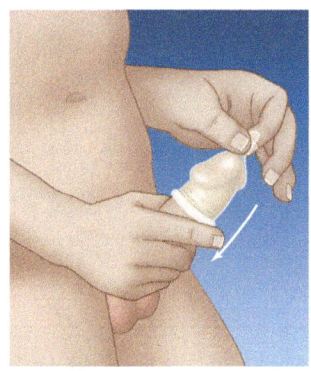 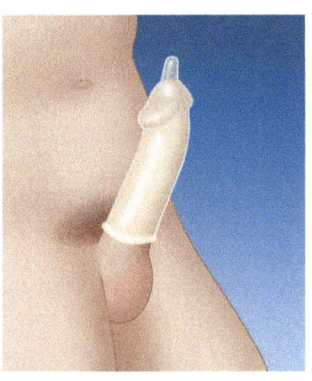 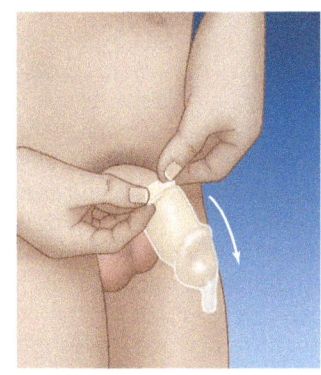

1. Pinch the tip of the condom to expel any air.
2. Keep the tip pinched with one hand. Use the other hand to roll the condom onto the penis.
3. Make sure the condom smoothly covers the entire penis.
4. After ejaculation, hold on to the base of the condom as you withdraw. Remove the condom carefully so that semen does not spill.

FIGURE 11.6 Using a Male Condom.

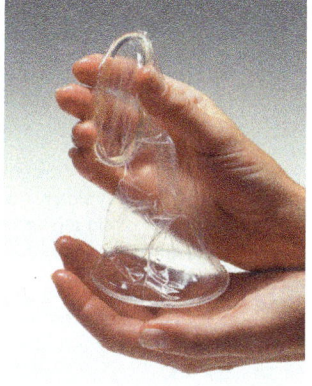 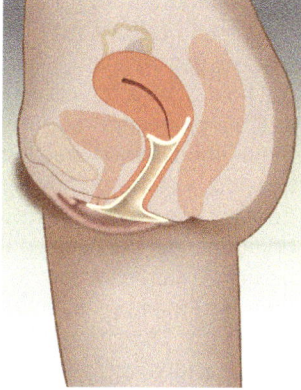

(a) Female condom (b) Female condom in place

FIGURE 11.7 **The Female Condom.** **(a)** The FC2 is made of synthetic latex. **(b)** A female condom properly inserted.

Diaphragm and Cervical Cap. The **diaphragm** and cervical cap are small, flexible, silicone cups that are filled with spermicide and inserted into the vagina **(Figure 11.8).** The devices must be fitted by a health-care provider, and some must be replaced annually. These devices must be left in place for at least 6 hours following intercourse and may be left in place for up to 24 hours. However, they do not reliably protect against STIs and are associated with an increased risk of urinary tract infection and toxic shock syndrome.

IUD. An **intrauterine device (IUD)** is a plastic, T-shaped device that is inserted by a health-care provider into the uterus for long-term pregnancy prevention. IUDs do not protect against STIs and can be expelled from the uterus. Four types are currently available in the United States, all of them highly effective in preventing pregnancy:

- The ParaGard Copper-T IUD continually releases copper, which works either by preventing sperm from reaching the fallopian tubes or by preventing implantation of a fertilized egg, should conception occur. It can be effective up to 10 years. The Copper-T can be inserted up to 5 days after unprotected sex to prevent pregnancy; it has the highest effectiveness rate of all contraceptive methods—99%. Side effects include cramps, nausea, severe menstrual pain and bleeding, painful sex, and anemia.[43]
- The Mirena hormonal IUD releases progestin, which works either by thickening the cervical mucus—blocking sperm transit—or by suppressing ovulation. It can be effective up to 5 years. Side effects include weight gain, acne, headaches, ovarian cysts, and abdominal pain.[44]
- Skyla and Liletta are newer hormonal IUDs that work by releasing a steady, very low dose of the hormone levonorgestrel. Women using these IUDs experienced decreased menstrual cramps and lighter periods. The most common side effects are abdominal pain, acne, headache, nausea, and breast tenderness.

Pharmaceutical Hormones. Synthetic hormones, including estrogen and progestin, are combined in **birth control pills,** typically referred to simply as "the pill" (**Figure 11.9**, next page). A progestin-only mini-pill is also available. Synthetic hormones are also available as a skin patch that is replaced weekly, a vaginal ring replaced monthly, injections given monthly or quarterly, and an under-the-skin implant that can last up to 3 years. To compare these hormonal methods, see **Table 11.1**.

Although hormonal methods are convenient and highly effective at preventing pregnancy, they do not protect against STIs; thus, condom use is still important. Also, because they release reproductive hormones into the body, these methods can provoke symptoms that mimic those of early pregnancy, including nausea, weight gain, breast tenderness, and moodiness.

> **diaphragm** A flexible silicone cup filled with spermicide and inserted in the vagina prior to sex to prevent pregnancy.
>
> **intrauterine device (IUD)** A plastic, T-shaped device inserted in the uterus for long-term pregnancy prevention.
>
> **birth control pills** Pills containing combinations of hormones that prevent pregnancy when taken regularly as directed.

In addition, women who have taken the pill for several months can experience long-term adverse effects. These include post-pill amenorrhea that can last for 3 to 6 months as well as increased blood pressure and an increased risk of cardiovascular disease, especially in smokers. Long-term use can also increase a woman's risk for cervical and liver cancers. On the upside, pill use can decrease a woman's risk for ovarian and endometrial cancer. The relationship between pill use and breast cancer is not clear.[45]

Other forms of hormonal contraceptives can have serious adverse effects. For example, the skin patch can increase the risk of blood clots, heart attack, and stroke, and the injection form can lead to reduced bone mineral density. Thus, anyone considering hormonal methods should carefully weigh the risks and benefits with her health-care provider.

In 2010, the Food and Drug Administration (FDA) approved the EC pill called *ella*. Unlike Plan B and related

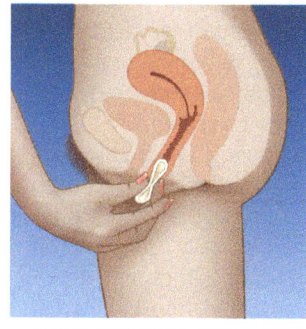 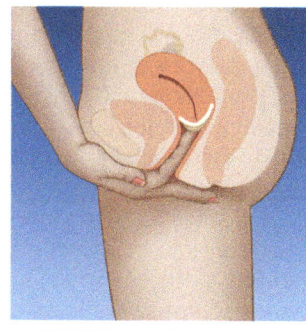

1 After filling the diaphragm with spermicide, hold it dome-side down and squeeze the opposite sides of the rim together.

2 Insert the diaphragm into the vagina, pushing it along the vaginal floor as far back as it will go. Make sure the diaphragm completely covers the cervix (the bump at the back of your vagina.) Tuck the front rim of the diaphragm up against your pelvic bone.

FIGURE 11.8 **Inserting a Diaphragm.**

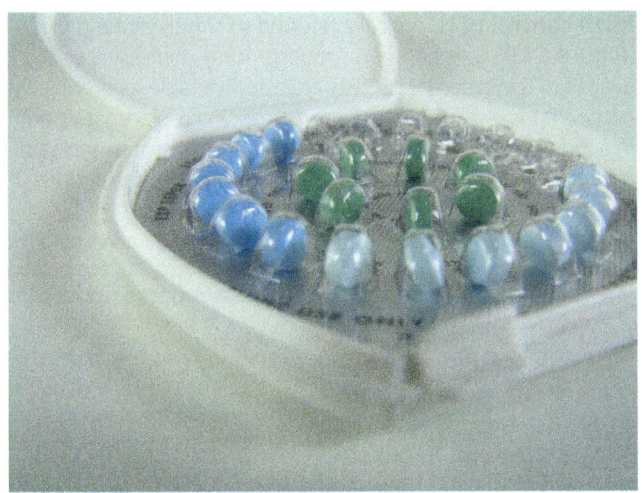

FIGURE 11.9 **A Typical Pack of Birth Control Pills.**

generics, which begin to lose effectiveness within 24 hours after sexual intercourse, *ella* is effective up to 5 days after unprotected sex.

Surgical Methods

The surgical methods discussed here are classified as *sterilization*; that is, they permanently prevent conception via surgical manipulation of the reproductive organs.

Tubal ligation is a surgical procedure in which a woman's fallopian tubes are tied off or sealed to prevent eggs from traveling toward the uterus. Sperm also cannot reach the eggs; thus, fertilization cannot occur. Tubal ligation can sometimes be reversed but should not be undertaken if a woman thinks she may change her mind.

A *hysterectomy* is a procedure in which a woman's uterus is surgically removed, sometimes along with the ovaries and fallopian tubes. It is considered to be permanent and irreversible sterilization; it is not an option for women who merely desire contraception. However, if other factors exist, such as excessive menstrual bleeding or benign or malignant uterine tumors, and she desires to permanently cease childbearing, then the procedure may be considered.

A *vasectomy* is a surgical procedure in which the male vas deferens are cut and then tied off or sealed. This makes it impossible for sperm (manufactured in the testes) to make their way into the semen. The man typically notices no difference in the quantity of semen he ejaculates, and although there is some swelling, bruising, and discomfort immediately after surgery, long-term complications are rare. The procedure is nearly 100% effective at preventing pregnancy and is difficult to reverse. Thus, men who choose vasectomy should consider the procedure permanent.[46]

Which Method Is the Best?

The answer to this question depends on each individual and each couple. When deciding which type of birth control to use, individuals and couples should consider how comfortable they are with the method, how many side effects it has, how well it works, and how likely they are to use it correctly.

It is important to note that although every method has a published **failure rate** (the percentage of women who typically get pregnant after using that method for 1 year), the figures are a bit misleading. That's because failure rates indicate pregnancy rates if the method is used exactly as directed, a concept known as "perfect use." In reality, couples do not always use birth control perfectly. Women forget to take their pills. Men put on condoms improperly. The end result is what is known as "typical use," which has substantially higher pregnancy rates. Another critical factor is the **continuation rate,** or the percentage of couples who continue to practice that form of birth control. Often, couples will stop using one method and, before choosing a new method, have unprotected sex.

> **failure rate** The percentage of women who typically get pregnant after using a given contraceptive method for 1 year.
>
> **continuation rate** The percentage of couples who continue to practice a given form of birth control.

When making a decision about the right birth control, either proactively on your own or as part of a couple, here are some factors to consider:

- Are you with one sexual partner? Or are you currently not in a committed relationship, or do you have more than one partner? Be sure your birth control considerations account for protection you may need against STIs as well as pregnancy.
- How good are you at sticking to routine? If you are a woman, will you remember to take a pill every day? Will you make a habit of keeping condoms available—and using them—when sexual encounters might be possible?
- Do you need or want a birth control method you can use without seeing a doctor? Some people, for reasons of cost or privacy, may prefer not to visit a doctor to seek birth control. However, as a student, you may have access to low-cost appointments and contraceptives through your student health center.
- Do you have any health risks, such as smoking? This is an especially important factor for women considering hormonal contraceptive methods such as birth control pills.
- Do you want to have children in the future? If so, you will want to rely on temporary methods of contraception.

If you are not yet in a sexual relationship but are considering one, talking to potential partners about contraception is another important step. For suggestions on how to make these conversations more effective and less awkward, see **Practical Strategies.**

>> Which contraceptive method is right for you? To find out, go to **www.mybirthcontrolapp.org.**

LO 11.6 QUICK CHECK

Where does fertilization of the egg normally occur?
a. ovary
b. fallopian tube
c. uterus
d. vagina

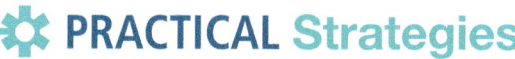

PRACTICAL Strategies

Communicating Effectively About Sex and Birth Control

If you are thinking about beginning a sexual relationship with someone, it's important to be able to communicate effectively about topics like sexual history, sexual health, contraceptive preferences, and how comfortable you each are with different types of sexual activity.

- **Know your preferences.** What do you hope for out of a sexual relationship? Are there certain sexual experiences that you aren't comfortable with? Do you know which type of contraception is right for you? Answer these types of questions for yourself first before you discuss them with a potential partner. Keep in mind that if you aren't ready for parenthood, contraception is a critical part of your decision making.

- **Prepare to talk.** Once your preferences are clear to you, jot down thoughts, concerns, and questions in advance. For instance, it's important to know your partner's sexual history. It's also important to share your own. What can you do to feel more comfortable asking about your partner's history, including experiences with contraceptives? Rehearsing the words in advance doesn't commit you to following a script, but it can help you frame your message in the moment with greater ease, clarity, and sensitivity.

- **Set a time to talk.** Once you're secure about the content of the conversation you want to have, reserve a time when you're both relaxed and not distracted and a place that's comfortable and private. You might want to tell your partner that there are some things you'd like to talk about and suggest that the two of you get together in a private place. Have the conversation before you are in a situation where you might have sex. Once you are "in the moment," it's especially hard to stop and have a detailed conversation about sexual history, STIs, and contraception.

- **Express your questions, concerns, and desires from a personal perspective.** Use "I" statements consistently, as in, "I'd like to know about your sexual history, and I will be honest in sharing mine." Pay attention to your partner's responses. Take in not only the words used but your partner's body language as well.

- **Be honest and clear.** Especially when it comes to deciding on a birth control method and agreeing on the sexual activities you're comfortable with, it's important that you stand up for your values and desires, even if they don't match your partner's. Make sure your partner understands your preferences.

- **Near the end of the conversation, recap any decisions you've mutually made.** Include steps that you'll take, such as, "Okay, so tomorrow we'll both schedule appointments at the campus health center to get screened for STIs." If you've made shared decisions about birth control, talk to make sure that necessary steps get followed up. If you decide you'll use condoms, for example, it's helpful to buy a few to keep in places where you are likely to have sex. Make sure that your words are followed up with actions that reflect the experiences and preferences the two of you have shared.

Source: Adapted from Alabama Medicaid Agency. (n.d.). *Talking with your partner about birth control.* www.medicaid.state.al.us; and Society of Obstetricians and Gynaecologists of Canada (2006). *Tips to talk to your partner about sex.* www.sexualityandu.ca.

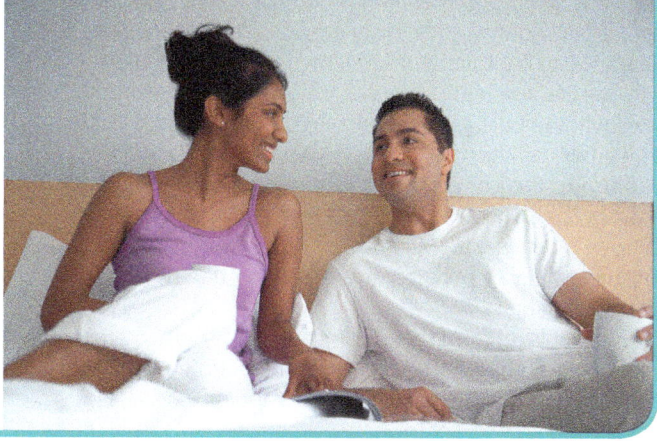

Abortion

LO 11.7 Discuss surgical and medical abortion.

Birth control failure and the failure to use birth control combine to create a large number of unintended pregnancies—about 3 million in the United States every year.[47] Many women experiencing unplanned pregnancies decide to keep their babies. Some—typically fewer than 2%—maintain the pregnancy but relinquish the baby for adoption. About 14% miscarry, and about 42% choose abortion each year.[48]

Abortion is a medical or surgical procedure used to terminate a pregnancy and involves removing the embryo or fetus from the uterus. The number of abortions performed has declined in recent years, and the abortion rate today is at its lowest since 1974. Nevertheless, an estimated 1.1 million abortions were performed in the United States in 2011, indicating that many couples still have difficulty avoiding unintended pregnancy.[49]

> **abortion** A medical or surgical procedure used to terminate a pregnancy.

Methods of Abortion

There are two types of procedures for terminating a pregnancy: medical and surgical abortion. *Medical abortion,* which involves the administration of medications (via pill or injection) to end a pregnancy, has been gaining in popularity since its approval by the U.S. Food and Drug Administration in 2000. In 2011, about 23% of women who underwent an abortion used the medical method, up from 17% just a few years before.[49] However, *surgical abortion* has a much longer history in the United States and remains the prevailing option.

Which method is advised? The World Health Organization has stated, "There is little, if any, difference between medical and surgical abortion in terms of safety and efficacy. Thus, both methods are similar from a medical point of view and there are only very few situations where a recommendation for one or the other method for medical reasons can be given."[50]

Medical Abortion

Medical abortions are intended for women in the earliest stages of pregnancy, within 9 weeks of the start of their last menstrual period (7 weeks of pregnancy). There is no surgery and no anesthesia. The medical route is recommended if the woman has health risks that make surgery unadvisable, such as obesity or uterine malformations.

The process starts with the administration—either by pill or injection—of the medication *mifepristone,* also known as *RU-486.* The medication blocks progesterone, which is needed to support a pregnancy. Two days later, the woman takes a pill containing the drug *misoprostol,* which causes the uterus to contract and expel the fertilized egg, along with the endometrial lining. The pregnancy usually terminates within hours after the second drug is ingested but sometimes can take up to 2 days. Women are instructed to return to their physician's office for a follow-up exam 2 weeks later. The procedure successfully terminates pregnancy in more than 96% of cases.[49] If the pregnancy was not successfully terminated, a surgical abortion is then recommended.

The expulsion from the uterus can cause severe cramping pain, nausea, heavy bleeding, fever, and diarrhea. Nevertheless, many women choose medical abortion because it allows them to end an unwanted pregnancy in privacy at home without the trauma of an invasive surgical procedure.

Surgical Abortion

Suction curettage, or vacuum aspiration, is the surgical abortion method most commonly chosen. Typically used in the first 6 to 12 weeks of pregnancy, it involves an injection to numb the cervix, followed by the insertion of a series of rods of increasing thickness to dilate (widen) the opening of the cervix. Once the cervix is adequately dilated, a hollow tube is inserted through the cervix into the uterus. The tube is attached to a pump, which generates suction to remove tissue from the uterine walls. Usually performed in a doctor's office or an outpatient clinic, suction curettage is a relatively quick procedure, often completed in just minutes.

Manual vacuum aspiration is similar to suction curettage but can be performed much earlier in the pregnancy. Doctors use thin flexible tubing attached to a handheld syringe and insert it through the cervix into the uterus. The syringe creates enough suction to strip the uterine lining and terminate the pregnancy.

For pregnancies that have progressed beyond 12 weeks, **dilation and evacuation (D&E)** may be performed. This procedure requires multiple trips to an outpatient clinic or hospital. During the first visit, an ultrasound scan is done to determine the status of the pregnancy and eligibility for the procedure. Then, 24 hours prior to surgery, the cervix is numbed and a medication administered that will dilate it slowly. At the final appointment, local anesthetic is administered (in some cases, spinal or general anesthesia), and the physician uses instruments and suction to remove the uterine contents. The procedure can cause pain and heavy bleeding, and there is a risk of surgical complications. Follow-up care is important.

> **suction curettage** A method of surgical abortion characterized by vacuum aspiration, typically used in the first 6 to 12 weeks of pregnancy.
>
> **dilation and evacuation (D&E)** A multistep method of surgical abortion that may be used in pregnancies that have progressed beyond 12 weeks.

STUDENT STORY

Open Talk About STIs

"**HI, I'M ABBEY.** I absolutely think that people have a responsibility to tell someone if they have a sexually transmitted disease before they have sex. That is definitely something that their partner should know ahead of time, and it's deceitful to hide that from them. If someone asked me if I had an STI right before sex, I would answer honestly. I wouldn't be put off. I would understand why they would want to know that and respect that they want to be safe and responsible with their body. How would I ask someone if they had an STI? I would just straightforwardly ask them."

What Do You Think?

1. Why is it so important to discuss sexual histories and exposure to sexually transmitted infections with a new partner prior to sex?
2. Do you think most college students are honest about their sexual history and STI status with new partners?
3. Why is it risky for sexually active individuals to skip regular medical checkups?

Physical and Psychological Complications of Abortion

The earlier an abortion is performed, the lower the risk of complications; however, at every gestational stage, abortion is safer than carrying the pregnancy to term.[51] When the procedure is performed by a qualified health professional, serious complications are extremely rare but may include hemorrhaging, fever, infection, adverse effects from anesthesia, perforation of the uterus, retention of blood in the uterus, bladder or intestinal injury, infection, and a blood coagulation disorder. In some cases, the embryo or fetus is not completely removed, and the procedure must be repeated. Deaths caused by abortion are rare. For example, of the more than 699,202 legally induced abortions in the United States in 2012, there were 2 known fatalities.[52]

For the vast majority of women who get an abortion, physical complications are not an issue. But what about the psychological effects? Abortion can be very stressful and can cause feelings of sadness or guilt. Just as the decision to have children is deeply personal, so is the choice to end a pregnancy. Emotional responses vary widely from one individual to another. After an abortion, some women feel a sense of relief. Others experience a sense of loss or guilt. If a woman chooses to terminate a pregnancy, it is important to recognize that a range of emotional reactions is possible and that she should seek support (and professional counseling) as needed.

While there is limited evidence that some women experience an increased risk of mental health problems after an abortion,[53] the American Psychological Association has concluded that terminating a single unwanted pregnancy creates no greater mental health risks for an adult woman than if she had opted to give birth.[54]

Legal Status of Abortion

Abortion has long been a contentious issue in the United States. Despite being legal during the nation's founding years, both abortion and contraception gradually fell out of favor. The federal Comstock Act of 1873 criminalized the distribution or possession of devices, medication, or even information used for abortion or contraception. For an entire century, many women who wanted to terminate an unwanted pregnancy resorted to "back-alley" abortions, performed in unsterile locations, often by untrained personnel using rudimentary instruments. These procedures were dangerous, and many women died as a result.

In 1973, the U.S. Supreme Court made a landmark decision in the case *Roe v. Wade* that all women have a constitutional right to an abortion in the first 6 months of their pregnancy. The legislation trumped all state laws limiting women's access to abortion and stipulated that individual states could only ban abortions during the final 3 months of pregnancy, when a fetus would have a chance of survival outside the womb. From the fourth through the sixth months of pregnancy, states can regulate the abortion procedure in the interest of maternal health.

Abortion continues to be legal in the United States, but a number of rulings have chipped away at *Roe v. Wade*, placing new restrictions on who can get an abortion and when. More than 30 states now require that minors notify their parents beforehand, often requiring parental permission to continue with the procedure. Others impose a mandatory waiting period, requiring women to read information on abortion alternatives before being allowed to terminate their pregnancy. Since 1976, the Hyde Amendment has severely restricted abortion coverage for Medicaid recipients. The 2010 Affordable Care Act continued these restrictions and also allowed private plans to prohibit abortion coverage, except when a pregnancy would endanger a woman's life or in cases of rape or incest. Women's rights advocates argue that abortions are really only available to those who can afford to pay for them.[55]

Some of the main arguments commonly advanced for and against abortion rights are presented in **Table 11.2**.

LO 11.7 QUICK CHECK

Which type of abortion is brought about by the administration of medications?

a. suction curettage
b. dilation and evacuation
c. vacuum aspiration
d. medical abortion

TABLE 11.2 Arguments Opposing and Supporting Abortion Rights

Opposition to Abortion Rights	Support for Abortion Rights
Life begins at conception, and abortion is therefore murder.	Legal abortion is performed when the embryo or fetus is not capable of sustaining life independently and is therefore not murder.
Performing an abortion violates medical ethics, which require health-care providers to promote and preserve life.	If safe clinical abortions were no longer legal, women would again resort to "back-alley" abortions, resulting in cases of permanent infertility, serious disease, and death.
Abortion exposes girls and women to significant risk of physical and psychological harm.	Carrying an unwanted pregnancy to term exposes girls and women to significant risk of physical and psychological harm.
Women with an unwanted pregnancy should relinquish their baby for adoption because many people are on waiting lists to adopt a child.	Carrying an unwanted pregnancy to term and then relinquishing the newborn for adoption can promote physical and emotional harm.
Highly reliable forms of contraception are readily available. Abortion should not be available as a form of birth control.	Among sexually active couples, no method of contraception is 100% reliable. Although the rate of unintended pregnancies can be reduced, some are inevitable, and women should not be forced to carry them to term.

Pregnancy and Childbirth

LO 11.8 Describe the key stages of pregnancy and childbirth.

Among the milestones in life that people cherish the most is the journey to becoming a parent and the birth of their child. The following sections provide an overview of the stages of pregnancy and childbirth and an examination of the choices available to couples struggling with infertility.

Pregnancy

Pregnancies are divided into three trimesters, each lasting about 3 months. Women may experience vastly different symptoms during each phase, with the second trimester often being referred to as the "golden age" because women tend to have more energy and less nausea at this point.

For young, healthy couples having unprotected sex, there is about a 20% chance of pregnancy during any given menstrual cycle.[56] A woman who suspects she might be pregnant can find out for certain by using a simple pregnancy test. There are two types on the market: a urine test available over the counter and a blood test offered only in physicians' offices. Both look for the presence of hCG, a hormone that is only made in the body during pregnancy.

The blood test can detect hCG about a week after ovulation. But many women opt for a home urine test, which is painless, inexpensive, and private. It's able to detect hCG levels about 2 weeks after ovulation—approximately the day a woman's period is due. For the most accurate results, health experts recommend waiting until a few days later before taking a home pregnancy test. In one study of six popular home pregnancy test kits, researchers found that only one, the First Response Early Result Pregnancy Test, was consistently able to provide correct results the day a woman's period was due.[57]

Because home pregnancy tests are not 100% accurate, women who get a negative result are encouraged to test again 1 week later if they still have not started menstruating.

Preconception Care

Many women recognize that **prenatal care,** including nutritional counseling and regular medical screenings throughout pregnancy, is important for the growth and development of the unborn baby. Prenatal vitamins containing a sufficient amount of folic acid are recommended because they significantly reduce the risk of birth defects.

Preconception care is also important. Obstetricians encourage patients who are attempting to start a family to first take care of any health problems that could affect the pregnancy, including type 2 diabetes and high blood pressure. During a preconception visit, a doctor may also suggest changes in a woman's nutrition or exercise routine and may advise prospective parents to not use tobacco, alcohol, or illegal drugs. Certain medications should also be avoided while attempting to conceive. It is critical to make positive lifestyle changes long before that faint positive sign first appears on a home pregnancy test.

> **prenatal care** Nutritional counseling and regular medical screenings throughout pregnancy to aid the growth and development of the fetus.

Early Signs of Pregnancy

Indications of pregnancy can appear before a woman even misses her period, although the first signs could also be indicative of illness or even impending menstruation. Women who experience many of the listed indicators should consider taking a home pregnancy test or visiting their gynecologist:

- A missed period
- An extremely light "period" that is actually implantation bleeding, which occurs when a fertilized egg implants itself in the uterus
- Frequent urination
- Nausea
- Swollen breasts and/or breast tenderness
- Fatigue
- Food aversions or cravings
- Mood swings
- Abdominal bloating or pressure
- Dizziness

Some women experience none of these symptoms in the early weeks of their pregnancy. Others may notice a few physical or emotional changes but not right away.

Changes in a Pregnant Woman's Body

A woman's body undergoes a series of physical changes throughout the course of pregnancy **(Figure 11.10)**. Some go unnoticed. For example, the heart begins to work harder, and a physician may notice fluctuations in the woman's blood pressure. Breathing patterns change slightly, with breaths becoming deeper and faster. The kidneys kick into high gear, filtering an increasing volume of blood. Ligaments and muscles stretch. The cervix becomes thinner and softer.

Myriad other changes, however, are difficult for women to miss. Hormonal changes, especially in the first trimester, can cause bouts of nausea and vomiting called "morning sickness," a misnomer because women afflicted with it often find that it persists throughout most of the day. Breasts become fuller and tender to the touch, as they get ready for milk production. The uterus enlarges as the fetus grows, ultimately extending up to the woman's rib cage. The growing uterus presses on the bladder, creating the constant urge to urinate. It also shifts the woman's center of gravity, exaggerating the curve in her lower back and giving her a characteristic "waddling" walk. The skin stretches to accommodate the growing breasts and abdomen and sometimes darkens at points on the face and in a thin line near the navel. During the last trimester, women may also develop heartburn and hemorrhoids. By the time the baby is born, the average woman will have gained between 25 and 30 pounds—and more if she is carrying twins or triplets. Not surprisingly, as a result of all these physical changes, many women report experiencing significant fatigue during pregnancy.

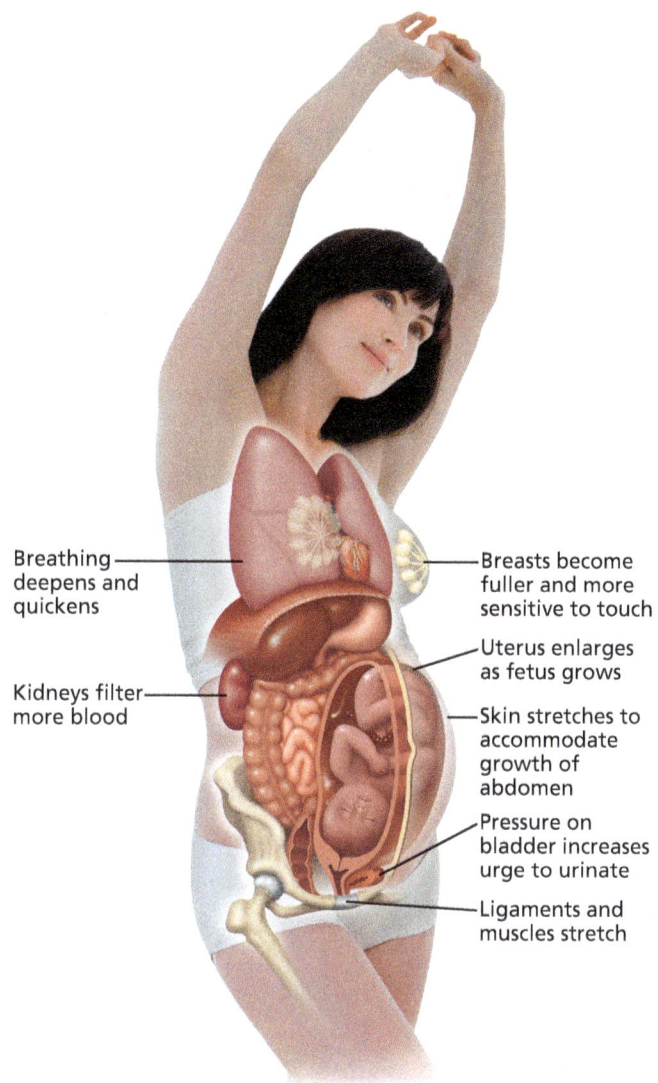

FIGURE 11.10 **Changes in a Pregnant Woman's Body.**

Development of the Fetus

The fetus also undergoes significant physical changes as it transforms from a microscopic fertilized egg into an average 7.5-pound newborn (**Figure 11.11**, next page).

First Trimester. The first trimester, the first 13 weeks of pregnancy, is the most critical period in the baby's development. At this stage, it is most susceptible to any substances a woman ingests, including drugs, alcohol, and certain medications, as well as any environmental toxins, from pesticides to the chemicals in cigarette smoke.

Recall that when an egg and sperm combine, they form a single-celled organism known as a *zygote*. As the zygote makes its way from a fallopian tube to the uterus, it rapidly divides and becomes a cluster of dozens of cells called a *blastocyst*. The blastocyst (no larger than a pinhead) implants itself in the uterine wall, where it begins to receive nourishment. About 2 weeks after fertilization—around the time a woman first misses her period—the growing collection of cells is known as an **embryo.**

The growing embryo has a powerful support system. It receives its nutrients and oxygen—and gets rid of its waste products—from the **placenta,** the tissue that connects mother and baby. The **umbilical cord** also plays a key role, linking the bloodstream of the placenta to that of the embryo and enabling the exchange of gases, nutrients, and wastes. The embryo is surrounded and protected by **amniotic fluid,** which keeps the baby's temperature regulated and allows it to move freely.

Eight weeks after fertilization, the embryo is called a **fetus,** a name it will keep until birth. By the end of the first trimester, the fetus is much larger, measuring 3 to 4 inches in length. Still, it weighs only the equivalent of 3 U.S. quarters. The majority of fetal growth will occur in the trimesters to come.

Second Trimester. The second trimester is an exciting time for many women. Fatigue and nausea tend to dissipate, and the fetus provides a few welcome signs of the life developing within. During this trimester, the woman begins to feel the fetus moving and kicking, and the fetal heartbeat can be heard through a stethoscope. All major organs and physiological systems become fully formed. The fetus continues its rapid growth; by the end of the second trimester it measures 13 to 16 inches and weighs about 2 or 3 pounds. A fetus might survive if born at the end of this trimester but would require lengthy hospitalization and could suffer long-term health effects.

embryo The growing collection of cells that ultimately become a baby.

placenta The tissue that connects mother and baby.

umbilical cord A vessel linking the bloodstream of the placenta to that of the baby and enabling the exchange of gases, nutrients, and wastes.

amniotic fluid Fluid that surrounds the developing fetus that aids in temperature regulation and allows the baby to move freely.

fetus The name given to a developing embryo 8 weeks after fertilization.

Third Trimester. During the last 3 months of pregnancy, the fetus gains most of its weight, including a layer of fat needed for insulation during the first weeks of life outside the womb. Its organs continue to mature, and it moves into position—head down—as it gets ready for birth. Throughout the last trimester, the mother may experience *Braxton Hicks contractions,* irregular movements of the uterus that may be confused with the signs of premature labor. These contractions are simply tightenings of the uterus, also known as "false labor."

Although a standard pregnancy lasts about 40 weeks, babies are considered full term if they are born between 37 and 42 weeks. Preterm babies (born before 37 weeks) are at risk for developmental delays and other complications. Babies born after 42 weeks' gestation are post-term and may stop growing in the uterus. In some instances, post-term pregnancies result in stillbirth.

Prenatal Care

The health of the baby depends in part on the health of the mother and the measures she takes during pregnancy to protect them both. Prenatal care, which includes regular

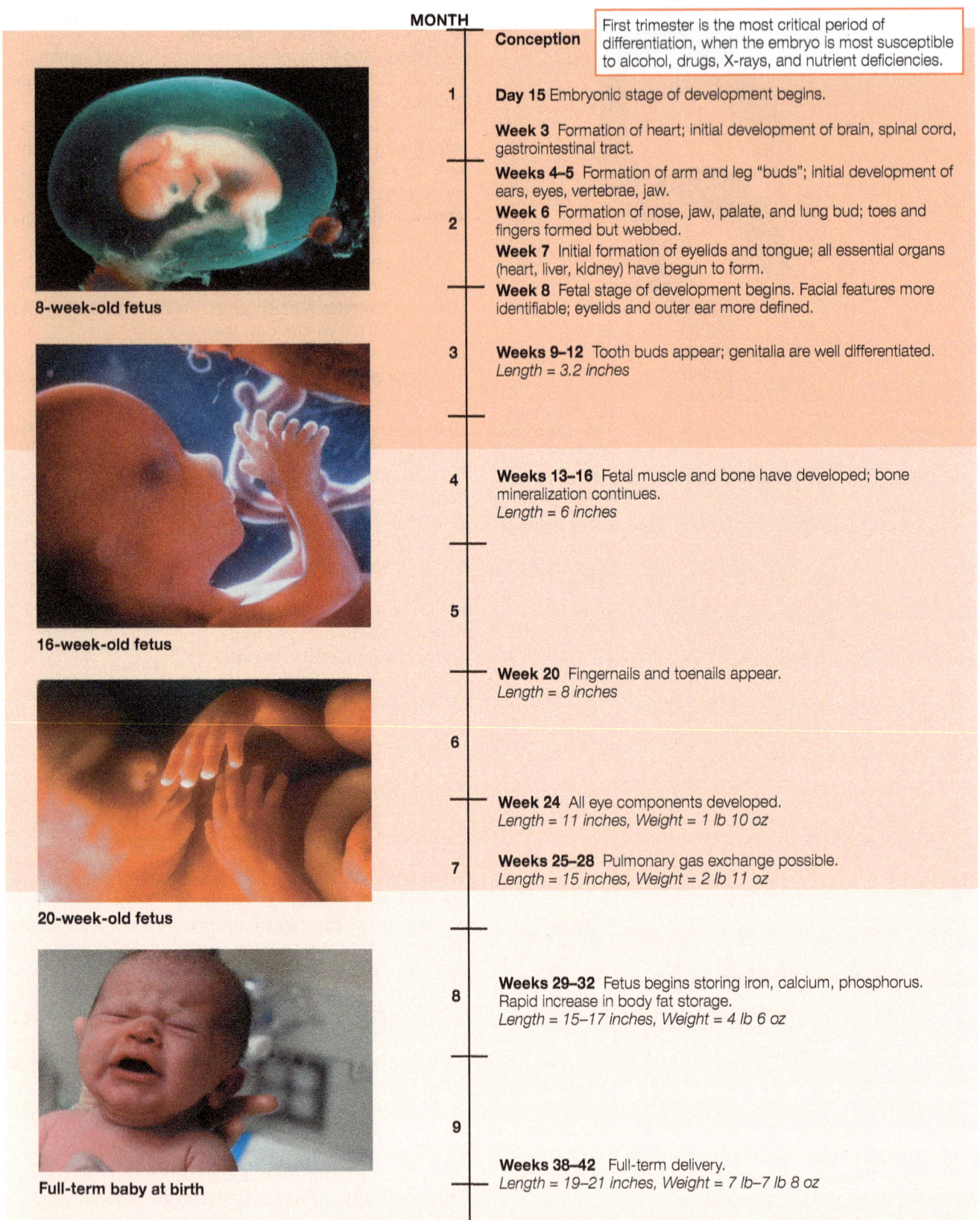

FIGURE 11.11 **Stages of Embryonic and Fetal Development.**

checkups during pregnancy and counseling about nutrition, exercise, sleep, and other topics, should be an integral part of every pregnancy. Babies born to mothers who receive no prenatal care are five times more likely to die than those whose mothers do get regular care.[58] As soon as a woman learns she is pregnant, she is encouraged to

- **Get regular checkups.** Select an obstetrician or certified nurse midwife and schedule an initial appointment. This is followed by regularly scheduled appointments at which the woman is monitored for many factors, including blood pressure, blood sugar, weight gain, and fetal well-being.
- **Follow sound nutrition advice.** It is commonly said that a pregnant woman is "eating for two," but that is only partially accurate. During pregnancy, the body needs only an extra 300 calories per day—not a double quantity of food. The quality of a pregnant woman's diet is what counts; she should eat nutrient-dense food and avoid poor-quality processed or fast food that provides calories but few or no nutrients.
- **Exercise regularly.** Fitness is important to the health of the mother and her growing baby. Exercise can help relieve some of the discomforts of pregnancy and may prevent gestational diabetes. It can also help prepare a woman for labor and childbirth.
- **Avoid drugs, including alcohol and tobacco.** These substances, including some prescription and over-the-counter medications, can be harmful to fetal growth and development. A pregnant woman should always check with her physician before taking any medications. The same holds true for dietary supplements, including herbs. Daily caffeine consumption should be limited to less than 200 mg (one 12-oz cup of coffee).[59]

Complications

Most pregnancies progress without a hitch, with the fetus developing properly and the birth being trouble free. For some women, there are complications; these are problems that pose risks to the health of the mother or baby or both.

Ectopic Pregnancy. An **ectopic pregnancy** occurs when a fertilized egg implants within a fallopian tube. It can also implant in the cervix or an ovary, although this occurs much less frequently. Between 2% and 3% of all pregnancies in the United States are ectopic, and that rate has increased slightly in recent years.[60]

As the mislocated embryo begins to grow, the woman may experience severe pain, and the fallopian tube may rupture. An ectopic pregnancy can never develop normally and survive—and it is a threat to the mother's life. The condition accounts for 3%-14% of all maternal deaths, with African American women and women over age 35 at the highest risk.[61] Ectopic pregnancies can also cause scarring in the fallopian tubes, creating future fertility problems. Risk factors include smoking, endometriosis, and having been infected with gonorrhea or chlamydia.

Miscarriage. A **miscarriage,** or *spontaneous abortion,* is a pregnancy that suddenly ends on its own before the 20th week. An estimated 10%-15% of known pregnancies end this way, but because many losses occur before a woman realizes she is pregnant, experts believe the true number could be closer to 40%.[62] Exactly what causes a pregnancy to terminate is not always clear, but the majority of miscarriages are thought to be caused by chromosomal problems in the fetus. The risk is higher in women who are over age 35, have a history of diabetes or thyroid disease, or have a history of miscarriages. Smoking, drinking alcohol, or using illicit drugs while pregnant may also increase a woman's risk of miscarriage.

Hypertension. A pregnant woman's blood pressure is normally checked at every prenatal visit to screen for hypertension (high blood pressure), which is the most common medical disorder in pregnancy.[63] If untreated, hypertension during pregnancy can progress to **preeclampsia,** a serious health condition that can threaten the life of both mother and fetus. Characterized by high blood pressure and protein in the urine, preeclampsia typically develops after the 20th week of pregnancy. Women may experience headaches, swelling of the hands and face, excessive weight gain, abdominal pain, and vision changes. Without skilled medical care, preeclampsia can result in seizures and multiple organ failure as well as fetal death.

About 5%-8% of pregnant women develop preeclampsia.[64] Unfortunately, there is no way to prevent it, and the only cure is childbirth. Physicians will often admit a woman with preeclampsia to the hospital so she and her fetus can be closely monitored. Although it can be harmful to the baby to be born prematurely, often it can be even more dangerous for a preeclamptic pregnancy to go full term. Doctors may decide to induce labor early in an effort to save both mother and child.

Low Birth Weight and Infant Mortality. Newborns weighing less than 5 pounds, 8 ounces at birth are called **low birth weight** babies and are at risk for serious health problems, including death. Currently, about 8% of babies born in the United States fall into this category. After being on the rise for decades, this percentage began declining after 2006.[65] Preterm labor and multiple births are the leading causes. Low-birth-weight babies are vulnerable to a host of health problems and disabilities, including learning disabilities, cerebral palsy, hearing loss, and vision problems. Women are more likely to have a low-birth-weight baby if they smoke, drink alcohol, or use illicit drugs during pregnancy.

Low birth weight and prematurity are two factors influencing the **infant mortality rate,** the ratio of infant deaths to live births in any given year. Congenital abnormalities, pregnancy complications, and

> **ectopic pregnancy** A pregnancy that occurs when a fertilized egg implants within one of the fallopian tubes instead of the uterus; considered a medical emergency.
>
> **miscarriage** A pregnancy that suddenly terminates on its own before the 20th week.
>
> **preeclampsia** A serious health condition characterized by high blood pressure in the pregnant woman.
>
> **low birth weight** Birth weight less than 5 pounds, 8 ounces.
>
> **infant mortality rate** A calculation of the ratio of babies who die before their first birthday and those who survive until their first birthday.

sudden infant death syndrome (SIDS) are also to blame. SIDS is the sudden death of a seemingly healthy infant while sleeping. Although researchers still do not entirely understand the phenomenon, they recognize that putting a baby to sleep on its stomach or side increases the risk for SIDS. The good news is that in 2014, the U.S. infant mortality rate declined to a record low of 5.8 deaths per 1,000 births.[66]

Childbirth

For expectant parents longing to meet their unborn baby, 40 weeks of waiting can seem like an eternity. Childbirth is a moment they await with anticipation—and sometimes apprehension—knowing that their lives are about to change forever.

Childbirth Options

Pregnant women have many choices about where to give birth, ranging from hospitals to alternative birthing centers to their own home. They must also decide who will be their care provider—an obstetrician, a certified nurse midwife, or a lay midwife known as a *doula*. Some parents-to-be even draft birth plans, documents that spell out their preferences on everything from the use of pain relievers during labor to the number of people they would like in the birthing room.

Even with so many choices, 99% of women still opt to have their baby in a hospital, attended by a physician or certified nurse midwife.[67] Fortunately, many U.S. hospitals today have birthing rooms designed to resemble a bedroom in a home, providing a more comfortable and soothing environment than the typical hospital room.

Women whose pregnancies are considered high risk because of their age, health problems, or concerns about the health of the baby may be encouraged to give birth in a medical center that has a neonatal intensive care unit. This is also true of women carrying twins, triplets, or quadruplets.

Labor and Birth

Anywhere from several hours to several days before labor begins, many women experience a discharge of copious, red-tinged mucus commonly called the "bloody show." This mucous plug has been blocking the cervix throughout the pregnancy, protecting it from bacteria and other harmful agents, and its discharge signals that the cervix is beginning to dilate in preparation for labor.

Onset of Labor. The precise events signaling the onset of **labor** differ for every woman and every pregnancy. Some women begin to experience regular, mild contractions—caused by the release of a hormone called oxytocin—that become more frequent and intense over several hours. Other women don't experience contractions until their "water breaks"—that is, until the sac holding the amniotic fluid ruptures, and amniotic fluid flows out from the vagina. Some women may experience vague abdominal cramps and lower back pain. Such symptoms are a sign that a woman is experiencing the first of three stages of the birth process **(Figure 11.12)**.

> **sudden infant death syndrome (SIDS)** The sudden death of a seemingly healthy infant while sleeping.
>
> **labor** The physical processes involved in giving birth.
>
> **transition** The final phase of the first stage of labor, characterized by the dilation of the cervix and strong, prolonged contractions.

First Stage of Labor. First-time mothers spend an average of 12 to 14 hours in labor, although some progress more quickly and others more slowly.[68] The first stage is the longest: 9 or more hours. Those who have already had one vaginal birth tend to experience a faster first stage during subsequent pregnancies.

During early labor, uterine contractions begin to move the fetus toward the birth canal. Contractions also cause the cervix to begin to open—dilate—and thin out, a process known as *effacement*. Between each contraction, the pain typically abates, and the woman can rest. If the sac holding the amniotic fluid has not already broken, it may do so now. During active labor, the cervix dilates further and contractions strengthen, lengthen, and become more frequent. Many women request pain medication during this time. The final phase of this first stage of labor is known as **transition.** Amid strong and prolonged contractions, the cervix dilates to about 10 centimeters, usually large enough for the baby's head to fit through. A woman may begin to feel shaky, sweaty, and weak. Physical and emotional

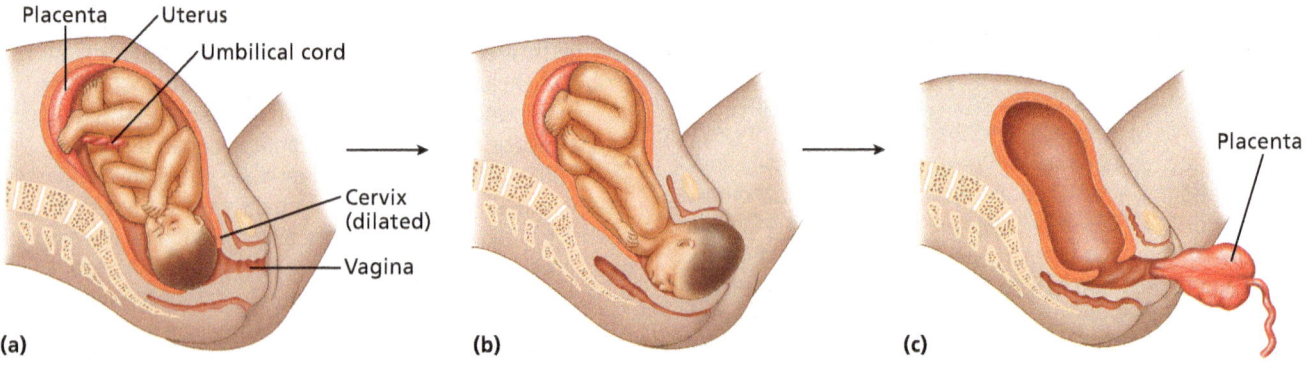

FIGURE 11.12 Stages of Childbirth. (a) The first stage is characterized by cervical dilation and contractions of the uterus that begin to move the baby toward the birth canal. **(b)** In the second stage, the woman pushes until the baby is born. **(c)** In the third stage, the placenta is expelled.

Source: From Stanfield, C. (2011). *Principles of human physiology*, 4th edition, Figure 22.24, p. 662. 2011. Pearson Education.

support from care providers and a partner, friend, or family member is important during this phase.

Second Stage of Labor. Once the cervix has dilated to 10 centimeters, the woman is encouraged to help move the fetus further into the birth canal by actively pushing, bearing down with each contraction. Many women find this stage of labor, which can last from 30 minutes to 3 hours, more rewarding than the first stage because they can feel that their efforts help the birth to progress.[68] Others view this as the hardest stage of labor. When the baby's head crowns (appears at the vaginal opening), labor is almost over. The woman stops pushing, and after one or two further contractions, the baby is born, slick and wet from the amniotic fluid. The birth attendant removes mucus and fluid from the newborn's mouth and nose and dries the baby with a towel. The umbilical cord, which still attaches the newborn to the placenta, is clamped and cut.

Third Stage of Labor. Although the baby has been born, the mother's body still has one important task to do: Expel the placenta. This is typically accomplished by a few more contractions. The woman continues to bleed, but massaging the abdomen or breast-feeding the newborn can control the bleeding within about 5 to 15 minutes. The final stage of labor is over.[68]

For the baby, the work has just begun. Just 1 minute after birth, the baby is given his or her first test, a measurement of how well he or she tolerated the stresses of birth. This test, known as the Apgar test,[69] is performed by a doctor, midwife, or nurse. The resulting score, from 1 to 10, is an **Apgar score**. Babies are assessed on five characteristics: muscle tone, heart rate, reflexes, skin coloration, and breathing. Five minutes after birth, the test is repeated to see if the baby's score has improved. A final score between 7 and 10 is considered normal. Babies who receive a lower score may need additional medical assistance.

Doctors also take a sample of blood from the infant's heel to test for hidden disorders that are not always apparent at birth. Rare metabolic disorders such as phenylketonuria (PKU) can be successfully controlled if detected early but can cause developmental disabilities or even death if left undiagnosed.

Cesarean Birth. In consultation with their health-care provider, some women decide to give birth via a scheduled **cesarean section (C-section).** This surgery involves making an incision through the woman's abdominal and uterine walls to extract the baby. A C-section may be necessary if the mother is experiencing hypertension or another disorder, if the placenta is covering the cervix, or if the fetus is very large or in the wrong position in the birth canal. Also, women who have had a prior C-section may be encouraged to have one during subsequent pregnancies to avoid the small but serious risk of uterine rupture. An emergency C-section may be performed if labor is not progressing properly or a vaginal delivery goes awry, placing the mother or baby in danger.

The rate of C-sections doubled between 1996 and 2006, according to national statistics.[70] Nearly 1 in 3 babies, 32.8%,[67] are now delivered via C-section, a rate more than double the World Health Organization's recommended limit of 15%.[71] Although the surgery is relatively safe, it has a higher rate of complications and involves a longer recovery time for mothers than a vaginal birth.

LO 11.8 QUICK CHECK

During which stage of labor is the baby actually born?
a. first stage
b. second stage
c. third stage
d. fourth stage

Infertility

LO 11.9 Discuss causes of and treatment for infertility.

Many couples attempt to get pregnant only to find that it is not always easy to do. An estimated 12% of women and 14% of couples in the United States experience **infertility,** or the inability to conceive after trying for 1 year.[72] The problem becomes more prevalent with age, and so doctors recommend that a woman in her 30s get checked for underlying health issues if she has been trying to get pregnant for more than 6 months without success. Doctors will also examine her partner because infertility can be caused by a low sperm count or other factors involving the male. Fortunately, there are many treatment options available, and about two-thirds of couples who have difficulty conceiving ultimately go on to have children who are biologically their own.[73]

> **Apgar score** A measurement of how well a newborn tolerated the stresses of birth and how well he or she is adapting to the new environment.
>
> **cesarean section (C-section)** A surgical procedure involving the incision of a woman's abdominal and uterine walls to deliver a baby.
>
> **infertility** The inability to conceive after trying for at least a year.

Causes of Infertility

Roughly one-third of infertility cases are due to health problems in the woman, another one-third are due to problems in the man, and the final one-third are either caused by problems in both partners or simply cannot be explained.[73]

For women, the most common causes of infertility are

- Blocked fallopian tubes, stemming from an ectopic pregnancy, surgery, or, most commonly, an untreated STI such as chlamydia or gonorrhea that caused scarring in the fallopian tubes and/or progressed into pelvic inflammatory disease (PID). Endometriosis also can block the tubes.
- Failure of ovulation prompted by hormonal problems, advanced age, premature menopause, or scarred ovaries.
- A deformed uterus, which can not only cause infertility but may lead to miscarriage.
- Uterine fibroids and other noncancerous growths, which can obstruct both the uterus and the fallopian tubes.

The most common causes of infertility in men include

- Low sperm count, defined as fewer than 10 million sperm per milliliter of semen. This can be caused by smoking cigarettes or marijuana.

- Incorrectly formed sperm, which are not able to penetrate the egg.
- Poor sperm motility, or the inability of sperm to move quickly and effectively.
- Prior infection. Contracting mumps during adulthood is a common culprit. STIs such as gonorrhea can also cause scarring that hinders sperm movement.
- Environmental exposure to pesticides, lead, and other substances that disrupt hormones in the body.

Options for Infertile Couples

The type of medical treatment ultimately chosen depends to a large degree on the root cause of the difficulty getting pregnant. Options include

- Surgery to repair blocked fallopian tubes, remove scarring or uterine growths, and treat endometriosis in women. Occasionally, surgery may be indicated if there is a problem with a man's sperm.
- Fertility drugs, which promote ovulation in women. Side effects can include headaches, nausea, hot flashes, and breast tenderness. Because the medications can spur the body to release more than one egg at a time, couples using fertility drugs have a higher chance of having twins, triplets, or quadruplets.
- Intrauterine insemination, to boost the odds that an egg will be fertilized. Sperm are collected from a woman's partner or a donor and processed in a laboratory, enabling a higher concentration of sperm to be injected into the vagina or uterus through a syringe.
- *In vitro fertilization (IVF)*, a procedure that dramatically transformed the field of fertility treatment when the first "test-tube baby" was born in 1978. Egg and sperm are retrieved from a woman and a man and combined in a laboratory dish (*in vitro* means "in glass"), where fertilization may occur. If eggs are fertilized, they are implanted in the uterus. When multiple eggs are transferred, multiple births may occur.
- *Gamete intrafallopian transfer (GIFT)*, a process similar to IVF, but the egg is not fertilized in a laboratory. Instead, sperm and several eggs are placed in a woman's fallopian tube. There is no guarantee that the sperm will penetrate at least one of the eggs.
- *Zygote intrafallopian transfer (ZIFT)*, fertilization of an egg or eggs in a laboratory setting. Unlike with IVF, the fertilized eggs are transferred to a fallopian tube rather than the uterus.
- *Intracytoplasmic sperm injection (ICSI)*, the direct injection of a single sperm into an egg. The fertilized egg is then implanted in the uterus using standard IVF technology. ICSI may be considered when men have low sperm counts or when fertilization failed to occur in previous IVF attempts.
- Surrogate motherhood, which requires an agreement with a third party—a fertile woman—to carry a pregnancy to term. In some cases the surrogate's egg is fertilized through intrauterine insemination with the prospective father's sperm. In other cases, she is impregnated through IVF with the couple's embryo. The surrogate is paid for her services, and immediately following the baby's birth, she relinquishes the infant to the parents.

Not all couples choose medical treatment. Many opt for adoption, either domestically or internationally. In 2014, there were 50,600 adoptions in the United States involving public child-welfare agencies.[74] Statistics on adoptions involving private agencies are not available because they do not have to be reported by states. The adoption experience can be as satisfying to parents as pregnancy and childbirth. It can also cost less—or much more. Adoptions from foster-care agencies typically cost very little or are free of charge. Domestic adoptions using private agencies can cost several thousand dollars. International adoptions can cost $30,000 or more, and the process can take several years. Not all couples who want to adopt a baby are successful.

Actions can be taken to prevent infertility. Although many couples in their late teens and early 20s are more interested in *avoiding* pregnancy, steps should be taken to preserve fertility for the years to come. Practicing safe sex can reduce the spread of STIs, which are often the cause of fertility problems. Getting timely treatment for an STI is also important. Because fertility drops and the risk of birth defects and miscarriages rises when a woman is in her 30s, couples who want to have a child are encouraged to start their family planning before the woman turns 35.

LO 11.9 QUICK CHECK

If a woman wants to reduce her chances of infertility, she is encouraged to start her family planning efforts before what age?
a. 30
b. 35
c. 40
d. 45

Change Yourself, Change Your World

LO 11.10 Consider ways of developing and promoting healthy sexuality.

We've presented a lot of facts about sexual health. But how do you integrate cold facts with the complex desires you feel? And how can the decisions you make about whether, when, and with whom to have sex stay aligned with your goals and your dreams? Healthy sexuality requires not only protecting the health of your body but also accepting and supporting your sexual orientation, contraception preferences, possible plans for children, and personal values.

Personal Choices

It's important to know yourself before you become intimate with others. You need to clarify what you want—and that requires you to distinguish your values from those of the people around you. Also, you should talk with your partner before things get physical. You can make an awkward situation easier by being the one to start the dialogue and share your experiences. Treat potential partners with the same respect you show yourself and be honest

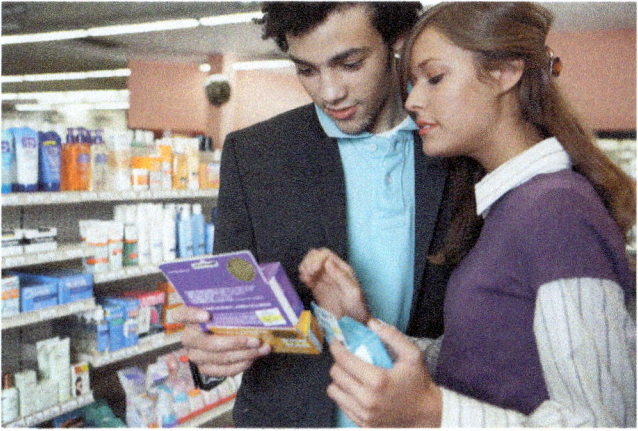

Choose a contraceptive with your partner and make sure you both understand how to use it.

about who you are and what you want. Discuss your expectations for the relationship, what you do and don't want physically, and the practical matters of your sexual history, STI prevention, and contraception. Also, if you become sexually active, consistently practice safe sex and have a backup plan if your primary method fails. Finally, if pregnancy occurs, the woman should visit a health-care provider right away, and couples should discuss their expectations and options.

Campus Advocacy

How can we avoid the trap of labeling ourselves or others based on our sexual histories, behaviors, or orientation? How can we develop tolerance and promote healthier sexuality in our community? Various methods have arisen on different college campuses. Here are a few ideas:

- More than 200 U.S. colleges and universities have programs fostering alliances among heterosexual and lesbian, gay, bisexual, or transgender (LGBT) students. These programs have names such as Safe Zone, Safe Space, Safe Harbor, and Safe on Campus. The hallmark of these "Safe" programs is the public identification of "allies" by placing a "Safe" symbol—usually a pink triangle or a rainbow—on doors or walls of offices or living spaces.
- Visit your campus health center and confirm that it offers a variety of low-cost contraceptives. In 2009, Congress reinstated a program enabling college health centers to purchase and sell prescription medications, including hormonal contraceptives, at a discounted rate.[1] Make sure your campus health center is taking advantage of this program.
- Consider supporting free condom distribution on your campus. Contact groups like the Great American Condom Campaign (GACC), whose members distribute millions of condoms to fellow students each year and work to educate their peers about sexual health. Find out more about GACC at www.amplifyyourvoice.org/gacc.

>> Watch videos of real students discussing sexuality, contraception, and reproductive choices at **Mastering**Health™

LO 11.10 QUICK CHECK

Before Craig and Chris become physically intimate, they want to discuss their expectations for the relationship. What topics should this conversation include?
a. sexual history
b. STI prevention
c. sexual activities they are and aren't comfortable with
d. all of the above

Choosing to Change Worksheet

To complete this worksheet online, visit **Mastering**Health™

Each safer sex method has pros and cons. Keep in mind that even the most effective methods can fail. But your chances of getting an STI or becoming pregnant are lowest if the method you choose always is used correctly and consistently every time you have sex.

Directions: Fill in your stage of change in step 1 and complete steps 2, 3, or 4, depending on which ones apply to your stage of change.

Step 1: Assess your stage of behavior change. Please check the following statement that best describes your readiness to follow your selected safer sex method correctly and consistently every time you have sex. Keep in mind that abstinence and intimacy without intercourse are forms of safer sex.

_____ I do not plan to practice safer sex consistently and correctly in the next six months. (Precontemplation)

_____ I might practice safer sex consistently and correctly in the next six months. (Contemplation)

_____ I am prepared to begin practicing safer sex consistently and correctly in the next month. (Preparation)

_____ I have been practicing safer sex consistently and correctly for less than six months. (Action)

_____ I have been practicing safer sex consistently and correctly for six months or longer. (Maintenance)

Step 2: Work the precontemplation and contemplation stages. What is holding you back from practicing safer sex correctly and consistently every time?

_____

_____

If a pregnancy or an STI were to occur due to inconsistent or incorrect use of a safer sex method, what would be the effects on you and your partner? Think of emotional, financial, school, and family effects.

_____

Even if you don't think you're ready, what could you do to move toward practicing safer sex correctly and consistently?

_____

_____

Step 3: Work the preparation, action, and maintenance stages. *Correct use:* Read the packaging of the contraceptive or safer sex method you are using. Or, for cost-free methods, reread the section of this chapter on these methods. Are you using the method correctly? If not, what have you been doing incorrectly, or what are you confused about? How can you begin to use the method correctly?

_____

_____

Consistent use: If you are in the preparation stage, write down a SMART goal for using this method consistently every time. If you are in the action or maintenance stages, how are you making sure you use the method consistently every time?

_____

_____

Step 4: Work the maintenance stage. What motivates you to continue practicing correct and consistent safer sex?

_____

_____

Are there obstacles you face in practicing safer sex correctly and consistently? If so, how are you dealing with them?

_____

_____

_____

CHAPTER 11 STUDY PLAN

CHAPTER SUMMARY

LO 11.1
- Good sexual health requires knowledge, effort, and appropriate medical care.
- Male and female sexual anatomy includes external and internal organs.
- Female organs include the ovaries, one of which releases an egg cell monthly, and the uterus, where a fertilized egg implants and grows.

MasteringHealth™
Build your knowledge—and health!—in the Study Area of **MasteringHealth**™ with a variety of study tools.

- Male organs include the testes, which constantly manufacture sperm that travel through a series of ducts to contribute to the man's semen.

LO 11.2
- The menstrual cycle is a monthly series of events in a nonpregnant woman of childbearing age. These events are controlled by hormones and include the buildup and shedding of the uterine lining and the maturation and release of an egg cell from an ovary.

LO 11.3
- The sexual response cycle consists of a series of phases from arousal to orgasm to resolution.
- Sexual dysfunction is fairly prevalent in the United States, with a sizable portion of men and women having difficulty enjoying sex at some point in their lives.

LO 11.4
- Abstinence is the avoidance of sexual intercourse; it has gained greater social acceptance in recent years.
- Sexual behavior includes sexual intercourse, along with various forms of non-intercourse sexual activity, including hugging, kissing, and masturbation; all are a healthy part of a sexually active lifestyle.

LO 11.5
- Humans develop their sexual orientation at a very early age. It is theorized that sexual orientation is a result of the interaction of biological, environmental, and cognitive factors.
- Heterosexuality, homosexuality, and bisexuality are variations of a broad spectrum of sexuality.
- A transgender person's biological sex is different from his or her gender identity.

LO 11.6
- Despite the wide variety of contraceptive options available, about half of all U.S. pregnancies are unplanned.
- Among contraceptive methods, only male and female condoms provide protection against STIs. Different methods offer varying rates of efficacy in preventing pregnancy.

LO 11.7
- Abortion is the purposeful termination of a pregnancy. There are two types: medical and surgical.
- Serious physical complications from abortion are rare, but it can cause feelings of sadness or guilt in some women.

LO 11.8
- Pregnancy involves three trimesters, each with unique stages of fetal development and physical effects for the mother.
- Women need preconception and prenatal health care to ensure a healthy pregnancy and healthy baby.
- The first stage of labor involves uterine contractions, cervical dilation, and fetal descent into the birth canal. During the second stage, the woman bears down with each contraction until the baby is born. The third stage is expulsion of the placenta.

LO 11.9
- Fertility declines with increasing age. Males and females have about an equal rate of infertility.

LO 11.10
- You can protect and promote your sexual health—and that of your partners and peers—by being honest about what you want out of sexual relationships, planning ahead for pregnancy and STI protections, and promoting open, tolerant conversations about sexual issues on campus.

GET CONNECTED

>> Visit the following websites for further information about the topics in this chapter:

- Planned Parenthood
  www.plannedparenthood.org
- FDA Birth Control Guide
  www.fda.gov (Search for "birth control")
- Abstinence
  www.stayteen.org/waiting

MOBILE TIPS!
Scan this QR code with your mobile device to access additional tips about *sexuality, contraception, and reproductive choices*. Or, via your mobile device, go to **http://chmobile.pearsoncmg.com** and choose by topic: sexuality, contraception, and reproductive choices.

- Go Ask Alice (advice about sexuality and sexual health)
  www.goaskalice.columbia.edu

Website links are subject to change. To access updated web links, please visit MasteringHealth

TEST YOUR KNOWLEDGE

LO 11.1
1. Which of the following is/are *not* part of the internal male genitals?
   a. glans penis
   b. epididymis
   c. vas deferens
   d. testes

LO 11.2
2. What is a woman's first period called?
   a. menstruation
   b. ovulation
   c. menarche
   d. menopause

LO 11.3
3. What is the name for the last phase of the sexual response cycle?
   a. finality
   b. resolution
   c. conclusion
   d. climax

LO 11.4
4. Which of the following is *not* considered non-intercourse sexual activity?
   a. oral sex
   b. anal sex
   c. mutual masturbation
   d. fantasy

LO 11.5
5. Which of the following best describes a transgender person?
   a. a person whose biological sex differs from the gender he or she identifies with
   b. a person born with both male and female genitalia
   c. a person who is equally attracted to both males and females
   d. a person who is only attracted to people of the opposite sex

LO 11.6
6. Of the following methods of birth control, which provide(s) protection against sexually transmitted infection?
   a. diaphragm
   b. female condom
   c. cervical sponge
   d. spermicides

LO 11.7
7. Which of the following statements is true about the legal status of abortion in the United States?
   a. Abortion is legal in some states but not in others.
   b. Recent Supreme Court decisions have made abortion legal only if the mother's life is at risk.
   c. Abortion is legal in the United States.
   d. Since 2014, women who want abortions must travel to Canada or Mexico.

LO 11.8
8. After the first 8 weeks of a pregnancy, what is the developing baby called?
   a. embryo
   b. blastocyst
   c. fetus
   d. zygote

LO 11.9
9. Which of the following is *not* an infertility treatment?
   a. ZIFT
   b. ICSI
   c. GIFT
   d. PIXY

LO 11.10
10. Which should happen before you become intimate with another person?
    a. Make sure he or she really likes you.
    b. Discuss where you want the relationship to go.
    c. Know yourself.
    d. Discuss your plans with your parents.

WHAT DO YOU THINK?

LO 11.4
1. What influence do you think social media has had on the sexual behavior of teens and young adults in the past 10 years?

LO 11.5
2. Many contend that today's college students are more accepting of homosexuality than their parents were. Do you believe this is true? Why or why not?

LO 11.6
3. In sexual relationships, what can men do to share responsibility for preventing an unwanted pregnancy?

LO 11.7
4. Should tax-supported programs such as Medicaid fund abortions for low-income women who want them? Why or why not?

LO 11.10
5. What are the most important steps a college student can take to protect his or her sexual health?

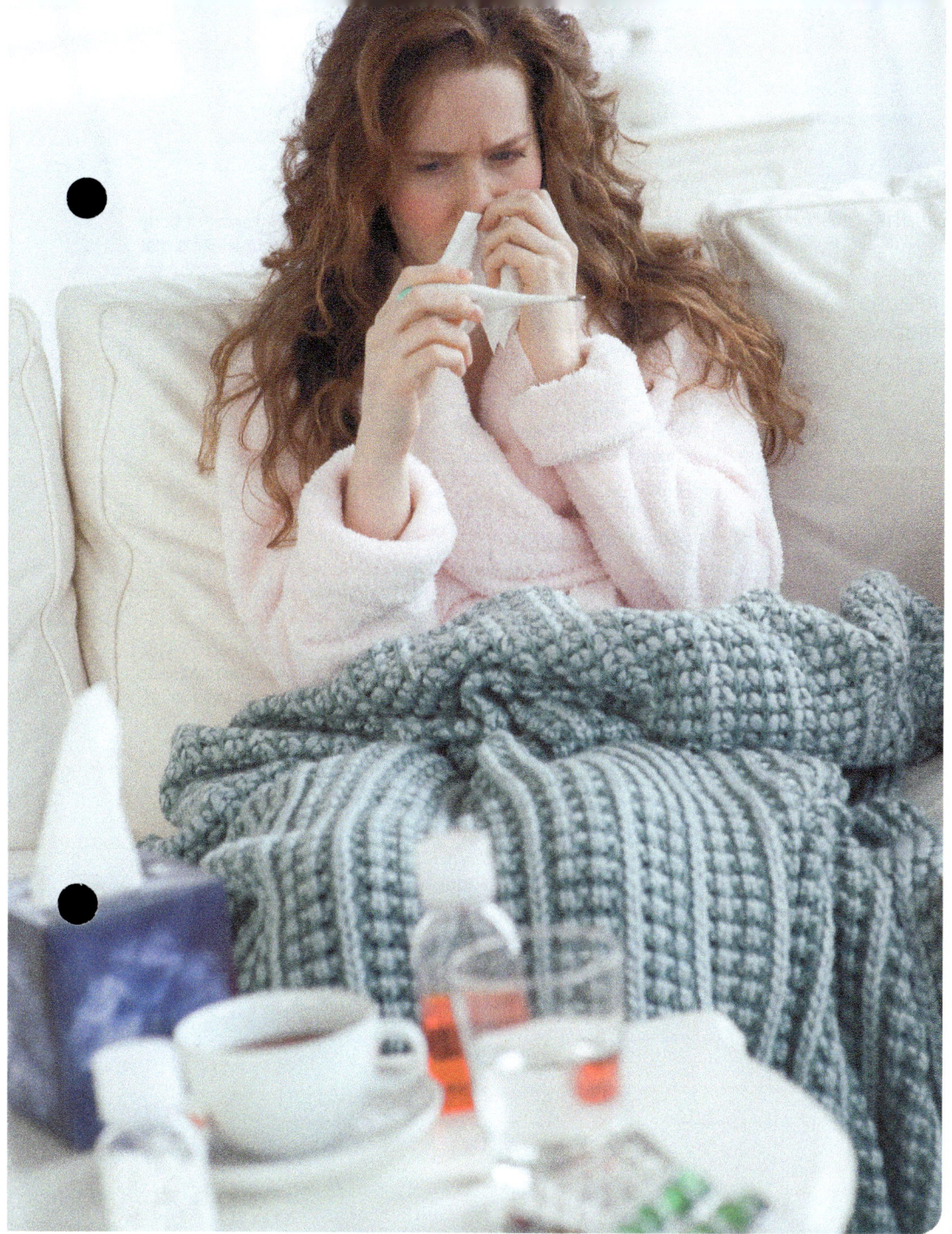

12

> Each year in the United States, 5% to 20% of the population gets the seasonal flu, resulting in 200,000 hospitalizations and as many as 49,000 deaths.[i]

> About 20 million people in the United States are infected each year with a sexually transmitted infection, and half of these cases occur in young people aged 15 to 24.[ii]

> Approximately 13% of the people in the United States infected with HIV do not realize it.[iii]

PREVENTING INFECTIOUS DISEASES AND SEXUALLY TRANSMITTED INFECTIONS

LEARNING OUTCOMES

LO 12.1 Identify the causes of infectious diseases and recognize how they are transmitted.

LO 12.2 Describe how the body's immune response works against infections and how immunization protects individuals and communities.

LO 12.3 Discuss the most common infectious diseases, their effects, and how to treat them.

LO 12.4 List common sexually transmitted infections (STIs), their causes, risk factors, symptoms, and treatment.

LO 12.5 Explain how to prevent infectious diseases and sexually transmitted infections.

The air we breathe, the food we eat, and even everyday items we touch

such as door handles and cell phones, carry tiny microorganisms. They may be small, but microorganisms have a large impact on human health. Some of these microbes are harmless or even helpful, but others are capable of causing disease. Millions of people die each year from infectious diseases such as influenza, malaria, tuberculosis, and acquired immunodeficiency syndrome (AIDS). Knowing how to protect yourself from infection is critical to your health.

How Are Infections Spread?

LO 12.1 Identify the causes of infectious diseases and recognize how they are transmitted.

Despite our best intentions to stay free of illness, it is impossible to make it to adulthood without ever having battled an infection. An **infection** is an invasion of body tissues by microorganisms that use the body's environment to multiply. In the process, these organisms damage and weaken the body and make us sick.

Pathogens are agents that cause disease. Common pathogens are harmful bacteria, viruses, fungi, protozoa, and parasitic worms. The natural environment for any particular pathogen, where it accumulates in large numbers, is called a **reservoir.** Pathogens move from a reservoir to a **host**—a person, a plant, or an animal in which or on which they can live and reproduce. The mode of transmission, or the way a pathogen moves from reservoir to host or from host to host, depends on the pathogen.

For infections to spread in a population, six conditions have to be met. These are collectively referred to as the **chain of infection (Figure 12.1).** Some of the ways infections are transmitted include:

Direct Transmission

- **Contact with infected people.** Close person-to-person contact with someone who has an infection is a common mode of disease transmission. Even if a person does not have any symptoms, he or she can still be infectious and considered a **carrier.** Many infections are spread sexually or even through simple touch. Contact with blood, saliva, or other bodily fluids can directly transmit infection from

> **infection** The invasion of body tissues by microorganisms that use the body's environment to multiply and cause disease.
>
> **pathogen** An agent that causes disease.
>
> **reservoir** The natural environment for any particular pathogen, where it accumulates in large numbers.
>
> **host** A person, a plant, or an animal in which or on which pathogens live and reproduce.
>
> **chain of infection** A group of factors necessary for the spread of infection.
>
> **carrier** A person infected with a pathogen who does not show symptoms but is infectious.

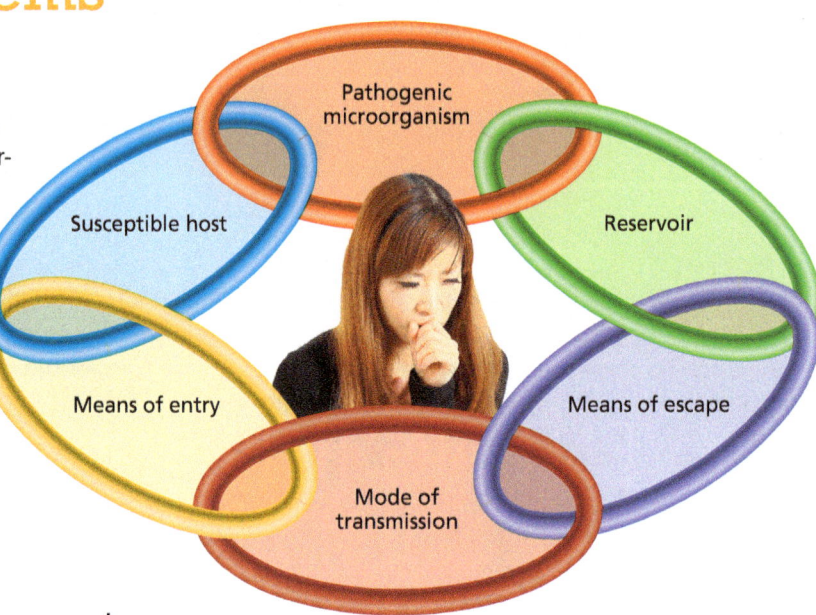

FIGURE 12.1 **Chain of Infection.** To cause infection, a pathogen such as a cold virus has to have a reservoir, such as a college student's body, in which to multiply and a means of escape, such as a cough. This enables the virus to be transmitted—for instance, by air to another student's eyes (the means of entry). If the student is susceptible—that is, if he or she has no immunity to the particular virus—he or she will experience infection.

one person to another as well. Follow safer sex practices, avoid kissing sick people or direct contact with blood, and thoroughly wash your hands often to reduce your risk of infection. See the **Practical Strategies** box on page 303 for tips on hand washing and hand sanitizer use.

- **Contact with infected animals.** Outbreaks of avian influenza showed us that people living and working closely with certain animals can risk catching infections from them. The Centers for Disease Control and Prevention (CDC) estimates that approximately 60% of human pathogens originated in animals and that 75% of emerging diseases involve transference from animals to humans.[1] It doesn't take an exotic animal to spread disease. Pets can carry rabies, meningitis, salmonella, or other infections passable to humans. Vaccinating your pets, washing your hands after handling animals, and avoiding contact with animal feces greatly reduce the risks of transmission.

Indirect Transmission

- **Touching contaminated objects.** If you have an infection and then cough or sneeze on an object—or touch it with your dirty hands—you leave pathogens behind for the next unwitting person to pick up. Bacteria adhere to both natural and manufactured surfaces, often as a survival mechanism, and once adhered, they can be harder to destroy than free-floating bacteria.[2] Touching a contaminated object and then touching your mouth, nose, or eyes can move pathogens into your body.

- **Breathing airborne pathogens.** When you cough and sneeze, tiny droplets of mucus tainted with pathogens waft in the air, which can be inhaled by another person. Viruses and bacteria that cause colds, influenza, and tuberculosis spread in this manner.

- **Bites from infected insects.** Pathogens can hitch a ride onboard a **vector,** an animal or insect that transports pathogens from one point to another. Classic examples of vectors are mosquitos, which transmit the malaria parasite, West Nile virus, and Zika virus, a growing global public health concern. (For more information on Zika virus, see the **Special Feature** on page 302) Deer ticks can transport the bacteria that cause Lyme disease.

- **Drinking or eating contaminated water or food.** Viruses, protozoa, and bacteria from animal or human feces can get into lakes, rivers, oceans, swimming pools, hot tubs, water slides, and public fountains. Chlorine can help kill pathogens but not entirely. Food can also become contaminated with pathogens when handled or processed in unsanitary ways.

> *"If you have an infection and then cough or sneeze on an object—or touch it with your dirty hands—you leave pathogens behind for the next unwitting person to pick up."*

LO 12.1 QUICK CHECK

For an infection to spread, how many conditions must be met?
a. 2
b. 6
c. 8
d. 10

Protecting Against Infections

LO 12.2 Describe how the body's immune response works against infections and how immunization protects individuals and communities.

Your body is not defenseless against infectious microorganisms. Even if you are exposed to pathogens, your body's defenses may protect you.

The Body's First Line of Defense

One of the most powerful barriers between you and pathogens is your skin. Your skin keeps the millions of bacteria that live on it from entering your body. Breaches can occur, however, if you get a cut, bad scrape, or puncture wound—one of the reasons doctors encourage you to thoroughly cleanse and cover a wound immediately after sustaining it.

> **vector** An animal or insect that transports pathogens from one point to another.
>
> **immune system** Your body's cellular and chemical defenses against pathogens.

Skin doesn't shield your entire body, of course. Openings such as your mouth and nose need other forms of protection. Mucous membranes line the mouth, airways, vagina, and digestive tract, trapping many unwanted microorganisms. *Cilia,* tiny hairlike projections, line the airways and help sweep away microscopic pathogens. Bodily fluids such as saliva, tears, earwax, vaginal fluid, and digestive acid trap and kill or expel many potential invaders. Coughing, sneezing, vomiting, and diarrhea are other ways the body expels foreign intruders.

If any of the systems that provide these first defenses becomes damaged—for instance, if your skin is severely burned or your cilia are damaged from smoking—you become more susceptible to infection. Even with healthy first defenses, however, pathogens can occasionally enter your body and infect you, at which point your immune response kicks in.

The Body's Immune Response

The **immune system** is the set of your body's cellular and chemical defenses against pathogens. Key players in the immune system are white blood cells, which patrol the circulatory system and body tissues, looking for microscopic enemies (**Figure 12.2,** next page).

Nonspecific Response

Some white blood cells respond to a broad range of foreign invaders and attack and destroy them in what is called a *nonspecific response*. These cells are neutrophils, natural killer (NK) cells, and macrophages. Neutrophils, the most common type of white blood cells, conquer bacteria and other foreign invaders traveling in the blood by ingesting

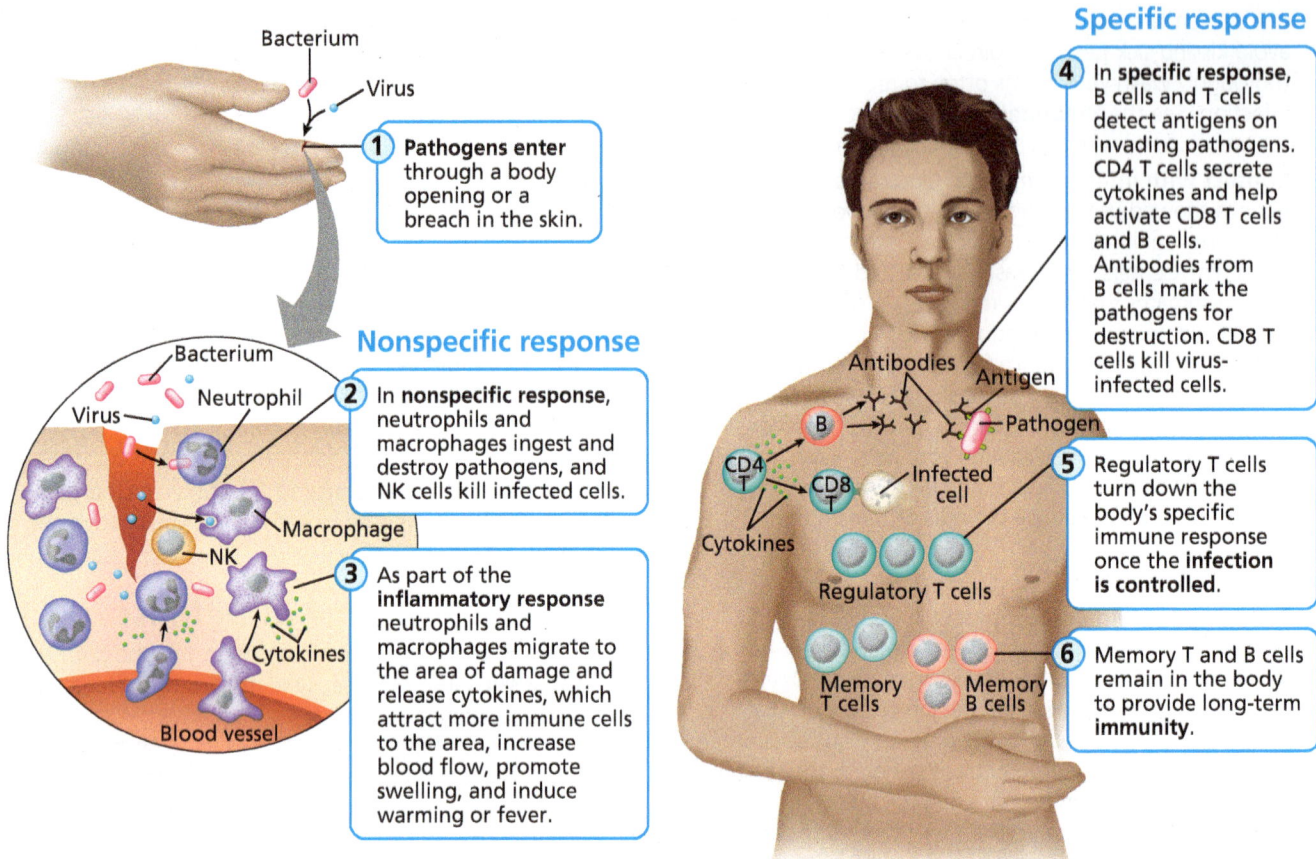

FIGURE 12.2 **Your Body's Immune Response.**

and destroying them. NK cells eliminate body cells that are infected by viruses. Macrophages survey our tissues and gobble up bacteria and wounded and dead cells.

Another essential component of nonspecific response is the **inflammatory response.** If body tissue is damaged, the inflammatory response kicks in. Neutrophils and macrophages migrate to the area of damage. They release chemical signals, called cytokines, which attract additional white blood cells to the location, increase blood flow to the area (promoting the delivery of immune cells), and induce fever. This response is designed to kill any pathogens that reside in the damaged tissue, promote healing, and prevent the spread of infection to other parts of the body.

Specific Response

Other white blood cell types, the lymphocytes, mount a *specific response* in which they recognize and attack specific pathogens. The lymphocytes consist of B cells and T cells and are mostly found in the body's lymph fluid, lymph nodes, and other lymph organs, such as the spleen. Both B cells and T cells bear surface receptors that detect **antigens,** tiny regions on the surface of a pathogen.

In response to an antigen, B cells release **antibodies,** proteins that bind tightly to invaders and mark them for destruction. In fact, the term *antigen* is a contraction of *anti*body-*gen*erator. Antibodies are highly specialized, with each type targeting only one specific antigen, just as a key fits only one lock.

How T cells respond to an antigen depends on the T cell type. There are three types of T cells. Cytotoxic T cells (CD8 T cells) kill virus-infected cells. Helper T cells (CD4 T cells) secrete cytokines that help activate B cells, cytotoxic T cells, and NK cells. Regulatory T cells help turn down the specific immune response once the infection is under control.

The antigen-activated B cells and T cells also create long-lived *memory B cells* and *memory T cells*. These cells stay in the body and quickly identify and attack that specific pathogen if it enters the body again in the future. This is why successfully defeating an infection leaves us with **acquired immunity,** which in some cases leads to lifelong protection against the same infection. For example, if you have ever had chickenpox, you are unlikely to get it again.

Immunization

Acquired immunity can protect you against infections that your immune system recognizes, but what about diseases that your body has never seen before? In the past, the

inflammatory response A response to damaged body tissues designed to kill any pathogens in the damaged tissue, promote healing, and prevent the spread of infection to other parts of the body.

antigen Tiny regions on the surface of an infectious agent that can be detected by B cells and T cells.

antibodies Proteins released by B cells that bind tightly to infectious agents and mark them for destruction.

acquired immunity The body's ability to quickly identify and attack a pathogen that it recognizes from previous exposure. In some cases acquired immunity leads to lifelong protection against the same infection.

STUDENT STORY

Germaphobe

"HI, I'M JESSICA. As a germaphobe, I'm constantly sanitizing my hands after touching doorknobs, ATMs, or anything in a store. I absolutely have to keep clean everywhere I go. I always have little hand sanitizer bottles in my bag, and I have a gigantic one in my room. I use it when I don't have access to a sink to wash my hands. It's really easy just to dab some on your hand and just go and it's quick. I also get the seasonal flu vaccine every year.

Living on campus, you're always around people and touching everything everyone else touches. Your chance of getting sick is always way higher than if you were to live on your own somewhere. So I'm just really careful to keep my hands clean—it's the best solution to prevent getting a cold every other week."

What Do You Think?

1. Will using hand sanitizer and getting a flu vaccine prevent Jessica from getting all infections? What other ways might Jessica get an infection?
2. Do you think Jessica is right that living on campus increases your chances of getting sick? Why or why not?
3. What are some infections that are more likely to be present on college campuses than other places?

---

primary way people developed immunity was by contracting a disease and surviving it, a process known as *naturally acquired immunity*. Many diseases such as polio, whooping cough, measles, mumps, and rubella commonly killed or crippled victims before their bodies could fight them off. Widespread adoption of immunizations turned that tide. The advent of immunizations has been recognized as one of the most monumental developments in modern medical history, effectively eradicating some diseases such as smallpox and limiting others significantly.

Immunization often involves exposing a person to a pathogen through a vaccine, which allows the body to develop immunity to the pathogen without actually falling ill. This is called *artificially acquired immunity*. Vaccines are composed of pathogens—or parts of pathogens—that have been killed or weakened. When they are introduced into the body, these dead or weakened microbes pose little threat, yet the body believes it is under attack and sounds the alarm to battle them. The immune system then produces memory B cells and memory T cells that can stave off that particular type of infectious disease for years to come, perhaps for a lifetime. This is known as *active immunity* because it induces an immune response.

> **immunization** Creating immunity to a pathogen through vaccination or through the injection of antibodies.

In other instances, injections can provide temporary *passive immunity*, when ready-made antibodies specific to a particular pathogen are introduced into the body to fight off an infection. Passive immunity is used, for example, in the case of exposure to the hepatitis A virus. The injected antibodies immediately target the virus for destruction. Passive immunity lasts only as long as the injected antibodies survive, a few months at most.

The Centers for Disease Control and Prevention has developed recommended immunization schedules for children, teens, and adults **(Table 12.1)**, and all states require certain

---

TABLE 12.1 Vaccines Recommended for College Students[a]

Vaccine	Number of Doses
Tetanus, diphtheria, pertussis (Tdap, Td)[a]	Single dose of Tdap then boost with Td every 10 years
Measles, mumps, rubella (MMR)[a]	2 doses recommended for college students
Polio (IPV)[a]	4 doses if given in childhood; 3 doses if given in adulthood
Varicella (Var) (chicken pox)[a]	2 doses
Human papillomavirus (HPV),[a,b]	3 doses
Hepatitis B (Hep B),[a]	3 doses
Meningococcal disease[c]	1 dose
Pneumococcal polysaccharide (PPV)[d]	1 dose with revaccination after 5 years for those with elevated risk factors
Hepatitis A (Hep A)[d]	2 doses
Annual influenza (and H1N1)[d]	1 dose annually

[a] Recommended for those who lack documentation of past vaccination with all recommended doses and have no evidence of prior infection.
[b] Recommended for those aged 26 and under.
[c] Recommended for previously unvaccinated college freshmen living in dormitories.
[d] Recommended if some other risk factor is present.

Source: Adapted from Centers for Disease Control and Prevention. (2016). *Recommended immunizations for adults.* www.cdc.gov.

MYTH OR FACT?

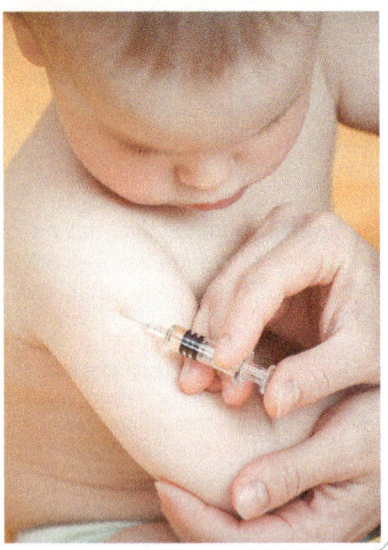

Do Vaccines Cause Autism?

In 1998, an article that appeared in the British medical journal *The Lancet* claimed that autism—a developmental brain disorder that causes problems in communication, social interaction, and behavior—was caused by the childhood vaccine for measles, mumps, and rubella (MMR).[1] In response, some parents' groups began a movement against vaccinations, and more and more parents stopped vaccinating their children.

Anti-vaccine groups claim that autism is linked to the recommended number and schedule of childhood vaccinations and the use of thimerosal, a preservative that contains mercury, in some vaccines. As evidence of the damage of vaccinations, parents of autistic children publicized "before" and "after" home videos of their children displaying autistic characteristics only after the date of vaccination. Celebrities such as Jenny McCarthy have advocated for vaccination reform.

However, much research has found no evidence of a link between autism and vaccines.[2] Thimerosal, which was never present in the MMR vaccines most blamed for autism, was removed from most common childhood vaccines by 2001, and rates of autism spectrum disorder have increased, not declined, since then.[3,4] And in February 2010 *The Lancet* retracted the original paper linking autism to the MMR vaccine, citing a recent British medical panel ruling that the lead author had been deceptive and violated basic research ethics in his study.

The causes of autism remain unknown. However, one thing is clear: It is dangerous to become infected with a disease that could be prevented by a vaccine.

What Do You Think?

1. Are there communities or groups where you live who don't vaccinate their children? If so, why not?
2. Should families who choose not to vaccinate be held responsible in some way if an infectious disease affects children in their community?
3. What are some steps that schools and public health officials can take to share accurate information about vaccines and infectious disease outbreaks?

Sources **1.** Wakefield, A. J., Murch, S. H., Anthony, A., Linnell, J., Casson, D. M., et al. (1998). Ileal-lymphoid-nodular hyperplasia, non-specific colitis, and pervasive developmental disorder in children. *The Lancet, 351*(9103), 637-641. **2.** American Academy of Pediatrics. (2013). *Vaccine safety: Examine the evidence.* www.aap.org. **3.** U.S. Food and Drug Administration. (2015). Table 1: Thimerosal content of vaccines routinely recommended for children 6 years of age and younger. In *Vaccines, Blood & Biologics.* www.fda.gov. **4.** Centers for Disease Control and Prevention. (2015). *Autism spectrum disorder (ASD).* www.cdc.gov.

---

immunizations before children can enter school. Exemptions to immunization laws can be given if a child has certain medical conditions, for religious reasons, and sometimes for other beliefs. In addition, some people are not immunized because they don't know or understand the recommendations, don't have access to health care, or cannot afford the shots. Groups of people not being immunized can compromise **herd immunity,** which occurs when greater than 90% of people in a community or group are fully vaccinated against a disease, leaving that disease little ability to spread through the population. Herd immunity is important because it offers some protection against the disease for individuals who cannot be vaccinated (due to medical conditions) or who haven't been vaccinated yet (such as newborns).

▶▶ *Frontline: The Vaccine War* explores both sides of the vaccine debate. Go to www.pbs.org/ and search for "The Vaccine War."

Immune Disorders

Not all immune systems are strong. Newborns do not yet have fully developed immune systems, and seniors tend to have weak ones, which grow less and less effective as they age. These groups are therefore more vulnerable than others to infection and disease. Chronic stress can also impair the immune system, a topic discussed in more detail in Chapter 3. In addition, the immune system can sometimes develop disorders. Two common problems are allergies and asthma.

Allergies

More than 50 million people in the United States have **allergies,** abnormal immune system reactions to substances that are otherwise harmless. Allergies are widespread on college campuses; in one survey, 19% of students stated that they had been treated for allergies in the past year.[3]

Allergies are caused by a hypersensitive immune system mistakenly perceiving substances such as pollen, peanuts, pet dander, and pest droppings to be serious threats.[4] If you

herd immunity The condition where greater than 90% of a community is vaccinated against a disease, giving the disease little ability to spread through the community and providing some protection against the disease to members of the community who are not vaccinated.

allergies Abnormal immune system reactions to substances that are otherwise harmless.

have allergies, you may suffer from itching, sneezing, coughing, watery eyes, difficulty breathing, and congestion. When allergic people come into contact with substances they are sensitive to, their immune systems begin to produce antibodies called immunoglobulin E (IgE). IgE molecules bind simultaneously to the allergen and to a **mast cell,** a type of cell in the skin and mucous membranes. As a result of these interactions, the mast cell releases powerful chemicals such as histamine into the bloodstream. It is these chemicals—and not the allergens themselves—that make allergy sufferers miserable.

In some instances, allergens cause a rare, serious allergic reaction known as *anaphylaxis*. In this case, the wave of histamine and chemicals released by mast cells occurs throughout the body and can cause **anaphylactic shock.** Blood pressure drops, and airways swell. If not treated immediately with an injection of epinephrine, a person can lapse into unconsciousness and even death.

Fortunately, there are strategies for coping with allergies. Allergists recommend you steer clear of the things you are allergic to whenever possible. Your doctor may recommend prescription or over-the-counter medications that can help alleviate symptoms. Immunotherapy, in which patients are given repeated shots containing increasing amounts of the allergen to desensitize them, is also an option.

>> The American Lung Association provides more information on how to manage asthma and minimize triggers of an asthma attack. Go to www.lung.org and search for "Asthma."

The incidence of allergies has increased steadily in recent years. Ironically, this increase may be the unintended result of our antiseptic, health-conscious lifestyle. A possible explanation, the *hygiene hypothesis,* contends that early childhood exposure to microbes can prevent the development of allergies, and, conversely, reduced exposure to microbes can increase the chances of developing allergies. Many factors in developed countries today reduce exposure to microbes: smaller family size (fewer siblings means fewer family members bringing microbes into the home); less exposure to animals, specifically farm animals; use of vaccines and antibiotics; and less exposure to general dirt and microorganisms.

The hygiene hypothesis may also contribute to the increasing rates of asthma, a condition that we'll look at next.

>> This video explores the hygiene hypothesis of developing allergies: www.pbs.org/wgbh/evolution/library/10/4/l_104_07.html.

Asthma

Asthma occurs when the airways of the lungs become constricted and inflamed, making breathing difficult. The symptoms and severity of asthma range from shortness of breath and wheezing (a whistling-type noise produced during exhalation) to the life-threatening inability to effectively move air into and out of the lungs. There are two general types of asthma. *Allergic asthma* is caused by exposure to allergens such as those in the air (e.g., pollen), in the blood (e.g., bee venom), or in food (e.g., peanuts). *Intrinsic asthma,* on the other hand, can be induced by exercise or cold temperatures and is not associated with an allergy. It isn't clear why some people have asthma and others do not, but it is likely a combination of genetics and the environment in which you live.

An asthma attack is a result of three main physiological changes: the constriction of the airway muscles, known as *bronchoconstriction,* the overproduction of mucus in the airway, and inflammation of the airway lining. All of these changes can lead to a terrifying result—the inability to breathe. Prevention of asthma includes avoiding known triggers and, in some cases, taking regular doses of medicines that prevent bronchoconstriction and inflammation. Once an attack has begun, fast-acting bronchodilators, administered through inhalers, and oral anti-inflammatory medicines help open the airways and ease breathing.

Nearly 1 in 10 school-aged children in the United States suffers from asthma, reflecting a doubling of asthma rates over the past 30 years.[5] Also notable is the racial disparity in asthma rates. About 17% of African American children have asthma, compared to about 11% of children of other racial and ethnic backgrounds. This is thought to reflect socioeconomic conditions, with children in lower-income households more likely to be exposed to mold, diesel soot, and air pollution.

> **mast cell** A type of cell in the skin and mucous membranes that releases histamine and other chemicals into the bloodstream during an allergic reaction.
>
> **anaphylactic shock** A result of anaphylaxis, where the release of histamine and other chemicals into the body leads to a drop in blood pressure, tightening of airways, and possible unconsciousness and even death.
>
> **asthma** Chronic constriction and inflammation of the airways, which makes breathing difficult and causes shortness of breath, wheezing, coughing, and chest tightness.
>
> **virus** A microscopic organism that cannot multiply without invading body cells.

LO 12.2 QUICK CHECK

What is the most common type of white blood cell?
a. natural killer (NK) cell
b. macrophage
c. mast cell
d. neutrophil

Infectious Diseases

LO 12.3 Discuss the most common infectious diseases, their effects, and how to treat them.

Even with advances in modern medicine, infections remain the world's leading killer of children and young adults. The burden on society from even minor infections is immense. Infectious disease costs the United States more than $120 billion per year.[6]

Infections can be categorized by the types of pathogens that cause them: viruses, bacteria, fungi, protozoa, and parasitic worms (**Table 12.2,** next page).

Viral Infections

Viruses are microscopic organisms that cannot multiply without invading body cells. They hijack the cellular machinery and force it to crank out duplicate viruses at the expense of the cells' normal functions—and at the expense of your

TABLE 12.2 Pathogens and the Diseases They Cause

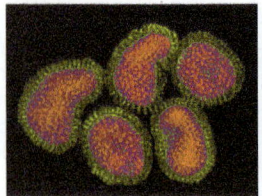 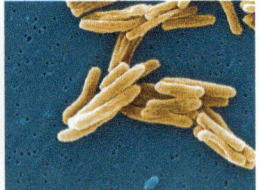 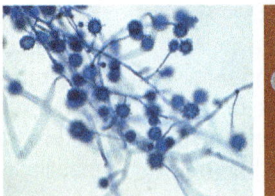 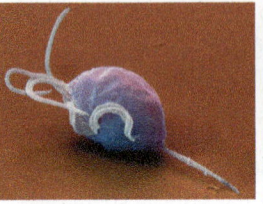 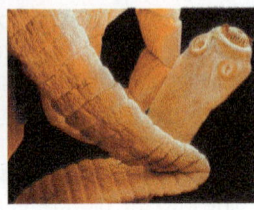

Influenza viruses (shown at 32,000 ×).	*Mycobacterium tuberculosis* bacteria (shown at 15,549 ×).	*Histoplasma capsulatum* (shown at 400 ×).	*Trichomonas vaginalis* (shown at 9,000 ×).	*Taenia* tapeworm (shown at 15 ×).
Pathogen: Viruses	**Pathogen: Bacteria**	**Pathogen: Fungi**	**Pathogen: Protozoa**	**Pathogen: Parasitic worms (helminths)**
Description: Microscopic infectious agents that are composed not of cells but of small amounts of genetic material covered by a protein coat. They cannot multiply unless they invade living cells and hijack those cells' metabolic machinery.	**Description:** Single-celled microorganisms that have genetic material but lack a distinct cell nucleus. They invade and reproduce inside a host, sometimes releasing toxic enzymes and chemicals.	**Description:** Organisms with sophisticated cellular structures, including a true nucleus and a strong, flexible cell wall. Fungi include yeasts and molds. They feed on organic matter, including human tissue.	**Description:** Single-celled parasites that rely on other living things for food and shelter.	**Description:** Multicellular parasitic creatures that are ingested as eggs or burrow through the skin and compete with a host body for nutrients.
Examples: Rhinoviruses; coronaviruses; influenza viruses; Epstein-Barr virus; hepatitis A-E; HIV; herpes simplex virus types 1 and 2 (HSV-1 and HSV-2); human papillomavirus	**Examples:** *Neisseria meningitidis, Staphylococcus aureus,* Group A *Streptococcus, Streptococcus pneumoniae, Borrelia burgdorferi, Mycobacterium tuberculosis, Chlamydia trachomatis, Treponema pallidum*	**Examples:** *Candida albicans, Histoplasma capsulatum, Trichophyton*	**Examples:** *Plasmodium, Toxoplasma gondii, Trichomonas vaginalis*	**Examples:** *Taenia solium, Taenia saginata, Hymenolepis nana, Enterobius vermicularis, Ancylostoma duodenale*
Diseases Caused: Common cold, flu, mononucleosis, hepatitis, AIDS, herpes (oral or genital), cervical cancer, warts, genital warts	**Diseases Caused:** Meningitis, staph infection, food poisoning, toxic shock syndrome, strep throat, pneumonia, Lyme disease, tuberculosis, sexually transmitted infections	**Diseases Caused:** Candidiasis (yeast infections), thrush, diaper rash, infections of nail beds, histoplasmosis, *tinea pedis* (athlete's foot), jock itch, ring worm, nail infections	**Diseases Caused:** Malaria, toxoplasmosis, trichomoniasis	**Diseases Caused:** Tapeworm, pinworm, hookworm infection

health. Viruses cannot survive for long periods outside a host, but once inside a host cell, they can multiply very quickly. For example, a cell infected with the common flu virus begins to release new flu viruses only 6 hours after the virus enters the cell, and it produces enough new viruses to infect another 20 to 30 cells. The infected cell dies about 11 hours after the virus entered.[7]

Colds

More than 200 different viruses cause cold symptoms. Common culprits are groups of viruses called *rhinoviruses* and *coronaviruses.* They are typically spread by touching contaminated objects, through personal contact, or by breathing airborne pathogens. Symptoms appear about two or three days after infection and can include a runny nose or congestion, sneezing, cough, sore throat, headache, and mild fever. There is no known cure, but over-the-counter pain relievers, antihistamines, and decongestants may provide some relief from symptoms.

Colds generally end in about a week and cannot be treated with antibiotics because antibiotics are designed to fight bacteria, not viruses. However, sometimes viral infections leave the body susceptible to secondary bacterial infections of the sinuses, ears, or respiratory tract, in which case antibiotics would be prescribed. Wash your hands frequently, keep your hands away from your face, and stay away from people who have colds to help keep from getting one.

Influenza

The flu is a contagious respiratory condition caused by a number of **influenza** viruses. Between 5% and 20% of the U.S. population get the flu every year, suffering from high fever, body aches, fatigue, and a dry cough. Although it often is a moderate illness, lasting a little longer and making people a little more miserable than the common cold, the flu can cause medical emergency in some infants, seniors, or people with weakened immune systems. The flu can also lead to bacterial pneumonia, dehydration, sinus infections, and ear infections and tends to exacerbate underlying medical conditions such as asthma and diabetes. Every year, more than 200,000 people in the United States are hospitalized with flu complications, and as many as 49,000 die from influenza infection.[8]

> **influenza** A group of viruses that cause the flu, a contagious respiratory condition.

As with colds, influenza viruses are spread through personal contact, airborne pathogens, or touching inanimate objects covered with a virus. There is no known cure—although antiviral medications may be prescribed to reduce symptoms—and so prevention remains the best medicine.

In addition to proper hand washing and coughing and sneezing into the bend of your arm rather than your hand, federal health officials recommend that children, pregnant women, health workers, people over age 65, and people of all ages with chronic medical conditions such as asthma and diabetes get an influenza vaccine annually. "Flu shots" are available at many campus health centers, doctors' offices, pharmacies, and even grocery stores every fall.

When a flu is able to pass quickly from person to person unchecked and eventually spreads worldwide, it is called a **pandemic.** Pandemics can occur when a new influenza virus emerges that humans have not been exposed to before. This lack of exposure leaves people with no acquired immunity to help defend against the virus, which can become very contagious. Often, animals are the reservoir for flu viruses that mutate into new strains that cause pandemics. The most recent pandemic, the 2009 H1N1 flu pandemic, was caused by a virus that started in pigs. When a pandemic virus is also deadly, the casualties can be staggering. In 1918, a global influenza pandemic killed approximately 40 million people.

>> This CDC video explains how to "Take 3" to avoid catching or spreading influenza. Go to www.cdc.gov and search for "CDCTV Take 3."

Mononucleosis

Infectious **mononucleosis,** or *mono,* which is often called "the kissing disease," is caused by the Epstein-Barr virus. It is transmitted through contact with an infected person's saliva, mucus, or tears. Sharing drinking glasses or straws, eating utensils, or toothbrushes can expose you to the Epstein-Barr virus. Common among teens and young adults, mono causes fatigue, weakness, sore throat, fever, headaches, swollen lymph nodes and tonsils, and loss of appetite. The condition usually is not serious, although some people may experience complications such as hepatitis or enlargement of the spleen. Most symptoms dissipate within two or three weeks, but the fatigue, weakness, and swollen lymph nodes can persevere for months. Blood tests may be used to diagnose mononucleosis, and the primary treatments are as basic as getting lots of rest and drinking plenty of fluids.

Hepatitis

Hepatitis is an inflammation of the liver. It causes **jaundice,** fatigue, fever, nausea, abdominal pain, and muscle and joint pain. In some cases it can be deadly. Viral infections are the primary cause of hepatitis, although alcohol, drugs, and some underlying medical conditions can be blamed. There are several types of hepatitis. Hepatitis A, hepatitis B, and hepatitis C are the most common forms in the United States, but there are also rarer hepatitis viruses, known as D and E. Hepatitis B is transmitted mostly through sexual contact in the United States, and is discussed on page 307.

Hepatitis A is the most widespread form of hepatitis. It is contracted through consuming microscopic amounts of feces that can lurk on contaminated fruits, vegetables, and ice cubes. The virus can also be spread during oral-anal sexual contact or by changing dirty diapers and failing to thoroughly wash your hands afterward. Symptoms can last for weeks or months, although some people never feel ill.

Although the virus can cause liver failure and death in a small portion of the population, most people make a full recovery, sustaining no permanent liver damage. Rates of hepatitis A have decreased in recent years. A vaccine for hepatitis A was introduced in 1995, and doctors recommend that children, travelers to certain countries, and other at-risk individuals get the vaccine, which has led to a reduction in infections.

Hepatitis C is the primary reason for liver transplants in the United States. More than three-fourths of those who are infected with this highly destructive virus go on to develop chronic infections that can last a lifetime, scarring the liver or triggering liver cancer. Unfortunately, early symptoms of this form of hepatitis are mild or nonexistent, and many people do not realize they have it until liver damage has occurred. About 3.5 million Americans are infected with hepatitis C, which is typically spread through sharing syringes and other drug-related paraphernalia.[9] It can also be passed on by unsterilized tattoo needles and piercing equipment or sexual contact. Before screening tests were developed and made available in the United States, it was also spread through blood transfusions and organ transplants. It is still possible to pick up the infection from needles or other medical instruments in other parts of the world where sterilization practices may not be as rigorous.

Treatment for hepatitis is usually nothing more than rest, fluids, and proper nutrition for acute cases, but chronic cases sometimes benefit from medications. If you have chronic hepatitis, your doctor should regularly screen you for liver disease.

> **pandemic** A worldwide epidemic of a disease.
>
> **mononucleosis** A viral disease that causes fatigue, weakness, sore throat, fever, headaches, swollen lymph nodes and tonsils, and loss of appetite.
>
> **hepatitis** Inflammation of the liver that affects liver function.
>
> **jaundice** A yellowing of the skin, mucous membranes, and sometimes the whites of the eyes, often caused by liver malfunction.
>
> **bacteria (singular** *bacterium***)** Single-celled microorganisms that invade a host and reproduce inside. Harmful bacteria release toxic enzymes and chemicals.
>
> **antibiotic resistance** A bacterium's ability to overcome the effects of an antibiotic through a random mutation or change in the bacterium's genetic code.

Bacterial Infections

Bacteria are single-celled microorganisms that are found throughout nature. They can exist independently or as parasites, drawing their nourishment from other forms of life. Harmful bacteria release toxins or damaging enzymes that disrupt the body. However, less than 1% of the many types of bacteria are actually harmful.[10] Some bacteria are even beneficial, helping us digest food, synthesize vitamins, and fight off disease. Manufacturers even add bacteria such as *Lactobacillus acidophilus* to many yogurt and cheese products because of their healthful properties.

Unlike viruses, bacteria are able to replicate on their own, without the help of a host cell, by dividing in two. Antibiotics help defeat bacteria by blocking key steps in this process. However, bacteria can also develop **antibiotic resistance** to these important drugs. This occurs when a random mutation, or change in a bacterium's genetic code, enables the bacterium to overcome the effects of the antibiotic. Perhaps only 1 bacterium in 10 million gains this advantage, but that cell rapidly grows and divides, even in the presence of the antibiotic, and the resistant bacteria take over.

The risk of antibiotic resistance makes it extremely important to take antibiotics only when they have been prescribed by a physician and to take them for the full course prescribed. Soaps and other cleaning products labeled "antibacterial" have also been linked to antibiotic resistance. While keeping your hands and surroundings clean can help reduce the risk of infection, regular soaps and cleansers are sufficient; you do not need to use antibacterial products. For hand washing and personal hygiene, regular soap is effective and doesn't increase the risk of creating resistant microbes.[11]

Meningitis

Meningitis is an infection of the meninges, the thin membranes that surround the spinal cord and brain. The infection can be caused by a number of viral and bacterial strains and is characterized by high fever, stiff neck, headaches, and confusion or seizures. When caused by a virus, meningitis tends to be much less severe and dissipates on its own. Bacterial meningitis, however, can be life threatening and may cause hearing loss, brain damage, and other disabilities. The bacteria that most commonly cause meningitis are *Streptococcus pneumoniae* and *Neisseria meningitidis*; most often, meningitis occurs when these bacteria have infected another part of the body and then enter the bloodstream and migrate to the meninges. Even when treated promptly with the proper antibiotics, bacterial meningitis kills between 5% and 10% of patients worldwide, usually within a day or two of the onset of symptoms. About 10% to 20% of survivors are left with hearing loss or brain damage.[12]

Adolescents and young adults account for nearly one-third of all cases of bacterial meningitis in the United States, and college students—especially those living in dormitories—are at moderately increased risk. To reduce their risk, the CDC recommends that all youths between the ages of 11 and 18 receive the meningococcal vaccine, an inoculation that protects against some but not all of the bacterial strains that cause meningitis. Several states now require that students receive a meningococcal vaccine before entering college or university.

Staphylococcal Infections

There are more than two dozen types of *Staphylococcus* bacteria, but one—*Staphylococcus aureus*—is responsible for the bulk of all "staph" infections. It causes boils and other minor skin ailments, especially in people with eczema (a chronic, itchy skin rash) or burned skin. Sometimes staph can cause more serious infections of the blood, lungs, heart, or urinary tract, most often in those whose immune system is compromised because of illness or other conditions.

Staphylococcus aureus also releases toxins that can trigger food poisoning and **toxic shock syndrome.** Toxic shock syndrome is a rare yet serious disease that resembles a bad cold or flu in the first few hours but can quickly progress to a medical emergency. Fever, chills, nausea, and diarrhea give way to seizures, low blood pressure, and organ failure and, in about 5% of cases, death.[13] In 1980, more than 800 menstruating women developed the condition, and 38 died from it. Federal investigators linked the cases to use of a highly absorbent tampon that was subsequently taken off the market. Menstruating women can avoid toxic shock syndrome by changing their tampons every 4 to 8 hours, using the lowest-absorbency tampon possible, and alternating between tampons and pads.

MRSA

Some staph bacteria are resistant to the antibiotics typically used to treat them. **Methicillin-resistant *Staphylococcus aureus* (MRSA)** is a strain that is resistant to the broad-spectrum antibiotics commonly used to treat staph infections. It is responsible for serious skin infections, which first appear as painful, red, pus-filled lesions, and can also cause other infections, including pneumonia. Because MRSA is not treatable with many antibiotics, it poses a threat to anyone who is infected.

The Centers for Disease Control and Prevention estimates that about 80,000 people in the United States develop a serious MRSA infection in any given year and that about 11,000 die from it.[14] Public health experts state that the development of bacteria like MRSA, which are resistant to multiple antibiotics, is in part due to the misuse of antibiotics.

The infection can be spread by direct skin-to-skin contact or by touching something that has been touched by an infected person. Most MRSA infections occur in hospital and other health-care settings. However, recent data indicate that following intensive infection control programs in many facilities, the number of MRSA cases acquired in health-care settings is declining. One study found that between 2005 and 2011, the number of MRSA infections originating in hospitals declined 54%.[15]

However, the rate of MRSA infection in the community has not undergone similar declines. In 2011, for the first time, more MRSA infections arose outside health-care facilities than inside them.[15] MRSA has been a persistent problem in schools and on college campuses. School athletes are especially susceptible due to frequent skin contact with others, the likelihood of cuts or abrasions on the skin, and the use of locker rooms, equipment, and facilities that may harbor MRSA.

Frequent hand washing, especially in a clinical setting, is critical to limiting the spread of this infection. In addition to hand washing, the following measures will help you avoid an MRSA infection:

- Keep open wounds covered with dry, sterile bandages.
- Shower immediately after exercise or participating in a contact sport.
- Do not share personal items such as towels or razors.
- If you have a skin infection that does not appear to be improving after 48 hours, see a doctor and request testing for MRSA.

> **toxic shock syndrome** A rare, serious illness caused by staph bacteria that begins with severe flu symptoms but can quickly progress to a medical emergency.
>
> **methicillin-resistant *Staphylococcus aureus* (MRSA)** A strain of staph that is resistant to the broad-spectrum antibiotics commonly used to treat staph infections.

Early detection is important, especially because some MRSA strains respond to the antibiotic vancomycin. Minor skin infections can be treated by cleaning and draining the lesion.

Streptococcus Infections

Chances are you or someone you know has been infected with the bacteria *Streptococcus,* perhaps more than once. Group A *Streptococcus* is behind all bouts of strep throat, a relatively mild illness that causes throat pain, swollen tonsils, fever, headache, and stomachache. Particularly common in children and teens, strep throat is highly contagious through airborne droplets or touching contaminated objects. Strep throat is usually treated with a course of antibiotics. If left untreated, it can lead to scarlet fever or rheumatic fever. Strains of *Streptococcus* bacteria can also cause other types of infections, including skin infections and pneumonia.

Lyme Disease

If you have ever been hiking in the northwestern, midwestern, or northeastern states, you may have seen warning signs about Lyme disease. The infection is caused by the bacterium *Borrelia burgdorferi* and is transmitted to people through the bite of infected deer ticks and blacklegged ticks. Early symptoms are headache, fatigue, fever, and muscle or joint pain. Within four weeks of infection, 70%-80% of victims also experience a bull's-eye-shaped skin rash that starts small and grows larger **(Figure 12.3)**. If the infection goes untreated, it can cause swelling and pain in the joints, rapid heartbeat or other heart problems, partial facial paralysis, and neurological problems such as memory loss, which can last for years. Antibiotics are usually successful at treating Lyme disease if used in the early stages, but some people have recurring symptoms of the disease for years. Prevention remains the best medicine. When hiking, wear long pants, long sleeves, and long socks to help keep ticks off your skin and avoid walking in wooded areas and overgrown grass and brush. Checking your body for ticks after being outdoors is also advised, and if you ever find one, pull it straight out with a pair of tweezers. Ticks normally do not transmit the bacterium until after they have fed, which can take anywhere from 36 to 48 hours.

Pneumonia

Pneumonia ranks as the eighth leading cause of death in the United States and the number-one cause of death for children worldwide.[16,17] Pneumonia is an inflammation of the lungs caused by bacteria, viruses, fungi, or parasites; the infection can vary from mild to deadly. Bacterial pneumonias are the most common in adults, and usually the most severe, causing high fever, chest pain, shortness of breath, chills, and a cough with green, yellow, or bloody mucus. Pneumonia tends to occur in conjunction with a cold or flu and is often mistaken by patients for these lesser infections. You should see a doctor immediately if you suddenly experience pneumonia symptoms.

The most common bacterial cause of pneumonia is the *Streptococcus pneumoniae* bacterium. Antibiotics are used to treat bacterial pneumonia infections, but as antibiotic-resistant strains have become more common, these drugs are less effective. Prevention remains the best measure. Health-care experts recommend that people get an annual flu shot to reduce their risk. Seniors and infants are at increased risk for pneumonia, as are younger people with asthma and other chronic respiratory problems, those with impaired immune systems, and those who have been exposed to certain chemicals and environmental pollutants. High-risk individuals are encouraged to get the pneumococcal vaccine.

Tuberculosis

Tuberculosis (TB) is a serious disease caused by the bacterium *Mycobacterium tuberculosis* that is spread through the air. The bacteria typically attack the lungs, where they create holes in the airways and hinder breathing. They can also settle into the brain, spine, or kidneys, and without proper treatment can prove fatal.

Symptoms of TB include weight loss, fatigue, fever, night sweats, and a persistent cough that does not go away after three weeks. But not everyone with a TB infection will become ill from it. Many have what is called a *latent* TB infection that does not cause any symptoms, is not infectious, and may never progress to active TB disease. In fact, only about 5%–10% of people with TB develop the active form of the disease.[18] Medication, taken for many months, can help keep latent TB infections from evolving into active TB disease, although drug-resistant strains of TB are emerging.

Once the leading cause of death in the United States, TB cases have been declining in recent years and reached an all-time low in 2014. Infection rates continue to be highest among immigrants and racial and ethnic minorities, the poor, the homeless, and those infected with HIV. Although there were only 9,421 new cases reported in 2014, millions of people in the United States are estimated to be living with a TB infection. Worldwide, about 9 million people were infected with TB in 2014, and about 1.5 million died from the disease.[19,20]

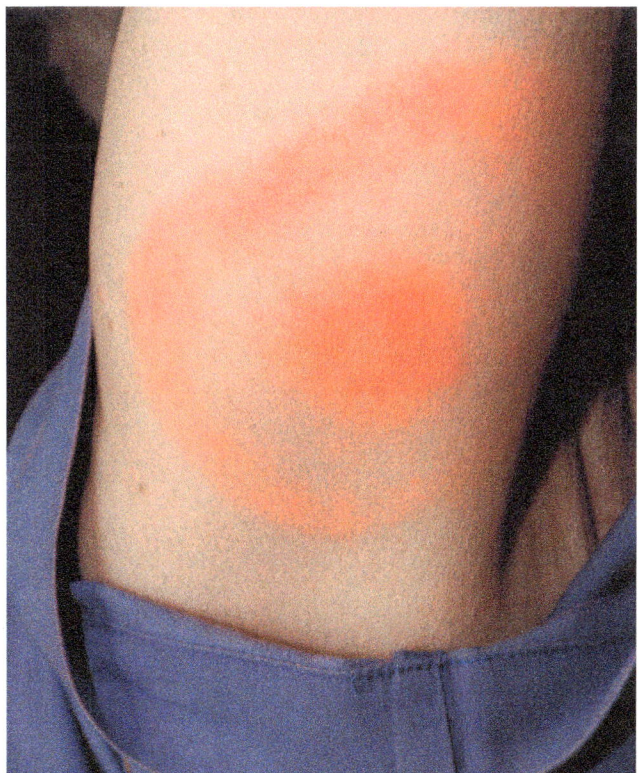

FIGURE 12.3 **Lyme Disease "Bull's-Eye" Rash.**

SPECIAL FEATURE

Emerging Mosquito-Borne Diseases
Zika Virus

Mosquitoes and the illnesses they spread, such as malaria and West Nile virus, have long plagued humankind. But that history doesn't stop mosquitoes—or the diseases they carry—from continuing to present new, unwelcome health threats. Worldwide travel brings extra urgency to the problem, giving mosquitoes and infectious diseases a broader, fast-moving reach. One emerging illness, *Zika virus,* provides a timely example of this type of global health threat.

Named after a forest in Angola, the Zika virus was first documented in Africa more than 70 years ago.[1] Zika-related illness appeared in relatively small, isolated outbreaks in Africa, the Pacific Islands, and Southeast Asia until 2015. At that time, public health officials in Brazil began noticing an alarming spike in the number of babies born with a condition called *microcephaly,* marked by small head size and a small, underdeveloped brain. As cases of this birth defect began to surge not only in Brazil but throughout Central and South America, scientists linked the rise in microcephaly to Zika virus and also found evidence linking the disease to a potentially fatal immune disorder called Guillain-Barrè, syndrome.[2] In early 2016, the World Health Organization declared Zika a global public health emergency, with 55 countries reporting ongoing mosquito-borne cases.[2]

In most people, Zika infection causes fever, muscle pain, and joint pain for about a week. While the infection itself is not fatal, its consequences can be severe. In pregnant women, the virus presents a serious danger to the brain of the developing fetus. In addition to being spread by mosquitoes, Zika can also be transmitted sexually, meaning that the sexual partners of pregnant women can spread the virus and put a developing baby at risk.[2]

Zika virus is most often spread by *Aedes* species mosquitoes, aggressive daytime biters most often found in warm climates.[3] While many parts of Central and South America see heavy mosquito activity year-round, more temperate regions are also prone to surges in disease-carrying mosquitoes during the warmer months. In the United States, health officials estimate that *Aedes* mosquitoes have a potential range that covers more than 30 states.[4] The Gulf Coast states, with their warm climate, are considered especially high risk areas as Zika makes its way northward.[5]

If you are in an area with an active Zika outbreak, you can take immediate steps to protect your health by shielding yourself from mosquito bites. Use repellant, stay indoors in air-conditioned or screened spaces as much as possible, and cover up with long-sleeved shirts and long pants. Remember that with *Aedes* mosquitoes, you'll need to guard against bites around the clock. If you are a man whose partner is pregnant, or if you are a pregnant woman, use condoms every time you have sex or abstain from sex until your baby is born.[6] There is currently no vaccine against Zika virus and no medicine to treat or cure it.[7]

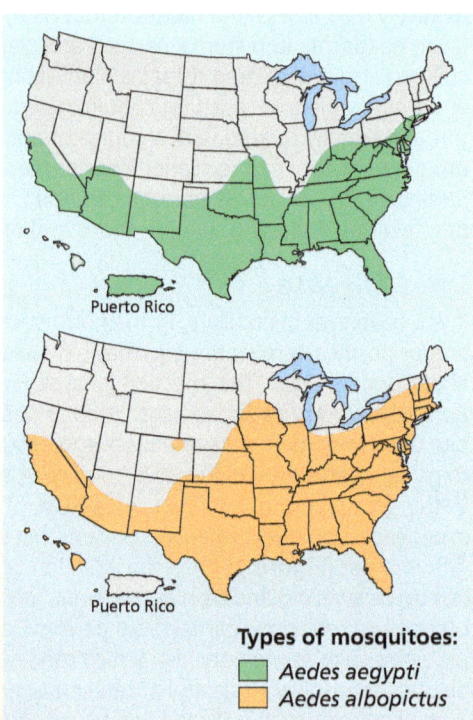

Types of mosquitoes:
- Aedes aegypti
- Aedes albopictus

References **1.** Centers for Disease Control and Prevention. (2016, April 15). *About Zika virus.* www.cdc.gov. **2.** World Health Organization. (2016, April 27). *Zika virus and complications.* www.who.int. **3.** Centers for Disease Control and Prevention. (2016, April 15). *Transmission and risks.* www.cdc.gov. **4.** Centers for Disease Control and Prevention. (2016, April 15). *About estimated range of* Aedes aegypti *and* Aedes albopictus *in the United States, 2016 maps.* www.cdc.gov. **5.** Centers for Disease Control and Prevention. (2016, January 28). *Transcript for CDC telebriefing: Zika virus travel alert.* www.cdc.gov. **6.** Centers for Disease Control and Prevention. (2016, January 28). *Prevention.* www.cdc.gov. **7.** Centers for Disease Control and Prevention. (2016, April 26). *Symptoms, diagnosis, & treatment.* www.cdc.gov.

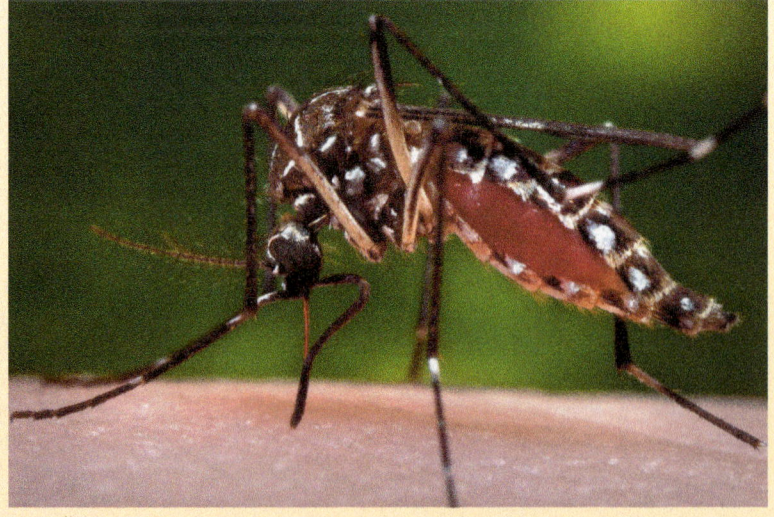

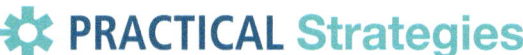

PRACTICAL Strategies

Protecting Yourself Against Infectious Diseases

To reduce your risk of contracting an infection:

- **Keep your hands clean.** The most effective method is to wash your hands with soap and water. Be sure to wash them thoroughly and frequently, especially during cold and flu season. Wet your hands with running water, lather up to your wrists with soap, and scrub for at least 20 seconds. Dry your hands using a clean towel or paper towel.

- **Use regular soap.** You do not need to use antibacterial soap when washing your hands. Regular soap is just as effective, and use of antibacterial soaps can lead to antibiotic resistance.

- **Hand washing** is most important before and after handling food, eating, treating wounds, and touching a sick person. It's also important after using the toilet, changing a diaper, touching an animal or animal waste, blowing your nose, coughing, sneezing, and handling garbage or anything else that could be contaminated with dirt or germs.

- **Use hand sanitizer.** If it isn't practical to wash your hands often, use hand sanitizer with at least 60% alcohol, applying enough to wet your hands completely and rubbing them together until dry. Unlike antibacterial soaps, alcohol-based hand sanitizers will not cause antibiotic resistance.

- **Keep your hands away from your eyes, nose, and mouth.** Touching your face is a common way to transmit pathogens from your hands into your body.

- **Avoid close contact** with people who are sick.

- **Routinely clean and disinfect surfaces**, including work areas, kitchen counters, keyboards, phones, and other electronic devices.

- **Keep up to date on your vaccinations** and get an annual flu shot.

- **Avoid contact with wild animals.** Rodents, bats, raccoons, skunks, and foxes can all spread harmful bacteria or viruses. Make sure your pets are up to date on their vaccinations as well.

- **Avoid mosquito bites.** In mosquito-dense areas, use repellent when you are outdoors, particularly at dusk and dawn; eliminate standing water in flower pots, bird baths, or other containers left outdoors; make sure you have intact window screens; and wear long-sleeved shirts and pants to avoid bites.

- **Avoid walking barefoot** in locker rooms or on dirt.

- **Don't smoke**; avoid secondhand smoke.

- **Don't drink alcohol** or drink only in moderation.

- **Get enough sleep.** Lack of sleep can impair the immune system.

- **Eat well.** Proper nutrition supports your immune system.

- **When you are sick, stay home.** If you are feeling under the weather, take steps to prevent infecting others. Rest at home, cover your mouth or nose with a tissue when you cough or sneeze, or cough or sneeze into the bend of your elbow, and wash your hands after coughing or sneezing.

Source: Mayo Clinic. (2014). *Hand washing: Do's and don'ts*. www.mayoclinic.com.

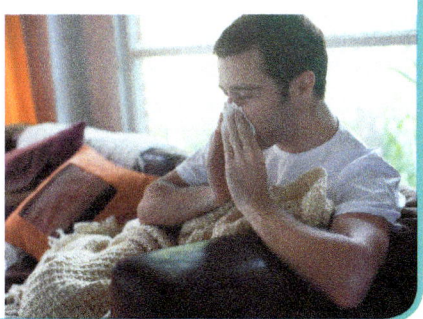

Fungal Infections

Fungi are organisms that obtain their food from organic matter, in some cases human tissue. Common examples of fungi are multicellular mold, mildew, and mushrooms, as well as single-celled yeast.

Some of the thousands of fungi that exist are quite beneficial. Penicillin, the powerful antibiotic used to treat a number of bacterial infections, is made from fungi. Yeast is used in making bread and cheese. Other types are not so helpful. Fungi are behind many minor infections of the skin, scalp, and nail beds but can also cause life-threatening systemic infections, especially for people with weakened immune systems.

Yeast infections are some of the most common types of fungal infections. Small amounts of a yeast called *Candida albicans* are always present in a person's body, but if imbalances occur—after taking antibiotics, for example, or, for women, during the normal hormonal changes that come with menstrual periods—this fungus is able to multiply out of control. It can cause infections in various parts of the body, such as the intestinal tract or vagina. Yeast infections, although uncomfortable and unpleasant, are usually not serious. In women, they are marked by itching in the vagina and around the genitals and are often accompanied by an abnormal vaginal discharge that can resemble cottage cheese. Sexual intercourse can also be painful. Treatment involves inserting a cream or suppository into the vagina or taking an oral medication. Other *Candida* infections include thrush (an overgrowth in the mouth), diaper rash, and infections of the nail beds.

fungi Multicellular or single-celled organisms that obtain their food from organic matter, in some cases human tissue.

protozoa Single-celled parasites that rely on other living things for food and shelter.

Protozoan Infections

Protozoa are single-celled organisms that, like fungi, obtain nutrients from feeding on organic matter. Although some are free-living, and even helpful—consuming harmful bacteria or serving as food for fish and other animals—protozoan parasites rely on other living things, such as humans, for food and shelter. These protozoa are capable of causing serious diseases in humans, especially in people living in developing countries. In the United States, where sanitation and food-handling standards have reduced our exposure to them, protozoan infections are less common.

One of the protozoan diseases of most concern is **malaria**, which kills almost half a million people every year, primarily infants, children, and pregnant women.[21] The infection is caused by the protozoa *Plasmodium* and is typically transmitted to humans through the bites of infected mosquitoes. Malaria is a serious threat throughout much of sub-Saharan Africa and parts of Latin America, Asia, and the Middle East, and fully 50% of the world's population is at risk of contracting it.[21] Since 2000, concentrated global health efforts have reduced the rates of disease and death from malaria. Many recent prevention campaigns have focused on sub-Saharan Africa, which continues to see the highest proportion of cases.[21] Although it was controlled in the United States more than five decades ago, occasional outbreaks still occur here.

Initial symptoms include fever, chills, vomiting, and headache. If not treated with antimalarial drugs promptly, the infection can be fatal. Some strains of malaria have become resistant to drugs, making treatment much more difficult. Malaria can be avoided by preventing mosquito bites. Antimalarial drugs can also be taken during trips to malaria-rich areas to reduce the risk of contracting the disease.

Parasitic Worm Infections

Parasitic worms (helminths) are creatures that compete with a host body for nutrients. Some tiny worms burrow through the skin, whereas others are contracted from eating microscopic eggs in undercooked foods. Once inside the body, some can grow up to 3 to 4.6 meters (10 to 15 feet) in length. Others can live for up to 15 years. They are most frequently found in tropical regions and are a problem in areas with poor sanitation. Infections are most common in travelers, refugees, migrant workers, children, and the homeless. Two of the most common parasitic worms in the United States are tapeworms and pinworms, both of which can be treated with oral medications.

LO 12.3 QUICK CHECK

What is the typical time frame for the acute phase of a mononucleosis infection?
a. two to three days
b. two to three weeks
c. two to three months
d. none of the above

Sexually Transmitted Infections

LO 12.4 List common sexually transmitted infections (STIs), their causes, risk factors, symptoms, and treatment.

Sexually transmitted infections (STIs) are commonplace. There are more than 30 different sexually transmissible bacteria, viruses, and parasites.[22] It is estimated that worldwide, nearly a million people acquire an STI every day, and there are approximately 20 million new cases of STIs every year in the United States, costing the U.S. health-care system nearly $16 billion.[22,23]

The CDC estimates that although 15- to 24-year-olds represent only 25% of the sexually active population, they account for half of all new STI cases.[23] The burden is especially high for teenage girls and young women; about 25% of sexually active teenage girls have an STI, and such infections cause about 20,000 women to become infertile each year.[24,25] Because many STI cases go unrecognized or untreated, and some STIs can be treated but not cured, the CDC estimates that there are more than 110 million STI cases overall among men and women nationwide, including new and existing infections.[23]

▶▶ These videos discuss STIs: Go to www.cdc.gov and search for "Be Well STD Videos."

Risk Factors for STIs

The college years can be a time of elevated risk for contracting STIs. Your likelihood of contracting an STI depends a lot on your behaviors. Some activities that increase risk are:

- Having unprotected vaginal, anal, or oral sex
- Having sex with multiple partners, especially strangers, and not discussing STIs before sex
- Exchanging sex for drugs or money
- Participating in sex while drunk or high on drugs
- Coming into direct skin-to-skin contact with someone who has infections such as human papillomavirus (HPV), herpes, pubic lice, or scabies
- Injecting drugs or steroids with dirty needles or syringes—or having unprotected sex with someone who has
- Sharing needles for tattoos and body piercings
- Failing to be vaccinated against HPV or hepatitis B

Are you at risk for a sexually transmitted infection? Take the **Self-Assessment** to find out.

Sexual Conduct and Risk

Only abstinence provides 100% protection from STIs. If you choose to have sex, the safest sex is between two completely monogamous partners who have been tested and are uninfected with any STIs. Although condoms are not 100% effective against STIs, when used correctly and consistently, they significantly reduce risk and make sex safer. If you or your partner is not monogamous or has not been tested, it is considered high risk to have vaginal, anal, or oral sex with that person without a condom. Unprotected anal sex carries the highest risk, especially for the receiving partner. Unprotected vaginal sex is next highest risk. Unprotected oral sex is also considered high risk, although it is less risky than unprotected anal or vaginal sex. If you or your partner has any type of STI, doctors recommend avoiding sex until treatment has been completed and symptoms are no longer present.

> **malaria** A serious disease that causes fever and chills that appear in cycles. In some cases malaria can be life threatening.
>
> **parasitic worms (helminths)** Multicellular creatures that compete with a host body for nutrients.
>
> **sexually transmitted infections (STIs)** Infections transmitted mainly through sexual activity, such as vaginal, anal, or oral sex.

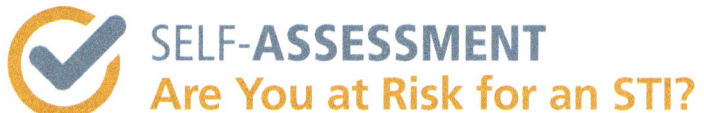

SELF-ASSESSMENT
Are You at Risk for an STI?

If you engage in sexual activity, then you are at risk for contracting an STI. However, your level of risk depends on certain behaviors.

"Sex" includes oral, vaginal, or anal sex, and a sexual partner is somebody with whom you have had oral, vaginal, or anal sex.

1. In the past 12 months, have you been diagnosed with any STI?*
   ☐ Yes ☐ No

2. In the past 12 months, have you had more than one sexual partner?
   ☐ Yes ☐ No

3. In the past 12 months, do you think your sexual partner(s) had any other partners?
   ☐ Yes ☐ Not sure ☐ No

4. In the past 12 months, have you had sex with a new partner?
   ☐ Yes ☐ No

5. Are you currently planning on having sex with a new partner?
   ☐ Yes ☐ Not sure ☐ No

6. In the past 12 months, how often have you used condoms during vaginal or anal intercourse or latex barriers during oral sex?
   ☐ Always ☐ Some of the time ☐ Most of the time ☐ Never

7. Do you discuss sexual history and testing with your partner(s)?
   ☐ Always ☐ Sometimes ☐ Never

HOW TO INTERPRET YOUR SCORE If you answered "Yes" or "Not sure" to questions 1–5 or anything other than "Always" to questions 6 and 7, you may be at increased risk for STIs.
Consider making an appointment at your campus health center for STI screening and/or to discuss prevention strategies.

To complete this Self-Assessment online, visit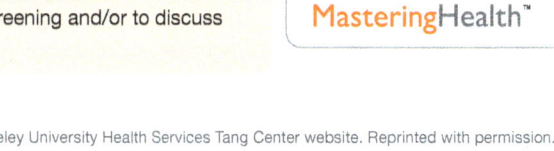

* Having had an STI recently may put you at increased risk for other STIs.

Source Adapted from UC Berkeley Sexually Transmitted Infection (STI) Risk Assessment, from UC Berkeley University Health Services Tang Center website. Reprinted with permission.

Talking About Safer Sex

It may feel awkward to talk about sexual history or STIs with a new partner, but it's important. Before you have sex with a new person, ask:

- Does he or she have any STIs?
- Has he or she participated in risky activities in the past?
- Has he or she been tested for STIs in the past? If so, has he or she participated in any risky activities since then?
- Is he or she prepared to use a condom? Are there any other safer sex measures he or she wants to take?

Be prepared to answer these questions yourself as well. In many cases, you will find that your partner is concerned about these issues, too. If your partner is unwilling to discuss safer sex or does not want to participate in the same level of safer sex that you do, reconsider sex with that person.

HIV and AIDS

Accounting for more than 1.2 million deaths worldwide every year, the human immunodeficiency virus (HIV) is the most serious of all sexually transmitted pathogens.[26] Worldwide, there are more than 36 million people with the infection, with the highest infection rates in sub-Saharan Africa **(Figure 12.4)**. In 2011, 70% of new HIV infections in adults and children were in sub-Saharan Africa.[26] Although intensive public health efforts in this region helped reduce new HIV infections there by more than 25% between 2001 and 2014, it remains the part of the world hardest hit by this devastating disease.[26] HIV was first identified in the United States in 1981, and today more than 1.2 million people in North America live with HIV infection and the condition it causes, acquired immunodeficiency syndrome, or AIDS (also called advanced HIV disease).[27] African Americans are disproportionately infected, as are sex workers, intravenous drug users, and men who have sex

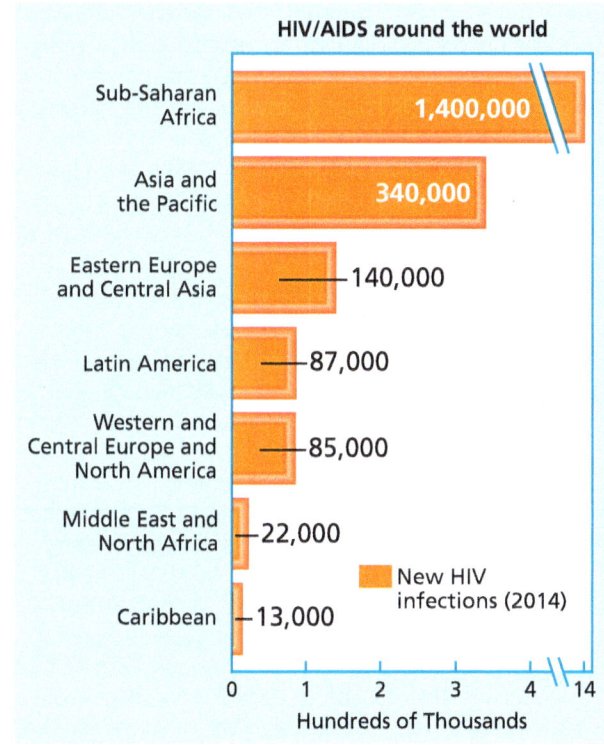

FIGURE 12.4 **HIV/AIDS Around the World.**
Source: Data from Joint United Nations Programme on HIV/AIDS (UNAIDS) and World Health Organization (WHO). (2015). AIDS by the numbers 2015. www.unaids.org.

with other men. Each year, 1.2 million people in sub-Saharan Africa die from AIDS-related illnesses. In North America, that number is about 7,000 people yearly.[27]

HIV infection severely damages the body's immune system. In particular, the virus infects and destroys helper T cells (CD4 T cells), important players in the body's specific immune response. HIV enters CD4 T cells and multiplies within them, generating millions of new HIV viruses and destroying the CD4 T cells in the process. The new viruses go on to infect more CD4 T cells and begin the replication process all over again. The immune system mounts a vigorous response, with B cells multiplying and secreting antibodies and CD4 T cells multiplying and secreting cytokines. After years or decades, however, CD4 T cell levels begin to decline, the immune system is progressively weakened, and the body loses its ability to fight off illness.

The first few weeks after contracting HIV are called the primary infection stage. During that period, some—but not all—people experience initial symptoms that resemble those of a cold or flu. Fatigue, fever, headache, sore throat, swollen lymph glands, and muscle aches are reported, as are diarrhea, yeast infections, rashes, and mouth sores. The primary infection is followed by an asymptomatic stage, and new symptoms may not occur for another 8 to 10 years. However, during this period the virus is still reproducing rapidly and the immune system is fighting it. Eventually, with the loss of CD4 T cells, the person will become more vulnerable to **opportunistic diseases**—infections and other disorders that take advantage of a weakened immune system—like pneumonia, tuberculosis, eye infections, yeast infections, and cancer, including Kaposi's sarcoma. An HIV-positive person is diagnosed with AIDS when at least one opportunistic disease has developed or when that person's CD4 T cell count drops below 200 cells per microliter of blood (a healthy CD4 count is between 450 and 1,200 cells per microliter). Once AIDS develops, additional complications can arise, including severe weight loss, dementia, brain tumors, and a protozoan infection called toxoplasmosis.

Transmission of HIV

Once infected with HIV, people can transmit it to others regardless of the stage of the disease or whether they have experienced symptoms. HIV is present in blood, seminal fluid, vaginal secretions, and breast milk. It can be transmitted during unprotected vaginal, oral, or anal sex or when sharing needles for intravenous drug use, tattoos, or piercing **(Figure 12.5).** You cannot catch the virus through sneezing, handshakes, insect bites, sharing food, or any other type of casual contact. Among the sexual transmission paths for HIV, unprotected anal sex is one of the most high-risk behaviors for spreading the virus. (See the "Sexual Conduct and Risk" section on page 304 for more about the relative risks of various sexual activities.) If you already have another STI, such as herpes or syphilis, your risk of becoming infected with HIV increases significantly. In the past, HIV was occasionally transmitted to recipients of blood transfusions; however, due to reforms, all donated blood in the United States is now screened for the virus and is considered safe.

Infected mothers are at risk of giving the virus to their infants, which is called *mother-to-child-transmission*

opportunistic diseases Infections and other disorders that take advantage of a weakened immune system.

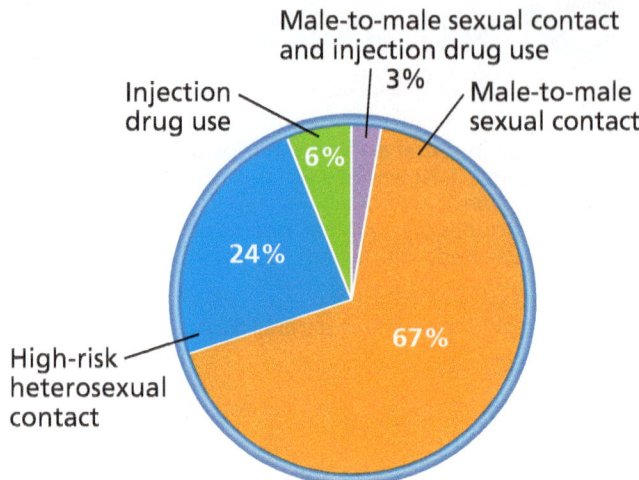

FIGURE 12.5 **Transmission Categories for New HIV/AIDS Cases in Adolescents and Adults in the United States.**

Source: Data from Centers for Disease Control and Prevention. (2015). *HIV/AIDS: Statistics overview.* www.cdc.gov.

(MTCT). This can occur during pregnancy, childbirth, and breast-feeding. The World Health Organization estimates that worldwide, 170,000 children are newly infected each year, the majority through MTCT.[28] Untreated, approximately 50% of these infected children will die before age 2. The rate of MTCT of HIV currently stands at about 14%, a number that is dropping due to intensive public health efforts targeting infected mothers and their babies. Between 2009 and 2014, international public health officials reported a 48% decrease in the number of new HIV infections among children.[29]

HIV Testing and Treatment

The CDC estimates that almost 15% of the people in the United States infected with HIV do not realize it. Because early HIV infections can have no or few symptoms, HIV screening is very important. Early diagnosis of HIV and prompt treatment is critical to slowing the virus's progression to AIDS. Knowing you have the virus can also help you take measures to avoid giving it to others.

The HIV test looks for the presence of antibodies to the virus rather than the virus itself; the presence of antibodies to HIV indicates that HIV is present in the body. The most common test is the EIA, or enzyme immunoassay, which is used to examine blood, saliva, or urine for antibodies to HIV. If an EIA test is positive, it is followed by an additional test such as the Western blot before a positive diagnosis of HIV infection is made. HIV antibody tests only work after a person's immune system has begun to develop antibodies to HIV. Because this can take up to six months in some people, testing too soon after potential exposure to the virus is considered ineffective.

The CDC recommends that all people between the ages of 13 and 64 be tested for HIV at least once. People at high risk for HIV (i.e., intravenous drug users, people engaging in unprotected sex or with multiple sex partners) should be tested annually, and pregnant women should be tested as part of their routine prenatal testing. Despite these recommendations, only 28.3% of college students report having ever been tested for HIV.[3]

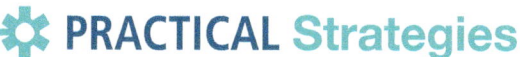

PRACTICAL Strategies

Reducing Your Risk of STIs

A few simple steps can dramatically reduce your risk of contracting an STI:

- **Use a condom or latex barrier.** Use latex or polyurethane condoms correctly and consistently for all vaginal or anal sexual encounters. Condoms, dental dams, or latex squares should be used for oral sex.
- **Be faithful.** If you have sex, do it with one uninfected partner who is not having sex with others.
- **Be picky.** Limit the number of sexual partners you have in your lifetime.
- **Talk with your partner.** Discuss STIs and prevention before you ever have sex. If you or your partner does not feel comfortable having that conversation, consider it a sign that you may not want to have sex with that person.
- **Get tested.** If you are sexually active, the only way to know for sure whether you have an infection is to be tested by a health practitioner. Many STIs have no noticeable symptoms and can go undetected for years, until treatment may be too late. It is a good idea for both partners to be tested before beginning a new sexual relationship.
- **Get annual checkups.** Annual checkups are a good time to discuss your sexual practices with your doctor.
- **Get vaccinated.** Ask your doctor about vaccines for HPV and hepatitis B. Men who have sex with other men should be vaccinated for hepatitis A as well.
- **Be alert to symptoms.** If you develop any signs of an STI, get checked out by a physician right away. Prompt treatment can make all the difference between an effective treatment and long-term problems.
- **Consider abstinence.** Abstinence from sexual intercourse is the most effective method for avoiding STIs.

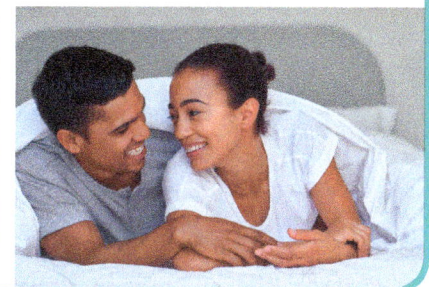

HIV and AIDS are not curable, but they are treatable. Treatments called antiretroviral therapies can dramatically slow the deterioration of a person's immune system and are responsible for a dramatic decrease in AIDS deaths in recent years. There are three main types of antiretroviral drugs: reverse transcriptase inhibitors, protease inhibitors, and fusion inhibitors. The medications are frequently prescribed in combinations of three or four, in a regimen often referred to as a *highly active antiretroviral therapy (HAART)*. For many living with HIV, HAART has changed the condition from a life sentence to a chronic manageable disease. The average life expectancy of a person newly diagnosed with HIV is approaching that of most uninfected people. Recent projection models suggest that a 39-year-old entering HIV care can expect to live until age 63.[30] Unfortunately, HIV drugs can be very expensive, have toxic side effects, and may not work for everyone. While as of 2015, international health efforts had brought HIV drugs to almost 16 million people, officials estimated that at least 22 million more HIV patients remained in need of retroviral therapy.[26]

Preventing HIV Infection

To avoid getting HIV and AIDS, you need to keep the blood, seminal fluid, vaginal fluids, or breast milk of an infected person from entering your vagina, penis, anus, mouth, or breaches in your skin. The surest way to protect yourself from HIV or any other STI is to avoid any sexual behavior that could transmit the disease. See **Practical Strategies: Reducing Your Risk of STIs** above for information on how to avoid STIs.

Intravenous drug users are at very high risk of contracting HIV if they share needles or syringes with other users. Efforts to sterilize equipment, including washing with bleach, are not always successful at killing HIV. Having sex while high on drugs is also risky because you are less likely to think clearly and practice safer sex.

>> These podcasts discuss HIV testing and prevention: Go to **www.cdc.gov** and search for "HIV AIDs podcasts."

Hepatitis B

Hepatitis B—which is more than 50 times as infectious as the virus that causes HIV—is most commonly spread through unprotected sex.[31] It can also be spread through sharing needles, razors, or syringes with an infected person and can be passed from an infected mother to her baby during childbirth. Symptoms generally occur two to three months after infection and involve abdominal and joint pain, nausea, dark urine, weakness and fatigue, and jaundice. Although the virus can cause immediate symptoms that go away on their own, for some people it can also remain in the body forever, resulting in long-term health problems ranging from liver damage to liver cancer and death. If you know you have been exposed to hepatitis B, contact your doctor right away. An injection of hepatitis B immune globulin (antibodies specific for hepatitis B; a passive immunization) within 24 hours of exposure may reduce your risk of developing hepatitis B. Because health-care providers began to routinely immunize children against hepatitis B in 1991, infection rates have dropped by an estimated 80%.[31] However, for as many as 1.4 million people in the United States currently living with a chronic hepatitis B infection, the vaccine became available too late.[31]

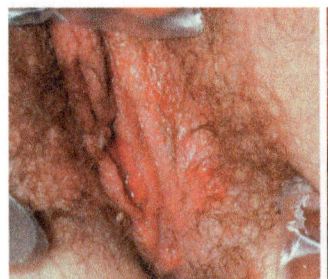 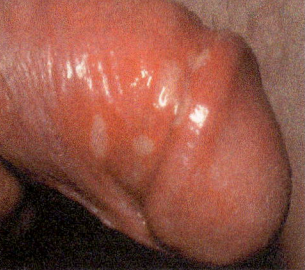

FIGURE 12.6 **Genital Herpes Sores.**

Genital Herpes

Genital herpes affects about 17% of people between the ages of 14 and 49 in the United States.[32] More than 80% of infected people do not realize they have the condition because they don't have symptoms or their symptoms are mild or mistaken for something else, such as jock itch, a yeast infection, or even insect bites. There are two types of herpes simplex virus: herpes simplex virus type 2 (HSV-2) and herpes simplex virus type 1 (HSV-1). Genital herpes is usually caused by HSV-2, whereas HSV-1 is the virus most often responsible for cold sores around the mouth. Herpes is extremely contagious. Genital herpes most often results from direct skin-to-skin contact, usually through vaginal, oral, or anal sex. Oral sex can pass both types of herpes virus back and forth between the mouth and the genitals. HSV-2 is almost always transmitted through sexual contact, so most people do not contract it until they have become sexually active, whereas many people are exposed to HSV-1 in childhood, through nonsexual kisses by family members or friends. HSV-1 is very common; 50%–80% of people in the United States have it, and as many as 90% of people have it by age 50.[33]

The hallmark of genital herpes is small, painful blisters or sores in the genital or anal area, although some people do not experience any symptoms at all **(Figure 12.6)**. The first outbreak usually occurs within two weeks of infection, is accompanied by flulike symptoms, and takes about three weeks to heal. Outbreaks can recur but tend to become less severe and less frequent over time. Stress, illness, poor diet, inadequate rest, and friction in the genital area can trigger outbreaks. The virus usually stays in the body forever, lying dormant in nerve cells, until the next recurrence. Herpes is most infectious when blisters or sores are present on an infected person. However, the herpes virus can be shed and passed on to others even when a person shows no symptoms. If you have ever had an outbreak of genital herpes, you should consider yourself contagious even if you have not had an outbreak for years. It is important to tell any potential partners that you have genital herpes and for both partners to remember that transmission, whether genital to genital or oral to genital, is possible even when the infection is in remission. Genital herpes can leave the body vulnerable to other STIs. The risk to a herpes patient of becoming infected with HIV if exposed to it is two to three times that of people who do not have herpes.[28] It can also make people with an HIV infection more infectious. Genital herpes can be fatal to a newborn baby if passed along during childbirth.

To diagnose herpes, a doctor takes a swab from a blister within the first 48 hours after it appears. If there is a sufficient amount of virus in the blister, it is possible to distinguish it as either HSV-1 or HSV-2. Tests are also available that look for antibodies to the herpes virus in the blood.

Treatments for genital herpes are targeted toward alleviating symptoms. Antiviral medications such as acyclovir can reduce pain, hasten the healing of sores, and reduce the number of recurrences. Sex should be avoided when one partner has visible herpes sores, but the partner can still be contagious even when the sores have healed. Condoms or dental dams should always be used if a partner has genital herpes. They can reduce the risk of passing on the virus but are not foolproof because contagious sores can appear on areas not covered by the barrier. When taken daily to suppress herpes outbreaks and viral shedding, antiviral medications can also reduce the risk of transmitting herpes to a sexual partner, although condoms or dental dams should still be used.

> **"Most sexually active Americans will become infected with HPV at some point in their lives."**

Human Papillomavirus

Human papillomavirus (HPV) causes all types of warts, wherever they may be on your body. There are over 100 types of HPV. More than 40 types can infect the genitalia, although only 4 are responsible for most genital HPV infections. HPV is the most reported STI on college campuses, and most sexually active Americans will become infected with HPV at some point in their lives.[34] An estimated 79 million people in the United States are currently infected with HPV, and an additional 14 million develop the infection every year.[35] The infection is spread through skin-to-skin contact, usually during vaginal, oral, or anal sex.

Most people do not realize they are infected with HPV. With the exception of the few HPV types that cause genital warts, HPV does not have any symptoms. For those who do experience warts, they can arise weeks or even months after infection. Warts can be raised or flat, pink or flesh-toned, and there may be only a single wart or multiple ones **(Figure 12.7)**. These warts can be treated with topical medications that are applied directly to the skin. They can also be frozen off through

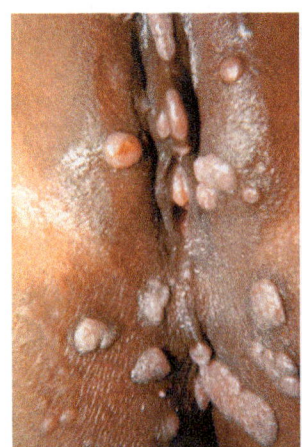 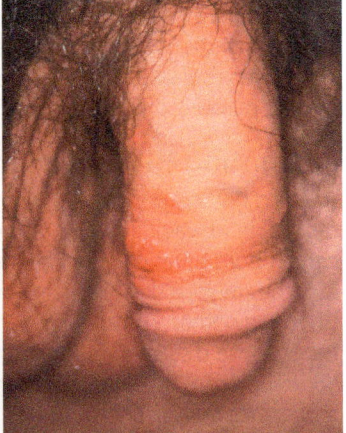

FIGURE 12.7 **Genital Warts.**

cryotherapy, burned off through electrocauterization, or removed by laser surgery. Warts can return even after treatment because these treatments do not cure HPV infection; they just alleviate symptoms.

In about 90% of cases, the body's immune system overcomes an HPV infection naturally. However, some infections linger and cause cells to become abnormal or even cancerous. The types of HPV that cause cancer of the cervix, vagina, throat, penis, and anus are called "high-risk" strains of HPV. These strains do not cause warts and must be tested for. Cervical cancer is the biggest concern. Highly treatable when detected early, it can be fatal when left undetected. That is why the Pap test, which is used to screen for abnormal and potentially cancerous cervical cells, now typically includes a test for HPV. More than 12,000 women are diagnosed with cervical cancer every year.[36]

In 2006, the Food and Drug Administration (FDA) approved the first vaccine for HPV, Gardasil, for females aged 9 to 26. A second brand, Cervarix, has recently been added to the market as well. The vaccines protect against the two most common types of HPV associated with high-risk cervical cancer (types 16 and 18) and the two most common types of HPV associated with genital warts (types 6 and 11). The vaccine is highly effective in women who were previously uninfected with those types of HPV. In 2009, the FDA also approved the use of Gardasil for the prevention of genital warts caused by HPV types 6 and 11 in males aged 9 to 26.[37]

Chlamydia

Chlamydia, which is caused by the bacterium *Chlamydia trachomatis*, is extremely common in the United States. In 2014, public health officials reported more than 1.4 million diagnosed chlamydia infections.[25] Young women are especially at risk; in 2014, females between the ages of 15 and 24 experienced more than three times the number of infections than males in the same age group.[38]

The infection can be spread during vaginal, anal, or oral intercourse, and it can be passed from mother to newborn baby during childbirth. Chlamydia can infect the vagina, penis, anus, cervix, urethra, and even the eyes or throat. Chlamydia is called the "silent disease" because the majority of those infected with it do not notice any unusual signs. Men, however, are more likely to show symptoms, often a burning sensation while urinating, as well as a discharge from their penis. Women who develop symptoms often notice an abnormal vaginal discharge and pain during urination. Symptoms usually develop within one to three weeks of infection.

If left untreated, chlamydia can have serious health consequences and lead to infertility. In 10%–15% of the women whose chlamydia is not treated promptly, pelvic inflammatory disease occurs.[39] This condition damages the fallopian tubes and uterus, resulting in pelvic pain, infertility, and **ectopic pregnancies** that can be deadly to mother and fetus. Chlamydia can also leave men infertile, inflaming the prostate gland and epididymis and scarring the urethra.

ectopic pregnancy A pregnancy in which the embryo implants outside the uterus, often in the fallopian tubes.

The U.S. Preventive Services Task Force recommends that all sexually active women aged 24 or younger undergo regular screening for chlamydia every year.[40] As a result, many pediatricians offer routine testing to their adolescent patients. Women who are 25 and older and at increased risk because of unsafe sex practices or intercourse with multiple partners are also encouraged to get screened regularly. A simple urine test or swab taken from the penis or cervix can detect a chlamydia infection. Chlamydia can be cured with antibiotics. All sexual partners should be treated at the same time to avoid reinfection.

Gonorrhea

Gonorrhea, sometimes referred to as "the clap," is a common and highly contagious sexually transmitted infection. It is caused by the bacteria *Neisseria gonorrhoeae* and most often affects young people aged 20 to 24.[25] As with chlamydia, U.S. health officials now recommend that all sexually active young women be screened for gonorrhea every year.[39] The bacteria are spread through intimate contact with an infected penis, vagina, anus, or mouth and can be passed on to a newborn baby during childbirth. Most women infected with gonorrhea experience no symptoms at all. Those who do may mistake the painful urination or increased vaginal discharge for a bladder or yeast infection. Men are more likely to have noticeable signs of the condition, including sore testicles, colored penile discharge, or a burning sensation while urinating. Symptoms usually occur within the first week after infection.

Without proper treatment, the bacteria can spread to the blood or joints, which can be life threatening. Pelvic inflammatory disease can also occur, causing pain and infertility. Women are at risk of having an ectopic pregnancy. Men can be left sterile. People with gonorrhea are also at greater risk of getting HIV.

Several laboratory tests can be used to diagnose gonorrhea, including a urine test or swab samples taken of the cervix, urethra, rectum, or throat. If you have the condition, your sexual partners should also be tested and treated. Antibiotics can often cure gonorrhea, but drug-resistant strains have been on the rise, making treatment more complicated. Because many people who have gonorrhea are infected with chlamydia at the same time, treatment often includes antibiotics for both. Avoid sexual contact until treatment is finished.

Pelvic Inflammatory Disease

Pelvic inflammatory disease (PID) is an infection of a woman's uterus, fallopian tubes, and other reproductive organs that occurs when bacteria travel up from the vagina and spread. It affects an estimated 750,000 women in the United States every year, causing infertility in about 10% to 15%.[41] PID is caused by bacteria, most often from the bacteria associated with two of the most common sexually transmitted infections, chlamydia and gonorrhea.

With PID, bacteria infect the fallopian tubes, turning normal tissue into scar tissue. This can cause chronic abdominal pain. It also may block eggs from moving into the uterus, causing ectopic pregnancies or leaving a woman infertile.

Women may have no idea that they have PID, even as their reproductive system is being damaged. When symptoms do occur, they may be subtle or vague, including fever, irregular menstrual bleeding, painful intercourse, or

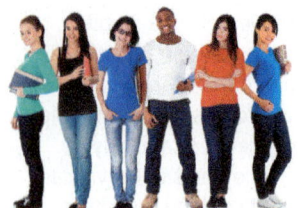

DIVERSITY & HEALTH

STIs Among Different Sexes, Races, and Sexual Orientations

STIs may affect people of various sexes, ages, races, and sexual orientations differently. Certain groups are at higher risk for particular STIs or STIs in general.

Sex

- Women are biologically more susceptible to becoming infected with STIs than men are. Young women, especially, are at high risk because the cells lining the cervix are less mature and are vulnerable to infection.
- Women are less likely than men to experience symptoms of STIs, which can postpone detection and treatment.
- Women are more likely than men to experience long-term, severe side effects of STIs, such as infertility and cervical cancer.

Race

- African Americans continue to experience an epidemic of HIV/AIDS, comprising 44% of all new infections of HIV in the United States in 2014.[1]
- African Americans—especially young African American women—are at disproportionately high risk for other STIs as well.
- Hispanics are disproportionately affected by HIV/AIDS, gonorrhea, chlamydia, and syphilis. Although Hispanics made up 17% of the U.S. population in 2009, they comprised 21% of new HIV/AIDS cases in the United States.[2]
- Asian and Pacific Islander groups are disproportionately affected by hepatitis B in the United States, accounting for more than 50% of Americans living with chronic hepatitis B.[3]

Sexual Orientation

- Young men who have sex with men, especially those of minority races or ethnicities, are at high risk for HIV infection, syphilis, and other STIs.
- The risk of female-to-female HIV transmission is low but possible, especially if one or both partners have sores on their genitals, if partners share sex toys, or if they participate in rough sex. Women can pass other STIs to one another as well.

What Do You Think?

1. Does young women's higher risk for contracting STIs make them especially motivated to follow safer sex practices and ask their partners to do the same? Why or why not?
2. Why do you think certain populations might experience disproportionally high rates of STIs?
3. What changes or new attitudes might encourage wider adoption of safer sex practices among young people?

Sources **1.** Centers for Disease Control and Prevention. (2016). *HIV among African Americans.* www.cdc.gov. **2.** Centers for Disease Control and Prevention. (2014). *Health disparities: Hispanics/Latinos.* www.cdc.gov. **3.** Centers for Disease Control and Prevention. (2013). *Asian Americans and hepatitis B.* www.cdc.gov.

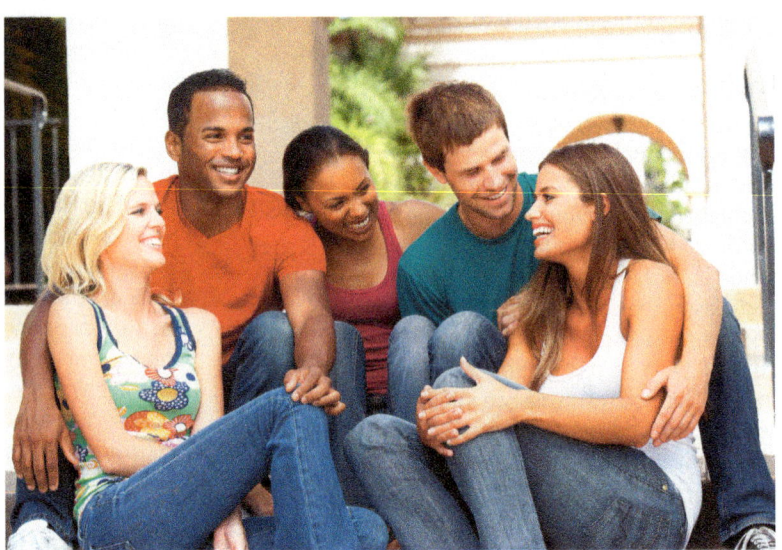

Young people are one of the groups at **elevated risk for STIs.**

---

lower abdominal pain. The condition often goes unrecognized by patients and physicians alike.

No single test detects the presence of PID. Doctors typically perform a pelvic examination and test for chlamydia and gonorrhea. However, an abdominal ultrasound and even laparoscopy (minimally invasive surgery) may be needed to confirm the diagnosis. Antibiotics can cure the infection but cannot undo any of the damage already done to a woman's reproductive organs. For that reason, prompt treatment is always critical. A woman's sex partners also should be treated—even if they have no symptoms—to avoid from spreading the bacteria that cause PID back and forth. In some cases, a woman may need surgery to reduce the scarring. Even so, she may still remain infertile.

Avoiding STIs—or getting immediate medical care if one occurs—will help protect women from developing PID. Because chlamydia and gonorrhea often have no noticeable symptoms, young sexually active women should undergo regular pelvic examinations and annual chlamydia testing.

Sexually active women under the age of 25 have a higher risk of PID. In addition, women increase their risk of PID by douching, having recently had an IUD for birth control inserted, and having multiple sex partners.

Syphilis

Although syphilis is less widespread than other STIs, almost 20,000 cases were reported in the United States in 2014, and the number of new cases has been climbing steadily each year since 2011.[38] Syphilis is especially prevalent in parts of the South and in urban areas, with men who have sex with men disproportionately affected. The infection can be transmitted from mother to child during pregnancy or childbirth. Syphilis is caused by the bacterium *Treponema pallidum,* which enters the body through irritated skin or mucous membranes, including the vagina, anus, penis, lips, and mouth.

If left untreated, syphilis can progress through three different stages. In the first stage, 10 days to three months after infection, primary syphilis appears. A painless sore called a *chancre* appears where the bacteria entered the body, around the genitals, inside the vagina or rectum, or on the lips or mouth **(Figure 12.8)**. The chancre will go away without treatment, but the infection itself will not. During the next stage, secondary syphilis, symptoms may include a rash on the hands or feet, neck, head, or torso; wart-like growths around the genitals; and grayish sores in the mouth. Hair loss may occur. The infection will then enter a latent stage, which lacks symptoms, and can last for years. If syphilis isn't treated, about 15% of people will develop the late or tertiary stage, where small tumor-like growths called *gummas* appear on internal organs and damage to the nervous system occurs. Tertiary syphilis can also cause severe problems with the heart, brain, and eyes, causing blindness, paralysis, brain damage, dementia, and even death. Syphilis also increases the chances of contracting HIV.

Examination of a fluid sample taken from a chancre or swollen lymph nodes can confirm infection during primary or secondary syphilis. Two types of blood tests are also available to detect the bacteria during any of its stages. Antibiotics are the first line of defense against syphilis. If treatment is not initiated until the final stage, the bacteria can be killed but the internal damage that has already occurred cannot be reversed.

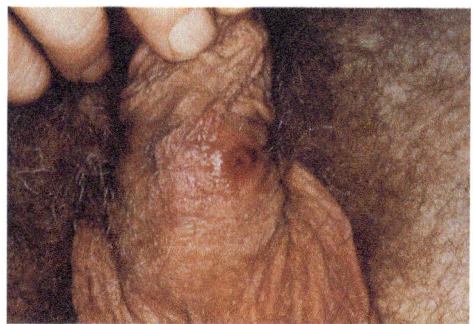

FIGURE 12.8 **A Syphilis Chancre.**

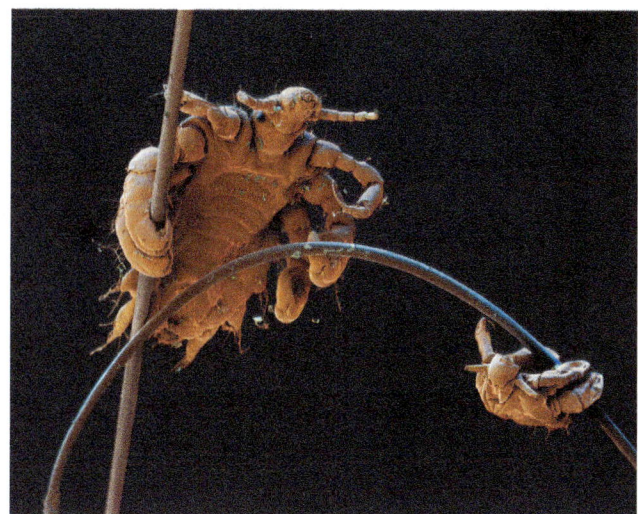

FIGURE 12.9 **Pubic Lice.**

Pubic Lice and Scabies

Pubic lice, or *Pthirus pubis,* are tiny six-legged creatures that infest pubic hair **(Figure 12.9)**. Commonly known as "crabs," they can also attach themselves to eyebrows, eyelashes, beards, mustaches, or chest hair. Scabies is caused by tiny, eight-legged mites that burrow into the top layer of a person's skin and lay eggs. Scabies generally occurs in and around folds of skin but can affect other parts of the body as well. Pubic lice and scabies are usually transmitted through sexual contact but occasionally are spread through contact with clothing, towels, sheets, or toilet seats that have been used by an infected person.

The most common symptom of pubic lice and scabies is itching, especially during the night. In some instances, the infested area also becomes inflamed, and scabies can sometimes cause allergic reactions. The pests themselves do not spread disease, but excessive scratching of the skin can lead to bacterial infection.

A pubic lice or scabies infestation can be easily diagnosed with a doctor's visit. Prescribed creams or lotions can usually clear up these conditions, although an oral medication may be needed for cases that are harder to treat.

Trichomoniasis

Trichomoniasis, or "trich," is caused by a protozoan called *Trichomonas vaginalis*. It is the most common curable STI in young women, and one study found the incidence to be even higher in women over age 40.[42] Men can be infected as well. More than 3.7 million Americans are believed to be infected.[43]

The most common route of transmission is vaginal-penile intercourse. However, an infected woman can transmit *T. vaginalis* to a female sex partner during vulva-to-vulva contact. Fortunately, women often experience symptoms, typically within 5 to 28 days, so they seek medical treatment. Symptoms include painful urination, pain during intercourse, vaginal itching and irritation, and a greenish-yellow, strong-smelling vaginal discharge. Men often do not experience symptoms, but if they do, they include irritation inside the penis and slight discharge. Infected women are at

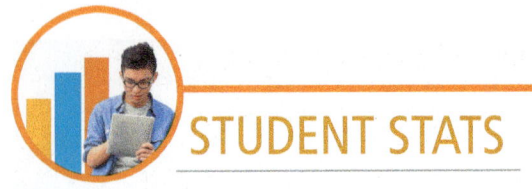

STUDENT STATS
STIs in People Aged 15-24

Of the total new syphilis, gonorrhea, and chlamydia cases in 2014, these charts show what percentages were in 15- to 19-year-olds and 20- to 24-year-olds.

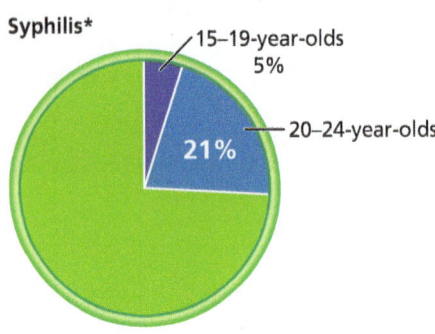

Syphilis*
- 15–19-year-olds: 5%
- 20–24-year-olds: 21%

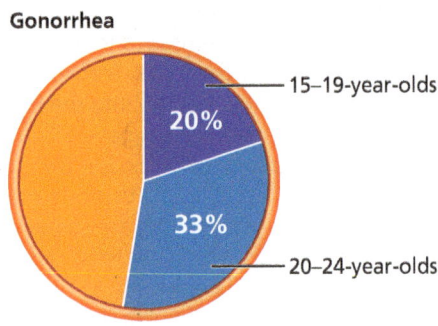

Gonorrhea
- 15–19-year-olds: 20%
- 20–24-year-olds: 33%

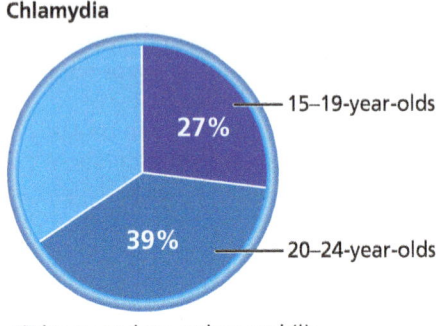

Chlamydia
- 15–19-year-olds: 27%
- 20–24-year-olds: 39%

*Primary and secondary syphilis.

Source: Data from Centers for Disease Control and Prevention. (2015). *2014 sexually transmitted diseases surveillance*. www.cdc.gov.

increased risk for HIV infection and are more likely to pass HIV to a partner. Studies also suggest that infected men and women are at increased risk for infertility.

Trich in women is diagnosed with laboratory analysis of a vaginal swab. In women, a pelvic exam will reveal small red sores on the vaginal wall or cervix. Infection can be cured with oral antimicrobial drugs, usually metronidazole. Both partners must be treated and must avoid sex until treatment is finished and all symptoms have cleared.

LO 12.4 QUICK CHECK

Which of the following accurately describes the treatment of genital herpes?
a. There are no treatments available.
b. Outbreaks can be controlled or reduced with medication.
c. The condition can be cured with medication.
d. None of the above.

Change Yourself, Change Your World

LO 12.5 Explain how to prevent infectious diseases and sexually transmitted infections.

Pathogens are all around us. This may leave you feeling that it's you against the world. But that's not true. When it comes to breaking the chain of infection, we work best when we work together.

Personal Choices

Help protect yourself from infections by keeping your immune system strong. Don't smoke. If you do, you're setting out the welcome mat for pathogenic microbes. Stay up to date on your vaccinations. Limit your alcohol. Eat right, don't short-change your sleep (short sleep reduces the number of functioning T cells), and exercise regularly.

When it comes to STIs, take these additional precautions:

- **Get vaccinated.** The CDC recommends that men who have sex with men receive the hepatitis A vaccine. All people need immunization against hepatitis B (HBV). The CDC also recommends vaccination against HPV for both males and females aged 9 to 26.

- **Use condoms.** One of the most important ways to protect yourself from STIs is to use latex condoms correctly and consistently—with every sex act. Always use a new condom. Never use an unapproved lubricant such as massage oil or petroleum jelly.

- **Get tested.** If you're sexually active, discuss STI testing with your health-care provider at each routine visit. If you don't have a regular health-care provider, visit your campus health center, which may offer free or low-cost testing. If you're concerned about high-risk exposure to HIV, see a doctor immediately! A course of treatment with HAART can significantly reduce your risk for developing an active infection.

If you find out that you've tested positive for any STI, tell your current partner and anyone you've had sex with during the past year. Encourage them to seek testing, too. If you're uncomfortable revealing your test results, talk with your health-care provider. Most states require that certain STIs be reported to public health authorities, who can then notify partners, anonymously and confidentially, about exposure to STDs. Some public health departments now use email notification.[44]

>> To find a local clinic where you can be tested for STIs; just type in your zip code at **https://gettested.cdc.gov**.

STUDENT STORY
Unprotected Sex

"**HI, I'M GABE.** Last weekend I did something really stupid. I went to a party with my friends and was flirting with this girl. We both got pretty drunk and ended up going back to my room and having sex. I was so drunk I didn't use a condom. She said it was OK, she's on the pill, but now I'm freaking out about STIs. She's friends with one of my friends, and he says he thinks she doesn't have anything, but I'm still worried. Do you think it makes it any better that it was only once?"

What Do You Think?

1. What could Gabe have done differently to reduce his risk for STIs?
2. Do you think Gabe can rely on his friend for information about whether his partner is healthy?
3. Do you think Gabe is at less risk because he had unprotected sex only once?

- **Get treated.** Bacterial STIs are usually curable with antibiotics. Trichomoniasis can also be cured with drug therapy. Taking the entire course of prescribed medication is essential, as is partner treatment. You must both avoid sex until the treatment is finished and you no longer have any symptoms.

In general, viral STIs are not curable, but antiviral medication can suppress herpes outbreaks, and HAART can keep HIV infection in check for many years. Both herpes and HIV can be transmitted while the person is taking medication, so condom use is still essential.

Because infections are spread among networks of people, the actions you take to reduce your own risk will benefit others in your campus community.

▶▶ Watch videos of real students discussing STIs and other infections at **Mastering**Health™

LO 12.5 QUICK CHECK

If you test positive for a sexually transmitted infection, whom should you inform?

a. all prior sexual partners
b. current sexual partners only
c. no sexual partners, as long as you take precautions to prevent transmission
d. current sexual partners and any prior partners over the past year

Choosing to Change Worksheet

To complete this worksheet online, visit **Mastering**Health™

Your likelihood of contracting an STI depends primarily on your behaviors. To reduce your risk of contracting an STI, follow the steps below.

Directions: Fill in your stage of change in step 1 and complete steps 2, 3, or 4, depending on which one applies to your stage of change.

Step 1: Assess your stage of behavior change. Please check one of the following statements that best describes your readiness to reduce your STI risk.

_____ I do not intend to reduce my STI risk in the next six months. (Precontemplation)

_____ I might reduce my STI risk in the next six months. (Contemplation)

_____ I am prepared to reduce my STI risk in the next month. (Preparation)

_____ I have been reducing my STI risk for less than six months. (Action)

_____ I have been reducing my STI risk for more than six months. (Maintenance)

Step 2: Work the precontemplation and contemplation stages. Increasing your knowledge of the risk factors for contracting an STI can help motivate you to change. If you answer "Yes" or "Don't know" to any of the 10 items below, you may be at increased risk for STIs.

1. I have had oral, vaginal, or anal sex without using a latex condom.   Yes   No

2. I have had sex with multiple partners and not discussed STIs before having sex.   Yes   No

3. I have had sex after consuming alcohol.	Yes	No	
4. I have had sex while under the influence of illegal drugs.	Yes	No	
5. I have exchanged sex for drugs or money.	Yes	No	
6. I have come into direct contact with someone who has infections such as HPV, herpes, pubic lice, or scabies.	Yes	No	Don't know
7. I have injected substances with dirty needles or syringes—or have had unprotected sex with someone who has.	Yes	No	Don't know
8. I have shared needles for tattoos or body piercings—or have had unprotected sex with someone who has.	Yes	No	Don't know
9. I have not been vaccinated against hepatitis A, hepatitis B, or human papillomavirus.	Yes	No	
10. I have had sex while infected with an STI.	Yes	No	Don't know

What might be some barriers holding you back from taking action on reducing your STI risk factors, and how could you overcome them?

Barrier	Strategy for Overcoming Barrier
Example: My partner doesn't want to wear a condom.	*I will explain to him why it is important to wear one and how I feel about his lack of wanting to use one.*
_____	_____

Step 3: Work the preparation and action stages. For each of the risk reduction guidelines listed below, indicate one action you can take (or have already taken) to meet that guideline in your own life. Be specific.

Reducing Your Personal STI Risk

STI Risk Reduction Guideline	Specific Action to Meet Guideline
Become more educated about the risks, symptoms, treatment, and prevention of STIs.	*Example: Talk to my nurse practitioner about safer sex practices and/or any STI symptoms I should watch out for.*
For STIs with an available vaccine (HPV and hepatitis B), get vaccinated.	
Be alert for signs or symptoms of STIs.	
Get tested.	
Communicate with sexual partners about your sexual histories, including histories of STIs.	
Don't impair your judgment before participating in sexual activity by using drugs or alcohol.	
Always use a latex condom from start to finish.	
Practice safe oral sex by using condoms, dental dams, or latex squares.	
Limit your number of sexual partners.	

Write down your **SMART goal** for reducing your STI risk, including a timeline, below.

_____
_____

Step 4: Work the maintenance stage. Your goal is to stay focused and maintain your commitment to preventing STIs. What benefits of practicing STI prevention are most important to you, and why?

_____
_____

How easy has it been to practice STI prevention? Is it truly a habit, or do you need to expend some effort to do it? How can you keep yourself on track?

_____
_____

CHAPTER 12 STUDY PLAN

CHAPTER SUMMARY

LO 12.1
- Pathogens are the agents that cause infections. Pathogens include viruses, bacteria, fungi, protozoa, and parasitic worms.
- Infectious diseases can be spread by personal contact with an infected person, touching inanimate objects that are contaminated with pathogens, inhaling airborne pathogens, or contact with infected animals, insects, water, or food.

LO 12.2
- Your body's first line of defense against infection is your skin, mucous membranes, cilia, and bodily fluids, which prevent pathogens from entering the body or trap and expel them if they do.
- Your immune system, a powerful network of cellular and chemical defenses, fights pathogens that enter the body. Neutrophils, natural killer cells, and macrophages are key nonspecific defenders. B cells and T cells target specific pathogens. Memory B cells and T cells play a role in long-term immunity.
- Sometimes the immune system mistakes common substances for harmful agents, triggering allergies. Allergic reactions range from relatively mild to very dangerous.

LO 12.3
- A wide range of pathogens, including viruses, bacteria, and fungi, cause both common and rare infectious diseases.
- Some general infectious diseases of concern to college students include the common cold, influenza, MRSA, meningitis, and hepatitis.

MasteringHealth™

Build your knowledge—and health!— in the Study Area of **MasteringHealth**™ with a variety of study tools.

- While many infectious diseases can be treated with medication, not all can be cured. Appropriate use of antibiotics is essential to reduce the risk of antibiotic-resistant pathogens.
- Some infectious diseases can be prevented through vaccination. Others can be prevented by personal hygiene practices such as effective hand washing.

LO 12.4
- HIV/AIDS is the most serious of the STIs. It targets and destroys the immune system and, left untreated, leads to death. Early detection is important because proper treatment can significantly prolong life.
- Other common sexually transmitted infections are hepatitis B, genital herpes, human papillomavirus (HPV), chlamydia, gonorrhea, syphilis, pubic lice, scabies, and trichomoniasis.
- Many STIs may not show symptoms until irreparable damage has been done, and some STIs can cause infertility or death. Prevention, safer sex practices, and appropriate health screenings are the best tactics for avoiding STIs.

LO 12.5
- You can take action to keep your immune system strong. Don't smoke, limit alcohol consumption, and get

adequate sleep. Get regular exercise and be sure your diet includes plenty of vitamin-rich fruits and vegetables. Stay up to date with your vaccinations.

- Protect your health and fertility by following safer sex practices. Show that you respect yourself and your potential partners by talking about STI history and risks before engaging in sexual activity.

GET CONNECTED

>> Visit the following websites for further information about the topics in this chapter:

- Mayo Clinic
  www.mayoclinic.com
- Medline Plus
  www.nlm.nih.gov/medlineplus
- Centers for Disease Control and Prevention
  www.cdc.gov
- American Sexual Health Association
  www.ashastd.org
- Planned Parenthood
  www.plannedparenthood.org/health-topics/stds-hiv-safer-sex-101.htm
- Center for Young Women's Health, College Health: Sexual Health, Relationships, and Resources
  www.youngwomenshealth.org/collegehealth10.html

MOBILE TIPS!
Scan this QR code with your mobile device to access additional tips about infections. Or, via your mobile device, go to **http://chmobile.pearsoncmg.com** and choose by topic: infections.

- The Body: The Complete HIV/AIDS Resource
  www.thebody.com
- Smartersex.org
  www.smartersex.org
- Go Ask Alice
  www.goaskalice.columbia.edu

Website links are subject to change. To access updated web links, please visit **Mastering**Health™

TEST YOUR KNOWLEDGE

LO 12.1
1. Pathogens
   a. cannot be stopped by your body's first line of defense.
   b. are agents that cause disease.
   c. infect animals but not humans.
   d. die once they enter your body.
2. A person who spreads infectious disease to others is called a
   a. reservoir.
   b. carrier.
   c. contaminator.
   d. pathogen.

LO 12.2
3. A first line of defense against infection is
   a. your immune system.
   b. antibiotics.
   c. immunization.
   d. your skin.
4. Acquired immunity
   a. develops when your body creates memory B cells and memory T cells.
   b. develops when your body creates regulatory T cells.
   c. only lasts a few months, at most.
   d. develops only when your body contracts a disease and survives it.

LO 12.3
5. Lyme disease is spread by
   a. fleas.
   b. ticks.
   c. mosquitoes.
   d. mice.
6. Antibiotics are appropriate treatments against
   a. bacteria.
   b. viruses.
   c. fungi.
   d. none of these pathogens.

LO 12.4
7. The most commonly reported sexually transmitted infection among college students is
   a. genital warts/HPV.
   b. genital herpes.
   c. chlamydia.
   d. HIV/AIDS.

8. What percentage of new STI infections in the United States each year occur in people between the ages of 15 and 24?
   a. 15%
   b. 25%
   c. 30%
   d. 50%

LO 12.4, 12.5

9. Which of the following practices will NOT reduce the risk of contracting HIV?
   a. correct use of condoms
   b. abstinence
   c. avoiding multiple partners and getting tested with new partners
   d. avoiding partners who look sick

LO 12.4

10. Cervical cancer is caused by
    a. pelvic inflammatory disease.
    b. vaccines.
    c. human papillomavirus (HPV).
    d. gonorrhea.

WHAT DO YOU THINK?

LO 12.3

1. When lives are at stake from infectious diseases, should pharmaceutical companies donate the medications they make to impoverished populations or countries? Why or why not?

LO 12.3

2. Should countries fighting infectious disease epidemics turn to genetically modified organisms such as genetically modified mosquitoes that might reduce the population of disease-carrying ones? Why or why not?

LO 12.3

3. Malaria is a preventable disease, and prevention efforts, including the use of insecticide-treated bed nets, have helped reduce malaria rates as much as 90% in some regions. Yet the organization Malaria No More reports that malaria still kills one child every minute worldwide. What actions could U.S. college students take to provide bed nets for poor families in malaria-ridden areas? (You can learn more at **www.malarianomore.org**.)

LO 12.4

4. If one sexual partner has a sexually transmitted infection, at what point should he or she tell the other person? What are some ways to make that awkward conversation easier?

LO 12.4

5. If a friend told you that he or she had an STI and asked for help, what kinds of questions would you ask? What next steps would you suggest for your friend?

13

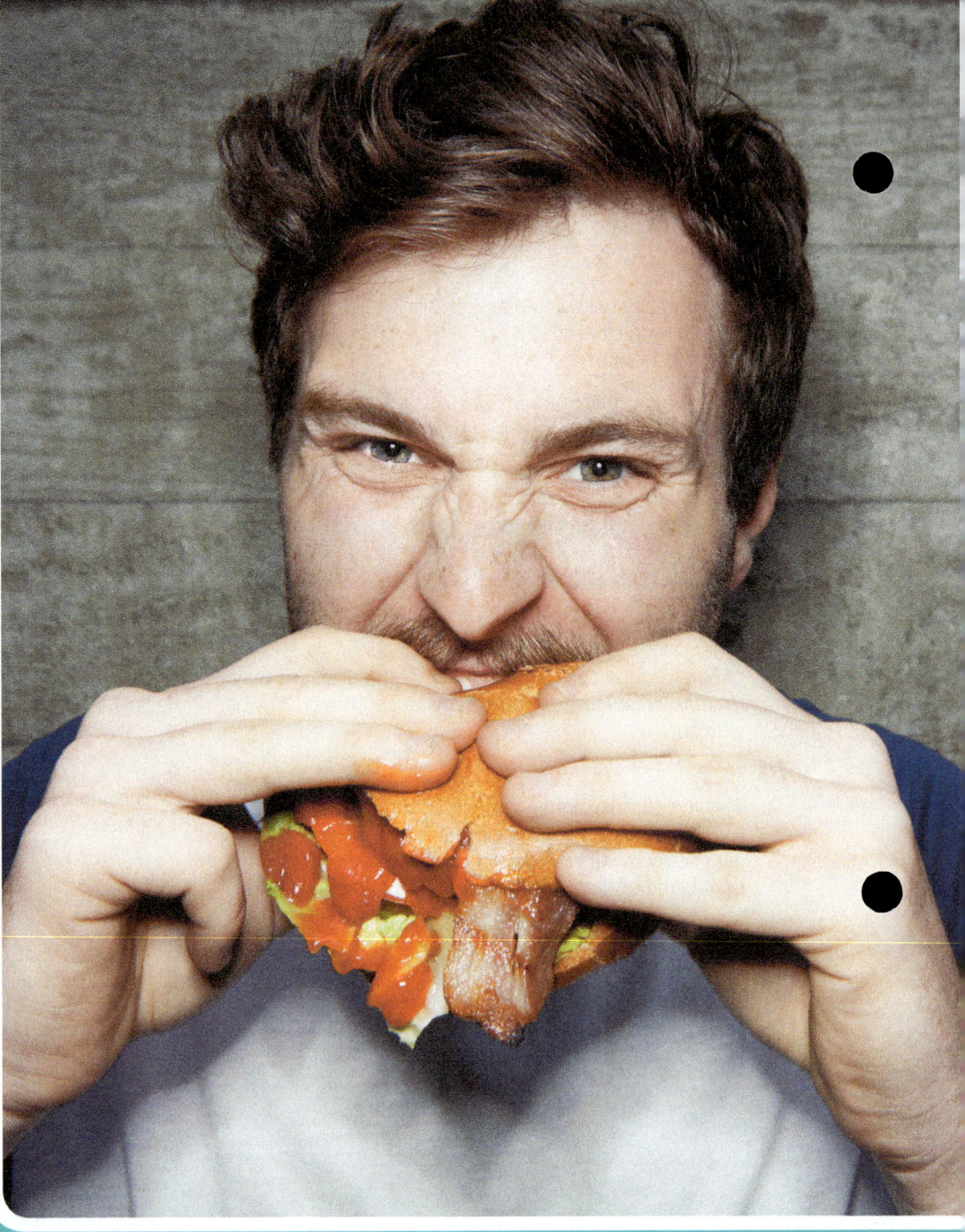

> More than 29 million Americans have diabetes.[i]

> Cardiovascular disease is the number-one cause of death in the United States.[ii]

> The five-year survival rate for Americans with cancer has now increased to 69%.[iii]

DIABETES, CARDIOVASCULAR DISEASE, AND CANCER

LEARNING OUTCOMES

LO 13.1 Discuss the burden of chronic disease in terms of personal health and costs to society.

LO 13.2 Identify the types, symptoms, complications, and risk factors associated with diabetes and explain how the disease is managed.

LO 13.3 Describe the cardiovascular system, the process of atherosclerosis, the four major types of cardiovascular disease, and the risk factors they share.

LO 13.4 List nine factors associated with cardiometabolic risk.

LO 13.5 Describe the initiation and progression of cancer and the most common types of cancer.

LO 13.6 Identify steps you can take to reduce your risk for chronic disease and its burden within your community.

Think you can avoid chronic disease?

The odds are against you. If 100 students were enrolled in your health course, and you all were to follow current U.S. health trends, here is where national statistics suggest you would wind up:

- About 16 people in your class would develop diabetes before reaching age 65.[1]
- About 30 class members would eventually die of either heart disease or a stroke.[2,3]
- Roughly 41 class members would develop cancer, and 21 would die of it.[4]

These numbers are sobering. But they're population statistics, so they don't necessarily predict your fate. Just as you can use your time in college to shape your career, you can also use these years to start beating the odds of developing a chronic disease.

Overview of Chronic Diseases

LO 13.1 Discuss the burden of chronic disease in terms of personal health and costs to society.

A **chronic disease** is a disease that comes on gradually and lasts a long time, causing either continual symptoms or recurring bouts of illness. The first two chronic diseases discussed in this chapter—diabetes and cardiovascular disease—usually resist complete cure. Instead, they're managed by a combination of lifestyle changes and medications focused on reducing the patient's *cardiometabolic risk*—that is, factors such as obesity, elevated blood pressure, and others that are associated with these two chronic diseases. We'll define cardiometabolic risk more precisely later in this chapter. Cancer, the third disease we'll focus on, can often be cured. The five-year survival rate for all cancers is now 69%.[5]

Scope of the Problem

About half of all adults in the United States have at least one chronic disease, and about one-fourth have two or more. In addition, chronic diseases cause 7 out of every 10 deaths in the United States each year.[6] Many of these deaths occur prematurely—that is, at an earlier-than-expected age. But chronic diseases reduce not only our years of life but also our *health-related quality of life* because of the discomfort, pain, psychological distress, and activity limitations that accompany them. If you've ever seen someone with advanced diabetes walking with crutches because of an amputated foot or heard someone struggling to speak because of the effects of a stroke, then you've witnessed some of the effects of reduced health-related quality of life.

Finally, the financial burden of chronic disease is tremendous: About 86% of all health-care spending in the United States is for people with chronic disease.[6] Between medical costs and lost productivity due to chronic disease, the cost to the U.S. economy is more than $700 billion annually.[6]

>> The Centers for Disease Control and Prevention has a comprehensive website covering chronic diseases, including strategies for prevention, statistics, fact sheets, and more: www.cdc.gov/chronicdisease/index.htm.

Influence of Four Key Behaviors

Diabetes, cardiovascular disease, and cancer might seem unrelated, but in fact they share some underlying physiological mechanisms and risk factors. That's because the functions of the body's chemicals, cells, and tissues are interrelated, and certain factors that promote disease in one type of tissue can promote disease in another. An example is chronic inflammation. Although inflammation is a natural and protective response to tissue injury, it causes changes throughout the body that are increasingly being recognized as factors in chronic disease.[7] Tobacco use, excessive alcohol consumption, and obesity all promote inflammation. Therefore, avoiding smoking, drinking alcohol in moderation if at all, consuming a healthful diet, and engaging in regular physical activity all contribute to reducing your risk for chronic disease.[6] If these four behaviors sound familiar, it's because we've discussed them throughout this text. How many college students practice these healthful behaviors? Check the **Student Stats** to find out.

Lifestyle choices cannot, of course, explain all cases of

chronic disease A disease that comes on gradually and lasts a long time; many chronic diseases can be managed but resist complete cure.

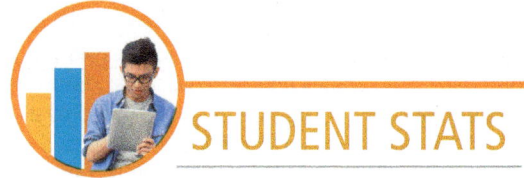

STUDENT STATS

College Students' Reported Participation in Key Health Behaviors

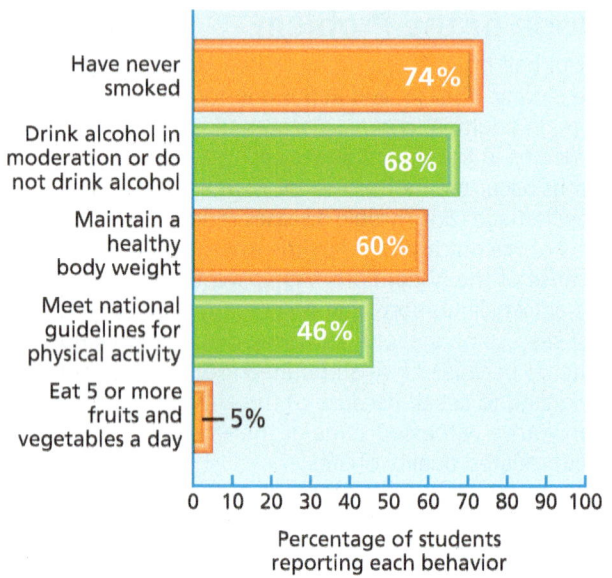

Behavior	Percentage
Have never smoked	74%
Drink alcohol in moderation or do not drink alcohol	68%
Maintain a healthy body weight	60%
Meet national guidelines for physical activity	46%
Eat 5 or more fruits and vegetables a day	5%

Source: Data from *American College Health Association National College Health Assessment (ACHA-NCHA II) Reference Group Executive Summary, Spring 2015,* by the American College Health Association, 2015, retrieved from http://www.acha-ncha.org.

chronic disease. As you learned in Chapter 1, genetics and biology contribute, as do social and physical determinants of health. Socioeconomic and racial and ethnic disparities also play roles in chronic disease incidence and mortality. For more information on these disparities, see the **Diversity & Health** box on page 322.

LO 13.1 QUICK CHECK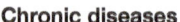

Chronic diseases

a. cannot be cured.
b. cost the United States nearly $7 billion annually.
c. do not usually reduce years of life but do reduce health-related quality of life.
d. are most likely to occur in people who smoke, abuse alcohol, or are obese.

Diabetes

LO 13.2 Identify the types, symptoms, complications, and risk factors associated with diabetes and explain how the disease is managed.

Do you know someone who has diabetes? Do you have it yourself? Your answer is far more likely to be "yes" than was your parents' reply at your age. That's because between

> **"** *About 21 million Americans have been diagnosed with diabetes, and another 8 million are estimated to have the disease but are not yet aware of it.*"

1973 and 2013, the percentage of Americans with diagnosed diabetes more than tripled, from 2% to over 7%.[8] About 21 million Americans have been diagnosed with diabetes, and another 8 million are estimated to have the disease but are not yet aware of it.[1]

Types of Diabetes

Diabetes, known formally as **diabetes mellitus,** is a broad term that covers a group of diseases characterized by high levels of sugar, or *glucose,* in the blood. In fact, the word *mellitus* is derived from the Latin word for "honey." These high levels of blood glucose arise from problems with **insulin,** a hormone produced by the **pancreas** that is necessary for transportation of glucose into the body's cells.

Normally, when our blood glucose levels rise after we eat a meal or snack containing carbohydrate, specialized cells in the pancreas, called *beta cells,* release insulin into the bloodstream (**Figure 13.1**, first panel). Insulin circulates throughout the body and binds to the outer membrane of body cells. There, it triggers proteins inside the cells to move to the membrane and take up glucose. In some people who have diabetes, the pancreas simply doesn't make enough insulin to adequately clear glucose from the bloodstream. In others, the pancreas makes enough insulin, but cells don't respond effectively. In either case, glucose builds up in the bloodstream, while the body's cells—unable to take in glucose—suffer from lack of nourishment.

> **diabetes mellitus** A group of diseases in which the body does not make or use insulin properly, resulting in elevated blood glucose.
>
> **insulin** A hormone necessary for glucose transport into cells.
>
> **pancreas** An abdominal organ that produces insulin as well as certain compounds that are helpful in digestion.
>
> **type 1 diabetes** A form of diabetes prompted by immune destruction of the beta cells of the pancreas, which impairs the production of insulin.

Type 1 Diabetes

Type 1 diabetes arises when the body's own immune system destroys the beta cells in the pancreas that make insulin (Figure 13.1, middle panel). Type 1 diabetes usually appears in childhood or adolescence, and researchers are investigating the role of specific genes in its development as well as the possible role of external factors such as viruses. People with type 1 diabetes must monitor their blood glucose level throughout each day and take supplemental insulin. For this reason, type 1 diabetes is often known as *insulin-dependent diabetes.*

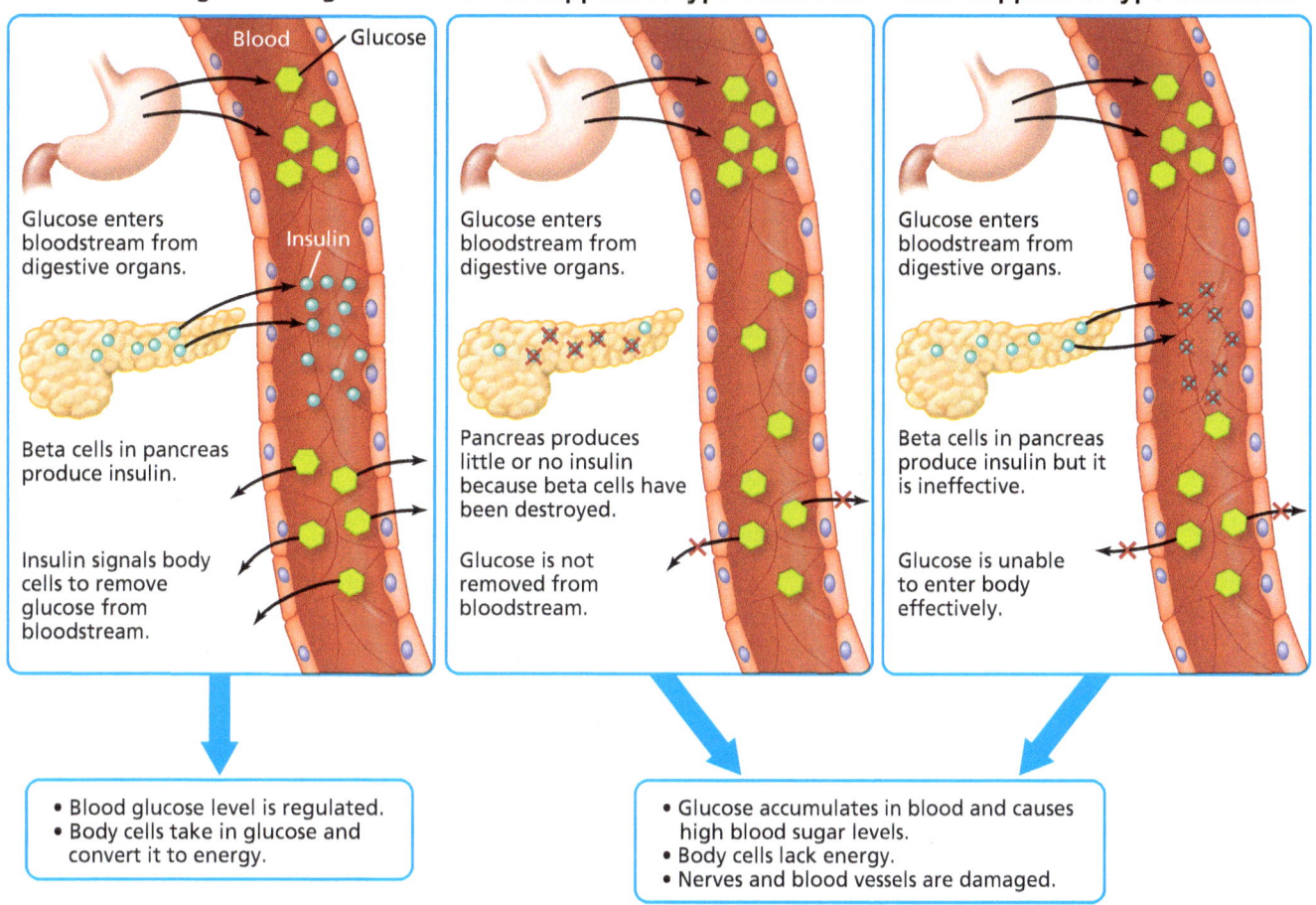

FIGURE 13.1 **Two Types of Diabetes.** In type 1 diabetes, the beta cells of the pancreas stop producing insulin entirely or produce an amount insufficient for normal body functioning. In type 2 diabetes, the body is unable to use insulin properly. In advanced cases, the pancreas becomes exhausted and, as with type 1 diabetes, stops producing insulin. In either case, the body's cells are unable to take in glucose from the bloodstream.

Type 1 diabetes accounts for the majority of diabetes in children and about 5% of diabetes cases in adults.[1] There is no cure for type 1 diabetes, but the condition is the focus of intense research, including studies into the use of stem cell therapy, which could replace the diabetic's non-functioning beta cells with beta cells that respond to glucose by producing insulin.

Type 2 Diabetes

Type 2 diabetes accounts for about 90%–95% of all adult diabetes cases.[1] Once known as *adult-onset diabetes,* type 2 diabetes used to be extremely rare among children and teens. Now, about 5,000 Americans younger than age 20 are diagnosed with type 2 diabetes annually.[1] The incidence is also rising among young and middle-aged adults.

Whereas in type 1 diabetes the beta cells of the pancreas stop making insulin, most cases of type 2 diabetes begin as *insulin resistance.* The pancreas makes normal amounts of insulin, but the body's cells don't respond to it properly; they resist its effects (Figure 13.1, third panel). A primary factor in this resistance is inflammation prompted by immune cells residing in fat tissue.[9,10] This explains why type 2 diabetes is especially common in people who are obese. Inflammatory chemicals impair the ability of body cells to respond to insulin and take up glucose; thus, glucose remains in the bloodstream. The resulting **hyperglycemia** (persistent high blood glucose) signals the pancreas to produce more insulin to get more glucose into the cells. As the demand for insulin continues to rise, the beta cells begin to fatigue. With continued high demand over time, they can lose their ability to produce insulin, just as in type 1 diabetes.

Other Forms of Diabetes

Less common varieties of diabetes resemble type 2 but also have differences that set them apart:

- *Gestational diabetes* develops in almost 6% of pregnant women. The condition usually disappears after childbirth, but researchers have learned that women who develop gestational diabetes have an increased risk of developing type 2 diabetes.[11]

> **type 2 diabetes** A form of diabetes that begins as insulin resistance and increased demand for insulin; as it progresses, the ability of the pancreas to produce insulin declines.
>
> **hyperglycemia** A persistent state of elevated levels of blood glucose.

DIVERSITY & HEALTH

Disparities in Chronic Disease

Even as broad public health efforts focus on reducing the risks of chronic diseases, significant disparities remain. Consider the following:

- Poverty is an obstacle to receiving quality health care. Poor Americans are more likely to lack health insurance, to lack access to health screenings and other preventive measures, and to engage in behaviors that increase chronic disease risk, such as smoking, physical inactivity, and poor diet. According to the U.S. Census Bureau's most recent five-year survey, 11.6% of Caucasian Americans and 11.7% of Asian Americans live in poverty. In contrast, 23.2% of Hispanic Americans, 25.8% of African Americans, and 27.0% of Native Americans live in poverty.[1]

- The prevalence of diabetes in these populations mirrors their rates of poverty: Caucasian Americans have the lowest prevalence of diabetes, at 7.6%. The rate for Asian Americans is 9.0%. Prevalence jumps to 12.8% for Hispanic Americans, then 13.2% for African Americans, and 15.9% for Native Americans.[2]

- African Americans have the highest rate of heart disease and stroke morbidity and mortality of all racial and ethnic groups. Their prevalence of hypertension is the highest in the world. Among African Americans, nearly 43% of adult males and 44% of adult females have been diagnosed with hypertension, and in 69% of these males and 47% of these females, their hypertension is uncontrolled.[3,4]

- The American Cancer Society (ACS) identifies poverty as the "overriding factor" explaining racial and ethnic disparities in cancer incidence and mortality. That is, people of lower socioeconomic status have higher cancer incidence and death rates than people who are more affluent, regardless of their race or ethnicity.[5] Their reduced survival is in part because poorer people are more likely to be diagnosed at an advanced stage and less likely to receive optimal treatment.

- African Americans have the highest rates of cancer overall and are the most likely to die of cancer. The cancer death rate among African American males, for example, is 27% higher than the rate among Caucasian males, and African American females have a cancer death rate 14% higher than that of Caucasian females. We noted above that the poverty rate is actually highest among Native Americans; unfortunately, cancer statistics among Native Americans are unreliable.[5]

If your socioeconomic status, race, or ethnicity puts you at increased risk for chronic disease, talk to your health-care provider. Maintaining a healthy weight, exercising, eating a nutritious diet, not smoking, and limiting your alcohol intake can go a long way toward reducing your risk.

What Do You Think?

1. Asian Americans have the lowest rates of obesity, binge drinking, and tobacco use of any ethnic group. How might these factors contribute to their risks for chronic disease, as identified here?

2. Chronic stress is a risk factor for diabetes and CVD. How might stress be related to some of the statistics discussed above?

3. Type 2 diabetes, CVD, and cancer are all complex, multifactorial diseases. How might social determinants, policy-making, and access to health services influence the differences in disease and death rates discussed here? (See Chapter 1.)

References: **1.** Macartney, S., Bishaw, A., & Fontenot, K. (2013, February). *Poverty rates for selected detailed race and Hispanic groups by state and place: 2007–2011: American Community Survey Briefs.* www.census.gov. **2.** Centers for Disease Control and Prevention. (2014). *National diabetes statistics report, 2014.* www.cdc.gov. **3.** American Heart Association. (2015, July). *African Americans and heart disease, stroke.* www.heart.org. **4.** Centers for Disease Control and Prevention. (2015, May). *Health, United States, 2014.* DHHS Publication No. 2015-1232. www.cdc.gov. **5.** American Cancer Society. (2016). *Cancer disparities. Cancer facts & figures 2016.* www.cancer.org.

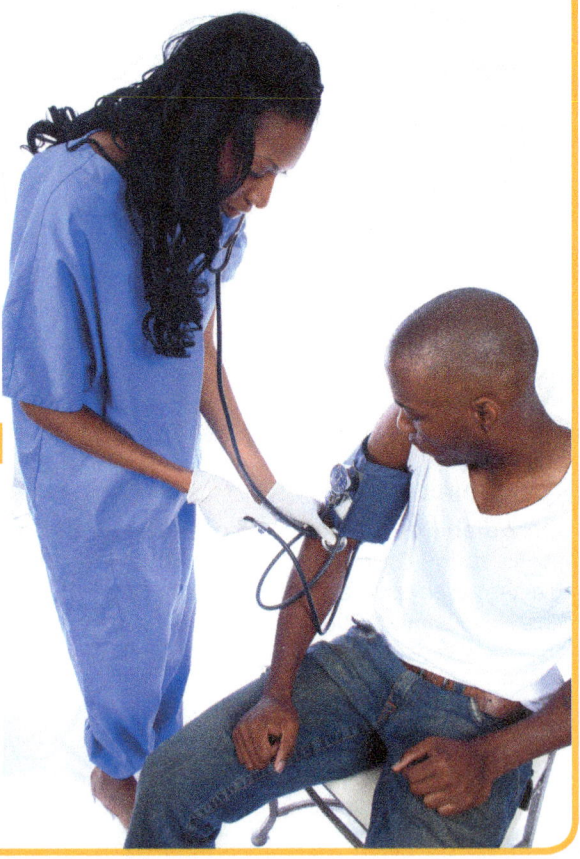

- Several other varieties of diabetes appear to blend aspects of type 1 and type 2. Sometimes referred to as "type 1.5," these variants include *latent autoimmune diabetes of adults (LADA)* and *maturity-onset diabetes of the young (MODY)*. Usually prompted by surgery, medications, or infections or other illnesses, they are often revealed when blood tests show some immune-system destruction of pancreatic beta cells—but healthy, insulin-producing beta cells as well. Researchers estimate that up to 5% of all diagnoses of diabetes are actually due to type 1.5.[11]

▶▶ Watch a video showing how diabetes affects blood sugar at **www.mayoclinic.com/health/blood-sugar/MM00641**.

Detecting Diabetes

The physical signs and symptoms of diabetes include

- Frequent urination
- Excessive thirst
- Hunger
- Tendency to tire easily
- Numbness or tingling in the hands and feet
- In women, a tendency to develop vaginal yeast infections

These manifestations, although common across all types of diabetes, can develop differently from person to person. Also, early stages of diabetes may not be accompanied by any symptoms at all.

Two simple laboratory tests can reveal whether you have—or are developing—diabetes. One of the most common is the *fasting blood glucose test (FBG)*, which requires you to fast (consuming nothing other than plain water) overnight. A technician then draws a blood sample, and the level of glucose in your blood is measured. Here is what the measurement values mean:[12]

- A blood glucose level below 100 mg/dL is normal.
- A blood glucose level between 100 and 125 mg/dL means that you have **prediabetes.** That is, your FBG is higher than normal but not high enough to warrant a diagnosis of diabetes. Prediabetes indicates that your body is struggling to regulate your blood glucose, and you are at significant risk for developing diabetes.

prediabetes A persistent state of blood glucose levels that are higher than normal but not high enough to qualify as diabetes.

- A blood glucose level of 126 mg/dL or higher indicates true diabetes.

A second test, known as the *glycated hemoglobin test,* or *A1C test,* is used to detect type 2 diabetes and prediabetes. The A1C test measures how much glucose is attached to the hemoglobin—the oxygen-carrying compound—in your red blood cells. This information reflects the average blood glucose level for the previous three months. Here is what the values mean:[12]

- An A1C level of about 5% is normal.
- An A1C level of 5.7% to 6.4% indicates prediabetes.
- An A1C level of 6.5% or higher on two separate occasions indicates that you have diabetes.[12]

If these tests suggest diabetes, the physician will order a further test to see whether there is evidence of an immune-system response against the beta cells of the pancreas. The urine may also be tested to look for waste chemicals suggesting that body cells, given their inability to use glucose for energy, are breaking down fats or proteins for energy.

Complications of Diabetes

Persistent hyperglycemia causes damage throughout the body, especially to blood vessels **(Figure 13.2)**. This damage can lead to a variety of complications:[1]

- Damage to the blood vessels that supply the heart and brain greatly increases the risk of heart attack and stroke. Moreover, death rates from cardiovascular disease are 1.7 times higher in patients with diabetes than in patients without diabetes.
- The kidneys have microscopic blood vessels that filter excessive glucose from the blood into urine. Hyperglycemia stresses this delicate filtration system, leading to kidney disease: diabetes is the primary cause of 44% of cases of kidney failure.
- Hyperglycemia also damages blood vessels that serve nerves, causing pain, loss of sensation, tissue breakdown, and poor wound healing, especially in the feet, ankles, and lower legs. This explains why about 60% of toe, foot, and lower leg surgical amputations occur among people with diabetes.
- Similarly, hyperglycemia damages the tiny blood vessels serving the retina of the eye, causing a form of vision impairment called *diabetic retinopathy*. Over 28% of diabetic adults age 40 and older have diabetic retinopathy, which is a leading cause of blindness among U.S. adults.

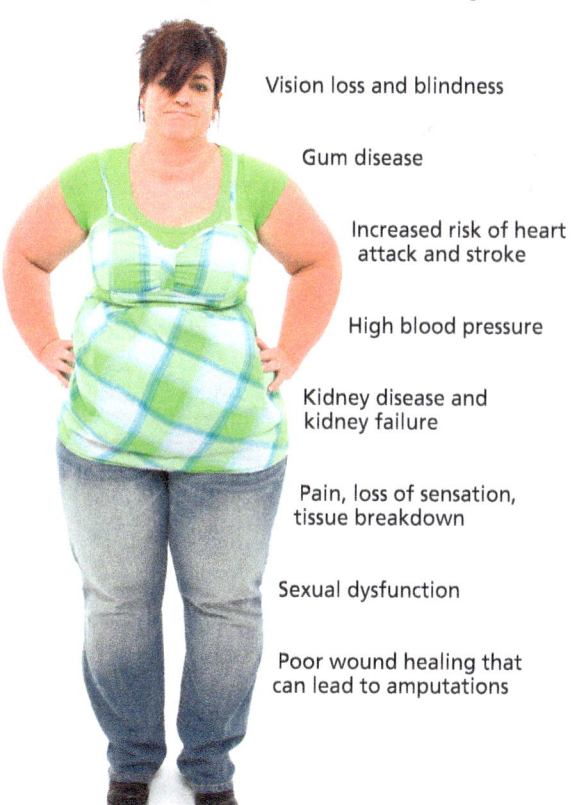

FIGURE 13.2 **Complications Associated with Diabetes.**

- Severe gum disease is also more common among people with diabetes.

Diabetes also increases the risk of cancer, as well as death from cancer,[13] infection, liver disease, hyperglycemic crisis, depression, and a variety of other disorders. Overall, diabetes is the seventh-most-common cause of death in the United States, and the death rate for people with diabetes is 1.5 times that of people without the disease.[1]

Risk Factors for Type 2 Diabetes

After age 50, body cells become increasingly less responsive to the effects of insulin. This explains in part the gradual increase in blood glucose levels that occurs as we age. But other risk factors are much more important than aging. These include

- **Overweight and obesity.** Almost 90% of people with type 2 diabetes are overweight or obese, and the rapid increase in diabetes rates over the past few decades parallels the rapid increase in obesity.[14] Abdominal obesity in particular is linked to diabetes and, as we discuss later in this chapter, is a key cardiometabolic risk factor.
- **Diet.** Many people wonder if particular foods play a role—independently of the number of calories—in the development of diabetes. Foods high in fiber are generally recommended because they slow the release of glucose into the bloodstream. What about sweets? Eating a diet high in added sugars does not directly cause type 2 diabetes because genetics, body weight, and many other factors play a role. However, epidemiological studies have revealed a relationship between the amount of sugar consumed within a population and that population's rate of diabetes.[15] Also, a diet high in added sugars is strongly associated with an increased risk for obesity.[16]
- **Lack of exercise.** When you have free time, do you opt for an activity like swimming or a bike ride? Exercise helps control weight, burns glucose, and makes your body cells more receptive to insulin. It also builds muscle mass, and muscle cells take up most of the glucose in your blood. In contrast, a sedentary lifestyle increases your risk for type 2 diabetes. A study that followed more than 1.5 million men for 26 years found that, regardless of body weight or family history, those who were unfit at age 18 (as measured by muscle strength and aerobic capacity) had three times the risk of developing diabetes by age 44 compared to men who had been fit at age 18.[17]
- **Smoking.** Smokers are 30%–40% more likely to develop diabetes than nonsmokers, and smokers are also at higher risk for poor management of their diabetes and for serious complications, including amputations and vision loss.[18]
- **Chronic stress.** Recent studies have associated a high level of the stress hormone cortisol, as measured in saliva or scalp hair, with a higher incidence of insulin resistance and diabetes.[19]
- **Genetic factors.** Do members of your family have type 2 diabetes? If so, you are at increased risk. Several common genetic variants increase a person's risk of type 2 diabetes. In addition, African Americans, Mexican Americans, Puerto Ricans, and Native Americans develop diabetes at higher rates than members of other racial and ethnic groups.[1]

You can also determine your risk for diabetes by completing the **Self-Assessment**.

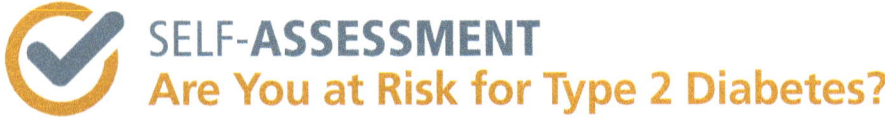

SELF-ASSESSMENT
Are You at Risk for Type 2 Diabetes?

For each question, find the correct answer and then write the corresponding number of points on the line.

1. Are you age 45 or older? _____
   Yes (1 point)   No (0 points)

2. What is your weight status? (See the BMI chart in Figure 7.1 on page 157.) _____
   BMI is less than 25 (0 points)
   BMI is 25–29.9 (1 point)
   BMI is 30–39.9 (2 points)
   BMI is 40 or above (3 points)

3. Do you have a parent, brother, or sister with diabetes? _____
   Yes (1 point)   No (0 points)

4. Is your family background African American, Alaska Native, American Indian, Asian American, Hispanic/Latino, or Pacific Islander American? _____
   Yes (1 point)   No (0 points)

5. For women: Have you had gestational diabetes? _____
   Yes (1 point)   No (0 points)

6. For women: Have you given birth to at least one baby weighing more than 9 pounds? _____
   Yes (1 point)   No (0 points)

7. Is your blood pressure 140/90 or higher, or have you been told that you have high blood pressure? _____
   Yes (1 point)   No (0 points)   Don't know (1 point)

8. Are your cholesterol levels higher than normal? Is your HDL, or good, cholesterol, below 35, or is your triglyceride level above 250? _____
   Yes (1 point)   No (0 points)   Don't know (1 point)

9. Are you fairly inactive? _____
   Yes (1 point)   No (0 points)

10. Do you have a history of cardiovascular disease? _____
    Yes (1 point)   No (0 points)

Add up your score: _____

HOW TO INTERPRET YOUR SCORE The higher your score, the higher your risk for type 2 diabetes. If you scored 3 or higher, it is recommended that you take immediate action to reduce your risk for type 2 diabetes. If you answered "Don't know" to any questions, visit your health-care provider to get checked.

To complete this Self-Assessment online, visit **MasteringHealth**™

Source: Based on *Am I at risk for type 2 diabetes?* by the National Institute of Diabetes and Digestive and Kidney Diseases, www.niddk.nih.gov; and *Type 2 diabetes risk test*, by the American Diabetes Association, www.diabetes.org.

Clinical Management of Diabetes

If you're diagnosed with diabetes or prediabetes, your doctor will work with you toward one central goal—stabilizing your body's use of glucose. The approach prescribed will depend on the type and severity of diabetes you have.

Glucose Monitoring

To stay healthy, people with diabetes must maintain a continual awareness of their blood glucose levels. That means measuring and recording blood glucose levels as often as three times a day. In the past, blood glucose monitoring required pricking the finger. Now, devices are available that can read glucose levels through the skin or from a small needle implanted in the body.

Weight Loss

Many studies have demonstrated that overweight or obese people with prediabetes can reduce their risk for developing type 2 diabetes with weight loss—and the amount of weight shed doesn't have to be dramatic. For example, a 2016 study of women with prediabetes found improvements in fasting insulin and other metabolic factors with a loss of just 4.4% of initial body weight.[20] In obese patients with diabetes, especially those with a body mass index (BMI) of 35 or higher who are at high risk for severe complications, bariatric (weight-loss) surgery may be an option. Bariatric surgery reduces the size of the stomach and may also bypass the first section of the small intestine, so weight loss can be dramatic. However, patients gradually begin to gain weight again if they overeat and fail to engage in regular exercise.

Exercise

During exercise, glucose is transported into body cells, especially muscle cells, for use as energy. Thus, building muscle improves blood glucose control. Exercise increases the sensitivity of body cells to insulin, so less insulin is needed to clear glucose from the bloodstream. For these reasons, a personalized program of aerobic exercise is typically prescribed.

Oral Medications

If someone with type 2 diabetes is not successful in losing weight, or if weight loss doesn't reduce blood glucose significantly enough, the physician may prescribe an oral medication. Diabetes medications work in a variety of ways. Some, for instance, prompt the pancreas to manufacture and release more insulin, whereas others help increase the cells' response to insulin. If A1C tests continue to show, however, that medication isn't reducing blood glucose levels effectively, the physician is likely to recommend the treatment approach used with type 1 diabetes, involving insulin therapy.

Insulin Therapy

All people with type 1 diabetes, and many with type 2, need insulin daily to survive. Insulin can't be taken by mouth because it is a protein and would be digested in the gastrointestinal tract. Many diabetics inject their insulin using a fine needle and syringe or an insulin pen—a device that looks like an ink pen, but the cartridge is filled with insulin. Others use an insulin pump worn on the outside of the body. A tube connects the reservoir of insulin to a catheter inserted under the skin of the abdomen. The person programs the pump to dispense specific amounts of insulin **(Figure 13.3)**. Most of the new devices are about the size and weight of an MP3 player, and some are even free of tubing, delivering insulin via skin absorption from a "pod" attached to the skin with a gentle adhesive.

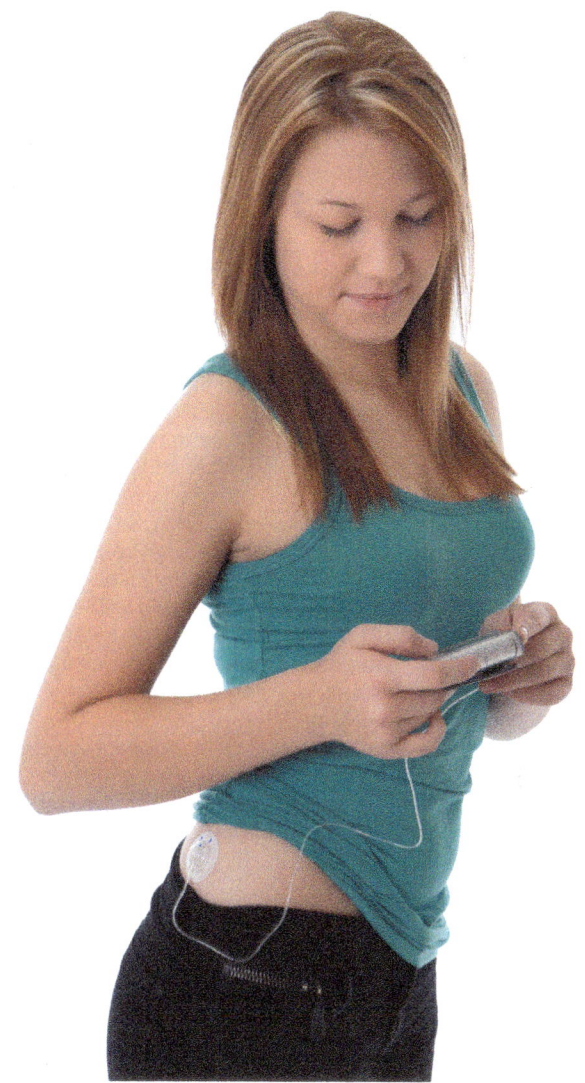

FIGURE 13.3 **Controlling Diabetes.** Insulin pumps allow many people to control their blood glucose levels throughout the day without painful injections.

As you've seen, controlling diabetes requires consistent attention to diet, exercise, body weight, blood glucose monitoring, and prescription therapies. But those who succeed in managing their diabetes are likely to avoid serious complications, live longer, and enjoy a better health-related quality of life.

LO 13.2 QUICK CHECK

Of the following risk factors, the one most strongly associated with the onset of type 2 diabetes is

a. alcohol consumption.
b. viral infection.
c. obesity.
d. a high-fat diet.

> **STUDENT STORY**

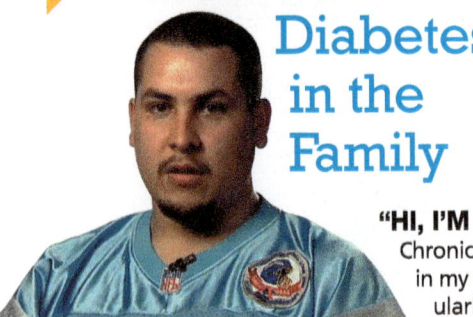

Diabetes in the Family

"HI, I'M MICHAEL. Chronic disease runs in my family, particularly diabetes on both my mom's and dad's sides. Just recently, my mom, my sister, and my dad were all diagnosed with type 2. It has affected me because I have to watch them take all their pills and recover from injuries and sicknesses and see the pain that they're going through, particularly with the circulation in their legs.

I am doing things to stop the risk of getting diabetes. I'm eating better. I'm exercising. I'm studying diabetes and other chronic diseases just to make sure that I protect myself to the fullest. I'm also teaching my mom and my dad about it.

I would tell other students to eat right, eat your fruits and vegetables, and exercise a minimum of 30 minutes every day, to help you fight against chronic diseases such as diabetes."

What Do You Think?

1. Michael mentions that "chronic disease" runs in his family, not just diabetes. What other form of chronic disease do you think he might be alluding to, and why?
2. Why is it that Michael's family members are having problems with pain and circulation in their legs? What are other short- and long-term effects of diabetes?
3. Michael is paying attention to his diet and staying physically active. What else could he do to lower his risk for developing diabetes?

Cardiovascular Disease

LO 13.3 Describe the cardiovascular system, the process of atherosclerosis, the four major types of cardiovascular disease, and the risk factors they share.

When an elderly acquaintance or loved one dies of a heart attack or stroke, you may not see any direct connection to your own health. After all, the person was a lot older than you. But even though heart attacks and strokes typically occur later in life, the conditions that trigger them begin to develop decades earlier.

Cardiovascular disease (CVD) is a large group of disorders affecting the heart or blood vessels. The four major types are hypertension (high blood pressure), coronary heart disease (including heart attacks), heart failure, and stroke. Diagnosed hypertension is present in 3% of college students, and nearly 25% have significant risk factors for heart disease.[21,22] However, the prevalence of CVD among young adults in general is over 10%, and as we age, it skyrockets: More than one-third of Americans in their 40s and 50s have CVD, and by age 80, the prevalence is about 85%.[23] Not surprisingly, CVD is the leading cause of adult mortality in the United States, responsible for nearly 3 in 10 deaths.[24]

A meaningful understanding of CVD requires that you become familiar with the structures and activities of your cardiovascular system.

The Healthy Cardiovascular System

The cardiovascular system is made up of blood vessels and the heart, which together form the blood-delivery network that keeps the body functioning. Blood, circulating through blood vessels, ferries oxygen, nutrients, and wastes to and from cells through **arteries,** which carry blood away from the heart, and **veins,** which carry blood to the heart **(Figure 13.4a)**.

At the center of this system is the heart, which is only about the size of a fist but is surprisingly strong. That's because it's almost entirely made up of a thick layer of muscle called the **myocardium.** The contractions of the myocardium keep blood moving, ensuring that it transports oxygen and nutrients to, and eliminates wastes from, every region of the body.

The interior of the heart consists of four hollow, muscular chambers **(Figure 13.4b)**. The two upper chambers are the **atria.** Each atrium is connected by a valve to one of the corresponding lower **ventricles.** A thick wall of tissue divides the right atrium and ventricle from the pair on the left, creating two side-by-side pumps. This division lets each side of the heart focus on a different task—either sending oxygen-poor blood to the lungs for replenishment or pumping that reoxygenated blood back out to the rest of the body.

Here's how the blood circulates. The right atrium receives oxygen-depleted blood from the superior and inferior vena cava, the largest veins in the body, and then releases it into the right ventricle, which sends it into the pulmonary artery, which takes it to the lungs. There, blood cells collect freshly inhaled oxygen and unload carbon dioxide (a metabolic waste), which we exhale. Then the pulmonary veins bring the oxygen-rich blood to the left atrium and ventricle, which receive this blood and pump it out into the body via the aorta, a large artery that branches off into smaller arteries. These include the coronary arteries, which sustain the heart muscle itself.

The body's blood vessels divide into a network of smaller branches, eventually fanning out into **capillaries,** tiny blood

> **cardiovascular disease (CVD)** A large group of disorders affecting the heart or blood vessels.
>
> **arteries** Vessels that transport blood away from the heart, delivering oxygen-rich blood to the body periphery and oxygen-poor blood to the lungs.
>
> **veins** Vessels that transport blood toward the heart, delivering oxygen-poor blood from the body periphery or oxygen-rich blood from the lungs.
>
> **myocardium** The heart's muscle tissue.
>
> **atria** The two upper chambers of the heart, which receive blood from the body periphery and lungs.
>
> **ventricles** The two lower chambers of the heart, which pump blood to the body and lungs.
>
> **capillaries** The smallest blood vessels, which deliver blood and nutrients to individual cells and pick up wastes.

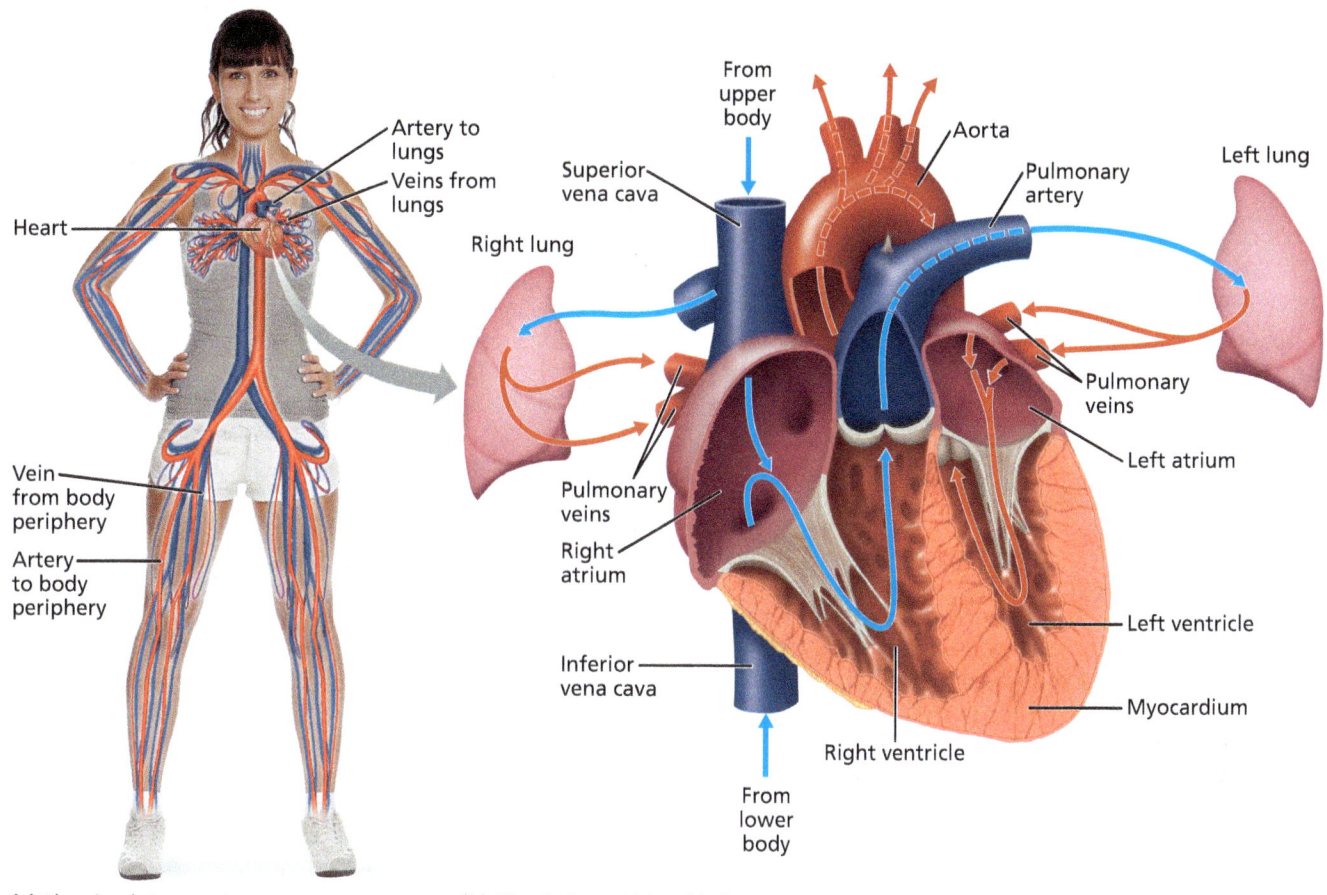

(a) The circulatory system (b) Circulation of blood in heart

FIGURE 13.4 **The Cardiovascular System.**

vessels that deliver oxygen and nutrients to individual cells and collect their wastes. Once blood in the capillaries has exchanged oxygen and nutrients for wastes, it is returned to the heart via the veins. As with any other system of pipes or tubes, the arteries, capillaries, and veins work best when they are free of blockage or damage, allowing blood to flow smoothly.

This complex process is remarkably quick. In adults at rest, the heart typically beats 60–120 times per minute, pumping a few ounces of blood with each beat. Within about 1 minute, all the blood—about 5 to 6 quarts in an average adult—has been circulated.

To keep up this rapid rhythm, the heart relies on electricity. A bundle of specialized cells in the heart's *sinus node*, located in the right atrium, generate electrical impulses and transmit them throughout the myocardium at a steady, even rate, setting the heart to beat about 100,000 times a day.

If your cardiovascular system is healthy, circulation generally runs smoothly. But if damage occurs to even one part of the system, it will begin to struggle to perform its functions. Next, we'll look at the physiological mechanism that most commonly damages the cardiovascular system: atherosclerosis.

>> Watch a video showing how the heart and blood vessels work at **www.mayoclinic.com/health/circulatory-system/MM00636**.

Atherosclerosis

Atherosclerosis is an arterial condition characterized by inflammation, scarring, and the buildup of mealy deposits along artery walls. In fact, the word's root, *athere*, is Greek for "porridge"! Together, these factors cause a narrowing of arteries, which restricts blood flow to cells and tissues "downstream" of the narrowed area. Cells starved of oxygen and nutrients cannot function; thus, when atherosclerosis affects the coronary arteries, the person can suffer a heart attack. When it affects arteries in the brain (cerebral arteries), the person can suffer a stroke.

Atherosclerosis begins when the delicate inner lining of an artery becomes damaged. Although the cause of this damage is not always known, in some cases it is thought to result when **blood pressure**—the force of blood pulsating against the artery walls—is excessive. In other cases, it reflects the lining's encounter with irritants, and as you now know, a high level of blood glucose is a major irritant of blood vessels. Excessive lipids in the bloodstream, including triglycerides and cholesterol, can also irritate the vessel lining. In addition, the toxins in tobacco smoke

> **atherosclerosis** A condition characterized by narrowing of the arteries as a result of inflammation, scarring, and the buildup of fatty deposits.
>
> **blood pressure** The force of blood moving against the arterial walls.

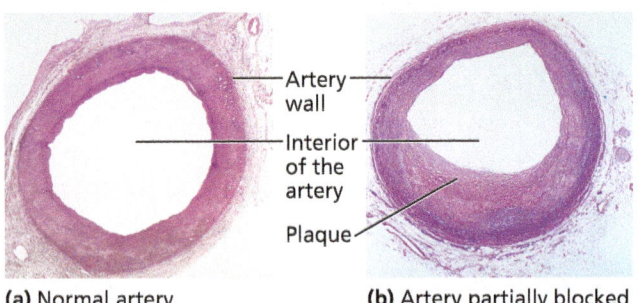

(a) Normal artery **(b)** Artery partially blocked with plaque

FIGURE 13.5 **Atherosclerosis.** These light micrographs show a cross section of (a) a normal artery allowing adequate blood flow and (b) an artery that is partially blocked with plaque, which can lead to heart attack or stroke.

and even certain types of infection can promote this initial damage.

The body responds to injury with inflammation, and at injured arterial sites, the resulting inflammation spreads into the artery wall. This leaves it weakened, scarred, and stiff (sclerotic). As a result, triglycerides and cholesterol circulating in the bloodstream can seep between the damaged lining cells and become trapped within the artery wall. Soon they are joined by white blood cells, calcium, and other substances. Eventually, this buildup, called *plaque*, narrows arteries significantly enough to impair blood flow **(Figure 13.5)**. When this occurs in a coronary artery, the person may experience chest pain (called *angina*), weakness, shortness of breath, and other symptoms.

Plaque may build up to the point where it significantly blocks or even stops the flow of blood through an artery. This causes death of the tissues that are normally served by that vessel. Sometimes plaque can become hardened and rupture, causing microscopic tears in the artery wall that allow blood to leak into the tissue on the other side. When this happens, blood platelets rush to the site to clot the blood, and the clot can quickly obstruct the artery. Alternatively, softer plaque can break off and travel through the bloodstream until it blocks a more distant, smaller artery. If either of these types of blockages occurs in a coronary or cerebral artery, the person will experience a heart attack or stroke.

As noted earlier, cholesterol, a lipid made by the body and found in certain foods, is a major component of plaque. We all need cholesterol for our bodies to function, but excessive amounts circulating in the blood can contribute to atherosclerosis. In a national survey, nearly 3% of college students reported that they had been diagnosed with unhealthful blood cholesterol levels.[21] We'll look more closely at types of cholesterol and what levels are considered healthful later in this chapter.

Atherosclerosis is difficult to detect without specific medical tests, and most people who are developing the condition are unaware it is occurring. Although it doesn't produce symptoms, atherosclerosis is dangerous because it directly contributes to the most common forms of CVD, which are discussed next: hypertension (high blood pressure), coronary heart disease, heart failure, and stroke. As you read about these disorders, bear in mind that they rarely develop in isolation; rather, one condition typically contributes to or occurs simultaneously with another. In addition, as noted earlier, the damage to the body's blood vessels caused by diabetes also contributes to CVD.

Hypertension (High Blood Pressure)

Hypertension, more commonly known as *high blood pressure,* is a chronic condition characterized by consistent blood pressure readings above normal. Hypertension in and of itself is considered a form of CVD. In addition, it's a risk factor for coronary heart disease, heart failure, and stroke.

> **hypertension** A persistent state of elevated blood pressure. Commonly called *high blood pressure*.

Factors Influencing Blood Pressure

The level of your blood pressure is determined, in part, by the pumping actions of your heart. When your heart contracts, an action called *systole,* the pressure of the blood in your arteries momentarily increases. When it relaxes, an action called *diastole,* your blood pressure drops.

Blood pressure is also affected by the *compliance*—the ability to stretch and recoil—of your arteries. We noted earlier that atherosclerosis can lead to both narrowing and stiffening of the arteries. When it does, blood pressure rises. To appreciate why, imagine the difference between trying to pump a pulsing stream of water into a network of wide, soft tubes versus narrow, stiff pipes. The tubing would stretch and bounce back with each pulsation, absorbing some of the pressure and allowing the turbulence to quickly settle down and the water to flow. In contrast, the stiff pipes would not accommodate the pulsating flow. This means the pump would have to work harder to propel the water against their resistance. When atherosclerosis has stiffened arteries and narrowed them with plaque, blood flow is impeded, and blood pressure goes up.

Blood pressure is also influenced by the volume of blood flowing through the vessels. Excessive glucose, sodium, or other solutes in the blood can increase its volume and stress the heart and blood vessels. In contrast, factors such as blood loss and dehydration can dangerously decrease the blood volume.

Signs and Symptoms of Hypertension

Most people with hypertension experience no symptoms. This fact, together with its contribution to heart attacks and strokes, explains the reputation of hypertension as a "silent killer." A very few people with dangerously advanced hypertension may experience headaches and dizziness.

Long-Term Effects of Hypertension

Left untreated, hypertension can lead to the other forms of CVD, including heart attack and stroke. Even in the absence of diagnosed heart disease or stroke, hypertension and hypertensive kidney disease combined are the 13th most common cause of death in the United States.[24] Hypertension can also promote vision loss and reduce your ability to think clearly, remember, and learn.

Risk Factors for Hypertension

Almost 30% of U.S. adults, or about 70 million people, have hypertension.[25] Although atherosclerosis contributes to hypertension in many people, usually the causes aren't entirely clear. Your age, weight, ethnic background, and diet all play a role, and a high-sodium diet is a significant risk factor for some people.

Clinical Management of Hypertension

Blood pressure is measured using a stethoscope and a device called a *sphygmomanometer.* Readings are recorded in millimeters of mercury (mm Hg). The systolic pressure—the pressure in your arteries as your heart contracts—is given first, and the diastolic pressure—the pressure when the heart is momentarily relaxed—is given second. So "125 over 70" means your systolic pressure is 125 and your diastolic is 70. Incidentally, this reading would qualify as prehypertension, even though, as you can see in **Table 13.1**, a diastolic reading of 70 is normal. In other words, if either number is elevated, the reading is considered abnormal.

Most physicians recommend that patients with hypertension follow a balanced, low-sodium diet. Sodium is an essential mineral, but if consumed in excess, it draws water out of cells and into the bloodstream. This increases the total volume of your blood and, therefore, the pressure that your blood exerts against the walls of your arteries. Sodium is bound to chloride in table salt but is also a prominent ingredient in most processed foods and fast food. The *2015–2020 Dietary Guidelines for Americans* suggests that everyone limit sodium intake to less than 2,300 mg per day.[26] People with hypertension, as well as African Americans and all Americans over age 50, should consume no more than 1,500 mg of sodium per day. To reduce your sodium intake, follow the DASH diet from the National Institutes of Health, which numerous studies have shown to reduce blood pressure.

>> Download a colorful guide to the DASH eating plan at www.nhlbi.nih.gov/health/public/heart/hbp/dash/new_dash.pdf.

In addition to eating a diet low in sodium, people with hypertension should follow a diet with an appropriate number of calories to help them achieve and maintain a healthy weight. Regular moderate exercise can also help reduce blood pressure and body weight. Smoking damages blood vessels, and anyone with hypertension who smokes should

TABLE 13.1 Blood Pressure Classification

Classification	Systolic Reading (mm Hg)		Diastolic Reading (mm Hg)
Normal	<120	and	<80
Prehypertension	120–139	or	80–89
Hypertension			
Stage 1	140–159	or	90–99
Stage 2	≥160	or	≥100

Source: Data from National Heart, Lung, and Blood Institute. (2005). *The seventh report of the Joint National Committee on Prevention, Detection, Evaluation, and Treatment of High Blood Pressure* (NIH Publication No. 03-5233). Bethesda, MD: National Institutes of Health.

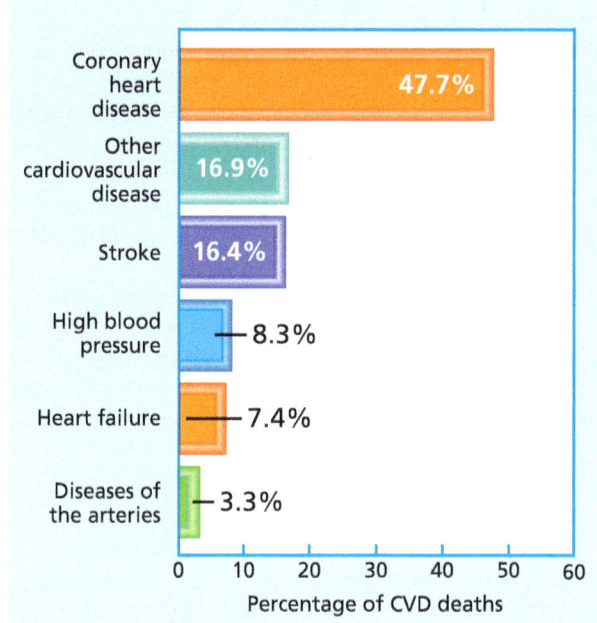

FIGURE 13.6 Deaths from Cardiovascular Disease in the United States. The majority of deaths result from coronary heart disease.

Source: Data from American Heart Association. (2015, December 16). Heart disease and stroke statistics—2016 update. *Circulation.* http://circ.ahajournals.org.

seek professional help to quit. Alcohol consumption should not exceed one drink per day for women and two drinks for men. Drinking in excess of this level raises blood pressure.[27]

Many patients with hypertension take prescription medications. Some of the most common medications are diuretics (commonly called "water pills"), which help the body eliminate sodium and water, reducing blood volume. Other medications work by helping relax and dilate blood vessels, and still others slow the heartbeat. Recently, the results of a large clinical trial found that, like patients with hypertension, patients with moderate prehypertension (average systolic pressure of 130 mm Hg) benefit from medication, as well.[28]

Coronary Heart Disease

Of all types of CVD, **coronary heart disease (CHD)** causes the most deaths; it was responsible for nearly 600,000 deaths in 2012 **(Figure 13.6)**.[24] In fact, CHD is the single leading cause of death in the United States.

Also called *coronary artery disease,* CHD arises when plaque in the coronary arteries builds up to the point that it impairs the heart's ability to function. Partial coronary artery blockages can cause *angina,* or chest pain, that occurs when the heart muscle doesn't get enough blood. Larger or even total blockages can trigger a *myocardial infarction* (heart attack) or a disruption in heart rhythm known as *sudden cardiac arrest.* We'll look at these conditions next.

> **coronary heart disease (CHD)** Disease characterized by atherosclerosis of the arteries that feed the heart, angina, and reduced blood supply to the myocardium. Also called *coronary artery disease.*

Angina

Narrowed coronary arteries can still deliver some blood to the heart—but not necessarily as much as this powerful muscle needs. Chest pain, or **angina pectoris,** occurs when the heart's need for nutrients and oxygen exceeds what the coronary arteries provide. Angina can feel like pressure or like a squeezing pain in the chest. These sensations can also radiate out to your shoulders, arms, neck, jaw, or back, and they may even resemble indigestion.

Angina itself may not be life-threatening, but it signals that a person is at significant risk of a life-threatening cardiac event. If angina isn't correctly recognized or treated, the arterial narrowing behind it may progress to a full blockage, leading to the next condition we'll discuss—heart attack.

Myocardial Infarction (Heart Attack)

An *infarct* is a region of dead tissue that develops as blockage of an artery deprives the region of its blood supply. When tissues of the myocardium die, the region stops working effectively, and the person experiences a **myocardial infarction (MI),** or *heart attack*. Each year, about 735,000 Americans have a heart attack.[2]

The more time that passes without treatment to restore blood flow, the greater the damage; thus, it's essential to know the warning signs of a heart attack. These include angina, which is a hallmark symptom in both men and women. Pressure or other discomfort in the chest or other parts of the upper body is also common, as are shortness of breath and breaking out in a cold sweat. Women are somewhat more likely than men to experience nausea, dizziness, or other less specific forms of pain and discomfort **(Figure 13.7)**.[29]

Arrhythmia and Sudden Cardiac Arrest

An **arrhythmia** is an irregularity in the heart's rhythm. The heart can beat too slowly, too quickly, or erratically. Arrhythmias have a variety of causes and can affect different aspects of the heart's function. Some are more serious than others. Millions of people in the United States live with some form of arrhythmia, and most cases are not serious.[30]

A slow heart rate of less than 60 beats per minute is called **bradycardia.** A fast heart rate—more than 100 beats per minute—is called **tachycardia.** An especially dangerous type of tachycardia is *fibrillation*. In fibrillation, an improper electrical signal causes either the atria or the ventricles to contract so quickly and unevenly that they quiver rather than pump, unable to move blood effectively. Many people live with atrial fibrillation and have no symptoms at all, or they have symptoms that are troubling but not life-threatening, such as palpitations or fainting spells. In contrast, *ventricular fibrillation* completely stops heart functioning and is a medical emergency. It is the most common type of arrhythmia seen in cases of **sudden cardiac arrest.** The person's heart must be restarted within six minutes via electrical shock to prevent

> **angina pectoris** Chest pain due to coronary heart disease.
>
> **myocardial infarction (MI)** A cardiac crisis in which a region of heart muscle is damaged or destroyed by reduced blood flow. Also known as *heart attack*.
>
> **arrhythmia** Any irregularity in the heart's rhythm.
>
> **bradycardia** A slow arrhythmia.
>
> **tachycardia** A fast arrhythmia.
>
> **sudden cardiac arrest** A life-threatening cardiac crisis marked by loss of heartbeat and unconsciousness.

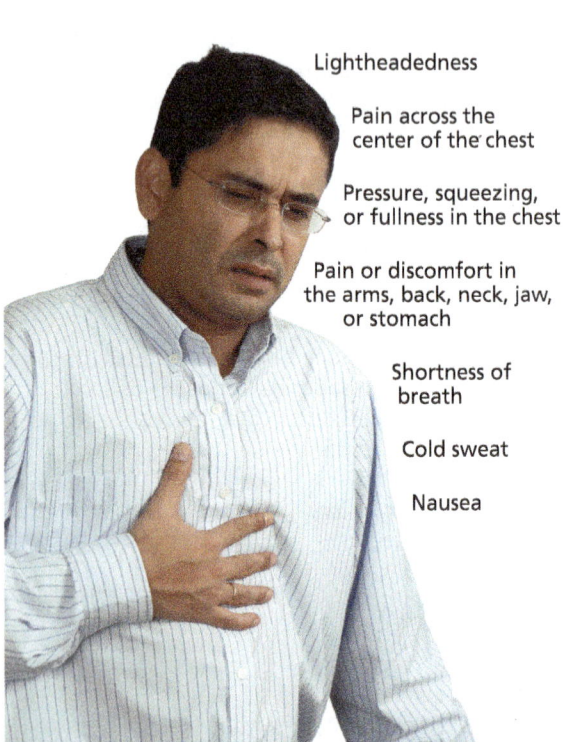

(a) Warning signs in men

Lightheadedness
Pain across the center of the chest
Pressure, squeezing, or fullness in the chest
Pain or discomfort in the arms, back, neck, jaw, or stomach
Shortness of breath
Cold sweat
Nausea

(b) Warning signs in women

Lightheadedness, dizziness, or fainting
Shortness of breath
Cold sweat
Pain or pressure across the center of the chest
Pain, pressure, squeezing, or fullness in the lower chest
Pain or discomfort in the arms, back, neck, jaw, or stomach
Abdominal pain or discomfort that can feel like indigestion
Nausea and/or vomiting
Weakness
Extreme fatigue

FIGURE 13.7 Warning Signs of a Heart Attack Differ Somewhat in Men and Women. These warning signs can occur individually, or several can occur simultaneously.

death. Even if the heart is restarted within six minutes, the patient may sustain irreversible brain damage from lack of oxygen to the brain. Each year, about 424,000 sudden cardiac arrests occur in the United States.[30]

Many factors increase the risk for arrhythmias. These include stress, smoking, genetic factors, heavy alcohol use, strenuous exercise, certain medications, and caffeine, which in high doses can disrupt electrical conduction in the heart and induce tachycardia. The U.S. Food and Drug Administration (FDA) has blamed consumption of energy drinks for at least 18 deaths due to fatal arrhythmias and other cardiovascular events, and the Center for Science in the Public Interest has linked energy drinks to at least 17 more deaths.[31]

If the heart is starved of oxygen and nutrients, electrical conduction in the heart can be affected. For this reason, an MI is a common cause of sudden cardiac arrest.[30]

Clinical Management of CHD

The diagnosis and treatment of CHD depends on the precise form it takes, so let's look at each separately.

Management of Angina. An **electrocardiogram**, also called an **ECG** (or **EKG**), measures the heart's electrical activity and is commonly used to detect arrhythmias as well as the restricted blood flow that causes angina. An ECG conducted with the patient resting provides a baseline measurement, or the test can be done while the patient is exercising. This form, called a *stress test*, shows how the heart performs under increased physical demands. An *echocardiogram* may be done during the stress test to produce images of the heart using sound waves.

Whether angina is mild or severe, lifestyle changes can help. These include weight loss, eating a healthy diet, engaging in prescribed exercise, avoiding smoking, and managing blood glucose levels. A physician might prescribe low-dose aspirin, which helps prevent blood clots and improves blood flow. You may also have heard of people with angina placing nitroglycerin tablets under their tongue or using a nitroglycerin spray: These work by dilating blood vessels. Medications may be prescribed to reduce blood cholesterol, slow the heartbeat, or relax the muscles of the blood vessel walls.

Management of an MI. When a person arrives in a hospital emergency department (ED) complaining of chest pains, the ED team typically hooks the person up to a heart monitor, administers oxygen so that the heart doesn't have to work as hard, and provides medication—typically intravenously (by IV)—to relieve the pain. A variety of tests may then be performed. A special blood test can determine if there is damage to the heart muscle indicative of an MI, and a test of the blood vessels, called *coronary angiography* (*angio-* means "vessel"), may be done to see how and where the blood is being blocked from flowing through the heart.[32]

electrocardiogram (ECG or EKG) A test that measures the heart's electrical activity.

angioplasty An arterial treatment that involves using a small balloon to flatten plaque deposits against the arterial wall.

coronary artery bypass grafting (CABG) A procedure to build new pathways for blood to flow around areas of arterial blockage.

heart failure Gradual loss of heart function.

In patients whose arteries are dangerously obstructed, procedures are available to open the arteries. **Angioplasty** involves threading a catheter through an artery and inflating a small balloon at the obstructed spot to flatten plaque against the arterial walls and open the vessel. **Coronary artery bypass grafting (CABG)** is a procedure used to circumvent a blocked vessel rather than open it. Using a healthy blood vessel from another part of the body, the surgeon creates an alternative route for blood to flow around the arterial obstruction. If more than one artery is blocked, multiple bypasses can be performed.[32]

Once the immediate crisis has been resolved, a special program of *cardiac rehabilitation* may be advised. In "cardiac rehab," patients learn to make lifestyle changes to improve their cardiovascular health. Exercise training is offered, as are counseling and support.

Management of Sudden Cardiac Arrest. In cases of sudden cardiac arrest, there is rarely time for transport to a hospital. The person's heart must be restarted within minutes with a device called an *automated external defibrillator (AED)* or the person will die. This device sends an electric shock to the heart and can restore a normal heartbeat, allowing time for transport to a medical center. Public places, including college campuses, usually have AEDs, and for obvious reasons, their location must be generally known and immediately accessible. Police, firefighters, and emergency medical technicians usually are trained and equipped to use a defibrillator.

If a person suddenly loses consciousness and fails to respond when asked if okay, tilt his or her head upright. If the person does not take a normal breath within five seconds, he or she may be experiencing a sudden cardiac arrest. If an AED is not available, the American Heart Association recommends that you call 911 and then begin hands-only CPR. The technique is simple, involving only pushing hard and fast in the center of the victim's chest until help arrives.

>> If you have two minutes to spare, you can learn hands-only CPR. Watch this video from the American Heart Association: **http://handsonlycpr.org**.

A person who survives a sudden cardiac arrest may have surgery to place an *implantable cardioverter defibrillator (ICD)*, which is similar to a pacemaker but transmits stronger electric pulses to help prevent further dangerous arrhythmias. For information on helping someone "on the scene" in a CVD emergency, see the **Special Feature** on page 333.

Heart Failure

In **heart failure,** the heart can no longer pump enough blood to meet the body's needs. As a result, blood may pool within the heart as well as in other areas of the body, such as the lungs, the abdomen, or the legs. This pooled blood quickly becomes depleted of oxygen and nutrients, so the affected regions become damaged and dysfunctional. More than 5 million Americans have heart failure.[33]

We noted earlier that the forms of CVD are interrelated, and indeed a common cause of heart failure is CHD, which damages heart muscle, reducing its ability to beat strongly. Persistent tachycardia may also cause the heart to work too hard, slowly wearing it out. In addition, hypertension, which forces the heart to work harder than it should to pump blood, is a common risk factor for heart failure, as is diabetes.[33]

A failing heart results in failing circulation. The arms and legs may swell with fluid. Pooling of fluid in the lungs may make breathing difficult. The abdomen may swell, and the person may gain "water weight." Heart failure also typically causes exhaustion, loss of appetite, and an inability to concentrate.

A low-sodium diet, smoking cessation, and maintenance of a healthful weight are all essential in slowing the progress of heart failure. A physician may prescribe diuretics and other medications to reduce the workload on the heart. Heart surgery may be necessary, either to open blocked coronary arteries or to insert a pacemaker or an ICD. However, most patients die within five years of diagnosis.[33]

Stroke

As you've learned in this chapter, a blockage in an artery that feeds the heart can cause a heart attack. What would happen if similar damage affected an artery serving the brain? The answer is a **stroke** (also called a *cerebrovascular accident* or sometimes a *brain attack*), a medical emergency in which the blood supply to a part of the brain ceases. More than 6 million Americans—2.6%—have suffered a stroke, and it is the fifth most common cause of death in the United States.[34]

Types of Stroke

Strokes can take either of two forms **(Figure 13.8)**.

Ischemic Stroke. The far more common form of stroke is **ischemic stroke,** in which either a cerebral artery or one of the carotid arteries that run through the neck into the brain becomes blocked. All brain tissues normally served by the blocked artery become starved of oxygen and nutrients.

Hemorrhagic Stroke. The term *hemorrhage* means "uncontrolled bleeding." In **hemorrhagic stroke,** a weakened cerebral artery leaks or ruptures, spilling blood into brain tissue. The blood compresses and damages the brain cells in the area of the spill; moreover, the brain regions that would normally have been served by the broken vessel are deprived of blood. In some cases, the bleeding seeps into the compartment between the brain and the skull (called the subarachnoid space). The two most common causes of hemorrhagic stroke are uncontrolled hypertension and the presence of an *aneurysm,* a weak spot in an artery wall that may rupture.

Signs and Symptoms of an Impending Stroke

Brain cells deprived of blood quickly die. Thus, a person having a stroke may suddenly feel weak, numb, or paralyzed in the arm, leg, or face, especially on one side of the body. Vision may become blurry, and speech may become slurred. A sudden and severe headache is also common and may be accompanied by dizziness or vomiting. The person may suddenly become confused or experience delusions.

Some people at risk for stroke may experience a fleeting episode of a milder version of these symptoms days, weeks, or months before having a full stroke. Such a mini-stroke, known as a **transient ischemic attack (TIA),** isn't always easy to recognize, but it is a clear warning sign of an impending stroke.

> **stroke** A medical emergency in which blood flow to or in the brain is impaired. Also called a *cerebrovascular accident* (*CVA*).
>
> **ischemic stroke** Stroke caused by a blocked blood vessel.
>
> **hemorrhagic stroke** Stroke caused by a leaking or ruptured blood vessel.
>
> **transient ischemic attack (TIA)** A temporary episode of strokelike symptoms that is indicative of high stroke risk.

Long-Term Effects of a Stroke

Prompt treatment can greatly reduce the long-term effects of a stroke. These effects include

- Paralysis, especially on one side of the body
- Impaired speaking, swallowing, and chewing
- *Aphasia,* which is difficulty understanding and expressing ideas in spoken or written words
- Loss of memory, impaired decision making, and personality changes
- Pain, cold, and other uncomfortable sensations

Rehabilitation efforts, including speech therapy and physical and occupational therapy, can help reduce some of these effects.

Clinical Management of a Stroke

Anyone showing signs of a stroke requires immediate medical attention to prevent or reduce brain damage. In an ischemic stroke, the goal of emergency treatment is to open the blocked cerebral artery and restore blood flow to that area of the brain. Believe it or not, aspirin, which impedes blood clotting, is the best-proven immediate treatment for ischemic stroke. The patient may be given an injection of a clot-busting drug, or the physician may

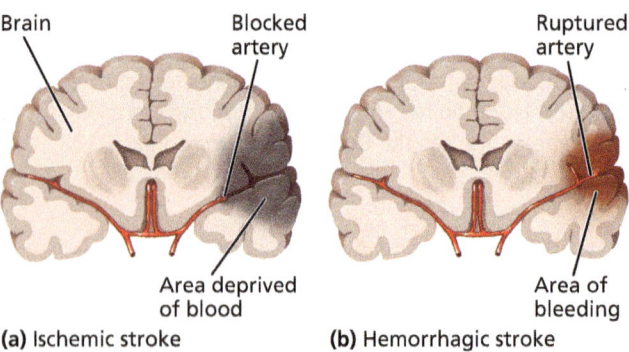

(a) Ischemic stroke   **(b)** Hemorrhagic stroke

FIGURE 13.8 **Two Types of Stroke.** (a) In an ischemic stroke, a blocked artery damages brain tissue by depriving it of blood. (b) In a hemorrhagic stroke, a weakened artery leaks or ruptures, releasing blood into and damaging the brain tissue as well as depriving brain cells beyond the rupture.

SPECIAL FEATURE

Helping Someone in a CVD Emergency

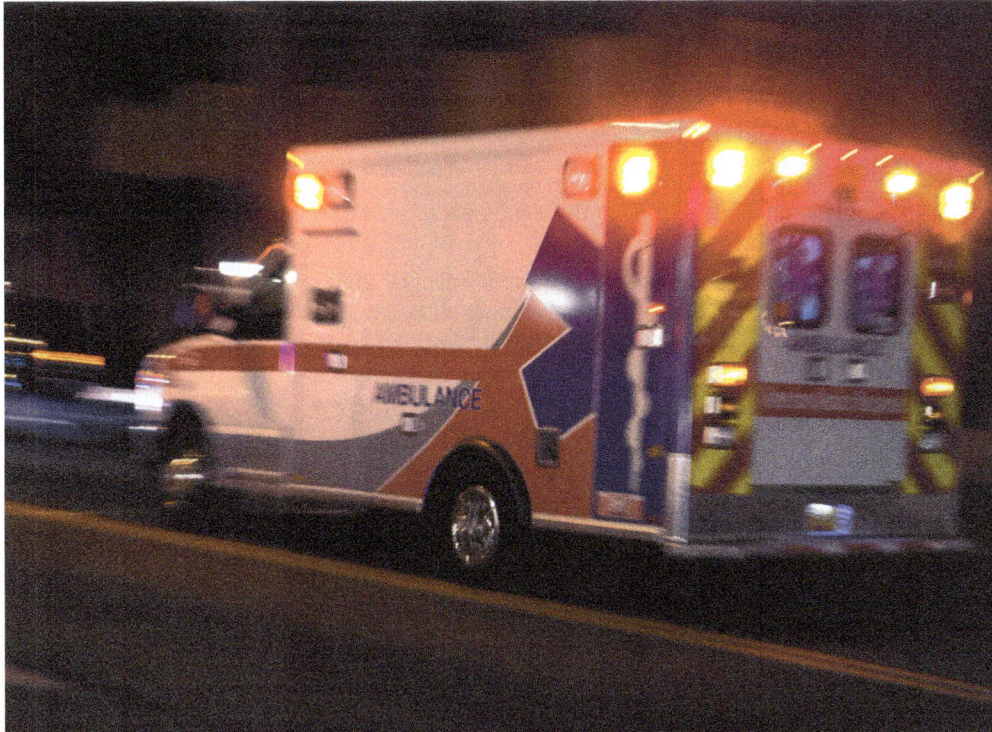

We all know that someone showing signs of a heart attack, sudden cardiac arrest, or stroke needs to head for the nearest hospital. But before the person is under medical care, you can take steps to help:

- If you see someone showing the signs of a heart attack, cardiac arrest, or stroke, the first thing you should do is call 911. If possible, make this call from a land line, not a cell phone. Land line calls to 911 are usually routed straight to local emergency dispatch centers, whereas calls from cell phones are often routed to local highway safety agencies, which must then reroute the call to the correct dispatch center, sometimes costing valuable time.
- Once you call 911, wait with the person until emergency medical services arrive rather than driving to the hospital yourself. Paramedic and ambulance units have life-saving equipment and skills that they can deploy immediately and sustain during the trip to the hospital. If you drive the person to the hospital, he or she can't benefit from this faster access to medical help.

In addition, here are ways you can help in specific types of emergencies:

Heart Attack

- Although the symptoms of a heart attack aren't always clear-cut, don't hesitate to call 911 if you suspect one is occurring. Trying a "wait and see" approach could cost the person's life.
- Have the person chew an aspirin, unless he or she is allergic to aspirin or is under medical orders to avoid it. Aspirin has blood-thinning properties that can help in a heart attack. The drug used must be aspirin, not another type of pain reliever.
- Have the person take nitroglycerin if already prescribed. This drug is often used in people with CVD.
- If the person falls unconscious, begin hands-only CPR. If you don't know how, ask the dispatcher to instruct you on the proper technique until help arrives.

Sudden Cardiac Arrest

- If you suspect cardiac arrest, call 911 immediately. People in cardiac arrest need their heart restarted within six minutes, or they will die.
- Check the unconscious person for a pulse *after* you call 911. The side of the neck is a more reliable place to feel for a pulse than the wrist.
- If you don't find a pulse, begin hands-only CPR. If you need help, the 911 dispatcher will instruct you on the proper technique until help arrives.
- If you are in a public place such as a campus or office building, an airport, or a shopping mall, ask someone nearby to look for a device called an *automated external defibrillator*, or AED. AEDs are electrical heart-starting machines, and they are designed for anyone to use. Just open the box and follow the instructions. Don't worry about shocking someone unnecessarily—AEDs are designed to scan for a heartbeat and not deliver a shock if a heartbeat is detected.

Stroke

- The classic signs of a stroke are face drooping, arm weakness, and slurred speech. If you suspect a stroke, call 911 immediately. The faster medical help arrives, the more likely it is that permanent brain damage can be avoided.
- Make note of the time you first noticed the symptoms. This information is vital for paramedics and doctors trying to provide treatment as fast as possible.
- While you wait for help, don't administer cardiac aid such as hands-only CPR unless the person goes into cardiac arrest. A person having a stroke may be disoriented or have trouble moving, but CPR should be reserved for people who are unconscious and have no pulse. Otherwise, it could be harmful.

Sources: Mayo Clinic. (2015). *Cardiopulmonary resuscitation (CPR): First aid.* www.mayoclinic.org; Medline Plus. (2014). *Heart attack first aid.* www.nlm.nih.gov; National Heart, Lung, and Blood Institute. (2011). *How to use an automated external defibrillator.* www.nhlbi.nih.gov; American Stroke Association. (2016). *Stroke warning signs and symptoms.* www.strokeassociation.org.

be able to thread a device into the brain that can grab and remove the clot.[35]

In a hemorrhagic stroke, aspirin is never given because it promotes bleeding. Instead, drugs are used to reduce the force of blood moving into the damaged area, to help control the bleeding, and to prevent seizures. Surgery can sometimes repair or isolate the ruptured vessel.[35]

Once a stroke patient is stabilized, rehabilitation can begin. This often requires admission to a special facility, where the patient works with a neurologist and speech and physical therapists.

Other Forms of Cardiovascular Disease

Less common types of CVD in the United States include the following:

- **Congenital heart disease.** About 8 in every 1,000 babies are born with some type of heart defect.[36] Some of the most frequently occurring defects include holes in the walls that divide the chambers of the heart, abnormal narrowing of the coronary arteries, and malformations of the arteries that connect the heart and lungs. Most congenital heart defects can be treated with drugs or surgery.
- **Heart valve disorders.** Blood flows through your heart in only one direction, from atrium to ventricle, because the chambers of your heart are gated with valves. These flaps of connective tissue swing open and shut like one-way doors, allowing blood to pass from atrium to ventricle but preventing it from pooling or streaming backward. Congenital defects, infections, or heart disease can damage the valves. In some cases, a valve may let too little blood pass. In other cases, a valve may leak. Medications can ease some valve problems, whereas more serious malfunctions may require surgical repair.
- **Hypertrophic cardiomyopathy.** About 1 in every 500 Americans has hypertrophic cardiomyopathy (HCM), a genetic disorder that results in a thick, stiffened muscle wall that cannot pump enough blood during vigorous activity.[37] Children with HCM are not allowed to play competitive sports because HCM can cause sudden cardiac arrest in an athlete.
- **Rheumatic heart disease.** A potentially fatal condition, rheumatic heart disease begins when a bacterial infection—caused by the same *Streptococcus* bacterium that causes strep throat—flares into rheumatic fever. Along with an elevated temperature, the illness causes inflammation of connective tissues throughout the body. Sometimes that damage includes the heart valves. Rheumatic heart disease is easily prevented by taking antibiotics in the early stages of a strep infection.

Risk Factors for Cardiovascular Disease

This section identifies the risk factors for CVD. We've encountered many of them already in our discussion of type 2 diabetes. And as we'll see shortly, several of them are defining factors in cardiometabolic risk:

- **Your age.** Most cases of heart attack, sudden cardiac arrest, and stroke occur in people older than 65. You can't stop yourself from aging, but you can work to make sure every year of life is as healthy as possible.
- **Your sex.** Men face greater heart attack risks than women, and they tend to have heart attacks earlier in life. However, CVD is still the top killer of women in the United States over the course of their lifetime, so women need to pay attention to CVD risks as well.
- **Your genetic inheritance.** Children of parents with CVD are more likely to develop the condition. Race is also a risk factor. (See the **Diversity & Health** box on page 322.) But inheritance isn't destiny. By reducing the CVD risks you can control, you can help make sure that your genes don't equal your fate.
- **Your blood pressure.** Have your blood pressure measured regularly. If your reading is 120 over 80 or higher, discuss your options with your primary care provider.
- **Your blood lipids.** Abnormal levels of various lipids circulating in your bloodstream, a condition known as **dyslipidemia,** puts the health of your heart and blood vessels at risk. A simple blood test can give you a variety of data about your blood lipid levels (**Table 13.2**). These include your total cholesterol score, the level of triglycerides circulating in your bloodstream, and your readings for two cholesterol-carrying protein compounds:
    - **LDL,** short for **low-density lipoprotein,** is a molecule that packs a lot of cholesterol with very little protein. It's often dubbed "bad" cholesterol because excess LDLs degrade over time, releasing their cholesterol load into your bloodstream, where it can become trapped in injured blood vessels. A high LDL score means there's a lot of cholesterol "littering" your bloodstream, so it increases your risk for CVD.
    - **HDL,** an abbreviation of **high-density lipoprotein,** is half protein with little cholesterol. It's often called "good" cholesterol because it picks up free cholesterol in the bloodstream and transports it to your liver for recycling. You can think of HDL as your arteries' "housekeeper." A high HDL score means a lower risk for CVD.

Some people with dyslipidemia may be prescribed medications called *statins*, which reduce the liver's ability to synthesize cholesterol, thereby reducing its level in the blood.

- **Your blood glucose.** A blood glucose level of 110 mg/dL or higher increases your risk for CVD. Notice that 110 is considered prediabetes; thus, even a modestly elevated blood glucose level increases your CVD risk.
- **Inflammatory markers.** As noted earlier, inflammation plays a key role in diabetes, CVD (specifically

> **dyslipidemia** A disorder characterized by abnormal levels of blood lipids, such as high LDL cholesterol or low HDL cholesterol.
>
> **low-density lipoprotein (LDL)** A cholesterol-containing compound that, as it degrades, releases its cholesterol load into the bloodstream; often referred to as "bad cholesterol."
>
> **high-density lipoprotein (HDL)** A cholesterol-containing compound that removes excess cholesterol from the bloodstream; often referred to as "good cholesterol."

TABLE 13.2 Classification of Blood Lipid Levels for Adults

LDL Cholesterol	Classification
<100	Optimal
100–129	Near optimal/above optimal
130–159	Borderline high
160–189	High
≥190	Very high

HDL Cholesterol	Classification
<40	Low
≥60	Optimal

Total Cholesterol	Classification
<200	Desirable
200–239	Borderline high
≥240	High

Triglycerides	Classification
<150	Normal
150–199	Borderline high
200–499	High
≥500	Very high

Source: Data from National Heart, Lung, and Blood Institute. (2005). *Third report of the Expert Panel on Detection, Evaluation, and Treatment of High Blood Cholesterol in Adults* (NIH Publication No. 05-3290). Bethesda, MD: National Institutes of Health.

---

atherosclerosis), and cancer. Physicians can detect inflammation in the body by measuring your blood level of a protein—called *C-reactive protein (CRP)*—which is produced by the liver during an inflammatory response. A high level of CRP (above 3.0 mg/L) indicates that inflammation is going on somewhere in the body, but not necessarily in the blood vessels. It's not likely that a physician would order a CRP test unless you had other significant risk factors, such as hypertension and dyslipidemia.

- **Homocysteine.** The amino acid homocysteine can only be metabolized by the body when we consume adequate amounts of the B vitamins folate, B_6, and B_{12}. High levels of homocysteine in the blood are associated with an increased risk of MI and stroke.
- **Your weight.** Obesity increases the risk for CVD and death from CVD. Several factors explain the link between obesity and CVD:[38]
  - Obesity increases the total volume of blood circulating in the body as well as the total metabolic demand of body cells. Therefore, the cardiac workload is greater.
  - The heart can grow excessively large in obese people, increasing the risk for ventricular dysfunction.
  - Fat cells can infiltrate and replace heart muscle, disturbing regions such as the sinus node, where the heart's electrical impulses are generated.
  - Fat cells—especially those stored in abdominal fat—manufacture and release into the bloodstream a variety of inflammatory chemicals and signaling molecules that can disrupt normal body functions. A recent study found that normal-weight men with abdominal obesity had more than twice the risk of cardiovascular death or death from any cause compared to men who were overweight or obese overall but did not have abdominal obesity. The risk for women with abdominal obesity was 48% increased.[39]
- **Your diet.** The association between a high intake of saturated fats and CVD risk is currently the subject of debate. In contrast, researchers agree that diets high in added sugars are uniquely harmful to cardiovascular health. That's because they promote many abnormalities linked to CVD, including insulin resistance, increased blood levels of LDLs and reduced HDLs, and abnormal blood platelet functions.[40] Thus, it's no wonder that a recent global assessment of the role of sugar-sweetened beverages (SSBs) in mortality rates estimated that, in a single year, 184,000 deaths worldwide were attributable to consumption of SSBs. The majority of these deaths were due to diabetes and CVD.[41]
- **Your level of physical activity.** Inactivity is a risk factor for CVD.[42] Regular exercise reduces blood glucose, increases HDL cholesterol, combats atherosclerosis, strengthens the heart muscle, and expends calories, helping you to maintain a healthful body weight.
- **Smoking.** Nicotine constricts the blood vessels, and carbon monoxide damages their walls, increasing their susceptibility to atherosclerosis. Smoking also increases blood pressure, increases the tendency for blood to clot, and decreases HDL cholesterol.
- **Alcohol intake.** As noted earlier, excessive alcohol consumption is associated with hypertension. In contrast, moderate alcohol consumption (no more than one drink per day for women and two drinks per day for men) is thought to offer some protection from CVD. Moderate alcohol intake appears to increase blood levels of "good" HDL cholesterol and decrease "bad" LDL cholesterol. It also reduces the risk of abnormal clot formation in the blood vessels.[43]
- **Drug abuse.** Researchers have found a connection between the abuse of prescription and illicit drugs and adverse cardiovascular effects, ranging from abnormal heart rate to heart attacks. For example, prescription stimulants can cause an irregular heartbeat and sudden heart failure, and marijuana increases blood pressure, quadrupling the risk of a heart attack within the first hour after use.[44]
- **Your level of stress.** A high level of stress can raise your CVD risk.[42] Chronically elevated blood levels of the stress hormone cortisol are associated with an increased risk for CVD and death from CVD, as well as reduced survival in patients following a heart attack.[45] Researchers speculate that these increased risks might be due in part to how some people deal with stress—such as by overeating, smoking, or drinking too much alcohol.
- **Your sleep.** Short sleep duration and poor-quality sleep increase your CVD risk in part by contributing to inflammation and hypertension.[46] Studies have also shown that lack of adequate sleep causes changes in the lining of blood vessels associated with atherosclerosis.[47]

SELF-ASSESSMENT
What's Your Risk for a Heart Attack?

Circle your answers.

1. Do you smoke?
   Yes   No

2. Is your blood pressure 140/90 mm Hg or higher OR have you been told by your doctor that your blood pressure is too high?
   Yes   No   Don't Know

3. Has your doctor told you that your LDL cholesterol is too high OR that your total cholesterol level is 200 mg/dL or higher OR that your HDL cholesterol is less than 40 mg/dL?
   Yes   No   Don't Know

4. Has your father or brother had a heart attack before age 55 OR has your mother or sister had one before age 65?
   Yes   No   Don't Know

5. Are you over 55 years old?
   Yes   No

6. Do you have a BMI of 25 or more? (See Figure 7.1 on page 157.)
   Yes   No   Don't Know

7. Do you get less than a total of 30 minutes of moderate-intensity physical activity on most days?
   Yes   No   Not Sure

8. Has a doctor told you that you have angina (chest pains) OR have you had a heart attack?
   Yes   No   Don't Know

HOW TO INTERPRET YOUR SCORE If you circled any of the "Yes" answers, you're at increased risk of having a heart attack. If you circled "Don't Know" for any questions, ask your doctor for help in answering them.

To complete this Self-Assessment online, visit **MasteringHealth**™

Source: Adapted from *The healthy heart handbook for women*, NIH Publication No. 07-2720, by the U.S. Department of Health and Human Services, National Heart, Lung, and Blood Institute (NHLBI), National Institutes of Health (NIH), 2007.

- **Your income.** Research shows that lower-income adults have an increased rate of CVD. (See the **Diversity & Health box** on page 322.)

▶▶ What's your risk for a heart attack or stroke? Complete the Self-Assessment or visit www.heart.org/gglRisk/locale/en_US/index.html?gtype=health.

LO 13.3 QUICK CHECK

A diet high in added sugars
a. increases blood levels of LDLs.
b. increases blood levels of HDLs.
c. reduces insulin resistance.
d. reduces atherosclerosis.

Cardiometabolic Risk

LO 13.4 List nine factors associated with cardiometabolic risk.

Now that you've learned about diabetes and CVD, you're ready to tackle a concept that has recently emerged as a critical public health concern: cardiometabolic risk. For decades, researchers have noted that abdominal obesity and insulin resistance together promote a variety of serious metabolic abnormalities. They use the term **metabolic syndrome** to refer to this cluster of abnormalities, which includes, for example, high fasting blood glucose and low HDL cholesterol. More recently, researchers have come to recognize that these abnormalities increase a person's risk not only for type 2 diabetes but also for CVD. As a result, many public health groups have expanded the concept of metabolic syndrome to include the risk factors traditionally associated with CVD, such as smoking. Their name for this expanded concept is cardiometabolic risk.[48]

In 2009, the Agency for Healthcare Research and Quality (AHRQ, part of the Department of Health and Human Services) published lengthy guidelines defining **cardiometabolic risk (CMR)** as a cluster of modifiable factors that identify individuals at increased risk for type 2 diabetes mellitus and cardiovascular disease.[49] CMR includes all five of the factors that make up the definition of metabolic syndrome, plus four additional factors. These are identified in **Figure 13.9**. All nine factors should be familiar to you, as we've discussed them all earlier in this chapter.

The first factor listed—abdominal obesity—is particularly dangerous. In fact, the International Chair on Cardiometabolic Risk refers to abdominal obesity as a "warning sign" of four underlying conditions linked to diabetes and CVD:[50]

- Elevated blood glucose and insulin resistance
- Blood lipid abnormalities—including high levels of "dense" LDL particles—strongly associated with atherosclerosis
- Increased tendency to form clots in the blood
- Inflammation

The AHRQ recommends that all males have an initial CMR screening at age 35 and females at age 45. If you have a waist circumference greater than 40 inches for males or 35 inches for females, or if you have already been diagnosed

metabolic syndrome A set of five unhealthy physical and metabolic conditions that are together linked to an increased risk for type 2 diabetes and other metabolic disease.

cardiometabolic risk (CMR) A cluster of nine modifiable factors that identify individuals at risk for type 2 diabetes and cardiovascular disease.

Cardiometabolic risk

Metabolic syndrome:
- Abdominal obesity (a waist circumference ≥ 40 inches for males and 35 inches for females)
- Elevated blood pressure (≥ 130/85 mm Hg)
- Elevated fasting blood glucose (≥ 110 mg/dL)
- Elevated blood triglycerides (> 150)
- Low HDL cholesterol (< 40)
- High LDL cholesterol (≥ 130)
- Smoking
- Inflammatory markers (notably CRP)
- Insulin resistance

FIGURE 13.9 **Cardiometabolic Risk.** These nine factors dramatically increase your risk of developing type 2 diabetes and cardiovascular disease.

with type 2 diabetes, hypertension, or dyslipidemia, you should have a CMR screening immediately and then annually. In addition, because depression is frequently associated with diabetes, you can anticipate that, if your physician determines that your CMR is high, he or she is also likely to screen you for depression.[51]

When college students are screened for CMR, studies show that one or more of the nine factors are already present in a significant percentage. For example, a 2012 study involving nearly 3,000 students found that 77% of males and 54% of females already had at least one risk factor, and nearly 10% of males and 3% of females met all five criteria for metabolic syndrome.[52] A 2014 assessment of college students on three U.S. campuses yielded similar findings: 12% of males and 6% of females met all criteria for metabolic syndrome.[53]

Individuals found to be at high CMR have a variety of clinical treatment options. However, lifestyle measures—discussed shortly—are essential.

LO 13.4 QUICK CHECK

Your cardiometabolic risk is your relative risk for
a. metabolic syndrome.
b. type 2 diabetes mellitus and cardiovascular disease.
c. abdominal obesity and atherosclerosis.
d. premature death.

Cancer

LO 13.5 Describe the initiation and progression of cancer and the most common types of cancer.

Few diseases evoke more fear than cancer. But recent developments in our understanding of cancer can also evoke another emotion—hope. Our ability to detect and treat cancer is improving rapidly, as is our understanding of how to prevent it.

To be sure, cancer remains a health priority for good reason. In a given year, about 1.7 million new cases of cancer will be diagnosed in the United States, and more than 595,000 people will die from the disease.[54] Cancer is the second most common cause of death in the United States. Statistics on cancer cases and deaths by body site are illustrated in **Table 13.3**.

Despite these disturbing figures, more people are surviving cancer than ever before. The 5-year survival rate for cancer is now 69%, up from 49% 35 years ago.[54] However,

TABLE 13.3 Leading Sites of Cancer Incidence/Deaths, 2016 Estimates

Estimated New Cases		Estimated Deaths	
Site	Incidence (% of all cases)	Site	Mortality (% of all cases)
Male		**Male**	
Prostate	180,890 (21%)	Lung and bronchus	85,920 (27%)
Lung and bronchus	117,920 (14%)	Prostate	26,120 (8%)
Colon and rectum	70,820 (8%)	Colon and rectum	26,020 (8%)
Urinary bladder	58,950 (7%)	Pancreas	21,450 (7%)
Melanoma of the skin	46,870 (6%)	Liver and intrahepatic bile duct	18,280 (6%)
Non-Hodgkin lymphoma	40,170 (5%)	Leukemia	14,130 (4%)
Kidney and renal pelvis	39,650 (5%)	Esophagus	12,720 (4%)
Oral cavity and pharynx	34,780 (4%)	Urinary bladder	11,820 (4%)
Leukemia	34,090 (4%)	Non-Hodgkin lymphoma	11,520 (4%)
Liver and intrahepatic bile duct	28,410 (3%)	Brain and other nervous system	9,440 (3%)
All sites	841,390 (100%)	All sites	314,290 (100%)
Female		**Female**	
Breast	246,660 (29%)	Lung and bronchus	72,160 (26%)
Lung and bronchus	106,470 (13%)	Breast	40,450 (14%)
Colon and rectum	63,670 (8%)	Colon and rectum	23,170 (8%)
Uterine corpus	60,050 (7%)	Pancreas	20,330 (7%)
Thyroid	49,350 (6%)	Ovary	14,240 (5%)
Non-Hodgkin lymphoma	32,410 (4%)	Uterine corpus	10,470 (4%)
Melanoma of the skin	29,510 (3%)	Leukemia	10,270 (4%)
Leukemia	26,050 (3%)	Liver and intrahepatic bile duct	8,890 (3%)
Pancreas	25,400 (3%)	Non-Hodgkin lymphoma	8,630 (3%)
Kidney and renal pelvis	23,050 (3%)	Brain and other nervous system	6,610 (2%)
All sites	843,820 (100%)	All sites	281,400 (100%)

Source: Data from American Cancer Society. (2016). *Cancer facts & figures 2016*. www.cancer.org.

significant health disparities persist, especially for African Americans, who are more likely to die of cancer than any other ethnic group.[54] Eliminating this disparity is a key focus of national cancer prevention efforts.

To reduce your own risk for cancer, it helps to have a basic understanding of how the disease arises and—in some cases—spreads. You'll also need to know about risk factors, early detection, and warning signs to watch for. After that, we'll provide a quick look at some common cancers and discuss treatment—and survival.

What Is Cancer?

Cancer is a group of diseases characterized by uncontrolled reproduction of abnormal cells and, in some cases, the spread of these cells to other sites in the body. These cells often don't start as abnormal, but for a variety of reasons, they undergo changes in their operating instructions that turn them into rogue agents of abnormal growth.

Understanding how this happens starts with a look at the body's genetic material, *DNA*. The structures and functions of just about every cell in the body are controlled by DNA because genes—precise segments of the DNA molecule—tell the cell which proteins to build and how to build them.

Genes can be damaged by a variety of external hazards. These include the toxins in tobacco and tobacco smoke, alcohol, many chemicals used in industry, radiation (including from sunlight and tanning beds), and even certain viruses.[55] When we come into contact with such agents—whether by absorbing them via our skin or breathing or ingesting them—they can cause dangerous *mutations*, or DNA changes, that can lead to cancer. These cancer-generating agents are known as **carcinogens**. Our body's defenses seek out cells with such mutations and repair the damage, cause the cells to self-destruct, or kill them. But some mutations are more severe than the body can fix, or the encounter with the carcinogen is so frequent that the body's defenses become overwhelmed. And, in some people, other features of their DNA actually diminish their body's ability to protect and repair its cells.

Two types of genes are important in the development of cancer. In a normal, healthy person, *proto-oncogenes* enable cells to grow and divide, ensuring that the body's tissues are as vital as possible. For instance, the cells lining your digestive tract are replaced every few days, and your skin cells are continually being shed and replaced. If you're injured, the cell replacement process speeds up to help you heal. Proto-oncogenes normally operate a bit like the accelerator and brakes on a car. If you need lots of new cells quickly, they accelerate their production. Once enough new cells are in place, the same genes slow the process back down to normal.

As you can imagine, if DNA mutations damage these genes, they will no longer be able to regulate cell reproduction appropriately. They will become cancer-causing **oncogenes,** issuing faulty orders for accelerated cell growth. As cells begin reproducing out of control, they form clusters of immature cells that serve no purpose. Their only function is to keep multiplying. Such clusters of cells eventually form clumps of abnormal tissue called **tumors.**

Tumor-suppressor genes are the second type of genes that have a significant role in cancer. These helpful genes slow tumor growth, repair DNA, or instruct old or damaged cells to self-destruct. These mechanisms protect against cancer. In people with mutated or weak tumor-suppressor genes, however, tumors can quickly grow out of control.

Not all tumors are cancerous. **Benign tumors** grow very slowly, do not invade surrounding tissues, and do not spread to other parts of the body. In contrast, **malignant tumors** are by definition cancerous **(Figure 13.10)**. They invade surrounding tissue, and frequently their cells break away and enter the bloodstream or lymphatic system, where they circulate and find new places to take root. This aggressive spreading process, called **metastasis,** makes treating the cancer far more challenging.

> **cancer** A group of diseases marked by the uncontrolled multiplication of abnormal cells.
>
> **carcinogen** A substance known to trigger DNA mutations that can lead to cancer.
>
> **oncogene** A mutated gene that encourages the uncontrolled cell division that results in cancer.
>
> **tumor** A mass of abnormal tissue made up of cells with no physiological function.
>
> **benign tumor** A tumor that grows slowly, does not spread, and is not cancerous.
>
> **malignant tumor** A tumor that grows aggressively, invades surrounding tissue, and can spread to other parts of the body; all cancers are malignant.
>
> **metastasis** The process by which a malignant tumor spreads to other body sites.

It's important to note that, whereas cancer can spread throughout the body, it cannot be spread from person to person. Although certain cancer-associated viruses, such as HIV or hepatitis, are contagious, cancer itself is not.

Risk Factors for Cancer

Given the complex series of interactions involved in cancer, it's no surprise that many different factors can influence cancer risk. These include genetic and biological factors, lifestyle factors, environmental exposure to carcinogens, and exposure to infectious agents. To get a sense of your level of risk, complete the **Self-Assessment**.

Genetic and Biological Factors

As you've learned, cancer is fundamentally a disease of the DNA. It involves not only the genes that become damaged in cancer but other genes involved in preventing this damage.

Some types of cancer run in families or are more common in certain ethnic groups. These include breast, ovarian, colon, prostate, stomach, skin, and lung cancers. But researchers are learning that these cancers are rarely due to a "cancer-causing gene." Instead, in many cases, such as with breast and ovarian cancer, the inherited risk is more closely linked to weaker versions of tumor-suppressor genes.[56] Again, cells with DNA mutations are more likely to multiply and lead to tumors in people who inherit weak tumor-suppressor genes.

Cancer can also be related to biological factors, such as the body's hormones. This is especially true for women. The age at which a woman had her first period and entered

SELF-ASSESSMENT
What's Your Risk for Cancer?

Next to each statement, check the answer that applies to you.

1. I eat a variety of vegetables, fruits, and whole grains every day.
   Always ☐   Sometimes ☐   Never ☐

2. If I eat red meat, I choose lean cuts and eat small portions.
   Always ☐   Sometimes ☐   Never ☐

3. I prepare meat, poultry, and fish by baking, broiling, or poaching rather than by frying, barbecuing, or grilling over a flame.
   Always ☐   Sometimes ☐   Never ☐

4. I limit my intake of processed meats, such as bacon, ham, deli meats, and hot dogs.
   Always ☐   Sometimes ☐   Never ☐

5. I get at least 150 minutes of moderate-intensity or 75 minutes of vigorous-intensity activity each week (or a combination of these), preferably spread throughout the week.
   Always ☐   Sometimes ☐   Never ☐

6. I limit sedentary behavior such as sitting, watching TV, and other screen-based entertainment.
   Always ☐   Sometimes ☐   Never ☐

7. I have maintained a healthy weight at all ages.
   Always ☐   Sometimes ☐   Never ☐

8. I avoid tobacco in all its forms.
   Always ☐   Sometimes ☐   Never ☐

9. I drink no more than one drink a day if I'm a woman or two drinks a day if I'm a man.
   Always ☐   Sometimes ☐   Never ☐

10. I avoid intense sunlight, or when in the sun, I wear protective clothing and a UVA and UVB sunscreen.
    Always ☐   Sometimes ☐   Never ☐

11. I am not exposed to environmental carcinogens (chemicals, radiation, airborne particles, air pollution, secondhand smoke, or pesticides) through work or at home.
    Always ☐   Sometimes ☐   Never ☐

12. I have access to quality health care and receive regular examinations by a health-care provider.
    Always ☐   Sometimes ☐   Never ☐

13. If I am a woman, I have been vaccinated against HPV.
    Yes ☐   No ☐

14. I have never been sexually active or I have always practiced safer sex to avoid exposure to STIs that can promote cancer.
    Yes ☐   No ☐

Totals: ___Always ___Sometimes ___Never ___Yes ___No

HOW TO INTERPRET YOUR SCORE For questions 1–12, the more "Always" responses, the better. For questions 13–14, each "No" answer increases your risk. Focus on improving the behaviors for which you selected "No," "Never," or "Sometimes." Those answers indicate that these are factors that can contribute to your risk of cancer. The **Choosing to Change Worksheet** at the end of the chapter will assist you in improving these areas.

To complete this Self-Assessment online, visit MasteringHealth™

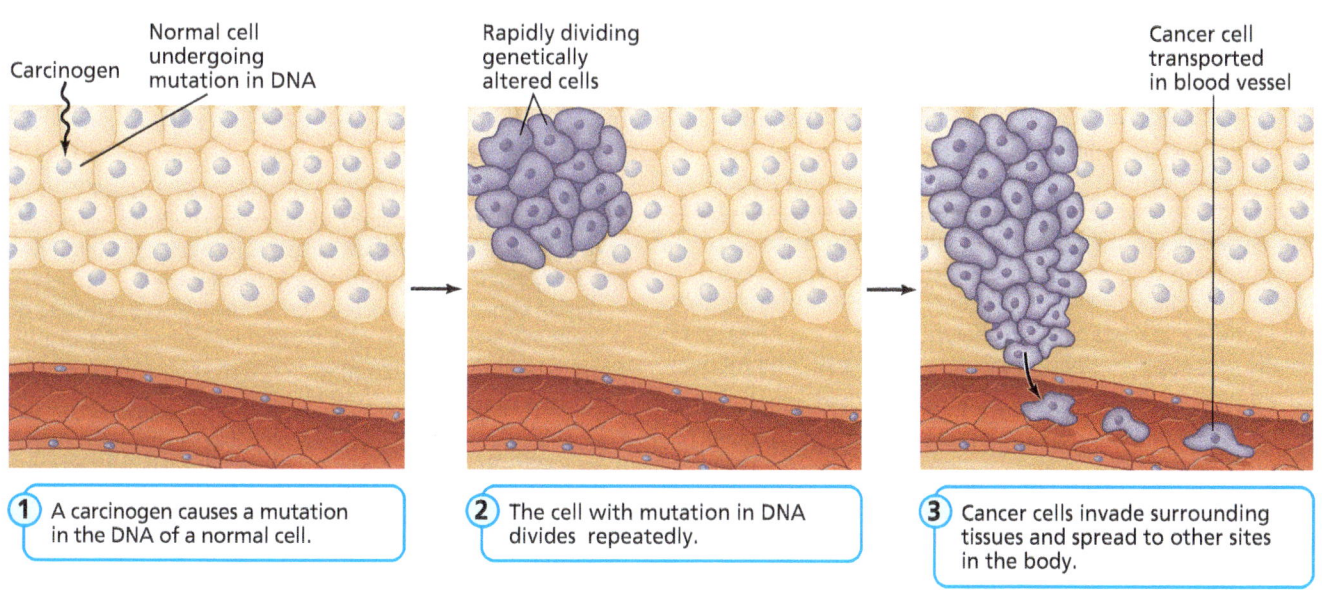

1. A carcinogen causes a mutation in the DNA of a normal cell.
2. The cell with mutation in DNA divides repeatedly.
3. Cancer cells invade surrounding tissues and spread to other sites in the body.

FIGURE 13.10 **Progression of Cancer.**
Source: From Thompson, J., Manore, M. & Vaughan, L. (2017). *The science of nutrition*, 4th ed., p. 405. © 2017. Reprinted and electronically reproduced by permission of Pearson Education, Inc., Upper Saddle River, NJ.

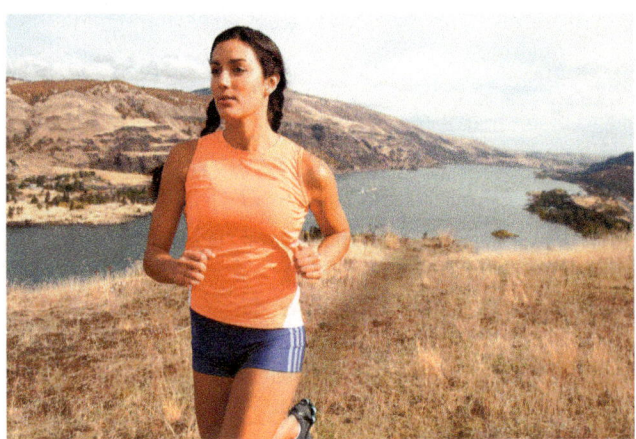

Regular exercise lowers your risk of cancer.

menopause, along with whether she used hormonal birth control, or had children (and if so, at what age) all factor into her risk for breast cancer.

Lifestyle Factors

How often do you exercise? Are your BMI and waist size within a healthful range? Do you smoke or spend time with someone who does? Do you drink alcohol, and if so, how much? The same basic lifestyle choices that are important in CMR also affect your risk of cancer. We identify healthy lifestyle choices later in this chapter.

Environmental Exposure to Carcinogens

Do you like to tan? Do you have a job that involves working with chemicals or radiation, or do you live in an area with high levels of air pollution? If so, you may be exposing your body—and your DNA—to carcinogens on a regular basis. Some of these risks are a matter of personal choice and are easier to control. For instance, you can opt to avoid sunbathing or visiting the tanning salon. But reducing your exposure to carcinogens in your workplace or neighborhood can be more challenging.

Many jobs involve working with chemicals or radiation, or produce airborne particles, such as wood dust from sanding, that are known carcinogens. Be sure you are aware of all safety procedures used at your workplace and follow them. State and federal laws lay out clear occupational safety requirements that companies must follow. If you devise your own summer job that requires you to work with chemicals—for instance, house painting, house cleaning, or landscaping—research the appropriate safety measures, such as wearing gloves and a mask, and follow them!

>> How safe is the environment at your summer job? Visit **www.osha.gov/SLTC/youth/summerjobs**.

If you live in an area known for air pollution, you can start reducing your risks by paying attention to public service announcements identifying days when pollution levels are especially high and avoiding outdoor exercise during those times. If pollutants from nearby industry or a landfill or other waste site are a concern, or if the safety of your public water supply is uncertain, consider getting involved in public pollution-reduction efforts. Many communities have environmental and health advocacy groups dedicated to reducing air, water, and land pollution.

Exposure to Infectious Agents

Certain infectious microorganisms are known carcinogens. Researchers theorize that they trigger cancer by causing persistent inflammation, suppressing a person's immune system, or stimulating cells into extended periods of growth. In the United States, some of the more common cancer-causing infectious agents include the following microbes:[55]

- **Helicobacter pylori.** Infection with this bacterium increases the risk for stomach cancer.
- **Hepatitis B and C.** These forms of the hepatitis virus can lead to liver cancer.
- **HIV.** The human immunodeficiency virus (HIV) suppresses the immune system, which can lead to certain types of cancer that are otherwise rare. These are called *opportunistic* cancers because they occur when reduced immune defenses give them the opportunity to develop.
- **HPV.** The human papillomavirus (HPV) is usually transmitted through sexual contact. Nearly all women with cervical cancer have evidence of HPV, although not all cervical HPV infections turn into cancer. A vaccine is now available that increases immunity against certain strains of HPV associated with cervical cancer. HPV is also linked to a rise in cases of throat cancer, most likely due to transmission during oral sex.

Detecting Cancer

Because cancer can occur in sites as varied as lungs, bones, and blood, no single test can detect all cancers. But an increasing variety of detection methods are allowing more cancers to be caught earlier, when they are easier to treat.

Some types of cancer can be found even before they cause any symptoms. Tests that screen large numbers of people to check for the presence of disease or conditions associated with disease are called *screening tests*. For instance, a colonoscopy is an examination of the colon (the large intestine) with a tiny camera. It allows a physician to find and remove precancerous growths called *polyps*. Screening tests are also used for many other types of cancer. Methods under development include screening tests that could analyze body fluids for signs of cancer-related DNA.

When cancer is suspected, either following the results of a screening test or because a patient has detected a suspicious mass, the physician may perform a **biopsy,** removing a small sample of the abnormal growth so that it can be studied for signs of cancer. In addition, lab tests of blood or other body fluids can check for the presence of substances called *tumor markers* that suggest cancer. Other detection methods rely on imaging technologies. These include ultrasound (US), magnetic resonance imaging (MRI), computed tomography (CT), and positron

biopsy A test for cancer in which a small sample of the abnormal growth is removed and studied.

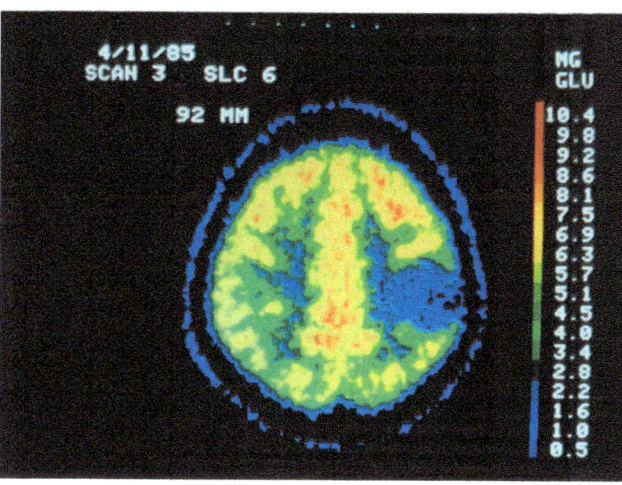

A PET scan of a cancerous growth in the brain. The cancer appears as the blue spot on the right.

emission tomography (PET), each of which has advantages and disadvantages for different types of tissues.

You should also be aware of five general signs and symptoms that the American Cancer Society (ACS) identifies as common early indicators of cancer. Most often, these *are not due to cancer*. However, if you notice any of them, and don't see an obvious reason for them, make an appointment with your doctor:[57]

- Unexplained weight loss
- Fever
- Fatigue
- Pain
- Skin changes, including darkened skin, yellowed skin and eyes (jaundice), reddened skin, itching, and excessive hair growth

Along with these general signs and symptoms, stay aware of changes in your health that may be due to specific cancers. For instance, a change in bowel habits is associated with colon cancer. Signs and symptoms of the most common types of cancer are identified later in this chapter.

Types of Cancer

Cancers can be grouped into five broad categories, according to the type of tissue in which the cancer arises:

- **Carcinomas** begin in the body's epithelial tissues, which include the skin and the tissues that line or cover internal organs. These are the most common sites for cancer, and cancers that occur here usually come in the form of solid tumors.
- **Sarcomas** start in the muscles, bones, fat, blood vessels, or other connective or supporting tissue. Sarcomas also take the form of solid tumors.
- **Central nervous system cancers** begin in the tissues of the brain and spinal cord. These form solid tumors and do damage both by directly altering nerve function and by growing large enough to interfere with the function of surrounding tissue.
- **Lymphomas** and **myelomas** involve different types of cells of the immune system. Lymphomas form tumors that invade the lymphoid tissues (lymph nodes, spleen, and bone marrow), whereas myelomas invade the bone marrow.
- **Leukemias** start in the tissues that make your blood. This type of cancer does not cause solid tumors but instead fills the blood with abnormal blood cells.

Common Cancers in Men and Women

Although cancer can arise in hundreds of different sites in your body, some sites are far more prone to cancer than others. We'll start with a look at cancers that affect both men and women and follow that with a separate overview of common sex-specific cancers.

Skin Cancer

More than 3 million people develop skin cancer each year.[54] The vast majority of these cancers are basal and squamous cell carcinomas, which typically are not aggressive and are easily treated. About 76,000 cases, however, are **malignant melanomas,** the most deadly form of skin cancer, resulting in more than 10,000 deaths each year.[54]

Risk Factors. Risk factors for all forms of skin cancer include[54]

- Fair skin and red or blonde hair
- Skin that sunburns easily and does not tan easily
- History of excessive sun exposure, including sunburns and use of tanning beds
- Past history of skin cancer

carcinoma Cancer of tissues that line or cover the body.

sarcoma Cancer of muscle or connective tissues.

central nervous system cancer Cancer of the brain or spinal cord.

lymphoma Cancer of the lymphoid tissues.

myeloma Cancer arising in plasma cells, which are a type of immune cells, and invading the bone marrow.

leukemia Cancer of blood-forming tissue.

malignant melanoma An especially aggressive form of skin cancer.

In addition, malignant melanoma is more common in people who have a family history of melanoma or numerous (more than 50) moles.

What should you watch for? Less serious forms of skin cancer look like bumps, colored spots, or scaly patches on the skin. These may bleed, itch, or ooze. In contrast, melanoma may arise as a new mole or other skin lesion or changes to an existing one. When examining any mole, use the ABCDE acronym shown in **Figure 13.11** (next page) to help remember the signs to look for.[54] The fifth letter, E, stands for *evolving;* that is, the lesion changes in size, shape, or color over the course of about a month. If you notice any of these skin changes, see your doctor as soon as possible.

If you have a family history of melanoma, many doctors recommend a yearly skin exam from a dermatologist. Otherwise, regular screenings are not necessary. But everyone's risk begins to increase at age 20, so it's a good idea to check your skin periodically for signs of change.

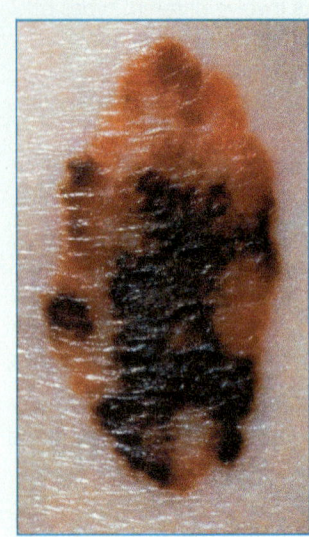

Asymmetry, where one side does not match the other.

Border irregularity, where edges are uneven or scalloped.

Color changes, where pigmentation is not uniform.

Diameter, where the size is more than 6 millimeters (about the size of a pea).

Evolving, where the appearance is changing in size, shape, or color over time.

FIGURE 13.11 **Malignant Melanoma.** This lesion shows the distinctive characteristics of malignant melanoma, the deadliest form of skin cancer.

Reducing Your Risk. Especially for people with fair skin, lots of unprotected sun exposure equals higher risks. Avoid extended time in the sun without a hat, protective clothing, and/or high sun protection factor (SPF) sunscreen. Avoid tanning, which is linked to an increased risk of melanoma and other forms of skin cancer. Tanning beds are classified as carcinogenic.[54] They emit doses of ultraviolet (UV) radiation far more powerful than those that come from the sun and are associated with a 75% increased risk of melanoma. The FDA requires tanning beds to have labels warning consumers of their dangers, which include burns, eye damage, premature aging of the skin, and skin cancer. The FDA is also proposing to ban the use of tanning beds by consumers under age 18.[58]

Lung Cancer

With more than 224,000 new cases diagnosed each year, lung cancer is the second most commonly diagnosed cancer in both men and women. Moreover, it accounts for more deaths than any other cancer—more than 158,000 in 2016, which is about 1 in every 4 cancer deaths.[54]

Risk Factors. Risk factors for lung cancer include

- A history of smoking or being exposed to secondhand smoke. About 80% of lung cancer deaths in the United States are caused by smoking. The longer you've smoked or been exposed to tobacco smoke, the higher your risk.
- Exposure to radon. In some areas, this naturally occurring radioactive gas exists in high concentrations in the soil and, over time, seeps into buildings or water supplies. Radon is the second most common cause of lung cancer.[54]
- Exposure to other carcinogens, such as asbestos or arsenic.
- Genetic factors.

What should you watch for? By the time any of the following symptoms have appeared, a case of lung cancer is usually fairly advanced:

- Spitting up blood-streaked mucus
- Chest pain
- A persistent cough
- Recurrent attacks of pneumonia or bronchitis

So far, this cancer has proven very difficult to detect early, and there are no established general screening guidelines. CT scans have been found effective at catching the disease early in people at high risk, but given the risks of radiation exposure with even low-dose CT scans, the ACS recommends shared clinician–patient decision making on a case-by-case basis.[54]

Reducing Your Risk. Smoking and regular exposure to secondhand smoke are the primary risk factors for lung cancer. If you smoke, get started on a plan to quit and, in the meantime, keep your smoke away from others. In addition, determine the radon levels in your home, workplace, and other buildings where you spend time.

Colorectal Cancer

About 95,000 cases of colon cancer and 40,000 cases of rectal cancer are diagnosed each year in the United States, making colorectal cancer the third most common cancer in both men and women. Nearly 50,000 Americans die of colorectal cancer annually.[54]

Risk Factors. Risk factors for colorectal cancer include

- A family history of colorectal cancer
- A family history of polyps, or precancerous growths, in the colon or rectum
- Being over the age of 50
- Obesity
- Presence of an inflammatory bowel disorder, such as colitis or Crohn's disease

What should you watch for? In its early stages, when it is easiest to treat, colorectal cancer often has no outward

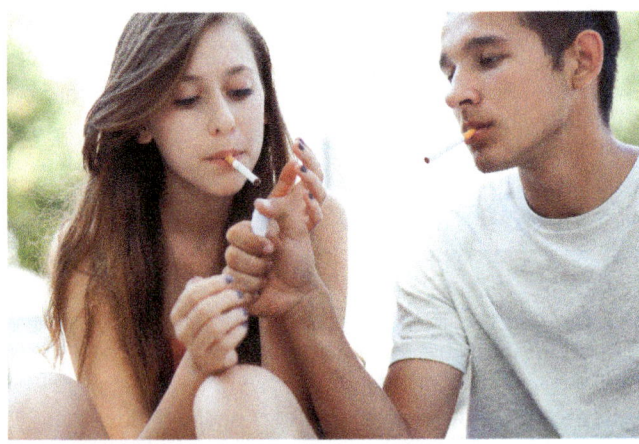

Lung cancer is the most deadly cancer in the United States, and smoking is its primary risk factor. Consider that before you light up.

symptoms. As the cancer progresses, warning signs include bleeding from the rectum, blood in the stool, and changes in bowel habits.

Screening is recommended for everyone once they reach age 50, using methods that include

- A yearly test that detects blood in the stool or a stool DNA test every 3 years
- Every 5 to 10 years, an internal imaging test that looks for polyps, such as a colonoscopy

For people at higher risk, such as those with a family history of colorectal cancer, doctors usually recommend a more frequent screening schedule.

Reducing Your Risk. The following measures may help to prevent colorectal cancer:

- Engaging in regular exercise
- Consuming a diet rich in fiber and plant-based foods and limiting your consumption of red and processed meats
- Maintaining a healthy weight
- Limiting alcohol consumption
- Avoiding smoking
- Following recommended screening guidelines because precancerous polyps can be removed during colonoscopy, and cancerous tumors can often be surgically removed if caught at early stages

Pancreatic Cancer

There are approximately 53,000 cases of pancreatic cancer diagnosed each year, and more than 41,000 deaths.[54] About 70% of patients die within a year of diagnosis, and just 7% survive for five years. The poor prognosis (estimated outcome) is due in part to the fact that pancreatic cancer typically goes undetected until it has advanced beyond the point at which treatment can be effective.

Risk Factors. Risk factors for pancreatic cancer include

- Smoking and use of smokeless tobacco
- Obesity
- Diabetes
- Chronic pancreatitis (inflammation of the pancreas)
- Genetic factors

What should you watch for? Signs of pancreatic cancer rarely appear until the disease is advanced. These include

- Abdominal discomfort and/or midback pain
- Jaundice, a yellowing of your skin and the whites of your eyes
- Unexplained weight loss

Currently, no standard screening guidelines exist for pancreatic cancer. Researchers are looking for ways to detect this cancer early and determine who would benefit most from screening.

Reducing Your Risk. Reduce your risk by following basic health guidelines, which include

- Not using any form of tobacco
- Maintaining a healthy weight
- Eating a healthy diet and exercising regularly

Oral Cancer

About 48,000 malignancies of the lips, tongue, mouth, and throat are diagnosed each year, and about 9,500 deaths result from oral cancers.[54]

Risk Factors. Risk factors include

- Smoking and use of smokeless tobacco
- Excessive drinking (A combination of heavy drinking and smoking increases risk of oral cancer 30-fold.)[54]
- HPV infection

What should you watch for? Symptoms include

- A sore that doesn't heal
- Red or white patches that don't heal or go away **(Figure 13.12)**
- An unexplained lump or thickening in the mouth, throat, or neck
- Ear pain
- Coughing up blood

Although there are no general screening guidelines, doctors and dentists usually make checking for oral cancer a routine part of any regular exam.

Reducing Your Risk. The best strategies are to avoid all types of tobacco products and excessive drinking and to use a dental dam or similar protection if engaging in oral sex.

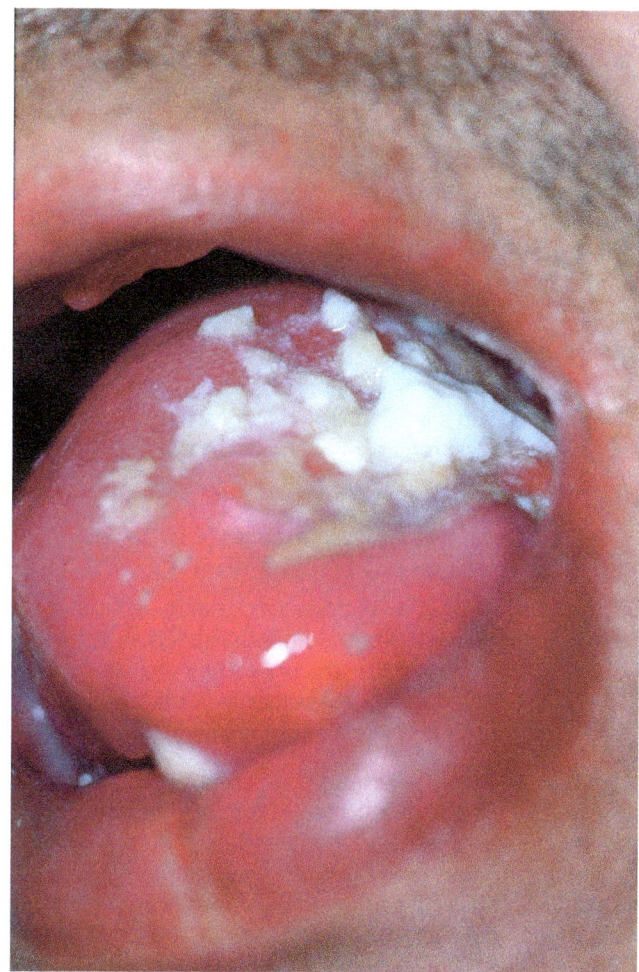

FIGURE 13.12 **Oral Cancer.**

Common Cancers in Men

Cancers affecting the male reproductive system include prostate cancer and testicular cancer. Although both are common, prostate cancer tends to occur in older men, whereas testicular cancer more commonly develops in younger men.

Prostate Cancer

The prostate is a gland in the male reproductive system that secretes a fluid that assists in the movement of sperm. It is located below the bladder. Prostate cancer is the most commonly diagnosed malignancy among men in the United States and the second most deadly. More than 180,000 cases are diagnosed each year, resulting in more than 26,000 deaths.[54]

Risk Factors. Risk factors include

- Age over 50
- Race (African American men are at increased risk of being diagnosed with prostate cancer and are more likely than others to have an aggressive form.)
- Family history

Detecting prostate cancer in its early stages can be difficult. Symptoms tend to develop in the disease's later stages and may include

- Difficulty urinating
- The urge to urinate frequently
- Blood in the urine
- Pain or burning with urination

Reducing Your Risk. There is no conclusive evidence of lifestyle changes that can lower your risk. Men over age 50 should speak with their health-care provider about whether it is advisable to have a prostate screening test (called a PSA test). African American men and men with a family history of prostate cancer should have this discussion at age 45.[54]

Testicular Cancer

Testicular cancer is a common malignancy in young men. About 8,700 men are diagnosed with it each year, and about 380 will die from it.[54]

Risk Factors. The risk factors for testicular cancer include

- Being a white male between the ages of 20 and 39
- Having a family history of cancer
- Having a history of an undescended testicle—that is, a testicle that did not descend from the abdomen into the scrotum before birth (The risk of cancer is increased for both testicles and remains whether or not the individual has had surgery to move the testicle into place.)

Reducing Your Risk. Because researchers still haven't uncovered the cause of testicular cancer, the most effective preventions aren't yet clear. Testicular self-exams can aid in detection, but there is no definitive evidence that they lead to a reduction in deaths from testicular cancer, and the ACS has no recommendation regarding them. If you are concerned about testicular cancer or have a family history of it, consult your doctor for advice on what to do.

>> If you decide to perform testicular self-exams, you can find instructions at the ACS website at **www.cancer.org**. (Search for "testicular self-exam.")

Common Cancers in Women

The most common cancers affecting the female reproductive system include breast cancer, ovarian cancer, and cervical and uterine cancers.

Breast Cancer

With more than 246,000 new cases and 40,000 deaths each year, breast cancer is the most common cancer among women in the United States and the second leading cause of cancer death in women.[54] Although more women are surviving breast cancer than ever before, prevention, detection, and treatment remain important.

Risk Factors. Risk factors include

- A family history of breast cancer, on either side of your family
- Inherited mutations in tumor suppressor genes identified as *BRCA1* and *BRCA2*
- Menstrual periods that started early and ended late in life

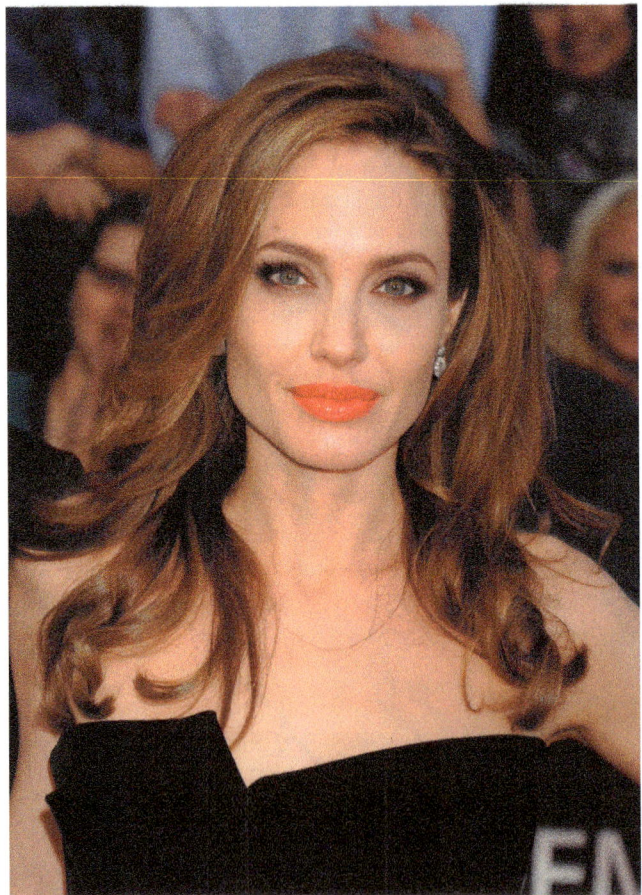

Angelina Jolie opted to have a preventive double mastectomy when she learned that she carries the BRCA1 gene, which increases the risk for breast and ovarian cancer. Two years later, she had her ovaries removed.

STUDENT STORY

Surviving Cancer

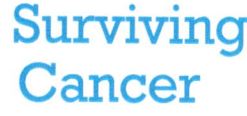

"HI, MY NAME IS AMANDA. I'm 19. I was diagnosed with acute lymphocytic leukemia at the age of 13. I was on chemo for about 3 years, had two surgeries, and had to miss about 2 years of school. The surgeries affected me socially because I basically had plastic tubes in my chest, so it was hard to give people hugs. People didn't understand, you know, when they would try to hug me—I'd be like, 'Oh you can't hug me, I'm a little bit fragile right here.' I've been in remission since 2007. I go for blood tests all the time just to make sure it hasn't come back.

My mother had breast cancer and shortly after she was in remission, she was diagnosed with ovarian cancer. Also, my mother's mother died of breast cancer, and her sister, my great-aunt, died of leukemia. So we have a lot of cancer in the women in our family.

I go for mammograms fairly regularly—I would say at least once a year. I am pretty young to be getting mammograms, but I do it because the frequency of cancer in my family is so high."

What Do You Think?

1. In what way might the genes Amanda inherited increase her risk for cancer? What might the mechanism be?
2. If you had been friends with Amanda when she was undergoing cancer treatment, how could you have supported her?
3. Do you have a family history of cancer? If so, are you taking extra precautions such as scheduling regular cancer screenings?

- Recent use of birth control pills or use of combined estrogen and progestin hormone replacement therapy
- Being overweight or obese (for postmenopausal women)
- Never having children, or having your first child after age 30
- Having dense breast tissue
- Heavy, long-term smoking
- Alcohol consumption

What should you watch for? Symptoms usually include changes in breast tissue, such as

- A typically painless lump or thickening in your breast or in the lymph nodes under your arm
- Dimpling, skin distortion, or skin irritation
- Unusual nipple appearance or discharge

Reducing Your Risk. A healthy lifestyle—including maintaining a healthful weight, limiting alcohol use, and engaging in regular moderate to vigorous exercise—is a good starting point for any woman who wants to reduce her risk.

Women who breast-feed for at least one year may also have a reduced breast cancer risk.[54]

Women whose family histories put them at increased risk should talk to their doctors about what to do. A doctor may advocate mammograms or other screenings at an earlier age or even genetic testing. Women at especially high risk may consider *chemoprevention* (the use of drugs to reduce cancer risk) or, in the most extreme cases, surgical mastectomy.

For women at average risk for breast cancer, the ACS recommends annual mammograms between ages 45 and 54 and annual or biennial mammograms for women aged 55 and older. Neither clinical breast exams nor breast self-exams are recommended; however, women are encouraged to become familiar with how their breasts normally look and feel and to report any changes to their health-care provider right away.[59]

Ovarian Cancer

More than 22,000 women are diagnosed with ovarian cancer each year, and 14,000 die from it.[54] Ovarian cancer causes more deaths among women than any other cancer of the female reproductive system. Like pancreatic cancer, it is usually advanced before it is detected; however, treatment has improved steadily in the past decade, and the death rate has correspondingly decreased.

Risk Factors. Risk factors for ovarian cancer include

- A family history of ovarian cancer or breast cancer
- Mutations in the BRCA1 or BRCA2 genes
- Being postmenopausal
- Never having children
- Infection that leads to pelvic inflammatory disease
- Obesity
- Use of estrogen-only or estrogen and progesterone hormone replacement therapy

Symptoms of ovarian cancer are nonspecific and mimic other common conditions, like bladder and digestive disorders, which can make diagnosis difficult. Women with ovarian cancer are likely to have a persistent feeling of abdominal bloating, urinary urgency, feeling full quickly after eating, and pelvic or abdominal pain.

Reducing Your Risk. Women between ages 35 and 40 who have the gene mutations associated with ovarian cancer may elect to have preventive surgery to remove their ovaries. There is currently no screening test available for ovarian cancer.[54]

Cervical and Uterine Cancers

About 60,000 women each year are diagnosed with cancer in the lining of the uterus, or endometrium.[54] Another 13,000 develop cancer in the cervix, at the base of the uterus. Uterine cancer results in more than 10,000 deaths each year, and cervical cancer results in approximately 4,000 deaths.[54]

Risk Factors. The risk factors for endometrial cancer are factors that increase the woman's exposure to estrogen. These include obesity, abdominal obesity, estrogen-only hormonal replacement therapy, late menopause, and never having children. The cause of most cases of cervical cancer is persistent infection with certain strains of HPV.[54] Other risk factors include a suppressed immune system, smoking, and long-term use of oral contraceptives.

What should you watch for? Signs of uterine or cervical cancer include unexplained vaginal bleeding or discharge. However, in most cases, cervical cancer develops silently. That's why a Pap test, performed during a woman's pelvic exam, is the most effective way to screen for cervical cancer. This swab of the cervix is used to look for precancerous cell changes. An HPV DNA test, which detects the presence of HPV strains associated with cancer, is also available.

The ACS recommends the following screening schedule:[54]

- Have your first Pap test at age 21.
- Continue getting tested every three years through age 29. From ages 30 to 65, continue screening every five years, using both the Pap test and the HPV test, or every three years if using the Pap test only. After age 65, if previous tests have been negative, screening may no longer be necessary.

Reducing Your Risk. Vaccination can protect against the most common types of HPV that cause cervical cancer. The vaccine may be administered as early as age 9 and through age 26. Some available vaccines also offer protection against HPV-associated anal cancer and genital and anal warts in both males and females and against vaginal and vulvar cancer in females.[60] A 2016 study found that, since the introduction of the HPV vaccination program, rates of HPV infection in females aged 14 to 19 have declined by 64% and in women aged 20 to 24 have declined by 34%.[61]

The HPV vaccines do not protect against all carcinogenic strains, so it's also essential to practice safer sex. If you have male partners, use a condom.

Treating Cancer

Over many decades, cancer treatment has evolved into a variety of methods that attempt to remove or shrink malignant tumors and impede metastasis:[62]

- Surgery offers the greatest chance for cure, especially if performed before the cancer has metastasized.
- Chemotherapy is the use of potent drugs to kill cancer cells, slow their growth, or keep them from spreading. It can also be used to relieve pain and other symptoms caused by a tumor.
- Radiation therapy uses high-energy subatomic particles or waves to damage or destroy cancer cells.
- Targeted therapy uses drugs or other substances to attack precise targets on cancer cells while sparing surrounding, healthy cells. The therapy may, for example, disrupt proteins that enable cancer cells to multiply, inhibit the ability of cancer cells to establish a blood supply, or induce cancer cells to self-destruct.
- Immunotherapy (also called biologic therapy) either stimulates the patient's immune system to increase its effectiveness against cancer cells or directly administers immune system proteins.

Many other types of treatment, including heat, light, and stem cell transplants, are also used, and more are in development.

LO 13.5 QUICK CHECK

Certain strains of HPV are
a. thought to initiate liver cancer.
b. known to cause oral, anal, and cervical cancer.
c. associated with the development of rare opportunistic cancers.
d. the only known risk factors for pancreatic cancer.

Change Yourself, Change Your World

LO 13.6 Identify steps you can take to reduce your risk for chronic disease and its burden within your community.

If you're feeling discouraged about your odds of developing a chronic disease, notice that all nine CMR factors are modifiable—meaning they are within your power to change! And many of the behaviors that can reduce your risk for diabetes and CVD can reduce your risk for cancer as well. To review these healthy behaviors, check out the **Special Feature** ahead. The sooner you start, the better for your body.

What if you're more worried about a loved one's risk for chronic disease than about your own? Maybe a parent or friend smokes, or abuses alcohol, or seems to be gaining more and more weight. If you're healthy, it can be tough to witness people you care about making poor choices. But it's important to recognize how hard it is to change. Your loved one might be addicted to nicotine or alcohol or have a disordered relationship to food. So try asking questions and offering your support—but avoid judgment. For instance: "I notice you've started smoking again. What's been stressing you out lately?" Or: "The new river walk just opened. Let's start walking Saturday mornings." Don't lecture and don't insist that what worked for you will work for them. Let them find their own way, and when they do, affirm their positive choices.

If a loved one has been diagnosed with diabetes, cardiovascular disease, or cancer, they might want to share their challenges, fears, and dreams. If so, listen not just to what is said but to how it's said. Ask questions about the condition—how it affects life day to day, what treatments seem helpful, and what the frustrations are. Directly ask what you can do to help—and then follow through. Whether it's driving your loved one to a medical appointment or going for a walk together, do your best to provide the help requested.

Honesty is of course crucial to all relationships, so it's important to acknowledge how your loved one's diagnosis is affecting you. Do you feel as if you can't indulge in a pastry whenever your friend with diabetes is around, or that you can't talk about your dreams for the future because your friend has a life-threatening cancer diagnosis? Opening

SPECIAL FEATURE

Reducing Your Risk for Chronic Disease

Making the following healthy choices can substantially reduce your odds of developing a chronic disease:

- **Don't smoke.** As you've learned, the ingredients in tobacco smoke constrict and irritate artery walls, trigger inflammation, promote atherosclerosis, and increase blood pressure. Moreover, smoking causes many types of cancer, not lung cancer alone.[1] If you smoke, visit your physician or your campus health center and ask for the help you need to quit. Do it *today*.

- **If you choose to drink alcohol, go easy.** Moderate alcohol intake—no more than two drinks per day for males and one drink per day for females—reduces your risk for cardiovascular disease. However, alcohol packs 7 calories per gram, which tend to be stored in the abdomen. Also, alcohol is a known human carcinogen, and heavy drinking is a significant risk factor for esophageal, stomach, liver, colorectal, and other cancers.[1]

- **Shed extra pounds.** Avoiding obesity—especially abdominal obesity—can reduce your CMR. And as you've read, obesity is a risk factor for many types of cancer; the ACS recommends being as lean as possible without being underweight.[1] So keep your BMI within the range for normal weight (18.5 to 24.9). And aim for a waist measurement of less than 40 inches if you are a man or less than 35 inches if you are a woman.

- **Pile your plate with plants.** Eat red meat less often and, when you do, keep the portion small and load your plate with vegetables. Avoid fatty and processed meats like pepperoni, bacon, sausage, low-grade ground beef, and luncheon meats. With fried or barbecued meats, remove any blackened regions because carcinogenic chemicals build up in these areas. Twice a week, choose fatty fish like salmon and tuna, which are high in heart-healthy omega-3 fatty acids. Make or choose vegetarian meals several times a week, with plant-based protein sources such as beans, lentils, tofu, and tempeh.

- **Decrease your sodium intake.** To reduce your risk for hypertension, limit your sodium intake to less than 2,300 mg/day. Cut back on processed foods, which tend to be high in sodium.

- **Eat yogurt.** Yogurt and other fermented dairy products contain *probiotics*, strains of bacteria that help reduce blood vessel inflammation and blood levels of LDL cholesterol.[2] Probiotics are also thought to reduce inflammation in the colon and thus may play some role in reducing your risk for colon cancer.[3]

- **Limit your exposure to pesticides.** Choose organic foods more often to reduce your overall exposure to pesticides, some of which are carcinogens. Scrub produce under running water to reduce the pesticide level and then peel if possible. Remove the outer leaves of lettuces. Trim off the fatty parts of meats, where pesticides and other residues consumed by animals tend to build up.[4]

- **Exercise.** Regular physical activity helps improve body weight, blood glucose levels, lipid levels, and blood pressure. It also strengthens the heart. Moreover, vigorous exercise releases adrenaline, which seems to boost immune surveillance for cancer cells, and increases levels of immune cells called *natural killer cells* that destroy cells with mutated DNA.[5] The ACS recommends a weekly minimum of 150 minutes of moderate-intensity physical activity or 75 minutes of vigorous physical activity spread throughout the week.[1] Balance aerobic activities that build heart and lung capacity with strength training.

- **Sleep.** Chronic short sleep duration is linked to hypertension, atherosclerotic changes, and inflammation. Aim for eight hours of sleep a night.

- **Manage your emotions.** A large review study found that heart attacks and strokes are significantly more common in the two hours following an outburst of anger.[6] Moreover, the National Cancer Institute reports that, although psychological stress has not been shown to directly cause cancer, it can weaken the immune system.[7] So if you need help managing your anger or stress levels, get it.

- **Reduce environmental risks.** Many air, water, and land pollutants are carcinogens. Find out what pollutants you might be exposed to and take steps to reduce your risk. Remember that one of the most harmful pollutants is tobacco smoke, so if you live with a smoker, insist that he or she take it outside.

- **Know your history.** Do you know your family's history of diabetes, CVD, and cancer? If not, ask. Becoming aware of inherited risks is important because it allows you to discuss them with your healthcare provider and to take the steps prescribed.

- **Get screened.** Visit your primary health-care provider to have your blood glucose, blood pressure, and blood lipids measured and to talk about any recommended cancer screenings. If you don't have a care provider, stop in at your campus health center and ask about the screenings you need.

Sources: **1.** American Cancer Society. (2016). *Cancer facts and figures, 2016.* www.cancer.org. **2.** DiRienzo, D. B. (2014). Effect of probiotics on biomarkers of cardiovascular disease: Implications for heart-healthy diets. *Nutrition Reviews, 72*(1), 18–29. **3.** Mendes, E. (2015, March 11). Colon health may rely on gut bacteria. *American Cancer Society: Research Updates.* www.cancer.org. **4.** U.S. Environmental Protection Agency (EPA). (2015, March 19). *Pesticides and food: Healthy, sensible food practices.* www.epa.gov. **5.** L. Pedersen, M., Idorn, G. H., Olofsson, B., Lauenborg, I., Nookaew, et al. (2016). Voluntary running suppresses tumor growth through epinephrine- and IL-6-dependent NK cell mobilization and redistribution. *Cell Metabolism, 23*(3), 554–562. **6.** Mostofsky, E., Penner, E. A. & Mittleman, M. A. (2014). Outbursts of anger as a trigger of acute cardiovascular events: A systematic review and meta-analysis. *European Heart Journal.* doi:10.1093/eurheartj/ehu033. **7.** National Cancer Institute. (2012, December). *Psychological stress and cancer.* www.cancer.gov.

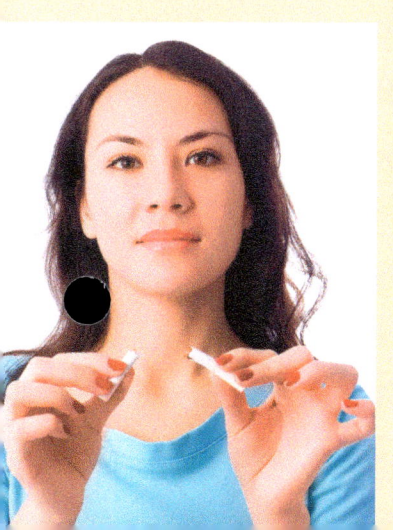

up about such feelings can help clear the air and allow you and your friend to support each other. However, try to avoid giving advice. Even if you've struggled with the same illness yourself, everyone's journey is different. Accept that your friend needs your presence, not your advice, and that's enough.

Just as you can help loved ones choose health and manage chronic disease, you can promote a healthier campus environment—by advocating for more healthful food choices in dining halls and neighborhood restaurants, lobbying for a tobacco-free campus, and volunteering at health-screening events. Also, make sure you find out the location of the AEDs on your campus, including in campus housing and in classrooms, labs, and other buildings you regularly use. If anyone were to suffer a sudden cardiac arrest, that information could enable you to save the person's life. Next time it's offered at your school, register for training in CPR. Both the American Red Cross and the American Heart Association offer certification classes, which are usually just a few hours long, scheduled for an evening or a Saturday, and are free or very low cost.

You might also consider getting a group of students together to sponsor a race, a "walk-a-thon," or another event to raise money for the American Diabetes Association, American Heart Association, American Cancer Society, or other reputable groups that work to prevent chronic disease and assist those who have been diagnosed. Or keep it simple: Next time your birthday comes around, ask family members and friends to make their gift a donation to the organization of your choice.

LO 13.6 QUICK CHECK

Among the behaviors recognized as reducing your risk for chronic disease

a. the majority are most effective for older adults and less effective or unrealistic for college students.
b. most are easy to maintain and rarely associated with relapse.
c. the most important are avoiding tobacco, alcohol, saturated fat, sodium, and a sedentary lifestyle.
d. the most important are avoiding tobacco, limiting alcohol, engaging in regular physical activity, and consuming a healthful diet.

>> Watch videos of real students discussing cardiovascular disease, diabetes, and cancer at **Mastering**Health™

 # Choosing to **Change** Worksheet

To complete this worksheet online, visit **Mastering**Health™

Remember that tobacco use, excessive alcohol consumption, inadequate physical activity, and poor nutrition significantly increase your risk for developing diabetes, cardiovascular disease, and cancer.

Directions: Fill in your stage of change in step 1 and complete step 2 with your stage of change in mind. Then complete steps 3, 4, or 5, depending on which ones apply to your stage of change.

Step 1: Assess your stage of behavior change. Please check one of the following statements that best describes your readiness to reduce your chronic disease risk:

_____ I do not intend to reduce my chronic disease risk in the next six months. (Precontemplation)

_____ I might reduce my chronic disease risk in the next six months. (Contemplation)

_____ I am prepared to reduce my chronic disease risk in the next month. (Preparation)

_____ I have been reducing my chronic disease risk for less than six months. (Action)

_____ I have been reducing my chronic disease risk for more than six months. (Maintenance)

Step 2: Recognize your risk. Now that you have read through the chapter, write down five risk factors you have for chronic disease. Next to each risk factor, indicate whether it is modifiable (you can change it) or not.

Risk Factor	Modifiable?

Step 3: Work the precontemplation or contemplation stages. What are some reasons to reduce your chronic disease risk factors?

_____
_____

Pick one of the *modifiable* risk factors from step 2. What obstacles might be holding you back from taking action to reduce this risk, and how can you overcome these obstacles? Fill in the grid below.

Obstacle to Reducing Risk	How Can You Overcome It?

Step 4: Work the preparation and action stages. In the **Special Feature** on page 347, you might find some strategies for reducing the risk you identified above. To find additional strategies, visit a valid and reliable government website such as the Centers for Disease Control and Prevention, at www.cdc.gov, to research strategies for reducing this risk. Select one strategy that you feel highly confident in implementing and set a start date: _____

Set a **SMART** goal and write it down: _____

Step 5: Work the action and maintenance stages. For one week, keep track of your progress in reducing the risk you identified. Evaluate your progress and explain whether you will modify your plan. _____

CHAPTER **13** STUDY PLAN

CHAPTER SUMMARY

LO 13.1
- A chronic disease comes on gradually, lasts a long time, and may resist complete cure. Chronic diseases cause 7 out of every 10 deaths in the United States, robbing Americans of years of life and health-related quality of life.
- Diabetes, cardiovascular disease (CVD), and cancer are three chronic diseases that share some underlying physiological mechanisms and risk factors, including tobacco use, excessive alcohol consumption, and obesity (related to poor diet and inadequate levels of physical activity).

LO 13.2
- Diabetes is a disorder in which blood glucose levels are consistently elevated above normal.
- Type 1 diabetes develops when the body's immune system destroys the beta cells in the pancreas that manufacture insulin. Type 2 diabetes develops when body cells resist the effects of insulin. Other forms include gestational diabetes and variants referred to as "type 1.5."
- Signs and symptoms of diabetes include frequent urination, excessive thirst and hunger, and fatigue. Poorly managed diabetes damages blood vessels, contributing to complications that include blindness, kidney failure, amputations, and increased risk for CVD.
- Risk factors for type 2 diabetes include age over 50, overweight and obesity (especially abdominal obesity), family history, chronic stress, and a sedentary lifestyle.
- Management includes weight loss if the person is overweight, glucose monitoring, medications, and insulin

MasteringHealth™

Build your knowledge—and health!— in the Study Area of **MasteringHealth**™ with a variety of study tools.

therapy in people with type 1 diabetes as well as many people with type 2 diabetes.

LO 13.3

- The cardiovascular system consists of the heart and blood vessels. It supplies the body with oxygen and nutrients and carries away wastes.
- Atherosclerosis is the development of plaque along the lining of an artery. It contributes to most forms of CVD, the four most common of which are hypertension, coronary heart disease, heart failure, and stroke.
- Hypertension is a blood pressure consistently higher than normal, which greatly increases the risk for heart attack, stroke, or heart failure.
- Coronary heart disease is characterized by atherosclerosis affecting a coronary artery. It can lead to angina (chest pain) and/or a heart attack or arrhythmia and sudden cardiac arrest.
- Heart failure is an inability of the heart to pump blood effectively.
- Stroke is a blockage or rupture of a cerebral artery. Permanent brain damage or death can result.
- CVD risk factors include age over 65, dyslipidemia, high blood glucose, inflammation, obesity, and tobacco use.

LO 13.4

- Cardiometabolic risk (CMR) is a cluster of nine modifiable risk factors associated with an increased risk for type 2 diabetes and CVD: abdominal obesity; elevated blood pressure, blood glucose, triglycerides, and LDL cholesterol; low HDL cholesterol; inflammatory markers; insulin resistance; and smoking.

LO 13.5

- Cancer, a group of diseases marked by uncontrolled growth of abnormal cells, is the second most common cause of death in the United States.
- Uncontrolled cell growth can be related to two types of genes: proto-oncogenes and tumor-suppressor genes.
- Cancer begins when the DNA in body cells undergoes a mutation that can occur as a result of exposure to carcinogens, including viruses, radiation, or toxic chemicals such as those in tobacco smoke.
- Malignant tumors invade nearby tissues, and metastasis is the spread of cancer cells to sites distant from the original tumor.
- Skin cancer is the most common cancer in men and women; only the least common form, malignant melanoma, tends to be invasive. Lung cancer is the second most common type of cancer affecting both men and women, and colorectal cancer is the third.
- Testicular cancer is the most common cancer in young males, and prostate cancer is the most common in men of all ages.
- A mutation in the BRCA1 or BRCA2 genes increases a woman's risk for breast cancer, the most common cancer in women, as well as for ovarian cancer. Sexually transmitted infection with a carcinogenic strain of the human papillomavirus (HPV) is a direct cause of cervical cancer.

LO 13.6

- Strategies for reducing your risk for chronic disease include avoiding all forms of tobacco, limiting alcohol consumption, maintaining a healthy weight, eating a nutritious diet, exercising regularly, limiting sun exposure, reducing your exposure to infection and toxic environmental chemicals, and getting adequate sleep.
- When a friend or family member is at risk for chronic disease or has been diagnosed with a chronic disease, you can help by listening without an agenda and offering your support.
- At the campus and community levels, you can advocate for smoke-free environments and more healthful food choices. Identify the AEDs on your campus, learn CPR, and/or sponsor or participate in a fund-raiser for reputable organizations that work to fight chronic disease.

GET CONNECTED

>> Visit the following websites for further information about the topics in this chapter:

- American Cancer Society
  www.cancer.org
- American Diabetes Association
  www.diabetes.org
- American Heart Association
  www.heart.org
- Centers for Disease Control and Prevention
  www.cdc.gov
- MedlinePlus
  www.nlm.nih.gov/medlineplus

MOBILE TIPS!

Scan this QR code with your mobile device to access additional tips about diabetes, cardiovascular disease, and cancer. Or, via your mobile device, go to **http://chmobile.pearsoncmg.com** and choose by topic: diabetes/cardiovascular disease/cancer.

- My Family Health Portrait, a tool from the U.S. Surgeon General
  https://familyhistory.hhs.gov/fhh-web/home.action
- National Cancer Institute
  www.cancer.gov

Website links are subject to change. To access updated web links, please visit MasteringHealth™

TEST YOUR KNOWLEDGE

LO 13.1
1. What percentage of deaths each year in the United States are due to chronic disease?
   a. 25%
   b. 50%
   c. 70%
   d. 90%

LO 13.2
2. What is the cause of type 1 diabetes?
   a. eating a high-sugar diet
   b. inability of body cells to respond to insulin properly
   c. absorption of excessive amounts of glucose across the small intestine into the bloodstream
   d. immune system destruction of insulin-secreting cells in the pancreas
3. Among American adults, diabetes is the most common cause of
   a. kidney failure.
   b. blindness.
   c. nontraumatic lower limb amputations.
   d. all of the above.

LO 13.3
4. Which form of CVD is known as a "silent killer"?
   a. hypertension
   b. coronary heart disease
   c. heart failure
   d. stroke
5. Which of the following statements about cardiovascular disease is true?
   a. Atherosclerosis increases the risk for hypertension, coronary heart disease, heart failure, and stroke.
   b. The best emergency treatment for a person experiencing the warning signs of myocardial infarction is to shock the heart using an automated external defibrillator (AED).
   c. A TIA is a warning sign of an impending heart attack.
   d. Heart failure is triggered when an arrhythmia such as ventricular fibrillation causes the heart to stop beating.

LO 13.4
6. Which of the following is one of the nine factors in cardiometabolic risk?
   a. having a body mass index (BMI) greater than or equal to 25
   b. drinking more than two alcoholic beverages a day for males and more than one for females
   c. smoking
   d. all of these

LO 13.5
7. Which of the following statements about cancer is true?
   a. Oncogenes are genes known to suppress the development of malignant tumors.
   b. Carcinogens are substances known to promote metastasis of malignant tumors.
   c. A malignant tumor is a tumor that has metastasized.
   d. Not all tumors are malignant.
8. One of the most common cancers affecting both men and women is
   a. oral cancer.
   b. malignant melanoma.
   c. pancreatic cancer.
   d. colorectal cancer.

LO 13.6
9. Which of the following behaviors has been shown to reduce your risk of developing diabetes, CVD, and cancer?
   a. taking fiber supplements
   b. engaging in regular physical activity
   c. drinking alcohol in moderation
   d. avoiding exposure to UV radiation
10. Which of the following actions is most appropriate for addressing the burden of chronic disease in your community?
    a. Limit your sodium intake to less than 2,300 mg a day.
    b. Enroll in a CPR class.
    c. When talking with a friend who has a chronic disease, listen for a short time and then change the subject to keep your friend's mind off it.
    d. Next time you and your friends go out to eat, order a soft drink instead of alcohol.

WHAT DO YOU THINK?

LO 13.2
1. An individual diagnosed with type 1 diabetes requires insulin therapy. Why can't this condition be managed through lifestyle changes such as exercise and a healthful diet?

LO 13.3
2. Distinguish between an ischemic stroke and a hemorrhagic stroke and explain why aspirin is an initial treatment for one type but not the other.
3. Why does obesity increase the risk for CVD? List at least four reasons.

LO 13.5
4. Why do you think that many people consider a cancer diagnosis a "death sentence"? Give at least two reasons. What information might counter that view?

LO 13.6
5. A moderate alcohol intake—no more than two drinks per day for males and one drink per day for females—is beneficial to your cardiovascular system, yet alcohol itself is a known human carcinogen. Is alcohol consumption a healthful choice for you? Why or why not?

14

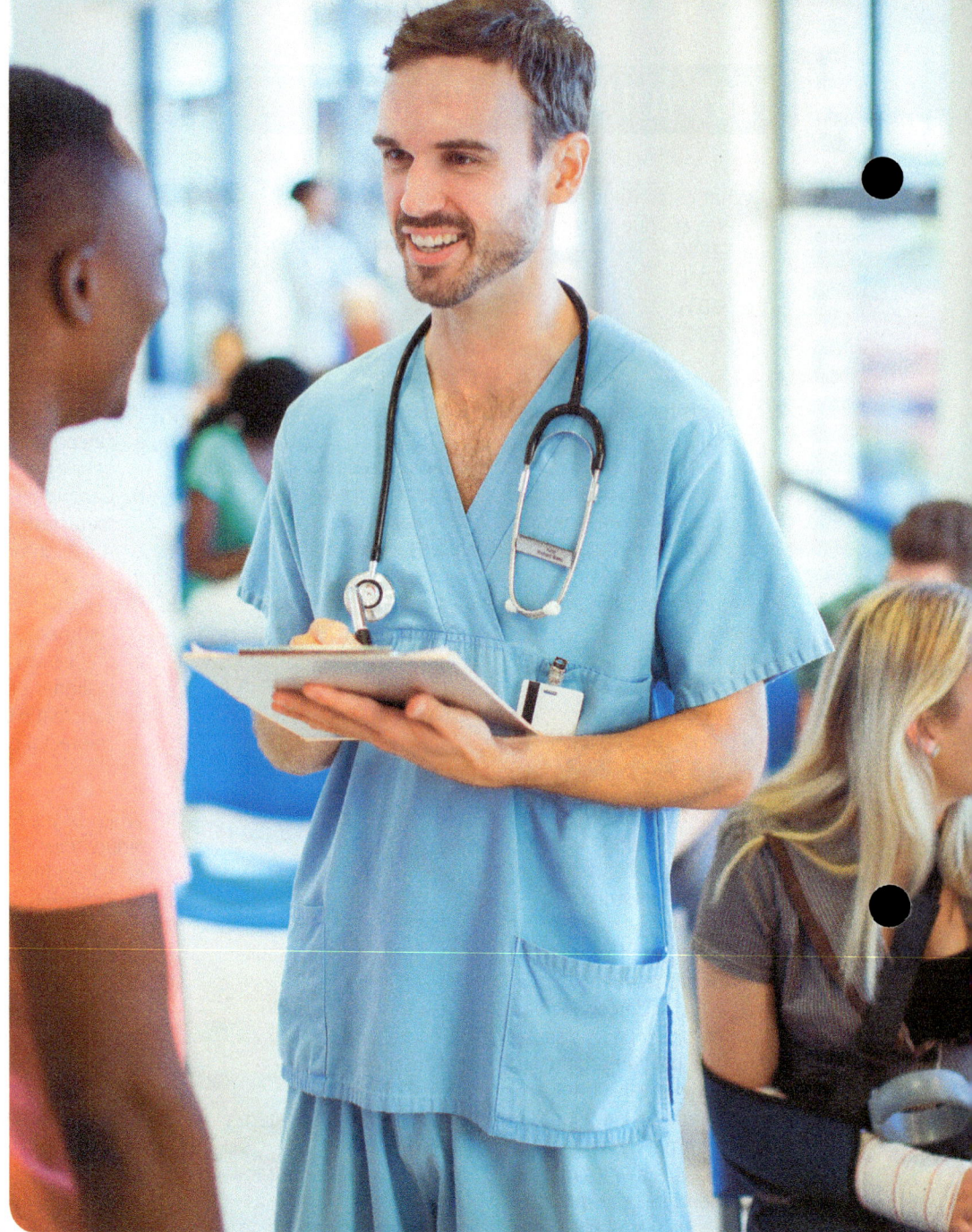

> **About 75% of Internet users have sought health information online.**[i]

> **Medical errors account for a significant number of deaths in the United States—about 250,000 per year.**[ii]

> **About 6.1 million young American adults aged 19 to 25 have gained health insurance since 2010.**[iii]

CONSUMER HEALTH

LEARNING OUTCOMES

LO 14.1 Describe different aspects of self-care.

LO 14.2 Explain how to determine when it's time to seek professional health care.

LO 14.3 Discuss the basis of conventional medicine, how to choose a provider, and how to be a smart patient.

LO 14.4 Describe common types of complementary and alternative medicine and how to evaluate them.

LO 14.5 Identify multiple methods of paying for health care.

LO 14.6 Discuss the genomic revolution and the future of personal health.

LO 14.7 Explain how to create your personal health-care plan.

It's near the end of the semester, and you've been feeling physically run-down.

Things got worse this morning, when you woke up with a bad sore throat, a fever, and—most troubling—a skin rash. What should you do?

Maybe you'll go online and do a search on your symptoms to decide whether they are serious enough to seek professional help. You might take an over-the-counter medicine for the sore throat and fever, and perhaps you'll ask a parent or friend for advice about the rash. If you decide to consult a doctor, things can quickly get more complicated: What doctor should you see? How will you pay for the health care? What if you don't have health insurance?

These are all examples of questions related to **consumer health.** In the United States today, we have more tools and options for taking care of our health than ever before. The Internet holds an unprecedented amount of health information. We can purchase a wide range of over-the-counter drugs and medications. We can choose to seek care at a traditional hospital, at a drugstore clinic, or at a campus health center. We can try alternative therapies like acupuncture or chiropractic, and we can select from a broad array of health-care professionals and insurance plans.

But this growing world of health choices also requires active and informed decision making. Increasingly, the burden is on you to research information, evaluate it, and make educated decisions that are best for you. You need to be a smarter health consumer than ever before. This chapter will help.

Choosing Self-Care

LO 14.1 Describe different aspects of self-care.

There are many things you can do on your own to stay healthy. As you've learned throughout this book, some of the most important health behaviors are preventive, promoting your overall wellness and reducing the likelihood that you will get sick in the first place. Maintaining basic wellness behaviors, learning how to critically evaluate health information (especially online), educating yourself about over-the-counter medications, using home health tests, and knowing when it's time to seek professional help are all examples of **self-care.**

> **consumer health** An umbrella term encompassing topics related to the purchase and consumption of health-related products and services.
>
> **self-care** Actions you take to keep yourself healthy.

Practicing Prevention

Prevention begins with the basic wellness behaviors you've learned about in this book, such as eating nutritiously, exercising, and refraining from unhealthful behaviors like smoking and excessive drinking. Regularly brushing your teeth and flossing, making sure you get enough sleep, keeping your stress level under control, and maintaining good relationships are additional aspects of self-care (**Figure 14.1**). Commonsense preventive behaviors—such as wearing a seat belt inside a car, wearing a helmet while riding a bike, and practicing safer sex—can protect you from serious injuries and illnesses. Similarly, the simple act of regularly washing your hands with soap and hot water can protect you from contracting infectious diseases. Prevention also means staying on top of regular health checks, including physicals and dental visits.

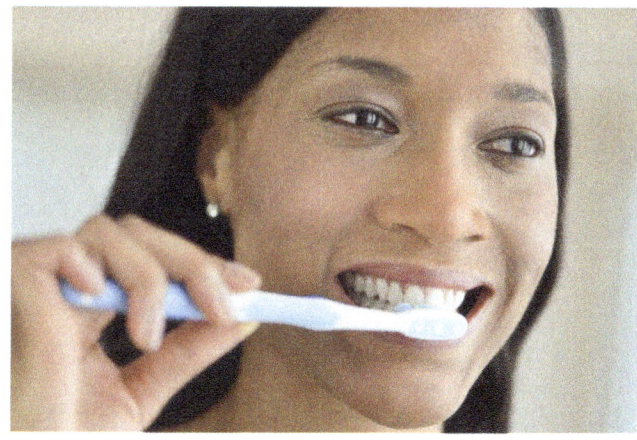

FIGURE 14.1 **Self-care.** Self-care includes basic wellness habits such as regularly brushing your teeth.

Finding Accurate Health Information

If you are living away from home for the first time, you have new responsibilities for making your own decisions about your care. Making any health-related decision intelligently starts with analyzing health information for yourself.

Evaluating Health Information and Tools

Using the Internet as a health resource has become so common that some health professionals joke that they've been replaced by "Dr. Google." Yet going online doesn't necessarily mean that one knows what to do with the health information found there. One study of college students found that although they use the Internet more than any other health information source, they also find other sources of information to be believable, including student health center medical staff, professors, coursework, and parents.[1]

As you know, the online world represents only one facet of all the health information you are likely to encounter each day. You may hear about scientific studies on news programs or see ads for health-related products in various media. A friend might recommend a new health-related app for your phone. Regardless of where you find information, you will be able to better evaluate it by first getting answers to a few basic questions:

- What is the source? Is the information provider a health expert or a group of such professionals? What are the source's credentials?
- What does the source have at stake? Is the information provider relatively unbiased? Will anyone benefit financially from how the information is perceived or used? If you are using a mobile app, does it have a one-time cost or ongoing fees?
- Is the information or tool supported by facts? Are those facts stated clearly, with supporting evidence to establish their credibility?
- Does the information or tool come with a timestamp? Does the site or app say when its underlying information was published or last updated, and is that date recent? If it relies on scientific studies, are those relatively recent or somewhat dated?
- Is the information presented in a balanced manner? Does it include and discuss other options or points of view, or does it pretend they don't exist?
- Does the information or tool offer something that sounds too good to be true? Achieving good health and wellness is a rewarding but ongoing process. Simplistic quick fixes may be of little actual substance.

In addition to answering these questions to evaluate health information in the news and other media, you can also watch for these "red flags":[2]

- The information is anonymous.
- There is a conflict of interest.
- The information is one-sided or biased.
- The information is outdated.
- There is a claim of a miracle or secret cure.
- No scientific evidence is cited.
- The grammar is poor and words are misspelled.

Much of the health information and tools you'll find online or in the media claim to rely on scientific research studies. The Internet has made these studies more accessible than ever before, and you don't need to be a scientist to read them. Next, we'll look at how you can make sense of scientific findings.

Understanding Research Studies

Reliable health information is supported by **evidence-based medicine**—practices that are based on systematic, scientific study. The process that supports quality research is called the "scientific method" and includes the following steps:

> **evidence-based medicine** Health-care policies and practices based on systematic, scientific study.

- First, the researcher makes an observation that prompts one or more questions about the factor observed.
- The researcher then formulates an educated guess (or hypothesis) that attempts to answer one or more of the original questions and conducts an experiment to test that educated guess. The experiment generates data that either challenges the hypothesis or supports it.
- Scientists typically share the results of their experiments with other researchers in the form of published research studies. Most studies undergo scrutiny by a team of independent reviewers before they can be published.

While the results of many studies may be published online, not all studies are equally reliable. To evaluate their validity and reliability, answer these questions:

- Is the description of this research specific and detailed? Credible research claims should include who conducted the study and their credentials, the research institutions involved, the question the study was trying to answer, and the dates the research was conducted and/or published.
- Who published this research? Quality science is published in *peer-reviewed journals,* publications where experts screen and evaluate all submissions. Research findings are also sometimes presented at meetings of scientific societies.

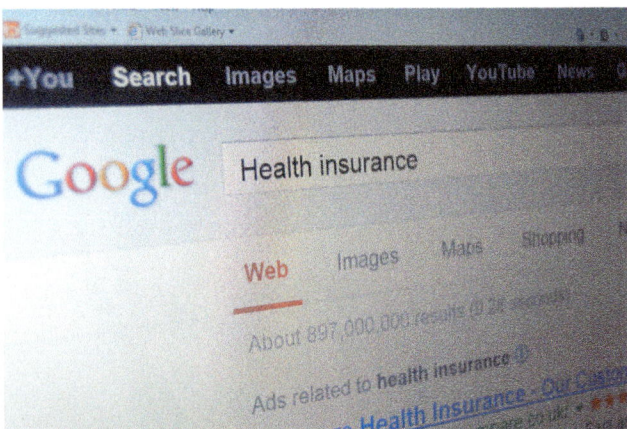

The Internet is increasingly the first place people turn to for health information.

- Who were the study participants? Was the research done on animals or people? Studies conducted on people usually have the greatest medical validity.
- How many people participated? The larger the pool of participants, the more significant the results. Especially significant studies often involve tens of thousands of people over several years.
- What were the profiles of the participants? How similar were they to you? The results of a health study of breast cancer prevention in 10,000 postmenopausal women may not be relevant if you are a woman in your 20s.
- Is the study the first of its kind? Scientific findings carry more weight if they have been replicated by other researchers.
- Do the people behind the study have any conflicts of interest? Credible studies disclose who paid for the research and whether the scientists involved have any financial or other interest in the outcome.

Credible health information sites highlight this type of scientific information. If a study has been made available online via a large public scientific library such as PubMed, that may indicate that the study has greater scientific legitimacy.

>> Use PubMed to look up reputable studies on a wide range of health and medical topics. Learn more at **www.nlm.nih.gov/services/pubmed.html.**

Options for Self-Care

In addition to practicing prevention and finding good health information, self-care means being your own caregiver from time to time. In order to care for yourself well, you need to understand the basic principles of commonly used medical products. We discuss those next.

Evaluating Over-the-Counter Medications

More than 80% of U.S. adults have typically purchased at least one type of medication in the past six months.[3]

over-the-counter (OTC) medication Medication available for purchase without a prescription.

The most readily available are **over-the-counter (OTC) medications,** which do not require a doctor's prescription. More than $40 billion worth of OTC drugs are sold in the United States each year.[4]

The U.S. Food and Drug Administration (FDA) regulates both prescription and OTC medications. The FDA defines OTC medications as those that[5]

- Have benefits outweighing their risks
- Have low potential for misuse
- Consumers can use for self-diagnosed conditions
- Can be adequately labeled
- Do not require consultation with health practitioners for safe and effective use of the product

About 74% of college students take at least one OTC drug a week, pain relievers being the most common.[6]

Many OTC drugs are effective, and they are often more affordable than prescription medications. One analysis showed that compared to the cost of prescription drugs, similar OTC medications save about $25 billion in the United States each year.[4] But OTC medications still carry risks and side effects. It is important not to exceed the recommended dosage, to use the medications for their intended purposes, and to talk to your doctor or pharmacist if you have any questions. (See **Consumer Corner** on page 356.)

>> Medicines in My Home at **www.accessdata.fda.gov/videos/cder/mimh/index.cfm** is an interactive presentation on how to choose and use OTC medications safely.

Taking Home Health Tests

Gone are the days when the only health-measuring instrument kept at home was a thermometer. Via drugstores and websites, we now have access to a wide range of medical devices that enable us to assess our health at home (**Figure 14.2**). Some of the most common include

- Pregnancy tests
- Blood pressure kits
- Fertility thermometers and apps
- Cholesterol tests
- Blood glucose monitors
- Colon cancer risk tests
- HIV tests (*Note: If you think you may have been exposed to HIV, consider taking the HIV test in a clinic or hospital setting where on-site counseling will be available. Taking this test at home is not ideal because there will be no medical professional present to advise you in the event that you have a positive result. In addition, some at-home HIV tests marketed online do not have FDA approval. Make sure any at-home HIV test you use is approved by the FDA.*)

When you take any kind of home health test, it is very important to follow the test instructions precisely. Not doing so can result in erroneous results. Also keep in mind that a number of external factors can cause test results to be inaccurate. For example, a pregnancy test may yield a "negative" result if the woman takes the test too early in her pregnancy. Drinking copious amounts of fluid or taking prescription medications may also interfere with the accuracy of some home health tests. If your test results indicate that you have a medical issue, consult a doctor immediately to confirm the results.

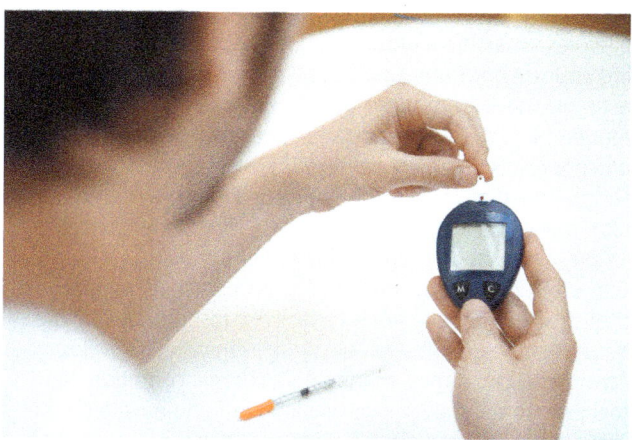

FIGURE 14.2 **Home Health Tests.** These are now available for everything from fertility testing to HIV detection.

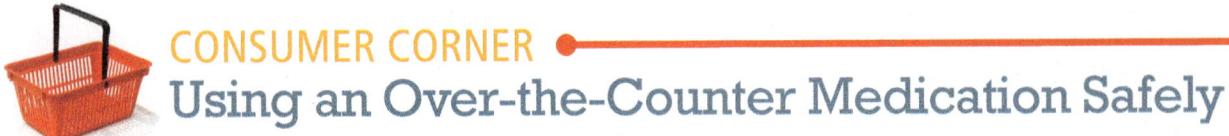

CONSUMER CORNER
Using an Over-the-Counter Medication Safely

A typical OTC medication label looks like the label on the right.

When you're using an OTC medication, be sure to read the label carefully and note the following:

- What is its active ingredient? Do you have any allergies to this ingredient, or any other ingredients in this medication? Are you taking any other medications that may interfere with or combine poorly with this ingredient?

- What is the medication's intended purpose or use? Are you using the medication properly?

- What are the warnings accompanying this medication? Could this medication be harmful to you?

- What are this medication's side effects? If it causes drowsiness or sleepiness, think twice before putting yourself in a situation where it is important to be alert (such as driving).

- What is the correct dosage? Keep in mind that dosage amounts can vary depending on age and other factors.

- How should the medication be safely stored? Improperly storing a medication may compromise its effectiveness.

Drug Facts

Active ingredient (in each tablet) — **Purpose**
Chlorpheniramine maleate 2 mg..................................Antihistamine

Uses temporarily relieves these symptoms due to hay fever or other upper respiratory allergies: ■ sneezing ■ runny nose ■ itchy, watery eyes ■ itchy throat

Warnings
Ask a doctor before use if you have
■ glaucoma ■ a breathing problem such as emphysema or chronic bronchitis
■ trouble urinating due to an enlarged prostate gland

Ask a doctor or pharmacist before use if you are taking tranquilizers or sedatives

When using this product
■ drowsiness may occur ■ avoid alcoholic drinks
■ alcohol, sedatives, and tranquilizers may increase drowsiness
■ be careful when driving a motor vehicle or operating machinery
■ excitability may occur, especially in children

If pregnant or breast-feeding, ask a health professional before use.
Keep out of reach of children. In case of overdose, get medical help or contact a Poison Control Center right away.

Directions

adults and children 12 years and over	take 2 tablets every 4 to 6 hours; not more than 12 tablets in 24 hours
children 6 years to under 12 years	take 1 tablet every 4 to 6 hours; not more than 6 tablets in 24 hours
children under 6 years	ask a doctor

Other Information ■ store at 20–25°C (68–77°F) ■ protect from excessive moisture

Inactive ingredients D&C yellow no. 10, lactose, magnesium stearate, microcrystalline cellulose, pregelatinized starch

- What should you do if you take an overdose of the drug? The label may offer instructions.

- In addition, look for an expiration date to be sure you are not purchasing or using a medication past its time.

Also, keep all medicines out of sight and reach of children.

Source for drug label: U.S. Department of Health and Human Services, U.S. Food and Drug Administration. (2014). *The new over-the-counter medicine label: Take a look.* www.fda.gov.

Managing Chronic Conditions

If you have a chronic health condition such as diabetes, allergies, or asthma, you'll often be responsible for providing your own routine care. Many people with diabetes, for example, have to monitor their blood glucose levels on a regular basis and use medication such as insulin to manage glucose levels. People with severe allergies—such as to bee stings—need to carry a special injection kit they can use to stop a severe allergic reaction in case of an emergency.

But although the daily management of a chronic condition often falls to the individual, it is important to remember that this type of self-care is never your responsibility alone. Your health-care provider will work with you to develop your care plan. Sometimes, managing a chronic condition can feel isolating and even overwhelming. If you have a chronic condition, seek out regular emotional and medical support. If you know someone with a chronic condition, offer to help and check in with them often.

LO 14.1 QUICK CHECK

Which of the following is NOT an example of a home health test?

a. pregnancy test
b. HIV test
c. colon cancer risk test
d. liver function test

When to See a Doctor

LO 14.2 Explain how to determine when it's time to seek professional health care.

Smart self-care includes knowing when it's time to seek professional help. Many of us call a doctor only when we are extremely sick. However, preventive checkups and exams are also important.

Checkups and Preventive Care

By working with your health-care providers to get regular screenings and checkups, you can prevent problems or catch them early, when they are often far easier to treat. See Table 14.1 for checkup and screening recommendations. Remember to schedule checkups for all aspects of your health, including oral health, vision, and vaccinations. For more information on vaccine recommendations for college students, see Chapter 12.

Health Problems Beyond Self-Care

Obviously, emergency situations require urgent care. Seek an emergency physician for yourself or someone else if any of the following situations arise:[7]

- Severe injuries, such as those sustained in a car accident
- Serious burns
- Sudden, severe pain anywhere
- Adverse reactions to a medication or an insect bite

TABLE 14.1 Recommended Health Screenings

Preventive Service	Who Needs It	How Often	Comments
General Screenings[1,3]			
Blood pressure measurement	All adults	Every 2 years for those with normal blood pressure	Those with elevated blood pressure (over 120/80) need to be under medical care.
Cholesterol measurement	All adults	At least once every 5 years; more often if results indicate risk	
General vision check	All adults	Every 2 years up to age 60; yearly thereafter	People at risk of vision damage or loss should consider starting yearly exams early in life.
Glaucoma screening	People at high risk, including those over 65 who are very nearsighted or diabetic, African Americans over age 40, and those with a family history of the disease	Talk with your vision care specialist	Many eye specialists advise screening all adults starting at age 40 or 50.
Dental checkup	All adults	Check with your dentist	Suggest checkup every 6 months.
Thyroid disease screening	Women aged 50 and older, those with high cholesterol, and those with other risk factors should discuss with their doctor	Check with your doctor	
Cancer Screenings[1]			
Pap test	All women starting at age 21	Between ages 21 and 29, at least every 3 years; between ages 30 and 65, every 5 years; for women over 65 who have had normal screenings for 10 years and are not at elevated risk, not necessary	
Mammogram	All women aged 50 to 75; women with a strong family history of the disease may start screenings earlier	Every 1 to 2 years	Other tests such as MRI may be suggested, depending on risk factors.
Colorectal cancer screening	Everyone aged 50 and over; earlier for those at higher risk, such as those with a family history of the disease	Occult blood test annually, sigmoidoscopy every 5 years; or colonoscopy every 10 years	
Prostate cancer screening	Men aged 50 and over	Digital rectal exam (DRE) yearly, prostate-specific antigen (PSA) on doctor's advice	Check with your doctor about PSA test.
Skin and mole exam	All adults	Check with your doctor	Can be done as part of a regular checkup; those with a personal or family history of skin cancer may also consider regular checkups with a dermatologist.
Vaccines[2]			
Tetanus/diphtheria booster	All adults	Every 10 years	
Influenza vaccine	Everyone aged 65 and over; people at higher risk, such as those with chronic health conditions	Every year in autumn	

TABLE 14.1 Recommended Health Screenings (continued)

Preventive Service	Who Needs It	How Often	Comments
Pneumococcal vaccine	Everyone aged 6 months and over, especially people at increased risk for complications and those who live with or care for others who are at increased risk for complications	Every 5 years	
Rubella vaccine	All women of childbearing age	Once	Avoid during pregnancy.
Hepatitis B vaccine	All young adults, as well as adults at high risk	Check with your doctor	
Meningococcal vaccine (MCV4 or MPSV4)	Includes college freshmen living in a dorm; military recruits; people traveling to or residing in countries where the disease is common	At least once every 5 years but more often if your results indicate risk	Of special concern to students living in high-density housing situations.

Sources: **1.** Centers for Disease Control and Prevention. (2015). *CDC prevention checklist.* www.cdc.gov. **2.** Centers for Disease Control and Prevention. (2015). *Adolescent and adult vaccine quiz.* www.cdc.gov. **3.** American Optometric Association. (n.d.). *Recommended eye examination frequency for pediatric patients and adults.* www.aoa.org.

- Other severe allergic reactions
- Heavy bleeding
- Difficulty breathing
- Signs of a heart attack (for specifics, see Chapter 13)
- Signs of a stroke (for specifics, see Chapter 13)
- Sudden worsening of a chronic health condition, such as diabetes or asthma

Keep in mind that the preceding list covers only some of the situations in which people need emergency care. Use common sense in deciding when a situation requires urgent attention and consult a health professional whenever you're not sure. If you are experiencing symptoms of any type that are severe, persistent, or unusual for you, check with your health-care provider.

Outside of emergencies, it's not always easy to know when a medical condition warrants professional care. *The Merck Manual,* a reputable guide to common health issues, suggests seeking care if any of the following situations arise:[8]

- Vomiting or inability to keep fluids down, painful swallowing, coughing that lasts more than two or three weeks, earache, symptoms that last more than seven days
- Black or bloody stools or more than six to eight watery stools in children (symptomatic of dehydration)
- A feeling that food is stuck in the throat, development of or change in heartburn, especially during exercise, frequent heartburn, persistent or severe abdominal pain, persistent nausea
- Symptoms that prevent participation in usual activities; unexplained weight loss; dizziness; persistent fatigue; sweating, especially heavy or cold sweats
- Severe headache that peaks in intensity within seconds; memory loss or confusion; blurred or double vision; slurred speech; loss of balance or dizziness; seizures; numbness in the arms, face, or legs; nausea
- Rapid or galloping heartbeats (palpitations); chest pain
- Pain in the calves that worsens when walking; swelling in the ankles or legs
- No periods by age 16; sudden stopping of periods; a period that lasts much longer than normal or is excessively heavy; a sudden feeling of illness while using tampons; severe cramps
- Fever of 100.4°F (38°C) or above; a rash that is painful, involves swelling, or oozes
- Swelling or redness in or around an eye; problems with vision
- Moderate or severe abdominal pain; symptoms of dehydration; green, black, or bloody vomit

▶▶ Use the iTriage app, created and reviewed by board-certified medical doctors, to check your symptoms and find nearby medical care. Download it from your app store or find it at **www.itriagehealth.com**.

LO 14.2 QUICK CHECK

Unexplained weight loss is a sign that you should do which of the following?
a. Make an appointment with your doctor.
b. Take a home health test.
c. Go to the emergency room.
d. none of the above

Conventional Medicine

LO 14.3 Discuss the basis of conventional medicine, how to choose a provider, and how to be a smart patient.

Conventional medicine, also called *allopathic medicine,* or *Western medicine,* is the predominant type of care in the U.S. health system. Although conventional medicine includes many complex, fast-developing types of care, a few key features shape its foundation:

- The use of science and the *scientific method.* Evidence-based medicine, which you learned about earlier in this chapter, is just one example of how science underlies all aspects of conventional medicine.

- A focus on physical causes and symptoms. Conventional medicine looks for physical causes of illness, such as injuries or pathogens, and assumes that each illness leads to a set of discernible symptoms that are similar in most people who suffer from that condition.
- An emphasis on physical exams, such as X-rays or blood tests, and physical treatments, such as drugs or surgery, to treat the physical causes of disease.
- A focus on public health. By controlling the spread of the microscopic physical causes of disease through programs such as improved sanitation and vaccination, conventional medicine has vastly improved health and life expectancy in the past century.

Practicing conventional medicine requires many years of education and training and a professional license. Some of the most common types of practitioners of conventional medicine include:

- **Medical doctors (M.D.s)** can either serve as *general practitioners* or *specialists* who focus on a particular type of care.
- **Doctors of osteopathic medicine (D.O.s)** are licensed physicians trained in the same areas of patient care as M.D.s; they also receive training in osteopathic manipulative treatment and usually have a holistic focus in regard to health and treatment.
- **Physician assistants (P.A.s),** also called physician associates, are licensed health professionals who practice under the supervision of a physician and provide a broad range of care.
- **Dentists** hold either doctor of dental surgery (D.D.S.) or doctor of medical dentistry (D.D.M.) degrees and specialize in care of the teeth, gums, and mouth.
- **Optometrists (O.D.s)** examine the eyes and provide vision care.
- **Podiatrists (D.P.M.s)** specialize in care of and surgery for the feet.
- **Nurses,** who may hold an R.N. or other degrees, provide a wide range of health services in many types of health-care settings. They often provide detailed or extensive care in times of greater medical need, such as when a patient is recovering from surgery in the hospital.
- **Nurse practitioners** are R.N.s who have undergone additional training and can perform some of the duties and provide some of the care of a medical doctor (**Figure 14.3** next page).

Where to Find Conventional Health Care

Conventional medicine was once offered primarily through doctor's offices and hospitals, but its availability has since expanded to better meet the needs of patients. The following are examples of facilities that offer conventional care:

- *Student health centers* serve students on campus. Some focus on basic primary care and student health needs, such as minor illnesses and contraception. Others feature a wider range of care, including substance abuse counseling, vision care, pharmacy, and dental services. Few offer emergency services. On most campuses, student health centers are available to all enrolled students, and most of the costs are covered by fees paid as part of student enrollment.
- *Primary care facilities* meet everyday medical needs, seeing patients for checkups, screenings, and minor ailments and providing referrals to more specialized care if needed. Costs are often covered by patient health insurance or a combination of insurance and patient payments.
- *Nonprofit clinics* provide primary care for free or at a reduced cost. They often focus on underserved communities and groups that would otherwise have little access to primary care.
- *Retail clinics,* also known as convenient care clinics, operate out of large stores and pharmacies (**Figure 14.4** on page 360). These clinics are designed to provide basic primary care in a timely manner for people who either don't have a primary care doctor, can't wait for an appointment at a primary care facility, and/or lack health insurance. Costs are lower than they would be at most traditional doctor's offices and are often paid directly by the patient or through insurance.
- *Urgent care centers* typically see patients with illnesses that need immediate attention but don't require the full resources of an emergency department. These centers often see many patients on evenings and weekends, when primary care centers are closed. Although not as expensive as emergency departments, urgent care centers often charge a premium for their services, which can either be covered by insurance or paid directly by the patient.
- *Specialists centers* focus on specific categories of medicine, such as obstetrics, cardiac care, or cancer. Most patients access specialists through referrals from a primary care center. Specialty care is an important part of the medical system but can be quite costly to patients if not covered by insurance.

---

conventional medicine Commonly called Western medicine, a system of care based on the scientific method; the belief that diseases are caused by identifiable physical factors and have a characteristic set of symptoms; and the treatment of physical causes through drugs, surgery, or other interventions.

medical doctor (M.D.) A physician trained in conventional medicine, with many years of additional formal education and training and a professional license.

doctor of osteopathic medicine (D.O) A licensed physician with similar training as an M.D. with additional training in osteopathic manipulative treatment; usually has a holistic focus.

physician assistant (P.A.) A licensed health professional who practices under the supervision of a physician and provides a broad range of care.

dentist (D.D.S.) A conventional medicine practitioner who specializes in care of the teeth, gums, and mouth.

optometrist (O.D.) A licensed professional who provides vision care.

podiatrist (D.P.M.) A licensed professional who specializes in the care of the feet.

nurse A licensed professional who provides a wide range of health-care services and supports the work of medical doctors.

nurse practitioner A registered nurse who has undergone additional training and can perform some of the care provided by a medical doctor.

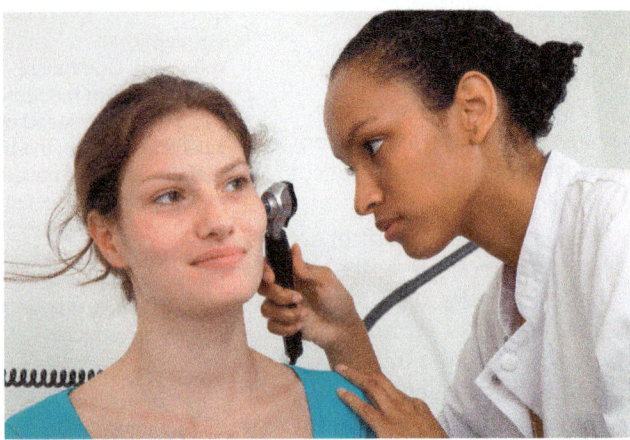

FIGURE 14.3 **Nurse Practitioners.** These health professionals are an example of conventional health care providers.

- *Hospitals* provide the highest level of care. Hospitals handle everything from emergencies to surgeries to complex screenings and cancer treatment. Patients can be seen on an *outpatient* basis, in which they visit the hospital but don't stay overnight, or on an *inpatient* basis, where care is provided for an extended period, including overnight stays.

Choosing a Provider

If you are the age of a traditional college student, you probably haven't had much say in the past over who served as your health-care provider, but at some point you will need to choose a primary care provider. Your primary care provider will see you for checkups and most screenings, answer your basic health questions, treat minor ailments, write prescriptions, and provide referrals for more complex health concerns.

To get started, check two resources—your insurance plan and your friends and family members. If your health insurance limits the providers you can see, start with providers from the plan's list. Then ask your friends and family members for their recommendations.

Once you have a list of providers to contact, start by calling their offices and ask a few questions of a nurse or other office staff:

- Is this provider accepting new patients? Some providers have a full roster and can't take more patients into their practice.
- What insurance plans does this office accept?
- If a physician, is this doctor *board certified*? Board certification means the physician has undergone extra training after medical school to specialize in an area such as family practice.
- How does the office handle lab work? Is there a lab in-house or nearby, or will you have to travel to a different location for a procedure such as a blood test?
- Is this a group practice? If so, will you mostly see your provider, or will you see all the providers in the group? Also if this is a group practice, how many doctors are there, and what are their specialties?
- Who will care for you if your provider is unavailable?
- Is this practice affiliated with any hospitals or specialty centers?

When you meet your provider in person, make sure that he or she listens to you, encourages you to ask questions, answers your questions completely, and treats you with respect. If you don't feel comfortable with a provider, shop around until you do.

Being a Smart Patient

Once you've chosen a provider, your visits will be more productive if you think of your provider as a partner. Your provider has the expertise to help you improve your health, but his or her work will be more effective if you are actively and constructively engaged in the process. In addition, it's important that you actively communicate with your doctor to help reduce the risk of medical errors.

Here are some suggestions from the American Academy of Family Physicians for how to get the most out of a medical appointment[9]:

- **Talk to your provider.** Be sure to tell your care provider any past or current health issues or concerns, even if they are embarrassing. Many medical appointments are only 15 minutes long, so effective communication is key to helping your doctor treat you.
- **Ask questions.** Let your provider know if you don't understand something. If you need more time to discuss an issue, be vocal about it.
- **Take information home with you.** Take notes during your appointment, ask your provider for handouts, or ask the office to supply background or reference materials.
- **Follow up with your provider.** Follow the instructions you receive, such as getting additional tests or seeing a specialist. If you've been given a new medication and feel worse or have problems with the drug, let your provider know right away. If you took a test and haven't received the results, let your provider's office know.

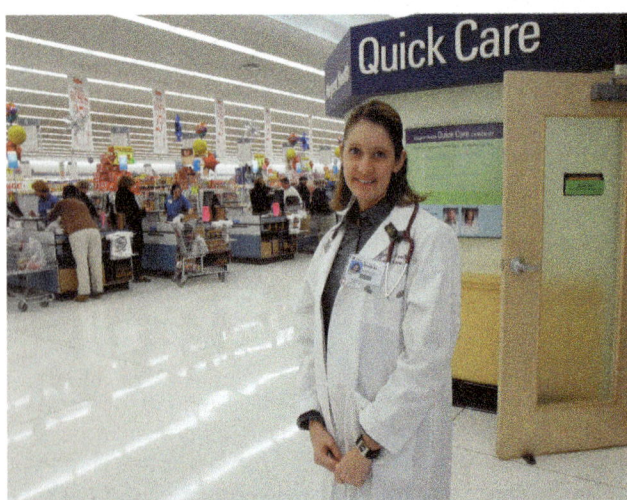

FIGURE 14.4 **Health Services Locations.** Large retail stores sometimes offer health services.

- **Help prevent medical errors through active communication.** While it's up to your medical team to provide high-quality care, you can help reduce the risk of medical errors through proactive communication. Let your provider know all the medicines, supplements, and other substances you may be taking (including alcohol) to help prevent risky drug interactions. Be proactive about sharing information with all members of your medical team, especially if you have more than one caregiver. Make sure you understand the side effects of any medication you are prescribed. If you are being discharged from care, make sure you understand any follow-up treatments to be done at home.

Many health-care providers and organizations offer information on your rights as a patient. While these rights vary from state to state and in regard to different types of providers, here are some basic patient rights, as outlined by the American Hospital Association:[10]

- **High-quality hospital care.** You have the right to receive the care you need, provided with compassion, skill, and respect.
- **A clean and safe environment.** Procedures should be in place to help prevent medical errors and reduce risks of complications such as infection.
- **Involvement in your care.** Your providers should discuss treatment options with you and actively communicate with you about your medical history, health-care goals, and personal values.
- **Protection of your privacy.** Providers should follow established policies and guidelines that protect the privacy of your personal health information.
- **Help when leaving the hospital.** You may need further support, such as medications, physical therapy, follow-up appointments, or other care. Your health-care team should make sure that you have a plan in place and know how to follow it.
- **Help with the medical claims process.** Health insurance and medical bills can be confusing. Your providers should help you by submitting accurate insurance claims and answering billing questions.

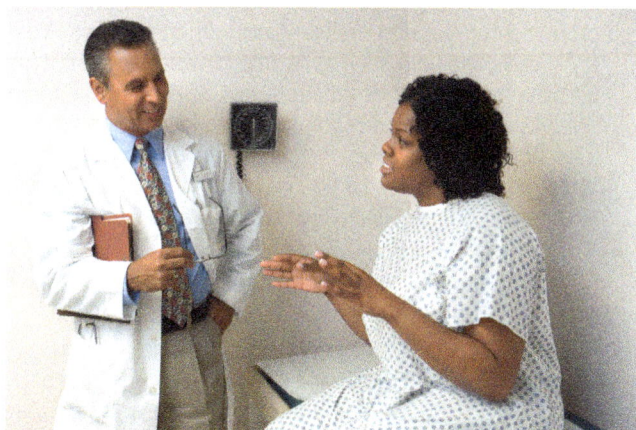

Ask your care provider questions to be sure you understand your care needs.

Handling Prescription Medications Properly

Prescription medications, which can only be obtained legally by receiving a prescription, or written order, from a health-care provider, cover a vast range of therapies, including everything from heart medication and painkillers to breathing aids and antibiotics. These medicines are typically more potent than OTC drugs—and also carry greater risks. Because prescription medications are powerful, it is especially important to use them properly. Unfortunately, some college students don't always follow the directions for taking prescription medications. In one recent survey, almost 14% of college students said they had taken a prescription medication not prescribed to them.[11]

Of special concern are prescription opioid painkillers. The rates of use and abuse of these medications have skyrocketed in recent years. Between 1999 and 2010, there was a fourfold increase in the amount of prescription painkillers such as oxycodone and codeine sold to pharmacies, hospitals, and doctors' offices.[12] The growing use of these opioid painkillers has led to huge increases in their misuse. Prescription painkillers often wind up in the hands of people who have become addicted or who were not prescribed them. The medications are especially dangerous when mixed with other prescription drugs, such as sleep aids or anti-anxiety medicines.[13] Because of this dangerous brew, prescription drugs are now the leading cause of drug overdose deaths in the United States, including more than 28,700 deaths in 2014.[14] As you learned in Chapter 8, some people who are addicted to prescription opioids eventually turn to heroin, an illegal opioid with extremely dangerous risks of its own.

To take prescription painkillers and other prescription drugs safely, be sure to do the following:[15]

- Use prescription drugs only as directed by a health-care provider. Don't take prescription medications that are not prescribed to you.
- Be sure you are the only one to use your prescription drugs. Don't share or sell them.
- Never take larger or more frequent doses of your medications, particularly prescription painkillers, to try to get faster or more powerful effects.
- Don't mix prescription painkillers with other medications unless specifically directed to do so by your physician.
- Store prescription painkillers in a secure place and dispose of them properly. For suggestions on medication disposal, see www.fda.gov/ForConsumers/ConsumerUpdates/ucm101653.htm.
- Get help for substance abuse problems, if needed.

LO 14.3 QUICK CHECK

A health-care practitioner with an O.D. degree is trained to provide

a. nursing care.
b. osteopathic medicine.
c. optometry and vision care.
d. dermatologic care.

Complementary and Alternative Medicine (CAM)

LO 14.4 Describe common types of complementary and alternative medicine and how to evaluate them.

Conventional medicine can be very effective, but it has limits. Conventional medicine's focus on physical ailments after they arise may sometimes overlook preventive steps and care that could have warded off illness. Some people are interested in health practices that take a broader, more holistic approach, looking beyond the body to include the mind and spirit as well.

These interests have led to the growth of **complementary and alternative medicine (CAM).** The term *alternative medicine* is used to refer to those practices and traditions not typically part of conventional Western medicine, including everything from herbal remedies and meditation to chiropractors and traditional Chinese medicine. *Complementary medicine,* also sometimes referred to as *integrative medicine,* refers to care combining conventional and alternative medicine. Many of us routinely practice complementary medicine without realizing it, perhaps trying an herbal remedy to treat a cold and seeing a traditional doctor for a serious injury. For a glimpse at how many college students use CAM, see the **Student Stats** box.

> **complementary and alternative medicine (CAM)** Health practices and traditions not typically part of conventional Western medicine, either used alone (alternative medicine) or in conjunction with conventional medicine (complementary medicine).

Alternative medicine has become such a common part of our approach to health that federal health officials now discuss and study it in a scientific way, and many states now require some CAM practitioners to be licensed. The National Center for Complementary and Alternative Medicine (NCCAM) groups CAM into five major domains:[16]

- *Whole medical systems* are built on theories and systems encompassing the totality of a person's health. These systems have typically evolved apart from and earlier than conventional Western medicine. Traditional Chinese medicine is a prime example (**Figure 14.5**).

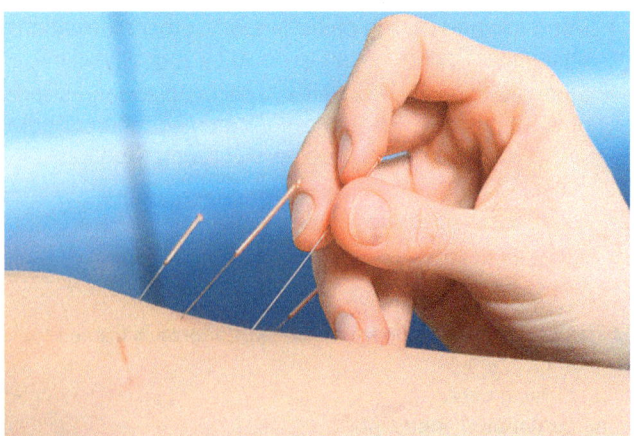

FIGURE 14.5 **Acupuncture.** A type of traditional Chinese medicine, acupuncture is an example of alternative health care.

STUDENT STATS

CAM Use Among College Students

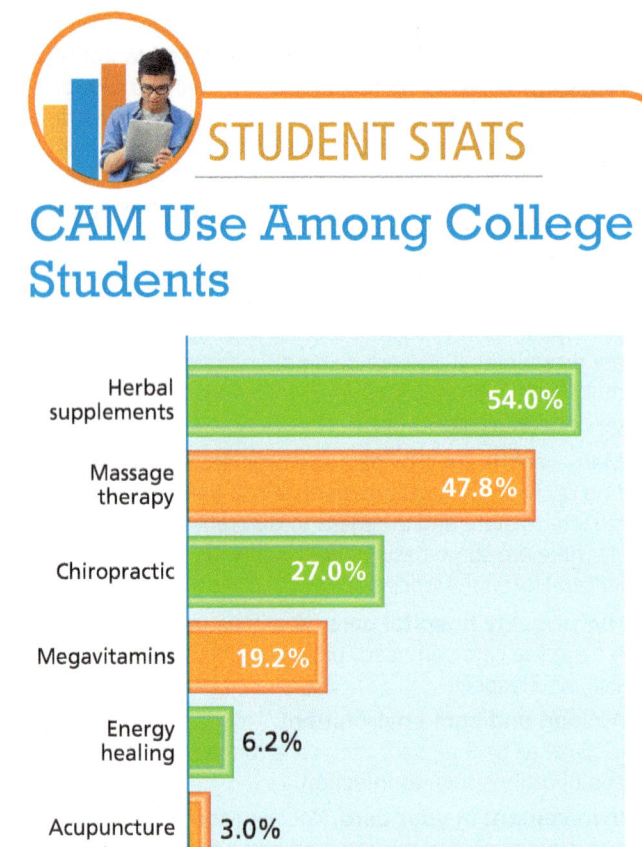

- Herbal supplements: 54.0%
- Massage therapy: 47.8%
- Chiropractic: 27.0%
- Megavitamins: 19.2%
- Energy healing: 6.2%
- Acupuncture: 3.0%

Percentage of students using in the past year

Data from LaCaille, R. A., & Kuvaas, N. J. (2011). Coping styles and self-regulation predict complementary and alternative medicine and herbal supplement use among college students. *Psychology, Health & Medicine, 16*(3).

- *Mind–body medicine* uses techniques designed to boost the mind's capacity to affect the body. Some of these techniques are now considered part of Western medicine, such as patient support groups. Others, such as prayer or meditation, are still considered CAM.
- *Natural products* rely on substances found in nature, such as vitamins and herbs. These practices focus on using plant-derived medicines called botanicals, dietary supplements, and sometimes even beneficial microbes such as probiotics to treat disorders ranging from the common cold to serious conditions such as depression and cancer. But just because these therapies are "natural" does not make them safe. As with any other medication, natural remedies may have side effects or dangerous interactions with other medicines, especially when taken in large amounts. (For more information on using supplements safely, see Chapter 5.)
- *Manipulative and body-based practices* are based on physical manipulation of the body and include therapies such as chiropractic medicine and massage.
- *Energy therapies* involve interaction with energy fields. These include biofield therapies, believed by practitioners to surround the body, and bio-electromagnetic–based therapies involving the alternative use of electromagnetic fields.

For a more detailed look at some of the better-known CAM practices, see **Table 14.2** on pages 363–364.

TABLE 14.2 Common Types of Complementary and Alternative Medicine

Practice	Description	Common Use	Risks	Scientific Evaluation
Acupuncture	This ancient system revolves around the concept of the free flow of qi (pronounced "chee"), or energy, through the body. Illness is believed to occur when qi is blocked or disrupted. Practitioners restore and rebalance qi not only to treat illness but to prevent it and increase overall energy.	Thin needles are inserted at key qi points in the body to balance or restore energy flow. A related technique, acupressure, uses firm touch at key energy points. In addition to being a common part of overall traditional Chinese care, acupuncture has also been used in Western settings for everything from pain relief to reducing nausea during cancer treatment.	Acupuncture appears to have relatively few side effects, although problems can arise when needles are not used or sterilized correctly.	Acupuncture appears to be effective in treating chronic pain, in treating women's health disorders such as PMS or painful periods, and in easing side effects of cancer care.[1]
Homeopathy	Homeopathy is based on the assumption that "like cures like." That is, a substance that produces symptoms or illness is thought to cure or alleviate symptoms of that same illness, if administered in very diluted quantities.	Homeopathy is used in an attempt to treat common health problems such as nausea, sinus infections, and fever.	Given the very diluted levels at which homeopathic substances are usually used, few side effects have been reported.	Several large studies have found that the practice offers no significant effect for any health condition.[2]
Naturopathy	Naturopathy incorporates traditional therapies and techniques from all over the world, from herbs to dietary changes and exercise, with an emphasis on supporting health rather than treating disease.	Naturopathy is especially popular with some people interested in an overall health approach that promotes wellness and prevents illness.	Some treatments, such as herbs, can have drug interactions and other side effects.	According to the NCCAM, scientific studies of the effectiveness of naturopathy are still preliminary.[3]
Ayurveda	One of the world's oldest medical systems, Ayurveda originated in India. It aims to integrate and balance the body, mind, and spirit to help prevent illness and promote wellness.	Ayurvedic medicine uses a variety of products and techniques to cleanse the body and restore balance. People who use Ayurveda, either on its own or in conjunction with conventional medicine, often choose it in the belief that it will help cleanse their body of harmful substances and energies and help restore vitality and overall health.	Some of the herbal and dietary substances, along with other practices meant to cleanse the digestive tract, can have drug interactions if used with conventional medicine, as well as other side effects. One NCCAM study of Ayurvedic medications found that some contained toxins such as mercury or lead.[4]	According to the NCCAM, scientific studies of the effectiveness of Ayurveda are still preliminary, and more research is needed.[4]
Natural products	These approaches focus on using herbs, other plant-derived medicines called *botanicals*, and dietary supplements to treat various conditions.	Botanicals, herbs, and supplements are used in an attempt to treat conditions ranging from the common cold to serious conditions such as depression and cancer. *Echinacea*, or coneflower, for example, is popularly used to treat colds and upper respiratory infections.	This group of alternative therapies is among the most risky, as these substances have the potential for harm if taken in high doses or for long periods of time, or if they interact badly with conventional drugs. For example, one botanical, *ephedra*, is now banned in the United States because of its harmful side effects.	Studies have found that these therapies have varying levels of usefulness, and physicians say that more research is needed on this broad and often popular CAM category.
Mind–body medicine	Mind–body medicines rely on the connection between the mental and physical realms and seek to create a more positive interaction between the two. Guided imagery, yoga, and meditation are popular forms of mind–body medicine.	Mind–body techniques are used to help prevent illness by reducing factors such as stress, and to help treat disorders such as depression, anxiety, and insomnia. These therapies are also sometimes used to support cancer patients by reducing patient anxiety, isolation, and stress.	Most mind–body therapies are considered relatively safe, although more strenuous forms, such as very active yoga, carry some risk of injury.	Some studies show some benefit, but most scientists caution that research is still preliminary. One study of the efficacy of meditation as a treatment for a variety of illnesses found some benefit but cautioned that more research remains to be done.[5]
Manipulative therapies	Manipulative therapies are remedies that focus on moving, stretching, or realigning sections of the body. These therapies focus on restoring overall wellness by correcting parts of the body that are out of alignment.	These techniques are often used to treat stiffness and pain. Chiropractic medicine, which focuses on structure and connections of joints and muscles, is an especially popular form.	Any intense physical manipulation of the body, especially of the spine, can be very dangerous, especially if a practitioner lacks training.	When administered correctly, chiropractic medicine has been shown to be effective for joint and bone pain, such as low back pain.[6]

TABLE 14.2 Common Types of Complementary and Alternative Medicine (continued)

Practice	Description	Common Use	Risks	Scientific Evaluation
Energy therapies	These forms of treatment focus on fields of energy originating within the body (biofields) or from external sources (electromagnetic fields). Changing or increasing the flow of the fields of energy, practitioners say, can have a variety of health benefits. Qigong, a movement-based component of traditional Chinese medicine, and magnet therapy are examples of energy treatments.	Energy fields are used for a variety of reasons, including stress reduction, pain relief, and improvement of cardiac health.	Risks appear to be relatively minor.	Research indicates that qigong may help improve balance and reduce pain.[7] One large analysis of the efficacy of qigong in reducing high blood pressure, for example, found some encouraging evidence but cautioned that further study is needed.[8]

Sources: 1. National Center for Complementary and Integrative Health. (2016). *Acupuncture: In depth.* https://nccih.nih.gov. 2. National Center for Complementary and Integrative Health. (2015). *Homoeopathy.* https://nccih.nih.gov. 3. National Center for Complementary and Integrative Health. (2016). *Naturopathy.* https://nccih.nih.gov. 4. National Center for Complementary and Integrative Health. (2016). *Ayurvedic medicine: In depth.* https://nccih.nih.gov. 5. Arias, A., Steinberg, K., Banga, A., & Trestman, R. (2006). Systematic review of the efficacy of meditation techniques as treatments for mental illness. *The Journal of Alternative and Complementary Medicine, 12*(8), 817–832. 6. Chou, R., Qaseem, A., Snow, V., Casey, D., Shekelle, K., et al. (2007). Diagnosis and treatment of low back pain: A joint clinical practice guideline from the American College of Physicians and the American Pain Society. *Annals of Internal Medicine, 147*(7), 478–491. 7. National Center for Complementary and Integrative Health. (2015). *Tai chi and qi gong: In depth.* https://nccih.nih.gov. 8. Lee, M., Pittler, R., Guo, M., & Ernst, E. (2007). Qigong for hypertension: A systematic review of randomized clinical trials. *Journal of Hypertension, 25*(8), 1525–1532.

Evaluating Complementary and Alternative Therapies

As you can see in Table 14.2, the effectiveness of many CAM therapies is still being studied, and research is inconclusive for many of these practices. If you are considering a CAM therapy, either on your own or through a practitioner, the NCCAM offers the following suggestions:[17]

- Be an informed consumer. Investigate the scientific evidence about any therapy's safety and effectiveness.
- Be aware that individuals respond differently to treatments, whether conventional or CAM. How a person might respond to a CAM therapy depends on many things, including the person's state of health, how the therapy is used, and the person's belief in the therapy.
- Keep in mind that "natural" does not necessarily mean "safe." (Think of mushrooms that grow in the wild; some are safe to eat, others are not.)
- Learn about factors that affect safety. For a CAM therapy that is administered by a practitioner, these factors include the training, skill, and experience of the practitioner. For a CAM product such as a dietary supplement, the specific ingredients and the quality of the manufacturing process are important factors.
- Tell all your health-care providers about any CAM practices you use. This will help ensure coordinated and safe care.

If you are considering using a CAM practitioner, the following guidelines, adapted from the NCCAM, may help:[18]

- Speak with your primary health-care provider regarding the therapy in which you are interested. Ask if he or she has a recommendation for the type of CAM practitioner you are seeking. If your provider isn't able to offer a recommendation, research reputable CAM practitioners using professional association websites and other credible sources.
- Make a list of CAM practitioners and gather information about each one before making your first visit. Ask basic questions about their credentials and practice. Where did they receive their training? What licenses or certifications do they have? How much will the treatment cost? How many treatments will be required to derive a benefit?
- Check with your insurer to see if the cost of therapy will be covered.
- After you select a practitioner, make a list of questions to ask at your first visit.
- Go to the first visit prepared to answer questions about your health history, as well as prescription medicines, vitamins, and other supplements you may take.
- Assess your first visit and decide whether the practitioner is right for you. Did you feel comfortable with the practitioner? Could the practitioner answer your questions? Does the treatment plan seem reasonable and acceptable to you?

LO 14.4 QUICK CHECK

Which of the following correctly describes supplements marked as "natural"?

a. always safe
b. certified as free of synthetic chemicals
c. plant-based
d. none of the above

Paying for Health Care

LO 14.5 Identify multiple methods of paying for health care.

In the United States, we are surrounded by highly advanced medical care—at a steep price. Our system is among the most expensive in the world, and our country spends the most on health as a percentage of gross domestic product.[19] According to the nonprofit California Health Care Foundation, health spending reached nearly $3 trillion in 2014,[20] or about $9,523 per person,[20] and costs for all of us continue to rise each year.[20] In 2015, the average annual cost for family insurance coverage obtained through work reached $17,545, a 68% increase from the $10,880 cost a decade earlier. In addition, each family's share of those costs climbed as well, with families picking up $4,995 of that price tag, compared with $2,713 in 2005.[21] Despite a rapidly changing insurance landscape, due in part to the national health-care reforms driven by the Affordable Care Act, insurance costs have held to a fairly stable rate of growth for the past decade, averaging about a 3% to 5% increase per year.[20]

As a student, you likely have access to basic care through your student health center, with costs covered by fees you pay as part of student enrollment. You may still be on your family's insurance plan, or your campus may offer a free or low-cost health insurance plan for students. No matter your coverage, it's important to understand what you need to pay for out of your own pocket.

Discount Programs

Does your student health center cover the cost of your prescriptions? If not, does it offer a program with nearby pharmacies that lets you fill your prescriptions at a reduced price? If so, you are taking part in a **health discount program.** These programs are increasingly offered by employers and large institutions that want to provide some level of assistance with medical costs but don't want to pay for full insurance. Discount programs typically offer prices from 5% to 25% lower than average, although some programs for students may provide deeper discounts.

Health Insurance

At its essence, **health insurance** is your buffer against medical costs. A health insurance policy is a contract between an insurance company and an individual or a group, in which the insurer agrees to cover a defined set of medical costs if the insured party pays a defined price. Insurers either pay your health-care providers directly or reimburse you for covered health-care expenses, although almost all plans limit the types of care covered. Although many plans cover primary care, for example, they may offer little or no coverage for services such as mental health services, substance abuse programs, or physical therapy. Alternative medicine is rarely covered. Many plans also restrict which doctors you can see and may place rules on seeing specialists. A few plans may refuse or limit your coverage if you already have an illness, or a **preexisting condition,** although this restriction has been gradually phased out because of national health-care reforms. Under the Affordable Care Act, people with preexisting medical issues cannot be denied health insurance when purchasing or joining a new insurance plan.

When it comes to paying for health insurance, there are several concepts you should understand: premiums, copays, and deductibles. A **premium** is the amount you pay an insurance company for an insurance policy. Premiums are usually charged monthly, and the amount of a premium depends on the level of health insurance benefits offered, your age, any preexisting conditions you may have, certain lifestyle habits (such as smoking), and even your sex.

A **copay** (copayment) is a flat fee charged at the time you receive a medical service or a medication. Copays are set at the time an insurance policy is offered, so before committing to an insurance policy, check the copay amount, which should be explicitly stated in the policy. Copays can vary widely with different policies and are usually set higher when the premium is lower.

A **deductible** is the total amount of out-of-pocket health-care expenses that a patient must pay before the health insurance begins to cover health-care costs. For example, if the deductible for your health insurance is $3,000, and you are in an accident that results in $20,000 in health-care costs, you must pay $3,000 out of pocket before your health insurance kicks in for the remainder of the bill. Deductibles are reset each year. As with copays, the amount of your deductible will be explicitly stated in the insurance policy, and deductibles are usually set higher when the premium for the policy is lower.

Insurance plans come in many forms. Some are created for groups, such as collections of people who work at the same company. Others are created for individuals who buy their insurance directly from an insurance company or through one of the Affordable Care Act's health insurance marketplaces. Common types of policies available to individuals and groups include *managed-care plans, public programs,* and *fee-for-service plans.*

> **health discount program** A system of health discounts given to members of groups, such as employees of a particular company or students attending a particular college.
>
> **health insurance** A contract between an insurance company and a group or an individual who pays a fee to have some level of health-care costs covered by the insurer.
>
> **preexisting condition** A health issue that existed prior to application to or enrollment in a health insurance plan.
>
> **premium** An amount paid to an insurance company for an insurance policy, usually in monthly installments.
>
> **copay** A flat fee charged at the time of a medical service or when receiving a medication.
>
> **deductible** The total amount of out-of-pocket health-care expenses that a patient must pay before health insurance begins to cover health-care costs.
>
> **managed-care plan** A type of health insurance in which the insurer contracts with a defined network of providers, which the consumer must use or face higher out-of-pocket costs.
>
> **health maintenance organization (HMO)** A type of managed care plan in which most health care is funneled through and must be approved by the primary care doctor.

>> Not sure what to look for in a health insurance policy? Consumer Reports can help: Go to **www.consumerreports.org/** and search for "Health Insurance Buying Guide."

Managed-Care Plans

Managed-care plans offer you lower costs but also less choice. In a managed-care plan, insurers have contracts with particular doctors, hospitals, and other health-care providers, and you must often limit your visits to these caregivers or face additional expense. Most people with employer-based insurance are in one of three types of managed-care plans:

- **HMOs,** or **health maintenance organizations,** restrict choice the most—requiring that all care be funneled

> STUDENT STORY

The Cost of Being Uninsured

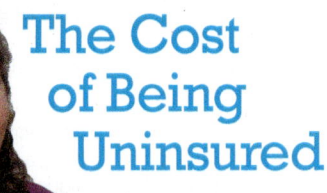

"MY NAME IS HOLLY. I am 45 years old. I was a single parent for about 12 years. I could not afford insurance for myself—it just wasn't in my budget. My kids always came first. If I got sick, I stayed at home and took care of myself. One time I had really bad abdominal pain and did not go to see the doctor because I didn't have any insurance. It got so bad that I couldn't stand up. I had to go to the emergency room and they did emergency surgery on me. My gall bladder had ruptured and the poison from that went through my system. I ended up being in the hospital for five days because of that. If I had gone to the doctor sooner, they would have caught it sooner. My doctor's bill ended up being a little over $12,000. That's a lot of money for a single mom."

What Do You Think?

1. Holly is a nontraditional-aged college student. What are some health insurance options that may be available to her now that she is in school?
2. Does your campus offer any health insurance options for students over age 26? If so, what are they?
3. What percentage of your income do you think you'll spend on medical care after you graduate? How do you plan to cover that cost?

through and managed by the primary care provider—but also usually cost the consumer the least.

- **PPOs,** or **preferred provider organizations,** offer more choice by letting the consumer see a wider range of providers without a referral but also usually carry a higher cost to the consumer.
- **POSs,** or **point-of-service plans,** offer some HMO members greater flexibility by letting them see outside physicians for an additional fee.

Managed-care plans can also be purchased on the individual insurance market or through one of the Affordable Care Act's health insurance exchanges. The price for such coverage varies, based on the selected level of coverage and how many people in your household are to be covered.

Public Programs

Public health insurance programs provide government-sponsored coverage for individuals and families who could otherwise not afford health coverage. These plans usually operate in a way similar to managed care, funneling services through primary care clinics whenever possible. Common types of public insurance include **Medicaid,** usually offered to low-income individuals and families through joint state–federal sponsorship; **Medicare,** a federal program that covers many health costs for Americans with certain disabilities or who are age 65 or older; and state and local children's health programs.

Fee-for-Service Plans

Fee-for-service plans allow you to use any medical provider you choose and then submit a bill to your insurance company, which pays part of it, leaving you to cover the rest. Many insurers offer a special version to younger people who may be out of college and find themselves without health insurance. These so-called **mini-med plans** often come at a more affordable monthly price than other types of individual coverage and pay for some health basics, such as primary care and trips to the emergency department. But they often don't cover other types of care, such as prenatal care and childbirth. If you are considering a mini-med plan, make sure you understand what the plan doesn't cover and see whether its limits fit your life for the next few years before you buy.

preferred provider organization (PPO) A type of managed care plan in which the consumer is encouraged to stay within an approved network of providers but can obtain care outside the network.

point-of-service (POS) plan A type of managed care plan that lets HMO members see a broader list of providers for an additional fee.

Medicaid A joint federal–state insurance program that covers low-income individuals and families.

Medicare A federal insurance program that covers people with long-term disabilities and individuals age 65 and older.

fee-for-service plan A type of health insurance in which you choose your providers, and you and your insurer divide the costs of care.

mini-med plan A type of managed-care plan, sold individually to younger people, which carries lower costs but does not cover many services.

Health Insurance and the Affordable Care Act

Major national reforms driven by the Affordable Care Act have made it easier for some people to afford health insurance. Beginning in 2014, many states and the federal government created "health insurance exchanges," in which people can shop for individual policies at competitive rates. See the **Special Feature.**

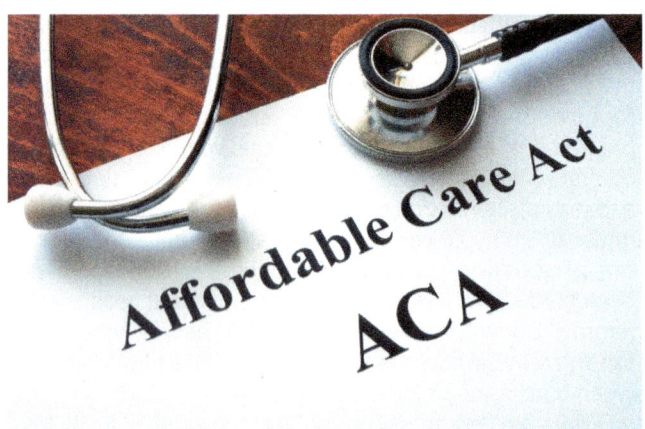

The Affordable Care Act, passed in 2010, remains a politically controversial issue even as it has helped bring health insurance to millions of Americans.

SPECIAL FEATURE

What the Affordable Care Act Means for You

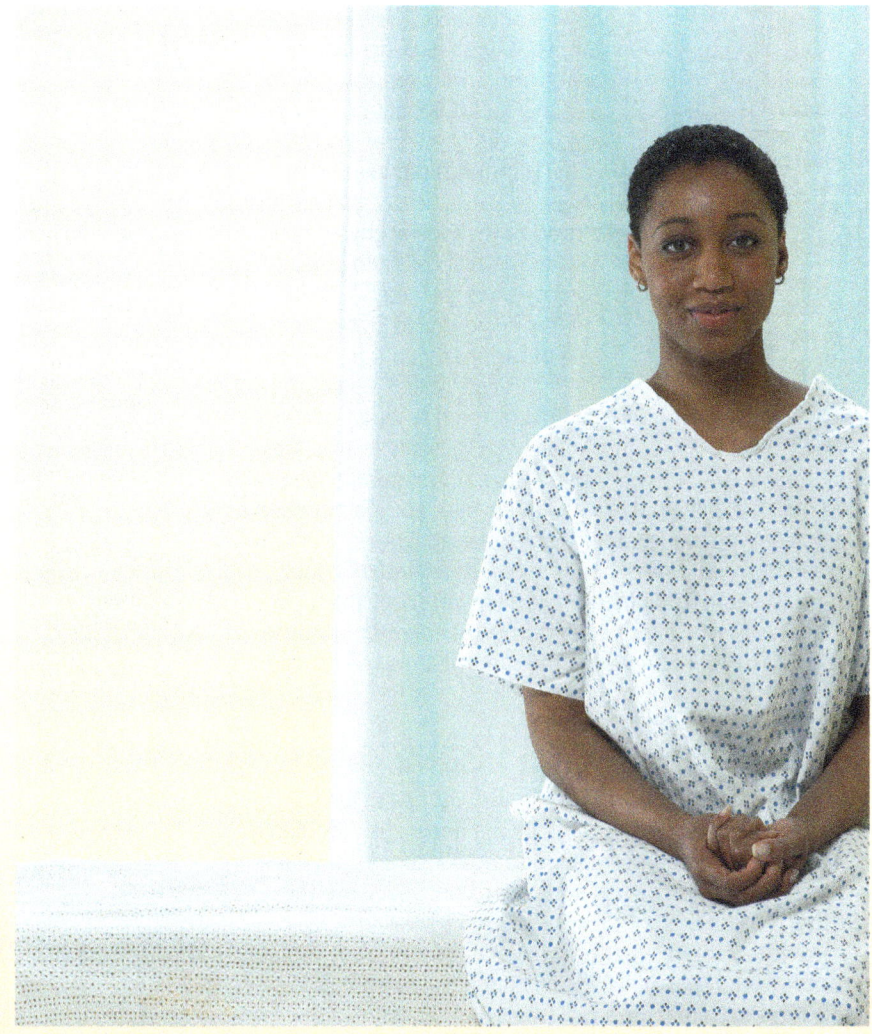

The Affordable Care Act, designed to increase health-care access for millions of Americans, has been in effect for almost a decade. The ACA remains the subject of political debate, and its application varies based on state decisions regarding health insurance marketplaces and Medicaid policies. However, many reforms are in place and are making a real difference for students and young adults. Here are some highlights:

- **For young adults, the magic number is 26.** You can now stay on a parent's insurance plan until your 26th birthday, if you and your parent so choose.[1]

- **A new requirement that many Americans be insured or pay a penalty.** This feature of the law, known as the "individual mandate," requires most Americans to have at least minimal health insurance to cover emergencies and serious conditions. The penalty for not having coverage went into effect in 2016, often equaling a fee of $695 per year for a single adult. However, some people are exempt from this requirement, including members of some religious groups and single people under age 65 who earn less than $10,000 a year.[2]

- **Health insurance exchanges.** To help Americans afford the cost of insurance being required by the individual mandate, these insurance marketplaces are intended to create large pools of insured individuals and small businesses, enabling them to compare health plans and enroll at a lower cost than would be possible if they sought insurance independently. Individuals and small companies have typically faced higher prices and other restrictions in the insurance market, and the exchanges are intended to reduce disparities and improve access to affordable coverage. Exchanges are already available in some states, with 24 states offering their own exchanges as of early 2016.[3] If you live in a state that doesn't operate its own marketplace, you can purchase coverage via the federal marketplace.

- **Better protections for people with preexisting conditions.** Children and adults enrolling in new private insurance plans, such as those offered through an employer, cannot be denied coverage because of preexisting conditions.[4]

- **Get sick, stay insured.** Health plans cannot cut off coverage if a person becomes sick, a practice known as rescission.[4]

- **No lifetime limits.** Insurers cannot place a lifetime cap on the insurance benefits you receive.[4]

- **Guaranteed coverage for women's health.** Certain preventive health services for women, including FDA-approved contraceptives, cervical cancer and HIV screenings, mammograms, and well-woman checkups, are now offered to women in newly created health plans without any out-of-pocket cost. Under the ACA, women are shielded from having to pay more for insurance than men.[4]

>> Learn more about the Affordable Care Act, including details about options for you, at **www.healthcare.gov**.

Sources: **1.** Health care.gov. (n.d.). *How to get or stay on a parent's plan.* www.healthcare.gov. **2.** Healthcare.gov. (n.d.). *The fee for not having health insurance.* www.healthcare.gov. **3.** Henry J. Kaiser Family Foundation. (2016). *State health insurance marketplace types, 2016.* http://kff.org. **4.** Office of Speaker Nancy Pelosi. (2010, May 3). *Affordable health care for America: Key provisions that take effect immediately.* http://docs.house.gov.

Health Savings Accounts and Flexible Spending Accounts

Special savings accounts can help you maximize your health dollars. Two of the most common are **health savings accounts (HSAs)** and medical **flexible spending accounts (FSAs)**.

HSAs can be offered through an employer, or individuals can set them up through a bank, an insurance company, or another trustee. HSAs were developed for people with high-deductible health insurance plans as a way to give them a tax benefit on savings accounts designated for medical costs. HSA funds can be used to cover medical expenses that are approved by the federal government, such as medical visits and prescription costs. An estimated 15% of families in the United States use this type of savings account to help pay for health-care costs.[22]

FSAs, offered through employers, allow employees to save pre-tax dollars to cover certain medical and health expenses. Unlike with an HSA, you do not need a particular type of insurance plan to use an FSA. To withdraw money from your FSA to pay for health-related expenses, you must show receipts to prove that you spent the funds for allowed medical or health purposes. You also must use the funds in your FSA within the same year as you contribute them, or you will lose them.

health savings account (HSA) A consumer-controlled savings account that can be used with a high-deductible health insurance plan to cover health-care costs not covered by insurance.

flexible spending account (FSA) A consumer-controlled account, usually offered through employers, that uses pre-tax dollars to cover approved health-related purchases.

Students and Health Insurance

Most college students have some form of health insurance, and the coverage picture is improving under the Affordable Care Act. For more information on how insurance availability has changed for young adults in recent years, see the **Student Stats** box.

However, improvements in rates of insurance for students do not mean that every college student is covered. Some states, for example, have not created their own health-care exchanges as part of the Affordable Care Act, or have not expanded state-level Medicaid coverage for low-income adults. These gaps, particularly in states that have opted not to expand Medicaid, left about 2.9 million adults under the age of 65 without insurance in 2016, and almost half those people were between the ages of 19 and 34.[23]

Even if you have insurance, no policy will cover all your health-care costs. See **Practical Strategies** for ideas about how to find health care that won't put you in debt.

What Happens When I Graduate?

When it's time to get your diploma, what happens to your health insurance? Students going straight to graduate school or a job offering health insurance may have little or no gap in their coverage. But if you face going without coverage for any length of time, you'll need to take steps to protect yourself.

If you have insurance through your parents, that coverage can continue until you reach age 26. If you have health insurance through your school, that coverage often ends around the time of your graduation. If you are covered through a public program, your insurance is less likely to be tied to your student status, but find out for sure.

When your coverage ends, you'll likely have options to extend it—but at a high price. College and university policies can often be extended, but the cost will likely be at least double the cost of the original premium. For example, if your campus policy costs $1,200 per year, you are likely to pay at least $2,400 per year for the extension. You may be able to

STUDENT STATS

An Improving Insurance Picture for Young American Adults

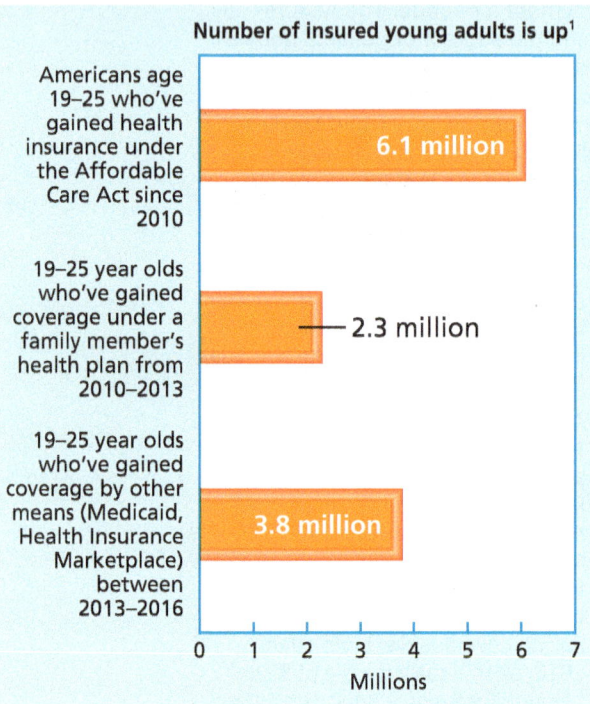

Number of insured young adults is up[1]

- Americans age 19–25 who've gained health insurance under the Affordable Care Act since 2010: **6.1 million**
- 19–25 year olds who've gained coverage under a family member's health plan from 2010–2013: **2.3 million**
- 19–25 year olds who've gained coverage by other means (Medicaid, Health Insurance Marketplace) between 2013–2016: **3.8 million**

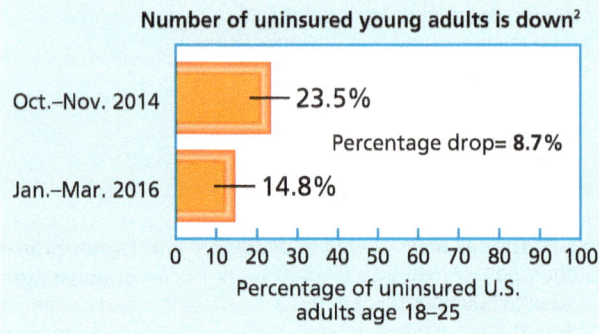

Number of uninsured young adults is down[2]

- Oct.–Nov. 2014: 23.5%
- Jan.–Mar. 2016: 14.8%
- Percentage drop = 8.7%

Percentage of uninsured U.S. adults age 18–25

Source: **1.** U.S. Department of Health and Human Services. (2016, March 3). *20 million people have gained health insurance coverage because of the Affordable Care Act, new estimates show.* www.hhs.gov. **2.** Gallup, Inc. (2016, April 7). *U.S. uninsured rate at 11.0%, lowest in eight-year trend.* www.gallup.com.

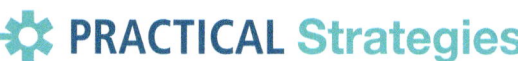

PRACTICAL Strategies

Tips for Affordable Health Care

No form of health-care coverage will pay for every penny of your health-care costs. To help ensure that you don't wind up with medical bills that you can't afford, keep these strategies in mind:

- If you have your own insurance, make sure you understand the basic limits of the policy. How much do you have to pay in deductibles? What copays or other out-of-pocket payments are you responsible for? Does your insurance restrict your care geographically? Does it have a separate prescription plan? What services or providers are excluded? Does it stop covering you when you reach a certain age? What are the rules on visiting a hospital in an emergency? Make sure you keep a current copy of your insurance card, which you'll need to show medical providers when you receive care.

- Learn about what services are offered at your college's student health center. If a service isn't provided, ask about discount arrangements the center may have with other providers. Student health centers may have arrangements with local pharmacies, dentists, and other types of health providers.

- Avoid heading to the emergency department or calling an ambulance unless you truly require emergency attention. Although emergency departments are required to treat all patients who enter their doors seeking help (even patients with minor illnesses who don't have insurance), the care they provide is expensive, and you may be billed directly. For less serious ailments, you can often receive the care you need at a much lower price from a community or retail clinic.

- Take care of your health preventively, which will help reduce the amount and cost of medical care you may need.

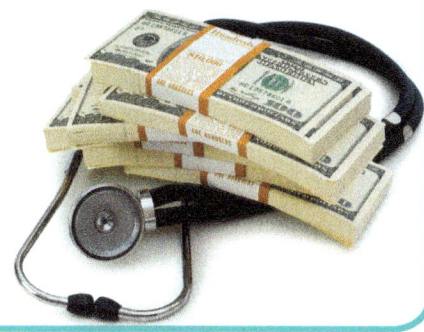

extend your coverage under your family or campus policy through a program called *COBRA*, but such policies often cost at least $3,600 per year.

You may also choose a policy on the individual insurance market by purchasing directly from a private insurer or through a state or federal health insurance marketplace. If your state doesn't operate its own marketplace, you can purchase insurance through the federal marketplace.

>> For information about state and federal health insurance marketplaces, including costs, coverage comparisons, and how to apply, go to **www.healthcare.gov**.

LO 14.5 QUICK CHECK

Which of the following correctly describes a health insurance deductible?

a. the price you pay each month for your health insurance
b. the amount that your health insurance requires you to pay per medical visit
c. a reduced price for health insurance, based on your health status or age
d. the amount you have to pay toward health-care costs each year before your insurance plan covers any costs

"Personalized Medicine" and the Future of Consumer Health

LO 14.6 Discuss the genomic revolution and the future of personal health.

New medical advances against major diseases such as cancer are made each year. In the coming years, however, few advances will have as much potential to fundamentally reshape how you think about your health as personal **genomics.** Defined broadly as the study of the human **genome** (the biological code that "builds" a human being), genomics once seemed largely confined to science fiction. But with the decoding of the human genome completed in 2003, our understanding of this "code of life" has made it possible for us to examine our own genomes and understand some of the information they hold about our health. The goal of this effort is **personalized medicine,** or health care based on the idea that because your individual DNA is unique, your health is as well, and your care and treatments should be tailored to you at the genomic level.

genomics The study of genomes and their effects on health and development.

genome The complete genetic code of an organism.

personalized medicine Health care based on the idea that because your individual DNA is unique, your health is as well, and your care and treatments should be tailored to you.

A Short Course in Genetics and Genomics

Genomics sounds complex—and it is—but to get a basic understanding of your own genome, you only need to know a few key concepts:

- DNA (*deoxyribonucleic acid*) is the material that carries the biological instructions that "build" us. These instructions are *genetic,* meaning that they are inherited from our parents and ancestors. For example, your DNA is genetic information because you inherited it from your mother and father, who passed their DNA on to you when you were conceived. If you have a *genetic disorder,* it means you have a health condition passed on in the DNA you inherited from someone in your family.

- *Genes* are packets of DNA that carry the code for specific building blocks in your body.
- *Chromosomes* are packets of genes and supporting DNA that make up your genome.
- *Your genome* is your entire collection of DNA, coiled in a tight double spiral. Copies of your genome are found in almost every cell in your body. Although all human beings share mostly the same DNA, everyone's genome contains a few unique differences, or *genetic variants*. Your variants make you distinct in many ways, including aspects that affect your health. Some variants may help you enjoy better health over time, while others may be connected to a higher risk for certain health problems, such as cancer or cardiovascular disease.
- *Your genome is not your destiny.* Although DNA is powerful, it is not the only factor that determines who you are or how healthy you may be. Environment and behavior choices are also powerful forces that can shape your health.

Uses of Genomic Information

As our understanding of the human genome evolves, this information is rapidly transforming health care. In the past, health has often been discussed in terms of "one size fits all" or "one size fits many." But genomic information increasingly enables people, either on their own or through their care providers, to find approaches more likely to work for them on an individual basis. Here are some of the ways genomic understanding is reshaping health.

Family Health Histories

Public health officials now encourage everyone in the United States to create a basic **family health history,** or a record of health conditions that have appeared in a family over time.

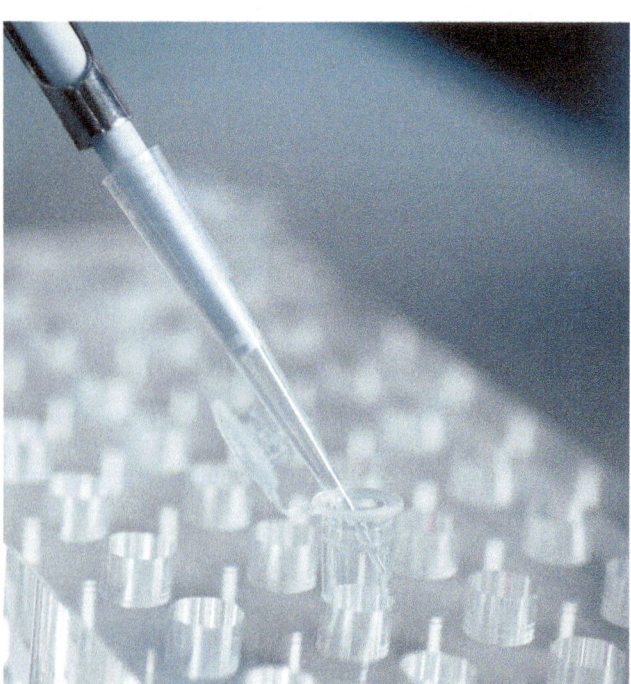

Advances in genomics are resulting in high-tech options for personalized health care.

Health histories used to be reserved for families with rare genetic conditions, such as the blood clotting disorder hemophilia. Now, however, genomic research has revealed that many common health conditions, such as type 2 diabetes, high cholesterol, and heart disease, have a genetic component. Creating a family health history enables you and your relatives to look for patterns of illness that might indicate genetic risk.

>> You can find information on creating a family health history at **www.hhs.gov/familyhistory**.

Targeted Testing

If you or your care provider thinks you are at risk for a genetic illness, you may opt to have genetic testing, or analysis of a certain gene or group of related genes. Such testing can tell you whether you carry DNA variants known to be linked to particular health conditions. Some women with particular family backgrounds, for example, choose to be tested for breast cancer–related variants in genes called *BRCA1* and *BRCA2*. If they find that they are at increased genetic risk, they may opt for medical treatments that reduce their risk.

These tests are powerful, and their cost is dropping rapidly. But they can also be medically and emotionally complex. Most such genetic testing is usually conducted with the help and support of a *genetic counselor*, a medical professional who helps patients understand genetic testing, assess their own feelings and beliefs about such testing, decide which genes to test, and determine how they will respond to the results.

family health history A detailed record of health issues in one's family that presents a picture of shared health risks.

whole exome sequencing A form of genetic testing that looks analyzes a person's exome, or the sections of their genome that carry the codes for making proteins.

whole genome sequencing The full decoding and readout of an entire genome.

Types of Genome Sequencing

Some genetic technologies analyze your whole genome, or sometimes large portions of it, at once and see what it says about your risk for a variety of health conditions. **Whole exome sequencing** is a form of testing that looks only at your *exome*, or all the portions of your genome that carry instructions for making your body's biological building blocks. Scientists can also decode and spell out every point on your genome, in a process called **whole genome sequencing.** The costs of whole exome sequencing and whole genome sequencing are decreasing rapidly as technologies improve.

If you find yourself thinking about any form of DNA testing, consider speaking with a genetic counselor first to help find options that are right for you. These health-care professionals are experts in explaining genetic options and helping people sort through health needs and personal values as they consider genetic testing or personalized medicine.

DNA Tests and Medical Choices

In addition to providing information about risks for certain illnesses, DNA information can sometimes help us decide how to treat problems in our bodies. Each of us, for example, carries DNA variants that affect how our bodies process certain medications. The study of this DNA–drug interaction,

> **pharmacogenomics** The use of DNA information to choose medications and make prescribing decisions.

called **pharmacogenomics,** has already changed the way some doctors prescribe certain blood thinners and other medications. In the case of some cancers, such as certain lung cancers, doctors now have the ability to analyze the DNA of tumors to determine which drugs offer the best treatment options.

Ethical, Social, and Legal Implications of Genomic Advances

Genomic advances can enable you to take a more personal approach to your health. But for many, they also raise doubts and fears. What about privacy? Will others use your genetic information to discriminate against you or to justify higher insurance premiums?

These questions are already shaping new laws designed to help build a lifetime of better health in the genomic era. In 2008, U.S. lawmakers enacted the *Genetic Information Nondiscrimination Act (GINA)*. This law strengthens the privacy of personal DNA information and prohibits genetic discrimination in health insurance and employment.

Still, other questions remain. Should genetic discrimination also be barred in other types of insurance, such as disability insurance? How widely should personal DNA information be shared? Will DNA knowledge make people feel more empowered about their health or more hopeless? These and other important questions will continue to drive discussion, regulation, and personal decisions as the genomic era unfolds.

LO 14.6 QUICK CHECK

Which of the following accurately describes the term "genetic variant"?

a. genetic change that makes an individual's DNA different from most other people's
b. genetic change that always causes disease
c. genetic change that equips an individual with an enhanced ability to resist disease
d. genetic change that makes each of your genes unique

Change Yourself, Change Your World

LO 14.7 Explain how to create your personal health-care plan.

"Be a smart patient? My own best health-care advocate? I'm just trying to get through this term!" The idea of being an active health consumer may feel a little daunting, but paying attention to just a few basic steps on a regular basis will go a long way. Investing a little time in these five areas will pay off—now and in the long run:

- **Practice prevention.** Use the information you've gained from this course and this book to build and maintain wellness. Take the **Self-Assessment** to see if you're practicing prevention enough.
- **Make informed choices.** Spend time learning about any new health option. If you don't have the information you need, ask. If you turn to online resources, make sure the information is credible and evidence based. Make sure you get all the details.
- **Find the right care before you need it.** Don't wait until you are sick to find a doctor. Learn about care providers on campus and in your community. That knowledge will make everything easier when you do need care.
- **Know when you need help.** When you have a busy schedule, it's easy to push health issues aside for later. But waiting can mean complications. Taking an hour to visit the student health center might make the difference between resting for a day or two and losing a bigger chunk of time to illness.
- **Know how you'll pay.** Few surprises can be as bad as a large medical bill that you didn't expect. Before you get sick, understand your health insurance, what it covers, and what costs it leaves in your hands. If you don't have health insurance now, talk to staff at your student health

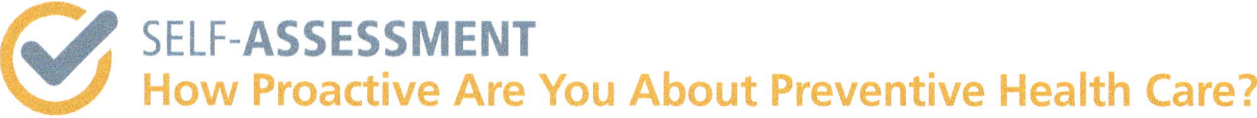

SELF-ASSESSMENT
How Proactive Are You About Preventive Health Care?

1. Have you visited a doctor for a physical exam in the past year? ___ yes ___ no
2. If female, have you had a gynecological exam (including a Pap test) in the past year? ___ yes ___ no
3. Do you regularly brush your teeth and floss? ___ yes ___ no
4. Have you visited a dentist in the past 6 months? ___ yes ___ no
5. Have you had a general vision exam in the past 2 years? ___ yes ___ no
6. Have you received a tetanus/diphtheria booster shot in the past 10 years? ___ yes ___ no
7. Have you received an influenza vaccination in the past year? ___ yes ___ no
8. Have you received a meningococcal vaccine in the past 5 years? ___ yes ___ no
9. If female and under 26, have you ever received an HPV vaccination? ___ yes ___ no
10. Do you have health insurance? ___ yes ___ no

HOW TO INTERPRET YOUR SCORE The more "yes" responses you gave, the more proactive you are about preventive health care. See Table 14.1 for a list of recommended health screenings.

To complete this Self-Assessment online, visit **MasteringHealth**™

center; they may be able to help you find viable insurance options. If you have an HSA or FSA, stay on top of your balance.

>> Watch videos of real students discussing consumer health at MasteringHealth™

LO 14.7 QUICK CHECK

How does an HSA or FSA help you cover health-related costs?

a. You can use these accounts to help pay for your insurance.
b. You can use these accounts to pay for certain medical costs that are not covered by insurance.
c. You can use these accounts to pay for anything that improves your overall health, such as a massage.
d. None of these answers are correct.

Choosing to Change Worksheet

To complete this worksheet online, visit MasteringHealth™

Many people avoid preventive care and thinking about health insurance until they get sick or injured. But a little planning can reduce your risk of illness and protect you if or when you need medical care.

Directions: Fill in your stage of change in Part I and complete the rest of the part with your stage of change in mind. Regardless of your stage of change, everyone should complete Part II.

PART I Becoming Proactive About Preventive Care

Step 1: Assess your stage of behavior change. Check one of the following statements that best describes your readiness to be proactive about your health care.

_____ I do not plan to take part in preventive care in the next six months. (Precontemplation)

_____ I might take part in preventive care in the next six months. (Contemplation)

_____ I am prepared to begin taking part in preventive care in the next month. (Preparation)

_____ I have been taking part in preventive care for less than six months. (Action)

_____ I have been taking part in preventive care for six months or longer. (Maintenance)

Step 2: Respond to the Self-Assessment. Complete the **Self-Assessment** on page 371.

1. Which questions did you answer "No" to? Based on this Self-Assessment, what can you do to be more proactive about your preventive care?

_____
_____
_____

2. What concerns or obstacles, if any, do you have about the preventive care behaviors described in this chapter? Write down who you could contact to ask questions about your concerns or how you could overcome these obstacles.

Example: I am concerned that having an eye exam will cost a lot of money. I could visit the campus health center to see if there are any low-cost programs for optometrist visits.

_____
_____
_____

PART II Scheduling Preventive Care Appointments

Use this worksheet to start becoming more proactive about your health.

	Past Behavior	Future Behavior
Physical exam	When was the last time you had a physical exam? _____	When will you schedule your next exam? _____
Gynecological exam with Pap test (for females)	When was the last time you had a gynecological exam? _____	When will you schedule your next exam? _____
Dental care	When was the last time you visited a dentist? _____	When will you schedule your next exam? _____
Vision care	When was the last time you had a general vision exam? _____	When will you schedule your next exam? _____
Protection from influenza	When was the last time you received an influenza vaccination? _____	If it's been over a year since your last vaccination, when will you schedule your next one? _____
Health insurance	Do you have health insurance? _____	If you do not have health insurance, when will you investigate the options available to you? _____

CHAPTER 14 STUDY PLAN

CHAPTER SUMMARY

LO 14.1
- Individuals have an abundance of health-care choices and also the responsibility of researching information, critically evaluating it, and making educated decisions.
- Self-care includes maintaining basic wellness habits, evaluating health information critically, using medications and home health tests properly, and knowing when it is time to see a doctor.

LO 14.2
- Preventive care, such as periodic screenings and checkups, can help prevent health problems or catch them early, when they are often easier to treat.

LO 14.3
- Conventional medicine is characterized by a focus on the physical aspects and treatment of disease; the presence of discernible, defined symptoms; the maintenance of public health; and the use of scientific evidence and the scientific method. Care is provided by a wide variety of facilities and health-care professionals.
- When choosing a health-care provider, find out whether he or she is covered by your insurance plan and ask friends and family members for recommendations. It is important to be informed and to have open communication with your provider; it is also important that your provider treat you with respect.
- Prescription medications are now the number-one cause of overdose deaths in the United States. It is very important to use prescription medications only as directed by a physician.

MasteringHealth™
Build your knowledge—and health!—in the Study Area of **MasteringHealth**™ with a variety of study tools.

LO 14.4
- Complementary and alternative medicine (CAM) encompasses therapies and practices outside those of conventional medicine. CAM practices often take a holistic approach, connecting mind, body, and spirit.
- Examples of CAM include traditional Chinese medicine, natural products such as herbs and botanicals, mind–body therapies, manipulative therapies, and energy therapies.
- Research any CAM therapy or provider you are considering and make sure that all health-care providers know your health history and the full range of care you are receiving.

LO 14.5
- Options for paying for health care include discount health programs, health insurance, health savings accounts, and flexible spending accounts.
- Health insurance coverage comes in many forms, including managed-care plans, fee-for-service plans, and government-funded plans. Individuals now have greater access to health insurance under the Affordable Care Act.

LO 14.6

- Genomics is the study of the human genome. Genomic research is spurring the development of personalized health care based on an individual's DNA.
- Examples of genomic applications in health care include prenatal testing, genetic testing, whole exome sequencing, and whole genome sequencing.

LO 14.7

- By evaluating health information carefully, communicating with your health-care providers, practicing prevention, and being aware of your health insurance coverage and health-care costs, you can create a personal plan that protects both your health and your finances.

GET CONNECTED

▶▶ Visit the following websites for further information about the topics in this chapter:

- The Medical Library Association's Top 100 List: Health Websites You Can Trust
  http://caphis.mlanet.org/consumer/index.html
- Evaluating Online Sources of Health Information (from the National Cancer Institute, part of the National Institutes of Health)
  www.cancer.gov/cancertopics/cancerlibrary/health-info-online
- Agency for Health Care Research and Quality (AHRQ)
  www.ahrq.gov

MOBILE TIPS!
Scan this QR code with your mobile device to access additional tips about consumer health. Or, via your mobile device, go to **http://chmobile.pearsoncmg.com** and choose by topic: consumer health.

- National Center for Complementary and Integrative Health
  https://nccih.nih.gov
- Genetics Home Reference
  https://ghr.nlm.nih.gov/primer

Website links are subject to change. To access updated web links, please visit MasteringHealth™

TEST YOUR KNOWLEDGE

LO 14.1, 14.7
1. What is NOT an example of preventive care?
   a. eating nutritiously
   b. wearing a seat belt
   c. scheduling regular physicals
   d. taking cold medicine correctly

LO 14.1
2. What are the typical characteristics of credible health-related research?
   a. publication in a peer-reviewed journal
   b. a large pool of study participants
   c. results that have been replicated by other scientists
   d. all of the above.

LO 14.2, 14.7
3. You should seek emergency care for all of the following EXCEPT
   a. cold symptoms.
   b. difficulty breathing.
   c. sudden, severe pain.
   d. adverse reactions to a medication or an insect bite.

LO 14.3, 14.4
4. Which of the following is NOT considered a practitioner of conventional medicine?
   a. medical doctor
   b. acupuncturist
   c. nurse practitioner
   d. dentist

LO 14.3, 14.7
5. Being a smart patient includes
   a. being honest and vocal with your doctor.
   b. asking questions when you don't understand something.
   c. following the instructions you receive from your doctor.
   d. all of these answers.

LO 14.4
6. Chiropractic is an example of which type of health care?
   a. alternative medicine
   b. conventional medicine
   c. energy therapy
   d. naturopathy

LO 14.5

7. Which of the following is characteristic of managed-care health insurance plans?
   a. The more flexibility you want, the more the insurance will cost.
   b. They don't cover medication.
   c. There are no out-of-pocket fees associated with them.
   d. They offer no flexibility for medical care outside of the plan's approved providers.

8. Under the Affordable Care Act, children can stay on their parents' insurance plans until what maximum age?
   a. 18
   b. 21
   c. 26
   d. 30

LO 14.6

9. Analyzing a certain gene to assess the risk of developing a specific disease is an example of
   a. whole-genome sequencing.
   b. single-gene testing.
   c. genomics.
   d. genetic variation.

10. The study of DNA–drug interaction is called
    a. pharmacogenomics.
    b. single-gene testing.
    c. alternative medicine.
    d. carrier testing.

WHAT DO YOU THINK?

LO 14.1

1. What are some reliable ways for you to learn more about new medical treatments and drugs? What about alternative therapies?

LO 14.3

2. What can you as a patient do to reduce your risk of medical errors when receiving treatment?

LO 14.5

3. Should government agencies help people obtain health insurance? If so, how? If not, why? What alternatives would you propose?

4. What information, if any, do you think health insurance companies should know about your health-related habits and lifestyle?

LO 14.6

5. If you discovered that you carried a genetic mutation related to an increased risk of disease, would you change how you live your life?

15

> About 74% of young adult (aged 20–24) deaths are caused by injuries[i]

> Injuries kill one American every three minutes.[ii]

> Each year, more than 3,300 Americans die and another 387,000 people are injured because of car crashes involving distracted driving.[iii]

> 1 in 4 women has been the victim of severe physical violence by an intimate partner.[iv]

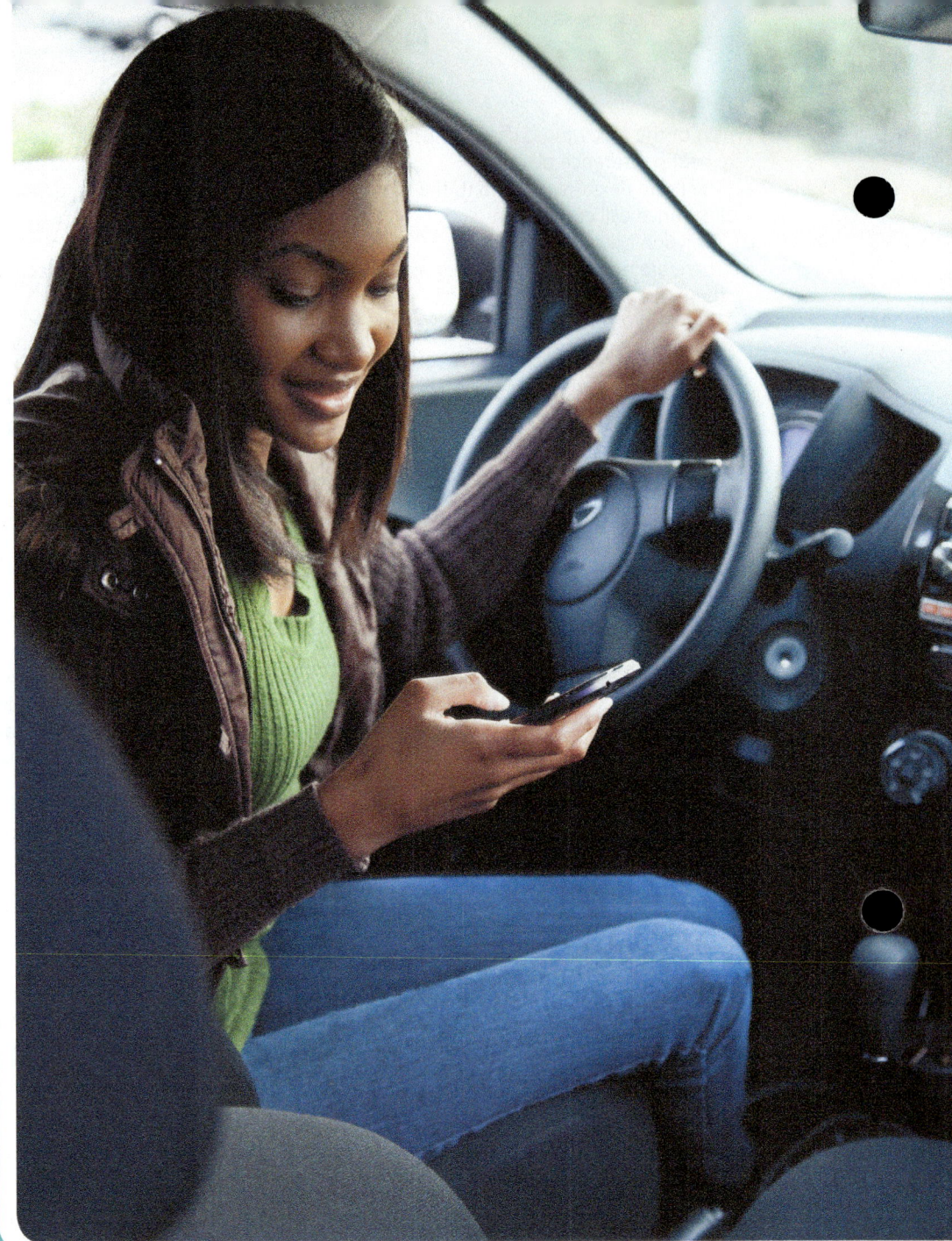

PERSONAL SAFETY AND INJURY PREVENTION

LEARNING OUTCOMES

LO 15.1 Name the most common types of unintentional injuries and their contributing factors.

LO 15.2 Discuss ways you can reduce your risk of motor vehicle accidents.

LO 15.3 Identify steps for staying safe while walking and cycling.

LO 15.4 Discuss contributing factors and prevention strategies for residential, recreational, and occupational injuries.

LO 15.5 Identify trends in the incidence of violent crime in the United States and common contributing factors.

LO 15.6 Discuss violence within communities, including school and campus violence.

LO 15.7 Define intimate partner violence and describe the factors that keep victims in abusive relationships.

LO 15.8 Identify types of sexual violence and strategies for preventing it.

LO 15.9 Explain how you can help improve campus safety.

Be Safe!

Did your parents ever shout this warning as you headed out the door? And if so, what did it mean to you? Driving within the speed limit? Wearing your seat belt? Staying sober at parties? In this chapter, we use the term **personal safety** to describe the practice of making decisions and taking actions that reduce your risk of injury and death.

Injuries are the number-one killer of Americans between the ages of 1 and 44.[1] They cause more deaths among people in this age group than all types of diseases combined. Injuries cost the U.S. economy over $671 billion in medical costs and work loss each year.[2] The good news is that a handful of simple choices can help you significantly reduce your injury risk.

An **unintentional injury** is any bodily damage not deliberately inflicted, such as injuries from motor vehicle accidents, falls, and fires. **Intentional injuries,** on the other hand, are purposefully inflicted through physical or sexual violence. Note that self-inflicted injuries and suicide are considered intentional injuries.

Overview of Unintentional Injuries

LO 15.1 Name the most common types of unintentional injuries and their contributing factors.

Unintentional injuries, or injuries that occur without intent to cause harm, send more than 30 million people to emergency departments in the United States each year.[3] In 2013, they caused more than 127,000 deaths among Americans of all ages.[1] The leading causes of unintentional injury death are as follows:

> **personal safety** The practice of making decisions and taking actions that reduce your risk of injury and death.
>
> **unintentional injury (accidents)** Bodily damage that is not deliberately caused.
>
> **intentional injury** Physical harm that is purposefully inflicted through violence.

- Motor vehicle accidents caused approximately 32,675 deaths in 2014, making them the primary cause of unintentional injury deaths.[4]
- Unintentional poisonings, including drug overdose, rank a close second, killing about 38,800 Americans annually.[1]
- Falls, drowning, and fires are other common causes of unintentional injury deaths. Together they account for more than 36,359 deaths each year.[1]

We tend to think of unintentional injuries as *accidents*, happening by chance. However, they typically involve one or more contributing factors, such as intoxication, fatigue, and distraction. For this reason, many of them are considered preventable. Although every type of unintentional injury has unique circumstances, as a group they share these risk factors:

- **Substance abuse.** Heavy alcohol consumption or other substance abuse increases the risk of unintentional injuries. Alcohol is a factor in 60% of fatal burn injuries and drownings and 40% of fatal motor vehicle accidents and falls.[5]
- **Sex.** Males account for almost 63% of the deaths attributed to unintentional injuries.[1]
- **Age.** Compared with other age groups, young people (aged 15 to 29) account for the largest proportion of overall injury death.[1]
- **Environmental factors.** Factors such as heavy traffic or poor weather can increase risk of automobile, motorcycle, bicycle, or recreational injury.
- **Divided attention.** Performing any type of potentially dangerous activity without completely focusing on the task at hand increases the risk of injury.

LO 15.1 QUICK CHECK

What is the leading cause of unintentional injury death in the U.S.?
a. fires
b. motor vehicle accidents
c. falls
d. shootings

CHAPTER 15 ■ Personal Safety and Injury Prevention   **377**

STUDENT STATS

Top Five Causes of Death in the United States Among People Aged 15–24

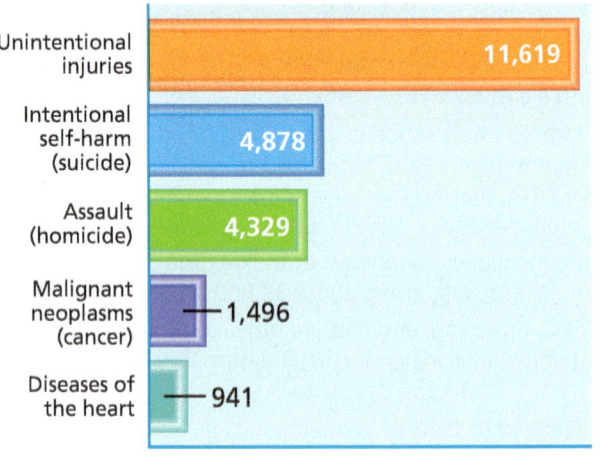

- Unintentional injuries: 11,619
- Intentional self-harm (suicide): 4,878
- Assault (homicide): 4,329
- Malignant neoplasms (cancer): 1,496
- Diseases of the heart: 941

Source: Data from Heron, M. (2016). Deaths: Leading causes for 2013. *National Vital Statistics Reports*, 65(2), 1–95.

Motor Vehicle Accidents

LO 15.2 Discuss ways you can reduce your risk of motor vehicle accidents.

On average each year, more than 2.5 million people in the United States are injured in motor vehicle accidents (MVAs) and nearly one-quarter of all deaths among people between the ages of 15 and 24 are due to MVAs.[1] No other single cause of death claims more young lives.

What Factors Increase the Risk for Motor Vehicle Accidents?

The National Safety Council identifies a number of key factors contributing to MVAs.[6]

Distracted Driving

Distracted driving includes any activity that diverts a person's attention away from the primary task of driving **(Figure 15.1)**. If you drive while distracted, your risk of being in an MVA greatly increases. Consider these statistics:

- In 2014, MVAs involving distracted driving caused the deaths of 3,179 people.[4] These crashes represent nearly 10% of all fatal MVAs that year.
- The risk of getting into a car accident that causes injury goes up fourfold when a driver is speaking on a cell phone.[7] A recent national study found that speaking on a hands-free cell phone, with no manual contact, does not increase crash risk; however, the same study noted that interfaces often require drivers to manipulate their phones in order to place and end calls and when voice recognition from remote devices fails.[7] Moreover, another national study challenged the claim that drivers are safe as long as their hands are on the wheel and their eyes on the road. It found that talking hands-free places a high "cognitive burden" on drivers that causes them to miss visual cues and slows their reaction times.[8] Thus, controversy remains over the level of distraction posed by use of hands-free devices.
- Because texting requires visual, manual, and cognitive attention from the driver, it is by far the most dangerous distraction. The risk of an MVA is 23 times higher than usual when texting while driving.[7] Texting takes a driver's eyes off the road for an average of 4.6 seconds, which at 55 mph is equivalent to driving the length of a football field blindfolded.[7] And some drivers videotaped while texting had their eyes off the road for nearly half a minute.[8] It's hardly surprising, then, that texting while driving has been outlawed in 46 states and the District of Columbia.[9] Prosecutions for vehicular homicide for texting-while-driving fatality cases are becoming more common.

Despite the dangers of distracted driving, the National Highway Traffic Safety Administration (NHTSA) reports that 71% of young drivers have composed and sent text messages while behind the wheel, and 78% have read messages while driving.[7]

Impaired Driving

Alcohol-impaired driving is responsible for about one-third of all highway fatalities each year in the United States, and driving with a blood alcohol concentration (BAC) of 0.08% or higher is illegal in all 50 states.[10] But drinking even a small amount of alcohol impairs your vision, motor skills, judgment, and alertness. That's why, in 2013, the National Transportation Safety Board recommended that states adopt a new, lower BAC limit of 0.05%. (For more on alcohol-impaired driving, see Chapter 9.) Illicit drugs, sleep medications, pain medications, anti-anxiety medications, and even over-the-counter cold remedies can also reduce driving skills.

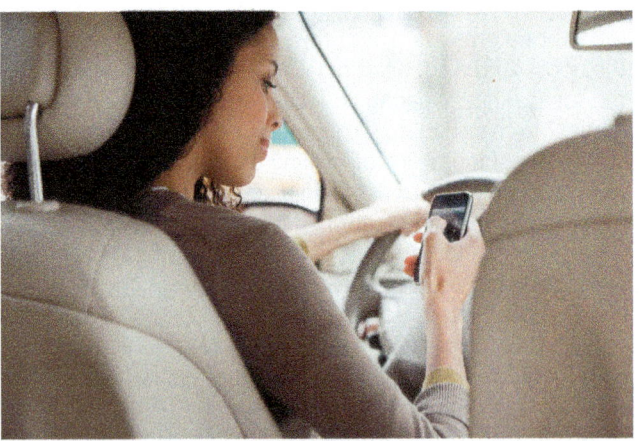

FIGURE 15.1 **Distracted Driving.** Distracted driving includes using a cell phone, reading or typing texts, eating, drinking, talking with passengers, grooming, reading maps or other materials, using a navigation system, watching a video, and adjusting a car stereo system or CD/MP3 player.

Consequently, most states have strict laws outlawing the presence of prohibited substances in the blood of drivers.[11]

Research studies have consistently found that drowsiness is a factor in about 1 out of 6 fatal MVAs.[12] Fatigue slows your reaction time and reduces your attention level, your ability to process information, and the accuracy of your short-term memory, all of which impair your driving. As of 2015, Arkansas, New Jersey, and New York had enacted laws specifically prohibiting driving while drowsy, and other states are considering similar legislation.[13]

Skipping Seat Belts

The NHTSA estimates that each year, seat belts save 12,804 lives.[14] Fortunately, seat belt use has continued to increase in the United States; in 2015, it was at 88.5%, the highest rate ever.[15] And college students do ever better. In a national survey, more than 95% of students report consistent seat belt use.[16]

Some people fail to buckle up in the belief that airbags provide sufficient crash protection, but seat belts are the single most effective prevention against injury or death in a car crash.[17] One benefit of seat belts is that they prevent you from being thrown from the car—an event that is five times more deadly than if you remain in the car during an accident.[18]

Speeding and Other Forms of Aggressive Driving

Aggressive driving is the operation of a motor vehicle in a manner that endangers people or property.[19] Examples of aggressive driving include speeding, driving too quickly for road conditions, tailgating, failing to yield the right-of-way, cutting off other vehicles, and abruptly or improperly changing lanes. Aggressive driving is estimated to be a factor in more than 55% of fatal car crashes.[4] Complete the **Self-Assessment** to evaluate your driving habits.

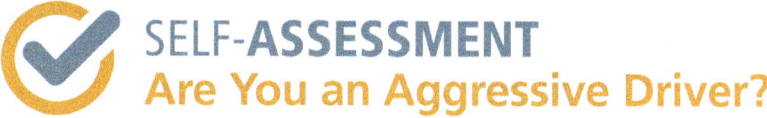

SELF-ASSESSMENT
Are You an Aggressive Driver?

Do you have aggressive habits that could threaten your safety or the safety of others on the road? Circle Yes or No for each question.

Do you . . .

1. Overtake other vehicles *only* on the left? Yes No
2. Avoid blocking passing lanes? Yes No
3. Yield to faster traffic by moving to the right? Yes No
4. Keep to the right as much as possible on narrow streets and at intersections? Yes No
5. Maintain appropriate distance when following other vehicles, bicyclists, or motorcyclists? Yes No
6. Provide appropriate distance when cutting in after passing a vehicle? Yes No
7. Use headlights in cloudy, rainy, or low-light conditions? Yes No
8. Yield to pedestrians? Yes No
9. Come to a complete stop at stop signs or before a right turn at a red light? Yes No
10. Stop for red traffic lights? Yes No
11. Approach intersections and pedestrians at slow speeds to show your intention and ability to stop? Yes No
12. Follow right-of-way rules at four-way stops? Yes No
13. Drive below posted speed limits when conditions warrant? Yes No
14. Drive at slower speeds in construction zones? Yes No
15. Maintain speeds appropriate for conditions? Yes No
16. Use turn signals for turns and lane changes? Yes No
17. Make eye contact and signal intentions where needed? Yes No
18. Acknowledge intentions of others? Yes No
19. Use your horn sparingly around pedestrians, at night, around hospitals, and at other times? Yes No
20. Avoid unnecessary use of high-beam headlights? Yes No
21. Yield and move to the right for emergency vehicles? Yes No
22. Refrain from flashing headlights to signal a desire to pass? Yes No
23. Drive trucks at posted speeds, in the proper lanes, using nonaggressive lane changing? Yes No
24. Make slow, deliberate U-turns? Yes No
25. Maintain proper speeds around roadway crashes? Yes No
26. Avoid returning inappropriate gestures? Yes No
27. Avoid challenging other drivers? Yes No
28. Try to get out of the way of aggressive drivers? Yes No
29. Refrain from momentarily using high occupancy vehicle (HOV) lanes to pass vehicles? Yes No
30. Focus on driving and avoid distracting activities (e.g., smoking, use of a cell phone, reading, shaving)? Yes No
31. Avoid driving when drowsy? Yes No
32. Avoid blocking the right-hand turn lane? Yes No
33. Avoid taking more than one parking space? Yes No
34. Avoid parking in a disabled space (if you are not disabled)? Yes No
35. Avoid letting your door hit the car parked next to you? Yes No
36. Avoid using a cell phone while driving? Yes No
37. Avoid stopping in the road to talk with a pedestrian or another driver? Yes No
38. Avoid inflicting loud music on neighboring cars? Yes No

HOW TO INTERPRET YOUR SCORE
0–3 "No" answers: Excellent
4–7 "No" answers: Good
8–11 "No" answers: Fair
12–38 "No" answers: Poor

To complete this Self-Assessment online, visit MasteringHealth™

Source: Adapted from *Are you an aggressive driver or a smooth operator?* from the New Jersey Office of the Attorney General, Division of Highway Traffic Safety website. Copyright © New Jersey Office of the Attorney General. Reprinted with permission.

Among people between the ages of 15 and 24, nothing claims more lives than motor vehicle accidents. To reduce your risk:

CHOOSE THIS.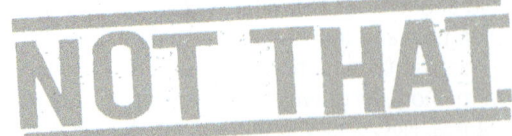

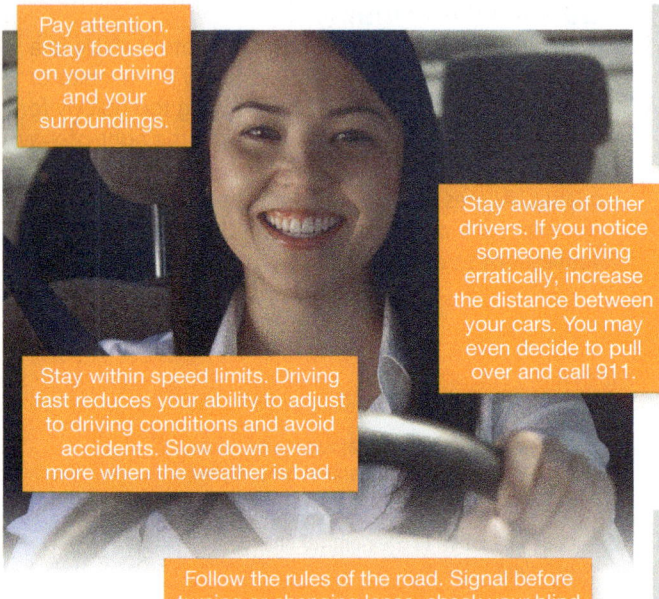

Pay attention. Stay focused on your driving and your surroundings.

Stay aware of other drivers. If you notice someone driving erratically, increase the distance between your cars. You may even decide to pull over and call 911.

Stay within speed limits. Driving fast reduces your ability to adjust to driving conditions and avoid accidents. Slow down even more when the weather is bad.

Follow the rules of the road. Signal before turning or changing lanes, check your blind spot, obey right-of-way rules, look both ways before entering an intersection, come to full stops, and obey traffic signals.

Don't tailgate. Make sure it takes at least 3 seconds for your car to cross a fixed reference point after the car in front of you crosses it.

Don't cut off other drivers or keep changing lanes. Every time you change lanes, you increase your risk of a crash.

Don't speed.

Don't drive if you've had alcohol or any other intoxicating drugs, including prescription medications.

Don't get distracted. Never call or text while driving. Set up your music before you start driving. Don't eat, shave, or put on make-up, even if you are stopped in traffic.

If you get drowsy, pull over for a 15- to 20-minute nap, a caffeinated beverage, and a few minutes of fresh air and exercise outside the car. On long drives, take a break every 2 hours.

Attentive and Defensive Driving:
The great majority of motor vehicle accidents could be prevented by attentive, defensive driving.

Distracted, Impaired, or Aggressive Driving:
Distracted, impaired, and aggressive driving are factors in a majority of fatal motor vehicle accidents. Avoiding these behaviors dramatically reduces your risk.

Speeding—driving at a rate above the posted speed limit—reduces the amount of time you have to react to conditions in the road in front of you, increases the distance needed to stop, and reduces the effectiveness of safety devices like seat belts and airbags. Speeding is a factor in 28% of all MVA fatalities.[4]

▶▶ The National Safety Council offers courses in defensive driving. Find out more at www.nsc.org.

Once you get on the road, drive defensively, not aggressively. See **Choose This, Not That** for specific strategies.

If you're considering buying a new or used car, make sure it has all recommended safety features, such as airbags, antilock brakes, and electronic stability control. Before you get behind the wheel, make sure you have enough gas to get where you're going and that your oil and windshield-washer fluid levels are adequate. Check the air pressure in your tires and check that your wipers and your headlights—both high and low beams—are in working order.

Motorcycle Accidents
Overall, the number of MVA injuries and fatalities, while still significant, has been declining—except among motorcycle riders. Between 2002 and 2012, the annual number of motorcycle injuries increased by 25%, and fatalities increased by 41%.[20] However, the latest findings show a 6% decrease from the 2012 fatality rate. In 2013, about 88,000 motorcycle riders and passengers were injured, and more than 4,600 died.[20] Per mile traveled, motorcycle-accident fatalities occurred 26 times more frequently than auto-related deaths.[20] In 2013, 40% of fatally

380 CHAPTER 15 ■ Personal Safety and Injury Prevention

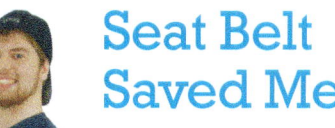

STUDENT STORY

Seat Belt Saved Me

"HI, MY NAME IS CALEB. When I was 16 years old, I got in my very first car accident. I've been in other car accidents since then, but this was by far the worst. I was in a rush one day, and I was going through an intersection that I thought was a four-way stop and just stopped at the stop sign, didn't really look either way and continued going. Well, it turns out it was a two-way stop and there was a guy going about 40 miles an hour, and all I heard was just the blare of his horn. Within an instant the guy hit me. I was able to keep control of the car and I was wearing my seat belt, so I wasn't hurt at all, but my back left passenger door was just obliterated. The window was shattered out. The door was dented in beyond repair. I know if I hadn't been wearing my seat belt, any number of injuries could have happened."

What Do You Think?

1. What personal and environmental factors increased Caleb's risk of getting into a car accident?
2. What could Caleb have done to prevent that car accident from occurring?
3. Do you think this accident had anything to do with the fact that Caleb was a 16-year-old inexperienced driver? Why or why not?

---

injured motorcyclists who died in a single-vehicle crash were alcohol impaired. Even though 37% of all motorcyclist fatalities could be prevented if riders were wearing a helmet, only 20 states require helmet use by all motorcyclists.[20]

LO 15.2 QUICK CHECK

Which of the following statements about seat belt use is true?
a. Seat belts are the single most effective prevention against motor vehicle crash injury and death.
b. College students use seat belts at a much lower rate than does the general population.
c. Seat belts don't actually prevent a passenger from being thrown from a car in a violent crash.
d. Seat belt use in the United States is at its lowest rate ever.

Pedestrian and Cyclist Safety

LO 15.3 Identify steps for staying safe while walking and cycling.

Accidents while walking, jogging, or cycling on roadways can cause injuries, one of the more common of which is **traumatic brain injury (TBI).** TBI is caused when the head is jolted or hit or when an object pierces the skull, resulting in a sudden injury that damages the brain. Although many TBI patients recover quickly, a significant number face a lifetime of disability, and some die. Each year, about 1.7 million Americans sustain TBIs.[21] Spinal cord injuries, fractures, and internal injuries are also common in MVAs involving pedestrians and cyclists.

> **traumatic brain injury (TBI)** Injury that disrupts normal functioning of the brain, caused by a jolt or blow to the brain or a penetrating head wound.

Accidents Involving Pedestrians and Cyclists

In 2013, more than 4,700 pedestrians were killed in traffic accidents and 66,000 were injured.[22] Nearly half of these accidents involved alcohol, and the majority occurred in the evening or at night. Thus, it's important to wear reflective clothing whenever you go out for an evening walk or run. Pedestrians distracted by listening to audio via headphones, looking at a cell phone screen, and/or texting are increasingly becoming a problem. Remember that the safest way to walk is to *look, listen, and be seen*. Unlike cyclists, pedestrians should always travel on the side of the road opposite the direction of traffic, facing oncoming vehicles. Wherever there are sidewalks, use them.

Bicycles may not pack the force or speed of a car or motorcycle, but riding one still carries risks. In 2013, around 48,000 Americans were injured cycling and 743 died.[23] The number of cycling-related fatalities has increased 19% since 2010.

Although cars need to make room on the road for bicycles, cyclists are responsible for road safety as well. Cyclists are required to travel in the same direction as the flow of vehicular traffic and obey all traffic signs, signals, and lane markings.[23]

In 21 states, children and teens are required by law to wear a helmet while riding a bike; however, in all 50 states, helmets are optional for adults.[24] In a national survey, about 71% of college students who ride a bike said they only sometimes, rarely, or never wear a bike helmet.[16]

For tips on reducing your risk of injury while cycling and during other activities, see the **Practical Strategies** box on page 382.

LO 15.3 QUICK CHECK

Which of the following is true for cyclists?
a. They are not required to obey traffic signals.
b. They are not required to adhere to lane markings.
c. They are required to travel in the same direction as the flow of vehicular traffic.
d. All bicycle riders are required to wear helmets.

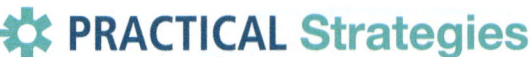

PRACTICAL Strategies

Reducing Your Injury Risk While . . .

Driving or Riding in a Motor Vehicle

- **Think prevention.** Don't get behind the wheel if you've been drinking—even a small amount—or using any other drugs. Pick a designated driver, use your campus "safe rides" program, or call a cab. Never get in a car with a driver who is impaired.
- **Be alert.** Don't drive if you haven't had adequate sleep. You might not feel sleepy, but many drivers in drowsy-driving MVAs report that they did not feel sleepy before they nodded off.
- **Slow down.** Don't set off if you haven't allowed enough time for your trip. If you can't get where you want to go by the time you want to get there, stay home, call, and reschedule.
- Before you set off, buckle up. It only takes a second. And in most states, it's the law.

Walking or Riding a Bike

- **Follow the rules of the road.** When on foot, cross in designated crosswalks and travel against the flow of traffic. When cycling, don't cut through lanes of traffic, run lights, or blow through stop signs. Ride with the flow of traffic.
- **Stay visible.** Don't assume that drivers can see you. Avoid cycling in a car's blind spot or passing quickly. Whether walking or cycling, wear brightly colored clothing on your upper body. At night, make sure your clothes, helmet, and/or bike are outfitted with reflectors.
- **Keep your eyes on the road.** Cyclists are considered vehicle operators and should avoid distraction. Pedestrians need to pay attention as well: Looking down to use your cell phone while crossing a busy street puts you at the mercy of drivers.
- **Wear a helmet every time you ride.** Wearing a helmet is the single most effective way to prevent TBI resulting from a bicycle crash.[24]
- **Don't drink and ride.** Nearly a quarter of cyclists killed in bike accidents are found to have blood alcohol concentrations at or above legal limits.[24] Impaired cyclists face the same increased risks of an accident as impaired drivers.

Residential, Recreational, and Occupational Injuries

LO 15.4 Discuss contributing factors and prevention strategies for residential, recreational, and occupational injuries.

A surprising number of accidents and injuries occur at home, at work, or during recreational activities. A few basic precautions will help keep you safe.

Unintentional Poisoning

Each year, more than 38,000 people in the United States die from unintentional poisoning.[1] We all know that certain toxic substances, such as cleaning products, solvents, and pesticides, are hazardous. However, more than 90% of unintentional poisoning deaths each year are due to drugs.[25] In fact, drug overdose was the leading cause of injury death in 2012, killing more Americans in the 25–64 age group than motor vehicle accidents.[26] In 2012, 53% of drug overdose deaths were caused by prescription medications. Of these, 72% involved opioid painkillers, such as oxycodone (OxyContin) and hydrocodone (Vicodin).[26] These drugs are highly addictive. When taken in excess, they suppress breathing, sometimes to a degree that is fatal. They are also associated with an increased risk for heart attack.[27]

If you think you or someone you are with has been poisoned, call the National Poison Control Center at 800-222-1222. To avoid poisonings, store all potential poisons in their original bottles and keep them in a locked closet or upper cabinet, out of the reach of children. Follow the label directions carefully. Never share or sell your prescription medications.

Choking and Suffocation

When a choking person's airway becomes blocked, oxygen can't reach the lungs. Permanent brain damage can occur within six minutes.[28]

Among young children, hot dogs cause the most food-related choking deaths, firmly and completely blocking the airway.[29] Grapes, cheese cubes and cheese "sticks," nuts, candies, and popcorn are other common causes of choking. If you're feeding young children, avoid foods likely to cause choking and cut other firm foods into small, thin pieces. Non-foods such as coins, buttons, and toys can be dangerous as well. Of all children's products, latex balloons cause the highest number of choking deaths.[29]

In adults, eating too fast, without chewing food properly, is the most common factor in choking. Consumption of even a small amount of alcohol increases the risk. Moreover, choking on vomit is a significant danger for anyone who has lost consciousness after binge drinking. Never leave the person alone to "sleep it off": If he or she can't be roused, seek emergency medical care immediately.

If you're dining with someone who begins coughing forcefully and can speak, leave the person alone because a strong cough can dislodge the food. If the person grabs at his or her throat (the universal sign of choking) and cannot cough forcefully or speak, public health experts recommend following these steps:

- First, try back blows. Stand behind the person and lean him or her forward onto your non-dominant hand **(Figure 15.2a)**. With the heel of your dominant hand, strike the person's upper back between the shoulder blades. This will often propel the food out of the person's mouth. If the first back blow is not successful, try up to four more, pausing between each to see if the blockage has cleared.

- If the person is still choking, try abdominal thrusts. Still standing behind the person, wrap your arms around his or her waist **(Figure 15.2b)**. Place your clenched fist just above the navel. With your other hand, grab the fist and pull up and in toward you. Stop to see if the blockage has cleared. If not, administer up to four more abdominal thrusts.
- If the person's airway is still blocked and you are the only rescuer, stop and call 911. If someone else is present, have that person call 911 while you continue cycles of back blows and abdominal thrusts.

You can take a class in basic emergency assistance from your local American Red Cross chapter or campus health center.

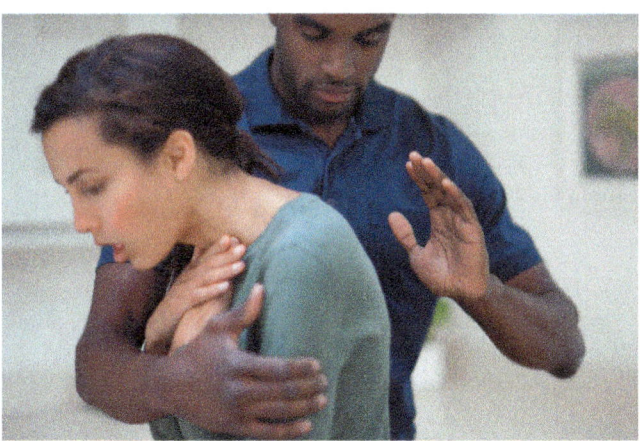

(a) Back blows

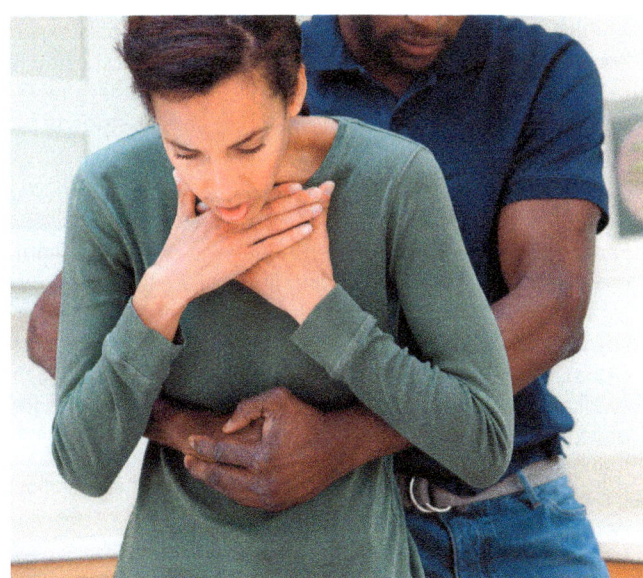

(b) Abdominal thrusts

FIGURE 15.2 **How to Help Someone Who Is Conscious but Choking.**

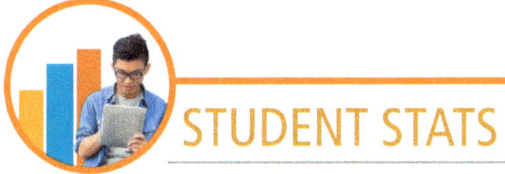

STUDENT STATS

Top Seven Causes of Death from Unintentional Injury in the United States Among People Aged 15–24

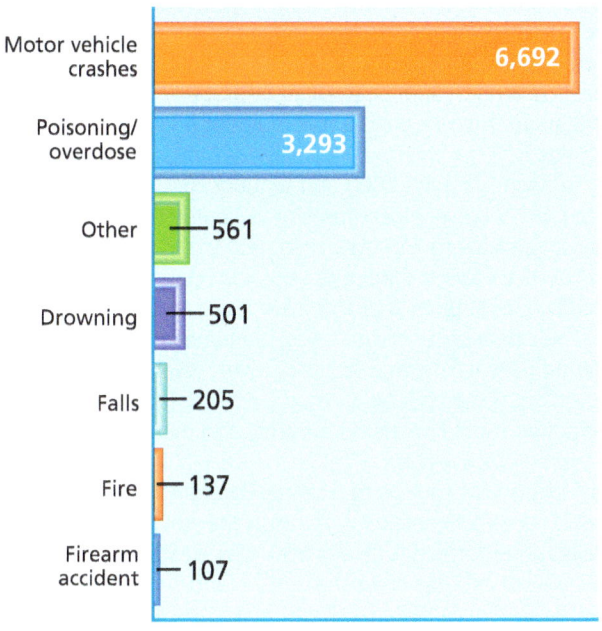

- Motor vehicle crashes: 6,692
- Poisoning/overdose: 3,293
- Other: 561
- Drowning: 501
- Falls: 205
- Fire: 137
- Firearm accident: 107

Source: Data from Heron, M. (2016). Deaths: Leading causes for 2013. *National Vital Statistics Reports, 65*(2), 1–95.

Drowning and Other Water Injuries

Drowning causes an average of 10 deaths a day, not including drownings due to boating accidents.[30] Two of these deaths each day are among children age 14 or younger. Children can die in less than five minutes in natural bodies of water, swimming pools, bathtubs, hot tubs, buckets, and even toilets. To protect them when they are around water, keep them within arm's reach at all times.

Drowning is also the second leading cause of unintentional injury death (after MVAs) among young people aged 10 to 19.[31] Among teens and adults, most drownings occur in natural water settings like lakes, oceans, or rivers. Consumption of alcohol is a factor in 60% of drowning deaths.[5]

The Centers for Disease Control and Prevention (CDC) offers the following water safety tips:

- Take swimming lessons!
- Swim with a companion, never alone. Whenever possible, swim at beaches and pools that have lifeguards on duty.
- Never drink alcohol when you are swimming or boating.
- Never dive or jump into an unknown body of water.
- Obey posted signs warning of unsafe swimming conditions.

- Know the signs of a rip current: water that is choppy, discolored, foamy, or filled with debris and moving in a channel away from shore. Don't go into such waters. If you are caught in a rip current, swim parallel to shore. Swim toward shore only once you're free of the current.
- Always wear a personal flotation device (life jacket) when riding in a boat or participating in other water sports like jet skiing or waterskiing.

Fire Injuries

About 85% of all fire deaths occur in the home.[32] In 2014, fires claimed the lives of more than 2,860 people in the United States—not including firefighters.[33] Most victims die from inhalation of smoke and toxic gases rather than from burns. The primary cause of fire-related deaths is smoking, but other common causes of residential fires include candles, cooking, malfunctioning or improperly used heaters, and arson. Alcohol plays a role in about 60% of fatal burn injuries.[5]

Between January 2000 and January 2013, 82 fatal fires occurred on college campuses or in nearby off-campus housing, claiming 119 lives.[34] So next time you're tempted to complain about the fire drills in your classroom building or dorm, remember that they save lives.

Fire safety isn't difficult if you plan ahead. Every home should have a smoke detector on every level, and every dorm room should have its own smoke detector. Smoke detectors should be tested monthly and the batteries replaced twice a year.

In campus fires, cooking causes more fatalities than smoking; so whenever you're using the stove or oven, don't leave it unattended. Candles should be in stable holders, away from curtains and other linens, and should be put out before you leave the area. Don't overload electrical outlets and make sure extension cords are used properly. If you use a portable space heater, keep it at least 3 feet away from anything flammable; never leave it unattended. If you smoke indoors, put out your cigarettes in ashtrays and never smoke in bed. Make sure you know at least two escape routes from your dorm room or apartment and participate in fire drills. Practicing in advance will help you in the chaos of a real fire.

What should you do if you see a fire or smoke or if you hear a fire alarm? The U.S. Fire Administration advises that you first feel the door for heat:[34]

- *If the door is hot*, fire may be on the other side. In that case, stay in the room, open a window, and scream for help.
- *If the door isn't hot,* leave the room and head for your planned exit. As you do . . .
- *Get down and stay low.* Smoke rises, so crouching and crawling will enable you to move underneath the smoke so you can see better, reduce smoke inhalation, and get out more quickly. If your planned exit is blocked, exit by your alternate route.

Work-Related Injuries

In 2014, more than 3.8 million U.S. workers were injured on the job and 4,679 died from these injuries.[35] If you

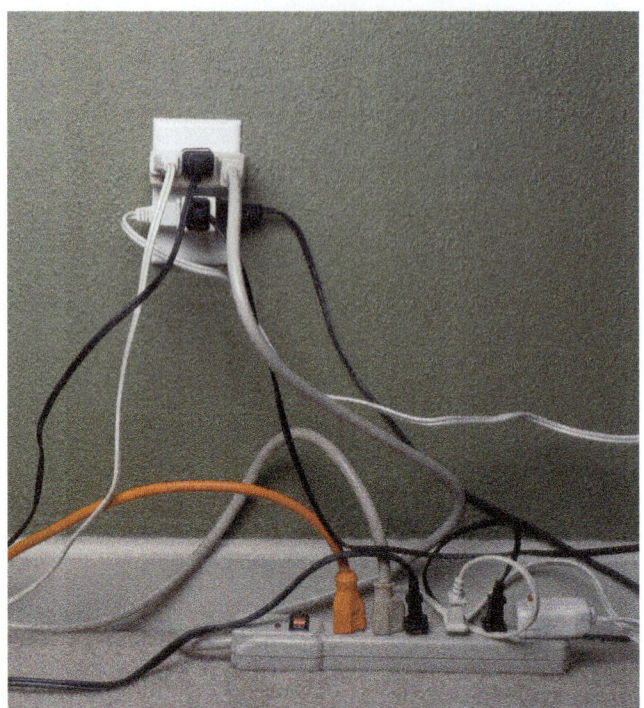

While **fires** in the home are caused, among other things, by smoking, cooking, candles, and improperly used heaters, they can also be started by overloading outlets with too many cords.

work at a job where safety equipment is provided, use it! Goggles, masks, gloves, and other devices take only a few moments to put on and provide invaluable protection. Learn and follow all safety measures required in your workplace, and if you aren't sure what they are, ask. Employers are required to provide necessary safety equipment, establish safety procedures, and provide training on both to all employees.

Even workers in offices, hospitals, and retail stores experience significant numbers of injuries each year, most often repetitive strain injuries and back injuries. Both of these types of injuries are also very common among college students, so let's take a closer look.

Repetitive Strain Injuries

Performing the same movements over and over, even slight movements with your hands and fingers, can injure and inflame your joints, connective tissues, and nerves. These **repetitive strain injuries (RSIs)** can lead to pain, swelling, numbness, loss of motion, and even permanent nerve damage. For example, an RSI called **carpal tunnel syndrome (CTS)** is characterized by pain in the thumb, fingers, palm, wrist, and forearm. It can develop when you're constantly typing, texting, or otherwise

> **repetitive strain injury (RSI)** Injury that damages joints, nerves, or connective tissue caused by repeated motions that put strain on one part of the body.
>
> **carpal tunnel syndrome (CTS)** A repetitive strain injury of the hand or wrist, often linked to computer keyboard use or other types of repetitive motion.

flexing your hand and wrist. The repetitive stress causes the tendons within the carpal tunnel of your wrist to swell and press on a nearby nerve.

The surge in mobile device use has resulted in RSIs and other overuse problems. Recent studies have linked excessive texting to the development of CTS and tendinitis of the thumb.[36] As we view mobile device screens, we tend to keep our neck and spine in unnatural positions, resulting in chronic neck and back strain or pain (called "tech neck"). See the **Practical Strategies** box on page 386 for more tips on how to use your devices safely.

>> For a video of seated stretches you can do while at your computer, check out **www.mayoclinic.com**. (Search for "seated stretches.")

Back Injuries

Lifting heavy objects is a leading cause of injury. If you need to pick up and carry a heavy box or other object, check out the instructions for lifting in **Figure 15.3**. Once you've lifted the item, keep it close to your body by holding your elbows close to your body. This helps keep strain off your spine. Don't twist your spine while carrying the load; if you need to change directions, change your foot placement. To release the object, lower it down by bending your knees, not your back.

LO 15.4 QUICK CHECK

Which of the following foods is responsible for greatest number of choking deaths in children?
a. hot dogs
b. cheese cubes
c. grapes
d. peanuts

Intentional Injuries and Violence

LO 15.5 Identify trends in the incidence of violent crime in the United States and common contributing factors.

Recall that intentional injuries are purposefully inflicted through **violence**, the use of force—threatened or actual—with the intent of causing harm. Violence is a serious health concern, especially for young people. Nonfatal injuries caused by violence account for more than 600,000 hospital emergency department visits annually by people between the ages of 15 and 24.[37]

According to the Federal Bureau of Investigation (FBI), **violent crime** includes murder, rape, sexual assault, robbery, and assault. Although levels of violent crime in the United States have fluctuated in recent years, the overall number of violent crimes has dropped in the past two decades[38] (**Figure 15.4**, next page). Still, in 2014, more than 3 million Americans were the victims of at least one violent crime.[39] Of these attacks

> **violence** Use of physical force—threatened or actual—with the intent of causing harm.
>
> **violent crime** Offenses involving force or the threat of force, including murder, rape, sexual assault, robbery, and assault.

- About 64% were aggravated assault, or an attack intended to cause serious injury, often involving a weapon.
- About 28% were robberies, or the taking of or attempt to take anything of value from a person by violence and/or by putting the victim in fear.
- Just over 7% were forcible rapes.
- Just over 1% were murders.

Many attacks have underpinnings in complex webs of personal, family, community, and social factors, including

- **Sex.** Males accounted for almost 80% of all arrests for violent crime in 2014. Men are also more often the victims of violent crime. See **Diversity & Health** on page 387 for some possible reasons men are at higher risk than women.
- **Age.** Teens and young adults experience the highest rate of violent crime.

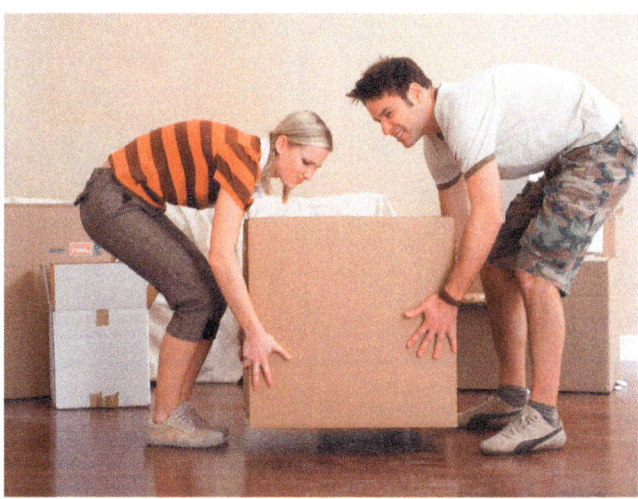

(a) The wrong way to lift

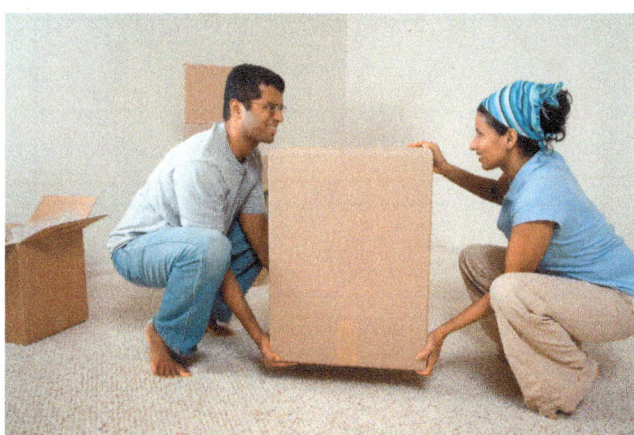

(b) The right way to lift

FIGURE 15.3 **Proper Lifting.** Rather than (a) bending over the object to be lifted, (b) stand near it and then bend your knees and hips. Bring the object as close as possible to your body and then hold onto it as you rise.

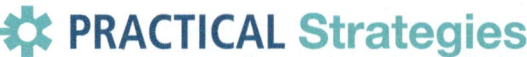

PRACTICAL Strategies

Preventing Tech Injuries

When Working on a Computer . . .

Knowing how to set up your computer for optimal posture can help you avoid RSI:

- Keep your neck in a neutral position by raising the top of the screen to about eye level.
- Angle the screen to avoid bending your head forward.
- Use a document holder so you don't have to bend your neck to look at papers.
- Allow for good hand and wrist posture by placing your keyboard and mouse on an adjustable keyboard tray that can be moved up or down. Correct position is slightly at or below elbow height.
- When typing, don't bend and twist your hand to reach awkward key combinations
- Keep your wrists straight with your fingers reaching down slightly to find the keys. Don't rest your palms on the keyboard.
- If a laptop is your main computer, set up a workstation with a standard-size external keyboard and mouse.
- Use a chair that supports a comfortable upright or slightly reclined posture. Prop your feet up to maintain a comfortable trunk–thigh angle, if needed.
- Position the screen at a right angle to windows to reduce glare. Keep it clean.
- Stop and stretch every 30 to 45 minutes.

When Using a Mobile Phone or Tablet . . .

- Be aware of when you are holding your head flexed and forward while looking down at your phone. This position can lead to muscle strain and even injury.
- Bring your phone up to eye level to view the screen rather than bending your neck downward.
- Limit the frequency with which you use small mobile devices. If you must use one for an extended time, take breaks. Set a timer to remind yourself to take a break every 15 to 20 minutes.
- Stretch your neck after using your mobile device.
- Whenever possible, use a tablet holder and place it at eye level.

Source: Based on U.C. Berkeley's Ergonomics Program for Faculty and Staff from the University Health Services Tang Center at Berkeley (2007). *Ergonomic tips for laptop users.* uhs.berkeley.edu and DeWitt, D. (2016). *How to avoid text neck overuse syndrome.* http://www.spine-health.com/.

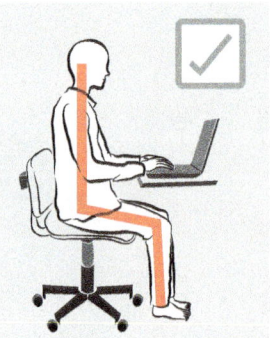
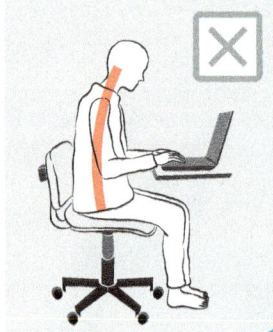

- **Guns.** The United States continues to have a high murder rate compared with other industrialized countries, and many experts link this phenomenon to the easy availability of firearms. In 2014, about 68% of the nation's murders, 41% of robberies, and 22% of aggravated assaults were committed with the use of guns.[38]
- **Poverty.** Communities that are distressed, with poor housing, high unemployment, and limited community services, often have increased rates of violence, especially among young people. Rates of violent crime also tend to be increased among disadvantaged socioeconomic groups. For example, African Americans are more likely to live in poverty than Caucasian Americans and are more likely to commit murder and to become murder victims.[38]
- **Interpersonal relationships.** Many crime victims know their attackers. About 22% of murders in 2011 occurred within families. Women are especially vulnerable to criminal acts at the hands of an acquaintance, a friend, an intimate partner, a family member, or a spouse.[40]
- **Drugs and alcohol.** Substances that disrupt judgment and impair your ability to control your emotions

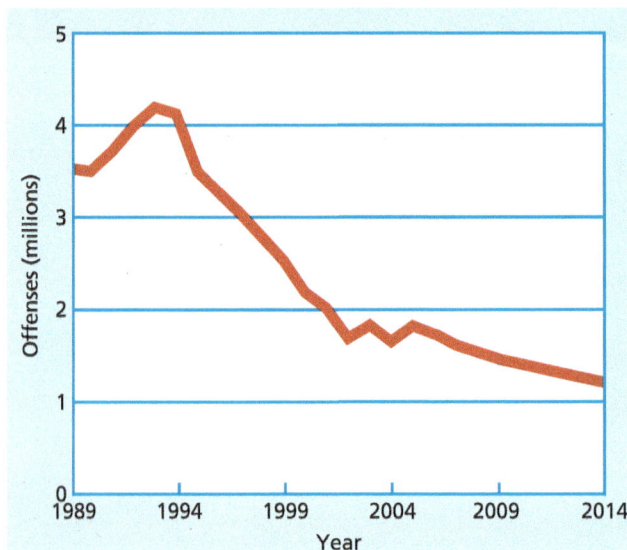

FIGURE 15.4 Violent Crime Rates Continue to Decline. The serious violent crimes included are murder, rape, robbery, and aggravated assault. Rates include estimates for crimes not reported to the police.

Source: Data from Federal Bureau of Investigation. (2015). *2014: Crime in the United States.* www.fbi.gov.

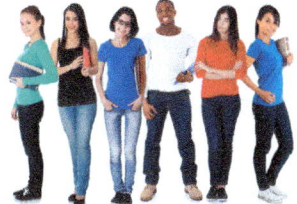

DIVERSITY & HEALTH

Injuries and Violence: Special Concerns for Young Men

Two of the biggest risk factors for injury and death due to accidents or violence are things none of us can control: age and sex. If you are young and male, your risk for traumatic injury and death is higher than that of women or any other age group. For example, males between the ages of 20 and 24 have the highest rate of nonfatal assault injuries, more than 50% higher than the rate for females of the same age.[1] Males of the same age also experience the highest rate of homicide deaths, more than six times higher than that of females.[1] Males also account for about 62% of alcohol-related emergency department visits in the 18–20 age group.[2] Sexual assault is one of the few situations where women are in more danger, but for most other types of violence and injuries, young men are at higher risk.

The reasons for these higher risks are widely debated among researchers. Some suggest that the influence of the male hormone testosterone leads to more aggression, anger, and risk taking. Some point to gender roles that encourage men, especially young men, to be tough, aggressive, risk taking, or confrontational. Males also have higher rates of substance use and abuse, as well as higher rates of participation in sports like football and hockey where injuries are common. Moreover, men are more likely to work in hazardous occupations, and they experience five times as many injury-related workplace fatalities as females.[3] Often, a mix of these factors puts young men in harm's way.

Reducing the risk of injury doesn't mean taking all the fun out of your life. Instead, experts suggest to channel your energies in ways less likely to get you hurt or killed. Here are just a few suggestions:

- Your car is no place for an adrenaline rush. Find thrills in sports, video games, or some other safe place—not behind the wheel.
- Watch how much you drink. As discussed throughout this chapter, alcohol is a significant risk factor for unintentional and intentional injuries and deaths. Whether you are the aggressor or the victim, you don't want to wind up a drinking-related statistic. (For more information on alcohol and its effects, see Chapter 9.)
- Anger can't help you solve problems. It's natural to get angry, but anger can quickly escalate a conflict into violence. Learning to manage anger and find other ways to resolve problems is one of the manliest things you can do. (For more information about managing anger and stress, see Chapters 2 and 3.)

What Do You Think?

1. This box identifies several factors that might contribute to males' higher risk for trauma. What others can you think of?
2. Can you propose any factors that might be protective for females—that is, factors that might reduce their risk?
3. Think of an incident among your own family members, friends, or high school or college classmates in which one or more males suffered traumatic injury. Identify the specific factors involved (e.g., alcohol, anger, etc.).

Sources: **1.** Centers for Disease Control and Prevention. (2013). *Youth violence: National statistics*. www.cdc.gov. **2.** Substance Abuse and Mental Health Services Administration. (2010). *News release: SAMHSA reports on hospital emergency department visits involving underage alcohol use*. www.samhsa.gov. **3.** Concha-Barrientos, M., Nelson, D. I., Driscoll, T., Steenland, N. K., et al. (2013). *Occupational health: Comparative quantification of health risks*. www.who.int.

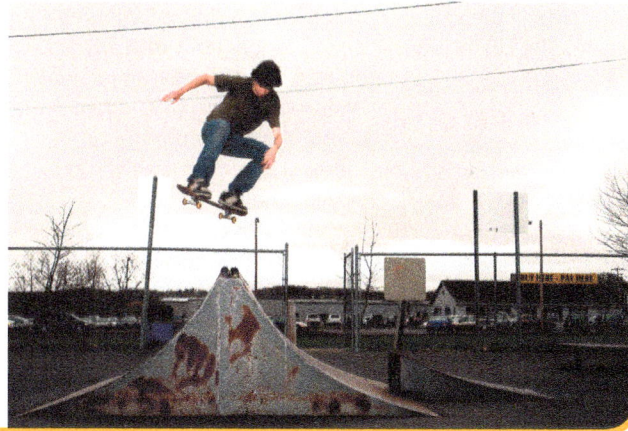

consistently emerge as a factor in violence. Alcohol is a factor in about 60% of homicides and 50% of sexual assaults.[5] Every year, nearly 800,000 college students reported being physically or sexually assaulted by another student who'd been drinking.[41] The use of illicit drugs is also a factor in many types of crime.

- **Childhood environment.** Researchers have consistently noted that children raised in violent surroundings are more likely to grow up to be violent adults.[42]
- **Violence in the media.** Most children and teenagers are exposed to thousands of violent messages each year in TV shows, movies, video games, and song lyrics.

Although most researchers agree that violence in the media contributes to an increased level of aggressive behavior and a perception that violence is normal, the strength of this association is still unclear.

- **Personal and cultural beliefs.** Some individuals hold values or religious beliefs that sanction violence.
- **Stress.** Think about the last time you were under a great deal of stress and how you were quicker to anger than you might have been otherwise. People who consistently experience high levels of stress are more likely to react violently.

LO 15.5 QUICK CHECK
All of the following are associated with an increased risk of committing violence EXCEPT
a. high levels of stress.
b. being a teen or young adult.
c. being from the southern United States.
d. alcohol use.

Violence Within Communities

LO 15.6 Discuss violence within communities, including school and campus violence.

Although even one violent crime is too many, our society has been making progress in reducing this threat to our communities. At the end of this chapter, we'll discuss ways you can get involved in these efforts.

Assault

Assault, a physical attack or threat of attack on another person, is one of the leading categories of violent crime. **Aggravated assault** is an assault committed with the intent to cause severe injury, often involving a weapon. Although just over 740,000 aggravated assaults were committed in 2014, this number represents a decline of more than 14% from 2005.[38] More effective prevention programs and tougher law enforcement appear to have helped reduce the number of assaults.

Homicide

Homicide is the willful (not negligent) killing of another person. The FBI includes in this category both **murder** and non-negligent manslaughter, which is the willful killing of another "without malice aforethought"—in other words, without having previously planned to do so.

Homicide is the third leading cause of death in the United States among people between the ages of 15 and 24, after unintentional injuries and suicides. Among all age groups nationwide, 14,249 people were murdered in 2014. This was almost a 15% decrease from 2005.[38] As noted earlier, the great majority of murder victims and perpetrators are male. More than two-thirds of murders involve firearms.[38] Mass murders, such as the 2016 shooting of 49 people at an Orlando, Florida nightclub, often involve assault rifles, weapons that were developed for military and law enforcement use. Mass shootings account for fewer than 1% of victims killed by firearms.

aggravated assault An attack intended to cause serious physical harm, often involving a weapon.

homicide The willful (not negligent) killing of another person; includes both murder and non-negligent manslaughter.

murder The act of intentionally and unjustifiably killing another person.

hazing Initiation rituals to enter a fraternity or other group that may be humiliating, hazardous, or physically or emotionally abusive, regardless of the person's willingness to participate.

School and Campus Violence

As of late 2015, there had been 144 deaths from mass shootings on U.S. school campuses since the 1999 murderous rampage at Columbine High School. However, despite high-profile tragedies, such as at Columbine and at Sandy Hook Elementary School in Newtown, Connecticut, in 2012, overall levels of school violence have dropped in the past decade. Moreover, a national analysis found that students are much more likely to be seriously hurt or killed off campus than while at school. For example, during the 2009–2010 school year, while there were 19 homicides of school-aged children within American schools, there were 1,396 homicides of school-aged children within their homes and communities.[43]

In 2007, a student at Virginia Tech killed 32 others and himself. In response to the tragedy, U.S. colleges and universities have developed new emergency response plans and procedures, upgraded communication systems, and implemented new safety techniques and services. Some are finding their policies to conflict with state laws; 28 states allow students to carry a concealed weapon on a college campus.

Another common problem on college campuses is **hazing,** a set of initiation rituals for fraternities, sports teams, or other groups. Hazing rituals typically involve humiliation, isolation, alcohol consumption, sleep deprivation, or physical or sexual abuse. Peer pressure or other power dynamics induce those being hazed to participate in high-risk activities that they wouldn't perform otherwise. Surveys suggest that more than half of college students involved in fraternities, clubs, teams, and similar organizations experience hazing.[44] According to one expert on hazing, there has been at least one hazing death a year since 1969. Alcohol poisoning and aggravated assault are usually the causes of death.[45]

All U.S. colleges and universities are required to disclose statistics about the crimes reported on and near their campuses. The legislation that mandates this disclosure is the Jeanne Clery Act, named after the Lehigh University student who, in 1986, was raped and murdered in her dorm room when dormitory security doors were propped open, allowing a perpetrator to enter. Unfortunately, many campus crimes

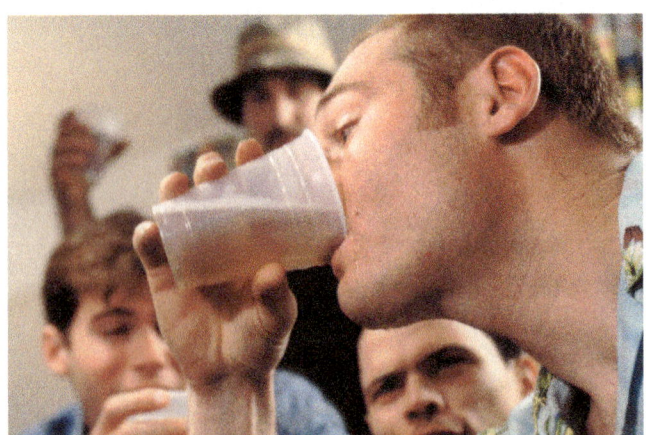

Hazing has been responsible for more than two dozen student deaths since 2008. Alcohol is often a factor in hazing incidents.

still go unreported, with victims often too embarrassed, ashamed, or afraid to step forward. Reporting a crime is the first step in addressing the problem and making a campus safer for everyone.

>> The Clery Center advocates for victims of campus crime. Contact them at http://clerycenter.org.

Hate Crimes

Certain crimes are fueled by bias against another person's or group's race or ethnicity, religion, national origin, sexual orientation, or disability. Any acts—whether physical assaults or vandalism against property—due to such prejudice have been classified as **hate crimes.** Almost 6,400 incidents involving such offenses were reported to the FBI in 2014. Of these, approximately 47% were racially motived. Religious bias and sexual orientation bias were involved in just under 19% of hate crimes.[46] About half of the hate crime incidents involved intimidation or destruction of property.

hate crime A crime fueled by bias against another person's or group's race or ethnicity, religion, national origin, sexual orientation, or disability.

terrorism Premeditated, politically motivated violence against noncombatant individuals, usually as a means of influence.

domestic violence An abusive situation in which a family member physically, psychologically, or sexually abuses one or more other family members.

intimate partner violence (IPV) An abusive situation in which one member of a couple or intimate relationship may physically, psychologically, or sexually abuse the other.

Terrorism

Terrorism is premeditated, politically motivated violence against nonmilitary people by subnational groups or clandestine agents, usually in an effort to influence a larger audience. The effects of terrorism are experienced on many levels: It can destroy property and injure or kill individuals, disrupt the patterns of daily life in a community, and cultivate widespread fear.

Since 2001, the year in which more than 3,000 Americans died in the September 11 attacks, the numbers of deaths and injuries due to terrorism in the United States have dropped. However, the global picture is much bleaker. In 2014, approximately 13,460 terrorist attacks occurred in 95 countries, causing more than 32,700 deaths. This represents an increase of 35% in terrorist attacks and an 81% increase in total fatalities from 2013 to 2014.[47] More than 60% of all terrorist attacks occurred in just five countries (Iraq, Pakistan, Afghanistan, India, and Nigeria).

The government agency responsible for defending the United States against terrorist threats is the Department of Homeland Security, which was created in response to the 2001 terrorist attacks. Other agencies, such as the FBI, the Central Intelligence Agency (CIA), the U.S. military, state and local law enforcement, and even the CDC, also guard against terrorism. Ongoing efforts work not just to disarm, catch, or kill terrorists but to discredit their tactics, diminish the perception of threats, and reduce their abilities to win public support and new recruits.

LO 15.6 QUICK CHECK

Hazing rituals typically involve all of the following EXCEPT
a. humiliation.
b. amputations.
c. sleep deprivation.
d. physical/sexual abuse.

Violence Within Relationships

LO 15.7 Define intimate partner violence and describe the factors that keep victims in abusive relationships.

We all desire relationships that are grounded in mutual support, respect, and affection, but sometimes we find ourselves in relationships characterized by abuse. In a phenomenon known as **domestic violence,** one or more members of a household experience physical, psychological, or sexual harm from another member. When the abuse is perpetrated by a current or former partner or spouse, it is known as **intimate partner violence (IPV).** Forms of IPV include physical and emotional abuse and sexual violence, such as rape, when it occurs between intimate partners. We discuss sexual violence later in this chapter.

Intimate Partner Violence

Victims of intimate partner violence can be married or not married, heterosexual, gay or lesbian, living together, separated, or dating. Many cases go unreported, so the exact scope of this problem is hard to pin down. The CDC estimates that 12 million Americans experience IPV each year.[48] Women are disproportionately affected:[48,49]

- 1 in 4 women has been the victim of severe physical violence by an intimate partner versus 1 in 7 men.
- Nearly 1 in 5 women has been raped versus 1 in 71 men.
- Women make up 70% of all deaths due to IPV versus 30% for men.

At its core, abuse in an intimate relationship arises from the abuser's need for control. This is thought to be related at least in part to a phenomenon called "anxious attachment": People who experience a high level of anxiety when forming and maintaining attachments have a high need to control their relationships. One way males do this is by identifying with rigid gender stereotypes. When a woman violates her partner's expectations of submission and dependence, the man may resort to violence to manage the perceived threat to his masculinity.[50]

The effort at control may take the form of emotional or physical abuse. Emotional abuse includes comments and actions that try to erode the other person's confidence, independence, and sense of self-worth, such as keeping a partner from contacting family member or friends or from getting a job. Physical abuse includes any type of physical assault or use of physical restraint. In most cases, emotional abuse accompanies physical abuse in a relationship.

Some people who find themselves the victim of an episode of abuse end the relationship and leave immediately. But other victims stay and may find themselves subject to

STUDENT STORY

From Control to Abuse

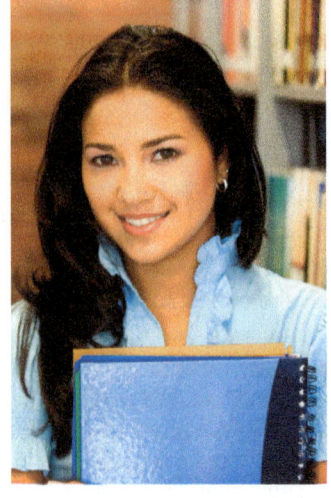

"HI, I'M JENNY. I was dating a guy for a few months who I really liked and everything seemed great at first, but he slowly started to get more and more controlling. First he didn't want to go out with my friends, then after a while he didn't want *me* to go out with my friends. He got really jealous any time he saw me talking to another guy and he started making me check in with him every day to let him know my schedule. He even checked my cell phone to see who I was talking to. One day we got into a fight about it and he grabbed me and pushed me into a wall. I got really scared and left immediately. I broke up with him by text and I've avoided him ever since."

What Do You Think?

1. What could have happened if Jenny had stayed with her abusive boyfriend?
2. What else could Jenny have done in response to her boyfriend's behavior along with breaking up with him?
3. Was Jenny right to break up with him with a text, or should she have met up with him to explain?

---

further and more severe abuse. This situation is referred to as *the cycle of violence*:

- **Tension building.** A phase in which relatively minor abuse occurs and the victim responds by trying to please the abuser and avoid provoking another attack.
- **Acute battering.** A phase in which the abuser lashes out more forcefully, no matter how accommodating or conciliatory the victim has been.
- **Remorse.** A phase in which the abuser may feel shock and denial over the abuse and swear it will never happen again. Over time, however, the tensions and need for control that started the cycle resurface, and abuse starts anew, often more seriously than before.

Victims stay in abusive relationships for a variety of reasons. Some are financially dependent on their partners or have children and don't want to break up their family. Some come from belief systems or cultures that forbid family separation or divorce. Some may still love their abuser. Others may lack the self-confidence to take action or don't know where to go. Some may be afraid of what their partner might do to them if they try to leave.

A variety of organizations provide counseling and shelter to victims of IPV. One annual survey of domestic violence groups found that on a given day, more than 64,000 adults and children received shelter or other types of support related to IPV.[51] More than 10,000 others seeking such help had to be turned away for lack of adequate resources.

IPV persists, in part, because of a broad lack of understanding of how and why it occurs. In one survey of college students, more than half agreed with IPV myths such as that some instances are caused by women picking physical fights with their partners or that most women can get out of an abusive relationship if they really want to.[52] College men taking the survey were more likely than college women to agree with these myths.

>> For one woman's story about the cycle of abuse and what kept her from leaving her abuser, listen here: **www.npr.org**. (Search for "domestic victims leave.")

Stalking and Cyberstalking

Stalking is a pattern of harassment or threats directed at a specific person that is intended to cause intimidation and fear, often through repeated, unwanted contact. Stalking may also take the form of contact through digital and online communications, a phenomenon called *cyberstalking*. Although both traditional stalkers and cyberstalkers are motivated by an obsession with having power and control over their victims, cyberstalkers are more likely to avoid detection, using tactics such as creating a variety of screen names at different sites to maintain their anonymity.

> **stalking** A pattern of harassment and threats directed at a specific person that is intended to cause intimidation and fear, often through repeated, unwanted contact.

Common stalking behaviors include

- Making unwanted phone calls
- Sending unwanted letters, emails, or text messages
- Following or spying
- Showing up at places where the victim would be, with no legitimate reason
- Waiting for the victim, with no legitimate reason
- Leaving unwanted items or presents for the victim
- Posting information or spreading rumors about the victim online, in a public place, or by word of mouth

According to a national survey, more than 5 million women are stalked each year in the United States.[48] Women were about three times as likely to be stalked as men, and men make up the majority of stalkers. Overall, 1 in 6 women has been stalked in her lifetime, versus 1 in 19 men.[49] Stalking and cyberstalking occur more frequently among college students than in the general population: In two recent surveys of college students, 5% and 12% reported that they had experienced stalking.[16,53] However, researchers have estimated the true prevalence at more than 40% of students.[53,54] Self-reported estimates are thought to be too low because many, if not most, incidents go unreported, in part because the victim doesn't recognize the behavior as stalking.[53,55]

College students also experience unique consequences of stalking victimization. In addition to the psychological distress felt by victims generally, they're at risk for academic consequences, including lower grades, additional time needed to graduate, and dropping out.[53]

If you are being stalked, don't try to reason with your stalker. Stalking is not rational behavior. Instead, start by letting the stalker know that the attention is unwelcome. Have someone else deliver this message for you—this thwarts the stalker's goal of trying to force contact with you. Avoid being alone as much as possible, vary your routines, and stop posting information about your location on social media sites. Also avoid revealing your whereabouts through GPS locator apps. Keep a record of all contacts with the stalker. Get a new phone number but leave the old one active. Ask a friend to screen and keep a record of calls to the old number. If the stalker persists, get help from your resident advisor, campus health center, campus security, or law enforcement.

Addressing Violence Within Relationships

If you find yourself attracted to someone, is there any way to tell—before you get in too deep—if the person has the potential for violence? Although there's no such thing as an IPV profile, the CDC has gathered a list of risk factors, including the following:[56]

- Low self-esteem
- Low academic achievement
- A history of aggressive or delinquent behavior
- A history of having been abused as a child
- Alcohol or other substance abuse
- Anger and hostility
- Depression and social isolation
- Belief in strict gender roles
- Desire for power and control

What if you're already in a relationship that's causing you to feel unsafe, or you've experienced one or more episodes of IPV? What if you're frightened by something you see in the relationship of a friend? Don't wait for things to "get better": Contact your student health center or the National Domestic Violence Hotline at 1-800-799-SAFE (7233) or at TTY ("text telephone" for the hearing impaired) 1-800-787-3224, or visit www.thehotline.org.

LO 15.7 QUICK CHECK

In the cycle of violence, during which stage does the abuser feel shock and denial over the abuse and swear it will never happen again?
a. tension-building stage
b. remorse stage
c. acute battering stage
d. wait-and-see stage

Sexual Violence

LO 15.8 Identify types of sexual violence and strategies for preventing it.

Although no standard definition of the term has emerged, **sexual violence** encompasses several forms of nonconsensual sexual activity, including noncontact sexual abuse, such as voyeurism or verbal harassment, unwanted touching, attempted but uncompleted sex acts, and completed sex acts. The common factor in all of these is the lack of consent of the victim, either because he or she refused consent or because he or she was threatened, coerced, intoxicated, underage, developmentally disabled, or otherwise legally incapable of either giving or refusing consent. Sexual violence is often referred to as sexual assault.

Risk Factors for Sexual Violence

Factors that increase the risk for sexual violence include the following:

- **Hostility toward women.** Men who report hostility toward or low opinions of women are more likely than others to show increased levels of sexual aggression.
- **Shared tolerance of sexual violence.** Membership in a fraternity or other male-only social group that holds attitudes tolerant of sexual violence—such as "Some women ask for it"—increases the likelihood that a man will engage in sexual violence.[57]
- **Low self-control.** Many studies point to low self-control as a personal characteristic of sexual offenders. This factor is thought to be especially potent when combined with membership in a male-only social group with attitudes tolerant of sexual violence.[58] In a sense, the man relinquishes control to the group ideology.
- **Substance abuse.** In one study of college students, about 15% of men reported having used some form of alcohol-related coercion to obtain sex.[58] According to the Core Institute, the nation's largest database of statistics on alcohol and other drug use on campus, nearly 78% of sexual assaults on campus involve alcohol or other drug use.[59]
- **"No" isn't always heard as "No."** Some men have problems understanding a woman's sexual refusals. Less direct refusals, such as "I don't think it's a good idea," may be misinterpreted as agreeing to sex.[60]

Sexual Harassment

Unwanted language or contact of a sexual nature that occurs in school or workplace settings is considered **sexual harassment** when it explicitly or implicitly affects a person's job or academic situation or work or school performance, or when it creates an intimidating, hostile, or offensive environment. Sexual harassment is a form of discrimination that violates the federal Civil Rights Act of 1964.

According to the U.S. Equal Employment Opportunity Commission (EEOC), sexual harassment can occur in a variety of circumstances, including but not limited to the following.

> **sexual violence** Any form of nonconsensual sexual activity.
>
> **sexual harassment** Unwelcome language or contact of a sexual nature that explicitly or implicitly affects academic or employment situations, unreasonably interferes with work or school performance, or creates an intimidating, hostile, or offensive work or school environment.

- The victim and the harasser may be a woman or man, and the two parties do not have to be of the opposite sex. According to the EEOC, in 2015, of the 6,822 charges of sexual harassment filed, just over 17% were filed by males.[61]

- The harasser can be the victim's supervisor (or teacher), an agent of the employer (or school), a coworker (or fellow student), or a nonemployee (or nonstudent).
- The victim does not have to be the person harassed but can be anyone affected by the offensive conduct.
- Harassment may occur even if the victim suffers no economic injury or stays on the job or at school.[62]

On campus, sexual harassment can take the form of everything from a student making sexually explicit remarks that make others uncomfortable to a professor demanding sexual favors from a student in exchange for a better grade. In one survey of college students, 62% of all students (male and female) reported having been sexually harassed while enrolled in school. About 80% of those harassed said their harasser was a student or former student. Among college males, 51% admitted to having sexually harassed someone, and about 22% said they had done so more than once. Only 10% of those harassed said they had reported the incident to a campus official.[63]

If you are being harassed, the first step is to confront your harasser. In person or in writing, tell the harasser to stop and state that you consider the actions to be sexual harassment. If direct communication has no effect, keep a record of all harassing contacts and behavior and report the problem to campus or workplace supervisors. They are required by law to investigate.

Title IX is federal civil rights legislation that prohibits sex discrimination in education. While it is often associated with equal opportunity in sports, it also addresses sexual harassment and sexual violence. As a college student, you have certain rights and protections under Title IX. Learn about your Title IX rights in the **Special Feature** on page 393.

rape Nonconsensual oral, anal, or vaginal penetration by body parts or objects, using force, threats of bodily harm, or taking advantage of circumstances that make a person incapable of consenting to sex.

statutory rape Any sexual activity with a person younger than the legally defined "age of consent," regardless of whether any coercion or force was involved.

date (acquaintance) rape Coerced, forceful, or threatening sexual activity in which the victim knows the attacker.

date rape drugs Drugs used to assist in a sexual assault, often given to the victim without his or her knowledge or consent.

Rape

The FBI defines **rape** as "penetration, no matter how slight, of the vagina or anus with any body part or object, or oral penetration by a sex organ of another person, without the consent of the victim."[38] Any sexual activity with a person younger than the legally defined "age of consent" is also considered a form of rape called **statutory rape,** regardless of whether any coercion or force was involved.

In 2014, FBI records showed that more than 116,600 rapes were reported in the United States.[38] As noted earlier, a large-scale national survey found that about 1 in 5 women and 1 in 71 men in the United States report having been raped at some point in their lives.[48] The same survey found that more than 1 million women had been raped the previous year. Among female victims, 79% of rapes occur before age 25. In one survey of college women, almost 20% said they'd been sexually assaulted during their undergraduate years.[58]

Rape and other forms of campus crime are especially common during the first few weeks of a new school year, a period referred to as the "red zone" when parental involvement abruptly ends and students are in new situations, often among people they've just met. As noted earlier, nearly 78% of sexual assaults on campus involve the use of alcohol or other drugs, which is especially common at parties and other social events early in a new academic year.[59]

Date Rape

Of rapes documented among college students, many take the form of **date (acquaintance) rape.** This form of coerced sexual activity, in which the victim knows the attacker, can have a severe long-term emotional impact because the victim is assaulted by someone who was trusted. A 2015 national survey of college students found that 9.7% of women had experienced nonconsensual sexual touching and 2.7% had experienced nonconsensual sexual penetration in the previous year.[16] Many cases of date rape go unreported. Drinking and drug use are factors, and in some instances the victim is unknowingly given a drug to facilitate rape.

Date Rape Drugs

Drugs used to assist in a sexual assault, known as **date rape drugs,** are powerful, dangerous, and difficult to detect once they've been slipped into a drink. They can

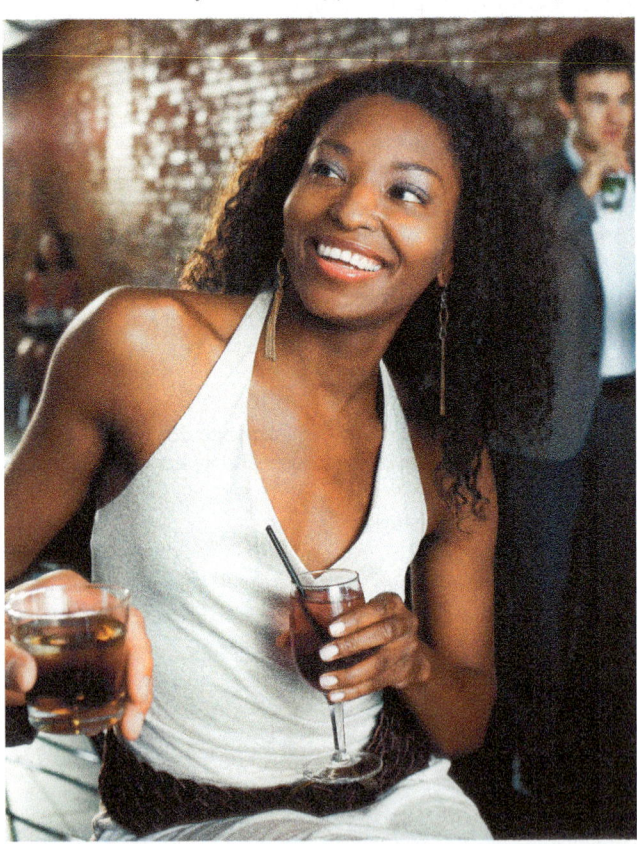

Date rape drugs can be difficult to detect once added to drinks.

SPECIAL FEATURE

Title IX
Know Your Rights

No person in the United States shall, on the basis of sex, be excluded from participation in, be denied the benefits of, or be subjected to discrimination under any educational program or activity receiving Federal financial assistance.

Signed into law in 1972, Title IX is a groundbreaking and comprehensive statute intended to end discrimination based on sex in any education program receiving federal funds. Because sexual harassment, including violence, can significantly interfere with a student's access to educational opportunities, Title IX mandates that colleges and universities take action to protect you from unwanted sexual behavior from peers, faculty, and university staff. Specifically, Title IX requires your school to:

- **Be proactive** in providing a campus that is free of sexual harassment, gender discrimination and sexual violence, including sexuality-based threats or abuse and intimate partner violence. If school officials know about discrimination, harassment, or violence, they must act immediately to eliminate it and to provide services to those who have been affected.

- **Protect everyone on campus from sex discrimination.** Protection must be provided to all—males, females, gender-nonconforming students, and faculty and staff.

- **Appoint a Title IX coordinator** to investigate all Title IX complaints in a timely manner. The Title IX coordinator's contact information should be widely publicized and easily accessible on the school's website.

- **Establish publicly accessible procedures for handling complaints** involving sexual discrimination, harassment, or violence. All Title IX complaints must be investigated within 60 days. Investigation findings must be provided to the victim in writing, and an appeals process must be available.

- **Conduct formal hearings for sexual violence complaints.** Schools may not allow mediation in sexual violence cases involving students.

- **Protect victims who file complaints from retaliatory harassment.** This protection can include a "no-contact directive," preventing accused students from interacting with their victims. Campus police are required to enforce these directives.

- **Pay the costs** of services or accommodations needed by sexual violence victims. If victims require counseling, changes in housing or class schedules, or tutoring to continue their education, the school must provide these at no cost.

For more information about your Title IX rights, visit www.knowyourix.org.

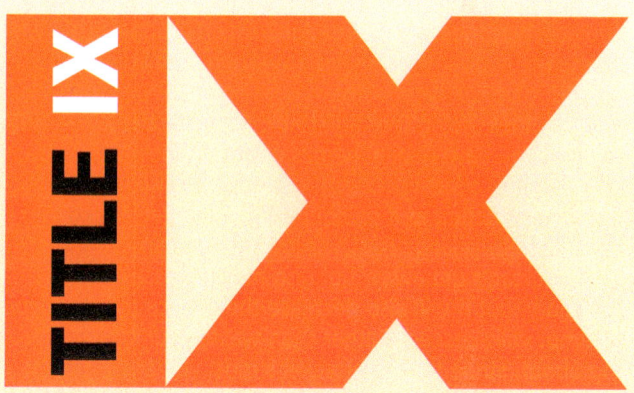

make a victim weak or confused or cause loss of consciousness—as well as make it difficult for the victim to remember later what happened while he or she was drugged. Under federal law, convicted rapists who use a date rape drug to incapacitate a victim automatically have 20 years added to their sentences.

Reducing the Risk of Date Rape

Preventing date rape requires joint efforts. To avoid becoming a victim, you can protect yourself in a number of ways:

- When dating someone you don't know well, stay in public or go out in a group. Arrange for your own transportation; don't rely on your date for transport.

- Watch out for coercive behavior. If your date tries to pressure you into activities you'd rather avoid, such as drinking heavily, you may face similar pressures for sex as well.

- Trust your instincts. If you feel uncomfortable with someone, leave.

- Stay sober. Drinking makes it harder for you to communicate clearly and set limits about sex.

- Don't accept drinks, including nonalcoholic ones, from other people. If you're at a club, even if someone offers to buy you a drink, go up to the bar yourself and watch as the bartender prepares it. Keep your drink with you at all times. If you've left it unattended, pour it out. And don't drink from a punch bowl or other open container.

- Be assertive and direct with both your words and your actions. If you are being pressured for sex and don't want to participate, say "No!" or "Stop it!" loudly. If the pressure persists or worsens, tell the other person that he or she is attempting rape. Yell, make a scene, and run away.

To avoid becoming an assailant, keep in mind the following:

- Accept that "No" means "No." Even if you think the person's flirtatious manner might mean "Yes," pay attention to the words and back off.
- Someone who is intoxicated cannot legally consent to sex. Again, sex with someone who is drunk or under the influence of drugs is rape.
- Drinking and using drugs make it harder for you to communicate clearly and set limits about sex, too.
- Remember what being together offers—and what it doesn't. It offers both of you a chance to get to know each other better in a social setting. It is not an automatic ticket to sex. You both have the right to set limits and refuse any level of sexual activity.

Defending Yourself Against Rape

What if you've followed all the precautions but still find yourself in a threatening situation? Experts suggest that, unless the assailant is carrying a weapon, immediate action on your part can be effective. Some potential victims think and talk their way out of an attack. For instance, you might say that you have genital herpes or are HIV-positive, or that your father is a local police officer. You can also try crying hysterically, acting as if you're having a mental breakdown, or repeatedly yelling "Fire!" as loud as you can.

If you can't get away, fighting may increase your risk for injury, but it will also decrease the chance that the rape attempt will succeed. Rather than waste your energy flailing about, strike for the attacker's most vulnerable areas: eyes, ears, temples, base of skull, windpipe (Adam's apple), spine, groin, and knees. Because thigh muscles are far more powerful than arm muscles, kicking can be more effective than hitting. Some self-defense experts advise dropping to the floor. This gives you a firm base from which to strike with your legs and can confuse an assailant used to upper-body fighting, giving you an extra second to roll out of reach and run.

If your attacker is armed, you may endanger your life by fighting. Every situation is different, so use your best judgment. Choosing not to resist does not equal consent.

>> Just Yell Fire is an award-winning video series teaching women practical self-defense. View the college version here: **www.justyellfire.com**.

If You Are Raped or Otherwise Sexually Assaulted

If you are raped or otherwise sexually assaulted, remember that you are not to blame. Sexual violence occurs because the attacker is hostile, not because of something you've said, done, or worn. It is a violent crime, and sex happens to be the weapon.

After an assault, go to a place where you feel safe and call someone you trust. Write down as many facts about the attack as you can remember. Try not to change your clothes or clean up; you'll destroy physical evidence that may be helpful if you report the attack to the police. Instead, go to a hospital to be treated for any injuries you've received and screened for sexually transmitted infections. If female, you can be monitored for pregnancy, and you may be offered emergency contraception. Physical evidence can be collected at that time, while you decide whether to report the attack. When you seek medical care, ask for referrals to a counselor who can help you deal with the many emotional and psychological challenges that can arise after a sexual assault.

The decision to report a rape or other sexual assault can be difficult. You may be reluctant to talk about the attack publicly. A classic study from the U.S. Department of Justice of sexual victimization among college students identified several barriers to reporting a sexual assault, including shame, guilt, and embarrassment; concerns about confidentiality; fear of reprisal from the assailant; fear of being treated with hostility by law enforcement officials; and concerns about not having sufficient evidence and not being believed.[64] Moreover, a year-long investigation of sexual assault on college campuses by the Center for Public Integrity revealed that, even when found guilty, perpetrators rarely face tough punishments such as expulsion and criminal proceedings, whereas many victims feel so traumatized that they drop out of school.[65] Reporting the crime, however, may help restore your sense of power and control. Sexual assailants tend to repeat their behavior. By reporting a sexual assault, you may prevent another attack in the future.

Effects of Sexual Violence

Sexual violence has immediate and long-term consequences on physical, psychological, and social health.[49] Victims are often physically injured, suffering cuts, bruises, or even fractures, head trauma, or internal bleeding. Many develop sexually transmitted infections. In the following days and weeks, victims often experience flashbacks, panic attacks, and sleep problems. Over time, they may develop low self-esteem, depression, eating disorders, and post-traumatic stress disorder. Their risk of suicide increases. They may try to cope with their trauma by drinking, using illicit drugs, or engaging in risky sex.[49] They may also have a decreased capacity to form intimate bonds with partners.

LO 15.8 QUICK CHECK

When a college student is subjected to sexual harassment, who is the perpetrator in the majority of cases?

a. a fellow or former student
b. a professor
c. a staff member at the college
d. a hometown boyfriend/girlfriend who doesn't attend the same college

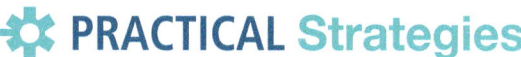

PRACTICAL Strategies

10 Tips for Campus Safety

1. Program numbers for campus safety services into your cell phone because most 911 calls from cell phones go to highway safety dispatchers, not local police. Also program in the direct line for the local police department. Sign up for email alerts from your campus safety services as well.
2. Whether you live in a dorm, a group house, or an apartment, know where the smoke detectors are and make sure they are working. Know where the emergency exits are and what your fire escape plan is, with two ways out.
3. To reduce your risk for falls, keep entryways, stairways, and hallways well lit and free of clutter. Don't stand on chairs, beds, or shelves to change ceiling lights or swat an insect above your reach. Instead, use a proper footstool or short ladder.
4. Drink in moderation, if at all. Alcohol is a factor in fires, falls, drownings, and many other injury situations, as well as in aggravated assaults, rapes, and other campus crimes.
5. Keep your valuables hidden. That's not always easy to do in a small dorm room, but it should still be possible to keep money, ATM cards, jewelry, and other valuables out of plain sight.
6. Protect your financial and personal data, too. If you make purchases online using your credit card, don't use a shared computer. If you own a smart phone, password-protect it. Also, make sure you know how to remotely lock it and erase personal data. If it's lost or stolen, you'll need to act fast.
7. Keep your doors locked when you're home and when you're out and don't loan out your keys. Never prop open access doors or let strangers in. Someone who has arrived to visit another occupant can get the person he or she is visiting to open the door.
8. Don't travel alone after dark. Take a shuttle, go with a friend, or use the security escorts who are available on many campuses.
9. Give friends or family members your schedule of classes, work, and other activities.
10. Know your surroundings and trust your instincts. If something doesn't seem right, get help by calling campus security.

Source: Based on Clery Center for Security on Campus, Inc. (2008). *Seven tips for campus safety.* http://clerycenter.org/; Livesecure.org. (2009). *College student safety tips.* http://livesecure.org; and Collegesafe.com. (2003). *College safety tips—Campus safety tips.* http://collegesafe.com.

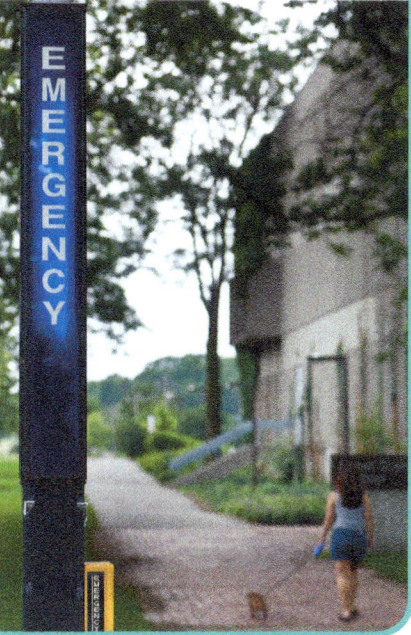

Change Yourself, Change Your World

LO 15.9 Explain how you can help improve campus safety.

By taking some basic injury-prevention precautions, knowing how to support a friend who has experienced violence, and encouraging others to look for nonviolent ways to resolve conflicts, you can help keep yourself from becoming a statistic and build a safer campus and community.

Personal Choices

Fires, falls, crimes, and abusive relationships unfortunately do occur on college campuses. For general tips on how to reduce your personal risk for unintentional and intentional injury on campus, see the **Practical Strategies** box. You can help make your whole campus safer by

- **Knowing your campus safety rules and resources.** Learn what they are and share that information with others.
- **Challenging social pressures that encourage violence.** You may encounter acquaintances or groups that encourage domination of others, hostility to outsiders, binge drinking, or sexual aggression. Don't play along.
- **Reporting crime.** If you see or hear about a crime, let campus security or police know.

Helping a Friend

The U.S. Department of Health and Human Services offers the following suggestions for helping a friend who's being abused:[66]

- Assuming that you're somewhere private, ask your friend to tell you about what she or he has been going through. Listen. Don't interrupt.
- Tell your friend you're concerned about her or his safety. Try to help your friend to see that what's going on isn't right and that she or he can do something about it and has your support.
- Offer specific assistance. For instance, offer to accompany your friend to your campus health center. Or invite your

friend to stay at your place while she or he figures out what to do.

- Stay involved. If your friend decides to leave the relationship, she or he may need your help working through feelings of sadness, anxiety, or regret. If your friend decides to stay, although it might be hard for you to understand, remind your friend that you're there no matter what.

To support a friend who has been sexually assaulted—or who believes that she or he was assaulted while intoxicated—the most helpful thing you can do is to listen. Give your friend time to explain what happened and explore what she or he wants to do next. Offer to accompany your friend to the campus health center or security office or to call the police or an advocacy agency in the community. Stay with your friend as long as you're needed. In the days and weeks that follow, continue to listen as your friend "processes" what's happened. Avoid suggesting that the incident was in any way your friend's fault. Even if substance abuse was involved, your friend was a victim of crime and was in no way to blame.

Campus Advocacy

Although it's easy to feel overwhelmed by issues of campus safety, the good news is that there are many ways you can help. Here are just a few:

- Students Against Violence Everywhere (SAVE) has more than 2,000 chapters in schools and colleges nationwide. SAVE works to promote personal safety and reduce violent crime and victimization. For more information, check out www.nationalsave.org.

- Join Students Active for Ending Rape (SAFER), the American Association of University Women's student group dedicated to fighting sexual assault on campus. Download the AAUW-SAFER Campus Sexual Assault Program in a Box from www.aauw.org (search for "sexual assault tool kit.")

- Men often feel as if their gender automatically makes them responsible for the problem of violence and excludes them from becoming part of the solution. Not so. A national organization called Men Can Stop Rape shifts the responsibility for violence prevention toward men by promoting healthy, nonviolent masculinity and engaging men as allies in proactive solutions to end violence against women. This organization is operating right now on college campuses across the nation. Find out more about its Campus Men of Strength Clubs at www.mencanstoprape.org .

>> Watch videos of real students discussing personal safety at MasteringHealth™

LO 15.9 QUICK CHECK

Beth's friend Jamie has been sexually assaulted. What is the most helpful thing Beth can do for Jamie?

a. Report the assault to the Title IX coordinator at her college.
b. Do things to help keep Jamie's mind off of the assault.
c. Listen to Jamie when she is able and willing to talk.
d. Insist that Jamie report the crime to the police.

Choosing to Change Worksheet

To complete this worksheet online, visit MasteringHealth™

PART I. Understanding Your Risk from Aggressive Driving

Complete the "Are You an Aggressive Driver?" Self-Assessment on page 379 and list each of your aggressive habits.

_____

_____

PART II. Avoiding Aggressive Driving

Directions: Fill in your stage of change in step 1 and complete steps 2, 3, or 4, depending on which one applies to your stage of change.

Step 1: Assess your stage of behavior change. Please check one of the following statements that best describe your readiness to make your driving safer.

_____ I do not intend to improve my driving in the next six months. (Precontemplation)

_____ I am contemplating improving my driving in the next six months. (Contemplation)

_____ I am planning on improving my driving in the next month. (Preparation)

_____ I have been improving my driving for less than six months. (Action)

_____ I have been improving my driving for six months or longer. (Maintenance)

Step 2: Work the precontemplation and contemplation stages. Consider what you can do to make your driving less aggressive. What are the advantages of adopting these behaviors to increase driving safety? (List at least three.)

___

___

___

What are some things that might get in the way of your efforts to implement these behaviors? (List at least two.)

___

___

What ideas do you have to overcome these obstacles?

___

Step 3: Prepare. How do you expect to benefit from increased driving safety?

___

___

List a SMART goal for improving your driving.

___

Step 4: Act and maintain. In what ways have you benefited from adopting these behaviors and actions?

___

___

What motivates you the most to continue practicing these behaviors, and why?

___

___

CHAPTER 15 STUDY PLAN

CHAPTER SUMMARY

LO 15.1
- Injuries are the leading cause of death among Americans between the ages of 1 and 44. One of the most significant risk factors for injuries is substance abuse.

LO 15.2
- Motor vehicle accidents (MVAs) claim more lives among Americans aged 15 to 24 than any other cause.
- Distracted driving, impaired driving, poor use of safety features, speeding, and other forms of aggressive driving are risk factors for MVAs.
- Motorcyclists are about six times more likely to die in a crash than are those driving or riding in a car. Motorcycle accidents kill more than 4,500 Americans each year.

MasteringHealth™
Build your knowledge—and health!—in the Study Area of **MasteringHealth**™ with a variety of study tools.

LO 15.3
- Thousands of pedestrians are injured or killed each year, and bicycle injuries cause several hundred deaths annually.
- Failure to wear a helmet while cycling increases the risk for disability and death.

LO 15.4
- An increasing number of Americans are dying from unintentional poisoning, and many of these deaths are due to overdose of legal and illicit drugs.

- In adults, eating too fast, without chewing food properly, is the most common factor in choking.
- Drowning is the second leading cause of unintentional injury death in people aged 10 to 19. Consumption of alcohol is a factor in 60% of drowning and fire fatalities.
- Repetitive strain injuries are common among those using computers and mobile devices.

LO 15.5

- Violence is a leading cause of death and injury among young people, especially young men. Murder is the third leading cause of death in the United States among those aged 15 to 24.
- Violent crimes include murder, forcible rape, robbery, and aggravated assault. The rate of violent crime in the United States has been declining.
- Hazing is a set of initiation rituals involving humiliation, isolation, alcohol consumption, sleep deprivation, and/or physical or sexual abuse.

LO 15.6

- Homicide, the willful killing of another person, is the third leading cause of death in the U.S. among those aged 15 to 24.
- The great majority of both murder victims and perpetrators are male.
- More that two-thirds of murders involve firearms

LO 15.7

- Intimate partner violence includes psychological abuse as well as physical and sexual assault. Victims stay in abusive relationships for a variety of reasons.
- Stalking is a pattern of harassment or threats directed at a specific person and intended to cause intimidation and fear. It includes cyberstalking, involving digital and online communications.

LO 15.8

- Sexual assault is a common problem on college campuses. Drinking and drug use are factors in more than three-quarters of these assaults.
- You can greatly reduce your risk for rape by staying sober, attending social gatherings with one or more friends, and communicating your choices firmly and clearly.

LO 15.9

- Declining rates of violent crime show that prevention works, including steps such as knowing and following campus safety rules, staying sober, encouraging a culture of respect, refusing to remain silent if you witness any aggressive act, and reporting crime.
- You can support a friend who has experienced violence by listening without judgment and encouraging actions such as using campus resources to get help.

GET CONNECTED

>> Visit the following websites for further information about the topics in this chapter:

- National Center for Injury Prevention and Control
  www.cdc.gov/injury/index.html
- National Safety Council
  www.nsc.org
- American Association of Poison Control Centers
  www.aapcc.org
- Injury Prevention Web
  www.injuryprevention.org
- Motorcycle Safety Foundation

MOBILE TIPS!
Scan this QR code with your mobile device to access additional tips about reducing your risk for intentional and unintentional injuries. Or, via your mobile device, go to **http://chmobile.pearsoncmg.com** and choose by topic: reducing risk of injury.

  www.msf-usa.org
- National Domestic Violence Hotline
  www.thehotline.org
- Rape, Abuse, & Incest National Network (RAINN)
  www.rainn.org

Website links are subject to change. To access updated web links, please visit MasteringHealth™

TEST YOUR KNOWLEDGE

LO 15.1

1. Of the following, which causes the most deaths in the United States?
   a. motor vehicle accidents
   b. violence, such as a fight or a gunshot
   c. drowning
   d. unintentional poisoning

LO 15.2

2. Which of the following behaviors is a contributing factor in the greatest number of motor vehicle accidents?
   a. feeling drowsy
   b. texting
   c. hands-free cell phone talking
   d. aggressive driving

LO 15.3

3. Safety experts advise that pedestrians reduce their risk of injury by
   a. wearing a helmet.
   b. walking with the flow of the traffic.
   c. wearing brightly colored clothing.
   d. waiting until they are within a crosswalk to use their cell phone.

4. Which of the following statements about unintentional injuries is true?
   a. Drowning is the second leading cause of unintentional injury death among people aged 10 to 19.
   b. Overdoses of prescription opioid painkillers now account for more than 40% of all unintentional drug overdose deaths.
   c. Alcohol consumption is a common contributing factor in choking deaths, drownings, and fatal fires.
   d. All of these answers are true.

LO 15.6

5. In the United States, violent crime
   a. has increased every year since 1980.
   b. is more common in schools than off campus.
   c. occurs most frequently in regions that are economically distressed.
   d. is more commonly committed by men, but women are more often the victims.

6. Which of the following is a common cause of death in hazing incidents?
   a. drowning
   b. alcohol poisoning
   c. aggravated assault
   d. alcohol poisoning AND aggravated assault

LO 15.7

7. Which of the following statements about intimate partner violence is true?
   a. Nearly 12 million Americans experience IPV yearly.
   b. Many cases of IPV go unreported.
   c. Women are more likely to be the victims of IPV.
   d. All of these answers are true.

LO 15.8

8. Date rape
   a. is more likely if one or both people on a date have been drinking.
   b. doesn't carry the same legal penalties as stranger rape.
   c. is legally known as statutory rape.
   d. All of these answers are true.

9. Sexual harassment
   a. occurs in both schools and workplaces.
   b. rarely occurs on college campuses.
   c. affects about twice as many women as men.
   d. can only occur between two members of the opposite sex.

LO 15.9

10. Which of the following is likely to be the most helpful strategy for supporting a friend experiencing intimate partner violence?
    a. Encourage your friend to break off the relationship.
    b. Tell your friend that you are concerned about her or his safety.
    c. Try to convince your friend to report the incident to the police.
    d. Discuss how her or his actions contributed to the incident.

WHAT DO YOU THINK?

LO 15.1
1. Explain the relationship between alcohol use and unintentional injuries.

LO 15.2
2. Would you support a ban on cell phone use while driving? Why or why not?

LO 15.5
3. The rate of violent crime has been dropping in America for the past two decades. Why do you think this has been occurring?

LO 15.7
4. A friend confides that she was sexually assaulted the night before. Explain how you would help her.

LO 15.9
5. What are some strategies a college student can adopt for staying safer on campus?

QUICK CHECK ANSWERS

Chapter 1
LO 1.1 c   LO 1.2 b   LO 1.3 d   LO 1.4 b
LO 1.5 a   LO 1.6 c   LO 1.7 a

Chapter 2
LO 2.1 b   LO 2.2 b   LO 2.3 c   LO 2.4 d
LO 2.5 d   LO 2.6 a   LO 2.7 b   LO 2.8 a
LO 2.9 c   LO 2.10 c

Chapter 3
LO 3.1 d   LO 3.2 a   LO 3.3 b   LO 3.4 c
LO 3.5 a   LO 3.6 d   LO 3.7 b

Chapter 4
LO 4.1 c   LO 4.2 d   LO 4.3 d   LO 4.4 b
LO 4.5 d   LO 4.6 a

Chapter 5
LO 5.1 b   LO 5.2 b   LO 5.3 a   LO 5.4 d
LO 5.5 c

Chapter 6
LO 6.1 a   LO 6.2 c   LO 6.3 d   LO 6.4 b
LO 6.5 a   LO 6.6 d   LO 6.7 b

Chapter 7
LO 7.1 d   LO 7.2 b   LO 7.3 d   LO 7.4 d
LO 7.5 b   LO 7.6 b   LO 7.7 d

Chapter 8
LO 8.1 c   LO 8.2 d   LO 8.3 b   LO 8.4 c
LO 8.5 b   LO 8.6 a   LO 8.7 b   LO 8.8 d

Chapter 9
LO 9.1 a   LO 9.2 a   LO 9.3 d   LO 9.4 b
LO 9.5 b   LO 9.6 c   LO 9.7 b   LO 9.8 b
LO 9.9 d   LO 9.10 a   LO 9.11 b

Chapter 10
LO 10.1 b   LO 10.2 c   LO 10.3 d   LO 10.4 a
LO 10.5 d   LO 10.6 c   LO 10.7 d

Chapter 11
LO 11.1 b   LO 11.2 b   LO 11.3 a   LO 11.4 d
LO 11.5 c   LO 11.6 b   LO 11.7 d   LO 11.8 b
LO 11.9 b   LO 11.10 d

Chapter 12
LO 12.1 b   LO 12.2 d   LO 12.3 b   LO 12.4 b
LO 12.5 d

Chapter 13
LO 13.1 d   LO 13.2 c   LO 13.3 a   LO 13.4 b
LO 13.5 b   LO 13.6 d

Chapter 14
LO 14.1 d   LO 14.2 a   LO 14.3 c   LO 14.4 d
LO 14.5 d   LO 14.6 a   LO 14.7 b

Chapter 15
LO 15.1 b   LO 15.2 a   LO 15.3 c   LO 15.4 a
LO 15.5 c   LO 15.6 b   LO 15.7 b   LO 15.8 a
LO 15.9 c

Chapter 16 (electronic chapter)
LO 16.1 c   LO 16.2 b   LO 16.3 a   LO 16.4 c
LO 16.5 c   LO 16.6 a   LO 16.7 c   LO 16.8 a
LO 16.9 b

Chapter 17 (electronic chapter)
LO 17.1 b   LO 17.2 c   LO 17.3 d   LO 17.4 a
LO 17.5 d   LO 17.6 c   LO 17.7 b

TEST YOUR KNOWLEDGE ANSWERS

Chapter 1
1. c 2. d 3. d 4. b 5. c 6. b 7. d
8. b 9. a 10. a

Chapter 2
1. d 2. b 3. b 4. c 5. d 6. a 7. c
8. d 9. c 10. a

Chapter 3
1. a 2. b 3. c 4. a 5. d 6. d 7. b
8. c 9. b 10. a

Chapter 4
1. c 2. b 3. a 4. b 5. d 6. c 7. d
8. a 9. d 10. b

Chapter 5
1. a 2. c 3. c 4. a 5. d 6. b 7. c
8. b 9. c 10. a

Chapter 6
1. d 2. d 3. c 4. c 5. b 6. d 7. b
8. a 9. c 10. a

Chapter 7
1. a 2. a 3. d 4. b 5. d 6. c 7. b
8. d 9. a 10. c

Chapter 8
1. b 2. d 3. c 4. a 5. d 6. a 7. d
8. d 9. b 10. c

Chapter 9
1. d 2. a 3. d 4. d 5. b 6. d 7. c
8. b 9. c 10. c

Chapter 10
1. d 2. b 3. b 4. d 5. d 6. b 7. c
8. d 9. a 10. c

Chapter 11
1. d 2. c 3. b 4. b 5. a 6. b 7. d
8. c 9. d 10. c

Chapter 12
1. b 2. b 3. d 4. a 5. b 6. a 7. a
8. d 9. d 10. c

Chapter 13
1. c 2. d 3. d 4. a 5. a 6. c 7. d
8. d 9. b 10. b

Chapter 14
1. d 2. d 3. a 4. b 5. d 6. a 7. a
8. c 9. b 10. a

Chapter 15
1. a 2. b 3. c 4. d 5. c 6. d 7. d
8. a 9. a 10. b

Chapter 16 (electronic chapter)
1. d 2. c 3. b 4. a 5. d 6. c 7. a
8. d 9. b 10. c

Chapter 17 (electronic chapter)
1. b 2. d 3. c 4. c 5. c 6. d 7. b
8. b 9. b 10. d

CREDITS

Photo Credits

Cover: Stellapictures/Blend Images; **Inside Front Cover:** Intellistudies. Shutterstock; **Visual Walkthrough p. 1:** Stellapictures/Blend Images; **Visual Walkthrough p. 2:** Biggie Productions/The Image Bank/Getty Images; **Visual Walkthrough p. 3, 1st top right:** Antonioguillem/Fotolia; **Visual Walkthrough p. 3, 2nd top right:** GoGo Images Corporation/Alamy; **Visual Walkthrough p. 3, left:** aslysun/Shutterstock; **Visual Walkthrough, p. 8:** Stellapictures/Blend Images; **p. iv, top:** Courtesy of April Lynch; **p. iv, middle:** Courtesy of Karen Vail-Smith; **p. iv, bottom:** Courtesy of Jerome Kotecki; **p. viii, left:** Sam Edwards/Getty Images; **p. viii, right:** Westend61/Getty Images; **p. ix:** Image Source/Getty Images; **p. x:** Biggie Productions/The Image Bank/Getty Images; **p. x, right:** MBI/Alamy Stock Photo; **p. xi, left:** VisualCommunications/E+/Getty Images; **p. xi, right:** Tetra Images/Getty Images; **p. xii, left:** Fuse/Getty Images; **p. xii, right:** Fotosearch/Getty Images; **p. xiii:** Tetra Images/Getty Images; **p. xiv, left:** Gallo Images-Hayley Baxter/Getty Images; **p. xiv, right:** Tetra Images/Getty Images; **p. xv, left:** Tara Moore/Getty Images; **p. xv, right:** Caia Images/Superstock; **p. xvi:** Susan Chiang/Getty Images; **p. xvii, left:** Blend Images/Superstock; **p. xvii, right:** ColorBlind Images/Getty Images; **p. xix:** Vasya Kobelev/Shutterstock; **p. xxi, top:** aslysun/Shutterstock; **p. xxi, bottom:** Piotr Marcinski/Shutterstock; **p. xxii:** paffy/Shutterstock

Chapter 1 opener: Sam Edwards/Getty Images; **p. 4:** Michael Jung/Fotolia; **p. 5:** John Panella/Shutterstock; **p. 6, top:** Piotr Marcinski/Shutterstock; **p. 6, bottom:** rocketclips/Fotolia; **p. 7:** aslysun/Shutterstock; **p. 8:** Friedrich Stark/Alamy Limited; **p. 10, top:** Fancy/Alamy Images; **p. 10, bottom:** blickwinkel/Alamy Stock Photo; **p. 11:** John Dawson/Pearson; **p. 12, top:** Vasya Kobelev/Shutterstock; **p. 12, bottom:** ollyy/Shutterstock; **p. 13:** Ghislain & Marie David de Lossy/Cultura Creative/Alamy; **p. 15, 1st from top:** Lissandra/Shutterstock; **p. 15, 2nd from top:** Tom Mareschal/Alamy; **p. 15, 3rd from top:** Monkey Business Images/Shutterstock; **p. 15, 4th from top:** Katrina Brown/Shutterstock; **p. 16:** glegorly/Getty Images; **p. 17, top:** Peter Bernik/Shutterstock; **p. 17, bottom:** Jeff Greenberg/Alamy Stock Photo

Chapter 2 opener: Westend61/Getty Images; **p. 27, top:** Monkey Business; **p. 27, bottom:** Rido. Shutterstock; **p. 30:** Tony Freeman/PhotoEdit; **p. 31:** Imaginechina/AP Images; **p. 32, top:** aslysun/Shutterstock; **p 32, bottom:** Darren Greenwood/Design Pics Inc./Alamy; **p. 35:** WavebreakMediaMicro/Fotolia; **p. 36, left:** Pearson Education; **p. 36, right:** Stephen VanHorn/Shutterstock; **p. 38:** Stockbroker/MBI/Alamy; **p. 39:** Blend Images/Alamy Stock Photo; **p. 41:** zdyma4/Fotolia; **p. 43, top left:** paffy/Shutterstock; **p. 43, top right:** Photographee.eu/Fotolia; **p. 44:** Tom Wang/Shutterstock

Chapter 3 opener: Image Source/Getty Images; **p. 53:** hektoR/Shutterstock; **p. 55, top:** Pearson Education; **p. 55, bottom:** Stockbyte/Getty Images; **p. 56:** Adam Gregor/Shutterstock; **p. 57:** aslysun/Shutterstock; **p. 58:** Samuel Borges Photography/Shutterstock; **p. 60, top:** Mehmet Dilsiz/Fotolia; **p. 60, bottom:** Minerva Studio/Shutterstock; **p. 61, top:** Piotr Marcinski/Shutterstock; **p. 61, bottom:** Miquel Llop/NurPhoto/Getty Images; **p. 64:** Pearson Education; **p. 65:** Commercial Eye/Getty; **p. 66:** Stockbyte/Getty Images; **p. 67, top:** wavebreakmedia/Shutterstock; **p. 67, bottom:** PhotoAlto/Alamy; **p. 68, left:** Samuel Borges Photography/Shutterstock; **p. 68, right:** Runzelkorn/Shutterstock

Chapter 4 opener: Biggie Productions/The Image Bank/Getty Images; **p. 76:** Pressmaster/Shutterstock; **p. 78:** Corbis Super RF/Alamy Stock Photo; **p. 79:** aslysun/Shutterstock; **p. 80, left:** Antonioguillem/Fotolia; **p. 80, right:** GoGo Images Corporation/Alamy; **p. 82, top:** Piotr Marcinski/Shutterstock; **p. 82, middle:** mariesacha/Fotolia; **p. 83:** Bubbles Photolibrary/Alamy; **p. 84:** Bubbles Photolibrary/Alamy; **p. 85:** Edhdar/Shutterstock; **p. 86:** Anthony-Masterson/FoodPix/Getty Images; **p. 87, top:** John Dawson/Pearson Education/Pearson Science; **p. 87, bottom:** Hank Morgan/Science Source; **p. 88, top left:** paffy/Shutterstock; **p. 88, top right:** Samantha Craddock/123RF; **p. 90:** JGI/Jamie Grill/Blend Images/Corbis

Chapter 5 opener: MBI/Alamy Stock Photo; **p. 98:** Tom Grill/Corbis; **p. 99:** Feng Yu/Shutterstock.com; **p. 100:** Corbis; **p. 101:** M. Unal Ozmen/Shutterstock; **p. 102:** sarsmis/Fotolia; **p. 103:** JJAVA/Fotolia; **p. 104, top 1st:** Barry Gregg/Keepsake/Corbis; **p. 104, top 2nd:** Barry Gregg/Keepsake/Corbis; **p. 104, top 3rd:** Barry Gregg/Spirit/Corbis; **p. 104, top 4th:** Barry Gregg/Spirit/Corbis; **p. 104, top 5th:** Barry Gregg/Keepsake/Corbis; **p. 104, top 6th:** Barry Gregg/Keepsake/Corbis; **p. 104, top 7th:** Barry Gregg/Keepsake/Corbis; **p. 105, top 1st:** Barry Gregg/Keepsake/Corbis; **p. 105, top 2nd:** Barry Gregg/Spirit/Corbis; **p. 105, top 3rd:** Barry Gregg/Spirit/Corbis; **p. 105, top 4th:** Barry Gregg/Keepsake/Corbis; **p. 105, top 5th:** Barry Gregg/Spirit/Corbis; **p. 105, top 6th:** Barry Gregg/Keepsake/Corbis; **p. 105, bottom 1st:** Barry Gregg/Keepsake/Corbis; **p. 105, bottom 2nd:** Barry Gregg/Spirit/Corbis; **p. 105, bottom 3rd:** Barry Gregg/Keepsake/Corbis; **p. 105, bottom 4th:** Barry Gregg/Spirit/Corbis; **p. 105, bottom 5th:** Morgan Lane Photography/Shutterstock; **p. 106:** Lana Langlois/Shutterstock; **p. 107, top left:** paffy/Shutterstock; **p. 107, top right:** hypedesign. Shutterstock; **p. 107, bottom:** Kati Molin/Shutterstock; **p. 108:** Jesse Kunerth/Alamy; **p. 109:** aslysun/Shutterstock; **p. 111, top:** Piotr Marcinski/Shutterstock; **p. 111, bottom:** Bernabea Amalia Mendez/Shutterstock; **p. 112, left:** Pearson Education; **p. 112, right:** Food & Drug Administration; **p. 113 left (all photos):** Pearson Education; **p. 113, right:** U.S. Department of Agriculture; **p. 114:** Gresei/Fotolia; **p. 115 (all photos):** Pearson Education; **p. 116, left:** Bonchan/Shutterstock; **p. 116, right:** Pixelbliss/Fotolia; **p. 118:** ksena32/Fotolia; **p. 119, top left:** paffy/Shutterstock; **p. 119, top right:** Regien Paassen/Shutterstock; **p. 121:** Image Source/Alamy

Chapter 6 opener: VisualCommunications/E+/Getty Images; **p. 128, top:** ranplett/E+/Getty Images; **p. 128, bottom:** Media Bakery/Shutterstock; **p. 129, left:** Ariwasabi/Shutterstock; **p. 129, right:** Apirut Siri/Shutterstock; **p. 132:** djma/Fotolia; **p. 133:** Pearson; **p. 134, top:** pressmaster/Fotolia; **p. 134, bottom left:** Maksim Šmeljov/Fotolia; **p. 134, bottom middle:** Doug Menuez/Photodisc/Getty Images; **p. 134, bottom right:** Stockbyte/Getty Images; **p. 135:** blue jean images/Getty Images; **p. 136:** Image Source/Getty Images; **p. 137 (all photos):** Elena Dorfman/Pearson Education; **p. 138 (all photos):** Elena Dorfman/Pearson Education; **p. 140 (all photos):** Elena Dorfman/Pearson Education; **p. 141, top-to-bottom, 1st-2nd-3rd-4th-5th:** Elena Dorfman/Pearson Education; **p. 141, top-to-bottom, 6th:** James Borchuck/Tampa Bay Times/Alamy; **p. 144:** aslysun/Shutterstock; **p. 146, top left:** paffy/Shutterstock; **p. 146, top right:** Kim Reinick/Shutterstock; **p. 147, top left:** Vasya Kobelev/Shutterstock; **p. 147, top right:** MJTH/Shutterstock; **p. 149, top:** Piotr Marcinski/Shutterstock; **p. 149, bottom:** Al Tielemans/Sports Illustrated/Getty Images; **p. 150:** Pearson Education

Chapter 7 opener: Tetra Images/Getty Images; **p. 156:** ssimone/shutterstock; **p. 158:** George Doyle/Stockbyte/Getty Images; **p. 159:** Imaginechina/AP Images; **p. 160:** aslysun/Shutterstock; **p. 161:** Mark Hayes/Shutterstock; **p. 163:** Pearson Education; **p. 164:** aslysun/Shutterstock; **p. 167 (all photos):** Pearson Education; **p. 169:** Jacek

Chabraszewski/Fotolia; **p. 171:** OLJ Studio/Shutterstock.com; **p. 172, left:** Samuel Borges/Shutterstock; **p. 172, right:** AmanaimagesRF/Getty Images; **p. 173, top:** Custom Medical Stock Photo/Alamy; **p. 173, bottom:** Albanpix Ltd/Rex Features/AP Images; **p. 176:** Pearson Education

Chapter 8 opener: Fuse/Getty Images; **p. 183:** Design Pics Inc./Alamy; **p. 184:** oneinchpunch/Fotolia; **p. 185:** aslysun/Shutterstock; **p. 186:** Piotr Marcinski/Shutterstock; **p. 188:** AP Photo/Victoria Will/Invision/AP; **p. 189:** Rommel Canlas/Shutterstock; **p. 190:** AJPhoto/Science Source; **p. 192, top:** Studio Pookini/Fotolia; **p. 192, bottom:** Multnomah County Sheriff/Splash/Newscom; **p. 193:** Nico Hermann/Westend61/Newscom; **p. 194:** Tom Wagner/Alamy; **p. 197, top:** Pearson Education; **p. 197, bottom:** Bill Cheyrou/Alamy; **p. 199:** WavebreakmediaMicro/Fotolia

Chapter 9 opener: Fotosearch/Getty Images; **p. 207, top:** Piotr Marcinski/Shutterstock; **p. 207, bottom:** Piotr Marcinski/Alamy; **p. 208:** aslysun/Shutterstock; **p. 210:** StockLite/Shutterstock; **p. 213:** Oleksii Nykonchuk/Fotolia; **p. 214:** Pearson Education; **p. 215:** Tatiana Popova/Shutterstock; **p. 219:** Jamie Grill Photography/Getty Images; **p. 220:** aslysun/Shutterstock; **p. 222:** gstockstudio/123RF; **p. 224:** Image Source/Alamy; **p. 225, top left:** paffy/Shutterstock; **p. 225, top right:** HALL PHILIP/SIPA/Newscom; **p. 226:** Vaclav Volrab/Shutterstock; **p. 227, top:** BSIP/UIG via Getty Images; **p. 227, middle:** Milos Luzanin/Shutterstock; **p. 228:** Pearson Education; **p. 229:** Milos Luzanin/Shutterstock

Chapter 10 opener: Tetra Images/Getty Images; **p. 236:** Zoonar GmbH/Alamy; **p. 237, left:** Robert Kneschke/Shutterstock; **p. 237, right:** Monkey Business Images/Shutterstock; **p. 239, top:** Pearson Education; **p. 239, bottom:** Randy Faris/Corbis; **p. 241:** Antonio Ovejero Diaz/Fotolia; **p. 242:** Pearson Education; **p. 244, top:** Hill Street Studios/G/AGE Fotostock; **p. 244, bottom:** Hill Street Studios/Blend Images/Getty Images; **p. 246:** amana images inc./Alamy; **p. 247, top:** Piotr Marcinski/Shutterstock; **p. 247, middle:** redkoala/Fotolia; **p. 248:** aslysun/Shutterstock; **p. 251:** Corbis/AGE Fotostock; **p. 254:** Dubova/Fotolia

Chapter 11 opener: Gallo Images-Hayley Baxter/Getty Images; **p. 259:** Mila Supinskaya/Shutterstock; **p. 261:** Fancy/Alamy; **p. 263:** Ardelean Andreea/Shutterstock; **p. 264:** aslysun/Shutterstock; **p. 266:** Tetra Images/AGE Fotostock; **p. 268:** JStone/Shutterstock.com; **p. 269:** Pearson Education; **p. 273:** aslysun/Shutterstock; **p. 275:** Exactostock/SuperStock; **p. 276:** Christy Thompson/Shutterstock.com; **p. 277:** Tammy Hanratty/Alamy; **p. 278:** Pearson Science; **p. 281:** Science Photo Library/Alamy; **p. 282, 1st from top:** SPL/Science Source; **p. 282, 2nd from top:** Nestle/Petit Format/Science Source; **p. 282, 3rd from top:** Neil Bromhall/Science Source; **page 282, 4th from top:** Mark Kurschner/Getty Images; **p. 287:** Fancy Collection/SuperStock

Chapter 12 opener: Tetra Images/Getty Images; **p. 292:** deep-blue-photographer/Shutterstock; **p. 295:** Pearson Education; **p. 296:** Dmitry Naumov/Shutterstock; **p. 298 top 1st:** Dr. Linda M. Stannard/Science Source; **p. 298 top 2nd:** Centers for Disease Control (CDC); **p. 298 top 3rd:** Centers for Disease Control (CDC); **p. 298 top 4th:** Centers for Disease Control (CDC); **p. 298 top 5th:** Andrew Syred/Science Source; **p. 301:** Centers for Disease Control (CDC); **p. 302, top:** Centers for Disease Control (CDC); **p. 302, bottom:** James Gathany/Centers for Disease Control (CDC) **p. 303:** OJO Images Ltd/Alamy; **p. 307:** Daxiao Productions/fotolia; **p. 308, top left:** Dr. P. Marazzi/Science Source; **p. 308, top right:** Biophoto Associates/Science Source; **p. 308, bottom left:** Centers for Disease Control (CDC); **page 308, bottom right:** Centers for Disease Control (CDC); **p. 310, top:** Piotr Marcinski/Shutterstock; **p. 310, bottom:** MBI/Alamy; **p. 311, top:** Eye of Science/Science Source; **p. 311, bottom:** Centers for Disease Control (CDC); **p. 312:** aslysun/Shutterstock; **p. 313:** Jack Hollingsworth/Getty Images

Chapter 13 opener: Tara Moore/Getty Images; **p. 320:** aslysun/Shutterstock; **p. 322, top:** Piotr Marcinski/Shutterstock; **p. 322, bottom:** Dewayne Flowers. Shutterstock; **p. 323:** Jaimie Duplass/Shutterstock; **p. 325:** hilleborg/fotolia; **p. 326:** Pearson Education; **p. 327:** Anton Gvozdikov/Shutterstock; **p. 328, top left:** Science Stock Photography/Science Source; **p. 328, top right:** Ed Reschke/Getty Images; **p. 330, left:** Ronald Sumners. Shutterstock; **p. 330, right:** BSIP SA/Alamy; **p. 333:** cleanfotos. Shutterstock; **p. 337:** michaeljung/Shutterstock; **p. 340:** Aurora Photos/Alamy; **p. 341:** National Cancer Institute/Science Source; **p. 342, top:** P. Marazzi/Science Source; **p. 342, bottom:** Edyta Pawlowska. Shutterstock; **p. 343:** BIOPHOTO ASSOCIATES/Getty Image; **p. 344:** Pictorial Press Ltd/Alamy; **p. 345:** Pearson Science; **p. 347:** Lana K/Shutterstock

Chapter 14 opener: Caia Images/Superstock; **p. 353:** Tetra Images. Shutterstock; **p. 354:** KW Photography/Alamy; **p. 355:** Moodboard/Cultura/Getty Images; **p. 356:** paffy/Shutterstock; **p. 360, top:** Simone van den Berg/Shutterstock; **p. 360, bottom:** Nati Harnik/AP Images; **p. 361:** Jupiterimages/Comstock Images/Getty Images; **p. 362, top:** aslysun/Shutterstock; **p. 362, bottom:** kreativwerden/Fotolia; **p. 366, top:** Pearson Education; **p. 366, bottom:** Shutterstock/designer491; **p. 367:** Siri Stafford/Photodisc/Getty Images; **p. 368:** aslysun/Shutterstock; **p. 369:** Africa Studio/Shutterstock; **p. 370:** Westend61/SuperStock

Chapter 15 opener: Susan Chiang/Getty Images; **p. 378, top:** aslysun/Shutterstock; **p. 378, bottom:** Image Source/SuperStock; **p. 380, left:** Dave & Les Jacobs/Blend Images/Getty Images; **p. 380, right:** Antonio Diaz/Fotolia; **p. 381:** Pearson Education; **p. 383, top:** aslysun/Shutterstock; **p. 383, middle:** Science Photo Library/Getty Images; **p. 383, bottom:** Science Photo Library/Alamy; **p. 384:** Big Pants Production/Shutterstock; **p. 385, top:** Radius Images/Alamy; **p. 385, bottom:** Sarah Fix Photography Inc/Blend Images/Alamy; **p. 386:** Ampon Akearunrung/Shutterstock; **p. 387, top:** Piotr Marcinski/Shutterstock; **p. 387, bottom:** Steve Olson/fStop/Alamy; **p. 388:** Chuck Savage/Getty Images; **p. 390:** WoodyStock/Alamy; **p. 392:** moodboard/Alamy; **p. 395:** woodygraphs/Shutterstock

Chapter 16 opener: Blend Images/Superstock; **p. 402:** Aurora Photos/Alamy; **p. 403:** aslysun/Shutterstock; **p. 404:** dbimages/Alamy; **p. 405:** National Geographic Image Collection/Alamy; **p. 409:** Jim West/Alamy; **p 411:** Car Culture/Getty Images; **p. 412:** 63814. Shutterstock; **p. 413, top left:** paffy/Shutterstock; **p. 413, top right:** Givaga/Fotolia; **p. 414:** riddypix/Alamy; **p. 415:** iodrakon.Shutterstock; **p. 416:** Stephen Gibson/Shutterstock.com; **p. 417, top:** Piotr Marcinski/Shutterstock; **p. 417, bottom:** Jeff Greenberg/AGE Fotostock; **p. 418, left:** Tomas/Fotolia; **p. 418, right:** Ronald Sumners/Shutterstock; **p. 420:** Pixland/Thinkstock; **p. 423:** Jupiterimages/Getty Images

Chapter 17 opener: ColorBlind Images/Getty Images; **p. 432:** Blend Images/Alamy; **p. 433:** Blend Images/Alamy; **p. 434, top left:** National Eye Institute; **p. 434, middle left:** National Eye Institute; **p. 434, bottom left:** National Eye Institute; **p. 434, bottom right:** Michael Klein/Peter Arnold/Getty Images; **p. 436:** Dr. Robert Friedland/Science Source; **p. 437:** Ellen Isaacs/Alamy; **p. 439:** Monkey Business Images/Shutterstock; **p. 440, top:** Piotr Marcinski/Shutterstock; **p. 440, bottom:** MBI/Alamy; **p. 442, top:** Vasya Kobelev/Shutterstock; **p. 442, middle:** Mark Bowden/E+/Getty Images; **p. 442, bottom:** Karen Gentry/Shutterstock; **p. 443:** Richard Ellis/Alamy; **p. 445:** iceteaimages/Alamy; **p. 447:** Mike Booth/Alamy; **p. 449:** Photolibrary RF/Getty Images

GLOSSARY

A

abortion A medical or surgical procedure used to terminate a pregnancy.

absorption The process by which alcohol passes from the stomach or small intestine into the bloodstream.

abstinence Avoidance of sexual intercourse.

acceptance and commitment therapy (ACT) An outgrowth of cognitive-behavioral therapy that increases patients' ability to engage in values-based, positive behaviors while experiencing difficult thoughts, emotions, or sensations.

accessory glands The glands (seminal vesicles, prostate gland, and Cowper's gland) that lubricate the reproductive system and nourish sperm.

acid rain A phenomenon in which airborne pollutants are transformed by chemical processes into acidic compounds; mix with rain, snow, or fog; and are deposited on Earth.

acquired immunity The body's ability to quickly identify and attack a pathogen that it recognizes from previous exposure. In some cases acquired immunity leads to lifelong protection against the same infection.

active stretching A type of static stretching in which you gently apply force to your body to create a stretch.

acute Characteristic of an illness or injury that comes on suddenly, progresses and resolves rapidly, and may or may not require medical treatment.

added sugars Sugars not naturally present in foods or beverages but added during processing or preparation.

addiction A chronic, progressive disease of brain reward, motivation, memory, and related circuitry characterized by uncontrollable craving for a substance or behavior despite both negative consequences and diminishment or loss of pleasure associated with the activity.

advance directives Formal documents that state a person's preferences regarding medical treatment and medical crisis management.

advocacy Working independently or with others to directly improve aspects of the social or physical environment or to change policies or legislation.

aerobic exercise Prolonged physical activity that raises the heart rate and works the large muscle groups.

age-related macular degeneration (AMD) An age-related vision disorder caused by deterioration of the macula that reduces central vision.

ageism Prejudice or discrimination against older adults.

aggravated assault An attack intended to cause serious physical harm, often involving a weapon.

Air Quality Index (AQI) An index for measuring daily air quality according to a list of federal air criteria, published by city or region.

alcohol abuse Drinking alcohol to excess, either regularly or on individual occasions, resulting in disruption of work, school, or home life and causing interpersonal, social, or legal problems.

alcohol intoxication The state of physical and/or mental impairment brought on by excessive alcohol consumption (in legal terms, a BAC of 0.08% or greater).

alcohol poisoning Dangerously high level of alcohol consumption, resulting in depression of the central nervous system, slowed breathing and heart rate, and compromised gag reflex.

alcoholism (alcohol dependence) A physical dependence on alcohol to the extent that stopping drinking brings on withdrawal symptoms.

allergies Abnormal immune system reactions to substances that are otherwise harmless.

allostatic overload A harmful state resulting from the cumulative burden of adapting, again and again, to stress.

altruism The practice of helping and giving to others out of genuine concern for their well-being.

Alzheimer's disease (AD) A progressive, fatal form of age-related dementia.

amenorrhea Cessation of menstrual periods.

amino acids Nitrogen-containing compounds that are the building blocks of proteins.

amniotic fluid Fluid that surrounds the developing fetus that aids in temperature regulation and allows the baby to move freely.

amphetamines Central nervous system stimulants that are chemically similar to the natural stimulants adrenaline and noradrenaline.

anaerobic exercise Short, intense exercise that causes an oxygen deficit in the muscles.

anal intercourse Intercourse characterized by the insertion of the penis into a partner's anus and rectum.

anaphylactic shock A result of anaphylaxis, where the release of histamine and other chemicals into the body leads to a drop in blood pressure, tightening of airways, and possible unconsciousness and even death.

andropause A period marked by a decline in the male reproductive hormone testosterone and its resultant physical and emotional effects; also referred to as *male menopause*.

angina pectoris Chest pain due to coronary heart disease.

angioplasty An arterial treatment that involves using a small balloon to flatten plaque deposits against the arterial wall.

anorexia athletica A mental disorder that involves using compulsive and excessive exercising as a purge.

anorexia nervosa A mental disorder characterized by extremely low body weight, body image distortion, severe calorie restriction, and an obsessive fear of gaining weight.

antibiotic resistance A bacterium's ability to overcome the effects of an antibiotic through a random mutation or change in the bacterium's genetic code.

antibodies Proteins released by B cells that bind tightly to infectious agents and mark them for destruction.

antigen Tiny regions on the surface of an infectious agent that can be detected by B cells and T cells.

antioxidants In nutrition, compounds (mainly nutrients and phytochemicals) that help protect the body from harmful chemicals called free radicals.

anxiety disorders A category of mental disorders characterized by persistent feelings of fear, dread, and worry.

Apgar score A measurement of how well a newborn tolerated the stresses of birth and how well he or she is adapting to the new environment.

appetite The psychological response to the sight, smell, thought, or taste of food that prompts or postpones eating.

arable Suitable for cultivation of crops.

arrhythmia Any irregularity in the heart's rhythm.

arteries Vessels that transport blood away from the heart, delivering oxygen-rich blood to the body periphery and oxygen-poor blood to the lungs.

arthritis Inflammation of one or more joints in the body, resulting in pain, swelling, and limited movement.

assertiveness The ability to clearly express your needs and wants to others in an appropriate way.

assortative mating The tendency to be attracted to people who are similar to ourselves.

asthma A chronic pulmonary disease in which the air passages become inflamed, making breathing difficult.

atherosclerosis A condition characterized by narrowing of the arteries as a result of inflammation, scarring, and the buildup of fatty deposits.

atria The two upper chambers of the heart, which receive blood from the body periphery and lungs.

attachment theory The theory that the patterns of attachment in our earliest relationships with others form the template for attachment in later relationships.

attention deficit/hyperactivity disorder (ADHD) A type of attention disorder characterized by inattention, hyperactive behavior, fidgeting, and a tendency toward impulsive behavior.

attention disorders A category of mental disorders characterized by problems with mental focus.

autonomy The capacity to make informed, uncoerced decisions.

autopsy A medical examination of a corpse that primarily attempts to identify the cause of death.

B

bacteria (singular *bacterium***)** Single-celled microorganisms that invade a host and reproduce inside. Harmful bacteria release toxic enzymes and chemicals.

ballistic stretching Performing rhythmic bouncing movements in a stretch to increase the intensity of the stretch.

barbiturates Types of central nervous system depressants prescribed to induce sleep or sedation.

bariatric surgery Weight-loss surgery using various procedures to modify the stomach or other sections of the gastrointestinal tract in order to reduce calorie intake or absorption.

basal metabolic rate (BMR) The rate at which the body expends energy for only the basic functioning of vital organs.

bath salts Any of a group of drugs containing a synthetic compound similar to cathinone, an amphetamine-like stimulant.

behavior change A sustained change in a habit or pattern of behavior that affects health.

behavior therapy A type of therapy that focuses on changing a patient's behavior and thereby achieving psychological health.

behavioral addiction A form of addiction involving a compulsion to engage in an activity such as gambling, sex, or shopping rather than a compulsion to use a substance.

benign tumor A tumor that grows slowly, does not spread, and is not cancerous.

benzodiazepines Medications commonly prescribed to treat anxiety and panic attacks.

binge drinking A pattern of drinking alcohol that results in a blood alcohol concentration of 0.08 or above (about five or more alcoholic drinks within two hours for men or four or more alcoholic drinks within two hours for women).

binge eating The rapid consumption of an excessive amount of food.

bioaccumulation A process by which substances increase in concentration in the fat tissues of living organisms as the organisms take in contaminated air, water, or food.

biomagnification A process by which certain contaminants become more concentrated in animal tissue as they move up the food chain.

biomonitoring Analysis of body tissues or specimens, including blood or urine, to measure chemical exposure in humans.

biopsy A test for cancer in which a small sample of the abnormal growth is removed and studied.

bipolar disorder (manic-depressive disorder) A mental disorder characterized by occurrences of abnormally elevated mood (or mania), often alternating with depressive episodes, with periods of normal mood in between.

birth control pills Pills containing combinations of hormones that prevent pregnancy when taken regularly as directed.

bisexuals People who are attracted to partners of the same and the opposite sex.

blood alcohol concentration (BAC) The amount of alcohol present in blood, measured in grams of alcohol per deciliter of blood.

blood pressure The force of blood moving against the arterial walls.

body burden The amount of a chemical stored in the body at a given time, especially a potential toxin in the body as the result of environmental exposure.

body composition The relative proportions of the body's lean tissue and fat tissue.

body dysmorphic disorder (BDD) A mental disorder characterized by obsessive thoughts about a perceived flaw in appearance.

body image A person's perceptions, feelings, and critiques of his or her own body.

body mass index (BMI) A numerical measurement, calculated from height and weight measurements, that provides an indicator of health risk categories.

bradycardia A slow arrhythmia.

brain death Cessation of brain activity, as indicated by various medical devices and diagnostic criteria.

bulimia nervosa A mental disorder characterized by episodes of binge eating followed by a purge behavior such as vomiting, laxative abuse, or extreme exercise.

burnout A phenomenon in which increased feelings of stress and decreased feelings of accomplishment lead to frustration, exhaustion, lack of motivation, and disengagement.

C

caffeine A widely used stimulant found in coffee, tea, soft drinks, chocolate, and some medicines.

calorie Common term for *kilocalorie*. The amount of energy required to raise the temperature of 1 kilogram of water by 1° Celsius.

cancer A group of diseases marked by the uncontrolled multiplication of abnormal cells.

capillaries The smallest blood vessels, which deliver blood and nutrients to individual cells and pick up wastes.

carbohydrates A macronutrient class composed of carbon, hydrogen, and oxygen that is the body's universal energy source.

carbon monoxide A gas that inhibits the delivery of oxygen to the body's vital organs.

carcinogen A substance known to trigger DNA mutations that can lead to cancer.

carcinogenic Cancer-causing.

carcinoma Cancer of tissues that line or cover the body.

cardiometabolic risk (CMR) A cluster of nine modifiable factors that identify individuals at risk for type 2 diabetes and cardiovascular disease.

cardiorespiratory fitness The ability of your heart and lungs to effectively deliver oxygen to your muscles during prolonged physical activity.

cardiovascular disease (CVD) A large group of disorders affecting the heart or blood vessels.

carpal tunnel syndrome (CTS) A repetitive strain injury of the hand or wrist, often linked to computer keyboard use or other types of repetitive motion.

carrier A person infected with a pathogen who does not show symptoms but is infectious.

carrying capacity The number of organisms of one species that an environment can support indefinitely.

cataracts An age-related vision disorder marked by clouding of the lens of the eye.

cause In health, a factor such as a genetic defect or virus that is directly responsible for a certain resulting condition.

cellular death The end of all vital functions at the cellular level, such as cellular respiration and other metabolic processes.

central nervous system cancer Cancer of the brain or spinal cord.

cesarean section (C-section) A surgical procedure involving the incision of a woman's abdominal and uterine walls to deliver a baby.

chain of infection A group of factors necessary for the spread of infection.

childbearing age The age range during which a woman can become pregnant.

cholesterol An animal sterol found in the fatty part of animal-based foods such as meat and whole milk.

chromosome In humans, one of 46 bundles of DNA carrying genes that determine heredity.

chronic Characteristic of a disease that typically comes on slowly, progresses gradually, and tends to persist despite medical treatment.

chronic bronchitis Inflammation of the main airways in the lungs that continues for at least three months.

chronic disease A disease that comes on gradually and lasts a long time; many chronic diseases can be managed but resist complete cure.

chronic obstructive pulmonary disease (COPD) A category of diseases that includes emphysema, chronic bronchitis, and asthma.

circadian rhythm A pattern of physical and behavioral changes that follows a 24-hour cycle, in accordance with the hours of darkness and light.

circumcision Surgical removal of the foreskin of the penis.

climate change A change in the state of the climate that can be identified by changes in the average and/or variability of its properties that persist for an extended period.

clinical death A medical determination that life has ceased according to medical criteria that often combine aspects of functional and neurological factors.

clitoris An organ composed of spongy tissue and nerve endings that is very sensitive to sexual stimulation.

club drugs Illicit substances, including MDMA (ecstasy), GHB, and many others that are commonly used at nightclubs and parties.

cocaine A potent and addictive stimulant derived from leaves of the coca shrub.

cognitive-behavioral therapy (CBT) A form of psychotherapy that emphasizes the role of thinking (cognition) in how we feel and what we do.

cohabitation Living together in the same household; usually refers to unmarried couples.

complementary and alternative medicine (CAM) Health practices and traditions not typically part of conventional Western medicine, either used alone (alternative medicine) or in conjunction with conventional medicine (complementary medicine).

complex carbohydrates Carbohydrates that contain chains of multiple sugar molecules; commonly called *starches* but also come in two non-starch forms: *glycogen* and *fiber*.

conception Fertilization of a female egg with male sperm.

condom (male condom) A thin sheath typically made of latex, polyurethane, or lambskin that is unrolled over an erect penis prior to vaginal penetration.

conflict avoidance The active avoidance of discussing concerns, annoyances, and conflict with another person.

conflict escalation Increasing conflict to a more confrontational, painful, or otherwise less comfortable level.

conflict resolution Resolving a conflict in a manner that both people can accept and that minimizes future occurrences of the conflict.

consumer health An umbrella term encompassing topics related to the purchase and consumption of health-related products and services.

continuation rate The percentage of couples who continue to practice a given form of birth control.

contraception Any method used to prevent pregnancy.

contraceptive sponge A flexible foam disk containing spermicide that is inserted in the vagina prior to sex.

conventional medicine Commonly called Western medicine, a system of care based on the scientific method; the belief that diseases are caused by identifiable physical factors and have a characteristic set of symptoms; and the treatment of physical causes through drugs, surgery, or other interventions.

copay A flat fee charged at the time of a medical service or when receiving a medication.

coronary artery bypass grafting (CABG) A procedure to build new pathways for blood to flow around areas of arterial blockage.

coronary heart disease (CHD) Disease characterized by atherosclerosis of the arteries that feed the heart, angina, and reduced blood supply to the myocardium. Also called *coronary artery disease*.

cortisol An adrenal gland hormone that is secreted at higher levels during the stress response.

counter-conditioning A behavior-change technique in which the individual learns to substitute a healthful or neutral behavior for an unwanted behavior triggered by a cue beyond his or her control.

cramp An involuntary contracted muscle that does not relax, resulting in localized intense pain.

cue control A behavior-change technique in which the individual learns to change the stimuli that provoked the lapse.

cunnilingus Oral stimulation of the vulva or clitoris.

D

danger zone Range of temperatures between 40° and 140° Fahrenheit at which bacteria responsible for foodborne illness thrive.

date (acquaintance) rape Coerced, forceful, or threatening sexual activity in which the victim knows the attacker.

date rape drugs Drugs used to assist in a sexual assault, often given to the victim without his or her knowledge or consent.

decibel A unit of measurement used to express sound intensity.

deductible The total amount of out-of-pocket health-care expenses that a patient must pay before health insurance begins to cover health-care costs.

dementia A group of symptoms caused by disorders that affect memory, cognitive function, personality, and social skills.

dentist (D.D.S.) A conventional medicine practitioner who specializes in care of the teeth, gums, and mouth.

dependence The state of being mentally attached to and/or physically needing a drug.

depressants Substances that depress the activity of the central nervous system and include barbiturates, benzodiazepines, and alcohol.

depressive disorder A mental disorder usually characterized by profound, persistent sadness or loss of interest that interferes with daily life and normal functioning.

determinants of health The range of personal, social, economic, and environmental factors that influence health status.

diabetes mellitus A group of diseases in which the body does not make or use insulin properly, resulting in elevated blood glucose.

diaphragm A flexible silicone cup filled with spermicide and inserted in the vagina prior to sex to prevent pregnancy.

diet The food you regularly consume.

Dietary Reference Intakes (DRIs) A set of energy and nutrient recommendations for supporting good health.

dietary supplements Products taken by mouth that include ingredients such as vitamins, minerals, amino acids, or herbs intended to supplement the diet.

dilation and evacuation (D&E) A multistep method of surgical abortion that may be used in pregnancies that have progressed beyond 12 weeks.

diminishing returns The principle that individuals adapt to a constant, static fitness routine and receive fewer benefits as a result.

disease An alteration in body structure or biochemistry that is significant enough to cause the body's regulatory mechanisms to fail. Symptoms may or may not be present.

disease prevention Activities such as vaccinations and cancer screenings to help prevent disease.

disordered eating A range of unhealthful eating behaviors used to deal with emotional issues that does not warrant a diagnosis of a specific eating disorder.

dissociative drug A medication that distorts perceptions of sight and sound and produces feelings of detachment from the environment and self.

distress Stress resulting from changes that are perceived as threatening.

DNA (deoxyribonucleic acid) A compound in the nucleus of living cells that transfers genetic information.

doctor of osteopathic medicine (D.O) A licensed physician with similar training as an M.D. with additional training in osteopathic manipulative treatment; usually has a holistic focus.

domestic partnership A legal arrangement in which a couple lives together in a long-term committed relationship and receives some, but not all, of the rights of married couples.

domestic violence An abusive situation in which a family member physically, psychologically, or sexually abuses one or more other family members.

dopamine A neurotransmitter that stimulates feelings of pleasure.

drug A chemical substance that alters the body physically or mentally for a non-nutritional purpose.

drug abuse The use (most often the excessive use) of any legal or illegal drug in a way that is detrimental to your health.

drug misuse The inappropriate use of a legal drug, either for a reason for which it was not medically intended or by a person without a prescription.

dynamic flexibility The ability to move quickly and fluidly through a joint's entire range of motion with little resistance.

dynamic stretching A type of slow movement stretching in which activities from a workout or sport are mimicked in a controlled manner, often to help "warm up" for a game or an event.

dyslipidemia A disorder characterized by abnormal levels of blood lipids, such as high LDL cholesterol or low HDL cholesterol.

dysmenorrhea Pain during menstruation that is severe enough to limit normal activities or require medication.

dysthymic disorder (dysthymia) A milder, chronic type of depressive disorder that lasts two years or more.

E

e-waste Hazardous waste generated by the production or disposal of electronic or digital devices.

eating disorders A group of mental disorders, including anorexia nervosa, bulimia nervosa, and binge eating disorder, that is characterized by physiological and psychological disturbances in appetite or food intake.

ecological footprint The collective impact of an entity on its resources, ecosystems, and other key environmental features.

ecological models Behavior-change models that acknowledge the creation of a supportive environment as being equally important to achieving change as an individual's acquisition of health information and development of new skills.

ecosystem A dynamic collection of organisms and their nonliving surroundings that function as a unit.

ectopic pregnancy A pregnancy in which the embryo implants outside the uterus, often in the fallopian tubes.

electrocardiogram (ECG or EKG) A test that measures the heart's electrical activity.

electroencephalograph (EEG) A device that monitors the electrical activity of different regions of the cerebral cortex of the brain, using electrodes placed on or in the scalp; a tracing of brain activity is called an *electroencephalogram*.

embryo The growing collection of cells that ultimately become a baby.

emergency contraception (EC; "morning after" pill) A pill containing levonorgestrel, a synthetic hormone used to prevent pregnancy after unprotected sex.

emotional health The "feeling" component of psychological health that influences your interpretation of and response to events.

emotional intelligence (EI) The capacity to perceive, express, and reason accurately with emotion and emotional information.

emphysema A chronic disease in which the air sacs in the lung become damaged, making breathing difficult.

empty calories Calories from solid fats or added sugars.

enabling factor A skill, social support, or resource that makes it possible (or easier) to succeed in changing a targeted behavior.

endocrine disruptor A substance that alters the production or use of hormones in the body and that can have harmful effects on health or development.

endometriosis A condition in which endometrial tissue grows in areas outside the uterus.

endorphins Hormones that act as neurotransmitters and bind to opiate receptors, stimulating pleasure and relieving pain.

energy balance The state achieved when energy consumed from food is equal to energy expended, maintaining body weight.

environmental health A discipline that addresses all the physical, chemical, and biological factors external to individual human beings, especially those that influence human health.

environmental mastery The ability to choose or create environments that suit you.

epididymis The coiled tube on top of each testicle where sperm are held until they mature.

erectile dysfunction (ED) Inability of a male to obtain or maintain an erection.

erection The process in which the penis fills up with blood as a result of sexual stimulation.

essential fatty acids (EFAs) Polyunsaturated fatty acids that cannot be synthesized by the body but are essential to body functioning.

estate A person's personal holdings, including money, property, and other possessions.

ethyl alcohol (ethanol) The intoxicating ingredient in beer, wine, and distilled liquor.

eustress Stress resulting from changes that are perceived as advantageous.

evidence-based medicine Health-care policies and practices based on systematic, scientific study.

excitement The first phase of the sexual response cycle, marked by erection in men and lubrication and clitoral swelling in women.

exercise A type of physical activity that is planned and structured.

F

failure rate The percentage of women who typically get pregnant after using a given contraceptive method for 1 year.

fallopian tubes The pair of tubes that connect the ovaries to the uterus.

family health history A detailed record of health issues in one's family that presents a picture of shared health risks.

fats (triglycerides) Lipids made up of three fatty acid chains attached to a molecule of glycerol; the most common types of food lipid.

fee-for-service plan A type of health insurance in which you choose your providers, and you and your insurer divide the costs of care.

fellatio Oral stimulation of the penis.

female athlete triad A multifaceted disorder typically seen in female athletes and characterized by disordered eating, amenorrhea, and osteoporosis

fertility awareness (rhythm or calendar method) Tracking of a woman's monthly menstrual cycle; may be used as a method of preventing pregnancy if the woman tracks carefully and has regular periods, although it is not fail-safe.

fertility rate Within a given population, the average number of births per woman.

fetal alcohol syndrome A pattern of mental and physical birth defects found in some children of mothers who drank excessively during pregnancy.

fetus The name given to a developing embryo 8 weeks after fertilization.

fiber A nondigestible complex carbohydrate that aids in digestion.

fight-or-flight response A series of physiological reactions to a stressor designed to enable the body to stand and fight or to flee.

FITT Exercise variables that can be modified in order to accomplish progressive overload: frequency, intensity, time, and type.

flexibility The ability of joints to move through their full ranges of motion.

flexible spending account (FSA) A consumer-controlled account, usually offered through employers, that uses pre-tax dollars to cover approved health-related purchases.

food allergy An adverse reaction of the body's immune system to a food or food component.

food intolerance An adverse food reaction that doesn't involve the immune system.

foodborne illness (food poisoning) Illness caused by ingesting foods or beverages contaminated by pathogenic microorganisms or their toxins.

functional death The end of all vital physiological functions, including heartbeat, breathing, and blood flow.

functional foods Foods thought to confer health benefits beyond those provided by their basic nutrients.

fungi Multicellular or single-celled organisms that obtain their food from organic matter, in some cases human tissue.

G

gamma-hydroxybutyric acid (GHB) A central nervous system depressant known as a "date rape drug" because of its use to impair potential victims of sexual assault.

gender Social, cultural, or psychological traits associated with identification as either male or female.

gender roles Behaviors and tasks society considers appropriate for men and for women.

gene A segment of DNA that codes for the assembly of a protein.

general adaptation syndrome (GAS) A homeostatic response to a stressor consisting of three stages: alarm, resistance, and exhaustion.

generalized anxiety disorder (GAD) An anxiety disorder characterized by chronic worry and pessimism about everyday events that lasts at least six months and may be accompanied by physical symptoms.

genome The genetic material of a living organism.

genomics The study of genomes and their effects on health and development.

glaucoma An age-related vision disorder arising from an increase in internal eye pressure that damages the optic nerve and reduces peripheral vision.

global warming A sustained increase in Earth's temperature due to an increase in the greenhouse effect resulting from pollution.

globalization The interaction and integration of regional phenomena globally.

glycemic index A measure of the potential of foods to raise the level of blood glucose.

groundwater The supply of fresh water beneath Earth's surface, which is a major source of drinking water.

H

hallucinogens Drugs that alter perception and are capable of causing auditory and visual hallucinations.

hangover Alcohol withdrawal symptoms, including headache and nausea, caused by an earlier bout of heavy drinking.

hate crime A crime fueled by bias against another person's or group's race or ethnicity, religion, national origin, sexual orientation, or disability.

hazardous waste Garbage or byproducts that can pose a hazard to human health or the environment when improperly managed.

hazing Initiation rituals to enter a fraternity or other group that may be humiliating, hazardous, or physically or emotionally abusive, regardless of the person's willingness to participate.

health More than merely the absence of disease, a state of well-being that encompasses physical, social, psychological, and other dimensions and is a resource for everyday life.

health belief model A model of behavior change that emphasizes the influence of personal beliefs on the process of creating effective change.

health discount program A system of health discounts given to members of groups, such as employees of a particular company or students attending a particular college.

health disparities Gaps in the rate and burden of disease and the access to and quality of health care among various population groups.

health insurance A contract between an insurance company and a group or an individual who pays a fee to have some level of health-care costs covered by the insurer.

health literacy The ability to evaluate and understand health information and to make informed choices for your health care.

health maintenance organization (HMO) A type of managed care plan in which most health care is funneled through and must be approved by the primary care doctor.

health promotion Information, programs, and services provided to help populations improve their health.

health savings account (HSA) A consumer-controlled savings account that can be used with a high-deductible health insurance plan to cover health-care costs not covered by insurance.

health-related fitness The ability to perform activities of daily living with vigor.

healthful weight The weight at which health risks are lowest for an individual; usually a weight that results in a BMI between 18.5 and 24.9.

Healthy Campus An offshoot of the Healthy People initiative specifically geared toward college students.

Healthy People initiative A federal initiative to facilitate broad, positive health changes in large segments of the U.S. population every 10 years.

heart failure Gradual loss of heart function.

heat exhaustion A mild form of heat-related illness that usually occurs as a result of exercising in hot weather without adequate hydration.

heatstroke A life-threatening heat-related illness that occurs when your core temperature rises above 105°F.

hemorrhagic stroke Stroke caused by a leaking or ruptured blood vessel.

hepatitis Inflammation of the liver that affects liver function.

herd immunity The condition where greater than 90% of a community is vaccinated against a disease, giving the disease little ability to spread through the community and providing some protection against the disease to members of the community who are not vaccinated.

heroin An illicit, highly addictive opioid.

heterosexuals People who are sexually attracted to partners of the opposite sex.

high-density lipoprotein (HDL) A cholesterol-containing compound that removes excess cholesterol from the bloodstream; often referred to as "good cholesterol."

homeostasis The physiological processes by which the body maintains its internal conditions within a narrow, healthful range.

homicide The willful (not negligent) killing of another person; includes both murder and non-negligent manslaughter.

homonegativity Negative attitudes toward homosexuality.

homophobia Irrational fear of, aversion to, or discrimination against homosexuals or homosexuality.

homosexuals People who are sexually attracted to partners of the same sex.

hormone A chemical secreted by a gland and transported through the bloodstream to a distant target organ, the activity of which it then regulates.

hospice A home-care program or facility that focuses exclusively on the dying and their loved ones, with a goal of providing comfort rather than facilitating cure.

host A person, a plant, or an animal in which or on which pathogens live and reproduce.

human sexual response cycle Distinct phases extending from the first moment of sexual desire until the calm after orgasm.

hunger The physiological sensation caused by the lack of food.

hyperglycemia A persistent state of elevated levels of blood glucose.

hypertension A persistent state of elevated blood pressure. Commonly called *high blood pressure*.

hypothermia A potentially fatal condition in which your core body temperature drops too low.

I

illicit drugs Drugs regulated by the U.S. Drug Enforcement Agency as unlawful substances, including prescription medications used unlawfully.

illness A subjective state in which a person feels unwell. Disease may or may not be present.

immune system Your body's cellular and chemical defenses against pathogens.

immunization Creating immunity to a pathogen through vaccination or through the injection of antibodies.

implantation Lodging of a fertilized egg in the endometrium of the uterus.

individuality The principle that individuals respond to fitness training in their own unique ways.

infant mortality rate A calculation of the ratio of babies who die before their first birthday and those who survive until their first birthday.

infection The invasion of body tissues by microorganisms that use the body's environment to multiply and cause disease.

infertility The inability to conceive after trying for at least a year.

inflammatory response A response to damaged body tissues designed to kill any pathogens in the damaged tissue, promote healing, and prevent the spread of infection to other parts of the body.

influenza A group of viruses that cause the flu, a contagious respiratory condition.

inhalants Chemical vapors that, when inhaled, produce mind-altering effects.

insomnia A condition characterized by difficulty falling or staying asleep, a pattern of waking too early, or poor-quality sleep.

insulin A hormone necessary for glucose transport into cells.

intentional injury Physical harm that is purposefully inflicted through violence.

intervention A technique used by family and friends of an addict to encourage the addict to seek help for a drug problem.

intestate Dying without leaving a legal will.

intimacy A sense of closeness with another person formed by being emotionally open and caring.

intimate partner violence (IPV) An abusive situation in which one member of a couple or intimate relationship may physically, psychologically, or sexually abuse the other.

intrauterine device (IUD) A plastic, T-shaped device inserted in the uterus for long-term pregnancy prevention.

ischemic stroke Stroke caused by a blocked blood vessel.

isometric exercise Exercise in which the muscle contracts but the body does not move.

isotonic exercise Exercise in which the muscle contraction causes body movement.

J

jaundice A yellowing of the skin, mucous membranes, and sometimes the whites of the eyes, often caused by liver malfunction.

jealousy A response to a threat to a relationship from an actual or imagined rival for a partner's attention.

L

labia majora The fleshy, larger outer lips surrounding the labia minora.

labia minora The thin, inner folds of skin, which rest protectively over the *clitoris,* the *vaginal opening,* and the *urethral opening,* through which urine is released from the body.

labor The physical processes involved in giving birth.

leukemia Cancer of blood-forming tissue.

leukoplakia White spots on the mucous membranes in the mouth that may become cancerous.

life expectancy The average number of years a person may expect to live.

locus of control A person's belief about where the center of power lies in his or her life; it can be external or internal.

loneliness A feeling of isolation from others, often prompted by a real or perceived loss.

long-lived greenhouse gases (LLGHGs) Gases that absorb and rerelease infrared energy from the atmosphere to Earth's surface, thereby contributing to global warming; the three most significant LLGHGs are carbon dioxide, methane, and nitrous oxide.

low birth weight Birth weight less than 5 pounds, 8 ounces.

low-density lipoprotein (LDL) A cholesterol-containing compound that, as it degrades, releases its cholesterol load into the bloodstream; often referred to as "bad cholesterol."

lymphoma Cancer of the lymphoid tissues.

lysergic acid diethylamide (LSD) A powerful hallucinogen manufactured from lysergic acid, a substance found in a fungus that grows on rye and other grains.

M

mainstream smoke Smoke exhaled from the lungs of smokers.

major depressive disorder (unipolar depression) A type of depressive disorder characterized by experiencing five or more symptoms of depression, including either depressed mood or loss of interest or pleasure, for at least two weeks straight.

malaria A serious disease that causes fever and chills that appear in cycles. In some cases malaria can be life threatening.

malignant melanoma An especially aggressive form of skin cancer.

malignant tumor A tumor that grows aggressively, invades surrounding tissue, and can spread to other parts of the body; all cancers are malignant.

managed-care plan A type of health insurance in which the insurer contracts with a defined network of providers, which the consumer must use or face higher out-of-pocket costs.

marijuana One of the most commonly used drugs in the United States; derived from the plant *Cannabis sativa*.

mast cell A type of cell in the skin and mucous membranes that releases histamine and other chemicals into the bloodstream during an allergic reaction.

masturbation Manipulation of one's own genitals for sexual pleasure.

Medicaid A joint federal–state insurance program that covers low-income individuals and families.

medical doctor (M.D.) A physician trained in conventional medicine, with many years of additional formal education and training and a professional license.

Medicare A federal insurance program that covers people with long-term disabilities and individuals age 65 and older.

menarche The first onset of menstruation.

menopause The permanent end of a woman's menstrual cycle and reproductive capacity.

menstrual cycle The monthly physiological cycle marked by *menstruation*.

menstrual phase The phase of the menstrual cycle characterized by menstrual flow, the release of follicle-stimulating hormone from the pituitary gland to the brain, and the release of estrogen into the bloodstream.

menstruation The cyclical discharge of blood and tissue from the vagina.

mental disorders Significant behavioral and psychological disorders that disrupt thoughts and feelings, impair ability to function, and increase risk of pain, disability, or even death.

mental health The "thinking" component of psychological health that allows you to perceive reality accurately and respond rationally and effectively.

metabolic equivalent of task (MET) A unit of measurement that describes the energy expenditure of a particular activity.

metabolic syndrome A set of five unhealthy physical and metabolic conditions that are together linked to an increased risk for type 2 diabetes and other metabolic disease.

metabolism The sum of all chemical reactions occurring in body cells, including those that break large molecules down into smaller molecules.

metastasis The process by which a malignant tumor spreads to other body sites.

methamphetamine A highly addictive and dangerous stimulant that is chemically similar to amphetamine but more potent and harmful.

methicillin-resistant *Staphylococcus aureus* (MRSA) A strain of staph that is resistant to the broad-spectrum antibiotics commonly used to treat staph infections.

methylenedioxymethamphetamine (MDMA) A synthetic drug, commonly called "ecstasy," that works as both a stimulant and a hallucinogen.

minerals Elements needed by the body to regulate functions and provide structure.

mini-med plan A type of managed-care plan, sold individually to younger people, which carries lower costs but does not cover many services.

miscarriage A pregnancy that suddenly terminates on its own before the 20th week.

mononucleosis A viral disease that causes fatigue, weakness, sore throat, fever, headaches, swollen lymph nodes and tonsils, and loss of appetite.

mons pubis The fatty, rounded areas of tissue in front of the pubic bone.

mood disorder Any chronic, pervasive emotional state that significantly alters the person's thoughts, behaviors, and normal functioning.

morbidity Clinical term for disease, specifically the level of disease within a population.

mortality Clinical term for death, typically the number of deaths in a certain population due to a certain cause.

municipal solid waste (MSW) Nonhazardous garbage or trash generated by industries, businesses, institutions, and homes.

murder The act of intentionally and unjustifiably killing another person.

muscular endurance The capacity of muscles to repeatedly exert force, or to maintain a force, over a period of time.

muscular strength The maximum force your muscles can apply in a single maximum effort of lifting, pushing, or pressing.

myeloma Cancer arising in plasma cells, which are a type of immune cells, and invading the bone marrow.

myocardial infarction (MI) A cardiac crisis in which a region of heart muscle is damaged or destroyed by reduced blood flow. Also known as *heart attack*.

myocardium The heart's muscle tissue.

N

narcolepsy A disorder in which the brain fails to regulate sleep–wake cycles normally.

near-death experience (NDE) A profound psychological event usually occurring in a person close to death and marked by a characteristic pattern of perceptions such as movement through space and perception of light.

neurotoxin A substance that interferes with or harms the functioning of the nervous system.

neurotransmitters Chemicals that enable the transmission of messages from one neuron to another across synapses.

nicotine An alkaloid derived from the tobacco plant that is responsible for smoking's psychoactive and addictive effects.

nocturnal eating disorder A condition characterized by significant food consumption at night and typically accompanied by depression, insomnia, and a daytime eating disorder.

non-REM (NREM) sleep A type of restful sleep during which the rapid eye movement characteristic of dreaming does not typically occur.

nonverbal communication Communication that is conveyed by body language.

nurse A licensed professional who provides a wide range of health-care services and supports the work of medical doctors.

nurse practitioner A registered nurse who has undergone additional training and can perform some of the care provided by a medical doctor.

nutrient-dense foods Any food in which the proportion of healthful nutrients is high relative to the number of calories.

nutrients Chemicals the body derives from food and requires for energy, growth, and survival.

nutrition The scientific study of food and its physiological functions.

O

obese A weight disorder in which excess accumulations of non-essential body fat result in increased risk of health problems. A weight resulting in a BMI of 30 or higher.

obsessive-compulsive disorder (OCD) An anxiety disorder characterized by repeated and unwanted thoughts (obsessions) that lead to rituals (compulsions) in an attempt to control the anxiety.

oncogene A mutated gene that encourages the uncontrolled cell division that results in cancer.

opioids Drugs derived from opium or synthetic drugs that have similar sleep-inducing, pain-reducing effects.

opportunistic diseases Infections and other disorders that take advantage of a weakened immune system.

optimism The psychological tendency to have a positive interpretation of life's events.

optometrist (O.D.) A licensed professional who provides vision care.

oral sex Stimulation of the genitals by the tongue or mouth.

orgasm The peak, or climax, of sexual response, characterized by rhythmic muscle contractions of the genitals and surrounding areas and ejaculation in men.

orthorexia nervosa Disordered eating characterized by a fixation with obsessively healthy eating.
osteoporosis A disease characterized by low bone mass and deterioration of bone tissue, leading to fragile bones and an increased risk of fractures.
outercourse Sexual intimacy without penetration of the vagina or anus.
ovaries The two female reproductive organs where ova (eggs) reside.
over-the-counter (OTC) medication Medication available for purchase without a prescription.
overload Increasing the stress placed on your body through exercise, which results in an improved fitness level.
overweight The condition of having a body weight that exceeds what is generally considered healthful for a particular height. A weight resulting in a BMI of 25 to 29.9.
ovulate To release an egg from the ovary.
ozone depletion Destruction of the stratospheric ozone layer, which shields Earth from harmful levels of ultraviolet radiation; results from pollution.

P

palliative care A type of care that focuses on reducing pain and suffering and caring for the whole person rather than prolonging life or curing disease.
pancreas An abdominal organ that produces insulin as well as certain compounds that are helpful in digestion.
pandemic A worldwide epidemic of a disease.
panic attacks Episodes of sudden terror that strike without warning.
panic disorder A mental disorder characterized both by recurring panic attacks and the fear of a panic attack occurring.
parasitic worms (helminths) Multicellular creatures that compete with a host body for nutrients.
parasomnia A condition in which unusual events accompany sleep.
particulates Minute quantities of harmful matter that can lodge in the lungs or deposit in the environment.
passive euthanasia Failure to begin or to maintain an intervention that is necessary to sustain a patient's life.
passive stretching Stretching performed with a partner who increases the intensity of the stretch by gently applying pressure to your body as it stretches.
pathogen An agent that causes disease.
penis The male sexual and reproductive organ.
Percent Daily Value (% DV) Nutrient standards that estimate how much a serving of a given food contributes to the overall intake of nutrients listed on the food label.
personal safety The practice of making decisions and taking actions that reduce your risk of injury and death.
personality type A set of behavioral tendencies.
personalized medicine Health care based on the idea that because your individual DNA is unique, your health is as well, and your care and treatments should be tailored to you.
pesticides Chemicals used to kill pests; in agriculture, chemicals used to help protect crops from weeds, insects, fungus, slugs and snails, birds, and mammals.
pharmacogenomics The use of DNA information to choose medications and make prescribing decisions.
phencyclidine (PCP) A dangerous synthetic hallucinogen that reduces and distorts sensory input and can unpredictably cause both euphoria and dysphoria.
phobia An extreme, disabling, irrational fear of something that poses little or no actual danger.
physical activity Bodily movement that substantially increases energy expenditure.
physical fitness The ability to perform moderate to vigorous levels of activity and to respond to physical demands without excessive fatigue.

physician assistant (P.A.) A licensed health professional who practices under the supervision of a physician and provides a broad range of care.
phytochemicals Naturally occurring plant substances thought to have health-promoting properties.
placenta The tissue that connects mother and baby.
plateau The second phase of the sexual response cycle, characterized by intense excitement, rapid heartbeat, genital sensitivity, the secretion of pre-ejaculatory fluid in men, and vaginal swelling in women.
podiatrist (D.P.M.) A licensed professional who specializes in the care of the feet.
point-of-service (POS) plan A type of managed care plan that lets HMO members see a broader list of providers for an additional fee.
pollution Contamination of the natural environment as a result of human activities.
polyabuser A person who abuses more than one drug.
polypharmacy Simultaneous use of several prescription medications that can interact in dangerous ways.
positive psychotherapy A recent field of psychology that focuses on increasing psychological strengths and improving happiness rather than on psychological problems.
post-traumatic stress disorder (PTSD) An anxiety disorder characterized by recurrent fear, anger, and depression occurring after a traumatic event.
prebiotics Nondigestible food ingredients that benefit human health by stimulating the growth and/or activity of beneficial bacteria in the large intestine.
prediabetes A persistent state of blood glucose levels that are higher than normal but not high enough to qualify as diabetes.
predisposing factor A physical, mental, emotional, or surrounding influence that affects the likelihood that a person will decide to change a current behavior.
preeclampsia A serious health condition characterized by high blood pressure in the pregnant woman.
preexisting condition A health issue that existed prior to application to or enrollment in a health insurance plan.
preferred provider organization (PPO) A type of managed care plan in which the consumer is encouraged to stay within an approved network of providers but can obtain care outside the network.
premature ejaculation (PE) A condition in which a male ejaculates earlier than he would like to.
premenstrual dysphoric disorder (PMDD) Severe and debilitating psychological symptoms experienced just prior to menstruation.
premenstrual syndrome (PMS) A collection of emotional and physical symptoms that occur just prior to menstruation.
premium An amount paid to an insurance company for an insurance policy, usually in monthly installments.
prenatal care Nutritional counseling and regular medical screenings throughout pregnancy to aid the growth and development of the fetus.
presbycusis Age-related hearing loss, which usually develops gradually, often due to damage to or changes in the inner ear.
presbyopia Age-related decline in the ability to focus on objects up close, especially in low light.
prevalence The proportion of a total population found to have a disease or other condition.
probiotics Living microbes present in fermented foods, the consumption of which improves the microbial balance in the large intestine.
progressive overload Gradual overloading of the body over time in order to avoid injury.
proliferative phase The phase of the menstrual cycle characterized by a thickening of the lining of the uterus and discharge of cervical mucus. This phase ends when luteinizing hormone triggers the release of a mature egg.

proof value A measurement of alcoholic strength, corresponding to twice the alcohol percentage (e.g., 13% alcohol equals 26 proof).

prostate gland The walnut-sized gland that produces part of the semen.

protein An energy-yielding macronutrient that helps build biological compounds and body tissues, including muscle, bone, skin, and blood.

protozoa Single-celled parasites that rely on other living things for food and shelter.

psilocybin A hallucinogenic substance obtained from certain types of mushrooms that are indigenous to tropical regions of South America.

psychoactive Capable of altering feelings, mood, perceptions, or psychological functioning.

psychoactive drugs Drugs that affect the user's mood, perceptions, or other aspects of the mental state.

psychodynamic therapy A type of therapy that focuses on the unconscious sources of a patient's behavior and psychological state.

psychological health A broad dimension of health and wellness that encompasses both metal and emotional health.

psychoneuroimmunology The study of interactions among psychological processes, the nervous system, hormones, and the immune system.

purging Behaviors such as vomiting, laxative abuse, or overexercising that are intended to reduce the calories absorbed by the body.

R

radiation Energy that travels in the form of rays, waves, or particles.

rape Nonconsensual oral, anal, or vaginal penetration by body parts or objects, using force, threats of bodily harm, or taking advantage of circumstances that make a person incapable of consenting to sex.

rational suicide Action taken deliberately by a reasoned, terminally ill patient to hasten his or her own death.

recovery The period necessary for the body to recover from exercise demands and adapt to higher levels of fitness.

reinforcing factor An influence that either rewards or opposes a change effort in progress. Positive reinforcers encourage individuals to continue their efforts to change; negative reinforcers discourage or block change.

relapse Returning to drinking after a period of sobriety.

religion A system of beliefs and practices related to the existence of a transcendent power.

REM behavior disorder (RBD) Parasomnia characterized by failure of inhibition of muscle movement during REM sleep.

REM sleep A type of sleep characterized by brain waves similar to those that occur while awake, during which rapid eye movement and dreaming occur.

repetitions The number of times you perform an exercise repeatedly.

repetitive strain injury (RSI) Injury that damages joints, nerves, or connective tissue caused by repeated motions that put strain on one part of the body.

replacement-level fertility The level of fertility at which a population exactly replaces itself from one generation to the next.

reservoir The natural environment for any particular pathogen, where it accumulates in large numbers.

resiliency The innate capacity to experience success and satisfaction following trauma or other stressors.

resolution The stage of the sexual response cycle in which the body returns to normal functioning.

restless legs syndrome (RLS) A nervous system disorder characterized by a strong urge to move the legs, accompanied by creeping, burning, or other unpleasant sensations.

reversibility The principle that fitness levels decline when the demand placed on the body is decreased.

risk factor A factor such as advanced age or alcohol abuse that increases the likelihood that an individual will experience a certain disease or injury.

Rohypnol A powerful sedative known as a "date rape drug" because of its use to impair potential victims of sexual assault.

S

sarcoma Cancer of muscle or connective tissues.

satiety Physical fullness; the state in which there is no longer the desire to eat.

saturated fats Fats that are typically solid at room temperature and that are generally found in animal-based foods.

schizophrenia A severe mental disorder characterized by delusions, hallucinations, and other aspects of psychosis.

scrotum The skin sac at the base of the penis that contains the testes.

secondhand smoke (environmental tobacco smoke) The smoke nonsmokers are exposed to when someone has been smoking nearby; a combination of sidestream smoke and mainstream smoke.

secretory phase The phase of the menstrual cycle characterized by the degeneration of the follicle sac, rising levels of progesterone in the bloodstream, and further increase of the endometrial lining.

self-acceptance A sense of positive and realistic self-regard, which results in elevated levels of self-confidence and self-respect.

self-actualization The pinnacle of Maslow's hierarchy of needs, which indicates truly fulfilling your potential.

self-care Actions you take to keep yourself healthy.

self-disclosure The sharing of honest feelings and personal information about yourself with another person.

self-efficacy The conviction that you can successfully execute the behavior required to make the change you desire.

self-medicating Using alcohol or drugs to cope with sadness, grief, pain, or mental health problems.

semen Male ejaculate, consisting of sperm and other fluids from the accessory glands.

sets Separate groups of repetitions.

sex Biological characteristics of males and females based on their genetic inheritance.

sexting The use of cell phones or similar electronic devices to send sexually explicit text, photos, or videos.

sexual dysfunctions Problems occurring during any stage of the sexual response cycle.

sexual harassment Unwelcome language or contact of a sexual nature that explicitly or implicitly affects academic or employment situations, unreasonably interferes with work or school performance, or creates an intimidating, hostile, or offensive work or school environment.

sexual orientation Romantic and physical attraction toward others.

sexual violence Any form of nonconsensual sexual activity.

sexuality The biological, physical, emotional, and psychosocial aspects of sexual attraction and expression.

sexually transmitted infections (STIs) Infections transmitted mainly through sexual activity, such as vaginal, anal, or oral sex.

shaping A behavior-change technique based on breaking broad goals into more manageable steps.

shyness The feeling of apprehension or intimidation in social situations, especially in reaction to unfamiliar people or new environments.

sidestream smoke Smoke emanating from the burning end of a cigarette or pipe.

signs Objective, often visible or measurable, indications that disease or injury is present.

simple carbohydrates The most basic unit of carbohydrates, consisting of one or two sugar molecules.

skills-related fitness The capacity to perform specific physical skills related to a sport or other physically demanding activity.

sleep A physiologically prompted, dynamic, and readily reversible state of reduced consciousness essential to human survival.

sleep apnea A disorder in which one or more pauses in breathing occur during sleep.

sleep bruxism Clenching or grinding the teeth during sleep.

sleep debt An accumulated amount of sleep loss that develops when the amount of sleep you routinely obtain is less than the amount you need.

sleep hygiene The behaviors and environmental factors that together influence the quantity and quality of sleep.

sleep terror Parasomnia characterized by the appearance of awakening in terror during a stage of NREM sleep.

sleepwalking Parasomnia in which a person walks or performs another complex activity while still asleep.

snoring A ragged, hoarse sound that occurs during sleep when breathing is obstructed.

social anxiety disorder (social phobia) An anxiety disorder characterized by an intense fear of being judged by others and of being humiliated by your own actions, which may be accompanied by physical symptoms.

social physique anxiety A mental disorder characterized by extreme fear of having one's body judged by others.

social support A sufficient quantity of relationships that provide emotional concern, help with appraisal, information, and even goods and services.

specificity The principle that a fitness component is improved only by exercises that address that specific component.

spermicide A substance containing chemicals that kill or immobilize sperm.

spirituality A lifelong quest for the answers to life's biggest questions.

stalking A pattern of harassment and threats directed at a specific person that is intended to cause intimidation and fear, often through repeated, unwanted contact.

standard drink A drink containing about 14 grams of pure alcohol (one 12-oz. can of beer, one 5-oz. glass of wine, or 1.5 oz. of 80-proof liquor).

static flexibility The ability to reach and hold a stretch at one endpoint of a joint's range of motion.

static stretching Gradually lengthening a muscle to an elongated position and sustaining that position.

status syndrome The disparity in health status and rates of premature mortality between the impoverished and the affluent within any given society.

statutory rape Any sexual activity with a person younger than the legally defined "age of consent," regardless of whether any coercion or force was involved.

stimulants A class of drugs that stimulate the central nervous system, causing acceleration of mental and physical processes in the body.

stress The collective psychobiological condition that occurs in response to a disruptive, unexpected, or exciting stimulus.

stressor Any physical or psychological event or other change that causes positive or negative stress.

stroke A medical emergency in which blood flow to or in the brain is impaired. Also called a *cerebrovascular accident* (*CVA*).

suction curettage A method of surgical abortion characterized by vacuum aspiration, typically used in the first 6 to 12 weeks of pregnancy.

sudden cardiac arrest A life-threatening cardiac crisis marked by loss of heartbeat and unconsciousness.

sudden infant death syndrome (SIDS) The sudden death of a seemingly healthy infant while sleeping.

Superfund A federal program that funds and carries out emergency and long-term identification, analysis, removal, and cleanup of toxic sites.

sustainability The ability to meet society's current needs without compromising future generations' abilities to meet their own needs; includes policies for ensuring that certain components of the environment are not depleted or destroyed.

symptoms Subjective experiences such as pain or fatigue that indicate disease or injury is present.

T

tachycardia A fast arrhythmia.

tar A sticky, thick brown residue that forms when tobacco is burned and its chemical particles condense.

target heart rate range The heart rate range to aim for during exercise. A target heart rate range of 64% to 91% of your maximum heart rate is recommended.

terminal illness An irreversible condition that will result in death in the near future.

terrorism Premeditated, politically motivated violence against noncombatant individuals, usually as a means of influence.

testes (testicles) Two reproductive glands that manufacture sperm.

tolerance Reduced sensitivity to a drug so that increased amounts are needed to achieve the usual effect.

toxic shock syndrome A rare, serious illness caused by staph bacteria that begins with severe flu symptoms but can quickly progress to a medical emergency.

toxicity The dosage level at which a drug becomes poisonous to the body.

trans fat A type of fat produced through the process of hydrogenation, which converts an oil into a solid.

transgender A person whose gender identity or gender expression is different from his or her biological sex.

transient ischemic attack (TIA) A temporary episode of strokelike symptoms that is indicative of high stroke risk.

transition The final phase of the first stage of labor, characterized by the dilation of the cervix and strong, prolonged contractions.

transsexual A person who has permanently changed or is transitioning to the opposite gender through clinical interventions such as hormone therapy and surgery.

transtheoretical model of behavior change A model of behavior change that focuses on decision-making steps and abilities. Also called the *stages of change* model.

traumatic brain injury (TBI) Injury that disrupts normal functioning of the brain, caused by a jolt or blow to the brain or a penetrating head wound.

tumor A mass of abnormal tissue made up of cells with no physiological function.

Twelve Step programs Addiction recovery self-help programs based on the principles of Alcoholics Anonymous.

type 1 diabetes A form of diabetes prompted by immune destruction of the beta cells of the pancreas, which impairs the production of insulin.

type 2 diabetes A form of diabetes that begins as insulin resistance and increased demand for insulin; as it progresses, the ability of the pancreas to produce insulin declines.

U

umbilical cord A vessel linking the bloodstream of the placenta to that of the baby and enabling the exchange of gases, nutrients, and wastes.

underweight A weight resulting in a BMI below 18.5.

unintentional injury (accidents) Bodily damage that is not deliberately caused.

unsaturated fats Fats that are typically liquid at room temperature and that generally come from plant sources.

urethra The duct that travels from the bladder through the shaft of the penis, carrying fluids to the outside of the body.

uterus (womb) A pear-shaped organ where a growing fetus is nurtured.

V

vagina A tube that connects a woman's external sex organs with her uterus.
vaginal intercourse Intercourse characterized by the insertion of the penis into the vagina.
values Internal guidelines used to make decisions and evaluate the world around you.
vas deferens The tube ascending from the epididymis that transports sperm.
vector An animal or insect that transports pathogens from one point to another.
veins Vessels that transport blood toward the heart, delivering oxygen-poor blood from the body periphery or oxygen-rich blood from the lungs.
ventricles The two lower chambers of the heart, which pump blood to the body and lungs.
violence Use of physical force—threatened or actual—with the intent of causing harm.
violent crime Offenses involving force or the threat of force, including murder, rape, sexual assault, robbery, and assault.
virus A microscopic organism that cannot multiply without invading body cells.
vitamins Compounds needed by the body in minute amounts for normal growth and function.
vulva All of the female external organs collectively. Also called *genitals*.

W

water A liquid composed of hydrogen and oxygen that is necessary for life.
wellness An active process through which people become aware of, and make choices toward, a more successful existence.
whole exome sequencing A form of genetic testing that analyzes a person's exome, or the sections of their genome that carry the codes for making proteins.
whole genome sequencing The full decoding and readout of an entire genome.
whole grains Unrefined grains that contain bran, germ, and endosperm.
will A legally binding document that states what should be done with a person's property after death.
withdrawal The process in which, and symptoms that develop when, a person stops using a drug.
withdrawal Withdrawal of the penis from the vagina before ejaculation.

Z

zygote A fertilized egg.

REFERENCES

Chapter 1

i. Xu, J., Murphy, S.L., Kochanek, K.D., & Bastian, B.A. (2016, February 16). *National vital statistics reports 64(2)*. Centers for Disease Control and Prevention. www.cdc.gov.

ii. Blair Johnson, N., Hayes, L. D., Brown, K., Hoo, E. C., & Ethier, K. A. (2014, October 31). CDC National Health Report: Leading causes of morbidity and mortality and associated behavioral risk and protective factors—United States, 2005–2013. *Morbidity and Mortality Weekly Report, 63*(4), 3–27. www.cdc.gov/mmwr.

1. World Health Organization. (1948). Preamble to the Constitution of the World Health Organization as adopted by the International Health Conference, New York, 19–22 June 1946; signed on 22 July 1946 by the representatives of 61 States (Official Records of the World Health Organization, no. 2, p. 100) and entered into force on 7 April 1948. www.who.int.

2. Dunn, H. L. (1959, June). High-level wellness for man and society. *American Journal of Public Health and the Nation's Health, 49*(6), 786–792. www.ncbi.nlm.nih.gov.

3. National Wellness Institute. (2015). *Definition of wellness*. www.nationalwellness.org.

4. Xu, J., Murphy, S.L., Kochanek, K.D., & Bastian, B.A. (2016, February 16). *National vital statistics reports 64(2)*. Centers for Disease Control and Prevention. www.cdc.gov.

5. Centers for Disease Control and Prevention. (2000). *Leading causes of death, 1900–1998*. www.cdc.gov.

6. Centers for Disease Control and Prevention. (2015, August 26). *Chronic disease overview*. www.cdc.gov.

7. Centers for Disease Control and Prevention. (2015, July 20). *Exercise or physical activity*. www.cdc.gov.

8. Centers for Disease Control and Prevention. (2014, June 4). *NCHS obesity data*. National Center for Health Statistics. www.cdc.gov.

9. Centers for Disease Control and Prevention. (2015, October 23). *Cigarette smoking in the United States*. www.cdc.gov.

10. Centers for Disease Control and Prevention. (2014, January 16). *Binge drinking*. www.cdc.gov.

11. U.S. Department of Health and Human Services. (2015). *About HHS*. www.hhs.gov.

12. U.S. Department of Health and Human Services. (2015, November 4). *About Healthy People*. www.healthypeople.gov.

13. American College Health Association. (2015). *ACHA-NCHA II: Reference group executive summary, spring 2015*. www.acha-ncha.org.

14. Joint United Nations Program on HIV/AIDS. (2014). *UNAIDS Fact Sheet 2014*. www.unaids.org.

15. World Health Organization. (2014, July). *Tuberculosis: Frequently asked questions—XDR-TB*. www.who.int.

16. Food and Agriculture Organization (FAO). (2015). *The state of food insecurity in the world, 2015*. FAO Media Centre. www.fao.org.

17. World Health Organization. (2015, January). *Fact Sheet no. 311: Obesity and overweight*. www.who.int.

18. U.S. Department of Health and Human Services. (2015, November 5). *Determinants of health*. www.healthypeople.gov.

19. Centers for Disease Control and Prevention. (2013, November 22). CDC health disparities and inequalities report—United States, 2013. *Morbidity and Mortality Weekly Report*, 62(Supplement). www.cdc.gov.

20. Calitz, C., Pollack, K. M., Millard, C., & Yach, D. (2015, April). National Institutes of Health Funding for Behavioral Interventions to Prevent Chronic Diseases. *American Journal of Preventive Medicine, 48*(4), 462–471.

21. Seeman, M., Merkin, S. S., Karlamangla, A., Koretz, B., & Seeman, T. (2014, October). Social status and biological dysregulation: The "status syndrome" and allostatic load. *Social Science and Medicine, 118*, 143–151. doi:10.1016/j.socscimed.2014.08.002.

22. Bosworth, B., Burtless, G., & Zhang, K. 2016. Later retirement, inequality in old age, and the growing gap in longevity between rich and poor. *Economic Studies at Brookings*, January, 2016. www.brookings.edu.

23. Martinez, M. E., & Cohen, R. A. (2015, November). *Health insurance coverage: Early release of estimates from the National Health Interview Survey, January–June, 2015*. National Center for Health Statistics. www.cdc.gov/nchs.

24. National Network of Libraries of Medicine. (2014, August 5). *Health literacy*. http://nnlm.gov.

25. Prochaska, J., & Velicer, W. (1997). The transtheoretical model of health behavior change. *American Journal of Health Promotion, 12*(1), 38–48.

26. Doran, G. T. (1981). There's a S.M.A.R.T. way to write management's goals and objectives. *Management Review, 70*(11), 35–36.

27. National Institutes of Health. (n.d.). *Guide to behavior change*. www.nhlbi.nih.gov.

28. Bandura, A. (1977). Self-efficacy: Toward a unifying theory of behavior change. *Psychological Review 84*(2), 191–215.

29. Rotter, J. B. (1954). *Social learning and clinical psychology*. Englewood Cliffs, NJ: Prentice Hall.

30. American Cancer Society. (2013, November 11). *Helping a smoker quit: Do's and don'ts*. www.cancer.org.

Chapter 2

i. American College Health Association. (2015). *ACHA-NCHA II: Undergraduate reference group executive summary, fall 2015*. www.acha.ncha.org.

ii. Goldberg, M. (2015). Understanding panic attacks: The basics. *WebMD*. www.webmd.com.

iii. National Center for Health Statistics. (2014). *Deaths, percent of total deaths, and death rates for 15 leading causes of death in 10-year age groups, by race and sex: United States 1999–2013*. www.cdc.gov.

1. Ryff, C. D. (1989). Happiness is everything, or is it? Explorations on the meaning of psychological well-being. *Journal of Personality and Social Psychology, 57*(6), 1069–1081.

2. Stinson, D., Logel, C., Zanna, M., Holmes, J., Cameron, J., et al. (2008). The cost of lower self-esteem: Testing a self- and social-bonds model of health. *Journal of Personality and Social Psychology, 94*(3), 412–428.

3. Maslow, A. H. (1998). *Toward a psychology of being*, 3rd ed. New York: John Wiley & Sons.

4. Greene, L., & Burke, G. (2007, Fall). Beyond self-actualization. *Journal of the Health and Human Services Administration*, 116–128.

5. Payne, W. L. (1985). A study of emotion: Developing emotional intelligence. The Union Institute. *Dissertation Abstracts International, 47*(01A), 203.

6. Mayer, J. D., Salovey, P., Caruso, D. R., & Cherkasskiy, L. (2011). Emotional intelligence. In Sternberg, R. J., & Kaufman, S. B. (Eds.), *The Cambridge Handbook of Intelligence*. Cambridge, UK: Cambridge University Press, 532, 545.

7. Day, A., Therrien, D., & Carroll, S. (2005). Predicting psychological health: Assessing the incremental validity of emotional intelligence beyond personality, type A behavior, and daily hassles. *European Journal of Personality, 19*, 519–536.

8. Seligman, M. (1998). *Learned optimism: Change your mind and change your life*. New York: Pocket Books.

9. Burris, J. L., Brechting, E. H., Salsman, J., & Carlson, C. R. (2009). Factors associated with the psychological well-being and distress of university students. *Journal of American College Health, 57*(5), 536–543.

10. Segovia, F., Moore, J. L., Linnville, S. E., Hoyt, R. E., & Hain, R. E. (2012). Optimism predicts resilience in repatriated prisoners of war: A 37-year longitudinal study. *Journal of Traumatic Stress, 25*(3), 330–336.

11. Geers, A. L., Wellman, J. A., Fowler, S. L., Helfer, S. G., & France, C. R. (2010). Dispositional optimism predicts placebo analgesia. *Journal of Pain, 11*(11), 1165–1171.

12. Rajandram, R. K., Ho, S. M., Samman, N., Chan, N., McGrath, C., & Zwahlen, R. A. (2011). Interaction of hope and optimism with anxiety and depression in a specific group of cancer survivors: A preliminary study. *BMC Research Notes, 4*, 519.

13. National Institutes of Health. (2011, September 26). Gene linked to optimism and self-esteem. *NIH Research Matters*. www.nih.gov.

14. Cecero, J. J., Beitel, M., & Prout, T. (2008). Exploring the relationships among early maladaptive schemas, psychological mindedness and self-reported college adjustment. *Psychology and Psychotherapy: Theory, Research, and Practice, 81*, 105–118.

15. Lereya, S. T., Copeland, W. E., Costello, E. J. & Wolke, D. (2015). Adult mental health consequences of peer bullying and maltreatment in childhood: Two cohorts in two countries. *Lancet Psychiatry*. doi: 10.1016/S2215-0366(15)00165-0.

16. Hefner, J., & Eisenberg, D. (2009). Social support and mental health among college students. *American Journal of Orthopsychiatry, 79*(4), 491–499.

17. Pew Research Center. (2015, May 12). *America's changing religious landscape*. www.pewforum.org.

18. Newport, F., Witters, D., & Agrawal, S. (2012, February 16). *In U.S., very religious have higher well-being across all faiths*. Gallup-Healthways Well-Being Index, Jan 2, 2010-Dec 30, 2011. www.gallup.com.

19. Seaward, B. L. (2013). *Health of the human spirit: Spiritual dimensions for personal health*, 2nd ed. Burlington, MA: Jones & Bartlett Learning.

20. Kaplun, A. (Ed.). (1992). *Health promotion and chronic illness: Discovering a new quality of health*. A. Kaplun, Ed. Geneva: World Health Organization.

21. Post, S. G. (2011). It's good to be good: 2011 fifth annual scientific report on health, happiness, and helping others. *International Journal of Person Centered Medicine, 1*(4), 814–829.

22. Johnstone, B., Yoon, D. P., Cohen, D., Schopp, L. H., McCormack, G., et al. (2012). Relationships among spirituality, religious practices, personality factors, and health for five different faith traditions. *Journal of Religion and Health, 51*(4), 1017–1041.

23. National Cancer Institute. (2011). *Spirituality in cancer care*. www.cancer.gov.

24. Kohls, N., Sauer, S., Offenbacher, M., & Giordano, J. (2011). Spirituality: An overlooked predictor of placebo effects? *Philosophical Transactions of the Royal Society B: Biological Sciences, 366*(1572), 1838–1848.

25. Weaver, A. J., & Koenig, H. G. (2006). Religion, spirituality, and their relevance to medicine: An update. *American Family Physician, 73*, 1336–1337.

26. Sieben, L. (2011, March 14). Nearly a third of college students have had mental health counseling, study finds. *The Chronicle of Higher Education*. http://chronicle.com.

27. Gonda, X., Fountoulakis, K. N., Rihmer, Z., Lazary, J., Laszik, A., & Akiskal, K. K. (2009). Towards a genetically validated new affective temperament scale: A delineation of the temperament phenotype of 5-HTTLPR using the TEMPS-A. *Journal of Affective Disorders, 112*(1–3), 19–29.

28. Eagan, M. K., Stolzenberg, E. B., Ramirez, J. J., Aragon, M. C., Suchard, M. R., & Hurtado, S. (2014). *The American freshman: National norms fall 2014*. Los Angeles: Higher Education Research Institute.

29. Lampert, R., Shusterman, V., Burg, M., McPherson, C., Batsford, W., et al. (2009). Anger-induced T-wave alternans predicts future ventricular arrhythmias in patients with implantable cardioverter-defibrillators. *Journal of the American College of Cardiology, 53*(9), 774–778.

30. Chida, Y., & Steptoe, A. (2009). The association of anger and hostility with future coronary heart disease: A meta-analytic review of prospective evidence. *Journal of the American College of Cardiology, 53*(11), 947–949.

31. Bagalman, E., & Napili, A. (2015). *Prevalence of mental illness in the United States: Data sources and estimates*. Congressional Research Service. www.fas.org.

32. Substance Abuse and Mental Health Services Administration. (2014). *Results from the 2013 National Survey on Drug Use and Health: Mental health findings*. NSDUH series H-49, HHS Publication No. (SMA) 14–4887. www.samhsa.gov.

33. Wilson, R. (2015, Fall). An epidemic of anguish. *The Chronicle of Higher Education*. http://chronicle.com.

34. American College Health Association. (2015). *ACHA-NCHA II: Undergraduate reference group executive summary, fall 2015*. www.acha.ncha.org.

35. Blanco, C., Okuda, M., Wright, C., Hasin, D. S., Grant, B. F., et al. (2008). Mental health of college students and their non-college-attending peers: Results from the National Epidemiologic Study on Alcohol and Related Conditions. *Archives of General Psychiatry, 65*, 1429–1437.

36. Kessler, R.C., Angermeyer, M., Anthony, J. C., De Graaf, R., Demyttenaere, K., et al. (2007). Lifetime prevalence and age-of-onset distributions of mental disorders in the World Health Organization's World Mental Health Survey Initiative. *World Psychiatry, 6*(3), 168–176.

37. CBS News. (2013, June 20). *Study shows 70% of Americans take prescription drugs*. www.cbsnews.com.

38. Organization for Economic Cooperation and Development. (2014). *Health at a glance: Europe 2014*. http://ec.europa.eu.

39. American Psychiatric Association. (2013). *Diagnostic and statistical manual of mental disorders*, 5th ed. Arlington, VA: American Psychiatric Publishing.

40. Angell, M. (2011, June 23). *The epidemic of mental illness: Why?* www.nybooks.com.

41. Bear, M. F., Connors, B. W., & Paradiso, M. A. (2007). *Neuroscience: Exploring the brain*, 3rd ed. Baltimore: Lippincott Williams & Wilkins.

42. Center for Behavioral Health Statistics and Quality. (2015). *2014 National Survey on Drug Use and Health: Mental health detailed tables*. www.samhsa.gov.

43. Breene, G., Webb, B. T., Butler, A. W., van den Oord, E. J., Tozzi, F., et al. (2011). A genome-wide significant linkage for severe depression on chromosome 3: The Depression Network Study. *American Journal of Psychiatry, 168*(8), 840–847.

44. Pergadia, M. L., Glowinski, A. L., Wray, N. R., Agrawal, A., Saccone, S. F., et al. (2011). A 3p26–3p25 genetic linkage finding for DSM-IV major depression in heavy smoking families. *American Journal of Psychiatry, 168*(8), 848–852.

45. Elyse, A. L., Inui, E. G., Turner, C. A., Hagenauer, M. H., Prater, K. E., et al. (2015). Fibroblast growth factor 9 is a novel modulator of negative affect. *Proceedings of the National Academy of Sciences of the United States of America, 112*(38), 11953–110958.

46. National Institute of Mental Health. (2011, July 27). *Depression*. www.nimh.nih.gov.

47. Centers for Disease Control and Prevention. (2008). Prevalence of self-reported postpartum depressive symptoms—17 states, 2004–2005. *Morbidity and Mortality Weekly Report, 57*(14), 361–366.

48. Murphy, S. L., Kochanek, K. D., Xu, J. Q., & Heron, M. (2015). Deaths: Final data for 2012. *National Vital Statistics Reports, 63*(9).

49. Kline, N. (1964). The practical management of depression. *Journal of the American Medical Association, 190*, 122–130.

50. Posternak, M. A., & Miller, I. (2001). Untreated short-term course of major depression: A meta-analysis of outcomes from studies using wait-list control groups. *Journal of Affective Disorders, 66*, 139–146.

51. Chen, S-Y., & Toh, S. (2011). National trends in prescribing antidepressants before and after an FDA advisory on suicidality risk in youths, *Psychiatric Services, 62*(7), 727–733.

52. Lu, C. Y., Zhang, F., Lakoma, M. D., Madden, J. M., Rusinak, D., et al. (2014). Changes in antidepressant use by young people and suicidal behavior after FDA warnings and media coverage; quasi-experimental study. *British Medical Journal, 348*, g3596.

53. Moran, M. (2014, Dec. 5). *Experts debate effects of antidepressant warning*. http://psychnews.psychiatry online.org.

54. Mayo Clinic. (2012, February 10). *Depression (major depression): Treatments and drugs*. www.mayoclinic.com.

55. Ioannidis, J. P. A. (2008). Effectiveness of antidepressants: An evidence myth constructed from a thousand randomized trials? *Philosophy, Ethics, and Humanities in Medicine, 3*, 14.

56. Kirsch, I. (2011). *The emperor's new drugs: Exploding the antidepressant myth*. New York: Basic Books.

57. National Institute of Mental Health. (2012, May 16). *Bipolar disorder*. www.nimh.nih.gov.

58. Spiegel, A. (2010, February 10). *Children labeled bipolar may get a new diagnosis*. www.npr.org.

59. National Institute of Mental Health. (2009). *Panic disorder*. www.nimh.nih.gov.

60. National Institute of Mental Health. (2013, January 3). *Social phobia (social anxiety disorder)*. www.nimh.nih.gov.

61. Cloos, J. M., & Ferreira, V. (2009, January). Current use of benzodiazepines in anxiety disorders. *Current Opinion in Psychiatry, 22*(1), 90–95.

62. McCarron. R.M. (2013). The DSM-5 and the art of medicine: Certainly uncertain. *Annals of Internal Medicine, 159*(5), 360–361.

63. U.S. Department of Veterans Affairs, National Center for PTSD. (2012, May 29). *What is PTSD?* www.ptsd.va.gov.

64. Mayes, R., Bagwell, C., & Erkulwater, J. (2008). ADHD and the rise in stimulant use among children. *Harvard Review of Psychiatry, 16*(3), 151–166.

65. DuPaul, G. J., Weyandt, L. L., O'Dell, S., & Varejao, M. (2009, November). College students with ADHD: Current status and future directions. *Journal of Attention Disorders, 13*(3), 234–250.

66. Weissman, J. M. (2013, January 15). *Study: Children with ADHD earn less, work less later in life*. www.theat lantic.com.

67. WebMD. (2010, April 12). *Stimulants for attention deficit hyperactivity disorder*. www.webmd.com.

68. Wolraich, M. L., McKeown, R. E., Visser, S. N., Bard, D., Cuffe, S., et al. (2014). The prevalence of ADHD: Its diagnosis and treatment in four school districts across two states. *Journal of Attention Disorders, 18*(7), 563–575.

69. Swartz, A. (2013, December 14). *The selling of attention deficit disorder*. www.nytimes.com.

70. Arria, A. M., & DuPont, R. L. (2010, October). Nonmedical prescription stimulant use among college students: Why we need to do something and what we need to do. *Journal of Addictive Diseases, 29*(4), 417–426.

71. National Institute of Mental Health. (2009). *Schizophrenia*. www.nimh.nih.gov.

72. Kane, J. M., Robinson, D. G., Schooler, N. R., Mueser, K. T., Penn, D. L., et al. (2015). Comprehensive versus usual community care for first-episode psychosis: 2-year outcomes from the NIMH RAISE Early Treatment Program. *American Journal of Psychiatry, 173*(4), 362–372.

73. International Society for the Study of Self-Injury. (2007). *Definition of non-suicidal self-injury*. www.itriples.org.

74. Batey, H., May, J., & Andrade, J. (2010, February). Negative intrusive thoughts and dissociation as risk factors for self-harm. *Suicide and Life-Threatening Behavior, 40*(1), 35–49.

75. Bresin, K., & Schoenleber, M. (2015). Gender differences in the prevalence of nonsuicidal self-injury: A meta-analysis. *Clinical Psychology Review, 38*, 55–64.

76. Muehlenkamp, J. J., Claes, L., Havertape, L., & Plener, P. L. (2012). International prevalence of adolescent non-suicidal self-injury and deliberate self-harm. *Child and Adolescent Psychiatric Mental Health, 6*, 10.

77. Centers for Disease Control and Prevention. (2015). *Web-based Injury Statistics Query and Reporting System, fatal injury reports, national and regional, 1999–2013*. www.cdc.gov.

78. Haas, A. P., Eliason, M., Mays, V. M., Mathy, R. M., Cochran, S. D., et al. (2010, December). Suicide and suicide risk in lesbian, gay, bisexual, and transgender populations: Review and recommendations. *Journal of Homosexuality, 58*(1), 10–51.

79. National Institute of Mental Health. (2010, September 27). *Suicide in the U.S.: Statistics and prevention*. www.nimh.nih.gov.

80. Kolanta, G. (November 2, 2015). *Death rates rising for middle-aged white Americans, study finds*. www.nytimes.com.

81. National Alliance on Mental Illness. (2012). *College students speak: Survey report on mental health*. www.nami.org.

82. Hunt, J., & Eisenberg, D. (2010, January). Mental health problems and help-seeking behavior among college students. *Journal of Adolescent Health, 46*(1), 3–10.

83. Hurtado, S., Eagan, M. K., Stolzenberg, E. B., & Suchard, M. R. (2014, December). *Research Brief: Findings from the 2014 college senior survey*. www.heri.ucla.edu.

84. Harvard Medical School. (2008, May). *Positive psychology in practice*. www.health.harvard.edu.

85. Simpson, H. B., Foa, E. B., Liebowitz, M. R., Huppert, J. D., Cahill, S., et al. (2013). Cognitive-behavioral therapy vs Risperidone for augmenting serotonin reuptake inhibitors in obsessive-compulsive disorder: A randomized clinical trial. *JAMA Psychiatry, 70*(11), 1190–1199.

86. Substance Abuse and Mental Health Services Administration. (2012, June 19). *Acceptance and commitment therapy (ACT)*. www.nrepp.samhsa.gov.

87. Ratanasiripong, P., Sverduk, K., Prince, J., & Hayashino, D. (2012). Biofeedback and counseling for stress and anxiety among college students. *Journal of College Student Development, 53*, 742–749.

88. Lowry, F. (2011, February 2). *FDA panel wants electroconvulsive therapy to retain high-risk class III status.* www.medscape.com.
89. Sarris, J., Logan, A. C., Akbaraly, T. N., Amminger, G. P., Balanzá-Martínez, V., et al. (2015). Nutritional medicine as mainstream in psychiatry. *The Lancet Psychiatry, 2*(3), 271.

Chapter 3

i. American College Health Association. (2015). *ACHA-NCHA II: Undergraduate reference group executive summary, spring 2015.* www.acha.ncha.org.
ii. American Psychological Association. (2014). *Stress in America: Paying with our health.* www.apa.org.
1. American Psychological Association. (2014). *Stress in America: Paying with our health.* www.apa.org.
2. Selye, H. (1980). *Selye's guide to stress research* (vol. 1). New York: Van Nostrand Reinhold.
3. Selye, H. (1974). *Stress without distress.* New York: Lippincott.
4. Nixon, P. G. (1982). The human function curve—A paradigm for our times. *Activitas Nervosa Superior, Suppl 3*(pt. 1), 130–133.
5. McEwen, B. S. (2013). The brain on stress: Toward an integrative approach to brain, body, and behavior. *Perspectives on Psychological Science, 8*(6), 673–675. doi: 10.1177/1745691613506907.
6. Merrifield, C., & Danckert, J. (2014). Characterizing the psychophysiological signature of boredom. *Experimental Brain Research, 232*(2), 481–491. doi: 10.1007/s00221-013-3755-2.
7. Manenschijn, L., Schaap, L., van Schoor, N. M., van der Pas, S., Peeters, G. M. E. E., et al. (2013). High long-term cortisol levels, measured in scalp hair, are associated with a history of cardiovascular disease. *Journal of Clinical Endocrinology & Metabolism, 98*(5), 2078–2083. doi: 10.1210/jc.2012–3663.
8. Daubert, D. L., Looney, B. M., Clifton, R. R., Cho, J. N., & Scheuer, D. A. (2014). Elevated corticosterone in the dorsal hindbrain increases plasma norepinephrine and neuropeptide Y, and recruits a vasopressin response to stress. *American Journal of Physiology: Regulatory, Integrative and Comparative Physiology, 307*(2), R212-R224. doi: 10.1152/ajpregu.00326.2013.
9. Marvar, P. J., & Harrison, D. G. (2012). Stress-dependent hypertension and the role of T lymphocytes. *Experimental Physiology, 97*, 1161–1167. doi: 10.1113/expphysiol.2011.061507.
10. Okutsu, M., Lira V. A., Higashida, K., Peake, J., Higuchi, M., & Suzuki, K. (2014). Corticosterone accelerates atherosclerosis in the apolipoprotein E-deficient mouse. *Atherosclerosis, 232*(2), 414–419.
11. DiDalmazi, G., Pagotto, U., Pasquali, R., & Vicennati, V. (2012). Glucocorticoids and type 2 diabetes: From physiology to pathology. *Journal of Nutrition and Metabolism.* doi: 10.1155/2012/525093.
12. Hackett, R. A., Kivimaki, M., Kumari, M., & Steptoe, A. (2015). Diurnal cortisol patterns, future diabetes and impaired glucose metabolism in the Whitehall II cohort study. *Journal of Clinical Endocrinology & Metabolism, 101*(2), 619–625.
13. Peters, A., & McEwan, B. S. (2015). Stress habituation, body shape and cardiovascular mortality. *Neuroscience and Biobehavioral Reviews, 56*, 139–150. doi: 10.1016/j.neubiorev.2015.07.001.
14. Paredes, S., & Ribeiro, L. (2014). Cortisol: The villain in metabolic syndrome? *Reviews of the Brazilian Medical Association, 60*(1), 84–92.
15. Sanghez, V., Razzoli, M., Carobbio, S., Campbell, M., McCallum, J., et al. (2013). Psychosocial stress induces hyperphagia and exacerbates diet-induced insulin resistance and the manifestations of the metabolic syndrome. *Psychoneuroendocrinology, 38*(12), 2933–2942. doi: 10.1016/j.psyneuen.2013.07.022.
16. American Psychological Association. (2012). *Stress in America: Our health at risk.* www.apa.org.
17. Khanfer, R., Carroll, D., Lord, J. M., & Phillips, A. C. (2012). Reduced neutrophil superoxide production among healthy older adults in response to acute psychological stress. *International Journal of Psychophysiology, 86*(3), 238–244.
18. Dhabhar, F. S. (2014). Effects of stress on immune function: The good, the bad, and the beautiful. *Immunologic Research, 58*(2–3): 193–210.
19. Houle, T. T., Butschek, R. A., Turner, D. P., Smitherman, T. A., Rains, J. C., & Penzien, D. B. (2012). Stress and sleep duration predict headache severity in chronic headache sufferers. *Pain, 153*(12), 2432–2440.
20. Blaauw, B. A., Dyb, G., Hagen, K., Holmen, T. L., Linde, M., Wentzel-Larsen, T., & Zwart, J. A. (2014). Anxiety, depression, and behavioral problems among adolescents with recurrent headache: The Young-HUNT study. *The Journal of Headache and Pain, 15*(1), 38.
21. American College Health Association. (2015). *ACHA-NCHA II: Undergraduate reference group executive summary, spring 2015.* www.acha.ncha.org.
22. Kalmbach, D. A., Pillai, V., Arnedt, J. T., & Drake, C. L. (2016). Identifying at-risk individuals for insomnia using the Ford Insomnia Response to Stress Test. *Sleep, 39*(2), 449–456. doi: 10.5665/sleep.5462.
23. Buck, A. A., & Neff, L. A. (2012). Stress spillover in early marriage: The role of self-regulatory depletion. *Journal of Family Psychology, 26*(5), 698–708. doi: 10.1037/a0029260.
24. Hamilton, L. D., & Julian, A. M. (2014). The relationship between daily hassles and sexual function in men and women. *Journal of Sex & Marital Therapy, 40*(5), 379–395. doi: 10.1080/0092623X.2013.864364.
25. Lynch, C. D., Sundaram, R., Maisog, J. M., Sweeney, A. M., & Buck Louis, G. M. (2014). Preconception stress increases the risk of infertility: Results from a couple-based prospective cohort study—The LIFE study. *Human Reproduction, 29*(5), 1067–1075. doi: 10.1093/humrep/deu032.
26. Kumar, M., Sharma, S., Gupta, S., Vaish, S., & Misra, R. (2014). Effects of stress on academic performance in medical students: A cross-sectional study. *Indian Journal of Physiology and Pharmacology, 58*(1), 81–86.
27. Strack, J., & Esteves, F. (2015). Exams? Why worry? Interpreting anxiety as facilitative and stress appraisals. *Anxiety, Stress, and Coping, 28*(2), 205–214. doi: 10.1080/10615806.2014.931942.
28. Slavich, G. M., & Irwin, M. R. (2014). From stress to inflammation to major depressive disorder: A social signal transduction theory of depression. *Psychological Bulletin, 140*(3), 774–815. doi: 10.1037/a0035302.
29. Johnson, P. L., Federici, L. M., & Shekhar, A. (2014). Etiology, triggers and neurochemical circuits associated with unexpected, expected, and laboratory-induced panic attacks. *Neuroscience & Biobehavioral Reviews, 46*(3), 429–454. doi: 10.1016/j.neubiorev.2014.07.027.
30. Friedman, M., & Rosenman, R.H. (1996). *Type A behavior: Its diagnosis and treatment.* New York: Plenum Press (pp. ix, 3, 4).
31. Bissonette, M. (1998, August). Optimism, hardiness, and resiliency: A review of the literature. *The Child and Family Partnership Project.* www.reachinginreachingout.com.
32. Kobasa, S. (1982). The hardy personality: Toward a social psychology of stress and health. In G. S. Sanders & J. Suls (Eds.), *Social psychology of health and illness.* Hillsdale, NJ: Lawrence Erlbaum Associates (pp. 3–12).
33. Jameson, P. R. (2014). The effects of a hardiness educational intervention on hardiness and perceived stress of junior baccalaureate nursing students. *Nurse Education Today, 34*(4), 603–607. doi: 10.1016/j.nedt.2013.06.019.
34. American Psychological Association. (2014). *The road to resilience.* www.apa.org.
35. Hartley, M. T. (2011). Examining the relationships between resilience, mental health, and academic persistence in undergraduate college students. *Journal of American College Health, 59*(7), 596–604. doi: 10.1080/07448481.2010.515632.
36. Komulainen, E., Meskanene, K., Lipsanen, J., Lahti, J. M., Jylhä, P., et al. (2014). The effect of personality on daily life emotional processes. *PLOS One, 9*(10), e110907. doi: 10.1371/journal.pone.0110907.
37. Poulin, M. J., & Haase, C. M. (2105). Growing to trust: Evidence that trust increases and sustains well-being across the life span. *Social Psychological & Personality Science, 6*(6), 614–621. doi: 10.1177/1948550615574301.
38. Ohio State University. (2015). *2014 national student financial wellness study.* http://cssl.osu.edu.
39. Castro-Diehl, C., Diez Roux, A. V., Seeman, T., Shea, S., Shrager, S., & Tadros, S. (2014). Associations of socioeconomic and psychosocial factors with urinary measures of cortisol and catecholamines in the Multi-Ethnic Study of Atherosclerosis (MESA). *Psychoneuroendocrinology, 41*, 132–141. doi: 10.1016/j.psyneuen.2013.12.013.
40. Haushofer, J., & Fehr, E. (2014). On the psychology of poverty. *Science, 344*(6186), 862–867. doi: 10.1126/science.1232491.
41. Davis, J. (2013, October). *School enrollment and work status: 2011.* U.S. Census Bureau. www.census.gov.
42. Lee, C. S., & Goldstein, S. E. (2016). Loneliness, stress, and social support in young adulthood: Does the source of support matter? *Journal of Youth and Adolescence, 45*(3), 568–580. doi: 10.1007/s10964-015-0395-9.
43. Cacioppo, S., Balogh, S., & Cacioppo, J. T. (2015). Implicit attention to negative social, in contrast to nonsocial, words in the Stroop task differs between individuals high and low in loneliness: Evidence from event-related brain microstates. *Cortex, 70*: 213–233. doi:10.1016/j.cortex.2015.05.032.
44. Phan, T. Q., & Airoldi, E. M. (2015). A natural experiment of social network formation and dynamics. *Proceedings of the National Academy of Sciences, 112*(21), 6595–6600. doi: 10.1073/pnas.1404770112.
45. Chen, W., & Lee, K. H. (2013). Sharing, liking, commenting, and distressed? The pathway between Facebook interaction and psychological distress. *Cyberpsychology, Behavior, and Social Networking, 16*(10), 728–734. doi: 10.1089/cyber.2012.0272.
46. Schilling, O. K., & Diehl, M. (2014). Reactivity to stressor pile-up in adulthood: Effects on daily negative and positive affect. *Psychology and Aging, 29*(1), 72–83. doi: 10.1037/a0035500.
47. Holmes, T. H., & Rahe, R. H. (1967). The Social Readjustment Rating Scale. *Journal of Psychosomatic Research, 11*, 213–218.
48. Radhu, N., Daskalakis, C. J., Arpin-Cribbie, C. A., Irvine, J., & Ritvo, P. (2012). Evaluating a web-based cognitive-behavioral therapy for maladaptive perfectionism in university students. *Journal of American College Health, 60*(5), 357–366. doi: 10.1080/07448481.2011.630703.
49. Chu-Lien Chao, R. (2012). Managing perceived stress among college students: The roles of social support and dysfunctional coping. *Journal of College Counseling, 15*(1), 5–21.
50. American Psychological Association. (2013). *Stress in America: Missing the health care connection.* www.apa.org.
51. Marti, S., King, J. R., & Dehaene, S. (2015). Time-resolved decoding of two processing chains during dual-task interference. *Neuron, 88*(6), 1297–1307. doi: 10.1016/j.neuron.2015.10.040.

52. Maier, S. U., Makwana, A. B., & Hare, T. A. (2015). Acute stress impairs self-control in goal-directed choice by altering multiple functional connections within the brain's decision circuits. *Neuron, 87*(3), 621–631. doi: 10.1016/j.neuron.2015.07.005.
53. American Council on Exercise. (2015). *Exercise can help control stress.* www.acefitness.org.
54. Jackson, E. M. (2013). Stress relief: The role of exercise in stress management. *ACSM's Health and Fitness Journal, 17*(3), 14–19. doi: 10.1249/FIT.0b013e31828cb1c9.
55. Chellew, K., Evans, P., Fornes-Vives, J., Perez, G., & Garcia-Banda, G. (2015). The effect of progressive muscle relaxation on daily cortisol secretion. *Stress, 18*(5), 538–544. doi: 10.3109/10253890.2015.1053454.
56. National Center for Complementary and Integrative Health. (2013, June). *Yoga for health.* www.nccih.nih.gov.
57. National Center for Complementary and Integrative Health. (2015, May). *Massage therapy for health purposes: What you need to know.* www.nccih.nih.gov.
58. National Center for Complementary and Integrative Health. (2014, December). *Relaxation techniques for health: What you need to know.* www.nccih.nih.gov.
59. National Center for Complementary and Integrative Health. (2014, November). *Meditation: What you need to know.* www.nccih.nih.gov.
60. Bradt, J., Dileo, C., & Potvin, N. (2013). Music for stress and anxiety reduction in coronary heart disease patients. *Cochrane Database of Systematic Reviews, 2*:CD006577. doi: 10.1002/14651858.CD006577.pub3.

Chapter 4

i. National Sleep Foundation. (2011, March 7). *2011 Sleep in America poll: Communications technology in the bedroom.* www.sleepfoundation.org.
1. American College Health Association. (2015). *ACHA-NCHA II: Undergraduate reference group executive summary, spring 2015.* www.acha.ncha.org.
2. Silverthorn, D. (2010). *Human physiology: An integrated approach,* 5th ed. San Francisco: Benjamin Cummings.
3. National Institute of Neurological Disorders and Stroke. (2015, December). *Brain basics: Understanding sleep.* www.ninds.nih.gov.
4. Bear, M. F., Connors, B. W., & Paradiso, M. A. (2007). *Neuroscience: Exploring the brain,* 3rd ed. Baltimore: Lippincott Williams & Wilkins (p. 596).
5. Watson, N. F., Badr, M. S., Belenky, G., Bliwise, D. L., Buxton, O. M., et al. (2015). Recommended amount of sleep for a healthy adult: A joint consensus statement of the American Academy of Sleep Medicine and Sleep Research Society. *Sleep, 38*(6), 843–844.
6. Harvard Health Publications. (2009, November). *Napping may not be such a no-no.* www.health.harvard.edu.
7. Bonnet, M. H., & Arand, D. L. (2010). How much sleep do adults need? *White paper: National Sleep Foundation.* www.sleepfoundation.org.
8. Jones, M. (2011, April 15). How little sleep can you get away with? *The New York Times.* www.nytimes.com.
9. Kamdar, B., Kaplan, K., Kezirian, E., & Dement, W. (2004). The impact of extended sleep on daytime alertness, vigilance, and mood. *Sleep Medicine, 5,* 441–448.
10. National Sleep Foundation. (2013, February 20). *2013 Sleep in America poll: Exercise and sleep.* www.sleepfoundation.org.
11. National Sleep Foundation. (2011, March 7). *2011 Sleep in America poll: Communications technology in the bedroom.* www.sleepfoundation.org.
12. Mann, D. (2011). *Can better sleep mean catching fewer colds?* www.webmd.com.
13. Ackermann, K., Revell, V. L, Lao, O., Rombout, E., Skene, D., & Kayser M. (2012). Diurnal rhythms in blood cell populations and the effect of acute sleep deprivation in healthy young men. *Sleep, 35*(7), 933–940.
14. Centers for Disease Control and Prevention. (2011, January 27). *Sleep and sleep disorders.* www.cdc.gov.
15. Luyster, F., Strollo Jr., P., Zee, P., & Walsh, J. (2012). Sleep: A health imperative. *Sleep, 35*(6), 727–734.
16. Regestein, Q., Natarajan, V., Pavlova, M., Kawasaki, S., Gleason, R., & Koff, E. (2010). Sleep debt and depression in female college students. *Psychiatry Research, 176*(1), 34–39.
17. Brooks, P. R., Girgenti, A. A., & Mills, M. J. (2009). Sleep patterns and symptoms of depression in college students. *College Student Journal, 43*(2), 464–472.
18. Ahrberg, K., Dresler, M., Niedermaier, S., Steiger, A., & Genzel, L. (2012). The interaction between sleep quality and academic performance. *Journal of Psychiatric Research, 46*(12), 1618–1622.
19. Patel, S. R., & Hu, F. B. (2008). Short sleep duration and weight gain: A systematic review. *Obesity, 16*(3), 643–653.
20. Mitchell, J., Rodriguez, D., Schmitz, K., & Audrain-McGovern, J. (2013). Sleep duration and adolescent obesity. *Pediatrics, 131,* e1428.
21. Asarnow, L. D., McGlinchey, E., Harvey, & A. G. (2015). Evidence for a possible link between bedtime and change in body mass index. *Sleep, 38*(10), 1523–1527.
22. Vail-Smith, K., Felts, W., & Becker, C. (2009). Relationship between sleep quality and health risk behaviors in undergraduate college students. *College Student Journal, 43*(3), 924–930.
23. Gilbert, S. P., & Weaver, C. C. (2010). Sleep quality and academic performance in university students: A wake-up call for college psychologists. *Journal of College Student Psychotherapy, 24*(4), 295–306.
24. Ridner, S. L., Newton, K. S., Staten, R. R., Crawford T. N., & Hall, L. A. (2015, December). Predictors of well-being among college students. *Journal of American College Health, 64*(2), 116–124.
25. Gaultney, J. F. (2010, September-October). The prevalence of sleep disorders in college students: Impact on academic performance. *Journal of American College Health, 59*(2), 91–97.
26. Thacher, P. V. (2008). University students and the "all nighter": Correlates and patterns of students' engagement in a single night of total sleep deprivation. *Behavioral Sleep Medicine, 6*(1), 16–31.
27. Becker, C. M., Adams, T., Orr, C., & Quilter, L. (2008). Correlates of quality sleep and academic performance. *Health Educator, 40*(2), 82–89.
28. American Academy of Sleep Medicine. (2010, November 7). Sleep: Nature's study aid. *Sleep Education.* http://sleepeducation.blogspot.com.
29. Rasch, B., & Born, J. (2013). About sleep's role in memory. *Physiology Reviews, 93,* 681–766.
30. Tamminen, J., Payne, J., Stickgold, R., Wamsley, E., & Gaskell, M. G. (2010, October). Sleep spindle activity is associated with the integration of new memories and existing knowledge. *The Journal of Neuroscience, 30*(43), 14356–14360.
31. National Sleep Foundation. (2011, July 27). *Drowsy driving prevention week highlights prevalent and preventable accidents.* http://drowsydriving.org.
32. Uehli, K., Mehta, A. J., Miedinger, D., Hug, K., Schindler, C., et al. (2014, Feb). Sleep problems and work injuries: A systematic review and meta-analysis. *Sleep Medicine Reviews, 18*(1), 61–73.
33. Guindalin, C., & Tufik, S. (2012). Genetic aspects of sleep in humans. *Sleep Science, 5*(4), 125–130.
34. Tomfohr, L., Pung, M. A., Edwards, K., & Dimsdale, J. E. (2012). Racial differences in sleep architecture: The role of ethnic discrimination. *Biological Psychology, 89*(1), 34–38.
35. National Sleep Foundation. (2015, March 2). *2015 Sleep in America poll: Sleep and pain.* www.sleepfoundation.org.
36. National Sleep Foundation. (2014, March 3). *2014 Sleep in America poll: Sleep in the modern family.* www.sleepfoundation.org.
37. Thompson, J., & Manore, M. (2012). *Nutrition: An applied approach,* 3rd ed. San Francisco: Benjamin Cummings (p. 85).
38. Fujiwara, Y., Arkawa, T., & Fass, R. (2012). Gastroesophageal reflux and sleep disturbances. *Journal of Gastroenterology, 47,* 760–769.
39. Edwards, S. J., Montgomery, I. M., Colquhoun, E. Q., Jordan, J. E., & Clark, M. G. (1992, September). Spicy meals disturb sleep: An effect of thermoregulation? *International Journal of Psychophysiology, 13*(2), 97–100.
40. U.S. Fire Administration. (2010, September 23). *Smoking and fire safety.* www.usfa.dhs.gov.
41. Orbeta, R. L., Overpeck, M. D., Ramcharran, D., Kogan, M. D., & Ledsky, R. (2006, April). High caffeine intake in adolescents: Associations with difficulty sleeping and feeling tired in the morning. *Journal of Adolescent Health, 38*(4), 451–453.
42. Ruxton, C. H. S. (2008). The impact of caffeine on mood, cognitive function, performance and hydration: A review of benefits and risks. *Nutrition Bulletin, 33,* 15–25.
43. WedMD Medical Reference. (2011, February 27). *Caffeine myths and facts.* www.webmd.com.
44. Substance Abuse and Mental Health Services Administration, Office of Applied Studies. (2015, September). *Behavioral health trends in the United States: Results from the 2014 national survey on drug use and health: Volume I: Summary of national findings.* http://samhsa.gov.
45. Clegg-Kraynok, M. M., McBean, A. L., & Montgomery-Downs, H. E. (2011). Sleep quality and characteristics of college students who use prescription psychostimulants nonmedically. *Sleep Medicine, 12,* 598–602.
46. Mann, M. (2013, January). *Alcohol and a good night's sleep don't mix.* www.webmd.com.
47. Myllymaki, T., Kyrolainen, H., Savolainen, K., Hokka, L., Jakonen, R., et al. (2011, March). Effects of vigorous late-night exercise on sleep quality and cardiac autonomic activity. *Journal of Sleep Research, 20*(1 pt. 2), 146–153.
48. American Academy of Sleep Medicine. (2014). *Sleep disorders.* www.sleepeducation.org.
49. American Academy of Sleep Medicine. (2015, March). *Insomnia.* www.sleepeducation.org.
50. American Academy of Sleep Medicine. (2014). *Snoring—Overview and facts.* www.sleepeducation.org.
51. National Institutes of Health. (2012, July). *What is sleep apnea?* www.nhlbi.nih.gov.
52. Young, T., Finn, L., Peppard, P., Szklo-Coxe, M., Austin, D., et al. (2008). Sleep disordered breathing and mortality: Eighteen-year follow-up of the Wisconsin sleep cohort. *Sleep, 31*(8), 1071–1078.
53. American Academy of Sleep Medicine. (2014). *Narcolepsy—Overview and facts.* www.sleepeducation.org.
54. American Academy of Sleep Medicine. (2014). *Nightmares—Overview and facts.* www.sleepeducation.org.
55. American Academy of Sleep Medicine. (2014). *Sleep terrors—Overview and facts.* www.sleepeducation.org.
56. American Academy of Sleep Medicine. (2014). *Sleepwalking—Overview and facts.* www.sleepeducation.org.
57. Mayo Foundation. (2011, May 19). *Sleep bruxism.* www.mayoclinic.com.

58. Winkelman, J. W. (2006). Sleep-related eating disorder and night-eating syndrome: Sleep disorders, eating disorders, or both? *Sleep, 29*(7), 876–877.
59. American Academy of Sleep Medicine. (2014). *Sleep eating disorder—Overview and facts.* www.sleepfoundation.org.
60. Postuma, R. B., Montplaisir, J. Y., Pelletier, A., Dauvilliers, Y., Oertel, W., et al. (2012). Environmental risk factors for REM sleep behaviour disorder: A multicenter case-control study. *Neurology, 79*(5), 428–434.
61. National Sleep Foundation. (2015). *Restless legs syndrome (RLS) and sleep.* www.sleepfoundation.org.
62. Hershner, S., & Chervin, R. (2014, June). Causes and consequences of sleepiness among college students. *Journal of Nature and Science of Sleep, 6*, 73–84.
63. Brown, F. C., Buboltz, W. C., & Soper, B. (2006). Development and evaluation of the sleep treatment and education program for students (STEPS). *Journal of American College Health, 54*(4), 231–237.
64. Kloss, J. D., Nash, C. O., Horsey, S., & Taylor, D. J. (2011). The delivery of behavioural sleep medicine to college students. *Journal of Adolescent Health, 48*(6), 553–561.
65. National Sleep Foundation. (2015). *Sleep aids and insomnia.* www.sleepfoundation.org.
66. American Academy of Sleep Medicine. (2015, June). *Choosing wisely: Sleeping pills for insomnia—They may not be the best treatment option.* www.sleepfoundation.org.
67. Austin, E. (2008). Addressing sleep deprivation in college students. *American Journal for Nurse Practitioners, 12*(6), 34.
68. Scripps Health. (2012, February 27). *Scripps study finds higher death risk with sleeping pills.* www.scripps.org.
69. Kripke, D., Langer, R., & Kline, L. (2012, January). Pharmacology and therapeutics: Hypnotics' association with mortality or cancer: A matched cohort study. *BMJ Open, 2*, e000850. doi: 10.1136/bmjopen-2012-000850.
70. U.S. Food and Drug Administration. (2013, January 10). *FDA requiring lower recommended dose for certain sleep drugs containing zolpidem.* www.fda.gov.
71. Kloss, J. D., Nash, C. O., Horse, S. E., & Taylor, D. J. (2011). The delivery of behavioral sleep medicine to college students. *Journal of Adolescent Health, 48*(6), 553–561.
72. Carney, C. E., & Waters, W. F. (2006). Effects of a structured problem-solving procedure on pre-sleep cognitive arousal in college students with insomnia. *Behavioral Sleep Medicine, 4*(1), 13–28.
73. National Center for Complementary and Alternative Medicine. (2014, April). *Sleep disorders and complementary health approaches: What you need to know.* https://nccih.nih.gov.
74. Caldwell, K., Harrison, M., Adams, M., & Triplett, N. (2009). Effect of Pilates and taiji quan training on self-efficacy, sleep quality, mood, and physical performance of college students. *Journal of Bodywork and Movement Therapies, 13*(2), 155–163.
75. Harmon, K. (2011, March 8). Short on sleep, the brain optimistically favors long odds. *Scientific American.* http://blogs.scientificamerican.com.
76. National Sleep Foundation. (2015). *Sleep hygiene.* www.sleepfoundation.org.

Chapter 5

i. U.S. Department of Agriculture. (2016, January 4). *Sugar and sweeteners yearbook tables.* Economic Research Service, USDA. www.ers.usda.gov.
ii. McDonald's USA. (2015, August 12). *McDonald's USA nutrition facts for popular menu items.* nutrition.mcdonalds.com.
iii. U.S. Food and Drug Administration. (2015, September 2). *Food allergies: What you need to know.* www.fda.gov.
1. U.S. Department of Agriculture. (2016, January 4). *Sugar and sweeteners yearbook tables.* Economic Research Service, USDA. www.ers.usda.gov.
2. Yang, Q., Zhang, Z., Gregg, E. W., Flanders, W. D., Merritt, R., & Hu, F. B. (2014). Added sugar intake and cardiovascular disease mortality among U.S. adults. *JAMA Internal Medicine, 174*(4), 516–524. doi: 10.1001/jamainternmed.2013.13563.
3. Lustig, R. H., Mulligan, K., Noworolski, S. M., Tai, V. W., Wen, M. J., et al. (2015). Isocaloric fructose restriction and metabolic improvement in children with obesity and metabolic syndrome. *Obesity, 24*(2), 453–460. doi: 10.1002/oby.21371.
4. Food and Nutrition Board, Institute of Medicine of the National Academies. (2005). *Dietary reference intakes for energy, carbohydrate, fiber, fat, fatty acids, cholesterol, protein, and amino acids.* Washington, DC: The National Academies Press. www.nap.edu.
5. Reicks, M., Jonnalogadda, S., Albertson, A. M., & Joshi, N. (2014). Total dietary fiber intakes in the US population are related to whole grain consumption: Results from the National Health and Nutrition Examination Survey 2009 to 2010. *Nutrition Research, 34*(3), 226–234. doi: 10.1016/j.nutres.2014.01.002.
6. Schulte, E. M., Avena, N. M., & Gearhardt, A. N. (2015). Which foods may be addictive? The roles of processing, fat content, and glycemic load. *PLOS One, 10*(2), e0117959. doi: 10.137/journal.pone.0117959.
7. Burris, J., Rietkerk, W., & Woolf, K. (2013). Acne: The role of medical nutrition therapy. *Journal of the Academy of Nutrition and Dietetics, 113*(3), 416–430. doi: 10.1016/j.jand.2012.11.016.
8. Goff, L. M., Cowland, D. E., Hooper, L., & Frost, G. S. (2013). Low glycaemic index diets and blood lipids: A systematic review and meta-analysis of randomized controlled trials. *Nutrition, Metabolism & Cardiovascular Diseases, 23*(1), 1–10.
9. American Heart Association. (2014, May 12). *AHA experts reiterate importance of limiting saturated fats.* www.americanheart.org.
10. U.S. Department of Agriculture and Department of Health and Human Services. (2015). *Dietary guidelines for Americans, 2015–2020*, 8th ed. Washington, DC: U.S. Government Printing Office.
11. U.S. Department of Agriculture. (2016, January 7). *All about the protein foods group.* www.choosemyplate.gov.
12. U.S. Food and Drug Administration. (2015, June 16). *Final determination regarding partially hydrogenated oils (removing trans fat).* www.fda.gov.
13. Gosby, A. K., Conigrave, A. D., Raubenheimer, D., & Simpson, S. J. (2014). Protein leverage and energy intake. *Obesity Reviews, 15*(3), 183–191. doi: 10.1111/obr.12131.
14. American College of Sports Medicine, American Dietetic Association, and Dietitians of Canada. (2009). Joint position statement. Nutrition and athletic performance. *Medicine and Science in Sports and Exercise, 41*(3), 709–731.
15. Phillips, S. M., & van Loon, L. J. (2011). Dietary protein for athletes: From requirements to optimum adaptation. *Journal of Sports Sciences, 29*(Suppl 1), S29-S38. doi: 10.1080/02640414.2011.619204.
16. Office of Dietary Supplements. (2014, November 10). *Dietary supplement fact sheet: Vitamin D.* http://ods.od.nih.gov.
17. Office of Dietary Supplements. (2012, December 14). *Dietary supplement fact sheet: Folate.* http://ods.od.nih.gov.
18. Food and Nutrition Board, Institute of Medicine of the National Academies. (2004). *Dietary reference intakes for water, potassium, sodium, chloride, and sulfate.* Washington, DC: The National Academies Press.
19. Thompson, J., Manore, M., & Vaughan, L. (2017). *The science of nutrition,* 4th ed. San Francisco: Pearson Education.
20. U.S. Food and Drug Administration. (2012, November 16). *Energy "drinks" and supplements: Investigations of adverse event reports.* www.fda.gov.
21. Rodriguez-Casado, A. (2014). The health potential of fruits and vegetables phytochemicals: Notable examples. *Critical Reviews in Food Science and Nutrition.* doi: 10.1080/10408398.2012..755149.
22. Firdous, S. M. (2014). Phytochemicals for treatment of diabetes. *EXCLI Journal, 13*, 451–453.
23. Gonzalez-Castejon, M., & Rodriguez-Casado, A. (2011). Dietary phytochemicals and their potential effects on obesity: A review. *Pharmacological Research, 64*(5), 438–455. doi: 10.1016/j.phrs.2011.07.004.
24. Liu, R. H. (2013). Health-promoting components of fruits and vegetables in the diet. *Advances in Nutrition, 4*(3), 384S-392S. doi: 10.3945/an.112.003517.
25. American College Health Association. (2015). *ACHA-NCHA II: Reference group executive summary, spring 2015.* www.acha.ncha.org.
26. Bull, M. J., & Plummer, N. T. (2014). Part 1: The human gut microbiome in health and disease. *Journal of Integrative Medicine, 13*(6), 17–22.
27. Hemarajata, P., & Versalovic, J. (2013). Effects of probiotics on gut microbiota: Mechanisms of intestinal immunomodulation and neuromodulation. *Therapeutic Advances in Gastroenterology, 6*(1), 39–51.
28. Zeratsy, K. (2014, October 15). *Do I need to include probiotics and prebiotics in my diet?* Mayo Foundation. www.mayoclinic.org.
29. Lieberman, H. R., Marriott, B. P., Williams, C., Judelson, D. A., Glickman, E. L., et al. (2015). Patterns of dietary supplement use among college students. *Clinical Nutrition, 34*(5), 976–985. doi: 10.1016/j.clnu.2014.10.010.
30. Office of Dietary Supplements. (2015, July 8). *Dietary supplement fact sheet: Multivitamin/mineral supplements.* http://ods.od.nih.gov.
31. MedlinePlus. (2016, January 13). *Nutrition and athletic performance.* www.nlm.nih.gov/medlineplus.
32. U.S. Food and Drug Administration. (2015, November 30). *How to understand and use the Nutrition Facts label.* www.fda.gov.
33. U.S. Food and Drug Administration. (2015, August 20). *Food labeling guide (8. Claims).* www.fda.gov.
34. U.S. Department of Agriculture. (n.d.) *Food groups.* www.choosemyplate.gov.
35. Centers for Disease Control and Prevention. (2014, January 8). *Estimates of foodborne illness in the United States.* www.cdc.gov.
36. Crim, S. H., Iwamoto, M., Huang, J. Y., Griffin, P. M., Gilliss, D., et al. (2014). Incidence and trends of infection with pathogens transmitted commonly through food—Foodborne Diseases Active Surveillance Network, 10 U.S. cities, 2006–2013. *Morbidity and Mortality Weekly Report, 64*(15), 328–332. www.cdc.gov/mmwr.
37. Centers for Disease Control and Prevention. (2013, July 26). *Norovirus: Overview.* www.cdc.gov/norovirus.
38. Centers for Disease Control and Prevention. (2015, December 17). *Salmonella.* www.cdc.gov/salmonella.
39. U.S. Department of Health and Human Services. (2016). *Check your steps.* www.foodsafety.gov.
40. U.S. Food and Drug Administration. (2015, September 2). *Food allergies: What you need to know.* www.fda.gov.
41. Lebwohl, B., Ludvigsson, J. F., & Gren, P. H. R. (2015). Celiac disease and non-celiac gluten sensitivity. *British Medical Journal, 351*, h4347. doi: 10.1136/bmj.h4347.

42. U.S. Environmental Protection Agency. (2015, March 19). *Pesticides and food: Healthy, sensible food practices.* www.epa.gov.
43. Goldrick-Rab, S., Broton, K., & Eisenberg, D. (2015, December). *Hungry to learn: Addressing food & housing insecurity among undergraduates.* Wisconsin HOPE Lab. http://wihopelab.com.

Chapter 6

i. Centers for Disease Control and Prevention. (2015). *Physical activity for everyone: Physical activity and health.* www.cdc.gov.
ii. Northwestern University. (2009, June 20). *Aerobically unfit young adults on road to diabetes in middle age.* www.sciencedaily.com.
iii. Liu-Ambrose, T., Nagamatsu, L. S., Graf, P., Beattie, B. L., Ashe, M. C., & Handy, T. C. (2010). Resistance training and executive functions: A 12-month randomized controlled trial. *Archives of Internal Medicine, 170*(2), 170–178.
1. Centers for Disease Control and Prevention. (2015). *Exercise or physical activity.* www.cdc.gov.
2. William, P. T. (2008). Vigorous exercise, fitness and incident hypertension, high cholesterol, and diabetes. *Medicine & Science in Sports & Exercise, 40*(6), 998–1006.
3. Kaminsky, L. A., Arena, R., Beckie, T. M., Brubaker, P. H., Church, T. S., et al. (2013). The importance of cardiorespiratory fitness in the United States: The need for a national registry: A policy statement from the American Heart Association. *Circulation, 127,* 652–662.
4. Lang, T. F. (2011). The bone-muscle relationship in men and women. *Journal of Osteoporosis,* article ID 702735, doi: 10.4061/2011/702735.
5. Ärnlöv, J., Ingelsson, E., Sundström, J., & Lind, L. (2010). Impact of body mass index and the metabolic syndrome on the risk of cardiovascular disease and death in middle-aged men. *Circulation, 121,* 230–236.
6. Lebrasseur, N., Achenbach, S., Melton, L., Amin, S., & Khosla, S. (2012). Skeletal muscle mass is associated with bone geometry and microstructure and serum insulin-like growth factor binding protein-2 levels in adult women and men. *Journal of Bone and Mineral Research, 10*(21), 59–69.
7. Knaepen, K., Goekint, M., Heym, E., & Meeusen, R. (2010). Neuroplasticity—Exercise-induced response of peripheral brain-derived neurotrophic factor: A systematic review of experimental studies in human subjects. *Sports Medicine, 40*(9), 765–780.
8. Williamson, J., & Pahor, M. (2010). Evidence regarding the benefits of physical exercise. *Archives of Internal Medicine, 170*(2), 124–125.
9. Lee, D., Sui, X., Artero, G., Lee, I., Church, T. S., et al. (2011). Long-term effects of changes in cardiorespiratory fitness and body mass index on all-cause and cardiovascular disease mortality in men. *Circulation, 124,* 2483–2490.
10. National Institutes of Health, National Institute of Diabetes and Digestive and Kidney Diseases. (2008, October). *Diabetes prevention program (DPP)* (NIH Publication No. 09–5099). Washington, DC: Government Printing Office.
11. Colberg, S., Sigal, R., Fernhall, B., Regensteiner, J., Blissmer, B., et al. (2010). Exercise and type 2 diabetes: The American College of Sports Medicine and the American Diabetes Association joint position statement. *Diabetes Care, 33*(12), 147–167.
12. Remon, J., Bertoni, A., Connelly, S., Feeney, P., Glasser, S., et al. (2010). Effect of the Look AHEAD study intervention on medication use and related cost to treat cardiovascular disease risk factors in individuals with type 2 diabetes. *Diabetes Care, 33*(6), 1153–1158.
13. Friedenreich, C., Neilson, H., & Lynch, B. (2010). State of the epidemiological evidence on physical activity and cancer prevention. *European Journal of Cancer, 46*(14), 2593–2604.
14. Dallal, C., Sullivan-Halley, J., Ross, R., Wang, Y., Deapen, D., et al. (2007). Long-term recreational physical activity and risk of invasive and in situ breast cancer: The California teachers study. *Archives of Internal Medicine, 167*(4), 408–415.
15. Nieman, D. C. (2012). Clinical implications of exercise immunology. *Journal of Sport and Health Science, 1*(1), 12–17.
16. Medline Plus. (2014). *Exercise and immunity.* www.nlm.nih.gov.
17. Gunter, K. B., Almstedt, H. C., & Janz, K. F. (2012). Physical activity in childhood may be the key to optimizing lifespan skeletal health. *Exercise & Sport Science Reviews, 40*(1), 13–21.
18. Rozanski, A. (2012). Exercise as medical treatment for depression. *Journal of the American College of Cardiology, 60*(12), 1064–1066.
19. Sui, X., Laditka, J. N., Church, T. S., Hardind, J. W., Chase, N., et al. (2009). Prospective study of cardiorespiratory fitness and depressive symptoms in women and men. *Journal of Psychiatric Research, 43*(5), 546–552.
20. Elliot, C., Kennedy, C., Morgan, G., Anderson, S., & Morris, D. (2012). Undergraduate physical activity and depressive symptoms: A national study. *American Journal of Health Behavior, 36*(2), 230–241.
21. Åberg, M. A. I., Pedersen, N. L., Torén, K., Svartengren, M., Bäckstrand, B., et al. (2009). Cardiovascular fitness is associated with cognition in young adulthood. *Proceedings of the National Academy of Sciences, 106,* 20906–20911.
22. Li, L., & Liu, L. (2012). Experimental studies of physical exercises to improve students' sleep quality and mental health. *Education and Educational Technology, 108,* 65–72.
23. Jespersen J. G., Nedergaard A., Andersen L. L., Schjerling P., & Andersen J. L. (2011). Myostatin expression during human muscle hypertrophy and subsequent atrophy: Increased myostatin with detraining. *Scandinavian Journal of Medicine & Science in Sports, 21*(2), 215–223.
24. American College of Sports Medicine. (2010). *ACSM's guidelines for exercise testing and prescription,* 8th ed. Baltimore, MD: Wolters Kluwer/ Lippincott Williams & Wilkins.
25. Centers for Disease Control and Prevention. (2009). *Physical activity for everyone: Target heart rate and estimated maximum heart rate.* www.cdc.gov.
26. Loprinzi, P., & Cardinal, B. (2013) Association between biologic outcomes and objectively measured physical activity accumulated in ≥10-minute bouts and <10-minute bouts. *American Journal of Health Promotion, 27*(3), 143–151.
27. Miyashita, M., Burns, S., & Stensel, D. (2008). Accumulating short bouts of brisk walking reduces postprandial plasma triacylglycerol concentrations and resting blood pressure in healthy young men. *American Journal of Clinical Nutrition, 88*(5), 1225–1231.
28. Page, P. (2012). Current concepts in muscle stretching for exercise and rehabilitation. *International Journal of Sports Physical Therapy, 7*(1), 109–119.
29. Garber, C., Blissmer, B., Deschenes, M., Franklin, B., Lamonte, M., et al. (2011). Quantity and quality of exercise for developing and maintaining cardiorespiratory, musculoskeletal, and neuromotor fitness in apparently healthy adults: Guidance for prescribing exercise. *Medicine & Science in Sports & Exercise, 43*(7), 1334–1359.
30. Hart, L. (2008). Which interventions prevent sport injuries? A review. *Clinical Review of Sports Medicine, 18*(5), 471–472.
31. Fradkin, A. J., Gabbe, B. J., & Cameron, P. A. (2006). Does warming up prevent injury in sport? The evidence from randomized controlled trials. *Journal of Sports Science and Medicine, 9,* 214–220.
32. Gergley, J.C. (2013). Acute effect of passive static stretching on lower-body strength in moderately trained men. *Journal of Strength and Conditioning Research, 27*(4), 973–977.
33. U.S. Department of Health and Human Services. (2016). *Physical activity guidelines for Americans.* www.health.gov.
34. McTiernan, A., Sorensen, B., Irwin, M., Morgan, A., Yasui, Y., et al. (2007). Exercise effect on weight and body fat in men and women. *Obesity, 15*(6), 1496–1512.
35. Centers for Disease Control and Prevention. (2011). *Physical activity guidelines: Appendix 1.* http://health.gov.
36. Patel, A., Bernstein, L., Deka, A., Feigelson, H., Campbell, P., et al. (2010). Leisure time spent sitting in relation to total mortality in a prospective cohort of US adults. *American Journal of Epidemiology, 172,* 419–429.
37. Centers for Disease Control and Prevention. (2008). *Physical activity guidelines for Americans: Be active your way: A guide for adults.* www.cdc.gov.
38. Mayo Clinic. (2014). *Eating and exercise: 5 tips to maximize your workouts.* www.mayoclinic.com.
39. Hackney, K., Cook, S., Fairchild, F., & Ploutz-Snyder, L. (2012). Skeletal muscle volume following dehydration induced by exercise in heat. *Extreme Physiology & Medicine, 1*(1), 1–9.
40. Hampton, T. (2006). Researchers address use of performance-enhancing drugs in non-elite athletes. *Journal of the American Medical Association, 295*(6), 607.
41. Partnership for Drug-Free Kids. (2014). *National study: Teens report higher use of performance enhancing substances.* www.drugfree.org.
42. MedlinePlus. (n.d.). *Creatine.* www.nlm.nih.gov.
43. Liu, H., Bravata, D., Olkin, I., Friedlander, A., Liu, V., et al. (2008). Systematic review: The effects of growth hormone on athletic performance. *Annals of Internal Medicine, 148*(10), 747–758.
44. National Center for Complementary and Integrative Health. (2013). *Ephedra.* http://nccih.nih.gov.
45. Vincent, J. B. (2003). The potential value and toxicity of chromium picolinate as a nutritional supplement, weight loss agent and muscle development agent. *Sports Medicine, 33*(3), 213–230.
46. Kumanyika, S., Wadden, T., Shults, J., Fassbender, J., Brown, S., et al. (2009). Trial of family and friend support for weight loss in African American adults. *Archives of Internal Medicine, 169*(19), 1795–1804.

Chapter 7

i. Ogden, C. L., Carroll, M. D., Kit, B. K., & Flegal, K. M. (2014). Prevalence of childhood and adult obesity in the United States, 2011–2012. *Journal of the American Medical Association, 311*(8), 806–814.
ii. Finkelstein, E., Trogdon, J., Cohen, J., & Dietz, W. (2009). Annual medical spending attributable to obesity: Payer- and service-specific estimates. *Health Affairs, 28*(5), 822–831.
iii. Murray, C., Vos, T., Lozano, R., Naghavi, M., Flaxman, A., et al. (2012). Disability-adjusted life years (DALYs) for 291 diseases and injuries in 21 regions, 1990–2010: A systematic analysis for the Global Burden of Disease Study 2010. *The Lancet, 380*(5859), 2197–2227.
iv. American College Health Association. (2015). *ACHA-NCHA II: Undergraduate reference group executive summary, fall 2015.* www.acha.ncha.org.
1. Ogden, C. L., Carroll, M. D., Kit, B. K., & Flegal, K. M. (2014). Prevalence of childhood and adult obesity in the United States, 2011–2012. *Journal of the American Medical Association, 311*(8), 806–814.
2. World Health Organization. (2015). *Global Health Observatory (GHO) data: Overweight and obesity.* www.who.int.
3. Centers for Disease Control and Prevention. (2012). Prevalence of underweight among adults aged 20 years and over: United States 1960–1962 through 2007–2010. *NCHS Health E-Stat,* www.cdc.gov.

4. American College Health Association. (2015). *ACHA-NCHA II: Undergraduate reference group executive summary, fall 2015.* www.acha.ncha.org.
5. Benowitz-Fredericks, C., Garcia, K., Massey, M., Vasagar, B., & Borzekowski, D. (2012). Body image, eating disorders, and the relationship to adolescent media use. *Pediatric Clinics of North America, 59*(3), 693–704.
6. Keel, P., Baxter, M., Heatheron, T., & Joiner, T. (2007). A 20-year longitudinal study of body weight, dieting, and eating disorder symptoms. *Journal of Abnormal Psychology, 116*(2), 422–432.
7. Forrest, K., & Stuhldreher, W. (2007). Patterns and correlates of body image dissatisfaction and distortion among college students. *American Journal of Health Studies, 22*(1), 18–25.
8. Arciszewski, T., Berjot, S., & Finez, L. (2012). Threat of the thin-ideal body image and body malleability beliefs: Effects on body image self-discrepancies and behavioral intentions. *Body Image, 9*(3), 334–341.
9. Eckler, P., Yalyago, Y., & Paasch, E. (2014, May 22–26). *Facebook and college women's bodies: Social media's influence on body image and disordered eating.* 64th Annual International Communication Association Conference, Seattle.
10. Ardern, C. I., Katzmarzyk, P. T., Janssen, I., & Ross, R. (2012). Discrimination of health risk by combined body mass index and waist circumference, *Obesity,11* (1), 135–142.
11. Freedman, D., Kettel Khan, L., Serdula, M., Dietz, W., Srinivasan, S., & Berenson, G. (2005). The relation of childhood BMI to adult adiposity: The Bogalusa heart study. *Pediatrics, 115*(1), 22–27.
12. Flegal, K., Kit, B., Orpana, H., & Graubard, B. (2013.) Association of all-cause mortality with overweight and obesity using standard body mass index categories: A systematic review and meta-analysis. *Journal of the American Medical Association, 309*(1), 71–82.
13. Sahakyan, K. R., Somers, V. K., Rodrigue-Escudero, J. P., Hodge, D. O., Carter, O. et al. (2015). Normal-weight central obesity: Implications for total and cardiovascular mortality. *Annals of Internal Medicine, 163*, 827–835.
14. Shape Up America! (2012). Everything you want to know about body fat. www.shapeup.org.
15. Centers for Disease Control and Prevention. (2012). *Overweight and obesity: Adult obesity facts.* www.cdc.gov.
16. Levi, J., Segal, LM, Rayburn, J., & Martin, A. (2015). *The state of obesity 2015.* http://stateofobesity.org.
17. Ng, M. M., Fleming, T., Robinson, Thomson, B., Graetz, N., et al. (2014). Global, regional, and national prevalence of overweight and obesity in children and adults during 1980–2013: A systematic analysis for the Global Burden of Disease Study 2013. *The Lancet, 6736*(14), 60460–60468.
18. Murray, C., Vos, T., Lozano, R., Naghavi, M., Flaxman, A., et al. (2012). Disability-adjusted life years (DALYs) for 291 diseases and injuries in 21 regions, 1990–2010: A systematic analysis for the Global Burden of Disease Study 2010. *The Lancet, 380*(5859), 2197–2227.
19. Economos, C. D., Hildebrandt, M. L., & Hyatt, R. R. (2008). College freshman stress and weight change: Differences by gender. *American Journal of Health Behavior, 32*(1), 16–25.
20. Gropper, S., Simmons, K., Connell, L., & Ulrich, P. (2012). Changes in body weight, composition, and shape: A 4-year study of college students. *Applied Physiology, Nutrition, and Metabolism, 37*(6), 1118–1123.
21. Jung, M., Bray, S., & Ginis, K. (2008). Behavior change and the "freshman 15": Tracking physical activity and dietary patterns in 1st-year university women. *Journal of American College Health, 56*(5), 523–530.
22. Kitahara, C. M., Flint, A. J., Berrington de Gonzalez, A., Bernstein, L., Brotzman, M., et al. (2014). Association between class III obesity (BMI of 40–59kg/m2) and mortality: A pooled analysis of 20 prospective studies. *PLoS Medicine, 11*(7), e1001673. doi: 10.1371/journal.pmed.1001673.
23. Centers for Disease Control and Prevention. (2014). *Age-adjusted percentage of adults aged 18 years or older with diagnosed diabetes who were overweight, United States, 1994–2010.* www.cdc.gov.
24. Nguyen, N. T., Magno, C. P., Lane, K. T., Hinojosa, M. W., & Lane, J. S. (2008). Association of hypertension, diabetes, dyslipidemia, and metabolic syndrome with obesity: Findings from the National Health and Nutrition Examination Survey, 1999–2004. *Journal of the American College of Surgeons, 207*(6), 928–934.
25. Olshansky, S. J., Passaro, D. J., Hershow, R. C., Layden, J., Carnes, B. A., et al. (2005). A potential decline in life expectancy in the United States in the 21st century. *New England Journal of Medicine, 352*, 1103–1110.
26. Finkelstein, E., Trogdon, J., Cohen, J., & Dietz, W. (2009). Annual medical spending attributable to obesity: Payer- and service-specific estimates. *Health Affairs, 28*(5), 822–831.
27. Cawley, J., & Meyerhoefer, C. (2012). The medical care costs of obesity: An instrumental variables approach. *Journal of Health Economics, 31*(1), 219–230.
28. Dor, A., Ferguson, C., Langwith, C., & Tan, E. (2010). *A heavy burden: The individual costs of being overweight and obese in the United States.* www.gwumc.edu.
29. Duyff, R. L. (2012). *American Dietetic Association complete food and nutrition guide,* 4th, revised and updated edition. New York: John Wiley and Sons.
30. Levi, A., Chan, K., & Pence, D. (2006). Real men do not read food labels: The effects of masculinity and involvement on college students' food decisions. *Journal of American College Health, 55*(2), 91–98.
31. Ball, D. (2013, March 28). *Men you're bigger than you think! (But women—you're thinner).* www.theguardian.com.
32. Power, M., & Schulkin, J. (2008). Sex differences in fat storage, fat metabolism, and the health risks from obesity: Possible evolutionary origins. *British Journal of Nutrition, 99*(5), 931–940.
33. Coutinho, T., Goel, K., Corrêa de Sá, D., Kragelund, C., Kanaya, A., et al. (2011). Central obesity and survival in subjects with coronary artery disease: A systematic review of the literature and collaborative analysis with individual subject data. *Journal of the American College of Cardiology, 57*, 1877–1886.
34. Mayo Clinic. (2011). *Belly fat in women: Taking—and keeping—it off.* www.mayoclinic.com.
35. Wang, K., Li, W., Zhang, C., Wang, Z., Glessner, J., et al. (2012). A genome-wide association study on obesity and obesity-related traits. *PLoS One, 6*(4), e18939.
36. Centers for Disease Control and Prevention. (2011). *Obesity and genetics: What we know, what we don't know and what it means.* www.cdc.gov.
37. Beydoun, M., & Wang, Y. (2009). Gender-ethnic disparity in BMI and waist circumference distribution shifts in US adults. *Obesity, 17*(1), 169–176.
38. Trasande, L., Blustein, J., Lui, M., Corwin, E., Cox, L. M., & Blaser, M. J. (2013). Infant antibiotic exposures and early-life body mass. *International Journal of Obesity, 37*, 16–23.
39. Cho, I., Yamanishi, S., Cox, L., Methe, B. A., Zavadil, J., et al. (2012). Antibiotics in early life alter the murine colonic microbiome and adiposity. *Nature, 488*, 621–626.
40. Duffey, K., & Popkin, B. (2011). Energy density, portion size, and eating occasions: Contributions to increased energy intake in the United States, 1977–2006. *PLoS Medicine, 8*(6), e1001050. doi: 10.1371/journal.pmed.1001050.
41. Wells, H., & Buzby. J. (2008). Dietary assessment of major trends in U.S. food consumption, 1970–2005. *Economic Information Bulletin No. (EIB-33),* 1–27. www.ers.usda.gov.
42. Newman, C. (2004). Why are we so fat? *National Geographic, 206*(2), 46–61.
43. McDonald's. (2015, August). *McDonald's USA nutrition facts for popular menu items.* http://nutrition.mcdonalds.com.
44. National Center for Health Statistics, Health Indicators Warehouse. (2010). *Leisure-time physical activity—none (percent).* www.healthindicators.gov.
45. Matthews, C. E., Chen, K. Y., Freedson, P. S., Buchowski, M. S., Bettina, M., et al. (2008). Amount of time spent in sedentary behaviors in the United States, 2003–2004. *American Journal of Epidemiology, 167*(7), 875–881.
46. The Neilson Company. (2014). *An era of growth: The cross-platform report.* www.tvb.org.
47. U.S. Census Bureau. (2011). *Commuting characteristics by sex. American community survey, 2011.* http://factfinder2.census.gov.
48. Moczulski, V., McMahan, S., Weiss, J., Beam, W., & Chandler, L. (2007). Commuting behaviors, obesity risk, and the built environment. *American Journal of Health Behaviors, 22*(1), 26–32.
49. O'Connor, D., Jones, F., Conner, M., & McMillan, B. (2008). Effects of daily hassles and eating styles on eating behavior. *Health Psychology, 27*(1), 20–31.
50. Food Research and Action Center. (2011). *Food insecurity and obesity: Understanding the connections.* http://frac.org
51. Larson, N., & Story, M. (2011). Food insecurity and weight status among U.S. children and families: A review of the literature. *American Journal of Preventive Medicine, 40*(2), 166–173.
52. Gustat, J., Rice, J., Parker, K., Becker, A., & Farley, T. (2012). Effect of changes to the neighborhood built environment on physical activity in a low-income African American neighborhood. *Preventing Chronic Disease, 9*, E57.
53. Physicians Committee for Responsible Medicine. (2011). *USDA's new MyPlate icon at odds with federal subsidies for meat, dairy.* http://pcrm.org.
54. Centers for Disease Control and Prevention. (2014). *Youth risk behavior surveillance system: 2013 national overview.* www.cdc.gov.
55. Dansinger, M., Gleason, J., Griffith, J., Selker, H., & Schaefer, E. (2005). Comparison of the Atkins, Ornish, Weight Watchers, and Zone diets for weight loss and heart disease risk reduction. *Journal of the American Medical Association, 293*(1), 43–53.
56. Mayo Clinic. (2011). *Trans fat is double trouble for your heart health.* www.mayoclinic.com.
57. U.S. Food and Drug Administration (2015). *FDA cuts trans fat in processed food.* www.fda.gov.
58. Ebbeling, C. B., Swain, J. F., Feldman, H. A., Wong, W. W., Hachey, D. L., et al. (2012). Effects of dietary composition on energy expenditure during weight-loss maintenance. *Journal of the American Medical Association, 307*(24), 2627–2634.
59. Marketdata Enterprises, Inc. (2011). *U.S. weight loss market worth $60.9 billion.* www.prweb.com.
60. Harring, H., Montgomery, K., & Hardin, J. (2010). Perceptions of body weight, weight management, strategies, and depressive symptoms among U.S. college students. *Journal of American College Health, 59*(1), 43–50.
61. Hackett, A., & Krska, J. (2012). Is it time to regulate over-the-counter weight-loss formulations? *International Journal of Pharmacy Practice, 20*(3), 199–202.
62. U.S. Food and Drug Administration. (2014). *Public notification: Magic Slim contains hidden drug ingredient.* www.fda.gov.
63. Weiss, F. (2004). Group psychotherapy with obese disordered-eating adults with body-image disturbances: An integrated model. *American Journal of Psychotherapy, 58*(3), 281–303.

64. American Society for Metabolic and Bariatric Surgery. (2012). *Fact sheet: Metabolic and bariatric surgery.* http://asmbs.org/asmbs-press-kit.
65. Ebell, M. (2008). Predicting mortality risk in patients undergoing bariatric surgery. *American Family Physician, 77*(2), 220–221.
66. Hagobian, T., Yamashiro, M., Hinke-Lipsker, J., Streder, K., Evero, N., & Hackney, T. (2013). Effects of acute exercise on appetite hormones and ad libitum energy intake in men and women. *Applied Physiology, Nutrition, and Metabolism, 38*(999), 66–72.
67. National Institute of Diabetes and Digestive and Kidney Diseases. (2013). *Weight-control information network: Choosing a safe and successful weight-loss program.* http://win.niddk.nih.gov.
68. Bair, C., Kelly, N., Serdar, K., & Mazzeo, S. (2012). Does the Internet function like magazines? An exploration of image-focused media, eating pathology, and body dissatisfaction. *Eating Behaviors, 13*(4), 398–401.
69. Mayo Clinic. (2010). *Body dysmorphic disorder.* www.mayoclinic.com.
70. Hart, E., Leary, M., & Rejeski, W. (1989). The measurement of social physique anxiety. *Journal of Sport Exercise Psychology, 11*(1), 94–104.
71. Hagger, M., & Stevenson, A. (2010). Social physique anxiety and physical self-esteem: Gender and age effects. *Psychology and Health, 25*(1), 89–110.
72. National Institute of Mental Health. (2011). *Eating disorders among children.* www.nimh.nih.gov.
73. National Institute of Mental Health. (n.d.) *Eating disorders among adults—Anorexia nervosa.* www.nimh.nih.gov.
74. Swanson, S., Crow, S., LeGrange, D., Swendsen, J., & Merikangas, K. (2011). Prevalence and correlates of eating disorders in adolescents: Results from the national comorbidity survey replication adolescent supplement. *Archives of General Psychiatry, 68*(7), 714–723.
75. Steinhausen, H. (2009). Outcomes of eating disorders. *Child and Adolescent Psychiatric Clinics of North America, 18,* 225–242.
76. Mayo Clinic. (2012). *Anorexia nervosa: Causes.* www.mayoclinic.com.
77. Gowers, S., Clark, A., Roberts, C., Byford, S., Barrett, B., et al. (2010). A randomised controlled multicentre trial of treatments for adolescent anorexia nervosa including assessment of cost-effectiveness and patient acceptability—The TOuCAN trial. *Health Technologies Assessment, 14*(15), 1–98.
78. U.S. Department of Health and Human Services, National Guideline Clearinghouse. (2011). *Practice guideline for the treatment of patients with eating disorders.* http://guideline.gov.
79. Salahi, L. (2012, April 19). *Internet crackdown on pro-anorexia sites.* http://abcnews.go.com.
80. National Institute of Mental Health. (n.d.) *Eating disorders among adults—Bulimia nervosa.* www.nimh.nih.gov.
81. National Institute of Mental Health. (2011). *Eating disorders: What are the different types of eating disorders?* www.nimh.nih.gov.
82. U.S. Department of Health and Human Services, Office on Women's Health. (2009). *Bulimia nervosa fact sheet.* http://womenshealth.gov.
83. National Institute of Mental Health. (n.d.) *Eating disorders among adults—Binge eating disorder.* www.nimh.nih.gov.
84. American Psychiatric Association. (2013). *Diagnostic and statistical manual of mental disorders,* 5th ed. Washington, D.C: American Psychiatric Association.
85. Eisenberg, D., Nicklett, E. J., Roeder, K., & Kirz, N. E. (2011). Eating disorder symptoms among college students: Prevalence, persistence, correlates, and treatment-seeking. *Journal of American College Health, 59*(8), 700–707.
86. Rand, C., Macgregory, A., & Stunkard, A. (1997). The night eating syndrome in the general population and among postoperative obesity surgery patients. *International Journal of Eating Disorders, 22*(1), 65–69.
87. Nolan, L., & Geliebter, A. (2012). Night eating is associated with emotional and external eating in college students. *Eating Behaviors, 13,* 202–206.
88. American College of Sports Medicine. (2011). *The female athlete triad.* www.acsm.org.
89. Deimel, J., & Dunlap, B. (2012). The female athlete triad. *Clinical Journal of Sports Medicine, 2,* 247–254.

Chapter 8

i. Substance Abuse and Mental Health Services Administration. (2015). *Behavioral health trends in the United States: Results from the 2014 National Survey on Drug Use and Health* (HHS Publication No. SMA 15–4927, NSDUH Series H-50). www.samhsa.gov.
ii. Rudd, R., Aleshire, N., Zibbell, J., & Gladden, M. (2016). Increases in drug and opioid overdose deaths—United States, 2000–2014. *Morbidity and Mortality Weekly Report, 64*(50), 1378–1382.
iii. National Institute on Drug Abuse. (2015). *Drugged driving.* www.drugabuse.gov.
1. Rudd, R., Aleshire, N., Zibbell, J., & Gladden, M. (2016). Increases in drug and opioid overdose deaths—United States, 2000–2014. *Morbidity and Mortality Weekly Report, 64*(50), 1378–1382.
2. Lawyer, S., Resnick, H., Bakanic, V., Burkett, T., & Kilpatrick, D. (2010). Forcible, drug-facilitated, and incapacitated rape and sexual assault among undergraduate women. *Journal of American College of Health, 58*(5), 453–460.
3. Substance Abuse and Mental Health Services Administration. (2015). *Behavioral health trends in the United States: Results from the 2014 National Survey on Drug Use and Health* (HHS Publication No. SMA 15–4927, NSDUH Series H-50). www.samhsa.gov.
4. National Council on Problem Gambling. (2014). *Help and treatment: FAQ.* www.ncpgambling.org.
5. American Society of Addiction Medicine. (2011, April 12). Definition of addiction. *ASAM Public Policy Statement.* www.asam.org.
6. American Psychiatric Association. (2012). *DSM-5 development.* www.dsm5.org.
7. National Center for Responsible Gaming. (2014). *Fact sheet: Gambling disorders among college students.* www.collegegambling.org.
8. Karila, L., Wery, A., Weinstein, A., Cottencin, O., Petit, A., et al. (2014). Sexual addiction or hypersexual disorder: Different terms for the same problem? A review of the literature. *Current Pharmaceutical Design, 20*(25), 4012–4020.
9. Maraz, A., Griffiths, M., & Demetrovics, Z. (2016). The prevalence of compulsive buying behavior: A meta-analysis. *Addiction, 111*(3), 408–419. doi: 10.1111/add.13223.
10. Cash, H., Rae, C., Steel, A., & Winkler, A. (2012). Internet addiction: A brief summary of research and practice. *Current Psychiatry Review, 8*(4), 292–298. doi: 10.2174/1573400 12803520513.
11. CTIA Media. (2011). *50 wireless quickfacts.* www.ctia.org.
12. Smith, A. (2011, September 19). *Americans and text messaging.* http://pewresearch.org.
13. Weinschenk, S. (2012, September 11). *Why We're all Addicted to Texts, Twitter, and Google.* https://www.psychologytoday.com.
14. National Drug Intelligence Center. (2011, April). *The economic impact of illicit drug use on American society.* www.justice.gov.
15. American College Health Association. (2015). *ACHA-NCHA II: Undergraduate reference group executive summary, spring 2015.* www.acha.ncha.org.
16. American Psychiatric Association. (2013). *Diagnostic and statistical manual of mental disorders,* 4th ed. Washington, DC: American Psychiatric Publishing.
17. U.S. Food and Drug Administration and the Consumer Healthcare Products Association. (2015). *Over-the-counter medicines: What's right for you?* www.fda.gov.
18. U.S. Food and Drug Administration. (2009, February 23). *A guide to safe use of pain medicine.* www.fda.gov.
19. U.S. Food and Drug Administration. (2012, October 22). *Consumer updates: Using over-the-counter cough and cold products in children.* www.fda.gov.
20. National Institute on Drug Abuse. (2016). *Abuse of prescription (Rx) drugs affects young adults most.* www.drugabuse.gov.
21. National Institute on Drug Abuse. (2014, October). *DrugFacts: Heroin.* www.drugabuse.gov.
22. Compton, W., Jones, C., & Baldwin, G. (2016). Relationship between nonmedical prescription-opioid use and heroin use. *New England Journal of Medicine, 374,* 154–163.
23. National Conference of State Legislatures. (2016). *Marijuana overview.* www.ncsl.org.
24. National Institute on Drug Abuse. (2015, September). *NIDA InfoFacts: Marijuana.* www.nida.nih.gov.
25. National Institute on Drug Abuse. (2015). *Drugged driving.* www.drugabuse.gov.
26. Rezkalla, S., & Kloner, R. (2014). Recreational marijuana use: Is it safe for your patient? *Journal of the American Heart Association, 3*(2), e000904.
27. Simon, S. (2012). *Study links marijuana use to testicular cancer.* www.cancer.org.
28. Weng, X., Odouli, R., & Li, D. (2008). Maternal caffeine consumption during pregnancy and the risk of miscarriage: A prospective cohort study. *American Journal of Obstetrics & Gynecology, 198*(3), 279e1–279e8.
29. National Institute on Drug Abuse. (2014, January). *NIDA InfoFacts: Methamphetamine.* www.drugabuse.gov.
30. National Institute on Drug Abuse. (2016, January). *DrugFacts: Synthetic cathinones ("bath salts").* www.drugabuse.gov.
31. National Institute on Drug Abuse. (2012, December). *Club drugs.* www.drugabuse.gov.
32. National Institute on Drug Abuse. (2013, September). *NIDA InfoFacts: MDMA (ecstasy).* www.drugabuse.gov.
33. National Institute on Drug Abuse. (2012, December). *Inhalants.* www.drugabuse.gov.
34. National Library of Medicine. (2013, February). *Barbiturate intoxication and overdose.* MedlinePlus. www.nlm.nih.gov.
35. The Partnership at Drugfree.org. (2011). *Preventing teen abuse of prescription drugs.* www.drugfree.org.
36. National Institute on Drug Abuse. (2010, August). *Drugs, brains, and behavior: The science of addiction.* www.drugabuse.gov.
37. Office of National Drug Control Policy. (2011). *National youth anti-drug media campaign.* www.mediacampaign.org.
38. Occupational Safety and Health Administration. (2011). *Workplace substance abuse.* www.osha.gov.
39. Executive Office of the President of the United States. (2016). *Addressing the epidemic of prescription opioid abuse and heroin use.* www.whitehouse.gov.
40. National Institute on Drug Abuse. (2016, January). *DrugFacts: Treatment approaches for drug addiction.* www.drugabuse.gov.
41. Narcotics Anonymous. (2010, May). *Information about NA.* www.na.org.
42. Augsburg College. (2011). *StepUP program: Outcomes.* www.augsburg.edu.
43. Substance Abuse and Mental Health Services Administration, Center for Behavioral Statistics and Quality. (2012, July 12). *The DAWN report: Outcomes of drug-related emergency department visits associated with polydrug use.* www.samhsa.gov.
44. National Institutes of Health. (2014, February). *Diet and substance use recovery.* www.nlm.nih.gov.
45. The Partnership at Drugfree.org. (n.d.). *5 things you need to know about relapse.* www.drugfree.org.
46. National Institute on Drug Abuse. (2012). *Principles of drug addiction treatment: A research-based guide,* 3rd ed. www.drugabuse.gov.

Chapter 9

i. National Institute on Alcohol Abuse and Alcoholism. (2010). *Rethinking drinking: Alcohol and your health.* http://rethinkingdrinking.niaaa.nih.gov.
ii. American College Health Association. (2016). *ACHA-NCHA II: Undergraduate reference group executive summary, fall 2015.* www.acha.ncha.org
iii. Centers for Disease Control and Prevention. (2012). *Fact sheet—Fast facts: Smoking and tobacco use.* www.cdc.gov.
1. Substance Abuse and Mental Health Services Administration. (2014). *Results from the 2013 National Survey on Drug Use and Health: Summary of National Findings*, NSDUH Series H-48, HHS Publication No. (SMA) 14–4863. Rockville, MD: Substance Abuse and Mental Health Services Administration. www.samhsa.gov.
2. National Institutes of Health. (2010). *Fact sheet: Alcohol-related traffic deaths.* www.nih.gov.
3. Carpenter, C., & Dobkin, C. (2011). The minimum legal drinking age and public health. *Journal of Economic Perspectives, 25*(2), 133–156.
4. McCartt, A. T., Hellinga, L. A., & Kirley, B. B. (2010). The effects of minimum legal drinking age 21 laws on alcohol-related driving in the United States. *Journal of Safety Research, 41*(2) 173–181.
5. Fell, J. C. (2008). The relationship of underage drinking laws to reductions in drinking drivers in fatal crashes in the United States. *Accident Analysis and Prevention, 40*(4), 1430–1440.
6. American College Health Association. (2016). *ACHA-NCHA II: Undergraduate reference group executive summary, fall 2015.* www.acha.ncha.org
7. National Institute on Alcohol Abuse and Alcoholism. (2004, Winter). Binge drinking defined. *NIAAA Newsletter, 3.* http://pubs.niaaa.nih.gov.
8. Silveri, M. M. (2012). Adolescent brain development and underage drinking in the United States: Identifying risks of alcohol use in college populations. *Harvard Review of Psychiatry, 20*(4), 189–200.
9. National Institute on Alcohol Abuse and Alcoholism. (2010). *Rethinking drinking: Alcohol and your health.* http://rethinkingdrinking.niaaa.nih.gov.
10. Hingson, R. W. (2010). Focus on: College drinking and related problems—Magnitude and prevention of college drinking related problems. *Alcohol Research Health, 33*(1), 45–54.
11. National Institute on Alcohol Abuse and Alcoholism. (2010). *Snapshot of annual high-risk college drinking consequences.* www.collegedrinkingprevention.gov.
12. Mikhailovich, K., George, A., Rickwood, D., & Parker, R. (2011). A duty of care: Non-drinkers and alcohol related harm among an Australian university sample. *Journal of Higher Education Policy and Management, 33*(6), 595–604.
13. Hingson, R. W., Zha, W., & Weitzman, E. R. (2009). Magnitude of and trends in alcohol-related mortality and morbidity among U.S. college students ages 18–24, 1998–2005. *Journal of Studies on Alcohol and Drugs*, Suppl. 16, 12–20.
14. Wechsler, H., & Nelson, T. F. (2008). What we have learned from the Harvard School of Public Health College alcohol study: Focusing attention on college student alcohol consumption and the environmental conditions that promote it. *Journal of Studies on Alcohol and Drugs, 69*(4), 481–490.
15. Courtney, K., & Polich, J. (2009). Binge drinking in young adults: Data, definitions, and determinants. *Psychological Bulletin, 135*(1), 142–156.
16. Turrisi, R., & Ray, A. E. (2010). Sustained parenting and college drinking in first-year students. *Developmental Psychobiology, 52*(3), 286–294.
17. Kerr, W. C., Greenfield, T. K., Tujague, J., & Brown, S. E. (2005). A drink is a drink? Variation in the amount of alcohol contained in beer, wine and spirits drinks in a U.S. methodological sample. *Alcoholism: Clinical and Experimental Research, 29*(11), 2015–2021.
18. Meier, P., & Seitz, H. K. (2008). Age, alcohol metabolism, and liver disease. *Current Opinion in Clinical Nutrition and Metabolic Care, 11*(1), 21–26.
19. Centers for Disease Control and Prevention. (2011). *Injury prevention and control: Motor vehicle safety—Effects of blood alcohol concentration.* www.cdc.gov.
20. Lembke, A., Bradley, K. A., Henderson, P., Moos, R., & Harris, A. (2011). Alcohol screening scores and the risk of new-onset gastrointestinal illness or related hospitalization. *Journal of General Internal Medicine, 26*(7), 777–782.
21. Rohsenow, D. J., & Howland, J. (2010). The role of beverage congeners in hangover and other residual effects of alcohol intoxication: A review. *Current Drug Abuse Reviews, 3*(2), 76–79.
22. Penning, R., van Nuland, M., Fliervoet, L. A., Olivier, B., & Verster, J. C. (2010). The pathology of alcohol hangover. *Current Drug Abuse Reviews, 3*(2), 68075.
23. Gapstur, S. M., Jacobs, E. J., Deka, A., McCullough, M. L., Patel, A. V., & Thun, M. J. (2011). Association of alcohol intake with pancreatic cancer mortality in never smokers. *Archives of Internal Medicine, 171*(5), 444–451.
24. Nelson, D. E., Jaman, D. W., Rehm, J., Greenfield, T. K., Rey, G., et al. (2013). Alcohol-attributable cancer deaths and years of potential life lost in the United States. *American Journal of Public Health, 103*(4), 641–648.
25. Yoon, Y., & Yi, H. (2012). *Liver cirrhosis mortality in the United States, 1970–2009.* National Institute on Alcohol Abuse and Alcoholism (Surveillance Report No. 93).
26. American Medical Association. (2010). *Harmful consequences of alcohol use on the brains of children, adolescents, and college students.* www.ama.assn.org.
27. SAMHSA Fetal Alcohol Spectrum Disorders Center for Excellence. (2013). *The FASD Center.* http://fasdcenter.samhsa.gov.
28. Substance Abuse and Mental Health Services Administration. (2012). *Results from the 2011 national survey on drug use and health: National findings.* www.samhsa.gov.
29. Ronksley, P., Brien, S., Turner, B., Mukamal, K., & Ghali, W. (2011). Association of alcohol consumption with selected cardiovascular disease outcomes: A systematic review and meta-analysis. *British Medical Journal, 342*, 671.
30. French, M. T., & Zavala, S. K. (2007). The health benefits of moderate drinking revisited: Alcohol use and self-reported health status. *American Journal of Health Promotion, 21*(6), 484–491.
31. Stockwell, T., Greer, A., Fillmore, K., Chikritzhs, T., & Zeisser, K. (2012). How good is the science? *British Medical Journal, 344*, e2276.
32. Allen, N. E., Beral, V., Casabonne, D., Kan, S. W., Reeves, G. K., et al. (2009). Moderate alcohol intake and cancer incidence in women. *Journal of the National Cancer Institute, 101*(5), 296–305.
33. National Highway Traffic Safety Administration. (2014, December). Alcohol-impaired driving. *Traffic Safety Facts* (DOT HS 812 102). www.nrd.nhtsa.dot.gov.
34. National Highway Traffic Safety Administration. (2009). *Ignition interlocks: What you need to know.* www.nhtsa.gov.
35. Wechsler, H., Lee, J. E., Kuo, M., Seibring, M., Nelson, T. F., & Lee, H. (2002). Trends in college binge drinking during a period of increased prevention efforts: Findings from 4 Harvard School of Public Health college alcohol study surveys: 1993–2001. *Journal of American College Health, 50*(5), 203–217.
36. Hingson, R., Heeren, T., Winter, M., & Wechsler, H. (2005). Magnitude of alcohol-related mortality and morbidity among U.S. college students ages 18–24: Changes from 1998 to 2001. *Annual Review of Public Health, 26*, 259–279.
37. Hufford, M. R. (2001). Alcohol and suicidal behavior. *Clinical Psychology Review, 21*, 797–811.
38. Grant, B., Dawson, D., Stinson, F., Chou, S., Dufour, M., & Pickering, R. (2004). The 12-month prevalence and trends in DSM-IV alcohol abuse and dependence in the United States, 1991–1992 and 2001–2002. *Drug and Alcohol Dependence, 74*(3), 223–234.
39. Moss, H. B., Chen, C. M., & Yi, H. Y. (2007). Subtypes of alcohol dependence in a nationally representative sample. *Drug and Alcohol Dependence, 91*(2–3), 149–158.
40. National Institute on Alcohol Abuse and Alcoholism. (2010, February). Alcoholism isn't what it used to be. *NIAAA Spectrum, 2*(1).
41. Cronce, J. M. (2011). Individual-focused approaches to the prevention of college student drinking. *Alcohol Research and Health, 34*(2), 210–221.
42. National Institute on Alcohol Abuse and Alcoholism. (1989). Relapse and craving. *Alcohol Alert*, No. 6; PH 277. http://pubs.niaaa.nih.gov.
43. National Institute on Alcohol Abuse and Alcoholism. (2010). *Rethinking drinking: Alcohol and your health: Tips to try.* http://rethinkingdrinking.niaaa.nih.gov.
44. American Boating Association. (2010). *Alcohol & BWI: Why we must get BADD.* www.americanboating.org.
45. University of Texas at Dallas. (2010). *How to help a friend.* www.utdallas.edu.
46. Students against Destructive Decisions. (2010). *SADD's mission.* www.sadd.org.
47. U.S. Department of Health and Human Services. (2014). *The health consequences of smoking—50 years of progress: A report of the surgeon general.* www.acha.ncha.org.
48. Centers for Disease Control and Prevention. (2014). Current cigarette smoking among adults—United States, 2005–2012. *Morbidity and Mortality Weekly Report, 63*(2), 29–34.
49. Center for Behavioral Health Statistics and Quality. (2015). *Behavioral health trends in the United States: Results from the 2014 National Survey on Drug Use and Health* (HHS Publication No. SMA 15–4927, NSDUH Series H-50). www.samhsa.gov/data.
50. Agrawal, A., & Lynskey, M. T. (2008). Are there genetic influences on addiction? Evidence from family, adoption and twin studies. *Addiction, 103*(5), 1069–1081.
51. Greenbaum, L., & Lerer, B. (2009). Differential contribution of genetic variation in multiple brain nicotinic cholinergic receptors to nicotine dependence: Recent progress and emerging open questions. *Molecular Psychiatry, 14*, 912–945.
52. Munafo, M. R., & Johnstone, E. C. (2008). Genes and cigarette smoking. *Addiction, 103*(6), 893–904.
53. Gilman, S., Rende, R., Boergers, J., Abrams, D., Buka, S., et al. (2009). Parental smoking and adolescent smoking initiation: An intergenerational perspective on tobacco control. *Pediatrics, 123*(2), 274–281.
54. Ling, P., Neilands, T., & Glantz S. (2009). Young adult smoking behavior: A national survey. *American Journal of Preventive Medicine, 36*(5), 389–394.
55. Campaign for Tobacco-Free Kids. (2009). *The path to smoking addiction starts at very young ages.* www.tobaccofreekids.org.
56. Song, A. V., Morrell, H. E. R., Cornell, J. L., Ramos, M. E., Biehl, M., et al. (2009, March). Perceptions of smoking-related risks and benefits as predictors of adolescent smoking initiation. *American Journal of Public Health, 99*(3), 487–492.
57. Helweg-Larsen, M., & Nielsen, G. A. (2009, January). Smoking cross-culturally: Risk perceptions among young adults in Denmark and the United States. *Psychology and Health, 24*(1), 81–93.

58. Koval, J. J., Pederson, L. L., Zhang, X., Mowery, P., & McKenna, M. (2008, September). Can young adult smoking status be predicted from concern about body weight and self-reported BMI among adolescents? Results from a ten-year cohort study. *Nicotine and Tobacco Research, 10*(9), 1449–1455.
59. National Cancer Institute. (2008). The role of the media in promoting and reducing tobacco use. *NCI Tobacco Control Monograph Series.* http://cancercontrol.cancer.gov.
60. Centers for Disease Control and Prevention. (2010). *How tobacco smoke causes disease: The biology and behavioral basis for smoking-attributable disease: A report of the Surgeon General.* www.cdc.gov.
61. Jha, P., Ramasundarahettige, C., Landsman, V., Rostron, B., Thun, M., et al. (2013). 21st-century hazards of smoking and benefits of cessation in the United States. *New England Journal of Medicine, 368,* 341–350.
62. American Cancer Society. (2009). *Cigarette smoking.* www.cancer.org.
63. Thun M. J., Carter, B. D., Feskanich, D., Freedman, N. D., Prentice, R., et al. (2013). 50-year trends in smoking-related mortality in the United States. *New England Journal of Medicine, 368*(4), 351–364.
64. American Cancer Society. (2016). *Cancer facts & figures 2016.* Atlanta, GA: American Cancer Society.
65. National Center for Health Statistics (2015). *Health, United States, 2014.* http://www.cdc.gov/nchs/
66. Centers for Disease Control and Prevention. (2008, November 14). Smoking-attributable mortality, years of potential life lost, and productivity losses: United States, 2000–2004. *Morbidity and Mortality Weekly Report, 57*(45), 1226–1228.
67. Centers for Disease Control and Prevention. (2009). *Tobacco use and pregnancy.* www.cdc.gov.
68. Salihu, H. M., Aliyu, M. H., Pierre-Louis, B. J., & Alexander, G. R. (2003). Levels of excess infant deaths attributable to maternal smoking during pregnancy in the United States. *Maternal and Child Health Journal, 7*(4), 219–227.
69. U.S. Department of Health and Human Services. (2006). *The health consequences of involuntary exposure to tobacco smoke: A report of the surgeon general.* www.surgeongeneral.gov.
70. California Environmental Protection Agency. (2005). *Identification of environmental tobacco smoke as a toxic air contaminant: Executive summary.*
71. American Cancer Society. (2009). *Cigar smoking.* www.cancer.org.
72. National Cancer Institute. (2009). *Cigar smoking and cancer (fact sheet).* www.cancer.gov.
73. Centers for Disease Control and Prevention. (2009). *Bidis and kreteks.* www.cdc.gov.
74. Severson, H. H., Klein, K., & Lichtenstein, E. (2005). Smokeless tobacco use among professional baseball players: Survey results, 1998 to 2003. *Tobacco Control, 14,* 31–36.
75. Nemeth, J. M, Lui, S. T., Klein, E., Ferketich, A. K., Kwan, M., & Wewers, M. E. (2012). Factors influencing smokeless tobacco use in rural Ohio Appalachia. *Journal of Community Health, 37*(6), 1208–1217.
76. National Center for Health Statistics. (2013). *National Health Interview Survey Public Use Data File 2012.* Atlanta, GA: Centers for Disease Control and Prevention.
77. U.S. Food and Drug Administration. (2016). *Deeming tobacco products to be subject to the Federal Food, Drug, and Cosmetic Act, as amended by the Family Smoking and Tobacco Control Act.* www.fda.gov.
78. Centers for Disease Control and Prevention. (2014). *New CDC study finds dramatic increase in e-cigarette-related calls to poison centers.* http://www.cdc.gov/
79. Centers for Disease Control and Prevention. (2012). Current cigarette smoking among adults: United States, 2011. *Morbidity and Mortality Weekly Report, 61*(44), 889–894.
80. Cosgrove, K. P. (2009). B2-nicotinic acetylcholine receptor availability during acute and prolonged abstinence from tobacco smoking. *Archives of General Psychiatry, 66*(6), 666–667.
81. U.S. Public Health Service. (2008). A clinical practice guideline treating tobacco use and dependence: 2008 update. A U.S. Public Health Service report. *American Journal of Preventive Medicine, 35*(2), 158–176.
82. National Cancer Institute. (2008, October). *Clearing the air: Quit smoking today* (NIH Publication No. 08–1647). www.smokefree.gov.
83. Harris, K. J., Stearns, J. N., Kovach, R. G., & Harrar, S. W. (2009, September/October). Enforcing an outdoor smoking ban on a college campus: Effects of a multicomponent approach. *Journal of American College Health, 58*(2), 121–126.
84. American College Health Association. (2011). *ACHA guidelines—Position statement on tobacco on college and university campuses.* www.acha.org.

Chapter 10

i. Facebook Newsroom. (2016). *Company info: Stats.* http://newsroom.fb.com.
ii. Centers for Disease Control and Prevention. (2015). *Key statistics from the National Survey of Family Growth.* www.cdc.gov.
iii. Wang, W., & Parker, K. (2014). *Record share of Americans have never married.* www.pewsocialtrends.org.
1. Jourard, S. M. (1971). *The transparent self.* New York: D. van Nostrand.
2. Berkeley Human Resources. (n.d.). *Resolving Conflict Situations.* http://hrweb.berkeley.edu.
3. Kimbrough, A. M., Guadgno, R. E., Muscanell, N. L., & Dill, J. (2012). Gender differences in mediated communication: Women connect more than do men. *Computers in Human Behavior, 29,* 896–900.
4. Tannen, D. (1991). *You just don't understand: Women and men in conversation.* New York: Ballantine Books.
5. Gray, J. (1992). *Men are from Mars, women are from Venus.* New York: HarperCollins.
6. Schuetz, A. (1998). Autobiographical narratives of good and bad deeds: Defensive and favorable self-description moderated by trait self-esteem. *Journal of Social and Clinical Psychology, 17,* 466–475.
7. Bellavia, G., & Murray, S. (2003). Did I do that? Self-esteem–related differences in reactions to romantic partners' moods. *Personal Relationships, 10*(1), 77–95.
8. Bowlby, J. (1982). *Attachment and loss: Vol. 1, attachment,* 2nd ed. New York: Basic Books.
9. Kilmann, P. R., Urbaniak, G. C., & Parnell, M. M. (2006). Effects of attachment-focused versus relationship skills-focused group interventions for college students with insecure attachment patterns. *Attachment & Human Development, 8*(1), 47–62.
10. Twenge, J., & Nolen-Hoeksema, S. (2002). Age, gender, race, socioeconomic status, and birth cohort differences on the children's depression inventory: A meta-analysis. *Journal of Abnormal Psychology, 4,* 578–588.
11. Katz-Wise, S. L., Priess, H. A., & Hyde, J. S. (2010). Gender-role attitudes and behavior across the transition to parenthood. *Developmental Psychology, 46*(1), 18–28.
12. Mayo Clinic. (2014). *Friendships: Enrich your life and improve your health.* www.mayoclinic.org.
13. Mundt, M., & Zakletskaia, L. (2014). That's what friends are for: Adolescent peer social status, health-related quality of life and healthcare costs. *Applied Health Economics and Health Policy, 12*(2), 191–201.
14. Swami, V., Chamorro-Premuzic, T., Sinniah, D., Maniam, T., Kannan, K., & Stanistreet, D. (2007). General health mediates the relationship between loneliness, life satisfaction and depression. *Social Psychiatry and Psychiatric Epidemiology, 42,* 161–166.
15. Anderson, M. (2015). *6 takeaways about teen friendships in the digital age.* www.pewresearch.org.
16. Hefner, J., & Eisenberg, D. (2009). Social support and mental health among college students. *American Journal of Orthopsychiatry, 79*(4), 491–499.
17. Ledbetter, A. M., Griffin, E. M., & Sparks, G. G. (2007). Forecasting "friends forever": A longitudinal investigation of sustained closeness between best friends. *Personal Relationships, 14*(2), 343–350.
18. Sternberg, R. J. (1986). A Triangular Theory of Love. *Psychological Review, 93,* 119–135.
19. Rhode, D. (2011). *The beauty bias.* New York: Oxford University Press.
20. Swami, V., Furnham, A., Chamorror-Premuzic, T., Akbar, K., Gordon, N., et al. (2010). More than just skin deep? Personality information influences men's ratings of the attractiveness of women's body sizes. *Journal of Social Psychology, 150*(6), 628–647.
21. Claxton, A., O'Rourke, N., Smith, J. Z., & Delongis, A. (2012). Personality traits and marital satisfaction within enduring relationships: An intra-couple discrepancy approach. *Journal of Social and Personal Relationships, 29*(3), 375–396.
22. Centers for Disease Control and Prevention. (2015). *Key statistics from the National Survey of Family Growth.* www.cdc.gov.
23. Bradshaw, C., Kahn, A. S., & Saville, B. K. (2010). To hook up or date: Which gender benefits? *Sex Roles, 62*(9–10), 661–669.
24. Roberson, P., Olmstead, S., & Fincham, F. (2015). Hooking up during the college years: Is there a pattern? *Culture, Health & Sexuality, 17*(5), 576–591.
25. Owen, J. J., Rhoades, G. K., Stanley, S. M., & Fincham, F. D. (2010). "Hooking up" among college students: Demographic and psychosocial correlates. *Archives of Sexual Behavior, 39,* 653–663.
26. Owen, J. J., & Fincham, F. D. (2011). Young adults' emotional reactions after hooking up encounters. *Archives of Sexual Behavior, 40,* 321–330.
27. Gates, G. (2014). *LGBT demographics: Comparisons among population-based surveys.* http://williamsinstitute.law.ucla.edu.
28. Gohn, L., & Albin, G. (2006). *Understanding college student subpopulations: A guide for student affairs professionals.* Washington, DC: National Association of Student Personnel Administrators.
29. Pew Research Center. (2013). *A survey of LGBT Americans.* www.pewsocialtrends.org.
30. Roisman, G. I., Clausell, E., Holland, A., Fortuna, K., & Elieff, C. (2008). Adult romantic relationships as contexts of human development: A multimethod comparison of same-sex couples with opposite-sex dating, engaged, and married dyads. *Developmental Psychology, 44*(1), 91–101.
31. Balsam, K. F., Beauchaine, T. P., Rothblum, E. D., & Solomon, S. E. (2008). Three-year follow-up of same-sex couples who had civil unions in Vermont, same-sex couples not in civil unions, and heterosexual married couples. *Developmental Psychology, 44*(1), 102–116.
32. Madureira, A. F. A. (2007). The psychological basis of homophobia: Cultural construction of a barrier. *Integrative Psychological & Behavioral Science, 41,* 225–247.
33. Cummings, E., El-Sheikh, M., Kouros, C. D., & Buckhalt, J. A. (2009). Children and violence: The role of children's regulation in the marital aggression–child adjustment link. *Clinical Child Family Psychological Review, 12,* 3–15.

34. MacMillan, H., & Wathen, C. (2014). Children's exposure to intimate partner violence. *Child & Adolescent Psychiatric Clinics of North America, 23*(2), 295–308.
35. Lyness, D. (n.d.). Am I in a healthy relationship? *TeensHealth from Nemours.* http://kidshealth.org.
36. Barelds, D. P. H., & Dijkstra, P. (2006). Reactive, anxious and possessive forms of jealousy and their relation to relationship quality among heterosexuals and homosexuals. *Journal of Homosexuality, 51*(3), 183–198.
37. National Health Service. (2014, March 21). *Overcoming Jealousy.* www.nhs.uk.
38. Lyness, D. (2010). Getting over a breakup. *TeensHealth from Nemours.* http://kidshealth.org.
39. Newport, F., & Wilke. J. (2013). *Most in U.S. want marriage, but its importance has dropped.* www.gallup.com.
40. Copen, C. E., Daniels, K., Vespa, J., & Mosher, W. D. (2012). First marriages in the United States: Data from the 2006–2010 national survey of family growth. *National Health Statistics Reports, 49,* 1–22.
41. Pew Research Center. (2010). *The decline of marriage and the rise of new families.* www.pewsocialtrends.org.
42. Hymowitz, K., Carroll, J., Wilcox, W., & Kaye, K. (2012). *Knot yet: The benefits and costs of delayed marriage in America.* The National Marriage Project at the University of Virginia. http://nationalmarriageproject.org.
43. Rhoades, G. K., Stanley, S. M., & Markman, H. J. (2009). The pre-engagement cohabitation effect: A replication and extension of previous findings. *Journal of Family Psychology, 23*(1), 107–111.
44. Goodwin, P. Y., Mosher, W. D., & Chandra, A. (2010). *Marriage and cohabitation in the United States: A statistical portrait based on cycle 6 (2002) of the national survey of family growth.* www.cdc.gov.
45. Wilcox, W. B., Doherty, W., Glenn N., & Waite, L. (2011). *Why marriage matters: Twenty-six conclusions from the social sciences,* 2nd ed. New York: Institute for American Values.
46. Koball, H. L., Moiduddin, E., Henderson, J., Goesling, B., & Besculides, M. (2010). What do we know about the link between marriage and health? *Journal of Family Issues, 31*(8), 1019–1040.
47. Rogers, A. (2014, March 28). *Study: Marriage is good for the heart.* http://time.com.
48. National Vital Statistics System, Centers for Disease Control and Prevention. (2013). *National marriage and divorce rate trends.* www.cdc.gov.
49. Amato, P. R., & Hohmann-Marriott, B. (2007). A comparison of high- and low-distress marriages that end in divorce. *Journal of Marriage and Family, 69,* 621–638.
50. Utah State University. (n.d.). *How common is divorce and what are the reasons?* www.divorce.usu.edu.
51. Kalmijn, M., & Monden, C. W. S. (2006). Are the negative effects of divorce on well-being dependent on marital quality? *Journal of Marriage and Family, 68,* 1197–1213.
52. Amato, P. A. (2010). Research on divorce: Continuing trends and new developments. *Journal of Marriage and Family, 72,* 650–666.
53. Riggio, H. R., & Fite, J. E. (2006). Attitudes toward divorce: Embeddedness and outcomes in personal relationships. *Journal of Applied Social Psychology, 36*(12), 2935–2962.
54. Copen, C., Daniels, K., & Mosher, W. (2013). First premarital cohabitation in the United States: 2006–2010 national survey of family growth. *National Health Statistics Reports, 64,* 1–16.
55. Seidman, G. (2015, August 21). *Why some people are just as happy being single.* www.psychologytoday.com.
56. Jiang, L., & O'Neill, B. C. (2007). Impacts of demographic trends on household size and structure. *Population and Development Review, 33*(3), 567–591.
57. U.S. Census Bureau. (2015). *Table CH1: Living arrangements of children under 18 years: 1960 to present.* www.census.gov.
58. Holzworth, A. N., & Radunovich, H. L. (2014). *Questions to ask as you consider parenthood: A couples' guide* (Publication no. FCS2271). Department of Family, Youth, and Community Sciences, Florida Cooperative Extension Service, IFAS, University of Florida, Gainesville.
59. McPherson, N., Fullston, T., Aitken, R., & Lane, M. (2014). Paternal obesity, interventions, and mechanistic pathways to impaired health in offspring. *Annals of Nutrition and Metabolism, 64*(3–4), 231–238.
60. Livingston, G. (2014, November 14). *Four-in-ten couples are saying "I do," again.* www.pewsocialtrends.org.
61. Lewis, J., & Kreider, R. (2015). *Remarriage in the United States.* www.census.gov.
62. National Stepfamily Resource Center. (n.d.). *Stepfamily fact sheet.* www.stepfamilies.info.
63. Speer, R. B., & Trees, A. R. (2007). The push and pull of stepfamily life: The contribution of stepchildren's autonomy and connection-seeking behaviors to role development in stepfamilies. *Communication Studies, 58*(4), 377–394.
64. National Center for Health Statistics. (2016). *Unmarried childbearing.* www.cdc.gov.
65. Williams, K., Sassler, S., & Nicholson, L. M. (2008). For better or for worse? The consequences of marriage and cohabitation for single mothers. *Social Forces, 86*(4), 1481–1511.
66. Amato, P. R. (2005). The impact of family formation change on the cognitive, social, and emotional well-being of the next generation. *The Future of Children, 15*(2), 75–96.
67. Jackson, M. (2007, November 4). *Going solo.* www.boston.com.
68. Riciutti, H. N. (2004). Single parenthood, achievement, and problem behavior in white, black, and Hispanic children. *Journal of Educational Research, 97*(4), 196–207.
69. Day, R. D. (2010). Stephen Gavazzi: Strong families, successful students: Helping teenagers reach their full potential. *Journal of Youth Adolescence, 39,* 704–705.
70. DeFrain, J., & Asay, S. M. (2007). Strong families around the world: An introduction to the family strengths perspective. *Marriage & Family Review, 41*(1/2), 1–10.
71. King, M. L., Jr. (1964). *Speech in St. Louis, Missouri, March 22, 1964.* Reprinted by permission of Writer's House LLC on behalf of the Estate of Martin Luther King, Jr.
72. Granovetter, M. (1973, May). The strength of weak ties. *American Journal of Sociology, 78*(6), 1360–1380.
73. Wickramasinghe, S. (2011, February 4). Learning to live together. *NDSU Spectrum.* www.ndsuspectrum.com.
74. Patchin, J. W., & Hinduja, S. (2012). School-based efforts to prevent cyberbullying. *The Prevention Researcher, 19*(1), 7–9.

Chapter 11

i. American College Health Association. (2015). *ACHA-NCHA II: Undergraduate reference group executive summary, fall 2015.* www.acha.ncha.org.
ii. Finer, L. B., & Zolna, M. R. (2014). Shifts in intended and unintended pregnancies in the United States, 2001–2008. *American Journal of Public Health, 104*(S1), S44-S48.
1. Centers for Disease Control and Prevention. (2002). Folate status in women of childbearing age, by race/ethnicity. *Morbidity and Mortality Weekly Report, 51*(36), 808–810.
2. American Congress of Obstetricians and Gynecologists. (2015, December). *Frequently asked questions: Cervical cancer screening.* www.acog.org.
3. American College Health Association. (2015). *ACHA-NCHA II: Undergraduate reference group executive summary, fall 2015.* www.acha.ncha.org.
4. National Women's Health Information Center. (2009). *Menstruation and the menstrual cycle.* www.womenshealth.gov.
5. American Congress of Obstetricians and Gynecologists. (2008). *Premenstrual syndrome.* www.acog.org.
6. Dennerstein, L., Lehert, P., & Heinemann, K. (2012). Epidemiology of premenstrual symptoms and disorders. *Menopause International, 18,* 48–51.
7. National Women's Health Information Center. (2010). *Premenstrual syndrome frequently asked questions.* www.womenshealth.gov.
8. National Women's Health Information Center. (2008). *Menstruation, menopause, and mental health.* www.womenshealth.gov.
9. Latthe, P. M., Champaneria, R., & Khan, K. S. (2011). *Dysmenorrhoea.* www.ncbi.nlm.nih.gov.
10. French, L. (2005). Dysmenorrhea. *American Family Physician, 71*(2), 285–291.
11. American Congress of Obstetricians and Gynecologists. (2008). *Endometriosis.* www.acog.org.
12. Masters, W. H., & Johnson, V. E. (1966). *Human sexual response.* New York: Bantam.
13. American Society for Reproductive Medicine. (2008). *Patient fact sheet: Sexual dysfunction and infertility.* www.asrm.org.
14. MedlinePlus. (2010). *Female sexual dysfunction.* www.nlm.nih.gov.
15. American College of Obstetrics and Gynecology. (2011). *When sex is painful.* www.acog.org.
16. Mayo Clinic. (2009). *Low sex drive in women.* www.mayoclinic.com.
17. Mayo Clinic. (2009). *Anorgasmia.* www.mayoclinic.com.
18. National Kidney and Urologic Diseases Information Clearinghouse. (2012). *Erectile dysfunction* (NIH Publication No. 09–3923). http://kidney.niddk.nih.gov.
19. MedlinePlus. (2008). *Premature ejaculation.* www.nlm.nih.gov.
20. Mayo Clinic. (2009). *Premature ejaculation.* www.mayoclinic.com.
21. American College Health Association. (2000). *ACHA-NCHA II: Undergraduate reference group executive summary, spring 2000.* www.acha.ncha.org.
22. Rosenbaum, J. E. (2009). Patient teenagers? A comparison of the sexual behavior of virginity pledgers and matched nonpledgers. *Pediatrics, 123*(1), 110–120.
23. Centers for Disease Control and Prevention. (2009). *Key statistics from the National Survey of Family Growth.* www.cdc.gov.
24. American Pregnancy Association. (2010). *Statistics.* www.americanpregnancy.org.
25. Caron, S. (2014). *The sex lives of college students: Two decades of attitudes and behaviors.* Orono, ME: Maine College Press.
26. O'Reilly, S., Knox, D., & Zusman, M. E. (2007). College student attitudes toward pornography use. *College Student Journal, 41,* 402–404.
27. Perkins, A. B., Becker, J. V., Tehee, M., & Mackelprang, E. (2014). Sexting behaviors among college students: Cause for concern? *International Journal of Sexual Health, 26*(2), 79–92.
28. Ward, B. W., Dahlhamer, J. M., Galinsky, A. M., & Joestl, S. S. (2014). Sexual orientation and health among U.S. adults: National health interview survey, 2013. *National Health Statistics Report, 77,* 1–12.
29. Mills, D. (2015, June 27). *Supreme Court ruling makes same-sex marriage a right nationwide.* www.nytimes.com.
30. Pew Research Center. (2009). *Majority continues to support civil unions.* www.pewforum.org.
31. Pew Research Center. (2015). *Changing attitudes on gay marriage.* www.pewforum.org.

32. Robinson, J. P., & Espelage, D. L. (2011). Inequities in educational and psychological outcomes between LGBTQ and straight students in middle and high school. *Educational Researcher, 40*, 315. doi: 10.3102/0013189X11422112.
33. Federal Bureau of Investigation. (2015). *Latest hate crime statistics available.* www.fbi.gov.
34. Ducker, D. J. (2012). Marking sexuality from 0–6: The Kinsey scale in online culture. *Sexuality & Culture, 16*, 241–262.
35. Diamond, L. M. (2008). Female bisexuality from adolescence to adulthood: Results from a 10-year longitudinal study. *Developmental Psychology, 44*(1), 5–14.
36. Humans Rights Campaign. (2016). *Sexual orientation and gender identity definitions.* www.hrc.org.
37. Bockting, W., Benner, A., & Coleman, E. (2009). Gay and bisexual identity development among female-to-male transsexuals in North America: Emergence of a transgender sexuality. *Archives of Sexual Behavior, 38*(5), 688–701.
38. Finer, L. B., & Zolna, M. R. (2014). Shifts in intended and unintended pregnancies in the United States, 2001–2008. *American Journal of Public Health, 104*(S1), S43-S48.
39. Daniels, K., Daugherty, J., & Jones, J. (2015). Current contraceptive status among women aged 15–44: United States, 2011–2013. *NCHS Data Brief, No. 173*. www.cdc.gov.
40. Dude, A., Neustadt, A., Martins, S., & Gilliam, M. (2013). Use of withdrawal and unintended pregnancy among females 15–24 years of age. *Obstetrics and Gynecology, 122*, 595–600.
41. Centers for Disease Control and Prevention. (2015). Sexually transmitted diseases treatment guidelines, 2015. *Morbidity and Mortality Weekly Report, 64*(3). www.cdc.gov.
42. McGuire, L. (2010). *New emergency contraceptive.* www.mayoclinic.com.
43. Mayo Clinic. (2010). *ParaGard (copper IUD).* www.mayoclinic.com.
44. Mayo Clinic. (2010). *Mirena (hormonal IUD).* www.mayoclinic.com.
45. Mayo Clinic. (2010). *Birth control pill FAQ: Benefits, risks and choices.* www.mayoclinic.com.
46. Mayo Clinic. (2009). *Vasectomy: Risks.* www.mayoclinic.com.
47. National Campaign to Prevent Teen and Unplanned Pregnancy. (2010). *National data.* www.thenationalcampaign.org.
48. National Campaign to Prevent Teen and Unplanned Pregnancy. (2008). *Policy brief: Thoughts for elected officials about teen and unplanned pregnancy.* www.thenationalcampaign.org.
49. Jones, R. K., & Jerman, J. (2014). Abortion incidence and service availability in the United States, 2011. *Perspectives on Sexual and Reproductive Health, 46*(1), 3–14
50. World Health Organization. (2006). *Frequently asked clinical questions about medical abortion.* www.who.int.
51. Raymond, E. G., & Grimes, D. A. (2012, February). The comparative safety of legal induced abortion and childbirth in the United States. *Obstetrics & Gynecology, 119*(2 Pt. 1), 215–219.
52. Pazol, K., Creanga, A. A., & Jamieson, D. J. (2015). Abortion surveillance—United States, 2012. *Morbidity and Mortality Weekly Report, 64*(SS10), 1–40.
53. Coleman, P. (2011). Abortion and mental health: Quantitative synthesis and analysis of research published 1995–2009. *British Journal of Psychiatry, 199*(3), 180–186.
54. American Psychological Association. (2008). *Report of the APA Task Force on Mental Health and Abortion.* Washington, DC. www.apa.org.
55. Boonstra, H. D. (2016). *On Roe anniversary, let's remember the U.S. women for whom abortion is a right on paper only.* www.guttmacher.org.
56. American Congress of Obstetricians and Gynecologists. (2012). *Treating infertility.* www.acog.org.
57. Cole, L. (2011). The utility of six over-the-counter (home) pregnancy tests. *Clinical Chemistry and Laboratory Medicine, 49*(8), 1317–1322.
58. U.S. Department of Health and Human Services. (2009). *A healthy start: Begin before baby's born.* http://mchb.hrsa.gov.
59. American Congress of Obstetricians and Gynecologists. (2015, April). *Nutrition during pregnancy.* www.acog.org.
60. Trabert, B., Holt, V. L., Onchee, Y., Van Den Eeden, S. K., & Scholes, D. (2011). Population-based ectopic pregnancy trends, 1993–2007. *American Journal of Preventive Medicine, 401*(5), 556–560.
61. Creanga, A., Shapiro-Mendoza, C., Bish, C., Zane, S., Berg, C., & Callaghan, W. (2011). Trends in ectopic pregnancy mortality in the United States 1980–2007. *Obstetrics and Gynecology, 117*, 837–843.
62. March of Dimes. (2009). *Miscarriage.* www.marchofdimes.com.
63. American Congress of Obstetricians and Gynecologists. (2011). *High blood pressure during pregnancy.* www.acog.org.
64. Young, B., Hacker, M. R., & Rana, S. (2012). Physicians' knowledge of future vascular disease in women with preeclampsia. *Informa Healthcare, 31*(1), 50–58.
65. Hamilton, B. E., Martin, J. A., Michelle, J. K., Osterman, M. H. S., Curtin, S. C., & Mathews, T. J. (2015). Births: Final data for 2014. *National Vital Statistics Report, 64*(12). www.cdc.gov.
66. Murphy, S. L., Kochanek, K. D., Xu, J., & Arias, E. (2015). *Mortality in the United States, 2014.* www.cdc.gov.
67. Martin, J. A., Hamilton, B. E., Osterman, J. K., Curtin, M.A., & Mathews. T. J. (2013). Births: Final data for 2012. *National Vital Statistics Reports, 62*(9), 1–88.
68. American Congress of Obstetricians and Gynecologists. (2011). *You and your baby: Prenatal care, labor and delivery, and postpartum care.* www.midtown.obgyn.com.
69. MedlinePlus. (2009). *Apgar.* www.nlm.nih.gov.
70. Martin, J. A., Hamilton, B. E., Sutton, P. D., Ventura, S. J., Menacker, F., et al. (2009). Births: Final data for 2006. *National Vital Statistics Reports, 57*(7), 1–104. www.cdc.gov.
71. The Commonwealth Fund. (2013). *Rate of Cesarean birth in the U.S. doubles the World Health Organization's recommended limit.* www.commonwealthfund.org.
72. Centers for Disease Control and Prevention. (2012). *National survey of family growth.* www.cdc.gov.
73. MedlinePlus. (2009). *Infertility.* www.nlm.nih.gov.
74. Children's Bureau. (2015). *Trends in Foster Care and Adoption: FY 2005-FY 2014.* www.acf.hhs.gov.

Chapter 12

i. Centers for Disease Control and Prevention. (2015). *Influenza-related questions & answers by topic.* www.cdc.gov.
ii. Centers for Disease Control and Prevention. (2015). *CDC fact sheet: Reported STDs in the United States 2014—National data for chlamydia, gonorrhoea, and syphilis.* www.cdc.gov.
iii. Centers for Disease Control and Prevention. (2016). *HIV/AIDS: Basic statistics.* www.cdc.gov.
1. Centers for Disease Control and Prevention. (2016). *CDC and zoonotic disease.* www.cdc.gov.
2. Busscher, H. J., & van der Mei, H. C. (2012). How do bacteria know they are on a surface and regulate their response to an adhering state? *PLoS Pathogens, 8*(1), e1002440. doi:10.1371/journal.ppat.1002440.
3. American College Health Association. (2015). *ACHA-NCHA II: Undergraduate reference group executive summary, spring 2015.* www.acha-ncha.org.
4. American Academy of Allergy, Asthma & Immunology. (n.d.). *Allergic reactions.* www.aaaai.org.
5. American Academy of Allergy, Asthma & Immunology. (2016). *Asthma statistics.* www.aaaai.org.
6. Directors of Health Promotion and Education. (n.d.). *Addressing infectious disease threats.* www.dhpe.org.
7. Baccam, P., Beauchemin, C., Macken, C., Hayden, F., & Perelson, A. (2006). Kinetics of influenza A virus infection in humans. *Journal of Virology, 80*(15), 7590–7599.
8. Centers for Disease Control and Prevention. (2015). *Influenza-Related questions & answers by topic.* www.cdc.gov.
9. Centers for Disease Control and Prevention. (2016). *Hepatitis C FAQs for the public.* www.cdc.gov.
10. National Institutes of Health. (2009). *Understanding microbes in sickness and in health.* www.niaid.nih.gov.
11. Mayo Clinic. (2014). *Hand washing: Do's and don'ts.* www.mayoclinic.com.
12. World Health Organization. (2015). *Meningococcal meningitis.* www.who.int.
13. Centers for Disease Control and Prevention. *Toxic shock syndrome (other than Streptococcal) (TSS). 2011 case definition.* www.cdc.gov.
14. Centers for Disease Control and Prevention. (2014). *National strategy for combating antibiotic resistant bacteria.* www.cdc.gov.
15. Dantes, R., Mu, Y., Belflower, R., Aragon, D., Dumyati, G., et al. (2013). National burden of invasive methicillin-resistant *Staphylococcus aureus* infections, United States, 2011. *Journal of the American Medical Association—Internal Medicine, 73*(21), 1978–1979.
16. Centers for Disease Control and Prevention. (2016). *Leading causes of death.* www.cdc.gov.
17. World Health Organization. (2015). *Pneumonia.* www.who.int.
18. Centers for Disease Control and Prevention. (2014). *The difference between latent TB infection and active TB disease.* www.cdc.gov.
19. Centers for Disease Control and Prevention. (2015). *Tuberculosis: Trends in tuberculosis, 2015.* www.cdc.gov.
20. World Health Organization. (2016). *Tuberculosis.* www.who.int.
21. World Health Organization. (2016). *Malaria.* www.who.int.
22. World Health Organization. (2015). *Sexually transmitted infections.* www.who.int.
23. Centers for Disease Control and Prevention. (2016). *CDC fact sheet—Incidence, prevalence, and cost of sexually transmitted infections in the United States.* www.cdc.gov.
24. Centers for Disease Control and Prevention. (2016). *STDs in adolescents and young adults.* www.cdc.gov.
25. Centers for Disease Control and Prevention. (2015). *CDC fact sheet: Reported STDs in the United States 2014—National data for chlamydia, gonorrhea, and syphilis.* www.cdc.gov.
26. Joint United Nations Programme on HIV/AIDS (UNAIDS) and World Health Organization (WHO). (2015). *AIDS by the numbers 2015.* www.unaids.org.
27. Centers for Disease Control and Prevention. (2016). *HIV/AIDS: Basic statistics.* www.cdc.gov.
28. World Health Organization. (n.d.). *Mother-to-child transmission of HIV.* www.who.int.
29. UNAIDS. (2015). *2015 progress report on the global plan.* www.unaids.org.
30. World Health Organization. (n.d.). *HIV/AIDS: Data and statistics.* www.who.int.
31. Centers for Disease Control and Prevention. (2015). *Hepatitis B FAQs for the public.* www.cdc.gov.

32. Centers for Disease Control and Prevention. (2016). *Genital herpes: CDC fact sheet.* www.cdc.gov.
33. American Social Health Association. (n.d.). *Treatment for oral herpes.* www.ashastd.org.
34. Centers for Disease Control and Prevention. (2015). *HPV and men: Fact sheet.* www.cdc.gov.
35. Centers for Disease Control and Prevention. (2014). *Genital HPV infection: Fact sheet.* www.cdc.gov.
36. Centers for Disease Control and Prevention. (2015). *Cervical cancer statistics.* www.cdc.gov.
37. U.S. Food and Drug Administration. (2009, October 16). *FDA approves new indication for Gardasil to prevent genital warts in men and boys* [News release]. www.fda.gov.
38. Centers for Disease Control and Prevention. (2015). *2014 sexually transmitted diseases surveillance.* www.cdc.gov.
39. Centers for Disease Control and Prevention. (2015). *STDs & infertility.* www.cdc.gov.
40. Centers for Disease Control and Prevention. (2016). *Chlamydia: CDC fact sheet.* www.cdc.gov.
41. Centers for Disease Control and Prevention. (2016). *Pelvic inflammatory disease: CDC fact sheet.* www.cdc.gov.
42. Ginocchio, C. C., Chapin, K., Smith, J. S., Aslanzadeh, J., Snook, J., et al. (2011, July). Prevalence of *Trichomonas vaginalis* and coinfection with *Chlamydia trachomatis* and *Neisseria gonorrhoea* in the USA as determined by the aptima *Trichomonas vaginalis* nucleic acid amplification assay. *Sexually Transmitted Infections, 87*(1), A72-A73.
43. Centers for Disease Control and Prevention. (2015). *Trichomoniasis—CDC fact sheet.* www.cdc.gov.
44. Tuller, D. (2009, January 19). *After hookups, e-cards that warn, "get checked."* www.nytimes.com.

Chapter 13

i. Centers for Disease Control and Prevention. (2014). *National diabetes statistics report, 2014.* www.cdc.gov.
ii. Murphy, S. L., Kochanek, M. A., Xu, J., & Heron, M. (2015, August 31). *National vital statistics reports 63*(9). Centers for Disease Control and Prevention. www.cdc.gov.
iii. American Cancer Society. (2016). *Cancer facts and figures 2016.* www.cancer.org.
1. Centers for Disease Control and Prevention. (2014). *National diabetes statistics report, 2014.* www.cdc.gov.
2. Centers for Disease Control and Prevention. (2015, August 10). *Heart disease facts.* www.cdc.gov.
3. Centers for Disease Control and Prevention. (2015, March 24). *Stroke facts.* www.cdc.gov.
4. American Cancer Society. (2014). *Lifetime risk of developing or dying from cancer.* www.cancer.org.
5. American Cancer Society. (2016). *Cancer facts and figures 2016.* www.cancer.org.
6. Centers for Disease Control and Prevention. (2016, February 23). *Chronic disease overview.* www.cdc.gov.
7. Stewart, A. G. & Beart, P. M. (2016). Inflammation: Maladies, models, mechanisms, and molecules. *British Journal of Pharmacology, 173*(4), 631–634.
8. Centers for Disease Control and Prevention. (2014, October). *Long-term trends in diabetes.* www.cdc.gov.
9. Boutens, L., & R. Stienstra. (2016). Adipose tissue macrophages: Going off track during obesity. *Diabetologia, 59*(5), 879–894.
10. Wensveen, F. M., Valentic, S., Sestan, M., Turk Wensveen, T., & Polic, B. (2015). The "Big Bang" in obese fat: Events initiating obesity-induced adipose tissue inflammation. *European Journal of Immunology, 45*(9), 2446–2456.
11. Centers for Disease Control and Prevention. (2015). *Diabetes report card, 2014.* www.cdc.gov.
12. National Institute of Diabetes and Digestive and Kidney Diseases. (2014, June). *Diagnosis of diabetes and prediabetes.* www.niddk.nih.gov.
13. Garg, S. K., Maurer, H., Reed, K., & Selagamsetty, R. (2014). Diabetes and cancer: Two diseases with obesity as a common risk factor. *Diabetes, Obesity and Metabolism, 16*(2), 97–110.
14. The Obesity Society. (2015, February). *Your weight and diabetes.* www.obesity.org.
15. Basu, S., Yoffe, P., Hills, N., & Lustig, R. H. (2013). The relationship of sugar to population-level diabetes prevalence: An econometric analysis of repeated cross-sectional data. *PLoS ONE, 8*(2), e57873.
16. Te Moranga, L., Mallard, S., & Mann, J. (2013). Dietary sugars and body weight: Systematic review and meta-analyses of randomized controlled trials and cohort studies. *BMJ, 346,* e7492.
17. Crump, C., Sundquist, J., Winkleby, M. A., Sieh, W., & Sundquist, K. (2016). Physical fitness among Swedish military conscripts and long-term risk for type 2 diabetes mellitus: A cohort study. *Annals of Internal Medicine, 164*(9), 577–584.
18. Centers for Disease Control and Prevention. (2015, September 1). *Smoking and diabetes.* www.cdc.gov.
19. Joseph, J. J., Wang, X., Spanakis, E., Seeman, T., Wand, G., et al. (2015). Diurnal salivary cortisol, glycemia and insulin resistance: The multi-ethnic study of atherosclerosis. *Psychoneuroendocrinology, 62,* 327–335.
20. Van Name, M. A., Camp, A. W., Magenheimer, E. A., Li, F., Dziura, J. D., et al. (2016). Effective translation of an intensive lifestyle intervention for Hispanic women with prediabetes in a community health center setting. *Diabetes Care, 39*(4), 525–531.
21. American College Health Association. (2015). *ACHA-NCHA II: Undergraduate reference group executive summary, spring 2015.* www.acha-ncha.org.
22. Arts, J., Fernandez, M. L., & Lofgren, I. E. (2014). Coronary heart disease risk factors in college students. *Advances in Nutrition, 5*(2), 177–187.
23. Mozaffarian, D., Benjamin, E. J., Go, A. S., Arnett, D. K., Blaha, M. J., et al. (2015). Heart disease and stroke statistics—2016 update. *Circulation, 133*(4), e38–e60.
24. Murphy, S. L., Kochanek, M. A., Xu, J., & Heron, M. (2015, August 31). *National vital statistics reports 63*(9). Centers for Disease Control and Prevention. www.cdc.gov.
25. Centers for Disease Control and Prevention. (2015, February 19). *High blood pressure facts.* www.cdc.gov.
26. U.S. Department of Health and Human Services and U.S. Department of Agriculture. (2015). *2015–2020 dietary guidelines for Americans,* 8th ed. http://health.gov.
27. National Heart, Lung, and Blood Institute. (2015, September 10). *How is high blood pressure treated?* www.nhlbi.nih.gov.
28. The SPRINT Research Group. (2015). A randomized trial of intensive versus standard blood-pressure control. *New England Journal of Medicine, 26*(373), 2103–2116.
29. American Heart Association. (2015, October 19). *Heart attack symptoms in women.* www.heart.org.
30. American Heart Association. (2014, November 18). *Arrhythmia.* www.heart.org.
31. Center for Science in the Public Interest. (2014). *Documents link more deaths to energy drinks.* www.cspinet.org.
32. National Heart, Lung, and Blood Institute. (2015, November 06). *How is a heart attack treated?* www.nhlbi.nih.gov.
33. Centers for Disease Control and Prevention. (2015, November 30). *Heart failure fact sheet.* www.cdc.gov.
34. Centers for Disease Control and Prevention. (2016, February). *FastStats: Cerebrovascular disease or stroke.* www.cdc.gov.
35. Mayo Foundation. (2016, January 20). *Stroke.* www.mayoclinic.com.
36. American Heart Association. (2015, October 26). *Understand your risk for congenital heart defects.* www.heart.org.
37. American Heart Association. (2015, August 21). *Hypertrophic cardiomyopathy.* www.heart.org.
38. Poirier, P., Giles, T. D., Bray, G. A., Hong, Y., Stern, J. S., et al. (2006). Obesity and cardiovascular disease: Pathophysiology, evaluation, and effect of weight loss. *Circulation, 113,* 898–918.
39. Sahakyan, K. R., Somers, V. K., Rodriguez-Escudero, J. P., Hodge, D. O., Carter, R. E., et al. (2015). Normal-weight central obesity: Implications for total and cardiovascular mortality. *Annals of Internal Medicine, 163*(11), 827–835.
40. DiNicolantonio, J. J., Lucan, S. C., & O'Keefe, J. H. (2016). The evidence for saturated fat and for sugar related to coronary heart disease. *Progress in Cardiovascular Diseases, 58*(5), 464–472.
41. Singh, G. M., Micha, R., Khatibzadeh, S., Lim, S., Ezzati, M., & Mozaffarian, D. (2015). Estimated global, regional, and national disease burdens related to sugar-sweetened beverage consumption in 2010. *Circulation, 132*(8), 639–666.
42. American Heart Association. (2015, July). *Understand your risk of heart attack.* www.heart.org.
43. Poli, A., & F. Visioli. (2015). Moderate alcohol use and health: An update a consensus document. *BIO Web of Conferences.* doi: 10.1051/bioconf/20150504001.
44. National Institute on Drug Abuse. (2012, December). *Medical consequences of drug abuse.* www.drugabuse.gov.
45. Jutla, S. K., Yuyun, M. F., Quinn, P. A., & Ng, L. L. (2014). Plasma cortisol and prognosis of patients with acute myocardial infarction. *Journal of Cardiovascular Medicine, 15*(1), 33–41.
46. Jackowska, M., & Steptoe, A. (2015). Sleep and future cardiovascular risk: Prospective analysis from the English Longitudinal Study of Ageing. *Sleep Medicine, 16*(6), 768–774.
47. Calvin, A. D., Covassin, N., Kremers, W. K., Adachi, T., Macedo, P., et al. (2014). Experimental sleep restriction causes endothelial dysfunction in healthy humans. *Journal of the American Heart Association, 3*(6), e001143.
48. International Chair on Cardiometabolic Risk. (2016). *Global cardiometabolic risk: Historical perspective.* www.myhealthyrisk.org.
49. Agency for Healthcare Research and Quality National Guideline Clearinghouse. (2012, April 13). *Cardiometabolic risk management in primary care.* www.guideline.gov.
50. International Chair on Cardiometabolic Risk. (2016). *The concept of CMR.* www.myhealthywaist.org.
51. Jani, B. D., Cavanagh, J., Barry, S. J. E., Der, G., Sattar, N., & Mair, F. S. (2014). Revisiting the J shaped curve, exploring the association between cardiovascular risk factors and concurrent depressive symptoms in patients with cardiometabolic disease: Findings from a large cross-sectional study. *BMJ Cardiovascular Disorders, 14,* 139
52. Morrell, J. S., Lofgren, I. E., Burke, J. D., & Reilly, R. A. (2012). Metabolic syndrome, obesity, and related risk factors among college men and women. *Journal of American College Health, 60*(1), 82–89.
53. Morrell, J. S., Byrd-Bredbenner, C., Quick, V., Olfert, M., Dent, A., & Carey, G. B. (2014). Metabolic syndrome: A comparison of prevalence in young adults at 3 land-grant universities. *American Journal of College Health, 62*(1), 1–9.

54. American Cancer Society. (2016). *Cancer facts and figures 2016*. www.cancer.org.
55. American Cancer Society. (2015, October 27). *Known and probable human carcinogens*. www.cancer.org.
56. National Cancer Institute. (2015, April 1). *National Cancer Institute fact sheet: BRCA1 and BRCA2: Cancer risk and genetic testing*. www.cancer.gov.
57. American Cancer Society. (2014, August 11). *Signs and symptoms of cancer*. www.cancer.org.
58. Food and Drug Administration. (2015, December 22). *Sunlamps and sunlamp products (tanning beds and booths). Radiation-emitting products*. www.fda.gov.
59. American Cancer Society. (2015, October 20). *American Cancer Society recommendations for early breast cancer detection in women without breast symptoms*. www.cancer.org.
60. American Cancer Society. (2015, February 2). *HPV and cancer*. www.cancer.org.
61. Markowitz, L. E., Liu, G., Hariri, S., Steinau, M., Dunne, E. F., & Unger, E. R. (2016). Prevalence of HPV after introduction of the vaccination program in the United States. *Pediatrics, 137*(3), e20151968.
62. American Cancer Society. (2016). *Treatment types*. www.cancer.org.

Chapter 14

i. Pew Internet & American Life Project. (2013). *Health fact sheet*. www.pewinternet.org.
ii. Makary, M., & Daniel, M. (2016). Medical error—The third leading cause of death in the US. *British Medical Journal, 353*, i2139.
iii. U.S. Department of Health and Human Services. (2016, March 3).*20 million people have gained health insurance coverage because of the Affordable Care Act, new estimates show*. www.hhs.gov.
1. Vader, A., Walters, S., Roudsari, B., & Nguyen, N. (2011). Where do college students get health information? Believability and use of health information sources. *Health Promotion Practices, 12*(5), 713–722.
2. University of California, San Francisco. (n.d.). *Evaluating health information*. www.ucsfhealth.org.
3. Nielsen and IMS Health. (2013). *Understanding trust in OTC medicines: Consumer and healthcare provider perspectives*. www.yourhealthathand.org.
4. Consumer Healthcare Products Association. (2015). *Statistics on OTC use*. www.chpa.org.
5. U.S. Food and Drug Administration, Center for Drug Evaluation and Research. (2015). *Regulation of nonprescription products*. www.fda.gov.
6. Stasio, M., Curry, K., Sutton-Skinner, K., & Glassman, D. (2008). Over-the-counter medication and herbal or dietary supplement use in college: Dose frequency and relationship to self-reported distress. *Journal of the American College Health Association, 56*(5), 535–547.
7. American College of Emergency Physicians. (n.d.). *Is it an emergency?* www.emergencycareforyou.org.
8. Merck. (2011). *The Merck manual, home health edition*. www.merck.com.
9. American Academy of Family Physicians. (2014). *Tips for talking to your doctor and 20 tips to help prevent medical errors*. http://familydoctor.org.
10. American Hospital Association. (2006). *The patient care partnership*. www.aha.org.
11. American College Health Association. (2015). *ACHA-NCHA II: Undergraduate reference group executive summary, spring 2015*. www.acha-ncha.org.
12. Centers for Disease Control and Prevention. (2011). *Vital signs—Prescription painkiller overdoses in the US*. www.cdc.gov.
13. Centers for Disease Control and Prevention. (2016). *Injury prevention and control. Opioid overdoses*. www.cdc.gov.
14. National Institute on Drug Abuse. (2016). *Abuse of prescription (Rx) drugs affects young adults most*. www.drugabuse.gov.
15. U.S. Food and Drug Administration. (2015). *A guide to safe use of pain medicine*. www.fda.gov.
16. National Center for Complementary and Integrative Health. (2016). *Complementary, alternative, or integrative health: What's in a name?* https://nccih.nih.gov.
17. National Center for Complementary and Alternative Medicine. (2016). *Safe use of complementary health products and practices*. http://nccam.nih.gov.
18. National Center for Complementary and Integrative Health. (2015). *How to find a complementary health practitioner*. https://nccih.nih.gov.
19. World Health Organization. (2015). *Health financing: Total expenditure on health as a percentage of gross domestic product: 2013*. http://gamapserver.who.int.
20. California Health Care Foundation. (2015). *Health Care Costs 101: Reaching a Spending Plateau?* www.chcf.org.
21. Kaiser Family Foundation. (2015). *2015 employer health benefits survey*. http://kff.org.
22. National Center for Health Statistics. (2009). *Consumer-Directed health care for persons under 65 years of age with private health insurance: United States, 2007*. www.cdc.gov.
23. Henry J. Kaiser Family Foundation. (2016). *Who is impacted by the coverage gap in states that have adopted the Medicaid expansion?* http://kff.org.

Chapter 15

i. Heron, M. (2016). Deaths: Leading causes for 2013. *National Vital Statistics Reports, 65*(2), 1–95.
ii. Centers for Disease Control and Prevention. (2011). *National intimate partner and sexual violence survey: Highlights of 2010 findings*. www.cdc.gov.
iii. National Highway Traffic Safety Administration. (2014). *Official US government website for distracted driving*. www.distraction.gov.
iv. Centers for Disease Control and Prevention. (2014). *Distracted driving. Injury prevention and control: Motor vehicle safety*. www.cdc.gov.
v. Centers for Disease Control and Prevention. (2011). *National intimate partner and sexual violence survey: Highlights of 2010 findings*. www.cdc.gov.
1. Heron, M. (2016). Deaths: Leading causes for 2013. *National Vital Statistics Reports, 65*(2), 1–95.
2. Centers for Disease Control and Prevention. (2015, September 30). *Cost of injuries and violence in the United States*. www.cdc.gov.
3. Centers for Disease Control and Prevention. (2013). *2011 Emergency department summary tables. National hospital ambulatory medical care survey*. www.cdc.gov.
4. National Highway Traffic Safety Administration. (2015, November). *2014 crash data key findings (Traffic safety facts, DOT HS 812 219)*. www-nrd.nhtsa.dot.gov.
5. National Institute on Alcohol Abuse and Alcoholism. (2010). *Rethinking drinking: Alcohol and your health*. http://rethinkingdrinking.niaaa.nih.gov.
6. National Safety Council. (2013). *Injury facts 2011 edition*. www.nsc.org.
7. National Highway Traffic Safety Administration. (2013, April). *The impact of hand-held and hands-free cell phone use on driving performance and safety-critical event risk (DOT HS 811 757)*. www.distraction.gov.
8. AAA Foundation for Traffic Safety. (2013, June). *Measuring cognitive distraction in the automobile*. www.aaafoundation.org.
9. Governors Highway Safety Association. (2013, May). *Distracted driving laws*. www.ghsa.org.
10. National Center for Statistics and Analysis. (2016, February). *Alcohol-impaired driving: 2014 data. (Traffic Safety Facts. DOT HS 812 231)*. www-nrd.nhtsa.dot.gov.
11. Governors Highway Safety Association. (2016, February). *Drug impaired driving laws*. www.ghsa.org.
12. AAA Foundation for Traffic Safety. (2012, March). *Two out of five drivers admit to falling asleep at the wheel, finds AAA Foundation study*. www.aaafoundation.org.
13. National Conference of State Legislatures. (2015, September). *Summaries of current drowsy driving laws*. www.ncsl.org.
14. National Center for Statistics and Analysis. (2015, November). *Lives saved in 2014 by restraint use and minimum-drinking-age laws (Traffic safety facts crash stats. Report No. DOT HS 812 218)*. www-nrd.nhtsa.dot.gov.
15. Pickrell, T. M. (2016, February). *Seat belt use in 2015—Overall results (Report No. DOT HS 812 243)*. Washington, DC: U.S. National Highway Traffic Safety Administration.
16. American College Health Association. (2015). *ACHA-NCHA II: Undergraduate reference group executive summary, fall 2015*. www.acha-ncha.org.
17. National Highway Traffic Safety Administration. (2010). *The top 5 things you should know about buckling up (DOT HS 811 257)*. http://trafficsafetymarketing.gov.
18. California Department of Motor Vehicles. (2010). Seat belts: Mistaken beliefs about seat belts. In *California Driver Handbook* (p. 19). www.dmv.ca.gov.
19. National Highway Traffic Safety Administration. (2013). *Aggressive driving*. www.nhtsa.gov.
20. National Highway Traffic Safety Administration. (2015, May). *Motorcycles. Traffic safety facts: 2013 data (DOT HS 812 148)*. www.nhtsa.gov.
21. Faul, M., Xu, L., Wald, M. M., & Coronado, V. G. (2010). *Traumatic brain injury in the United States: Emergency department visits, hospitalizations, and deaths*. Centers for Disease Control and Prevention. www.cdc.gov.
22. National Highway Traffic Safety Administration. (2015, February). *Pedestrians. Traffic safety facts: 2013 data (DOT HS 812 124)*. www.nhtsa.gov.
23. National Highway Traffic Safety Administration. (2015, May). *Bicyclists and other cyclists. Traffic safety facts: 2013 data (DOT HS 812 151)*. www.nhtsa.gov.
24. Governors Highway Safety Association. (2013, June). *Helmet laws*. www.ghsa.org.
25. Paulozzi, L. J. (2012). Prescription drug overdoses: A review. *Journal of Safety Research, 43*(4), 283–289.
26. Centers for Disease Control and Prevention. (2014). *Web-based Injury Statistics Query and Reporting System (WISQARS)*. www.cdc.gov.
27. Solomon, D. H., Rassen, J. A., Glynn, R. J., Garneau, K., et al. (2010, December). The comparative safety of opioids for nonmalignant pain in older adults. *Archives of Internal Medicine, 170*(22), 1979–1986.
28. National Institutes of Health. (2011, July 16). Choking: Adult or child over 1 year. *MedlinePlus*. www.nlm.nih.gov.
29. American Academy of Pediatrics. (2010, March 1). Prevention of choking among children. *PEDIATRICS, 125*(3), 601–607.
30. Centers for Disease Control and Prevention. (2012, November 29). *Unintentional drowning: Fact sheet*. www.cdc.gov.
31. Sleet, D. A., Ballesteros, M. F., & Borse, N. N. (2010). A review of unintentional injuries in adolescents. *Annual Reviews, 31*, 195–212.

32. Centers for Disease Control and Prevention. (2011, October). *Fire deaths and injuries: Fact sheet.* www.cdc.gov.
33. U.S. Fire Administration. (2015). *2014 residential fire civilian facilities map.* http://apps.usfa.fema.gov.
34. U.S. Fire Administration. (2013, January 29). *Campus fire safety: Tips for students and parents.* www.fema.gov.
35. U.S. Bureau of Labor Statistics. (2015). *Census of fatal occupational injuries summary, 2014.* www.bls.gov.
36. Berolo, S., Wells, R. P., & Amick, B. C. (2011). Musculoskeletal symptoms among mobile handheld device users and their relationship to device use: A preliminary study in a Canadian university population. *Applied Ergonomics, 42*(2), 371–378.
37. Centers for Disease Control and Prevention. (2013, March 14). *Youth violence: National statistics.* www.cdc.gov.
38. Federal Bureau of Investigation, Criminal Justice Information Services Division. (2015, September). *2014 crime in the United States.* www.fbi.gov.
39. Bureau of Justice Statistics. (2015, August). *Criminal victimization, 2014.* www.bjs.gov.
40. Bureau of Justice Statistics. (2012, April 17). *National crime victimization survey.* www.bjs.gov.
41. National Institute on Alcohol Abuse and Alcoholism. (2012, April). *College drinking.* http://niaaa.nih.gov.
42. Krug, E. G., Dahlberg, L. L., Mercy, J. A., Zwi, A. B., & Lozano, R. (Eds.). (2010, June). *World report on violence and health.* World Health Organization. www.who.int.
43. Bureau of Justice Statistics & National Center for Education Statistics. (2012). *Indicators of school crime and safety: 2012.* www.bjs.gov.
44. Allan, E. J., & Madden, M. (2011). The nature and extent of college student hazing. *International Journal of Adolescent Medicine and Health, 24*(1), 83–90.
45. Newer, H. (2012). *The hazing reader.* Bloomington: Indiana University Press.
46. Federal Bureau of Investigation, Criminal Justice Information Services Division. (2015). *Hate crime statistics, 2014.* www.fbi.gov.
47. U.S. Department of State. (2015). *Country reports on terrorism 2014.* www.state.org.
48. Centers for Disease Control and Prevention. (2013, May 10). *National intimate partner and sexual violence survey: Highlights of 2010 findings.* www.cdc.gov.
49. Centers for Disease Control and Prevention. (2012). *Understanding intimate partner violence: Fact sheet 2012.* www.cdc.gov.
50. McDermott, R. C., & Lopez, F. G. (2013). College men's intimate partner violence attitudes: Contributions of adult attachment and gender role stress. *Journal of Counseling Psychology, 60*(1), 127–136.
51. National Network to End Domestic Violence. (2013). *National summary: Domestic violence counts 2012: A 24-hour census of domestic violence shelters and services.* www.nnedv.org.
52. Nabors, E., Dietz, T., & Jasinski, J. (2006). Domestic violence beliefs and perceptions among college students. *Violence and Victims, 21*(6), 779–795.
53. McNamara, C. L., & Marsil, D. F. (2012). The prevalence of stalking among college students: The disparity between researcher-and self-identified victimization. *Journal of American College Health, 60*(2), 168–174.
54. Reyns, B. W., Henson, B., & Fishers, B. S. (2012). Stalking in the twilight zone: Extent of cyberstalking victimization and offending among college students. *Deviant Behavior, 33*(1), 1–25.
55. Kraft, E. M., & Wang, I. (2010). An exploratory study of the cyberbullying and cyberstalking experiences and factors related to victimization of students at a public liberal arts college. *International Journal of Technoethics, 1*(4), 74–91.
56. Centers for Disease Control and Prevention. (2010, September). *Intimate partner violence: Risk and protective factors.* www.cdc.gov.
57. Franklin, C. A., Bouffard, L. A., & Pratt, T. C. (2012). Sexual assault on the college campus: Fraternity affiliation, male peer support, and low self-control. *Criminal Justice and Behavior, 39*(11), 1457–1480.
58. Krebs, C., Lindquist, C., Warner, T., Fisher, B., & Martin, S. (2009). College women's experiences with physically forced, alcohol- or other drug-enabled, and drug-facilitated sexual assault before and since entering college. *Journal of American College Health, 57*(6), 639–647.
59. Core Institute. (2013, April 24). *Core alcohol and drug survey: 2011 data.* http://core.siu.edu.
60. O'Byrne, R., Hansen, S., & Rapley, M. (2007). If a girl doesn't say "no" . . .: Young men, rape, and claims of "insufficient knowledge." *Journal of Community and Applied Social Psychology, 18*, 168–193.
61. U.S. Equal Employment Opportunity Commission. (2016). *Sexual harassment charges: FY 2015.* www.eeoc.gov.
62. U.S. Equal Employment Opportunity Commission. (2016). *Sexual harassment.* www.eeoc.gov.
63. Hill, C., & Silva, E. (2005). *Drawing the line: Sexual harassment on campus.* American Association of University Women Educational Foundation. www.aauw.org.
64. U.S. Department of Justice. (2000). *The sexual victimization of college women.* www.ncjrs.gov.
65. Center for Public Integrity. (2010, February 24). *Sexual assault on campus: A frustrating search for justice: Key findings.* www.publicintegrity.org.
66. U.S. Department of Health and Human Services. (2011, May 18). *Violence against women: How to help a friend who is being abused.* http://womenshealth.gov.

Chapter 16

i. Population Reference Bureau. (2015). 2015 World Population Interactive Map. www.prb.org.
ii. National Aeronautics and Space Administration (NASA). (2016, March 10). Consequences of climate change: Effects. Global climate change: Vital signs of the planet. http://climate.nasa.gov.
iii. Environmental Protection Agency. (2016, March 27). Municipal solid waste. www.epa.gov.
1. World Health Organization. (2016). *Environmental health.* www.who.int.
2. World Health Organization. (2016, March). 10 facts on preventing disease through healthy environments. www.who.int.
3. Environmental Protection Agency. (2015, September 29). About EPA: Our mission and what we do. www.epa.gov.
4. Lin, J., Pan, D., Davis, S., Zhang, Q., He, K., et al. (2014). China's international trade and air pollution in the United States. *Proceedings of the National Academy of Sciences, 111*(5), 1736–1741.
5. Wong, E. (2013, April 1). Air pollution linked to 1.2 million premature deaths in China. The New York Times. www.nytimes.com.
6. Lewis, J. (1985, November). The birth of EPA. EPA Journal. www.epa.gov.
7. National Aeronautics and Space Administration (NASA). (2016, March 10). Consequences of climate change: Effects. Global climate change: Vital signs of the planet. http://climate.nasa.gov.
8. Ocko, I. (2016, February 16). 3 reasons the Zika outbreak may be linked to climate change. Environmental Defense Fund. www.edf.org.
9. United Nations Environment Programme. (2014, June). Emerging issues for small island developing states. Results of the UNEP Foresight Process. www.unep.org.
10. World Health Organization. (2015, September). Climate change and health. www.who.int.
11. United Nations Department of Economic and Social Affairs, Population Division. (2015). World population prospects: The 2015 revision. New York: United Nations.
12. Food and Agricultural Organization of the United Nations. (2015). The state of food insecurity in the world. www.fao.org.
13. International Energy Agency. (2016). Energy poverty. www.iea.org.
14. U.S. Energy Information Administration. (2016). International energy statistics: Total primary energy consumption. www.eia.gov.
15. World Bank. (2016). Data: Fertility rate: 2011–2015. http://data.worldbank.org.
16. U.S. Department of Homeland Security. (2014, August). Yearbook of immigration statistics: 2013. www.dhs.gov.
17. Population Reference Bureau. (2015). 2015 world population data sheet—with a special focus on women's empowerment. www.prb.org.
18. Sen, A. (2015, November 2). Amartya Sen: Women's progress outdid China's one-child policy. www.nytimes.com.
19. Peters, G. L. (2012). Depopulation in some rich nations: Good news for planet earth? Yearbook of the Association of Pacific Coast Geographers, *74*, 122–140.
20. Lee, R., Mason, A., & members of the NTA Network. (2014). Is low fertility really a problem? Population aging, dependency, and consumption. *Science, 346*(6206), 229–234.
21. The National Academies. (2016). Our energy sources: Fossil fuels. What you need to know about energy. http://needtoknow.nas.edu.
22. Environmental Protection Agency. (2016, February 23). Pollutants and sources. www3.epa.gov.
23. Environmental Protection Agency. (2016, February 23). Climate change science overview. www3.epa.gov.
24. Marcott, S. A., Shakun, J. D., Clark, P. U., & Mix, A. C. (2013, March 8). A reconstruction of regional and global temperature for the past 11,300 years. *Science, 399*(6124), 1198–1201.
25. Kopp, R. E., Kemp, A. C., Bittermann, K., Horton, B. P., Donnelly, J. P., et al. (2016). Temperature-driven global sea-level variability in the common era. *Proceedings of the National Academy of Sciences, 113*(11), e1434–e1441.
26. Hansen, J., Sato, M., Hearty, P., Ruedy, R., Kelley, M., et al. (2016). Ice melt, sea level rise and superstorms: Evidence from paleoclimate data, climate modeling, and modern observations that 2° C global warming could be dangerous. *Atmospheric Chemistry and Physics, 16*, 3761–3812.
27. DeConto, R. M., & Pollard, D. (2016). Contribution of Antarctica to past and future sea-level rise. *Nature, 531*, 591–597.
28. Environmental Protection Agency. (2016, February 24). Weather and climate. www.epa.gov.
29. World Meteorological Organization. (2015, November 9). Greenhouse gas bulletin. http://library.wmo.int.
30. Environmental Protection Agency. (2016, May 12). EPA's actions to reduce methane emissions from the oil and natural gas industry: Final rules and draft information collection request. www3.epa.gov.
31. Environmental Protection Agency. (2016, February 24). Overview of greenhouse gases: Nitrous oxide emissions. www3.epa.gov.
32. Environmental Protection Agency. (2014, September 21). Good up high bad nearby: What is ozone? http://cfpub.epa.gov.
33. American Lung Association. (2016). State of the air 2015. www.stateoftheair.org.
34. Environmental Protection Agency. (2016, February 22). What is acid rain? www3.epa.gov.
35. Environmental Protection Agency. (2016, March 12). Sulfur dioxide. www3.epa.gov.

36. Environmental Protection Agency. (2016, February 23). Light-duty automotive technology, carbon dioxide emissions, and fuel economy trends, 1975 through 2015. www3.epa.gov.
37. United Nations Framework Convention on Climate Change. (2015, December 12). Adoption of the Paris Agreement. https://unfccc.int.
38. Clark, P. U., Shakun, J. D., Marcott, S. A., Mix, A. C., Eby, M., et al. (2016). Consequences of twenty-first-century policy for multi-millennial climate and sea-level change. *Nature Climate Change, 6*, 360–370.
39. United Nations World Water Assessment Programme. (2015). The United Nations World Water Development Report 2015: Water for a sustainable world. www.unesco.org.
40. Food and Drug Administration. (2015, July 25). FDA explores impact of arsenic in rice. www.fda.gov.
41. Environmental Protection Agency. (2016, March 17). Basic information about lead in drinking water. www.epa.gov.
42. Environmental Protection Agency. (2015, December 10). Learn about dioxin. www3.epa.gov.
43. Environmental Protection Agency. (2016, March 21). Learn about polychlorinated biphenyls (PCBs). www3.epa.gov.
44. International Agency for Research on Cancer. (2015, March 20). Evaluation of five organophosphate insecticides and herbicides. www.iarc.fr.
45. International Bottled Water Association. (2014, December 4). Bottled water sales expected to increase in 2015, expected to be the number one packaged drink by 2016. www.bottledwater.org.
46. International Bottled Water Association. (2016, March 21). Recycling. www.bottledwater.org.
47. National Oceanic and Atmospheric Administration Marine Debris Program. (2016, March 31). Types and sources. http://marinedebris.noaa.gov.
48. Environmental Protection Agency. (2016, March 27). Municipal solid waste. www3.epa.gov.
49. San Francisco Department of the Environment. (2016). Zero waste FAQ. www.sfenvironment.org.
50. Acaroglu, L. (2013, May 4). Where do old cellphones go to die? *The New York Times*. www.nytimes.com.
51. Environmental Protection Agency. (2015, October 14). Fiscal year 2014 Superfund national accomplishments summary. www.epa.gov.
52. Food and Drug Administration. (2016, February 5). Questions and answers on bisphenol A (BPA) use in food contact applications. www.fda.gov.
53. Environmental Protection Agency. (2015, October 14). Phthalates. www.epa.gov.
54. Luz, C. (2012, June). Our food: Packaging and public health. *Environmental Health Perspectives, 120*(6), A232–A237.
55. Food and Drug Administration. (2015, December 31). FDA revokes food additive approval for the use of long-chain perfluorinated compounds as oil and water repellents for paper used in food packaging. www.fda.gov.
56. Environmental Working Group. (2016, January 4). FDA bans three toxic chemicals from food wrapping—too little, too late. www.ewg.org.
57. Environmental Protection Agency. (2015, December 24). Asbestos: Protect your family. www.epa.gov.
58. National Cancer Institute. (2011, December 6). Radon and cancer. www.cancer.gov.
59. Centers for Disease Control and Prevention. (2016, February 1). Carbon monoxide (CO) poisoning prevention. www.cdc.gov.
60. Environmental Protection Agency. (2016, January 28). Volatile organic compounds' impact on air quality. www.epa.gov.
61. Centers for Disease Control and Prevention. (2015, February). Fourth national report on human exposure to environmental chemicals: 2015 updated tables. www.cdc.gov.
62. National Institute on Deafness and Other Communication Disorders. (2014, June 24). Hearing loss and older adults. www.nidcd.nih.gov.
63. National Institute on Deafness and Other Communication Disorders. (2015, May 15). Noise-induced hearing loss. www.nidcd.nih.gov.
64. Sulaiman, A. H., Husain, R., & Seluakumaran, K. (2015). Hearing risk among young personal listening device users: Effects at high-frequency and extended high-frequency audiogram thresholds. *Journal of International Advanced Otology, 11*(2), 104–109.
65. Harrison, R. V. (2012). The prevention of noise-induced hearing loss in children. *International Journal of Pediatrics*. www.hindawi.com.
66. Orr, D. W. (2007). Optimism and hope in a hotter time. *Conservation Biology, 21*(6), 1392–1395.
67. Association for the Advancement of Sustainability in Higher Education. (2012). Resources for campus sustainability: Resources for students. www.aashe.org.

Chapter 17

i. Administration on Aging, Administration for Community Living. (2014, December). *A profile of older Americans: 2014*. www.aoa.acl.gov.
ii. Saul, D. J. (2014, January 15). *2014 Facebook demographic report*. https://isl.co.
1. Administration on Aging, Administration for Community Living. (2014, December). *A profile of older Americans: 2014*. www.aoa.acl.gov.
2. National Council on Aging. (2015, June 5). *Connections with community and family—not money—most important for seniors' quality of life*. www.ncoa.org.
3. Centers for Medicare & Medicaid Services. (2015). *National health expenditure projections 2014–2024: Forecast summary*. www.cms.gov.
4. Murphy, S. L., Kochanek, K. D., Xu, J., & Arias, E. (2015, December). Mortality in the United States, 2014. *NCHS Data Brief No. 229*. www.cdc.gov.
5. Ekelund, U., Ward, H. A., Norat, T., Luan, J., May, A. M., et al. (2015). Physical activity and all-cause mortality across levels of overall and abdominal adiposity in European men and woman: The European Prospective Investigation into Cancer and Nutrition Study (EPIC). *American Journal of Clinical Nutrition, 101*(3), 613–621.
6. O'Doherty, M. G., Cairns, K., O'Neill, V., Lamrock, F., Jorgensen, T., et al. (2016). Effect of major lifestyle risk factors, independent and jointly, on life expectancy with and without cardiovascular disease: Results from the Consortium on Health and Ageing Network of Cohorts in Europe and the United States (CHANCES). *European Journal of Epidemiology, 18*, 1–14.
7. Chetty, R., Stepner, M., Abraham, S., Lin, S., Scuderi, B., et al. (2016). The association between income and life expectancy in the United States, 2001–2014. *Journal of the American Medical Association, 315*(16), 1750–1766.
8. Central Intelligence Agency. (2016, April). Country comparison: Life expectancy at birth, 2015 estimates. *CIA World Factbook*. www.cia.gov.
9. Centers for Disease Control and Prevention. (2016, March 14). *Current cigarette smoking among adults in the United States, 2014*. www.cdc.gov.
10. Kaiser Family Foundation. (2015, March 31). *Gender differences in health care, status, and use: Spotlight on men's health*. www.kff.org.
11. American Academy of Ophthalmology. (2016). *Eye health statistics*. www.aao.org.
12. Glaucoma Research Foundation. (2015, May 5). *Glaucoma facts and stats*. www.glaucoma.org.
13. McCusker, M. M., Durrani, K., Payette, M. J., & Suchecki, J. (2016). An eye on nutrition: The role of vitamins, essential fatty acids, and antioxidants in age-related macular degeneration, dry eye syndrome, and cataract. *Clinics in Dermatology, 34*(2), 276–285.
14. Centers for Disease Control and Prevention. (2016, April 14). *Arthritis: Data and statistics*. www.cdc.gov.
15. Centers for Disease Control and Prevention. (2015, September 29). *Osteoporosis*. www.cdc.gov.
16. National Institute on Aging. (2015, September 8). *Hormones and menopause*. www.nia.nih.gov.
17. Cosman, F., de Beur, S. J., LeBoff, M. S., Lewiecki, E. M., Tanner, B., et al. (2014). Clinician's guide to prevention and treatment of osteoporosis. *Osteoporosis International, 25* (10), 2359–2381.
18. Dimopoulou, C., Ceausu, I., Depypere, H., Lambrinoudaki, I., Mueck, A., et al. (2016). EMAS position statement: Testosterone replacement therapy in the aging male. *Maturitas, 84*, 94–99.
19. Lee, D. M., Nazroo, J., O'Connor, D. B., Blake, M., & Pendleton, N. (2016). Sexual health and well-being among older men and women in England: Findings from the English Longitudinal Study of Ageing. *Archives of Sexual Behavior, 45* (1), 133–144.
20. Minichiello, V., Rahman, S., & Hawes, G. (2012). STI epidemiology in the global older population: Emerging challenges. *Perspectives in Public Health, 132* (4), 178–181.
21. Chakrabati, S., & Mohanakumar, K. P. (2016). Aging and neurodegeneration: A tangle of models and mechanisms. *Aging and Disease, 15* (7), 111–113.
22. National Institute on Aging. (2016, March 10). *Alzheimer's disease fact sheet*. www.nia.nih.gov.
23. Burke, S. L., Maramaldi, P., Cadet, T., & Kukull, W. (2016). Associations between depression, sleep disturbance, and apolipoprotein E in the development of Alzheimer's disease: Dementia. *International Psychogeriatrics, 29*, 1–16.
24. Centers for Disease Control and Prevention. (2013, August 14). *Healthy places terminology*. www.cdc.gov.
25. Social Security Administration. (2015, September). *Facts and figures about Social Security, 2015*. www.socialsecurity.gov.
26. Rhee, N. (2013, June). The retirement savings crisis: Is it worse than we think? *National Institute on Retirement Security*. www.nirsonline.org.
27. Substance Abuse and Mental Health Services Administration. (2016, March 2). *Specific populations: Older adults*. http://samhsa.gov.
28. Curtain, S. C., Warner, M., & Hedegaard, H. (2016, April). *Increase in suicide in the United States, 1999–2014*. www.cdc.gov.
29. National Institutes of Health. (2015, August). *Alcohol and aging*. http://nihseniorhealth.gov.
30. Charlesworth, C. J., Smit, E., Lee, D. S., Alramadhan, F., & Odden, M. C. (2015). Polypharmacy among adults aged 65 years and older in the United States: 1988–2010. *Journals of Gerontology. Series A, Biological Sciences and Medical Sciences, 70* (8), 989–995.
31. Maher, R. L., Hanlon, J. T., & Hajjar, E. R. (2014). Clinical consequences of polypharmacy in elderly. *Expert Opinions on Drug Safety, 13* (1), 57–65.
32. Govindaraju, D., Atzmon, G., & Barzilai, N. (2015). Genetics, lifestyle and longevity: Lessons from centenarians. *Applied and Translational Genomics, 4*, 23–32.
33. Vaillant, G. E. (2002). *Aging well: Surprising guideposts to a happier life from the landmark Harvard Study of Adult Development*. Boston: Little, Brown.
34. Harvard Study of Adult Development. (2016). *Publications*. www.adultdevelopmentstudy.org.
35. Loprinzi, P. D., Loenneke, J. P., & Blackburn, E. H. (2015). Movement-based behaviors and leukocyte telomere length among US adults. *Medicine and Science in Sports and Exercise, 47* (11), 2347–2352.

36. Gradari, S., Palle, A., McGreevy, K. R., Fontan-Lozano, A., & Trejo, J. L. (2016). Can exercise make you smarter, happier, and have more neurons? A hormetic perspective. *Frontiers in Neuroscience, 10,* 93.

37. Swain, R. A., Berggren, K. L., Kerr, A. L., Patel, A., Peplinski, C., & Sikorski, A. M. (2012). On aerobic exercise and behavioral and neural plasticity. *Brain Science, 2,* 709–744.

38. Tsai, S. F., Chen, P. C., Calkins, M. J., Wu, S. Y., & Kuo, Y. M. (2016). Exercise counteracts aging-related memory impairment: A potential role for the astrocyte metabolic shuttle. *Frontiers in Aging Neuroscience, 8,* 57.

39. Chen, W., Zhang, X., & Huang, W. (2016). Role of physical exercise in Alzheimer's disease. *Biomedical Reports, 4* (4), 403–407.

40. Centers for Disease Control and Prevention. (2015, June 4). *Physical activity for everyone: How much physical activity do older adults need?* www.cdc.gov.

41. Clifford, J., & Bellows, L. (2015, July). *Nutrition and aging.* http://extension.colostate.edu.

42. Centers for Disease Control and Prevention. (2015, June 5). *Health effects of overweight and obesity.* www.cdc.gov.

43. Ja, P., Ramasundarahettige, C., Landsman, V., Rostron, B., Thun, M., et al. (2013). 21st-century hazards of smoking and benefits of cessation in the United States. *The New England Journal of Medicine, 368* (4), 341–350.

44. Karama, S., Ducharme, S., Corley, J., Chouinard-Decorte, F., Starr, J. M., et al. (2015). Cigarette smoking and thinning of the brain's cortex. *Molecular Psychiatry, 20* (6), 778–785.

45. Friedrich, M. J. (2013, February 20). Tobacco smoke and dementia. *Journal of the American Medical Association, 309* (7), 649.

46. Roberts, R. O., Cha, R. H., Mielke, M. M., Geda, Y. E., Boeve, B. F., et al. (2015). Risk and protective factors for cognitive impairment in persons aged 85 years and older. *Neurology, 84* (18), 1854–1861.

47. Tomioka, K., Kurumatani, N., & Hosoi, H. (2016). Relationship of having hobbies and a purpose in life with mortality, activities of daily living, and instrumental activities of daily living among community-dwelling elderly adults. *Journal of Epidemiology, 26* (7), 361–370.

48. Bak, T. H., Nissan, J. J., Allerhand, M. M., & Deary, I. J. (2014). Does bilingualism influence cognitive aging? *Annals of Neurology, 75* (6), 959–963.

49. Steptoe, A., Deaton, A., & Stone, A. A. (2015). Subjective wellbeing, health, and ageing. *Lancet, 385* (9968), 640–648.

50. Gawande, A. (2014). *Being mortal.* New York: Metropolitan Books.

51. Speece, M. W. (1995). Children's concepts of death. *Michigan Family Review, 15* (1), 1.

52. Howarth, G. (2011). Dying as a social relationship. In D. Oliviere, B. Monroe, & S. Payne (Eds.), *Death, dying, and social differences* (pp. 9–10). London: Oxford University Press.

53. Broom, A. (2016). *Dying: A social perspective on the end of life.* New York: Routledge.

54. Sleutjes, A., Moreira-Almeida, A., & Greyson, B. (2014). Almost 40 years investigating near-death experiences: An overview of mainstream scientific journals. *Journal of Nervous and Mental Disease, 201* (11), 833–836.

55. U.S. Department of Health and Human Services. (2015). *The need is real: Data.* www.organdonor.gov.

56. Reeves, J. (2016, April 26). Plan ahead: 64% of Americans don't have a will. *USA Today.* www.usatoday.com.

57. Hall, M. J., Levant, S., & DeFrances, C. J. (2013). *Trends in inpatient hospital deaths: National hospital discharge survey, 2000–2010* (NCSH Data Brief 118). Hyattsville, MD: National Center for Health Statistics.

58. National Hospice and Palliative Care Organization. (2015). *NHPCO's facts and figures: Hospice care in America, 2015 edition.* www.nhpco.org.

59. Tarzian, A. J., & ASBH Core Competencies Update Task Force. (2013). Health care ethics consultation: An update on core competencies and emerging standards from the American society of bioethics and humanities' core competencies update task force. *The American Journal of Bioethics, 13* (2), 3–13.

60. Stöppler, M. C. (2015, June). *Autopsy (post-mortem examination, necropsy).* www.medicinenet.com.

61. Maciejewski, P., Zhang, B., Block, S., & Prigerson, H. (2007). An empirical examination of the stage theory of grief. *Journal of the American Medical Association, 297* (7), 716–723.

62. Neimeyer, R.A. (2011). Reconstructing meaning in bereavement. *Rivista Psichiatria, 46* (5–6), 332–336.

63. Hibberd, R. (2013). Meaning reconstruction in bereavement: Sense and significance. *Death Studies, 37* (7), 670–692.

64. National Alliance for Grieving Children. (2013). About childhood grief. www.childrengrieve.org.

65. Allegra, J., Ezeamama, A., Simpson, C., & Miles, T. (2015). Population-level impact of loss on survivor mortality risk. *Quality of Life Research, 24* (12), 2959–2961.

66. Kübler-Ross, E. (1997). *On death and dying.* New York: Collier Books.

67. Byock, I. (2014). *The four things that matter most.* New York: Atria Books.

68. National Center for Education Statistics. (2015, May). *Table 303.40: Total fall enrollment in degree-granting postsecondary institutions, by attendance status, sex, and age: Selected years, 1970 through 2024.* http://nces.ed.gov.

69. Centers for Disease Control and Prevention. (2016, February 23). *Chronic disease overview.* www.cdc.gov

INDEX

Note: Page references in *italics* refer to figures and tables.

A

AARP (formerly the American Association of Retired Persons), 453
Abdominal aortic aneurysm, tobacco use and, 223
Abortion, 277–279, *279*
    legal status of, 279
    physical and psychological complications, 279
Absorption, alcohol, 209
Abstinence, 264, 304
    website, 289
Academic performance
    impediments to, 57
    sleep and, 80–81
Academic pressure, 59
Academy of Nutrition and Dietetics, 124, 179
Acamprosate, 218
Acceptable Macronutrient Distribution Range (AMDR), 110, *110*
Acceptance and commitment therapy (ACT), 43–44
Accessory glands, 258
Accidents, *5*, 377–381
Acetaldehyde, 209
Acetaminophen, 188
Acid rain, 408
Acquired immunity, 294
ACTH (adrenocorticotropin hormone), 53–54
Action, behavior change, 14
Active euthanasia, 445
Active immunity, 295
Actively Moving Forward, 448–449
Active Minds, 45
Active stretching, 139
Activity, physical
    aging and, 439
    cardiorespiratory fitness, 127
    diabetes, risk of, 127
    Dietary Guidelines for Americans, 114, 124
    fitness, components of, 127–128
    fitness training principles, 131–132
    flexibility, 128, 136, 139
    frequency recommendations, 142, 144
    muscular strength and endurance, 127–128, 135–139
    safety issues, 145–148
    weight management, 130
Acupuncture, *362*, *363*
Acute, defined, 3
Acyclovir, 308
Adaptation, 53
Adderall, 40, 82–83, 188, 189
Addiction
    behavioral, 183–184
    coping with, 195, 197
    defined, 182
    to technology, 183–184, *184*
    warning signs of, 183
Addictive behaviors. *See* Alcohol use and abuse
Additive interactions, 187
    drugs, 187
Adequate Intake (AI), 110
Administration on Aging, 453
Adoption, 286
Adult neurogenesis, 439
Adult-onset diabetes, 321
Advance directives, 444
Advertising, smoking and, 221, 222
Advocacy, 18
Aedes species mosquitoes, 302

Aerobic exercise, 132
Affordable Care Act, 11, 365, 366, 367, *367*, 368
African-Americans
    aging population, 431
    alcohol and tobacco use, 207
    cancer, 322, 338
    cardiovascular disease, 322
    diabetes, 322
    health disparities, 6
    HIV/AIDS and, 305
    hypertension, 9
    life expectancy, 432
    overweight and obesity, 162
    poverty, 322
    sexually transmitted infections, 310
    sleep, 82
    stress among, 61
    tobacco use, 207
Age
    alcohol and tobacco use, 207
    alcohol use and abuse, 216–217
    basal metabolic rate, 162
    cardiovascular disease, 334
    causes of death among people aged 15-24, *4*
    drug use, 184
    health and, 9
    infertility, 286
    sexually transmitted infections, 310
    stress and, 59
    tobacco use, 207, 220
    unintentional injuries, 377
    violent crime, 385
    weight gain and, 162
Ageism, 436
Agency for Healthcare Research and Quality (AHRQ), 336, 374
Age-related macular degeneration (AMD), 434, *434*
Aggravated assault, 385, 388
Aggressive driving, 379
Aging
    in Blue Zones, 439, 440
    body composition changes, 433, *433*
    campus advocacy, 448–449
    chronic disease, 434–435
    cognition and memory, 436–437
    current trends, 430, 431–433
    end-of-life issues, 441–443
    gender and longevity, 432–433
    grief, 447, *449*
    hearing loss, 433
    life expectancy, 431, 432
    personal choices, 448–449
    psychosocial changes, 437
    sexuality, 436
    statistics on, 430
    successful, tips for, 438–441
    trends in health and health care, 431–432
    in United States, 431–433, *431*
    vision loss, 433–434
    weight management, 439–440
Aging in place, 438
Agoraphobia, 37
AIDS, 8, *8*, 264, 292, 305–307
Airborne pathogens, 293
Air pollution, 340, 402, *402*, 405–411
    national efforts, 409–410
    personal choices, 409
Air Quality Index (AQI), 409–410
Alanon and Alateen, 232
Alarm stage, stress response, 53–54, *53*
Alcohol dehydrogenase (ADH), 209
Alcohol dependence, 216

Alcoholic cirrhosis, 213
Alcoholic hepatitis, 213
Alcoholics Anonymous, 218, 232
Alcohol intoxication, 211
Alcohol poisoning, 212, 215
Alcohol use and abuse, 66, 68, *68*
    abuse defined, 216
    age and, 210, 216–217
    alcohol, metabolizing, 209–210
    alcohol, metabolizing of, *210*
    alcoholism, 216–217
    behavioral effects, 214–215
    binge drinking on campus, 206–208
    blood alcohol concentration, 209–210, *211*
    burn injuries, 384
    campus advocacy, 219–220
    campus use statistics, 208
    chronic disease, 319, 347
    driving and, 214–215, 377–378
    effects on body, 211–213, *212*
    friends, 219
    gender and, 210, 216
    health benefits of alcohol, 214
    heart health, 335
    hypertension, 329
    injuries and, 377
    intoxication, 211
    makeup of alcohol, 208–209
    media and, 222
    neurological effects, 213–214
    older adults, 438
    peer pressure, 208, 219
    pregnancy, 213–214, 283
    prevention strategies, 218–220
    serving sizes, 209, *209*
    sexual violence, 214–215, 391, 392–393
    sleep and, 83, 89
    statistics, 205, 206
    treatment options, 217–218
    violent crime, 386–387
    why students drink, 208
Alcohol use disorders identification test (AUDIT), 217
Allergens, 297, 419
Allergic asthma, 297
Allergies, 96, *118*, 296–297
    food, 117–118
Alli diet drug, 168
Allopathic medicine, 358–360
Allostatic overload, 54
Alternative medicine, 362–364
Altruism, 31, *31*
Alzheimer's Association, 453
Alzheimer's disease (AD), 436, *436*
Ambien, 87
Amenorrhea, 262
American Academy of Family Physicians, 360
American Academy of Sleep Medicine, 87
American Academy of Sleep Medicine's Consumer Information Site, 94
American Association for Marriage and Family Therapy, 253
American Association of Poison Control Centers, 398
American Association of University Women, 396
American Cancer Society (ACS), 18, 221, 341, 348, 350
American College Health Association (ACHA), 7, 187, 229
American College of Sports Medicine (ACSM), 132, 142, *142*, 145, 152, 179
American Congress of Obstetricians and Gynecologists (ACOG), 257

I-1

American Council on Exercise, 152
American Diabetes Association, 348, 350
American Heart Association, 127, 329, 331, 348, 350
American Hospital Association, 361
American Lung Association, 224, 408
   Freedom from Smoking Online, 232
American Medical Association, 213
American Psychiatric Association (APA), 33, 37, 183, 187, 267
American Psychological Association, 49, 58, 72, 253, 279
   Active Minds, 45
   Psychologist Locator, 49
American Sexual Health Association, 316
American Society of Addiction Medicine, 182
Amino acids, 102
Amniotic fluid, 281
Amphetamines, 192, *192*, *196*
Anabolic steroids, 148
Anaerobic exercise, 135
Anal intercourse, 264, 306, 308
   See also Sexually transmitted infection
Anaphylactic shock, 118, 297
Anaphylaxis, 297
Andropause, 435–436
Androstenedione, 148
Aneurysm, 332
Anger, 32–33, *32*
Angina, 328, 330
   management, 331
Angina pectoris, 330
Angioplasty, 331
Animals, infections from, 293, 301, 303
Anorexia athletica, 175
Anorexia nervosa, 172–174, *173*
Antagonistic interactions, drugs, 187
Antibiotic resistance, 299
Antibodies, 294
Anticonvulsant medications, 37
Antidepressant medications, 35–36, 38, 435
Antigens, 294
Antioxidants, 107, *107*
Antiretroviral drugs, 307
Anxiety, procrastination, 60
Anxiety and Depression Association of America, 49
Anxiety disorders, 25, 37–38
   stress and, 56, 57
Apgar score, 285
Aphasia, 332
Appetite, 164–165
Apple-shaped fat patterning, 156, *156*
Arable land, 404
Arrhythmia, 330, 331
Arsenic, 412
Arteries, 326, 328, *328*
   See also Cardiovascular disease
Arthritis, 434
Artificially acquired immunity, 295
Artificial sweeteners, 169
Asbestos, 419
Asbestosis, 419
Asian Americans
   aging population, 431
   alcohol and tobacco use, 207
   cancer, 322
   cardiovascular disease, 322
   diabetes, 322
   health disparities, 6
   life expectancy, 432
   overweight and obesity, 162
   poverty, 322
   sexually transmitted infections, 310
   sleep, 82
   tobacco use, 207
Assault, 388
Assertiveness, 27
Association for the Advancement of Sustainability in Higher Education (AASHE), 424
Assortative mating, 242
Asthma, 223, 297
   exercise choices, 149

Atherosclerosis, 159, 327–328, *328*
   tobacco use, 223
Athletes. *See also* Exercise
   ergogenic aids, 109
   nutrition needs, 110, 145
   performance-enhancing drugs, 148
Athletic shoes, 146, *146*
Atkins, Robert, 167
Atkins diet, 165, *165*
Atria, 326, *327*
Attachment theory, 238
Attention deficit hyperactivity disorder (ADHD), 39–40, 188, 189
Attention disorders, 39–40
Attraction, 242
Autism, 296
Automated external defibrillator (AED), 331, 333
Autonomy, 27, *27*
Autopsy, 446
Aversion therapy, 43
Avian influenza, 293
Ayurveda, 66, *363*

B

BACCHUS Network, 220
Back extension, *138*
Back injuries, 384, 385
Bacteria, *298*, 299
   foodborne illness, 117
   infections from, 293
Bacterial infection
   chlamydia, 285
   gonorrhea, 264
   HIV/AIDs, *306*
   immunizations, 294–296
   Lyme disease, 301, *301*
   meningitis, 300
   overview of, 299–300
   pelvic inflammatory disease, 285, 309–311
   pneumonia, 301
   Staphylococcus, 300
   Streptococcus, 301
   syphilis, 311
   tuberculosis, 292, 301, 306
Ballistic stretching, 139
Bandura, Albert, 16
Barbiturates, 194, *196*
Bariatric surgery, 168, 325
Basal metabolic rate (BMR), 161–162
Bath salts, 192
B cells, 294, 306
Behavioral addictions, 183
Behavior change
   building, 16–17, *17*
   factors related to, 13
   models of, 14–15
Behavior-change contract, 18, 21–22
   improving your sleep, 91–93
   stress overload, 69–70
Behavior therapy, 43
Beliefnet, 49
Belviq, 168
Benign tumors, 338
Benzene, tobacco, 223
Benzodiazepines, 38, 194–195
Beta-carotene, 107
Beta cells, 320
Beverages
   caffeine content of, *191*
   pollutants in, 416–417
Bianchi, Suzanne, 249
Biceps curl, *137*
Bicycle accidents, 381
Bicycling, 132, *134*, 149
Bidis, 225–226, *226*
Binge drinking, 206–208
   See also Alcohol use and abuse
Binge eating disorder, 174
Biofeedback, 38, 44

Biofuels, 410
Biologic therapy, 346
Biology, health and, 9
Biomagnification, 418, *418*
Biomonitoring, 419
Biopsy, 340
Biotin, *105*
Bipolar disorder, 25, 36–37
Birth control, 269–276, *276*, *277*
   cost-free methods, *270*, 272–273
   methods available by prescription, *271–272*, 274–276
   over-the-counter methods, *270*, 273–274
   summary of methods, *270–273*
   surgical methods, *272*, 276
Birth control pills, *271*, 275–276, *276*
Bisexuality, 243, 268
Bisphenol A, 418–419
Blastocyst, 281
Blended families, 249
Blood alcohol concentration (BAC), 206, 209–210, 211, 214, 378
   intoxication, 211
Blood glucose, 334
   See also Diabetes
Blood glucose monitors, 355
Blood lipids, 334, *335*
   overweight and, 159
Blood pressure, 327, *329*, 334
   screenings, *357*
Blood pressure kits, 355
Blue Zones, aging in, 439, 440
Boating accidents, 383
Body, The: The Complete HIV/AIDS Resource, 316
Body burden, 419
Body composition, 128, 157
Body dysmorphic disorder (BDD), 171–172
Body image
   defined, 155
   disorders, 171–172
   factors related to, 155–156
   positive, developing, 176
   support and, 172, 175
Body language, 236, *236*
Body mass index (BMI), 156, *157*, 158, 325
Body measurements, 156
Body weight
   healthful, defining, 156–157
   statistics, 154
   websites, 179
   weight trends, 158–159
Bone-building medications, 435
Borrelia burgdorferi, 301
Botanicals, 362, *363*
Botanical supplements, 109
Bottled water, 104, 413
Botulism, 117
BPA, 418–419
Bradycardia, 330
Brain
   cancer in, *341*
   cell phone and, 423
   drugs and effects on, 186
Brain death, 442
Brain fitness, 441
Brain stem, sleep and, 75, *76*
Braxton Hicks contractions, 281
BRCA1 gene, 344, 370
BRCA2 gene, 344, 370
Breast cancer, 130, 212–213, 338, 370
   See also Cancer
Bronchitis, tobacco use and, 223
Bronchoconstriction, 297
Bruxism, 85
Build-Your-Budget Worksheet, 72
Built environment, 10, 164, 401
Bulimia nervosa, 175
Bupropion, 228, 229
Burial, 446
Burn injuries, 384

Burnout, 54
Byock, Ira, *448*

C

Caffeinated alcoholic beverages (CABs), 213
Caffeine, 52, 82, 89, 90, 105–106, 191, *191*
    pregnancy, 283
Calcium, 104, *105*
Calendar method, *270*, 272, 272–273, *273*
California Health Care Foundation, 365
Calories. *See also* Energy
    defined, 97
    dietary guidelines, 114
    empty, 115
    energy and, 97
    healthful weight gain diet, 169–170, *170*
    reducing, 169
    sweetened beverages, *107*
    weight gain, causes of, 163
    weight-loss diets, 166
Campus Men of Strength Clubs, 396
Campus Pride, 251
Campylobacter, 117
Cancer
    activity, benefits of, 130
    aging and, 434, 440
    alcohol abuse, 212–213
    breast cancer, 344–345, 370
    colorectal cancer, 342–343
    defined, 338
    detecting, 340–341
    excess body weight and, 160
    lung cancer, 342, *342*, 419
    oral cancer, 343, *343*
    ovarian cancer, 345
    overview of, 337–338
    pancreatic cancer, 343
    progression of, *339*
    prostate cancer, 344
    risk factors for, 338, 340
    skin cancer, 341–342, *342*
    statistics on, 318, *337*
    survival rates for, 319
    testicular cancer, 344
    tobacco use and, 223
    treating, 346
    types of, 341
    uterine cancer, 345–346
    websites, 350
Cancer screenings, *357*
Candida albicans, 303
Cannabis, *196*
Cannon, Walter B., 52, 54
Capillaries, 326–327
Carbohydrates, 98–100, *99*
    complex, 98, *99*
    defined, 98
    fiber, 99
    glycemic index, 99–100
    low-carbohydrate diets, 167
    recommended intake, 100
    simple, 98
    whole grains, 99, *99*
Carbon dioxide, 407, *407*
Carbon emissions, 403
Carbon footprint, 407
Carbon monoxide (CO), 221, 223, 404, 419
Carcinogenic, smoking and, 221
Carcinogens, 338, *339*, 340
    reducing environmental risks, 347
Carcinomas, 341
Cardiac rehabilitation, 331
Cardiometabolic risk (CMR), 160, 319, 336–337, *337*, 346–347, *347*
Cardiomyopathy, alcohol use, 213
Cardiorespiratory fitness, 127, 130, 132
Cardiovascular disease (CVD). *See also* Cardiovascular system
    aging and, 434, 439–440

alcohol use, 213
    forms of, 328, *328*, 329–336
    overview of, 326
    physical inactivity and, 127
    risk factors for, 319, 326, 334–336
    saturated fats and, 101
    statistics, 318, *329*
    tobacco use and, 223
Cardiovascular system, *327*
    chronic stress, 55
    normal functions, 326–327
    target heart rate, 132
    tobacco use and, 223
Caring Connections, 453
Carotenoids, 107
Carpal tunnel syndrome (CTS), 384–385
Carrier, infection transmission, 292
Carrying capacity, 404
Carson, Rachel, 402
Cataracts, *434*
Cathinone, 192
Caucasians
    alcohol and tobacco use, 207
    alcohol use, 206
    cancer, 322
    cardiovascular disease, 322
    diabetes, 322
    health disparities, 6
    life expectancy, 432
    overweight and obesity, 162
    poverty, 322
    sleep, 82
    suicide, 41
    tobacco use, 207
Cause, defined, 5
CD4 T cells, 306
Celibacy, 264
Cell phones, 62, 378, *378*, 415, 423
    preventing tech injuries, 386
Cellular death, 442
Center for Effective Government, 417
Center for Public Integrity, 394
Center for Science in the Public Interest, 124
Center for Young Women's Health, 316
Centers for Disease Control and Prevention (CDC), 5, 23, 79, 164, 226, 229, 232, 264, 293, 295, 316, 350
    websites, 179, 427
Central Intelligence Agency (CIA), 389
Central nervous system cancers, 341
Central obesity, 162
Central sleep apnea, 84
Cerebral cortex, 75
Cerebrovascular accident, 332
Cerebrum, sleep and, 75, *76*
Cervarix, 309
Cervical cancer, 257, 309, 340, 345–346
Cervical cap, *271*, 275
Cervical mucus, 260
Cesarean section (C-section), 285
Chain of infection, 292, *292*
Chamomile, 88
Chancre, syphilis, 311, *311*
Chantix, 228
Checkups, medical, 357
Chemical imbalance theory, of mental disorders, 33
Chemoprevention, 345
Chemotherapy, 346
Chewing tobacco, 226
Chickenpox, 295
Childbearing age, 257
Childbirth, 284–285, *284*
Children, 225, 248–249
    body image, 155
    choking incidents, 382
    grief in, 447
China
    air pollution, 402, *402*
    "one child policy," 405

Chinese medicine, traditional, 362
Chiropractic medicine, 362, *363*
Chlamydia, 285, 309, *311*
Chlamydia trachomatis, 309
Chlorofluorocarbons (CFCs), 408
Choking, 382–383, *383*
Cholera, 8
Cholesterol, 100, 328
    healthy diet, 166–167
    home tests, 355
ChooseMyPlate.gov, 113, *115*
Choose This, Not That
    conflict resolution, 237
    exercise vs. alcohol, 68
    fitness level, 129
    healthful *vs.* high-fat lunch, 116
    healthy food choices, 172
    safe driving, 380
Chromium picolinate, 148
Chromosomes, 370
    defined, 9, *9*, 370
Chronic, defined, 3
Chronic disease. *See also* Cancer; Cardiovascular disease (CVD); Diabetes
    aging and, 431–432, 434–435, 439–440
    campus advocacy, 348
    cardiometabolic risk factors for, 319
    defined, 319
    diversity and disparities in, 322
    four key behaviors, 319–320
    management of, 356
    overview of, 319–320
    personal choices, 346–348
    risk factors for, 319
    self-care, 356
    sleep difficulties and, 79
    statistics, 319
    supporting friends with, 346, 348
    websites, 350
Chronic obstructive pulmonary disease (COPD), 223
Chronic severe subtype alcoholism, 217
Chronic stress, health effects, 55–57, *55*
Cigars/cigarettes
    aging and, 439, 441
    chemical contents, 221
    forms of, 225–226, *226*
    "light" cigarettes, 225
Cilia, 293
Circadian rhythm, 75
Circumcision, 258, *258*, 259
Cirrhosis, liver, 213
Civil Rights Act of 1964, 391
Clean Air Act of 1963, 410
Cleaning products, environmentally friendly, 416
Climate change, 402, *403*, 406–407
    choosing to combat, 409
    statistics, 400
Clinical death, 442
Clitoris, 256, *257*
Clostridium botulinum, 117
Clothing, physical activity, 146
Clove cigarettes, 225, *226*
Club drugs, 193–194, *196*
COBRA, 369
Cocaine, 191, *192*, *196*
    See also Drug use and abuse
Cochlear hair cells, 420
Codeine, 188, 361
Cognition, aging and, 436–437, 442
Cognitive-behavioral therapy (CBT), 38, 42–43, 87–88
Cognitive distortion, 43
Cohabitation, 246
Coitus, 264
Coitus interruptus, 273
Colds, 298
Cold virus, 292
College and University Food Bank Alliance, 121

Colon cancer, alcohol use, 213
Colonoscopy, 340
Colorectal cancer, 130, 338, 342–343
    home tests, 355
Columbine High School, Colorado, shooting at, 388
Commitment, 240, *240*
Communication skills
    relationships and, 235–238, *236*
    sex, communication about, 277
    social media, 241
Compact fluorescent light bulbs, 409
Companionate love, 240, *240*, 242
Complementary and alternative medicine (CAM), 88, 362–364
    defined, 362
    evaluating therapies, *363–364*, 364
    types of, *363–364*
Complementary medicine, 362
Complete proteins, 102
Complex carbohydrates, 97, 99
Compliance, blood pressure and, 328
Composting, 415
Comprehensive Environmental Response and Liability Act, 415–416
Compulsive spending, 183
Comstock Act, 279
Conception, 268–269
Concerta, 40, 189
Condoms, 264, *270*, 274, *275*, 276, 308, 312
    female, *270*, 274 *275*
    male, *270*, 274, *274*
Conflict avoidance, 236
Conflict escalation, 236–237
Conflict Management Information Source, 253
Conflict resolution, 236, 237
Congeners, 212
Congenital heart disease, 334
Consumer Corner
    athletic shoes, 146
    beverages, 107
    bottled water, 413
    choosing a therapist, 43
    "light" cigarettes, 225
    organic, local, all natural, and fair trade choices, 119
    over-the-counter medications, 356
    sleep aids, 88
Consumer health
    being smart patient, 360–361
    checkups and preventive care, 357
    defined, 353
    emergency situations, 357, 358
    genomics, 369–371
    herbal and dietary supplements, 362
    home health tests, 355, *355*
    information sources, evaluating, 354–355
    paying for care, 364–369
    personal choices, 371
    physicians, when to seek help, 356–358
    providers, choosing, 360
    providers, complementary and alternative medicine, 362–364, *363–364*, 364
    providers, conventional, 359–360
    screenings, recommended, *357–358*
    self-care, defined, 353
    self-care, 353–356
    statistics, 352
    vaccinations, 357, *357–358*
    website evaluation, 354
    websites, 374
Consummate love, *240*, 242
Contaminated objects, infections from, 293
Contemplation, behavior change, 14
Continuation rate, birth control, 276
Contraception, 269–276, *275*, 276, 287, 405
    summary of methods, 270, *270–273*
Contraceptive sponge, *270*, 274
Conventional health care, finding, 359–360
Conventional medicine, 358–360
Cool-down, physical activity, 145
Copays, medical services, 365

Core muscle strength, building, 135
Coronary angiography, 331
Coronary arteries
    atherosclerosis, 328
    coronary heart disease, 329–331
    normal function, 326–327
Coronary artery bypass grafting (CABG), 331
Coronary artery disease, 329–331
Coronary heart disease (CHD), 329–331
    angina, 330
    clinical management of, 331, 334
    excess body weight and, 159
    sudden cardiac arrest, 330–331
    tobacco use and, 223
Coronaviruses, 298
Corpus luteum, 260
Cortisol, 54
Cotinine, 224
Counselors, 42
Counter-conditioning, 18
Cowper's glands, 258, *258*
CPAP machine, sleep apnea, 84, *84*
CPR, 331, 333
Crack, 191
Cramps, 147
Craving, drug addiction, 182, 183, 187
C-reactive protein (CRP), 335
Creatine, 148
Credit card debt, 60
Cremation, 446
Crossfit, 135
Crystal meth, 192
Cue control, 18
Cues to action, behavior change, 14
Cunnilingus, 264
Curl-up, *138*
Cyber-bullying, 241
Cyberstalking, 390–391
Cycle of violence, 390
Cytokines, *294*
Cytotoxic T cells, 294

D

Dairy foods, 115
Danger zone, food-borne illness, 117
DASH diet, 328
Date (acquaintance) rape, 392
Date rape drugs, 194, *194*, 392–393, *392*
Dating, 242–243
Day of the Dead, Mexico, 443, *443*
DDT, 402
Death
    definitions of, 441–443
    developing concepts of, 443
    end-of-life issues, 444–446
    grief, 447
    leading causes of, 1, 4, 7
Decibels, noise pollution, 421, *421*
Deductibles, health care, 365
Deep breathing, 67
Deforestation, 407
Dehydration, 211
Dehydroepiandrosterone, 148
Delusions, 40
Dementia, 436
Dental hygiene, *353*
    screening, *357*
Dentists, 359
Department of Homeland Security, 389
Dependence, drugs, 187
Depressants, 194–195, *196*
Depression, 25, 57, 79, 81
    older adults, 438
Depressive disorders, 34–35
Destructive thoughts, 44
Determinants of health, 8–12
    biology and genetics, 9, *9*
    individual behaviors, 9–10
    physical determinants, 10–11
    social determinants, 10

Detroiters Working for Environmental Justice (DWEJ), 424
Diabetes, 56
    chronic disease, overview, 320–326
    chronic stress and, 324
    clinical management of, 325
    complications of, 323–324, *323*
    detecting, 323
    diabetes mellitus, 320
    excess body weight and, 159, 324
    exercise and, 325
    exercise choices, 149
    managing, 356
    overweight, 324
    statistics, 318
    types of, 320–323
    websites, 350
Diabetic retinopathy, 323
Diagnostic and Statistical Manual of Mental Disorders (DSM), 33
Diaphragm, *271*, 275, *275*
Diastolic pressure, 328
Diencephalon, sleep and, 75, *76*
Diet. *See also* Nutrients; Weight management
    chronic disease and, 347
    complex carbohydrates, 99
    cutting calories, *167*
    defined, 97
    diabetes, 324
    drug addiction, 199
    for healthful weight gain, *170*
    healthy food choices, 172
    heart health, 335
    low-calorie, 166
    low-sodium, 329
    popular, *165–166*
    premenstrual syndrome, 261
    stress and, 65
    vegetarian, 111
    weight-loss, 166–167
Dietary Guidelines for Americans, 113, 114, 124, 329
Dietary Reference Intakes (DRIs), 110, *110*
Dietary supplements, 106–109, 108–109, 362
    guidelines, 109
Diethylpropion, 168
Dieting, on campus, 160
Diet pills, 167–168
Digestive system
    digestive process, *98*
    stress response, 55–56
Dilation and evacuation (D&E), 278
Diminishing returns, in physical activity, 132
Dioxins, 411–412, 412–413
Diphtheria, *295*
Disease
    definition of, 2
    health *vs.*, 2–3
Disease prevention, defined, 5
Disordered eating, 174
Disorganized thinking, 40
Dissociative drug, 193
Distillation, 208–209
Distracted driving
    motor vehicle accidents, 378
    statistics, 376
    texting, 378, *378*
Distress, 52
Distribution half-life, drugs, 187
Disulfiram, 218
Diuretics, 329
Diversity & Health
    aging in the Blue Zones, 439, 440
    alcohol and tobacco use, 207
    chronic disorders, 322
    drug use and overdose, 185
    health disparities among groups, 6
    heart disease, 322
    injuries and violence, 387
    safe exercise for special populations, 149
    same-sex marriage, 247

sexually transmitted infection, 310
sleep, 82
stress in minority populations, 61
tobacco use, 207
vegetarian diets, 111
working for environmental justice, 417
Divided attention, 377
Divorce, 247
DNA (deoxyribonucleic acid), 9, *9*, 269, 338, 369
Doctors of osteopathic medicine (D.O.s), 359
Dodson, John, 54
Domestic partnerships, 248
Domestic violence, 389
Do Not Resuscitate (DNR) order, 444
Dopamine, 33, 186, 190, 191
  tobacco use, 221
Doula, 284
Dreaming sleep, 76, 77, *77*
Driving
  alcohol use and, 214–215
  drowsy, 79, 81
  texting and, 378, *378*
Drought, 407
Drowning, 377, 383–384
Drowsiness, 76
Drug Enforcement Agency (DEA), 184
Drugs
  defined, 184
  misuse, defined, 186
  overdose rates, *185*
Drugs of Abuse Information, 203
Drug testing, 195
Drug use and abuse
  abuse and misuse defined, 186
  amphetamines, 192
  body response to, 186–187
  caffeine, 191, *191*
  campus advocacy, 200
  cardiovascular disease, 335
  club drugs, 193–194
  cocaine, 191, *192*
  commonly abused drugs, 187–195, *196*
  common methods of drug administration, *186*
  date rape drugs, 194, *194*
  depressants, 194–195
  hallucinogens, 193
  heroin, *196*
  how drugs leave the body, 187
  inhalants, 194
  injuries and, 377
  LSD, 193
  marijuana, 190–191, *190*
  MDMA (ecstasy), 193–194
  methamphetamine, 192, *192*
  older adults, 438
  overview of addiction, 182
  PCP, 193
  personal choices, 198–199
  prescription and over-the-counter medications, 187–188
  prevention and treatment, 195, 197
  statistics on, 181, 182
  stimulants, 82–83, 191–192
  "study drugs," 189
  violent crime, 386–387
  websites, 203
Durable power of attorney for health care, 444
DWI, 214–215
Dynamic flexibility, 136, 139
Dynamic muscular endurance, 128
Dynamic stretching, 139
Dyslipidemia, 334
Dysmenorrhea, 261
Dysphoria, 261
Dysthymic disorder, 34

E

Early-onset Alzheimer's, 436
Ears

aging, hearing loss, 433
noise pollution, 420–421
Eartheasy Non-Toxic Home Cleaning, 427
Eating disorders, 172–174, *173*
  amenorrhea and, 262
  anorexia nervosa, *134*, 172–174
  bulimia nervosa, 174
  getting help for, 173–174, *175*
  sleep-related, 86
Eat Right for Your Type diet, *165*
Ebola virus, 7–8
ECG (EKG), 331
Echocardiogram, 331
E-cigarettes, 226, *227*
Ecological footprint, 404
Ecological models, behavior change, 14–15, *15*
Ecosystem, 400, 401
Ecstasy, club drugs, 193–194, *196*
Ectopic pregnancy, 283, 309
Education level
  alcohol and tobacco use, 207
Edwards, John, 189
Effacement, 284
Ejaculation, premature, 263
Ejaculatory duct, 258
EKG, 331
Electricity usage, 409
Electric vehicles (EVs), 411
Electrocardiogram (ECG or EKG), 331
Electroconvulsive therapy (ECT), 44
Electroencephalograph (EEG), 75
Electrolytes, 145
Electromagnetic spectrum, 422
Electronic cigarettes, 226, *227*
Ella prescription-only emergency contraception, 274, 275–276
Embryo, development of, 281, *282*
Emergency contraception (EC), *270*, *271*, 274, 275–276
Emergency response, cardiac events, 333
Emotional abuse, 389
Emotional health. *See also* Psychological health
  chronic disease and, 347
  defined, 26
  heart health, 335
  premenstrual dysphoric disorder, 261
  premenstrual syndrome, 261
  schizophrenia, 40
  stress and, 67
Emotional intelligence (EI), 29
Emphysema, tobacco use and, 223
Employment, aging and, 438
Empty calories, 115
Empty love, 240, *240*
Empty nest syndrome, 437
Enabling factors, behavior, 13
Endocrine disruptors, 412–413
End-of-life issues, 444–446
Endometrial cancer, 345–346
Endometriosis, 261–262, 285
Endometrium, 257
Endorphins, 199
Energy, calories and, 97–98
Energy balance, 161, *161*
Energy consumption, reducing, 409
Energy drinks, 106
Energy therapies, 362, *364*
Enteric nerves, 55
Environment, defining, 401–402
Environmental health, 4, *4*
  air pollution, 405–410, *410*
  campus advocacy, 424
  defined, 401
  evolution of, 402–403
  as global concern, 402
  land pollution, 414–416
  noise pollution, 420–421
  overpopulation, 403–405
  overview, 400–403
  personal choices, 424

pollution at home, 416–420
population growth, *403*, *404*
radiation, 422–423, *422*
statistics, 400
sustainability, 403
trash, 400
water pollution, 411–414, *414*
websites, 427
Environmental justice, 417, *417*
Environmental mastery, 27–28, *27*
Environmental Protection Agency (EPA), 118, 402, 409, 414, 417
  website, 427
Environmental stressors, 62
Environmental tobacco smoke, 224
Environmental Working Group, 427
Enzyme immunoassay (EIA), 306
Ephedra, 148
Epididymis, 258, *258*
Epstein-Barr virus, 299
Erectile dysfunction (ED), 263
Erection, 258
Ergogenic aids, 109
Escherichia coli (E. coli), 117
Essential fatty acids (EFAs), 101
Estate, 444
Estimated Average Requirement (EAR), 110
Estimated Energy Requirement (EER), 110
Estrogen, 275, 345, 434
Ethanol, 208
  See also Alcohol use and abuse
Ethics, genomics and, 371
Ethnicity
  alcohol and tobacco use, 207
  chronic disease, 322
  health, 9
  health disparities, 322
  life expectancy, 432
  pollution burden, 417
  sleep, 82
  stress and, 61
  suicide, 41
  tobacco use, 207
  weight gain, 162
Ethyl alcohol, 208
  See also Alcohol use and abuse
Eudemonic well-being, 441
Eustress, 52
Euthanasia, active and passive, 445–446
Evaluating Online Sources of Health Information, 374
Evidence-based medicine, 354, 358
e-waste, 415, *416*
Excitement phase, human sexual response cycle, 262
Exercise, 45, 67, *67*, 114
  See also Physical activity
  ACSM guidelines, *142*
  aerobic, 132, 134
  aging and, 439, *439*, 440
  anaerobic, 135
  benefits of, 129–130
  body composition and, 128
  cancer, reducing risk of, 340, *340*
  cardiorespiratory fitness and, 127, 131, 132
  chronic disease, preventing, 347
  defined, 127
  diabetes, management of, 325
  diabetes, risk of, 324
  fitness training principles and, 131–132, *131*
  flexibility, 128, 136, 139
  frequency recommendations, 142, 144
  goal setting, 149
  heart health, 335
  intensity levels, *134*
  isometric and isotonic, 135–136
  menopause and, 435
  muscular strength and endurance, 127–128, 135–139, 139
  nutrition and, 114

Exercise (cont.)
  personal choices, 148–150
  pregnancy, 283
  safety issues, 145–148
  for special populations, 149
  stress and, 65–66, 66
  websites, 152
  weight gain, causes of, 163
  weight loss and, 169
Exhaustion stage, stress response, 53, 54
Exposure therapy, 38, 43
External locus of control, 17
Eye contact, 236
Eyes
  aging and, 433–434
  cataracts, 433
  diabetes, 323

F

Facebook, 60, 234, 241
  older adults, 430
Failure rate, birth control, 276
Fair trade, 119
Fallopian tubes, 257, 257, 285
Falls, 377
Family health history, 9, 370
  preventing chronic disease, 347
Family life
  aging and, 437
  choosing children, 249
  happy families, characteristics, 250
  single parenthood, 249
  stepfamilies, 249
Fantasy, sexual, 265
Fasting blood glucose test (FBG), 323
Fatigue, 379
Fats, dietary, 100–103
  consumption statistics, 96
  as food lipids, 101
  "good," 167
  healthful, 102, 169
  recommended intake of, 101–102
  saturated, 101
  trans fats, 101, 102, 166–167
  unsaturated, 101
Fat soluble, 416
Fat-soluble vitamins, 103, 104–105
"Fat Studies," 171
Fatty acids, 101
Fatty liver, 213
Fatty liver disease, 160
Fatuous love, 240, 242
Federal Bureau of Investigation (FBI), 385, 389
Federal Uniform Drinking Age Act (FUDAA), 206
Fee-for-service plans, 366
Fellatio, 264
Female athlete triad, 175
Female sexual anatomy, 256–258, 257
Fermentation, 208
Fertility, 160, 249, 273
Fertility awareness method, 270, 272–273, 273
Fertility drugs, 286
Fertility rate, 404, 405
Fertilization, 269, 269
Fetal alcohol syndrome, 214
Fetal development, 281, 282
Fetus, 281
Fiber, dietary, 99, 108, 343
Fibrillation, 330
Fight-or-flight response, 53, 53, 54
Financial stressors, 59, 60
Fire injuries, 384, 384
First Response Early Result Pregnancy Test, 280
Fitness apps, 147
FITT principle, 131, 131
Flat affect, 40
Flavonoids, 107
Flexibility, 128, 136, 139
Flexible spending accounts (FSAs), 368
Flexitarians, 111

Flint, Michigan water supply, 412, 417
Fluid balance, 438
Fluorescent light bulbs, 409
Fluoride, 104
Flu shots, 357
Folic acid, 103
Follicle-stimulating hormone (FSH), 260
Food
  allergies, 118
  caffeine content of, 191
  groups, 115
  intolerances, 118
  labels, 111–113, 112, 113
  pollutants in, 416–417
  residues, 118
  supply, safety of, 116–117
Food addictions, 100
Food allergies, 117–118
Food and Drug Administration (FDA), 5, 35, 101, 109, 113, 116, 124, 148, 166, 168, 188, 226, 275, 278, 289, 355, 418
Foodborne illness, 116–117
"Food insecurity–obesity paradox," 163
Food poisoning, 116–117
Foodsafety.gov, 124
Forcible rape, 385
Foreplay, 264
Foreskin, 258, 258, 259
Fossil fuels, 405, 407
Fractures, osteoporosis and, 434
Freebase cocaine, 191
Free radicals, 107
Frequency, FITT principle, 131, 131
Freud, Sigmund, 26, 29, 43
Friedman, Meyer, 57
Friendships, 45, 171, 239–240, 239, 395–396
  See also Relationships
Fructose, 98
Fruits, 107, 107, 115
Fuel economy, 410
Functional death, 442
Functional foods, 106
Functional subtype, alcoholism, 217
Funerals, 446
Fungal infections, 303
Fungi, 298, 303
Fusion inhibitors, 307

G

Galactose, 98
Gallbladder disease, 160
Gambling, pathological, 183
Games, high-tech, 442
Gamete intrafallopian transfer (GIFT), 286
Garbage, 414–415
Garbage patch in ocean, 413
Gardasil, 309
Gastric banding, 168
Gastric bypass, 168
Gastroesophageal reflux disease (GERD), 81–82
Gastrointestinal system, alcohol, effects of, 211
Gay people, 41, 243
Gender
  alcohol and tobacco use, 207
  alcohol use and abuse, 210, 216
  body image, 155
  building muscle, 128, 128
  cardiovascular disease, 334
  communication and, 237–238
  death and dying, 443
  defined, 6
  depressive disorders, 35
  drug use, 185
  generalized anxiety disorder, 37
  health, 9
  heart attacks, 330
  longevity, 432–433
  mental health, 35
  roles, relationships and, 238–239
  sexually transmitted infections, rates of, 310

  sleep, 82
  stress and, 54–55, 58–59
  tobacco use, 207
  violent crime, 385
  weight gain, 162
Gender dysphoria, 268
Gender expression, 268
Gender identity, 268
Gender identity disorder, 268
Gender transition, 268
Gene, defined, 9
General adaptation syndrome (GAS), 53, 53
Generalized anxiety disorder (GAD), 37
Genes
  cancer and, 338
  defined, 370
Genetically modified foods, 119
Genetic counselor, 370
Genetic factors
  Alzheimer's disease, 436
  bipolar disorder, 36–37
  cancer, 338, 340
  cardiovascular disease, 334
  depressive disorders, 34–35
  diabetes, risk of, 324
  genomics, 369–371, 370
  health and, 9, 9
  schizophrenia, 40
  sleep patterns, 81
  weight gain, 162
Genetic Information Nondiscrimination Act (GINA), 371
Genetics Home Reference, 374
Genetic variants, 370
Genital herpes, 308, 308
Genitals, 256
Genome, defined, 9, 369
Genome sequencing, 370
Genomics, 369–371, 370
  defined, 369
  targeted testing, 370
  uses of information, 370–371
Geography
  alcohol and tobacco use, 207
  drug use, 185
  tobacco use, 207
Germ theory of disease, 402
Gestational diabetes, 321
GHB (gamma-hydroxybutyric acid), 194, 196, 215
Glaucoma, 433, 434
Globalization, 404
Global warming, 406
"Globesity," 8
Glucose, 53, 98, 100, 320
Glucose monitoring, 325
Gluteal stretch, 141
Glycated hemoglobin test (A1C test), 323
Glycemic index, 99–100
Glycogen, 98
Glyphosate (RoundUp), 413
Goal setting, 16
Go Ask Alice, 23, 253, 289
Gonorrhea, 264, 285, 309, 311
Google Plus, 241
Grains, 115
"Granny pods," 437
Granovetter, Mark, 250
Great American Condom Campaign (GACC), 287
Green burials, 446
Greenhouse effect, 406
Greenhouse gases, 406, 410
Grief, 447, 449
Ground-level ozone, 407
Groundwater, 411
Growth hormone, 76
Guillain-Barré syndrome, 302
Gum disease, diabetes and, 324
Gummas, 311
Guns, 386

H

H1N1 flu pandemic, 299
Habits, 1, 353–354, *353*
  See also Self-Assessment
Hallucinations, 40
Hallucinogens, 192–193, *196*
Hamstrings stretch, *141*
Hand washing, 117, 293
Hand washing and hand sanitizers, 303
Hangover, 211–212
Hardiness, 58
Hate crimes, 389
Hazardous waste, 415–416
Hazing, 388
HDL, 166
Headaches, stress and, 56
Health
  across America, 4–6
  aging and trends in, 431–432
  care paying for, 364–369
  definitions of, 2–3
  determinants of, 8–12
  disease *vs.*, 2–3
  global, 7–8
  keys to, *5*
  older adults, statistics, 430
  trends in, 432
  wellness and, dimensions of, 3–4, *4*
  wellness *vs.*, 3
Health belief model, 14
Health-care directive, 444
Health-care proxy, 444
Health discount program, 365
Health disparities, 6
Health equity, 6
Health exchanges, state, 367
Healthful weight, 156
Health history, 9
  weight gain and, 162–163
Health information
  accurate, 354–355
  in media, evaluating, 12
Health insurance, 11, 322, 360
  defined, 365
  statistics, 352
  for students, 368
  youth, 352
Health insurance exchanges, 367
Health insurance marketplaces, 367
Health literacy, 11
Health maintenance organizations (HMOs), 365–366
Health promotion, defined, 5
Health-related fitness, 127
  See also Exercise; Physical fitness
Health-related quality of life, 319
Health savings accounts (HSAs), 368
Health services, access to, 11
Healthy Campus Initiative, 7
Healthy Hunger-Free Kids Act, 164
Healthy People Initiative, 5–6
  defined, 5
Hearing loss, 420–421, 433
Heart, 326, *327*
  activity, benefits of, 129–130
  cardiorespiratory fitness, 127, 131
  normal cardiovascular function, 327–328
  target heart rate, 132, *133*
Heart attack, 323, 326, 330, 331, 333
  warning signs of, *330*
Heart disease, 55, 329
  excess body weight and, 159
  genomes and, 370
  omega-3 and omega-6 fatty acids, 101
  sleep difficulties and, 79
  tobacco use and, 223
  trans fats and, 101
Heart failure, 331–332
Heart valve disorders, 334
Heat exhaustion, 146

Heatstroke, 146
Heavy episodic drinking, 206
Heavy metals, 415
Helicobacter pylori, 56, 340
Helmets, 381, 382
Helminths, 304
Helper T cells, 294, 306
Hemorrhagic stroke, 332, *332*
Hepatitis, 213, 299
Hepatitis A, *295*, 299
Hepatitis B, 264, *295*, 307, 340
  vaccine, *358*
Hepatitis C, 299, 340
Herbal supplements, 362
Herbicides, 413
Herbs, 109
Herd immunity, 296
Heroin, 188, 190, *196*
  See also Drug use and abuse
Herpes, genital, 308, *308*
Hertz, Rosanna, 249
Heterosexuality, 243, 267
Hierarchy of needs (Maslow), 28, *28*
High blood pressure, 104, 328–329, *329*
  obesity, 159–160
High-density lipoprotein (HDL), 334
High-fructose corn syrup (HFCS), 98, 105
Highly active antiretroviral therapy (HAART), 307
High-tech games, 442
Hip flexor stretch, *141*
Hip stretch, *141*
Hispanics
  aging population, 431
  alcohol and tobacco use, 207
  cancer, 322
  cardiovascular disease, 322
  diabetes, 322
  health disparities, 6
  overweight and obesity, 162
  poverty, 322
  sexually transmitted infections, 310
  tobacco use, 207
Histamine, 297
HIV (human immunodeficiency virus), 8, *8*, 264, 340
  incidence of, 305–306, *305*
  preventing, 307
  statistics, 291
  testing and treatment, 306–307, 355
  transmission of, 306, *306*
Hoffman, Philip Seymour, 188
Holmes, Thomas, 61
Home, pollution in, 416–420, *420*
Home care, end of life, 444
Home health tests, 355, *355*
Homeopathy, *363*
Homeostasis, 52–53
Homicides, 388
Homocysteine, 335
Homonegativity, 243, 267
Homophobia, 243, 267
Homo sapiens, 404
Homosexuality, 243, 267–268
Hookahs, 226
Hooking up, 242–243
Hormones
  birth control pills, 275–276
  childbirth, 284
  depressive disorders, 35
  menstrual cycle, 259–260, *260*
  pregnancy, 280
  stress response, 53–54
  weight gain, 162
Hormone therapy (HT), 435
Hospice, 444
Hospitals, 360, 444
Hot flashes, 435
Household hazardous waste, 416
Human chorionic gonadotropin (hCG), 260, 280
Human genome, 369

Human growth hormone (HGH), 148
Human papillomavirus (HPV), 257, *295*, 308–309, 340, 346
Human Rights Campaign, 253
Human sexual response cycle, 262
Humor, 67
Hunger, 8, 81–82, 164
Hybrid electric vehicles (HEVs), 411
Hydration, 145–146
  See also Fluid balance
Hydrochlorofluorocarbons (HCFCs), 408
Hydrocodone, 188
Hydrogenation, oils, 101
Hygiene hypothesis, 297
Hyperglycemia, 321, 323
Hypersexual disorder, 183
Hypersomnia, 79
Hypertension, 159–160, 283, 326, 328–329
Hypertrophic cardiomyopathy (HCM), 334
Hypnic myoclonia, 76
Hypoglycemia, 212
Hypothalamus, 53, 75, *76*
Hypothermia, 146, 212
Hysterectomy, *272*, 276

I

Illicit drugs, 184
Illness, defined, 2
Illness-wellness continuum, *3*
Immune disorders, 296–297
Immune response, *294*
Immune system
  activity, benefits of, 130
  defined, 293
  response, overview, 293–294
  stress effects on, 56
Immunizations, 294–296
Immunoglobulins, 297
Immunotherapy, 346
Implantable cardioverter defibrillator (ICD), 331
Implantation, 269, *269*
Implants, contraceptive, *272*
Incomplete proteins, 102
India, *404*
Individuality, fitness training, 132
Infant mortality, 283–284
Infatuation, 240, *240*
Infections, defined, 292
Infectious agents, cancer and, 340
Infectious disease, 7–8
  See also Sexually transmitted infection
  bacterial infections, 299–301
  emerging, 302
  fungal infections, 303
  immunizations, 294–296
  parasitic worm infections, 304
  protection against, 293–297, 303
  protozoan infections, 303–304
  sleep and, 79
  spread of, 292–296
  viral infections, 297–299
Infertility, 285–286
Inflammation atherosclerosis and, 328, 334–335
  chronic, 319
Inflammatory markers, 334–335
Inflammatory response, 294
Influenza, 291, 292, *295*, 298–299, *298*
Ingestion, drugs, *186*, *196*
Inhalation, drugs, *186*, 194, *196*
Injection, drugs, *186*, *196*
Injections, contraceptive, *272*
Injury
  activity, benefits of, 130
  bicycling, 381
  campus advocacy, 394
  care for, 147–148
  choking and suffocation, 382–383, *383*
  drowning and other water injuries, 383–384
  fire injuries, 384, *384*
  intentional, 377, 385–387

Injury (cont.)
　motor vehicle accidents, 377–381
　personal choices, 395
　poisoning, 382
　sleep problems, 79, 81
　statistics on, 134, 376, 377
　traumatic brain injury, 381
　unintentional, overview of, 377
　violence, 385–387, 388
　websites, 398
　work safety, 384–385
Injury Prevention Web, 398
Inner-thigh butterfly stretch, *141*
Insecticides, 402, 413
Insects, infections from, 293
Insomnia, 83, *84*
Insulin, 320, *321*
Insulin-dependent diabetes, 320–321
Insulin pump, 325, *325*
Insulin resistance, 321, 335
Insulin therapy, 325
Integrative medicine, 362
Intellectual health, 3, *4*
Intensity, FITT principle, 131, *131*
Intentional injury, 377
Intercourse, 264. *See also* Sexual health; Sexually transmitted infection
　painful, 263
Intergovernmental Panel on Climate Change (IPCC), 402
Intermediate familial subtype, alcoholism, 217
Internal locus of control, 17
Internal stressors, 62
Internet
　addiction to, 183–184
　health information, 352
　information on, 11, 354, *354*
Intersex, 243
Intervention, drug treatment, 199–200
Intestate, 444
Intimacy, 26–27, 240, *240*
Intimate partner violence (IPV), 376, 389–390
Intracytoplasmic sperm injection (ICSI), 286
Intrauterine device (IUD), *271*, 275
Intrauterine insemination, 286
Intrinsic asthma, 297
In vitro fertilization (IVF), 286
Iodine, 104
Ionizing radiation, 422, *422*
Iron, 104, *105*
Ischemic stroke, 332, *332*
Isometric exercise, 135–136
Isotonic exercise, 135–136
It (iliotibial band) Stretch, *141*

J

Jaundice, 299
Jealousy, 244–245
Jeanne Clery Act, 388
Jed Foundation, 49
Jenner, Caitlin, *268*
Jenny Craig, *165*
Jet lag, 75, 88
Jobs
　injuries, 384–385
　stress and, 59
Jogging, 132
Johnson, Virginia E., 262
Jolie, Angelina, *344*
Jourard, Sidney M., 235
Journaling, stress and, 66

K

Kaposi's sarcoma, 306
Karate, 132
Kegel exercises, 263
Kickboxing, 132
Kidneys, diabetes and, 323

Kilocalories, 97
King, Martin Luther, Jr., 250
Kinsey, Alfred, 264
Kinsey Scale, 267, 268
Kobasa, Suzanne, 58
Kreteks, 225
Kübler-Ross, Elisabeth, 448

L

Labels
　claims, 113
　food, 111–113
　OTC medications, *356*
Labia majora, 256, *257*
Labia minora, 256, *257*
Labor, childbirth, 281, 284–285, *284*
Lactobacillus acidophilus, 299
Lacto-ovo-vegetarians, 111
Lactose, 98
Land pollution, 414–416
LAP-BAND, 168
Latent autoimmune diabetes of adults (LADA), 323
Latinos
　alcohol and tobacco use, 207
　cardiovascular disease, 322
　diabetes, 322
　health disparities, 6
　overweight and obesity, 162
　sexually transmitted infections, 310
　tobacco use, 207
Laughter, 67
Lead, 420
　in drinking water, 412
Learning, sleep and, 80
Leg abduction, *137*
Legumes, 106, 115
Leisure, stress and, 66
Lesbian, gay, bisexual, transgender, queer or questioning, or intersex (LGBTQI), 243
　stress among, 61, *61*
　suicide, 41
Lesbians, 41, 243
Leukemias, 341
Leukoplakia, 226
LGBT. *See* Lesbian, gay, bisexual, transgender, queer or questioning, or intersex (LGBTQI)
Life expectancy, 1, 431
　defined, 4
　economics and, 438
　obesity, 160
Lifestyle
　Alzheimer's disease and, 437
　cancer and, 340
　coronary heart disease and, 331
　effect on health, 2
　health and, 2
　longevity and, 439
　stress and, 65–66
Lifting, proper *vs.* improper, 385
Liking, 240, *240*
Liletta IUD, 275
Lipids, 100
Listening, 236
Lithium, 37
Liver
　alcohol, effects of, 211, 213
　hepatitis, 213, 299
Living wills, 444
Local food, 119
Locus of control, 17
Loneliness, 32, 239
Longevity, 78, 439
Longevity revolution, 431
Long-lived greenhouse gases (LLGHGs), 406, 407, 410
Lorcaserin (Belviq), 168
Lose It, 169
Love, 235, 438, 446
　See also Relationships
　Sternberg's triangular theory of, 240, 242

Loveisrespect.org, 253
Low birth weight, 283
Low-carbohydrate diets, 167
Low-density lipoproteins (LDLs), 166, 334
Low-fat diets, 166–167
LSD (lysergic acid diethylamide), 193, *196*
Lung cancer, 223, 338, 342, *342*, 347, 371, 419
Lunge, *137*
Lungs, 326, *327*
　activity, benefits of, 129–130
　cardiorespiratory fitness, 127
Luteinizing hormone (LH), 260
Lyme disease, 301, *301*, 402
Lymphocytes, 294
Lymphomas, 341
Lysergic acid diethylamide (LSD), 193, *196*

M

Macronutrients, 97
Macrophages, 293
Macula, 434
Magic Mushrooms, 193, *193*
Magnesium, 104, *105*
Mainstream smoke, 224
Maintenance, behavior change, 14
Major depressive disorder, 34
Major life events, stress and, 61–62
Malaria, 292, 304, 402
Male menopause, 435
Male sexual anatomy, 258–259, *258*
Malignant melanoma, 341, *342*
Malignant tumors, 338
　See also Cancer
Maltose, 98
Mammograms, 345
Managed-care plans, 365–366
Manganese, 104
Mania, 36
Manic-depressive disorder, 36–37
Manipulative therapies, 362, *363*
Manual vacuum aspiration, 278
Marijuana, 190–191, *190*, *196*, 335
　See also Drug use and abuse
Marriage, 57, 234
Maslow, Abraham, hierarchy of needs, 28, *28*
Massage, 66, 362
Mast cells, 297
Masters, William H., 262
Masturbation, 265
Mature adults, 59
　See also Aging
Maturity-onset diabetes of the young (MODY), 323
Maximum heart rate, 133
Mayo Clinic, 23, 316
McCarthy, Jenny, 296
MDMA (Ecstasy), 193–194, *196*
Measles, 295
Meat, 103
Meat consumption, 409
Media
　alcohol and tobacco use and, 222
　smoking and, 221, 222
　violence in, 387
Media and aging, high-tech games, 442
Media and fitness, fitness apps, 147
Media and health, evaluating health information, 12
Media and sexuality, pornography, 266
Media and violence, studies on, 387
Media Literacy Project, 23
Medicaid, 11, 366, 368
Medical abortion, 278
Medical devices, 355
Medical doctors (M.D.s), 359
Medical errors
　preventing, 361
　statistics, 352
Medical Library Association's Top 100 List: Health Websites You Can Trust, 374
Medical marijuana, 190

INDEX **I-8**

Medicare, 11, 366, 432
Medications. *See also* Over-the-counter (OTC) medications; Prescription medications
　bone-building, 435
　diabetes, 325
　driving and, 378
　heart, 331
　hypertension, 329
　menopause, 435
　over-the-counter medications, 355, 356
　pain, 445
　proper handling of, 361
　sleep, 87, 88
　stimulants, 82–83
　testosterone therapy, 435–436
Meditation, 45
　stress and, 66, *67*
MedlinePlus, 23, 316, 350
Melanoma, 341, 408, 422
Melatonin, 75, 88
Memorial Day, 443
Memorial services, 446
Memory, aging and, 436–437
Memory B cells, 294
Memory consolidation, 81
Memory T cells, 294
Men
　alcohol and tobacco use, 207
　alcohol use and abuse, 210, 216
　body image, 155
　building muscle, 128, *128*
　caloric needs of, 97
　communication, 237–238
　contraception, 269–276, *270–273, 274, 275*
　depression, 35, *35*
　fiber intake, 99
　heart disease, 334
　infertility, 285–286
　life expectancy, 432–433
　obesity, 160
　prostate cancer, 344
　sexual anatomy, 258–259, *258*
　sexual dysfunctions, 262, 263
　sexually transmitted infections, rates of, 310
　sleep, 82
　steroid use, 148
　stress, 59
　testicular cancer, 344
　tobacco use, 207
　unintentional injuries, 377
　violent crime, 385
　warning signs of heart attack, *330*
　weight gain, 162
Menarche, 259
Men Can Stop Rape, 394
Meningococcal disease, *295*
Menopausal transition, 435
Menopause, 260, 340, 345, 435
Menstrual cycle, 257, 259–262, *260, 260*
Menstrual phases, 260, *260*
Menstruation, 259
Mental disorders
　attention disorders, 39–40
　bipolar disorder, 25, 36–37
　mood disorders, 34–37
　obsessive-compulsive disorder (OCD), 38
　overview, 33–34
　schizophrenia, 40
Mental health. *See also* Psychological health
　chronic stress and, 57
　defined, 26
　statistics on, 25, 33
Mental Health America, 49
Men who have sex with men, sexually transmitted infections, 310
The Merck Manual, 358
Mercury, 415, 420
Metabolic equivalent of task (MET), 143–144
　of common activities, *145*

Metabolic syndrome, 160, 336–337
Metabolism
　activity, benefits of, 130
　alcohol, 209–210, *210*
　defined, 97
Metastasis, 338
　See also Cancer
Methamphetamine, 192, *192*, 196
Methane, 407
Methicillin-resistant *Staphylococcus aureus* (MRSA), 300–301
Methylenedioxymethamphetamine (MDMA), 193–194
Methylmercury, 401
Microcephaly, 302
Micron filtration, 413
Micronutrients, 97
Microorganisms, 292
Midwife, 284
Mifepristone, 278
Migraine headaches, 56
Milk and milk substitutes, 105, *106*
Millennials, stress, 59
Minamata, Japan, 401
Mind-body medicine, 362, *363*
Minerals, 104, *105*
　major, 104
　trace, 104
Mini-med plans, 366
Mini-pill, *271*
Minority stress model, 61
Mirena IUD, 275
Miscarriage, 283
Misoprostol, 278
Modeling, 17
Models, of behavior change, 14–15
Modified push-ups, *138*
Mold, 420
Money, financial stress, 51
Mononucleosis, 299
Monosaturated fats, 101
Mons pubis, 256, *257*
Monterey Bay Aquarium Seafood Watch App, 427
Mood changes, aging and, 438
Mood disorders, 34–37
Morbidity, 5
Morning after pill, *270*, 274
Morning sickness, 280
Morphine, 188
Mortality, 4
Mosquito-borne diseases, 8, 293
Mothers Against Drunk Driving (MADD), 215
Mother-to-child transmission (MTCT), HIV, 306
Motorcycle accidents, 380–381
Motorcycle Safety Foundation, 398
Motor vehicle accidents (MVA), 81, 377–381
Movement disorders, 40
Mucosal absorption, drugs, *186*
Multivitamin/mineral supplements (MVMs), 108–109
Mumps, 295
Municipal solid waste (MSW), 414–415
Murder, 385, 388
Muscle confusion, 132
Muscular endurance, 128, 135
Muscular strength, 127–128, *128*, 135
Music, 66–67
Mutations, cancer, 338, *339*
Mycobacterium tuberculosis, 301
Myelomas, 341
My Family Health Portrait, 350
MyFitnessPal, 169
Myocardial infarction (MI), 329, 330, 331
　management of, 331
Myocardium, 326, *327*
　See also Cardiovascular disease (CVD)
My Physical Activity & Exercise Pyramid, *143*
MyPlate for Older Adults, *441*
MyPlate website, 124
MySpace, 241
Myth or Fact?

caffeinated alcoholic beverages, 213
cell phone and your brain, 423
circumcision, need for, 259
electric vehicles, 411
stress and ulcers, 56
vaccines and autism, 296

N

NA. *See* Narcotics Anonymous
Naltrexone, 218
Naps, 78, 89
Narcolepsy, 85
Narcotics, 188
　See also Drug use and abuse
Narcotics Anonymous, 197, 203
National Aging in Place Council, 438
National Alliance on Mental Illness (NAMI), 45
National Association to Advance Fat Acceptance (NAAFA), 171
National Cancer Institute (NCI), 222, 225, 228, 232, 347, 350, 419, 423
National Center for Complementary and Alternative Medicine (NCCAM), 362
National Center for Complementary and Integrative Health, 374
National Center for Environmental Health (NCEH), 427
National Center for Injury Prevention & Control, 398
National Center on Addiction and Substance Abuse at Columbia University, 203
National Domestic Violence Hotline, 391, 398
National Educational Association of Disabled Students (NEADS), 251
National Institute of Mental Health, 49, 179
National Institute on Alcohol Abuse and Alcoholism, 206, 217
National Institute on Drug Abuse, 193, 195
National Institutes of Health (NIH), 5, 10, 158
National Institutes of Health Senior Health, 453
National Oceanic and Atmospheric Administration, 409
National Park Service, 409
National Poison Control Center, 382
National Safety Council (NSC), 378, 398
National Sleep Foundation, 82, 94
National Student Campaign Against Hunger and Homelessness, 121
National Suicide Prevention Lifeline, 49
National Survey on Drug Use and Health, 190
National Traffic Safety Administration (NHTSA), 378
National Transportation Safety Board, 378
National Wellness Institute, 3
Native Americans
　alcohol and tobacco use, 207
　cardiovascular disease, 322
　diabetes, 322
　health disparities, 6
　overweight and obesity, 162
　suicide, 41
　tobacco use, 207
Natural foods, 119
Natural killer (NK) cells, 293
Naturally acquired immunity, 295
Natural products, 362, *363*
Natural Resources Defense Council, 424
Naturopathy, *363*
Near-death experiences (NDEs), 443
Neck stretches, *140*
Negative population growth, 405
Neisseria gonorrhoeae, 309
Neisseria meningitidis, 300
Nervous system, 212
Neural tube development, 103
Neuromotor exercise, 139
Neurotoxins, 412–413
Neurotransmitters, 33–34, 53, 189
　defined, 33
　drug abuse, 186

Neutrophils, 293
Newtown, Connecticut, school violence in, 388
Niacin, *105*
Nicotine, 220, 223, 224, 226, 335
Nicotine replacement therapies, 228, 229
Night blindness, 8
Night-eating syndrome, 86, 174–175
Nitrogen oxides, 408
Nitroglycerin, 331
Nixon, Peter, 54
Nixon, Richard, 409
Nocturnal eating disorder, 85–86, *86*
Noise pollution, 420–421
Non-ionizing radiation, 422, *422*
Nonlove, 240, *240*, 242
Nonoxynol-9, 274
Nonprofit clinics, 359
Non-REM (NREM) sleep, 76, *77*
Nonspecific immune response, 293–294, *294*
Non-suicidal self-injury (NSSI), 40
Nonverbal communication, 236
Norepinephrine, 53, 55
Norovirus, 117
Nurse practitioners, 359, *360*
Nurses, 359
Nursing homes, 437
Nutrient-dense fast foods, 121
Nutrient-dense foods, 115
Nutrients
    antioxidants, 107–108
    carbohydrates, 98–100, *99*
    defined, 97
    fats, dietary, 100–103
    fiber, 99
    minerals, 104, *105*
    phytochemicals, 107–108
    prebiotics and probiotics, 108
    proteins, 102–103
    vitamins, 103–104
    water soluble, *105*
Nutrition
    aging and, 439, 440, *441*
    campus advocacy, 121
    ChooseMyPlate.gov, 113, *113*
    chronic disease and, 319, 347
    defined, 97
    Dietary Reference Intakes (DRIs), 110, *110*
    food labels, reading, 111–113, *112*
    personal choices, 120
    physical activity, 145
    pregnancy, 283
    shopping smart, 120–121
    statistics on, 96
    stress and, 65
    variation for different groups, 115
    websites, 124
Nutrition Facts panel, 111–112, *112*
Nuts, food allergies, 118, *118*

O

Obesity, 8
    aging and, 439–440
    on campus, 159, 160
    cardiometabolic risk, 336, *337*
    cardiovascular disease, 335
    central obesity, 162
    chronic disease and, 347
    clinical options for, 168–169
    definition of obese, 155
    financial burden of, 160–161
    healthful weight, defining, 156
    health risks with, 159–161, *160*
    physical activity, 144–145
    physical factors, 164
    public policy, 164
    sleep difficulties and, 79
    statistics on, 154, 158, *159*
    type 2 diabetes and, 321
    weight gain, causes of, 161–164
Obesogenic environments, 164

Obsessive-compulsive disorder (OCD), 25, 38
Obstructive sleep apnea, 84, *84*
Occupational health, 4, *4*
Oils, 115
Older adults. *See* Aging
Omega-3 fatty acids, 2, 101
Omega-6 fatty acids, 101
Oncogenes, 338
On Death and Dying (Kübler-Ross), 448
Online dating, 243
Online information, evaluating, 354
Opioids, 188, *188*, 190, 196
    painkillers, warnings, 361
Opportunistic diseases, 306
Optimism, 29, 58
Optometrists, 359
Oral cancer, 343, *343*
Oral hygiene, *353*
    screenings, *357*
Oral sex, 242, 264, 306, 308, 343
    See also Sexually transmitted infection
Organ donation, 444
Organic foods, 119
Organosulfur compounds, 107
Orgasm, 262
    inability to achieve, 263
Orgasmic platform, 262
Orlistat, 168
Ornish diet, 165
Orr, David, 424
Orthorexia nervosa, 175
Osteoarthritis, 160, 434
Osteoporosis, 106, 130, 223, 434–435, *434*
Ounce-equivalent, 115, *115*
Outercourse, 265
Ovarian cancer, 130, 338, 345
Ovaries, 257, *257*, 269
Overdose, drug, 188, 195, 198
    prescription painkillers, 361
    statistics, 382
Overeaters Anonymous, 170
Overload, fitness training, 131
Over-the-counter (OTC) medications, 187–188, 355, 356
    See also Medications
    sleep, 88
Overweight, 155
    on campus, 159, 160
    chronic disease and, 347
    diabetes, risk of, 324
    financial burden of, 160–161
    healthful weight, defining, 156
    physical activity, 144–145
    physical factors, 164
    public policy, 164
    social factors, 163–164
    statistics on, 154
    stress and, 56
    weight gain, causes of, 161–164
Ovulation, 260, 269, 286
Oxidation reactions, 107
Oxycodone, 188, 361
OxyContin, 188
Oxytocin, 284
Ozone (O_3), 406, 407, 410
Ozone depletion, 408

P

Pacific Islanders, sexually transmitted infections, 310
Pain medications, end of life, 445
Palliative care, 444
Pancreas, 320, *321*
Pancreatic cancer, 343
Pandemics, 299
Panic attacks, 37, 57
Panic disorder, 25, 37
Pantothenic acid, *105*
Pap test, 257, 346
ParaGard Copper-T IUD, 275

Parasitic worm infections, 304
Parasomnias, 85–86
Paris Agreement, 410
Particulates, 408
Passion, 240, *240*
Passive euthanasia, 445–446
Passive immunity, 295
Passive smokers, 224
Passive stretching, 139
Pathogens, 117, 292, 293, *294*, 295
Patient rights, 361
Payne, Wayne Leon, 28
PCBs, 412
PCP (phencyclidine), 193, *196*
Pear-shaped fat patterning, 156, *156*
Pedestrian safety, 381
Peer mentoring associations, 200
Peer pressure, 18, 219
Peer-reviewed journals, 355
Pelvic inflammatory disease (PID), 285, 309–311
Penicillin, 303
Penis, 258, *258*
Perceived benefit, behavior change, 14
Perceived severity, behavior change, 14
Perceived threat, behavior change, 14
Percent daily value (%DV), 112–113
Percocet, 188
Percodan, 188
Performance-enhancing drugs, 109, 148
Perimenopause, 435
Persistent vegetative state, 445–446
Personal growth, *27*, 28
Personality types, stress and, 57–58
Personalized medicine, 369
Personal safety
    assault, 388
    defined, 377
    domestic and intimate partner violence, 376, 389–390
    hate crimes, 389
    murder, 385, 388
    school and campus violence, 388–389
    sexual violence, 391–394
    websites, 398
    work safety, 384–385
Personal values, 30–31
Pertussis, 295
Pesco-vegetarians, 111
Pesticides, 118, 413, *420*
    chronic disease prevention, 347
Pets, infection from, 293
Pharmacogenomics, 371
Pharmacologic therapy, 44
Phencyclidine (PCP), 193, *196*
Phentermine-topiramate, 168
Phobias, 36–37
Phospholipids, 100
Phosphorus, 104
Phthalates, 419
Physical abuse, 245, 389–390
Physical activity. *See also* Exercise
    ACSM guidelines, *142*
    aerobic exercise, 132, 134
    aging and, 439, *439*, 440
    benefits of, 129–130
    body composition, 128
    cardiorespiratory fitness, 127, 131, 132
    chronic disease, 319, 347
    defined, 127
    diabetes, risk of, 127
    fitness, components of, 127–128
    fitness training principles, 131–132, *131*
    flexibility, 128, 136, 139
    frequency recommendations, 142, 144
    heart health, 335
    intensity levels, *134*
    muscular strength and endurance, 127–128, 135–139, 139
    personal choices, 148–150
    safety issues, 145–148
    statistics on, 126, 127

websites, 152
weight loss and, 169
Physical Activity Guidelines for Americans, 142
Physical dependence, drugs, 187
Physical fitness. *See also* Exercise; Physical activity
    defined, 127
    Rating of Perceived Exertion (RPE) Scale, *134*
    statistics, 126
Physical health, 3, *4*
Physical inactivity
    cancer and, 130
    diabetes, risk of, 324
    weight gain, causes of, 163
Physician-aid-in-dying (PAD), 445
Physician assistants (P.A.s), 359
Physician-assisted suicide, 445
Physicians, 359
Phytochemicals, 107–108
Phytoplankton, 408
Pilates, 128, 139
Pineal gland, sleep and, 75, *76*
Pinworms, 304
Pituitary gland, 53
Placebo, 29
Placenta, 281, *284*, 285
Plan B, 274
Plank, *138*
Planned Parenthood, 289, 316
Plaque, 328, 331
Plasmodium, 303
Plateau, human sexual response cycle, 262
Plyometrics, 128
PMAs. *See* Peer mentoring associations
Pneumococcal polysaccharide (PPV), *295*
Pneumonia, 301
Podiatrists, 359
Point-of-service plans (POSs), 366
Poisoning, unintentional, 377, 382
Policy-making, 11
Polio, 295, *295*
Pollution. *See also* Environmental health
    air, 340, 402, *402*, 405–411, *410*
    defined, 400, 401
    at home, 416–420, 420
    land, 414–416
    noise, 420–421
    water, 411–412, *414*
Polyabusers, 198
Polychlorinated biphenyls (PCBs), 412
Polypharmacy, 438
Polyps, 340
Polysomnogram, 84
Polyunsaturated fats, 101
Polyvinyl chloride (PVC), 419
Pons, REM sleep and, 75, 77
Population growth, *403*, *404*
    overpopulation, 403–405
    statistics, 400
Pornography, 266
Portion control, 163
Positive psychotherapy, 43
Positive relations with others, 26–27, *27*
Postmenopause, 435
Postpartum depression, 35
Post-traumatic stress disorder (PTSD), 38–39
Potassium, 104, *105*
Poverty, 322, 386
Practical Strategies
    affordable health care tips, 369
    bicycle helmets, 382
    building self-esteem, 27
    campus safety, 395
    choosing to combat climate change, 409
    communicating effectively about sex and birth control, 277
    cutting calories, not nutrition, 169
    fiber-rich carbohydrates, 100
    financial stress, 59
    go lean with protein, 103
    grief, 449
    hand washing and hand sanitizers, 303
    healthful fats, 102
    infectious diseases, 303
    medications for mental health issues, 36
    naps, 78
    nutrient-dense fast foods, 121
    preventing tech injuries, 386
    promoting clean water, 414
    quitting smoking, 229
    reducing pollution at home, 420
    reducing risk of STIs, 307
    risky alcohol-related behavior, 215
    safe weight lifting, 136
    spotting destructive thoughts, 44
    stress overload, 58
    strong relationships, 244
    warning signs of addiction, 183
Prebiotics, 108
Precontemplation, behavior change, 14
Prediabetes, 323
Predisposing factors, behavior, 13
Preeclampsia, 283
Pre-existing condition, 365
Preferred provider organizations (PPOs), 366
Prefrontal cortex, 80
Pregnancy, 260
    alcohol and, 215
    changes in a woman's body, 280, *281*
    complications, 283–284
    early signs of, 280
    ectopic, 309
    excess body weight and, 160
    exercise choices, 149
    gestational diabetes, 321
    home tests, 280, 355
    overview of, *282*
    preconception care, 280
    prenatal care, 280, 281, 283
    sleep and, 81
    smoking and, 223–224, 281
    stages, 280–285
    trimesters, 280, 281
    unintended, 255, 268–269, 277
    weight gain, 160, 162
    Zika virus, 8, 302, 402
Premature ejaculation (PE), 263
Premenstrual dysphoric disorder (PMDD), 261
Premenstrual syndrome (PMS), 261, *261*
Premium, health insurance, 365
Prenatal care, 280, 281, 283
Preparation, behavior change, 14
Presbycusis, 433
Presbyopia, 433
Prescription medications. *See also* Medications
    abuse of, 438
    antidepressants, 435
    driving and, 378
    obesity and overweight, 168
    proper handling of, 361
    sleep medications, 87
    stimulants, 82–83
    unintentional poisoning, 382
Prescription painkillers, 361
Prescription stimulants (PS), 188, 189
President's Challenge Program: The Active Lifestyle Activity Log, 152
Preterm babies, 281
Prevalence, 4
Prevention, practicing, 353, *353*
Primary care facilities, 359
Probiotics, 108, 347, 362
Problem solving, 67
Prochaska, James O., 14
Procrastination, 60
Professional trainers, 145
Progestin, 274, 275
Progressive muscle relaxation (PMR), 66
Progressive overload, fitness training, 131, *131*
Proliferative phase, menstrual cycle, 260, *260*
Proof value, 209
Prostaglandins, 261
Prostate cancer, 338, 344
Prostate gland, 258
Protease inhibitors, 307
Protein, dietary, 102–103, 115, 145, 167
Protein-leverage hypothesis, 102–103
Proto-oncogenes, 338
Protozoa, *298*, 303
Protozoan infections, 293, 303–304
Psilocybin (magic mushrooms), 193, *193*
Psychiatrists, 42
Psychoactive drugs, 33, 34, 184
Psychoanalysis, 43
Psychodynamic therapy, 43
Psychological dependence, drugs, 187
Psychological health, 3, *4*. *See also* Emotional health
    activity, benefits of, 130
    aging and, 438–441
    anger, 32–33, *32*
    anxiety disorders, 37–38
    attention disorders, 39–40
    bipolar disorder, 36–37
    campus advocacy, 45
    components of, 26
    defined, 26
    depressive disorders, 34–36
    emotional intelligence, 28
    facets of, 26–28
    factors related to, 29–31
    family history, 29
    helping others, 45
    loneliness, 32
    mental disorders, overview, 33–34
    optimism, 29
    overview, 26
    physical activity benefits, 130
    professional help, 42–44
    reaching out, 45
    schizophrenia, 40
    self-care, 45
    self-esteem, 45
    shyness, 31–32
    social support, 29
    spirituality, 29–31
    statistics on, 25, 32, *32*
    suicide and self-injury, 40–41
    websites, 49
Psychologists, 42
Psychoneuroimmunology, 56
Psychosis, 40
Psychotherapy, 35, 168
Pthirus pubis, 311–312, *312*
Pubic lice, 311–312, *312*
Public health, 4, 359
Public health insurance programs, 366
Purging, 174
Purpose in life, *27*, 28, 31
Push-ups, modified, *138*

Q

Qsymia, 168
Quadriceps stretch, *141*
Queer or questioning, 243

R

Race
    alcohol and tobacco use, 207
    chronic disease, 322
    drug use, 185
    health, 9
    health disparities, 6
    life expectancy, 432
    sexually transmitted infections, rates of, 310
    suicide, 41
    tobacco use, 207
    weight gain, 162

Radiation, 422–423
Radiation exposure, 340, 422–423, *422*
Radiation sickness, 422
Radiation therapy, 346
Radon, 342, 419, 420
Rahe, Richard, 61
Random drug testing, 195
Rape, Abuse, & Incest National Network (RAINN), 398
Rape, 215–216, 385, 392–394
Rapid eye movement (REM) sleep, 76, 77, *77*, 81
Rating of Perceived Exertion (RPE) Scale, *134*
Rational suicide, 445
Real Food Challenge, 171
Recommended Dietary Allowance (RDA), 110
Recovery, exercise, 136
Recycling, 414–415, *414*
   reducing water pollution, 414
Refractory period, sexual response cycle, 262
Regulatory T cells, 294
Reinforcing factors, behavior, 13
Relapse, 18
   alcohol abuse, 218
   drug abuse, 199
   tobacco use, 228
Relationships
   attraction, causes of, 242
   campus advocacy, 250–251
   cohabitation, 246, *246*
   committed, 245–248
   communication in, 235–238
   conflict resolution, 236–237
   dating, 242–243
   developing, 238–239
   domestic partnerships, 248
   dysfunctional, 244–245
   early, 238
   ending, 245
   friendships, maintaining, 239–240, *239*
   gender roles, 238–239
   healthy, 243
   intimate, 240–241
   marriage, 246–247
   personal choices, 250
   same-sex relationships, 243
   single, remaining, 248
   statistics on, 234, 248
   stress and, 59
   stress effects on, 57
   Triangular Theory of Love, 240, *240*, 242
   violence within, 389–390
   websites, 253
Relaxation techniques, 43
Reliability, of research studies, 354–355
Religion, 30, *30*
REM behavior disorder (RBD), 77, 86
Repetitions, 136
Repetitive strain injuries (RSIs), 384–385, *386*
Replacement-level fertility, 404
Research studies, understanding, 354–355
Reservoir, infection transmission, 292
Residence changes, aging and, 437–438
Resiliency, 29, 58
Resistance stage, stress response, *53*, 54
Resistance training, *128*, 135
Resolution phase, human sexual response cycle, 262
Respiratory disease, tobacco use and, 223
Resting metabolic rate (RMR), 162
Restless legs syndrome (RLS), 86
Retail clinics, 359, *360*
Rethinking Drinking: Alcohol and Your Drinking, 232
Reticular activating system (RAS), 75
Retirement, 438
Reuse, 414
Reverse curl, *138*
Reverse osmosis, 413
Reverse transcriptase inhibitors, 307
Reversibility, fitness training, 131

Rewards, 18
Rheumatic heart disease, 334
Rhinoviruses, 298
Rhythm method, *270*, 272–273, *273*
RICE protocol, 147–148
Riciutti, Henry, 249
Risk factors, defined, 5
Ritalin, 40, 82–83, 188, 189
Robbery, 385
Roe v. Wade, 279
Rohypnol, 194, *196*, 215
Romantic love, 240, *240*
Rosenman, Ray, 57
Rotter, Julian B., 17
RU-486, 274, 278
Rubella, 295
Ryff, Carol D., 26
Ryff Scales of Psychological Well-Being, 26, *27*

S

"Safe" programs, 287
SafeRides programs, 382
Safety
   assault, 388
   domestic and intimate partner violence, 376, 389–390
   hate crimes, 389
   murder, 385, 388
   physical activity, 145–148
   school and campus violence, 388–389
   sexual violence, 391–394
   work safety, 384–385
Safe Zone, campus, 287
Salmonella, 117
Same-sex marriage, 246, 247
Sarcomas, 341
Satiety, 165
Saturated fats, 101
Scabies, 311–312
Schedule II drugs, 192
Schizophrenia, 40
School and campus violence, 388–389
ScienceDaily: Mind & Brain, 49
Science of Addiction, The, 203
Scientific method, 354, 358
Screenings, recommended
   cancer, 340–341
   preventing chronic disease, 347, *357–358*
Scrotum, 258, *258*
Seat belts, 379
Seaward, Brian Luke, 30
Secondhand smoke, 224–225, 342
   statistics, 205
Secretory phase, menstrual cycle, 260, *260*
Sedentary lifestyle, 144, 163
Selenium, 104
Self-acceptance, 26, *27*
Self-actualization, 28
Self-Assessment
   aggressive driving, 379
   alcohol use disorders identification test, 217
   anxiety assessment, 39
   cancer risk, 339
   death, 449
   eating disorders, 175
   eating well, 120
   health of current lifestyle, 19–20
   healthy relationships, 245
   heart attack risk, 336
   loud music, 422
   maximum heart rate and target heart rate range, 133
   negative event scale for university students, 63
   preventive health care, 371–372
   readiness for sex, 265
   seeking drug treatment, 198
   sexually transmitted infections, 305
   sleep, 89
   type 2 diabetes, 324
   weight-related health risks, 158

Self-care, 45, 353–356
   information sources, 352, 354–355
   options, 355–356
   practicing prevention, 353, *353*
   understanding research studies, 354–355
   wellness habits, *353*
Self-disclosure, 235
Self-efficacy, 16
   building, 17
Self-esteem, 45, 67, 238
   building, *27*
Self-exams, testicular, 344
Self-injury, 40–41
Self-medicating, alcohol, 216
Self-monitoring, 17
Self-perception, relationships and, 238
Seligman, Martin, 29
Selye, Hans, 52, 53, 54
Semen, 258
Seminal fluid, 258
Seminal vesicles, 258
Semivegetarians, 111
Separation and divorce, 247
September 11, 2001, terrorist attacks, 389
Serious mental illness (SMI), 33
Serotonin, 33
Serving sizes, estimating, *113*
Sets, 136
Sex, defined, 9
Sexting, 265–267
Sexual desire, low level of, 263
Sexual harassment, 391–392
Sexual health. *See also* Sexually transmitted infection
   abortion, 277–279
   abstinence and celibacy, 264
   aging and, 436
   alcohol and tobacco use, 208
   alcohol use and abuse, 215–216
   campus advocacy, 287
   common problems in females, 257–258
   communicating about sex, 265
   conception and contraception, 268–276, *269*, *270–273*, *275*
   health problems in males, 259
   hooking up, 246–247
   infertility, 285–286
   intimacy without intercourse, *270*, 272
   menstrual cycle, 259–260, *260*
   non-intercourse sexual activity, 265
   personal choices, 286–287
   pregnancy and childbirth, 280–285, *281*, *282*, *284*
   readiness for sex, 265
   sexual anatomy, 256–259
   sexual dysfunctions, 262–263
   sexual intercourse, 264
   sexual orientation and gender identity, 267–268
   sexual response cycle, 262
   statistics on behavior, 255
   stress and, 57
   understanding sexuality, 256
Sexually transmitted infection, 259, 265
   See also Infectious disease
   aging and, 436
   asking potential partner about, 278
   chlamydia, 285, 309
   condoms and, 274, 304, 307
   diaphragm and cervical cap, 275
   genital herpes, 308, *308*
   gonorrhea, 285, 309
   hepatitis B, 307
   HIV/AIDS, 305–307
   hooking up, 243
   human papillomavirus, 308–309
   incidence of, 304
   infertility, 285–286
   intrauterine device, 275
   oral sex, 264
   pelvic inflammatory disease, 309–311
   personal choices, 312–313

pubic lice and scabies, 311–312, *312*
risk factors for, 304–305
statistics, 291
syphilis, 311, *311*
trichomoniasis, 312
Sexual orientation, 266–267, 310
Sexual violence, 391–394
Shaping, 16
Shopping, compulsive, 183
Shoulder stretch, *140*
Shyness, 31–32
Sidestream smoke, 224
Signs, defined, 2
Silent Spring (Carson), 402
Simple carbohydrates, 98
Single parenthood, 249
Sinus node, 217
Skills-related fitness, 127
Skin, 293
Skin cancer, 338, 341–342, *342*, 408
Sklyla IUD, 275
Sleep
    academic performance, 80–81
    activity, benefits of, 130
    alcohol, effects of, 89, 211
    alcohol and, 83
    in America, 79, *79*
    cardiovascular disease, 335
    chronic disease prevention, 347
    chronic stress and, 56
    complementary and alternative medicine, 88
    cycles of, 77, *77*
    defined, 75
    disorders, 83–86
    health effects, 79–80
    individual behaviors and, 81–83
    personal choices, 88–89
    physical activity benefits, 130
    regions and rhythms of, *77*
    short and long, research on, 78
    sleep debt, 77–78
    snoring, 83–84
    stages of, 76–77, *77*
    statistics on, 74
    stress and, 65, 66, *66*, 81, 83, *83*
    websites, 94
Sleep apnea, 81, 84–85, *84*
    defined, 84
    diagnosis of, 84
    excess body weight and, 160
    treatment of, 84
    types of, 84
Sleep bruxism, 85
Sleep debt, 77–78
Sleep disorders
    diagnosis of, 86–87
    websites, 94
Sleep hygiene, 89
Sleep initiation, 89
Sleep maintenance, 89
Sleep-related eating disorder, 86
Sleep studies, 87, *87*
Sleep terrors, 85
Sleep Treatment and Education Program for Students (STEPS), 86
Sleepwalking, 85
Slim-Fast diet, *165*
Slow-wave sleep, 76
Smartersex.org, 316
SMART goal, 16
Smart Grid, 410
Smog, 408
Smoke detectors, 384
Smokeless ("spit") tobacco, 226
Smoking, tobacco
    age and, 220
    benefits of quitting, *227*
    birth control pills and, 276
    on campus, 220–221
    campus advocacy, 229
    cancer and, 223, 342, *342*

cardiovascular disease and, 335
cessation programs, 227–228, *228*, 229
chemical contents, 221
chronic disease and, 319, 347
diabetes and, 324
fire-related deaths, 384
health effects, 221–225, *224*
hypertension, 329
longevity and, 432
media and, 222
menopause and, 435
personal choices, 228–229
pregnancy and, 223–224, 283
sleep and, 82
statistics on, 205, 220
stress and, 220–221
treatment options, 227–228
Snoring, 83–84
Snuff, 226
Social anxiety disorder, 37, *38*
Social environment, 401
Social health, 3–4, *4*
Social media, 241
    stress and, 51, 59
Social physique anxiety, 172
Social Readjustment Rating Scale (SRRS), 61–62
Social Security, 438
Social stressors, 59
Social support, 17–18, 29, 45, 218
    for managing stress, 62
Social withdrawal, 40
Socioeconomic status
    cardiovascular disease, 336
    life expectancy, 438
Sodium, 104, 329
    preventing chronic diseases, 347
South Beach Diet, *166*
Special Feature
    Affordable Care Act, 367
    core strengthening, 135
    CVD emergency, 333
    dietary guidelines, 114
    peer pressure: alcohol use and abuse, 219
    reducing risk of chronic disease, 347
    sleep, 90
    social media, communication, and cyber-bullies, 241
    Title IX: antidiscrimination rights, 393
    Zika virus, 302
Specialists centers, 359
Specific immune response, 294, *294*
Specificity, fitness training, 131
Speeding, 379–380
Sperm, 258, 269, 286
Spermicides, *270*, 274
Sphygmomanometer, 329
Spicy foods, sleep and, 82
Spiritual health, 3, *4*
    See also Psychological health
Spirituality, 30–31
Spiritual well-being, Seaward's pillars of, 30, *30*
Sponge, contraceptive, *270*
Spontaneous abortion, 283
Sports beverages, 104–105
Spotlight, feeding your bones, 106
Squat, *137*
Stalking, 390–391
Standard drink, 209, *209*
Stanford University, Center for Sleep and Dreams Sleep Guide, 94
Staphylococcus aureus, 300
Starches, 99
Static flexibility, 136, 139
Static muscular endurance, 128
Static stretching, 139
Statins, 334
Status syndrome, 10, *10*
Statutory rape, 392
Stepfamilies, 249
Sterilization, 276
Sternberg, Robert, 240

Steroids, anabolic, 109, 148
Sterols, 100–101
Stimulants, 188, 189
    amphetamines, 192, *192*
    caffeine, 191, *191*
    cocaine, 191, *192*
    commonly abused drugs, *196*
    defined, 191
Stomach cancer, 338
Stratosphere, 406
Strength training, 128, 135
Streptococcus, 301
Streptococcus pneumoniae, 300, 301
Stress
    academic pressure, 59–60
    aging and, 440
    body's response to, 52–54
    cardiovascular disease, 335
    cardiovascular system and, 55
    changing thinking, 67
    chronic, health effects of, 55–57, *55*
    common causes of, 59–63
    daily hassles, 62
    defined, 52
    diabetes, risk of, 324
    digestive system and, 55–56
    environmental, 62
    exercise, 65–66, *67*
    financial, 59, 60
    general adaptation syndrome, 53, *53*
    grief and, 447
    help on campus, 62, 64
    immune system and, 56
    internal, 62
    job-related, 59
    lifestyle and, 65–66
    major life events, 62–63
    managing, 62–68
    mental health and, 57
    overload, signs of, 58
    personality types and, 57–58
    personalized stress management plan for, 68
    physical activity benefits, 130
    post-traumatic stress disorder, 38–39
    relationships and, 57
    self-assessment, 62
    sleep and, 56, 65, *66*, 81, 83
    smoking and, 220–221
    social, 59
    statistics on, 51
    tension relievers, 66
    test-taking skills, 65–66, *65*
    thought process and, 67
    ulcers and, 56
    violent crime and, 387
    websites, 72
    weight and, 56
Stressors, 52, 58
Stress response, 53
Stress test, 331
Stretching, 136, 139, *140–141*
    exercises, *140–141*
Stroke, 55, 101, 159, 323, 326, *329*, 332, 333, 334
    atherosclerosis and, 159
    tobacco use, 223
Student health centers, 359
Student loans, 59
Students, health insurance and, 368
Students Active for Ending Rape (SAFER), 394
Students Against Destructive Decisions (SADD), 220
Students Against Violence Everywhere (SAVE), 394
Student Stats
    alcohol use on campus, 208
    CAM use among college students, 362
    causes of death among people aged 15–24, 378
    causes of death from unintentional injury, 383
    common health problems, 7

Student Stats (*cont.*)
 contraception and college students, 273
 dieting and exercising on campus, 164
 drug use among young adults, 186
 herb and supplement use, 109
 impediments to academic performance, 57
 overweight, obesity, and dieting on campus, 160
 physical activity on campuses, 144
 psychological health on campus, 32
 reported participation in key health behaviors, 320
 sex and the college student, 264
 sexually transmitted infections in people aged 15-24, 311
 sleepless on campus, 79
 smoking on campus, 220
 students and relationships, 248
 thinking green, 403
Student Story
 abusive relationship, 390
 adapting exercise to my needs, 150
 aging, 437
 avoiding infections, 295
 balancing school and family, 55
 birth control pills, 269
 car accident, 381
 cardiorespiratory fitness, 132
 car *vs.* campus shuttle, 412
 coping with addiction, 197
 cost of being uninsured, 366
 dealing with depression, 36
 drinking's darker side, 214
 eating disorders, 176
 family history of diabetes, 326
 fixing a poor diet, 108
 friend's suicide, 41
 good friends, 239
 grieving, 447
 health coverage, 368
 healthy couples, 242
 pressure to succeed, 64
 quitting smoking, 228
 recycling cell phones, 415
 scars and self-acceptance, 11
 sleep apnea, 85
 sleep deprivation, 87
 surviving cancer, 345
 talking honestly about STIs, 278
 unprotected sex, 313
 vegetarianism, 112
 weight loss, 163
Subarachnoid space, 332
Substance abuse. *See also* Alcohol use and abuse; Drug use and abuse
 injuries and, 377
Substance Abuse and Mental Health Services Administration, 5, 199
Substance use disorder, 187
Sucrose, 98
Suction curettage, 278
Sudden cardiac arrest, 329, 330–331, 333
 management of, 331
Sudden infant death syndrome (SIDS), 224, 284
Sudden sniffing death, 194
Suffocation, 382–383
Sugars
 added, 98
 consumption statistics, 96
Suicide, 25, 35, 36, 41, *42*, 189, 267, 394, 438, 445
 alcohol use, 208
Sulfur, 104
Sulfur dioxide, 408
Sun protection factor (SPF), 342
Superfund, 415–416
Superweeds, 119
Support groups, *13*, 14
Surgery

birth control methods, 276
 infertility options, 286
 weight-loss, 168–169
Surgical abortion, 278
Surrogate motherhood, 286
Sustainability, environmental, 403
Sustainable Endowments Institute, 424
Sustained sitting, avoiding, 144
Sweetened beverages, 105, *107*
Swimming, 132, *134*
Symptoms, defined, 2
Synapses, 34
Syphilis, 310, 311, *311*
Systematic desensitization, 38
Systole, 328
Systolic pressure, 329

T

Tachycardia, 330
Tai chi, 66, 128, 139
Talk therapy for alcoholism treatment, 218
Tapeworms, *298*, 304
Tar, tobacco, 221, 224
Targeted therapy, 346
Target heart rate range, 132, 133
T cells, 294
Technology
 addiction to, 183–184, *184*
 sleep and, 81, *83*
Temperature inversion, 408
Temporal lobes, 81
Tendinitis, 385
Tension headaches, 56
Tension relievers, 66
Terminal illness, 444, 448
Termination, behavior change, 14
Terrorism, 389
Testes (testicles), 258, *258*
Testicular cancer, 259, 344
Testosterone, 435
Test-taking skills, 65–66, *65*
Tetanus, 295
Tetanus booster, *357*
Texting, 241
 addiction to, 184, *184*
 distracted driving, 378, *378*
 repetitive strain injuries, 384–385
THC (tetrahydrocannabinol), 190
Therapists, mental health, 42, 43
Therapy, types of, 42–44
Thimerosal, 296
Thought disorders, 40
Thought process, stress and, 67
Thrush, 303
Ticks, 301
Time, FITT principle, 131, *131*
Time management, 64–65, 150
Time Management for Students, 72
Tobacco use and abuse
 aging and, 441
 cancer and, 223, 338
 cessation programs, 227–228, *228*, 229
 chronic disease, 319
 health effects, 221–225, *224*
 pregnancy and, 223–224
 statistics on, 205
Tolerable Upper Intake Level (UL), 110
Tolerance, promoting, 251
Tolerance
 alcohol use and abuse, 216
 drugs, 186–187, 191
Topical administration, drugs, *186*
Topiramate, 218
TOPS (Take Off Pounds Sensibly), 170
Torso twist, *140*
Toxicity, drugs, 187
Toyota Prius, 411
Trace minerals, 104
Transdermal patch, *271*

Trans fats, avoiding, 101, 102, 166–167
Transgender, 268
Transgenderism, 243
Transient ischemic attack (TIA), 332
Transition, labor, 284
Transparent Self, The (Jourard), 235
Transsexual, 268
Transtheoretical model of behavioral change, 14, *14*
Traumatic brain injury (TBI), 381
Traumatic injury, short sleep and, 81
Treatment programs
 alcohol abuse, 217–218
 drug abuse, 195, 197
Treponema pallidum, 311
Triangular Theory of Love, 240–241, *240*, 242
Tricep stretch, *140*
Trichomonas vaginalis, *298*, 312
Trichomoniasis, 312, 313
Triglycerides, 101, 328
Trimesters, pregnancy, 281
Tubal ligation, *272*, 276
Tuberculosis, 292, *298*, 301, 306
Tumor markers, 340
Tumors, 338
Tumor-suppressor genes, 338
Twelve step programs, 197, 199
Twin studies, sleep patterns, 81
Twitter, 241
Type, FITT principle, 131, *131*
Type 1 diabetes, 320–321, *321*
 See also Diabetes
Type 1.5 diabetes, 323
Type 2 diabetes, 79, 100, 130, 321, *321*, 323–324, 337, 370, 432, 434, 440
 See also Diabetes
Type A personality, 57–58
Type B personality, 58
Type C personality, 58
Type D personality, 58

U

Ulcers, stress and, 56
Ultraviolet (UV) radiation, 342, 408, 422
Umbilical cord, 281
Undernourishment, 8
Underweight, 154, 155, 172–174, *173*
Uninsured population, 11
Unintentional injury, 377
Union of Concerned Scientists, 411
Unipolar depression, 34
United Nations Environment Program, 402
United Nations Framework Convention on Climate Change (UNFCCC), 410
United Nations Programme on HIV/AIDS, 8
Unsaturated fats, 101
Upper-back stretch, *140*
Urethra, 258
 female, *257*
 male, 258, *258*
Urgent care centers, 359
U.S. Census Bureau, 322
U.S. Department of Agriculture, Nutritional Database, 179
U.S. Department of Agriculture (USDA), 110
U.S. Department of Energy, 410
U.S. Department of Health and Human Services (HHS), 5, 8, 23, 395
U.S. Department of Justice, 394
U.S. Equal Employment Opportunity Commission, 391
U.S. Preventive Services Task Force, 309
U.S. Public Health Service (PHS), 5
Uterine cancer, 345–346
Uterus, 256–257, *257*

V

Vaccines, 294–296, *296*, 346, 357, *357*–358
 recommended, *295*

Vacuum aspiration, 278
Vagina, 256, *257*
Vaginal estrogen, 435
Vaginal intercourse, 255, 264, 306, 310
Vaginal ring, *271*
Validity, of research studies, 354–355
Valium, 38, 87
Values, personal, 30–31
Varenicline, 228
Varicella, *295*
Vas deferens, 258, *258*
Vasectomy, *272*, 276
Vector, infectious disease, 293
Vector-borne diseases, 402
Vegans, 111
Vegetables, 108, 113, 115
Vegetarianism, 111, 112
Veins, 326, *327*, 328
   See also Cardiovascular disease
Ventricles, 326, *327*
   See also Cardiovascular disease
Ventricular fibrillation, 330
Vicodin, 188
Vietnam War, 402
Violence
   alcohol use and abuse, 208, 215–216
   assault, 387
   defined, 385
   domestic and intimate partner violence, 376, 389–390
   hate crimes, 389
   injuries and, 388–389
   media and, 387
   murder, 388–389
   relationship, addressing, 391
   school and campus violence, 388–389
   sexual violence, 391–394
   stalking and cyberstalking, 390–391
   terrorism, 389
Violent crime, 385, *386*
Virginia Tech shootings, 388
Viruses
   cancer and, 338
   colds, 298
   defined, 297
   foodborne illness, 117
   genital herpes, 308, *308*
   hepatitis, 299, 307
   HIV/AIDS, 305–307
   infections from, 293
   influenza, 298–299
   mononucleosis, 299
   Zika, 8, 302, 402
Visceral fat, 56
Vision, diabetes and, 323
Vision, screening, *357*
Vision loss, aging and, 433–434, *434*
Vitamin D, bone health and, 103, 106
Vitamins, *104–105*
   bone health, 103, 106
   deficiencies and toxicities, 103
   defined, 103
   fat-soluble and water-soluble, 103–104, *104–105*
   functions and sources of, *104–105*
Volatile organic compounds (VOCs), 408, 419, 420
Volumetrics, *166*
Volunteering, 45, 438
Vulva, 256, *257*

W

Waist circumference, 156, 158, 336, *337*
Waist-to-hip ratio, 156, 158
Wakes, 446
Walking, 132, *134*, 150
Warm-up, physical activity, 145
Warts, genital, 308–309, *308*
Water, 169
   bottled, 413, 419
   as nutrient, 97, 104
   physical activity and, 145–146
   promoting clean water, 414
   recommended intake, 104
   sources of, 104
Water injuries, 383–384
Water pills, 329
Water pollution, 411–414, *414*
Water-soluble vitamins, 103, *104–105*
Weather, physical activity and, 146
Websites, 23, 174, 203, 232, 253
   AARP (formerly the American Association of Retired Persons), 453
   abstinence, 29
   Academy of Nutrition and Dietetics, 124, 179
   Administration on Aging, 453
   Agency for Healthcare Research and Quality (AHRQ), 374
   Alanon and Alateen, 232
   Alcoholics Anonymous, 232
   alcoholism treatment, 218
   alcohol use and abuse, 214
   Alzheimer's Association, 453
   American Academy of Sleep Medicine's Consumer Information Site, 94
   American Association for Marriage and Family Therapy, 253
   American Association of Poison Control Centers, 398
   American Cancer Society, 350
   American College of Sports Medicine (ACSM), 152, 179
   American Council on Exercise, 152
   American Diabetes Association, 350
   American Heart Association, 350
   American Psychological Association, 49, 72
   American Sexual Health Association, 316
   Anxiety and Depression Association of America, 49
   BeliefNet, 49
   Body, The: The Complete HIV/AIDS Resource, 316
   Budget Worksheet for College Students, 72
   Caring Connections, 453
   Center for Science in the Public Interest, 124
   Center for Young Women's Health, 316
   Centers for Disease Control and Prevention, 23, 179, 232
   chronic disease, 350
   Conflict Management Information Source, 253
   consumer health, 374
   Dietary Guidelines for Americans, 124
   domestic violence, 398
   Drugs of Abuse Information, 203
   Eartheasy Non-Toxic Home Cleaning, 427
   environmental health, 427
   Environmental Working Group, 427
   evaluating health information and tools, 354
   Evaluating Online Sources of Health Information, 374
   exercise, 152
   FDA Birth Control Guide, 289
   Food and Drug Administration (FDA), 124
   Foodsafety.gov, 124
   Freedom from Smoking Online, 232
   Genetics Home Reference, 374
   Go Ask Alice, 23, 253, 289
   Health Websites You Can Trust, 374
   Human Rights Campaign, 253
   injury prevention and personal safety, 398
   Injury Prevention Web, 398
   Jed Foundation, 49
   Kiplinger.com Build-Your-Budget Worksheet, 72
   Loveisrespect.org, 253
   malaria, 317
   Mayo Clinic, 23
   Media Literacy Project, 23
   Medical Library Association's Top 100 List: Health Websites You Can Trust, 374
   MedlinePlus, 350
   Mental Health America, 49
   Motorcycle Safety Foundation, 398
   My Family Health Portrait, 350
   MyPlate, 124
   Narcotics Anonymous, 203
   National Cancer Institute (NCI), 232, 350
   National Center for Complementary and Integrative Health, 374
   National Center for Environmental Health (NCEH), 427
   National Center for Injury Prevention & Control, 398
   National Center on Addiction and Substance Abuse at Columbia University, 203
   National Domestic Violence Hotline, 398
   National Institutes of Health Senior Health, 453
   National Safety Council, 398
   National Sleep Foundation, 94
   National Suicide Prevention Lifeline, 49
   online dating, 243
   Overweight and Obesity website (CDC), 179
   Planned Parenthood, 289
   President's Challenge Program: The Active Lifestyle Activity Log, 152
   psychological health, 49
   Psychologist Locator, 49
   Rape, Abuse, & Incest National Network (RAINN), 398
   rape and sexual assault, 398
   relationships, 253
   Rethinking Drinking: Alcohol and Your Drinking, 232
   safety issues, 398
   ScienceDaily: Mind & Brain, 49
   Science of Addiction, The, 203
   sexually transmitted infection, 316
   sleep, 94
   Smartersex.org, 316
   Stanford University, Center for Sleep and Dreams Sleep Guide, 94
   stress management, 72
   Stress Management Techniques, 72
   Time Management for Students, 72
   USDA Nutritional Database, 179
   U.S. Department of Health and Human Services, 23
   violence, 398
   weight management, 179
   World Health Organization (WHO), 23
Weight-bearing exercise, 130
Weight lifting, 136
Weight management
   activity, benefits of, 169
   aging and, 439–440
   angina, 331
   campus resources, 171
   chronic disease and, 347
   chronic stress, 56
   diabetes, 325
   diet pills, 167–168
   healthful, maintaining, 170–171
   healthful body weight, assessing, 156–157
   heart health, 335
   hypertension, 329
   personal factors, 156–157
   physical activity, 130
   popular diets, 164–168, *165–166*, *165–166*
   smoking and, 221
   support for, 170
   weight gain, factors contributing to, 161–164
   weight gain diet, 169–170
   weight trends, 158–159
Weight Watchers, 165, *166*
Wellness, health and, dimensions of, 3, *4*
Wellness, defined, 3
Wellness-illness continuum, *3*
Western medicine, 358

White blood cells, 293
Whole-exome sequencing, 370
Whole-genome sequencing, 370
Whole grains, 99, *99*
Whole medical systems, 362
Whooping cough, 295
Wills, 444
Withdrawal
    alcohol use and abuse, 216
    drugs, 186, 187
    nicotine, 221, 227
Withdrawal method, *270*, *272*, 273
Women
    alcohol use and abuse, 207, 208, 210, 214, 216
    body image, 155–156
    breast cancer, 344–345, *344*
    building muscle, 128, *128*
    caloric needs of, 97
    cervical cancer, 345–346
    communication and, 237–238
    contraception, 269–276, *270–273*, *274*, *275*, *276*
    depression, 35
    fiber intake, 99
    heart disease, 334
    infertility, 285, 286
    intimate partner violence, 376, 386, 389–390
    life expectancy, 432–433, *433*
    obesity, 160
    osteoporosis, 434–435
    ovarian cancer, 345
    pregnancy and childbirth, 280–285, *281*, *282*, *284*
    sexual anatomy, 256–258, *257*
    sexual dysfunctions, 262–263
    sexually transmitted infection, 311
    sleep, 82
    steroid use, 148
    stress, 55, 58–59
    tobacco use, 207
    uterine cancer, 345–346
    warning signs of heart attack, *330*
    weight gain, 162
Work-related injuries
    back injuries, 384, 385
    repetitive strain injuries, 384–385
World Health Organization (WHO), 2, 8, 30, 33, 179, 278, 285, 400, 401, 403
World Meteorological Organization, 402, 407

X

Xanax, 38
Xenical, 168

Y

Yeast infections, 303
Yerkes, Robert, 54
Yerkes-Dodson law, 54
Yoga, 66, 128, 139
Yogurt, 347
Young adult subtype, alcoholism, 216
Young antisocial subtype, alcoholism, 216–217
YouTube, 241

Z

Zero population growth, 405
Zika virus, 8, 302, 402
Zinc, 104, *105*
Zone diet, 165
Zuckerberg, Mark, 241
Zyban, 228
Zygote, 269, *269*, 281
Zygote intrafallopian transfer (ZIFT), 286